This book is dedicated to the premise that, as a profession, we could do better by our patients if we were more humble about the knowledge that underlies our clinical judgment, aware of its limitations, and appreciative of the power of billions of years of evolution on earth.

CONTENTS

PREFACE

OUR GOAL IN WRITING this book is to help make basic medical physiology become much more useful to students and health care professionals than is generally the case today. We do this, first, by approaching basic medical physiology from a generalist's clinical perspective, emphasizing its application to medicine. Second, we showcase some new roles for basic physiology, which we have found valuable in our clinical practices, and which provide a new motivation and importance for understanding physiology. Third, we present physiological knowledge in a way that emphasizes how it is ever changing; an approach that we believe will enhance its long-term utility by corresponding better with reality.

Most clinicians greatly underutilize basic physiology in clinical practice. In part, this is a consequence of the static, encyclopedic, and clinically disconnected way in which medical physiology is usually presented. Traditional medical physiology courses often leave students with "book knowledge" that is rapidly forgotten, difficult to apply to the "real world" of clinical practice, and quickly overtaken by new developments at the cutting edge of research. This causes students to become cynical and exclaim "just tell us what we need to know to pass the exam!"—and study accordingly. Knowledge assimilated for such short-term purposes is often not well retained and not very useful in clinical practice. Instead, we attempt to entice students to learn physiology by highlighting its potentially powerful applications to clinical medicine—which is the reason for their study of the subject in the first place. By learning to effectively apply physiology to clinical medicine, students will be better equipped than were their predecessors to meet the challenges of clinical practice in the next millennium.

Physiology has many potential roles in clinical medicine. The classical role of physiology in medical education is that of a foundation for understanding the pathophysiology of disease. While valid, this may not be its most important role. We will showcase three additional ways in which physiology can be powerfully applied to clinical practice. First, it is an adjunct to differential diagnosis in the initial management of patients' medical conditions. Second, it facilitates communication with patients. Third, it is useful in articulating an effective case for doing or not doing tests or treatments for individuals whose circumstances fall outside the norms addressed by guidelines and other standardized criteria whose application has become quite fashionable. Let us consider each of these new roles further.

How can physiology help in the initial management of a patient's medical condition? Even before a conclusion is reached as to a patient's diagnosis, a teleological consideration of normal physiology can often provide an immediate "road map" for prioritization of treatment. Thus, instead of trying to remember an arcane list of interventions to carry out for any given clinical condition (from which it is easy to forget one or two items over time), the clinician can view the patient's illness as a deviation from normal organ system function. This way, the crucial therapeutic and diagnostic maneuvers are more easily remembered as the logical and engaging path from organ system dysfunction, back to normal organ system function. Students who have learned to use physiology in this way, may have greater facility in avoiding some of the simple, common, practical errors and oversights, which occur so often in the face of complex clinical conditions today.

Furthermore, since homeostasis is a fundamental principle of physiology, this way of thinking emphasizes diet and lifestyle interventions as ways to restore normal physiology where appropriate and mitigates the knee-jerk reliance on pharmaceuticals so prevalent in medical practice today. This approach is not applicable to all patients in every clinical setting, but it helps with many, especially at the most cost-effective point of intervention—before they get really sick. Thus, a physiological approach to health and disease is a valuable tool for students and practicing clinicians alike.

Another powerful and underutilized role for physiology is to facilitate communication with patients. Following a careful history, the development of a teleological narrative including the normal physiology of the system of concern in a particular patient, how and why this is likely to be (or become) disordered in the patient, and how and why various prescribed treatments are believed likely to help the patient, has great therapeutic potential. It can facilitate patient acceptance of, and cooperation with, a treatment plan. It can empower the patient to be more involved in his or her medical care. It can help the patient process the experience of illness in a way that favors healing at many levels. This book fosters students' learning of physiology

in a way that is readily conveyed to patients. Thus, physiology, which has traditionally been taught as part of the science of medicine, has something to contribute to the reinforcement and rejuvenation of medicine's art.

The final new role for physiology highlighted in this book is its utility in explaining why particular tests or treatments have been recommended in an environment in which care must be justified to be obtained. Large corporate health care insurance and delivery systems, increasingly the model worldwide, often rely on guidelines, algorithms, and authorization criterion to judge quality of care and to approve expenditures. These evaluation tools are (at best) developed from population-based norms, statistical probability, and current views on disease mechanisms and appropriate treatment that are subject to change. Scientific evidence backing these tools may be limited or even non-existent. Furthermore, population-based evidence usually does not apply to every individual or all circumstances. Clinical judgment, as it applies to individual patients, must be based on more than just what goes into guidelines and algorithms. Clinical judgment also must utilize individual experience, context, common sense—and physiologic knowledge, which increasingly must be articulated well and with good basis, in order to secure patients the care a clinician feels they need.

This book takes a different approach than do most physiology textbooks, to the nature of physiological knowledge. Viewing physiological knowledge as a fixed body of facts rather than as an ongoing, ever-changing work-in-progress, is a serious mistake. A common approach is to assume that what we think today is what is true, and that our current understanding is "the way things work." Thus, traditional courses in physiology tend to present current understanding (read "best guess") as more akin to stable facts than operational working hypotheses. This imbues the student with the impression of certainty in medical knowledge, a myth that can do great harm (see Chap. 1).

We believe that knowledge, including the level of detail at which it is presented, depends on what it is to be used for. While we do emphasize the current, consensus view on most subjects, to the level of detail that is clinically useful, we present this not as the "facts" or the "truth," but rather as a useful device. We recognize explicitly that, at best, today's facts are but a snapshot in an evolving understanding that is almost certain to be substantially revised, more likely completely overturned, in years to come. We believe that addressing uncertainty directly, as it applies to the physiological "foundations" of medicine, will help the student better develop a mental framework that can adapt to, and incorporate into itself, future change in medical practice—as the facts themselves change. Furthermore, since we present the current view of how things work as valid only to the extent that it is useful clinically, we do not shy away from the use of teleology, that is, the assumption of purpose in physiological mechanisms, as a didactic tool—even though such an approach has no role in physiological science per se.

In addition, this approach facilitates the important, but difficult, communication of uncertainty to patients. Acknowledgment of profound uncertainty by clinicians, both as individuals and as a profession, when done tactfully, sympathetically, with humility, and in a supportive manner, need not be unsettling to patients. In our experience, patients with complex medical problems are frequently relieved to know that difficulties in diagnosis or treatment often stem from our imperfect understanding of how the body is "supposed to work." Indeed, they can find quite gratifying the realization that their individual experience (e.g., with respect to side effects of therapy or ameliorating and exacerbating factors) provides extremely valuable clues as to health and disease, which

should be conveyed to their health care providers for the optimal management of their condition.

This book approaches basic medical physiology from a generalist clinical perspective, in order to help students, when they become clinicians, to better apply physiological knowledge to the delivery of improved medical services. In part, this book puts into didactic form much of what we have learned as generalist clinicians and medical educators about the ways physiology can and should do this. We both have active clinical practices, one as a general internist (VL) and one as a family practitioner (KF). Our fundamental commitment is not to the discipline of physiology, but to meeting the needs of our patients. Both of us are involved in the teaching of medical and other health professional students during their pre-clinical and clinical years and house officers during their residency training. Over the last two decades, one of us (VL) has directed and the other (KF) has taught in a first-year medical school physiology course at the University of California, San Francisco. One of us (VL) also has an active, grant-supported basic research program in cellular physiology, which facilitates the balanced, concurrent presentation of physiological knowledge as both everchanging working hypotheses and a teleological narrative.

Some of the distinctive features of this book are as follows:

• The opening of each chapter with a clinical case, allows the student to appreciate how the organ system in question can present itself in clinical practice. Toward the end of the chapter the initial case is revisited and the key physiological concepts, as they affect clinical practice, are pointed out. Likewise, each chapter closes with another case that illustrates a different aspect of physiology as it can be used to improve the practice of medicine.

- Clinical Pearls highlight the practical implications of basic physiology for medical practice, which are interspersed throughout the text. These serve as a constant reminder of the applicability of physiology to medicine—and serve to pique the student's interest.
- Simple, section-by-section review questions allow readers to monitor whether they have been awake and have assimilated the key points.
- Frontiers in each chapter highlight areas of controversy, excitement, and even heresy, some of which are new and breaking as the book goes to press. This illustrates the important theme that physiological knowledge, and its application to medicine, is in flux.
- There is a chapter-by-chapter summary of the main points, and a glossary of terms appears at the end of the book.

- Suggested readings provide the citations for the specific articles in Frontiers, as well as particularly thought-provoking background articles and other sources.

Physiology, appropriately applied to the medical thought process and to practical therapeutics and communication in the healing relationship, has a special role to play in facilitating the practice of medicine. It is our hope that this book will help its readers better utilize physiology in both the art and science of their practice of medicine and delivery of health care.

Vishwanath R. Lingappa, MD, PhD
Krista Farey, MD, MS

ACKNOWLEDGMENTS

Writing a textbook of medical physiology from a generalist's perspective has proven a more challenging task than we realized at the outset. Without the guidance, critique, encouragement and support of a huge number of individuals, including some of our former teachers, current and former colleagues at the University of California, San Francisco (UCSF) and elsewhere, students, friends, family, and others, we would never have completed this work. Some of these individuals provided important critique of VL's endocrinology syllabus from which parts of this book are derived; Others read early drafts of particular chapters, providing innumerable suggestions both small and large that improved the subsequent product. Still others provided ideas and general comments that inspired one or more aspects of this approach to teaching medical physiology. Of course, any errors that remain are our responsibility and ours alone. However, the number of such errors would have been far greater without their input. Individuals, to whom we wish to express our deepest gratitude are listed here.

William Amend, MD
Professor of Medicine
University of California, San Francisco
San Francisco, California

Richard Auchus, MD
Assistant Professor of Internal Medicine
Division of Endocrinology and Metabolism
University of Texas, Southwestern
Dallas, Texas

Hal Barron, MD
Assistant Clinical Professor of Medicine
University of California, San Francisco
San Francisco, California

Gregory Barsh, MD, PhD
Assistant Professor of Pediatrics and
  Genetics
Stanford University School of Medicine
Palo Alto, California

Amanda E.M. Browne, BS
Research Fellow
University of California, San Francisco
San Francisco, California

Lucy Candib, MD
Professor of Family and Community
  Health
University of Massachusetts Medical
  School
Worcester, Massachusetts

Tony M. Chou, MD
Associate Clinical Professor of Medicine
University of California, San Francisco
San Francisco, California

Gregory Conner, PhD
Associate Professor of Cell Biology,
  Anatomy, and Medicine
University of Miami
Miami, Florida

Mary F. Dallman, PhD
Professor of Physiology
University of California, San Francisco
San Francisco, California

Michael Ennis, MD
Associate Professor of Family and
    Community Health
University of Massachusetts Medical
    School
Worcester, Massachusetts

Arden Farey, BA
Menlo Park, California

Gwen Farey, BA
Menlo Park, California

Alicia Fernandez, MD
Assistant Clinical Professor of Medicine
University of California, San Francisco
San Francisco, California

Scott Friedman, MD
Professor of Medicine
Mount Sinai School of Medicine
New York, New York

David Gardner, MD
Professor of Medicine
University of California, San Francisco
San Francisco, California

Nora Goldschlager, MD
Professor of Clinical Medicine
San Francisco General Hospital
University of California, San Francisco
San Francisco, California

Gary D. Hammer, MD, PhD
Assistant Professor of Medicine
University of Michigan Medical School
Ann Arbor, Michigan

Ann Harvey, MD
Assistant Clinical Professor of Family and
    Community Medicine
University of California, San Francisco
San Francisco, California

Michael Humphreys, MD
Professor of Medicine
San Francisco General Hospital
University of California, San Francisco
San Francisco, California

B.T. Lingappa, PhD
Professor of Biology, Emeritus
College of the Holy Cross
Worcester, Massachusetts

Jairam Lingappa, MD, PhD
Centers for Disease Control
Atlanta, Georgia

Yamuna Lingappa, PhD
Worcester, Massachusetts

Daniel Lowenstein, MD
Professor of Neurology
Harvard Medical School
Boston, Massachusetts

Umesh Masharani, MD
Assistant Clinical Professor of Medicine
University of California, San Francisco
San Francisco, California

James Mastrianni, MD
Assistant Professor of Neurology
University of Chicago School of Medicine
Chicago, Illinois

Carolyn M. Ott, BS
Graduate Student
University of California, San Francisco
San Francisco, California

D. Thomas Rutkowski, BS
Graduate Student
University of California, San Francisco
San Francisco, California

Paul Sarvasy, MD
Richmond Health Center
Contra Costa County Health Services
Richmond, California

Richard Schuldenfrei, PhD
Professor of Philosophy
Swarthmore College
Swarthmore, Pennsylvania

Barry Schwartz, PhD
Professor of Psychology
Swarthmore College
Swarthmore, Pennsylvania

Dean Sheppard, MD
Professor of Medicine
San Francisco General Hospital
University of California, San Francisco
San Francisco, California

Dolores Shoback, MD
Professor of Medicine,
Veteran's Administration Hospital, San
    Francisco
University of California, San Francisco
San Francisco, California

Michael Slott, PhD
Rutgers University
Newark, New Jersey

Robert N. Taylor, MD, PhD
Professor of Obstetrics and Gynecology
University of California, San Francisco
San Francisco, California

Jeanine Weiner-Kronish, MD
Associate Professor of Anesthesia
University of California, San Francisco
San Francisco, California

C. Spencer Yost, MD
Associate Professor of Anesthesia
University of California, San Francisco
San Francisco, California

Daniel F. Zlogar, BA
Medical Student
Duke University School of Medicine
Durham, North Carolina

PRINCIPLES OF PHYSIOLOGICAL AND MEDICAL KNOWLEDGE

1

1. AN INTRODUCTION TO PHYSIOLOGICAL AND MEDICAL KNOWLEDGE

The importance of epistemology for physiology and medicine

Epistemology is the study of knowledge, including what it is and how it is acquired. In their daily lives, people often take the "ground rules" for what constitutes knowledge for granted. Hence, this issue may appear to some readers as obvious or trivial. However, it is neither. An extensive discussion of the epistemology of physiology and medicine is beyond the scope of this book (see Ref. 1). Nevertheless, epistemology has an enormous (though often overlooked) impact on clinical practice, affecting what clinicians do, how they do it, and the quality of their interactions with patients. For these reasons it must be considered here at least briefly, before discussing physiological knowledge and its utility for clinical practice.

The importance of medical epistemology is particularly apparent in the all-too-frequent occurrence that treatments prescribed for a given patient don't seem to be working (or stop working after a period of time). Then the patient often becomes angry or despairing, and clinicians often become frustrated, sometimes losing confidence in their own judgment or blaming the patient. This happens far more often than clinicians would like to admit — just speak with your friends and family about their experiences with health care providers. Clinicians as a group would be far better able to deal with such situations if they looked more critically at the knowledge that treatments are based on and the basis for belief in treatment efficacy.

A less apparent way in which an appreciation of epistemology can influence medical practice is in tempering the overexuberant application of scientific breakthroughs to patient care. Sometimes, side effects and idiosyncratic reactions to new therapies occur on a delayed time scale or at an incidence and in specific subpopulations that were not identified in the initial studies. Sometimes, limitations to particular therapies become clear only with an expanded base of experience. Just because something is the latest innovation does not mean it is necessarily the greatest treatment for a particular patient. It is important to understand where our knowledge comes from and what its limitations are, if we are to provide the best care for our patients. This is true not only for physiological knowledge but also for medical knowledge in general.

Case Presentation

Mr. F. A. is a 54-year-old father and office worker who transferred himself to your clinic's primary care area seeking more satisfying care than he had received in the past. His underlying medical problems included ulcerative colitis, chronic obstructive pulmonary disease, hypertension, diabetes mellitus, and depression. He articulated many reasons for his anger and mistrust. He has a long history of unanticipated side effects of drugs that were rarely fully effective at treating his complaints. Explanations by health care providers as to what they thought was wrong with him were inadequate. The potential limitations of the therapies they prescribed were never clearly presented. Often, the provider's pronouncements came down as inscrutable edicts from above, or their idea of involving him in decision making meant providing statistical data on therapeutic efficacy — and expecting him to choose between clinical approaches whose pros and cons were not obvious. Although he had sought and seen a series of new health care providers over the years, he was often frustrated that they assumed they understood his illnesses (without listening to his experience of failure with the very therapies they were about to prescribe! His illnesses terrified him and have wreaked havoc in his life.

Trying to understand his concerns and to build his trust, you start by taking some time to listen to Mr. A., asking questions about his experience with interventions that may have made his symptoms better or worse. Then, following a careful physical examination and inspection of laboratory results, you provide him with a physiological framework in which to view his diseases, including plausible explanations for why previously tried therapies did not work, and why it might be worth trying them, or a variation of them, again.

As part of your approach, you acknowledge that modern medicine's understanding of his diseases is limited and that he may have a disease variant that is uncommon, has been misdiagnosed, or is particularly poorly understood. You assure Mr. A. that, while you cannot guarantee either improvement or cure, you will work with him to devise a strategy for managing his illnesses that optimizes the quality of his life.

First, you make some adjustments to his diabetes and lung disease pharmaceutical regimens. Then you proceed to make recommendations regarding some of his symptomatic complaints. These include nonpharmaceutical measures to address the underlying disturbances of homeostasis whose symptoms will exacerbate any illness (e.g., diet, exercise, and other recommendations to ameliorate his diabetes mellitus and various symptoms such as diarrhea or constipation, difficulty sleeping, and headache). You inform him about likely and possible side effects of any medications you prescribe and ask him to keep a careful log of things that he associates with exacerbations and remissions of his various diseases.

Mr. A. leaves your office more empowered and more confident in you as his new health care provider than he has been with anyone in years. Some of the nonpharmaceutical measures may well make him feel better. In the long run, the relationship he builds with you will likely have a powerful beneficial effect. It remains to be seen how effectively the measures you have initiated, or will institute in the future, will treat his chronic underlying medical conditions. What you are trying may work no better than the therapies instituted by Mr. A.'s previous health care providers. Nevertheless, he is subjectively better already, and will almost certainly be no worse than he would be otherwise, as a result of this more accurate, honest, humble, homeostatic, and collaborative approach.

Data, working hypotheses, scientific method, and "facts"

Humans have an extraordinary capacity to reason. Sometimes we reason by deduction from accepted first principles, as in mathematics. From this we reach conclusions that are truly timeless, as seen in the continued validity and utility today of the conclusions reached by Pythagoras on geometry over 2500 years ago. Other times, we reason empirically, that is, by induction from experiments on the environment. This is the basis for conclusions about the physical, chemical, and biological worlds. Induction is not without its limitations. A great philosopher once noted that a person who jumped off the Empire State Building and counted stories while falling, might conclude by induction that nothing bad would happen as a result (. . . 97, 98, 99, so far, so good).

Data are empirical findings about some aspect of the environment. Alone, data provide no insight into how a system works. For this, we must formulate working hypotheses, based on data and our current concepts about what might be going on. We use these working hypotheses to interpret additional data, revising our working hypothesis. When the data is particularly compelling, our conceptual framework or paradigm must be revised as well. Thus data and hypotheses are interrelated (see Figure 1.1). Data are largely meaningless without a hypothesis in which to interpret them. Conversely, a hypothesis is largely at the mercy of the data — if it does not fit, it must be revised or discarded. This process of moving back and forth, from data to hypothesis to new data with which to reevaluate the hypothesis, is known as the scientific method. The term *Occam's razor* refers to the notion that, all else being equal, the simplest hypothesis that fits the data is the most appropriate one. This is not because a simple hypothesis is necessarily more likely to be correct than a complex hypothesis, but rather because the simpler hypothesis is easier to test.

When a working hypothesis stands the test of time and experimentation long enough, it is elevated to a theory. This occurs mainly when a hypothesis has a major impact on the way data are interpreted in a variety of related but distinct fields. Darwin's theory of evolution, for example, provides a framework that makes integrated sense of data from diverse scientific disciplines, including population biology, individual physiology, cell biology, genetics, and molecular biology, for both plants and animals. That is not to say that the theory of evolution, or any other human construct, is beyond revision in either detail or fundamental principle. Rather it just means that, in the opinion of the vast majority of scientists at work today, it is the best framework in which to view and interpret all of the data on the physical, chemical, and biological world that is presently in hand.

At face value, a fact is something that we are confident is true. But the preceding discussion suggests that, to be precise, science deals not with facts but rather with interpretations of data. That interpretation occurs within the framework of a particular working hypothesis that seems likely to be valid. Scientific knowledge, then, is best not viewed as a fixed body of facts, such as some kind of foundation of bricks upon which the future will be built. Rather, it is more useful to view scientific knowledge as a far more fluid conglomeration of data and working hypotheses. These data and hypotheses are derived by the scientific method and reinforced by our honest willingness to subject them to reinspection in light of new data, technology, or other sources of insight to the best of our abilities in the future. What is certain is not any particular interpretation of the data, but rather that the most meaningful interpretation and assessment of the data at any point in time will flow from application of the scientific method to the data, hypotheses, and technology available at that time.

This point is potentially elusive and extremely important. In casual parlance people frequently use the terms *fact* and *information* to refer to specific interpretations of data within a generally accepted paradigm that seem likely to be valid. The words *fact* or *information* are not really used to refer to an unchanging truth, but rather to the current best informed guess. The reason this is a crucial distinction is that the facts in this sense do change, sometimes rapidly, often within the course of a remarkably short period (see Figure 1.2). Sometimes this change is driven by new concepts and ideas, sometimes by new

FIGURE 1.1. The scientific method. Revision of scientific hypotheses involves more than new data. Reinterpretation of data is a crucial component of the process.

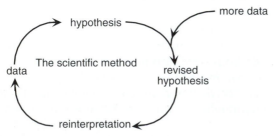

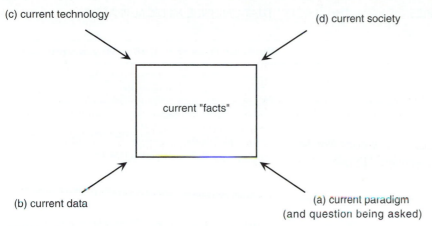

FIGURE 1.2. The genesis of "facts." What is believed to be true in science and medicine is influenced by *(a)* working hypotheses within the current paradigm and conceptual framework, *(b)* data from experimentation, *(c)* current technology, and *(d)* the economic, political, and social context of the time. When the generally accepted hypothesis changes, one or more of these factors are usually contributory and are the basis for "reinterpretation" within the scientific method diagrammed in Figure 1.1.

technology, sometimes by new data, often by a complex mix of the three.

The notions depicted in Table 1.1 are generally accepted today but would have been considered outrageous and inconceivable 20 years ago when the authors were in medical school. New data underlie, to some extent, each of these new views. However, in some cases new technology made collection of the new data possible. In other cases it is hard to understand why this conclusion had not been arrived at earlier. Perhaps no one thought to ask the right question — or if they did, it was ignored. In these cases, "blinders" that derive from hegemonic economic, social, and political forces may well have played an important role in influencing, consciously or unconsciously, what science was viewed as interesting or worthwhile.

If changes in what are commonly referred to as facts were driven solely by new concepts, technology, and data, the historical record would be far more logical than it actually has been. For better or for worse, scientists and clinicians are human and thus can be influ-

enced by other forces such as social custom, political ideology, and economic imperatives, which can sometimes contribute to the definition of generally accepted facts. Science and medicine in Nazi Germany or Stalinist Russia provide clear historical examples of this. There are other examples that are closer to home and to our present time, which would be correspondingly more controversial. The tension between objective and subjective influences on what we view as scientific or medical knowledge is real. What is crucial is that we be aware of this tension and as self-conscious as possible of how it may be influencing us.

The principal intellectual tool scientists have is the scientific method. The questions are: How well has it been applied, based on the available data, technology, and conceptual framework, as the basis for knowledge at any given point in time? How have those parameters (i.e., data, technology, and conceptual framework) changed since the scientific method was last brought to bear on the issue? If you keep these in mind you will be

TABLE 1.1   SOME EXAMPLES OF HOW THE "FACTS" THAT UNDERLIE MEDICAL PRACTICE CAN CHANGE

Popular view in 2000	Outdated views of 1, 5, 10 or 20 years previous
Human prion diseases are due to transmissible protein conformations.	Scrapie, Creutzfeldt-Jakob disease, and related disorders were believed to be due to slow viruses.
Oxidation is a key contributor to human disease; consumption of antioxidants is protective.	The role of antioxidants in human disease was not generally considered and those promoting antioxidant intake as preventive medicine were subject to ridicule.
Steroids are useful during treatment of certain acute infectious diseases: this is because we now realize the importance of endogenous cytokines as the cause of both good and harm.	Steroids, being immunosuppressive, were not given during severe, acute infectious processes. Little was known about cytokines.
Peptic ulcers (and possibly gallstones, atherosclerosis, and heart disease) are due to infectious diseases.	Peptic ulcer was believed to be due to excess acid; infection was not believed to be a relevant consideration for ulcers, gallstones, or heart disease.
β-adrenergic blockers are useful for treatment of some patients with heart failure; sometimes slowing the heart can make it pump more efficiently.	β-adrenergic blockers decrease the force of cardiac contractions and, therefore, exacerbate heart failure and should not be given to such patients.
Low protein diets are recommended for patients in renal failure; high protein results in glomerular hyperfiltration and a more rapid rate of nephron loss.	Patients with renal failure typically have proteinuria, a high protein diet was viewed as replacing the protein lost.
A key role of chloride channels in cystic fibrosis is to allow endogenous antibiotic peptides to function; the high salt environment that occurs without these chloride channels impairs an important line of host defense.	Lack of chloride channel function in cystic fibrosis results in sticky mucus and impaired ciliary function, which predispose to lung infections.
The best diet for blood glucose control in diabetes mellitus is low in protein and high in complex carbohydrates.	Since diabetes is a disorder of carbohydrate metabolism, the best diet for diabetic patients is high in protein and low in carbohydrates of all sorts.
Vitamin metabolism (e.g., resulting in elevated blood levels of homocysteine) may be a major risk factor in the development of heart disease.	Vitamin metabolism was not believed relevant to heart disease.
Hormone replacement therapy is not the only way to prevent clinically significant osteoporosis and does not protect against cardiovascular disease in postmenopausal women.	Hormone replacement therapy is mandatory to prevent osteoporosis and to lower the risk of cardiovascular disease in postmenopausal women.
Diuretics rather than calcium channel blockers should be first line therapy for hypertension: diuretics decrease the likelihood of stroke, while calcium channel blockers do not.	Diuretics cause hypokalemia and predispose to arrythmias, whereas calcium channel blockers are more effective at lowering blood pressure.

less upset in the future when something you thought you were sure about comes unglued and is radically reinterpreted (see Ref. 2).

Another flaw in thinking about our current knowledge as facts is that it assumes that history has ended. In the past, prevailing ways of thinking have been superseded by very different new ways of thinking. Often these changes were driven by a transformation in technology, economics, or politics. Even the facts fundamental to our present biomedical worldview, such as the roles and mechanisms of genes, DNA, RNA, proteins, membranes, cells, organ systems, or particular disease states, are all likely to have aspects that are historically specific. That is, it is likely that the future will view these facts quite differently than we do today. Humans arrived at these concepts using the scientific method. These concepts have thrived because they have been useful. A time may well come when their usefulness is superseded by other ways of viewing the world, as a consequence of new data, new concepts, new technology, or new ideologies.

There is yet another reason why the fruits

of scientific inquiry are best not viewed as "facts." This is because the significance of would-be facts is tremendously influenced by the way a question involving them is asked, and the sophistication of the context in which the question is posed. With scientific progress, the questions we ask encompass a larger and larger body of experimental data, more complex conceptual frameworks, more sophisticated technology, and so on. As a result, the possible answers become more contingent — there is no longer one correct answer, but rather various correct answers that address different dimensions of a question now realized to be far more complex than was appreciated in the past. It makes little sense to say that the questions that interest us now are less important than the questions that were the focus at some previous time. And yet, the questions that interest us today often could not have even been conceived until attempts were made to address the earlier simpler questions.

Remembering these points is crucial when (a) an investigator comes upon new data that do not easily fit into the prevailing scheme; (b) there is a change in paradigm that throws the basis for previous clinical practice out the window; or (c) a clinician is faced with a difficult case with features that do not lend themselves easily to the prevailing modes of thinking or treatment.

The relation of science and art in medicine

In some sense, the working hypotheses of basic science and their corollaries from the study of disease are the "data" that must be woven into meaning as the scientific contribution to clinical practice. For some situations, this is relatively straightforward. A patient with a particular infection, for example, not given antibiotics, may be likely to die or suffer permanent damage, while the similar patient given antibiotics may be more likely to recover and survive. In many other cases, how-

ever, the relation between science and medicine is far less clear. These decisions take medicine beyond the realm of science and into the realm of what we will call, for lack of a better term, *art*.

The art of medicine includes many issues that could be studied scientifically (such as when to start treatment, how often to treat, and when to stop treatment), but have not yet been so studied. The benefit of therapy to the patient is usually offset, to some degree, by complications of therapy in the short or long term. Often, effectiveness diminishes with high-dose therapy, especially in the long term (see Adaptation, Chap. 3). It is particularly hard to measure this balance when the patient who is at risk for a complication of therapy might not have been alive without that therapy. This is where the issue of the quality of life becomes particularly significant.

In addition, issues such as the speed with which complications are recognized are not easily amenable to productive scientific investigation. This will depend not only on the attentiveness of the clinician, but also on the extent to which the patient is attentive to changes in his or her body, feelings, or symptoms, etc. This is, in turn, influenced by the art of communication with patients: of two equally qualified professionals, one may be more skilled or gifted than the other at communication skills. As a result, the patient may be more or less willing to be engaged in his or her own health care, in response to interactions with one clinician versus the other.

Finally, one must always remember that, even for those issues that have been studied scientifically, the individual patient may or may not fit some statistical norm with respect to physiological process or response to treatment. Treatment recommendations and algorithms aimed at the "statistically typical patient" may not be useful for any given individual patient (see discussion of biochemical individuality in Frontiers of Chap. 2).

Thus, the art of medicine is more than just

the ability to communicate well with the patient, or the ability of some clinicians to make technical decisions better than others with similar training, be it due to experience, greater attention to detail, intuition, or some other skill. The art of medicine includes all aspects that are not a straightforward application of the scientific method to clinical practice. We do not understand the nuances of the art of medicine. Some aspects surely can be taught, as with other arts. Perhaps even the virtuoso will be more likely to flourish with the best teachers than left to his or her own devices to develop and hone particular skills.

One approach to combining the science and art of medicine is to recognize the fluidity between these two themes and traditions. Nothing prevents us, as individual clinicians, from integrating both traditions and being willing to use each of them separately or together, depending on what seems most effective or useful in the care of any given individual patient. Similarly, one size does not fit all in terms of interaction or communication with patients. While openness of communication with patients is an appropriate general rule, pragmatism should prevail in the specific instance. For example, some patients want to hear only "the truth" from their health care provider, whom they believe to be all-knowing. While the clinician may be uncomfortable with, or concerned by, this view, there is no need to cause unnecessary anguish to such patients by endless reminders of uncertainty.

A further challenge to the application of science to clinical practice occurs when one includes approaches from outside the Western allopathic medical tradition. These approaches may or may not have data tested scientifically to support them, but may have validity in the eyes of individual patients. It may sometimes be most helpful to work with another cultural paradigm or find a compromise between the cultural paradigm and that in which we have been trained. Whether due to a placebo effect or to knowledge yet to be understood by Western allopathy, a broad variety of treatment approaches may be effective. Treatments from any therapeutic paradigm, Western or otherwise, need to be selected cautiously and used with the same consideration for both their potential efficacy and possible complications.

This is a textbook of medical physiology, not of medical care, allopathic or otherwise. However, in order to be most effective in the care of patients via the allopathic model, it is necessary for clinicians (and when possible, patients), to recognize the limitations of science and the incompleteness of our current understanding of human physiology and other sciences. Similarly, we need to acknowledge the potential value of approaches that are part of the art of medicine, including those that are outside of Western medical traditions. Thus the current paradigm of physiology in particular, and modern science in general, while valuable as a basis for the care of many patients, does not necessarily indicate the most appropriate care for any individual patient.

Dealing with change in an uncertain world

Change is treacherous for clinicians in a number of different ways:

- The laboratory values from blood samples drawn yesterday or even just an hour ago may no longer provide a valid basis for the decision you are about to make now (for example, in patients with a falling blood glucose due to an insulin overdose, or a falling red blood cell count due to a gastrointestinal hemorrhage, or a rising blood urea nitrogen and creatinine level due to renal failure).
- The patient's underlying clinical condition could have fundamentally changed, even when a particular blood test is still valid (for

example, the comatose patient in diabetic ketoacidosis who is now having a silent myocardial infarction).

• New data can undermine our understanding of what is going on or the rational basis for our therapy (whether or not that therapy actually works). Sometimes this can leave clinicians in the awkward position of continuing treatment that no longer has a rational scientific basis, simply because it seems to be working (presumably for some other reason than is currently known). New data, when particularly compelling, can sometimes lead us to change therapy to something that has not yet stood the test of time. Sometimes patients bring to our attention an oversimplified caricature of new data (e.g., from the local newspaper) about which we may not be aware, which leads them to question the treatment we recommend.

Several principles can facilitate the application of physiology in particular and scientific knowledge in general to medicine in a world subject to these (and many other) kinds of change (see Figure 1.3):

• Pay meticulous attention to detail. Look for changes in the history or physical examination that suggest that the patient's condition may have changed. For example, consider the time at which the laboratory studies were drawn. Be attentive to whether the specimens were left sitting out and thus may be invalid (e.g., blood gas determinations need to be kept on ice; cultures for infectious organisms need to be plated expeditiously). Know the limitations of the kinds of studies you order (e.g., the pitfalls of radioimmunoassays as a basis for determination of blood levels of hormones and other substances; see Chap. 3).

• Be forthcoming with your patients as to the current limits of knowledge, both personally and on the part of the health professions as a whole. This does not require frightening them or suggesting that you personally or the profession as a whole is stupid. Nor does it mean abdicating the role of providing patients with clearly articulated recommendations. After all, despite uncertainty or ignorance, you are still in a better position to make a recommendation than most of your patients would be on their own. Indeed, as a professional, you have a solemn responsibility to provide the best advice you can. Often, an effective approach is to indicate the pros and cons of different courses of action. In doing so, it is often useful to clarify for the patient your assumptions. It is also

FIGURE 1.3. Roles of physiology in the practice of medicine. The critical interpreter applies physiological knowledge conservatively, in order to come to recommendations for therapy. Physiology is just one contributor toward the final conclusion, which may also include contributions from clinical epidemiology, personal experience, and alternative medical systems. The functional storyteller uses physiological knowledge as a tool to empower and engage patients in their own health care. The imaginative hypothesizer uses physiological knowledge to design new testable hypotheses that may one day change the conclusions reached by the critical interpreter.

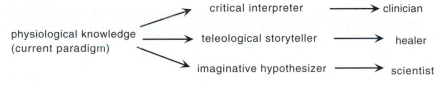

important to acknowledge your ignorance on particular aspects and affirm a plan to consult with colleagues, study the subject, and get back to the patient later, with your updated (and possibly revised) opinion based on current knowledge. Feigned knowledge, exposed, greatly undermines credibility.

• Be open to utilizing physiological knowledge in different ways, depending on the circumstances. The critical examiner of data (e.g., when reading a medical journal) is different from the functional storyteller (e.g., when explaining the current paradigm's view of the illness to a patient). In the former mode, you focus on the "holes" and the weaknesses in a hypothesis in order to better test it and perhaps replace it with a preferred one. In the latter mode, your goal is coherence — you want the patient, or yourself, to have a simple and convenient way of remembering the big picture. Inconsistencies are appropriately downplayed for the sake of a more engaging story. Both of these modes are different from that of the "imaginative hypothesizer," in which mode physiological knowledge is used more creatively: By a clinician to step back and think more broadly about a desperately ill patient who is not responding to conservative therapy; By a scientist brainstorming to go beyond the confines of conventional thinking. Each of these three ways of using physiological knowledge is a valid role for the clinician. Each has its uses, limitations, and risks. The goal of your study of medical physiology should be to cultivate the ability to use each of these approaches, individually and in combination, as appropriate for the best care of your patients.

• Remember that compassion and caring count for a lot in medicine — more than you can probably imagine. Telling the physiological story of their illness in a sympathetic way can give your patients insight, understanding, and motivation to participate in overcoming their illness — whether or not the treatment itself effectively alters the disordered physiology.

Clinical Pearls

○ The flux of medical knowledge is seen most clearly in the constant drumbeat of results from clinical trials and other studies, many of which propose new ways of approaching the care of particular subsets of patients.

○ Besides the specific merits or limitations of the study in question, one must always ask: What about the individual history of my particular patient might suggest that he or she is a different subset from that which benefited from a particular new therapy? Are there compelling reasons why the therapy currently in place should be changed?

○ A good rule of thumb, with respect to the care of the stable patient, is never to be the first or last clinician to change your practice in response to new information. The first clinician may be exposing patients to too many unknown long-term risks of recently developed treatments. The last clinician to move to new standards may simply not have kept up.

Review Questions

1. What is epistemology? What are two scenarios in which it is a valuable tool for clinicians?
2. What is the scientific method?
3. If the simplest hypothesis is not more likely to be correct than a complex hypothesis, why do scientists favor simple hypotheses?
4. What is scientific knowledge, and what kinds of things can result in its change?
5. What are three different ways to use scientific knowledge?

6. What are four principles to remember in the application of scientific knowledge to the practice of medicine in a changing world?

2. A FRAMEWORK FOR THE STUDY OF HUMAN PHYSIOLOGY

Having pointed out the changing nature of knowledge over time, let us focus on the different perspectives on an area of knowledge that can exist at any given time.

Human physiology is the study of the organ systems of the human body and their interactions over the course of the human life cycle.

Physiological knowledge is the set of reproducible observations as to how organ systems normally respond to various stimuli over time, which is organized into working hypotheses about organ system function (see Ref. 3).

Pathophysiological knowledge deals in the same way with organ system dysfunction. These working hypotheses on normal and abnormal organ system function have a valuable role to play in making sense of both epidemiological findings and clinical observations related to disease, as will be discussed later.

Physiological (or pathophysiological) knowledge can be presented at many different levels of detail, from the molecular to the cellular to that of organ systems as a whole. The difference between textbooks of physical chemistry, biological chemistry, cell biology, and physiology is, fundamentally, the level of detail at which they attempt to describe phenomena. Physiological mechanisms can, more and more, be described in considerable molecular detail. However, more commonly, the level of detail is limited, with consideration of only those molecular features that are needed to make sense of the organ system as a whole.

Physiological knowledge and biological plausibility

Physiological knowledge, derived from the study of organ systems, forms the basis for much of the "biological plausibility" of various hypotheses in pathophysiology and epidemiology. When a disease state is observed or studied, the most appealing conclusions in epidemiology or pathophysiology are those that are also consistent with what we know about the normal physiological function of relevant organ systems. This applies equally to analysis of specimens from individual humans, to animal models believed to be relevant to human disease (the domain of basic pathophysiology), or to variables that correlate to clinical findings in human populations (clinical epidemiology).

Sometimes, insights from disease models or from clinical epidemiology are not consistent with, or are tangential to, the current view of physiological mechanism. Those circumstances suggest the existence of important gaps in physiological, pathophysiological, or epidemiological thinking that await new information or perspectives. Physiological, pathophysiological, and epidemiological knowledge, like all knowledge, is not certain. However, it need be neither certain nor entirely consistent with the conclusions from other sources of information in order to make a valuable contribution to the care of patients.

Consider the hypothetical situation in which physiology, pathophysiology, and clinical epidemiology suggest very different answers to a clinical issue. In these circumstances, which line of evidence do you follow? There is no simple answer to this question. Physiology does not necessarily inform us as to how disease comes about, or how the functioning of an organ may change once the disease is established. Pathophysiology does not inform us about the potential homeostatic mechanisms that might be called upon to rescue organ system function, especially early in a disease. Clinical epidemiological studies may miss correlations because they lump together what should be categorized as different diseases due to differences in physiological mechanisms that are dysfunctional. Conversely, they may pick up phenotypic commonalities that come about as a result of very different physiological or pathophysiological mechanisms.

Part of clinical judgment includes learning, from experience as much as anything else, what information to act upon and what to ignore or hold, at least temporarily, in abeyance. In contrast, knowing that you have set aside some information in making a particular decision should leave you more open to revising that decision in the face of new information suggesting another course of action. This is reality, lamentable as it may seem to the student trying to learn what is going on.

Conceptual organization of the body

We have considered how knowledge can change over time, with new information, new technology, and new ideas. However, even within any given paradigm, knowledge can be viewed from different disciplines and perspectives. Consider the human body and how it functions. It can be conceptualized in many different ways involving the fundamental principles of the mathematical, physical, chemical, and biological sciences.

- From the most abstract mathematical perspective, the body, and indeed all of life, can be thought of as a means of storing, copying, and transferring information.
- From a purely physical and chemical perspective, life can be viewed in terms of the laws that apply to all matter, under the conditions of temperature and pressure at which life occurs. This approach is particularly useful for converting observations about living systems into a form in which

conclusion from physics and chemistry can be applied. Thus, for example, chemical reactions occur between different substances (termed *reactants*) resulting in the creation of other substances (termed *products*). The laws of physics and chemistry determine whether particular substances will react chemically, what substances they may form as a result of their reaction, the extent to which the reactants are converted to products, and the factors that influence that conversion.

Typically, at temperatures and pressures compatible with life, reactions have a certain likelihood of occurring on their own and a certain extent to which they will proceed in the direction of forming products, when they occur. Kinetics is the study of the rate at which reactions occur. Biological and physiological systems have special means of altering the kinetics of various chemical reactions, which is one of the reasons why life, as we know it, is possible. Thermodynamics is the study of the distribution between reactants and products, or equilibrium, which is achieved when a reaction has gone to completion (see Chap. 2). Living systems fully obey the laws that apply to the physical world — but take advantage of some "tricks." An example is the ability to couple thermodynamically unfavorable reactions to thermodynamically favorable ones. As a result, limitations on the extent to which certain reactions proceed spontaneously in the nonliving world can be overcome (see Chap. 2).

- A number of different biological perspectives can be used to conceptualize the body and life itself. Historically, the body was first understood in anatomic terms, a heritage that, for example, probably accounts for the anatomic organization of the titles of most of the chapters in this book. Later, within the anatomic framework, the body was conceptualized and studied in terms of the similarities and differences in composition between anatomic structures. Thus, cells are the smallest unit of life, defined as the smallest scale of organization at which the capacity to carry out functions needed for reproduction can occur. In multicellular organisms such as humans, cells are organized into tissues (groups of cells of similar structure and function) and organs (groups of tissues that work together to carry out a particular role in the survival of the organism). Finally, several organs often work together to make an organ system. Thus, for example, individual cardiac muscle cells comprise cardiac muscle tissue capable of beating spontaneously. Together with connective tissue (e.g. comprising the cardiac valves) they make up the organ known as the heart which is capable of pumping blood. The cardiovascular system is an organ system that includes the heart, blood vessels, and regulatory mechanisms of blood circulation (see Chaps. 7 and 10) which pumps the right amount of blood at the right pressure to meet all of the body's needs, under normal circumstances.

• The last half century has seen the rise of a biochemical and molecular perspective on biological systems. In many ways this is a synthesis of the mathematical, physical, chemical, cellular, and anatomic perspectives on life, with a focus on specific macromolecules that play unique roles in biological systems, such as deoxyribonucleic acid (DNA), ribonucleic acid (RNA), and proteins (see Chap. 2). Many proteins serve as biological catalysts or enzymes. By altering the kinetics of chemical reactions and, in some cases, by coupling thermodynamically unfavorable chemical reactions to favorable ones, enzymes are a major reason why life is possible (see Chap. 2).

As described earlier in contrasting the disciplines of physiology to pathophysiology or epidemiology, no one scientific perspective within physiology (e.g., the molecular, cellular, or whole animal) is, by itself, intrinsically more "accurate" or "useful" than the others, in terms of how they inform clinical medicine. They are each different. Their value depends, as was pointed out earlier, upon the question being asked, the use to which the knowledge is applied, and the skill of the practitioner at applying a particular perspective.

Thus, if you are a clinician-scientist developing new products in the pharmaceutical industry, a molecular and structural perspective may be crucial in allowing you to sort among many possible candidate drugs. This is the basis of the concept of rational drug design into which pharmaceutical companies are investing hundreds of millions of dollars in the hope of developing future new products (see Ref. 4). Such knowledge does not, however, predict efficacy or toxicity. This is why animal experimentation and human clinical trials will most likely always be a part of the drug development process. In contrast, a primary care clinician might not use the molecular mechanism of action of a drug in choosing to prescribe that agent to a patient. Instead, he or she may rely primarily on knowledge of clinical epidemiological studies to provide the rational underpinning for the use of that drug in clinical practice.

Nevertheless, it stands to reason that an understanding of many different perspectives provides the clinician's knowledge base with the maximum degree of flexibility in terms of remembering what to do, answering his or her own questions, and in explaining the disease and the treatment to the patient. Thus, in presenting physiological knowledge, as it is relevant to medical practice, reference will be made to insights at various levels and from various perspectives, including the molecular, cellular, and organ systems.

In Table 1.2 explanation (1) shows the simplest response to the question of the mechanism of blood glucose control, describing the hormones and their overall effects. A slightly

TABLE 1.2   MULTIPLE LEVELS OF DETAIL IN PRESENTATION OF PHYSIOLOGICAL MECHANISMS
What is the primary mechanism by which the body controls blood glucose?

Explanation of mechanism	Goal of answer
1. Blood glucose is controlled by the pancreatic hormones insulin and glucagon. Insulin causes blood glucose to go down, while glucagon causes blood glucose to go up. When you do not make enough insulin, your body is unable to keep the blood glucose in the normal range, so you need to take insulin or drugs that make your body make more insulin.	This is a very simple mechanical answer, good enough to satisfy a patient wondering about the blood test you are ordering for assessment of his or her mild diabetes mellitus.
2. Insulin stimulates insulin receptors on the liver, fat, and muscle cells, activating various signal transduction pathways whose net effect is to lower blood glucose. One of insulin's effects on fat and muscle is to induce glucose uptake by signaling intracellular vesicles bearing glucose transporters to fuse to the plasma membrane and thereby allow an increase in glucose transport. Insulin also stimulates glycogen, fatty acid, and protein synthesis in liver, fat, and muscle, respectively, to allow storage of the glucose as glycogen, fat, and protein. Insulin's effects in the liver include activation of signaling pathways that regulate pathways of glucose utilization including glycogen synthesis, glycolysis, and fatty acid synthesis (for lipoprotein production and export). Glucagon, the most important of several counter-regulatory hormones that oppose insulin's action, raises blood glucose by antagonizing insulin's effects on the aforementioned pathways in the liver. It thereby stimulates the opposing pathways of gluconeogenesis and glycogenolysis and increases fatty acid uptake into mitochondria and subsequent oxidation.	This is a more sophisticated answer, with the kind of detail that is needed for modern clinical practice, but not sophisticated enough for basic research on diabetes.
3. Upon insulin binding of the insulin receptor, the receptor is autophosphorylated on a critical tyrosine residue that triggers a cascade of phosphorylation events. As a result of these phosphorylation reactions, various second messenger pathways are activated. These in turn affect transcription, translation, and posttranslational modification of various proteins including allosteric activation and inactivation of key enzymes in the pathways of glucose formation and disposal (mentioned earlier). Glucagon acts on numerous enzymes to antagonize and oppose the actions of insulin, including activation of glycogen phosphorylase, and activation of acylation of fatty acids to carnitine. This serves to carry them, via the carnitine shuttle, into mitochondria, for oxidation. Paracrine interactions between α, β, and δ cells in the islets of Langerhans govern the phases of insulin secretion. . . .	This is the highlight of a far more complex answer that would be the starting point for research into the mechanism of insulin and glucagon action. Note that the level of sophistication of the answer given by someone interested in rational drug design focusing at the angstrom level of resolution or the answers needed to mimic a normal endocrine pancreas are both far beyond even this level of detail.

more complex version (2) describes some biochemical and cell biological features but still does not define the pathway. The highlights of a still more complex version (3) provides substantial biochemical detail but still is not as detailed as would be needed for rational drug design or to duplicate the function of the normal endocrine pancreas (see Chap. 6).

Physiological knowledge will be most useful for the student if it is integrated with other realms of knowledge, including pharmacology and clinical epidemiology, and in the context of practical clinical issues (hence the Clinical Pearls). However, it is important to recognize that there is no limit that we can foresee in our lifetimes to the degree of complexity that can be added to a description of the molecular mechanism of any particular physiological pathway. Which level and angle of sophistication you use depends on your purpose in asking the question — Is it to explain the suggested treatment to a patient? Is it to guide your own thinking in coming up with a therapeutic approach? Is it to develop new medicines that intervene in different ways in the pathogenesis of disease? The requirements for each are different.

Organ systems and their interaction

The precise subdivision of the body into organ systems is somewhat arbitrary, and is based in part on the current understanding of what these structures do. It is often striking to pick up a copy of the latest issue of research journals at the frontier of a particular medical specialty and notice how the topics covered are different from the topics in a chapter on the physiology of that organ (in this book or any other basic textbook). The journal articles tend to reflect the subset of areas where rapid progress is being made, e.g., the application of immunology and molecular biology to aspects of the more traditional body of knowledge. Inevitably, subjective opinions affect decisions as to what is more or less important and, therefore, subsumable within another category — or are simply bypassed in a general text such as this. Having made this disclaimer, we can categorize the major organ systems of the body to include:

• The liver, involved in filtering blood for many different purposes including defense and metabolism (see Chap. 4). The liver also provides substances such as many of the serum proteins found in blood.
• The gastrointestinal tract, including the esophagus, stomach, small and large intestines, and accessory organs of gastrointestinal function, such as the pancreas and gallbladder (see Chap. 5).
• The endocrine system, including the endocrine pancreas, pituitary, thyroid, adrenal, and parathyroid glands (see Chaps. 4, 11, 12, 13, 16, respectively).
• The cardiovascular system, including the heart and blood vessels (see Chap. 7).
• The respiratory system, including the lungs, diaphragm, and accessory muscles of respiration, and blood (insofar as blood plays a crucial role in transport of oxygen into the body and between tissues and in transport of carbon dioxide out of the body, see Chap. 8).
• The kidneys (also termed *the renal system*), urinary bladder, and the mechanisms of formation and regulation of urine (Chaps. 9 and 10).
• The reproductive system, including the various structures involved in production, storage, and delivery of germ cells and, in the female, the growth of the fetus (see Chaps. 15 and 16).
• The nervous system, which comprises the brain, spinal cord, peripheral nerves, and tissues in other organ systems that are specialized for rapid transmission of signals (see Chap. 18). Within the nervous system are the "special senses" of sight, hearing, taste, and smell.
• The immune system, including the spleen, bone marrow, lymph nodes, and specialized immune cells that reside in most organs or travel between organs and in blood (see Chap. 19).
• Blood, a crucial fluid by which the diverse organ systems communicate and exchange materials and energy. Blood is essential to the function of just about every other organ system (see Chap. 19).

- The skeleton, the hard matrix around which organ systems are suspended (see Chap. 14). The bones that make up the skeleton provide crucial support for all other organ systems.
- Muscles, cartilage, and connective tissue. Muscles and cartilage make possible movement of the body as a whole and of individual organ systems, often working in concert with bones. Connective tissue serves to protect, delimit, and demarcate various tissues.
- The skin, the outer covering of the body. Skin not only protects the internal environment from external physical assault (e.g., evaporation and dehydration) but also is a barrier to invasion of pathogens.

Each of these organ systems is comprised of many different tissues and is involved in many different functions. The liver, for example, includes both specialized hepatocytes that carry out many of the functions that we uniquely associate with the liver and reticuloendothelial cells that have structural, immunological, and other host defense functions. Furthermore, based on its functions, including the products it makes, the liver can be considered part of the gastrointestinal, cardiovascular, renal, reproductive, immune, mineral metabolism, and blood systems (see Chap. 20). To one degree or another, most organ systems function in concert with other organ systems. This is why disorders of one organ system often cause problems involving other organ systems. Conversely, for the same reason, a certain type of disorder (e.g., autoimmune disease) can manifest in many different organ systems.

Review Questions

7. What is physiology? What is physiological knowledge?

8. What are some of the organ systems of the body?

9. What is biological plausibility, and how does it serve to relate physiology to epidemiology and pathophysiology?

3. PRINCIPLES OF FEEDBACK

Physiological systems are characterized by the property of feedback (see Ref. 3. and Figure 1.4). For example, cells often signal other cells in response to a stimulus. The response typically shuts off further generation of the signal that triggered it. This is negative feedback, the most common form of feedback in biological systems. It occurs when an increase in any sort of output from a system triggers a decrease in whatever input triggered the output in the first place. A crucial consequence of negative feedback is that it allows biological systems to resist deviation of a particular parameter from some preset range. Feedback systems in the body have many layers of complexity built in, compared to the simplest framework (see Figure 1.4A).

- Feedback systems can utilize an external sensor allowing them to respond in anticipation of a signal. For example, this is why more of the hormone insulin is released in response to an oral glucose load than to an intravenous one (see Chap. 6). One effect of such an adaptation is to apply even more stringent controls on deviation from the normal range than would be otherwise possible.
- Feedback systems can involve signals directly from cell to cell or via activation of specialized signaling machinery (e.g., neural reflex arcs or endocrine glands). This allows several organ systems to be notified of a change in a crucial parameter at once and for the message to be sent in different ways, some short acting but fast, others long lasting but slow.
- Feedback systems can involve an integration center that processes many different

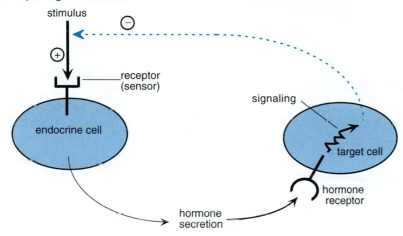

A Simple negative feedback

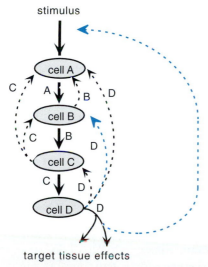

B Complex negative feedback

target tissue effects

FIGURE 1.4. Feedback. *A.* In simple negative feedback, a change in the blood concentration of some metabolite is detected by a receptor (sensor) on an endocrine cell that then responds with hormone secretion. The hormone is recognized by a receptor on a target cell which responds by altering the level of the metabolite in the bloodstream in a direction opposite that of the initial change. Thus, homeostasis is reestablished. *B.* In complex negative feedback, a set of hormones are placed in series (A, B, C, D), comprising an interlocking system wherein cells respond to both "feedforward" signals that trigger further secretion and feedback signals that shut it off. Typically, the feed-forward signal to activate secretion at one level is also a feedback signal to inhibit secretion at all previous levels. Thus, cell A secretes hormone A that stimulates cell B to secrete hormone B. Hormone B stimulates cell C to secrete hormone C. Hormone B also feeds back to inhibit secretion of hormone A.

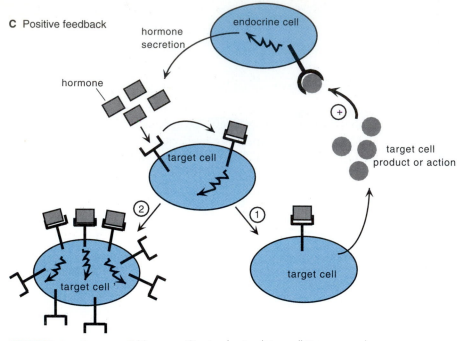

C Positive feedback

FIGURE 1.4. — *(continued)* Hormone C not only stimulates cell D to secrete hormone D, it also feeds back onto both cells A and B, inhibiting their secretion of hormones. Hormone D not only has target tissue effects elsewhere in the body, it also feeds back to inhibit hormone secretion by cells A, B, and C. The advantage of complex negative feedback over simple negative feedback is that a far more intricate set of instructions can be accommodated. Thus, programs that alter responsiveness to feedback can be used to selectively alter hormone secretion at any level. *C.* In positive feedback, a consequence of signaling by one hormone (solid rectangles) includes stimulation of further signaling and increased hormone secretion, rather than its termination, as occurs in simple negative feedback. Two ways by which this can occur are (1) having the first hormone induce the target cell to secrete a second hormone (solid circles) that itself is a trigger for secretion of the first hormone or (2) have the first hormone induce more receptors for itself on the target cell, thereby increasing target cell sensitivity to the first hormone. Either way, in positive feedback, the consequence of interaction of endocrine and target cells is not to achieve homeostasis, but rather, to drive a change in gene expression (e.g., development or maturation) of target cells.

kinds of inputs and determines what response is in the organism's best interests. Various regions in the hypothalamus play this role for a number of physiological functions (see Chap. 11).

Feedback occurs both between cells and within them. The preceding discussion refers to examples of feedback between cells. However, even within a single cell, enzymes that carry out the individual chemical reactions that make up biochemical pathways also display feedback (see Chap. 2). Thus the final product of a series of enzymes often inhibits the activity of the earlier enzymes in the pathway, thereby shutting off the enzyme when its action is not needed because its product is plentiful. Once the concentration of that product starts to fall, signifying that more of it needs to be made again, its lack disinhibits the enzyme, allowing enzyme activity to increase again.

Occasionally, usually as part of a developmental program, feedback is positive rather than negative. By definition, positive feedback is an unstable situation that often culminates in cell death. Often, cell death resulting from positive feedback has been programmed into the behavior of a cell and occurs via one of the many pathways of apoptosis (see Chap. 2).

4. HOMEOSTASIS AND THE NORMAL RANGE

No concept is more central to normal physiology than that of homeostasis, the tendency of physiological systems to resist deviations from a normal range (see Refs. 3 and 4). The "robustness" of homeostasis reflects the many nuances and levels of feedback, as noted earlier. Homeostatic physiological systems are not generally based on a single molecular mechanism. More typically, multiple mechanisms have evolved at different levels of organization to reinforce a particular physiological response. New mechanisms used by cells and organs to reinforce and regulate feedback and homeostasis are still being discovered (see Frontiers of Chap. 2). Circadian rhythms, by which parameters such as temperature and basal secretion of various hormones change significantly over the course of a 24-hour day, most likely have been selected because they further optimize various mechanisms of homeostasis.

The adaptive value of homeostasis should be clear: Life is a fragile and transient property of matter that can be extinguished by deviations from rather narrow ranges of many parameters including temperature, ox-

ygen, and acidity. Only those systems that were sufficiently able to maintain themselves within these limits were selected during the course of evolution. Surely one of the most amazing stories in the course of evolution has been the building of layer upon layer of regulation, reinforcing the organisms ability to establish homeostasis, sometimes at the expense of individual cells that commit suicide for the good of the organism as a whole (see Chap. 2).

Of course, the degree to which various adaptations and specializations are effective at maintaining homeostasis is itself contingent on many other variables, including:

• The particular point in the life cycle of the organism
• The nature of the environment
• The range of other genes that directly or indirectly affect expression of a particular homeostatic adaptation

There is no single optimum set point for every parameter that applies to all humans. Thus, because of differences in our genes, differences in the environment in which we were raised or currently live, and differences in our ages and emotions, we are each likely to display differences in optima and set points around which homeostasis occurs. This notion is further developed under the concept of biochemical individuality in Chapter 2 (see Frontiers).

5. CYCLES OF DEVELOPMENT

Development, homeostasis, and evolution

Anything more than a mention of developmental biology goes beyond the scope of this book. However, because development is a crucial variable in the behavior of physiological systems, it must be briefly included, with reference to more detailed sources (see Ref. 5). Biological systems are born, develop, mature, grow old, and finally die. This life cycle is played out in individual organ systems and in the whole organism. To understand a physiological system and try to predict its behavior, it is crucial to specify when during this cycle one is looking. An immature animal or organ system will not display the full range of functions observed in the adult, and may even display certain immature forms that will later regress and not be apparent in the adult.

Development and homeostasis may, at first, seem like contradictory concepts in that one is programmed change while the other is programmed resistance to change. One of the powerful features of the modern theory of evolution is that it can explain in molecular terms how a system can integrate both programmed change and programmed resistance to change in continuity over time. Thus:

• Evolution is the story of how the program of life has changed over geological and historical time (see Refs. 6 and 7).
• Development is a dynamic program in place for the lifetime of an individual.
• Homeostasis is the effect of forces in operation at any given moment, until a developmental change alters the program that put those forces in motion.

Aging and physiological function

Aging has manifestations in both normal development and disease and can be viewed as occurring both at the level of the whole organism and at the level of individual organs. It is a normal part of the human life cycle and developmental program (e.g., growing old); however, for individual organ systems, aging can be inappropriately accelerated under pathological conditions.

The underlying mechanisms of aging, manifest as gradual, progressive loss of a particular physiological function that was the domain of a particular organ system, are poorly understood in molecular terms. Earlier hypotheses included accumulation of errors in protein synthesis and accumulation of random mutations in various important genes. Thus far, these notions have not been proved. Other hypotheses include the notion that aging is, in part, a consequence of cell death, either in a programmed fashion termed *apoptosis* (see Chap. 2) or due to repeated small insults and illnesses, manifest as inflammation and cell necrosis (see Chap. 19). When specialized cells die, they are often replaced with cells such as fibroblasts that lack those specialized functions (i.e., formation of a scar).

Aging is associated with changes in gene expression that can affect organ system function, quite apart from the actual loss of a functional mass of cells. Thus, for example, amyloid deposits in the islet of Langerhans in patients with diabetes mellitus or fibrosis in the liver of patients with cirrhosis can compromise organ system function and may contribute to a vicious cycle of loss of homeostasis, inadequate compensation, and, in effect, accelerated aging.

Another way to think about aging is in terms not of molecular mechanisms, but rather, of aggregate residual functional capacity of the organ system in question. Most of our organ systems are built with a far greater capacity, roughly 90% excess, than is minimally necessary for homeostasis in the nonstressed state. This is why donation of one kidney for transplant is possible without ill effect on a relatively young and healthy donor. This built-in excess capacity may serve several purposes:

• It allows us to comfortably meet transient extremes of need, as may occur during times of stress when the body makes a greater than usual demand on an organ system's function.

- It allows some function to be lost (e.g., due to illness or injury) without compromising the survival of the organism.
- It allows homeostasis to proceed uncompromised until well into old age.

When a disease process is not self-limited, or if it recurs repeatedly, it can accelerate the underlying rate at which organ system function is lost. When this happens, a crucial threshold will be reached at which the inability to maintain homeostasis will first appear during the brief times of stress or other periods when more than usual capacity is required. As the disease progresses, physiological reserves may fall below that needed to maintain homeostasis even in the nonstressed state (see Figure 1.5).

Mechanisms activated in response to an illness can sometimes restore homeostasis adequately in the short term, but initiate accelerated loss of organ system function in the long term. Examples of this are seen in many of the organ systems to be discussed, including the endocrine pancreas in diabetes mellitus, the kidney in renal failure, and the heart in dilated cardiomyopathy (see Chaps. 6, 9, and 7, respectively).

Clinical Pearls

Often, the dimension of time is neglected in clinical situations, resulting in misdiagnoses and inappropriate therapy. For example:

○ The patient on insulin or other therapy for diabetes mellitus, who has worsening hyperglycemia in the morning, may, in fact, be rebounding as a compensatory overreaction to hypoglycemia in the middle of the night. The tip-off is often that the patient relates having nightmares or

unusually weird or vivid dreams, a sign of nocturnal hypoglycemia (see Chap. 6).
○ The patient who has hypertension in the acute setting of a stroke may not need chronic antihypertensive therapy if baseline blood pressure is normal. The question is which of the following scenarios applies: chronic hypertension culminating in a stroke versus a stroke triggering an acute episode of hypertension. Immediately after the stroke it is difficult to sort out these two possibilities. Only later can the distinction be made (see below).

Review Questions

10. What is the role of feedback in homeostasis?
11. Why is time an important variable in physiology?
12. What is the relation of evolution to development and to homeostasis?
13. Why do we have approximately 90% excess capacity over basal needs, in the case of many organ systems?

6. TIME AND SPACE

The dimension of time

Physiological systems exist in real time. Deviations from the optimum and the body's attempts to correct these deviations have a beginning, a middle, and an end. Hormonal systems have actions on various time scales, some immediate (in seconds to minutes), some delayed (occurring over hours), and some very delayed (occurring over days). In order to understand a physiological system, one needs to chart its response to a stimulus over time. This is addressed explicitly for various hormonal systems (see Chap. 6).

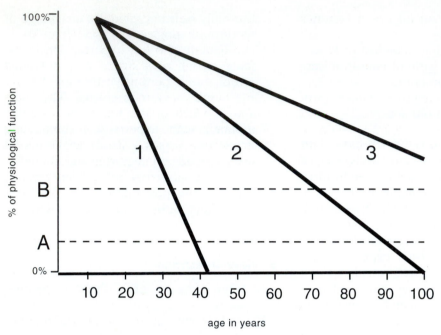

FIGURE 1.5. Loss of physiological function of a hypothetical organ system with age. X axis is age in years; y axis is level of physiological function. A, minimum level of physiological function needed at rest. B, maximum level of physiological function needed in stress. 1, Decay rate of function in severe underlying disease process. 2, Decay rate of physiological function with normal aging. 3. Maintenance of adequate physiological function throughout life due to optimal diet, lifestyle, genes and absence of disease. Note that this graph is not meant to imply any particular mechanism for the loss of physiological function, or whether the mechanisms involved in 1, 2, and 3 are the same or different.

The dimension of space: anatomy and physiology

Physiological function has evolved in concert with anatomic form. Here are some striking examples:

- The nuances of the anatomy of the pituitary portal blood supply are what make the neuroendocrine axes that govern thyroid, adrenal, reproduction, and other functions work.
- The implications of insulin delivered normally into the portal vein, where it is seen first by the liver and then, at lower concentrations, by the rest of the body, are central to the proper action of insulin and normal glucose homeostasis.
- Paracrine interactions are implicated in the fine-tuned function of practically every organ. These are tailored to the local environments and, most likely, to features we have yet to be aware of (see Frontiers).

7. CONCEPTS RELATED TO MEASUREMENT

The study of physiology requires that we measure various things including concentration of substances in solution. A fundamental concept in measurement is molarity. A mole refers to a certain number of molecules of a particular substance (6.0235×10^{23} to be precise, also known as Avogadro's number). This number of molecules turns out to be equal in weight, expressed in grams, to the molecular weight of the substance. When expressed in terms of moles per volume, molarity gives us a measure of the concentration of a substance. The important implications of concentration of substances in physiology are seen in the central role of receptor-ligand interactions in organ system function and communication. Changes in the concentrations of receptors and ligands can make events happen or prevent them from happening, as will be seen in phenomena such as "down-regulation" and the effects of "spare" receptors (see Chap. 3).

Clinical Pearls

○ Measurements are only as good as their range of error. A common mistake in clinical practice is a failure to appreciate this point. Thus, in a patient who has been bleeding, a change in hematocrit from 32 (+/− 3 points) to 28 (+/− 3 points) is not necessarily an indication of active bleeding. It could simply be laboratory error, since the initial value of 32 really was 29-35 and the later value of 28 was really 25-31, which overlap and, hence, may or may not really be significantly different. Given such a result, the appropriate approach is to treat the second result as raising the possibility that there is active bleeding in progress, to be followed up with: (a) close monitoring of blood pressure and heart rate, lying down and standing (loss of blood volume would drop blood pressure and raise heart rate upon standing), and signs of acute bleeding (e.g., blood upon flushing the stomach with saline, gross blood in stools), and (2) another check of hematocrit, within one or two hours after the possible fall in hematocrit was noted to see if the possible trend had continued.

○ Measurements are only as good as your ability to know what to measure. Consider a patient who is comatose and may have ingested a poison. We typically screen urine and sometimes serum for blood levels of common poisons in cases where a patient presents in coma for unknown reasons. But what if the poison is an uncommon one? As soon as a comatose patient arrives in the emergency room and the airway, breathing, and circulation have been stabilized, a tube is placed in his or her stomach to wash out and collect any pill fragments whose analysis might give a clue as to a possible ingestion overdose. Clinicians often measure the "anion gap," the difference between total anions and bicarbonate and chloride (the major normal anions). When elevated, this suggests that there is something (e.g., the poison) in the blood stream that should not be there and whose presence may account for the patient's comatose state. This is also why talking to family members or looking for circumstantial clues (e.g., empty pill bottles) is crucial in this setting.

8. COMPLEXITY AND REDUNDANCY LEAD TO RESILIENCE

Physiological systems are complex. Simple presentation of the essence of a pathway conveys the core concept in the least confusing manner. However, it should not be forgotten that the biochemical pathways through which physiological systems work are enormously more complex than their simplest representations (see Figure 1.6). Not only are regulatory pathways complex, they are strikingly redun-

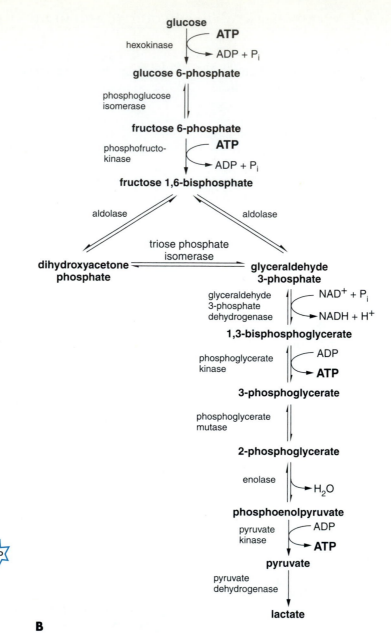

FIGURE 1.6. The pathway of glycolysis viewed in simple terms *(A)*, in more complex terms *(B)*, and in very complex terms *(C)*. It can be seen that there are many levels of complexity at which any given phenomenon can be explained. The question that must be asked is: For what purpose is this explanation? A functional storyteller may only need to describe the starting material, a crucial intermediate and the end product, as in A, to make his or her point about what the pathway does for the body. However, the critical interpreter may use the additional information in B to use this knowledge practically, while the imaginative hypothesizer focuses on aspects of C needed to explore frontiers of regulation of the pathway that may, ultimately, lead to new treatments or diagnostic tools. *(B, Adapted, with permission, from Stryer, L. Biochemistry, 4th ed. New York, Freeman, 1995, p. 484. C, Adapted, with permission, from Salway, J.G. Metabolism at a glance. Malden, MA, Blackwell Science, 1994, p. 67.)*

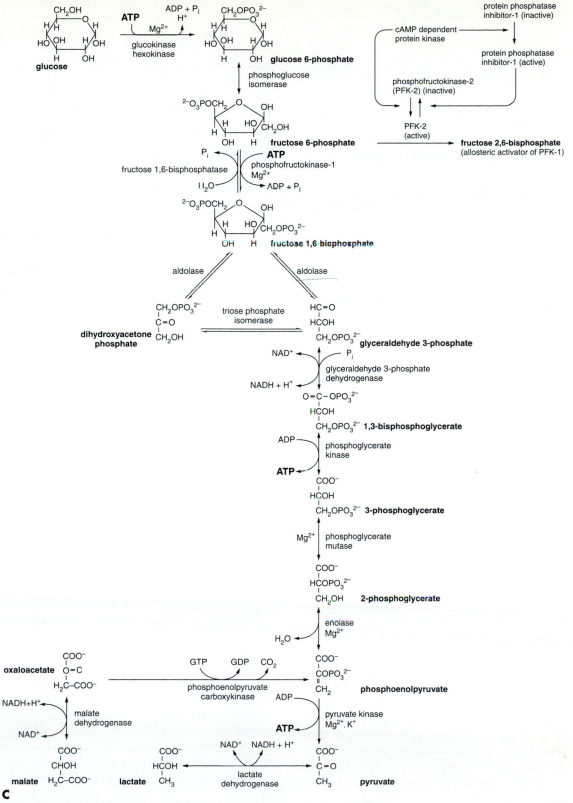

C

FIGURE 1.6 — (continued)

25

dant, but in a peculiar sort of way. In the healthy state multiple mechanisms reinforce one another. When one of them is impaired, for one reason or another, backup mechanisms fill-in almost as well.

This lesson has been particularly apparent in recent years with the development of gene "knockout" technology, whereby, through molecular genetic manipulations, it is possible to delete both copies of a particular gene from a mouse. A recurring theme from these studies is that the defects are often less profound than would have been expected, based on the importance of those functions. Most likely, this reflects the large number of genes that serve overlapping functions and are therefore able to partially compensate for lack of a particular product. Interestingly, the gene-deficient animals are generally altered in some ways suggesting that the redundant systems are not perfect ones. Rather, the back-up systems are able to function when needed, but are not tailored as perfectly as the primary system, and hence defects may be more readily manifest in times of stress.

Table 1.3 shows some cases where the knockout mouse phenotype is entirely consistent with the known function of the eliminated gene. However, in a remarkable number of cases, the phenotype could never have been predicted from the known functions of the missing protein. Either the phenotype is unexpectedly tissue- or organ-specific, or it is milder than would have been expected for loss of a crucial gene, presumably due to the presence of partially redundant back-up systems. These cases illustrate that our current understanding of pathways is quite limited. Furthermore, it is noteworthy that these experiments were all carried out on inbred mouse lines, in an attempt to limit the effects of other genes. It is likely that many of these phenotypes would be further accentuated, attenuated, or changed in minor or major ways by simply crossing them with outbred strains

that would more closely mimic the genetically more diverse situation in humans. Thus far we have only considered those aspects of systems that we know enough about to categorize as being involved in a particular biochemical pathway or physiological function. What of pathways, products, and even entire concepts about which we have not yet discovered any connection?

Indeed, it seems likely that what we are missing is more than just the completion of the process of filling in regulatory details in pathways. Entirely new concepts of cellular and subcellular functions are likely to emerge in the coming years. One implication of this is that the resilience of biological systems is far more robust than we can currently fathom. Conversely, drugs prescribed for a given indication may be more or less effective or have mild or more severe side effects in one person than they do in another. This may be because of individual genetic and/or environment-induced differences in patterns of gene expression, or by other mechanisms of which we are currently unaware. Further discussion of this concept of biochemical individuality can be found in the Frontiers section of Chapter 2.

Clinical Pearl

○ Never underestimate the significance of individual variation in medicine: Often an individual patient taking a nonsteroidal anti-inflammatory drug for treatment of arthritis or another chronic pain condition will swear by one medicine or another (e.g., ibuprofen vs. naprosyn). Often an antihypertensive medication that is efficacious without side effects in one patient will be inefficacious or will be associated with intolerable side effects in another. In general, these sorts of differences are not well understood and, in large part, their

TABLE 1.3   EFFECTS OF VARIOUS GENE KNOCKOUTS ON PHENOTYPE IN MICE

Gene	Protein function	Human syndrome	Knockout mouse phenotype
Pms2	DNA mismatch repair	HNPCC	Lymphoma
Msh2	DNA mismatch repair	HNPCC	Microsatellite instability (dinucleotide repeats, 5-10%) Lymphoma, colon cancer
Mlh1	DNA mismatch repair	HNPCC	Male and female sterility, microsatellite instability
XPA	DNA repair	Xeroderma pigmentosum	Hypersensitivity to ultraviolet light and 7,12-dimethylbenz[a]anthracene
XPC	DNA repair	Xeroderma pigmentosum	Hypersensitivity to ultraviolet light
ADPRT	ADP-ribosyl transferase	None	Epidermal hyperplasia
DNA-MT	DNA methyltransferase	None	Increase in sensitivity to alkylating agents
HR6B	DNA repair ubiquitin conjugating enzyme	None	
ATM	Unknown	Ataxia-telangiectasia	Pleiotropic; ataxia, spermatogenesis arrest
ERCC1	DNA repair	None	Growth arrest, nuclear abnormalities, lethality
RAD51	DNA repair	None	Embryonic lethality
E2F1	Transcription activator	None known	Lymphoma
Wt-1	Zinc fingers	Wilms' tumor/aniridia	Homozygous lethal, urogenital defects
c-fos	Leucine zipper	None known	Homozygous lethal, defective spermatogenesis
c-jun	Leucine zipper	None known	Osteopetrosis, altered B-cell development, behavioral defects
fosB	Leucine zipper	None known	Normal
Apc	Binds b-catenin	Adenomatous polyposis coli	Polyps and adenomas
Mom-1	Phospholipase A2	?	Modification of APC
DCC	N-CAM homology	Colon cancer	Normal
E-cadherin	Cell adhesion	Breast cancer	Homozygous lethal
Neurofibromatosis-1	Ras-GAP cytoskeletal protein	Neurofibromatosis	Homozygous embryonic lethal, cardiac abnormalities; heterozygotes develop tumors
Inhibin-α	Morphogenic protein	?	Interstitial ovarian and testicular tumors
Inhibin-β	Morphogenic receptor protein	?	Cachexia and adrenal tumors
Cox-1	Mediates inflammation	None	Normal
Cox-2	Mediates inflammation	None	Renal development
TO53	Transcription factor	Li-Fraumeni syndrome	High incidence of spontaneous tumors
Rb	Nuclear phosphoprotein	Retinoblastoma	Embryonic homozygous lethal, pineal tumors in heterozygotes
p16^{INK4a} p15	Cyclin/cdk inhibitor	Familial melanoma	Sensitivity to carcinogens, spontaneous sarcomas and lymphomas
p21	Cyclin/cdk inhibitor	None	Lack of radiation response
p27	Cyclin/cdk inhibitor	None	Growth regulation, larger mice
Cyclin D	G$_1$ cyclin	None	Aberrant mammary and retina growth

Adapted, with permission, from Rosenberg, M.P. Gene knockout and transgenic technologies in risk assessment: the next generation. *Mol. Carcinogenesis* 20:262-274, 1997.

basis remains unknown. It seems plausible that biochemical individuality accounts for at least some of these differences (see Chap. 2).

9. A PLETHORA OF CONTINGENCIES LEADS (BACK) TO UNCERTAINTY

At the outset of this chapter, the argument was made that physiological and medical knowledge is, by definition, neither certain nor timeless. Rather, knowledge is the product of the scientific method applied at a given time to a given body of data, with a given technology, in a given society.

An independent argument for uncertainty as a fundamental characteristic of physiological knowledge suggested by the preceding discussion is that evolution has introduced more variables into physiological systems than we can ever hope to track. Given the complexity and redundancy of underlying mechanisms that reinforce homeostasis, and given added variables such as the stage of development and effects from the environment, how can we be certain of anything? The answer is that we cannot — but that certainty need not be a cornerstone of either physiology or medicine, and we need not feel paralyzed without it.

This leads us to emphasize once again the diverse roles of physiology in medicine. Physiology, applied to medicine, tells a story that provides a plausible scenario, perhaps even what is believed to be the most likely scenario, but one that need not be the only possible scenario. Thus, when dealing with a clinical problem, our knowledge of physiology often suggests a likely means of treating a disorder but not necessarily the only one or the best one. Whether following physiologically based therapy or not, the patient's condition needs to be monitored, and the patient's observations of possible side effects

should be taken seriously. Although less than certain, a physiological approach is superior to the alternative for the three reasons presented previously:

1. Physiology provides an operational framework in which to place other information related to making a diagnosis.
2. Physiology provides a starting point for consideration of what therapies might work in the short term to correct aspects of organ system dysfunction that are apparent even in the patient whose specific diagnosis is awaiting the results of further diagnostic studies.
3. Physiology provides a ready means of engaging the patient in the story of his or her disease, in a way that is empowering and facilitates the patient's adherence to and participation in treatment.

Review Questions

14. Describe simple and complex views of a biochemical process and identify the strengths and weaknesses of each.
15. How has the intimate connection between anatomic form and physiological function been achieved?
16. How do gene knockout experiments illustrate the principle of complexity and redundancy through the course of one billion years of animal evolution?
17. What is the role of certainty in physiology or medicine?

10. FRONTIERS IN PHYSIOLOGY AND MEDICINE

A theme of this chapter has been the changing nature of knowledge that makes currently accepted views more akin to rafts at sea rather than buildings on a firm foundation.

Here are three examples of the way knowledge is in flux.

Clinical epidemiology of progesterone and estrogen therapy for secondary prevention of coronary heart disease in women

Studies have shown a statistically significant correlation between postmenopausal estrogen and progesterone replacement and a decrease in heart attacks in women with known coronary artery disease. The assumption has been that this is because estrogen and progesterone result in a favorable change in blood lipids that lowers the risk of heart attacks. Indeed, since the "lipid hypothesis" for heart disease risk has been in favor for decades, these findings were felt to be highly consistent with the existing paradigm and, hence, extremely likely to be correct.

While some cautioned that other explanations for this observation were possible, others argued that the likelihood of other explanations was implausible and that further study was not really necessary. Despite this criticism, some epidemiologists persevered with formal, prospective, randomized controlled trials, in an attempt to address the concern of other sources of bias. What was found was that, contrary to expectations, estrogen and progesterone do not seem to protect postmenopausal women from heart attacks, at least initially. Suddenly, a different "biological plausibility" is in favor: that estrogen and progesterone have opposing effects on lipids and blood clot formation. The "protective" effect of estrogen and progesterone in lowering blood lipids is offset, at least in the short term, by the tendency to increase formation of blood clots, which can cause heart attacks. These findings serve as a stark reminder that we most certainly do not have a certain grasp of extremely fundamental aspects of human physiology (see Refs. 9 and 10).

Homocysteine and cardiovascular risk

A good example of the uncertainty that characterizes science and medicine is the recent thinking regarding the amino acid homocysteine as a risk factor for vascular thrombosis (inappropriate blood clot formation) and coronary artery disease (see Chaps. 7 and 20). The association was first suggested 30 years ago, based on the increased vascular disease in children with inherited disorders (genetic defects) in homocysteine metabolism (50% of these individuals have an inappropriate blood clot, a heart attack, or a stroke by age 30). Subsequently, clinical epidemiology confirmed an association between elevated blood homocysteine and increased heart disease risk. However, there is currently no evidence that folic acid intake (known to lower homocysteine levels) prevents the consequences. This has prompted more studies to identify a biological mechanism to account for these associations, in order to direct drug development. Indeed, studies with cells in culture suggest an effect of homocysteine on vascular endothelium that would be expected to promote clot formation.

Nevertheless, where does homocysteine act and how does it produce these bad effects? There is a vast amount of literature on the first question. Some studies implicate an effect on plasma coagulation factor levels and activity, or in impairment of fibrinolysis, the mechanism by which clots are naturally lysed (see Chap. 19). Other studies suggest effects on platelets (enhanced aggregation), vascular endothelium (increased thrombosis), or smooth muscle (increased proliferation). Any or all of these could contribute to disease, but many of these effects are difficult to reproduce or are seen clearly only at far higher concentrations than are believed to occur in vivo. Perhaps new technology or new ways of thinking about thrombosis will help make sense of these contradictions.

Two general hypotheses have been put forward to explain the possible mechanisms of the action of homocysteine (see Refs. 11-14). The first is that oxidation of homocysteine may generate reactive oxygen species (ROS), such as superoxide, hydrogen peroxide, and hydroxyl radicals. These compounds have a range of effects on proteins that are consistent with homocysteine pathophysiology (see Figure 1.7A).

A second hypothesis is based on the observation that homocysteine is a tightly regulated part of the mechanism by which methyl groups are transferred from one compound to another within cells (see Fig. 1.7B). Alteration of methyl group transfer could result in an increased risk of thrombosis in at least two very different ways. First, a decrease in methylation activity decreases methylation of certain proteins including the important signal transduction protein Ras (see Chap. 3), which affects the growth and repair potential of cells (e.g., the vascular endothelium). Second, in some cases, for example, when an excess of the amino acid methionine is consumed, increased methylation results in inhibition of nitric-oxide-mediated relaxation of vascular smooth muscle (see Chap. 10). This, in turn, could compromise the blood flow to ischemic tissues.

Which of these competing notions will prove to be true? Perhaps none. For example, it is possible that the relevant effect of oxidation is not on the substrates currently under suspicion. Oxidation also affects the lipids, through a process termed *lipid peroxidation.* The possibility that this is the cause of ROS toxicity remains to be explored.

More recent clinical epidemiological studies suggest that the apparent association of heart attacks to elevated homocysteine is less dramatic than previously thought. Thus, elevated blood homocysteine levels may not be an independent risk factor for coronary artery disease, but rather, may prove to be largely a consequence rather than a cause of these conditions (see Refs. 13 and 14), or may prove to be associated only indirectly. More studies are clearly needed, but what do we tell our patients about homocysteine in the meantime? Perhaps the best interim recommendation is one that applies to so much else: a diet relatively lower in protein and fat and higher in fiber, with a variety of different antioxidants, when compared to the standard American diet would decrease sources of oxidative stress (including homocysteine) and promote homeostasis.

Treatment and risk: where is the balance?

Every medical treatment that is effective in prolonging life also subjects the patient to the potential risks of complications. Consider diabetes mellitus (see Chap. 6): prior to the discovery of insulin and other modalities of treatment, patients who were insulin-dependent had a rapid demise in childhood, while those with adult-onset disease died relatively quickly of complications. Now, patients survive and live largely normal lives — until chronic complications result in blindness, kidney failure, neuropathy, and other disabilities.

A growing body of data has suggested that close monitoring of blood glucose, with intensive insulin or other drug therapy to maintain blood glucose as close to the norm as possible, delays complications and improves the patient's quality of life. Now, the flip side of the coin is coming to light (see Ref. 16). It seems that patients with intensive medical regimens that normalize blood glucose are also at greater risk of dying from exacerbation of a subset of diabetes-associated complications compared to patients with moderate control of blood glucose (see Figure 1.7). One possible explanation is that tight control is associated with weight gain, which results in more problems than would occur with moder-

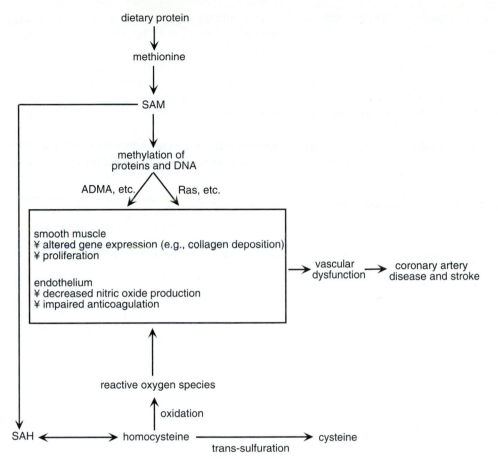

FIGURE 1.7. Some hypothetical mechanisms for the association of elevated blood homocysteine with increased risk of coronary artery disease and stroke. One hypothesis (upper half) implicates altered protein methylation (e.g., of ADMA and RAS) due to the effects of a high dietary methionine load on pathways of intermediary metabolism. Another hypothesis implicates reactive oxygen species. Both mechanisms converge on altered smooth muscle and/or altered endothelial activity resulting in vascular dysfunction that predisposes to coronary artery disease and stroke. Possibly, the two mechanisms are related by virtue of the connection between SAM and SAH. Asymmetric dimethyl arginine (ADMA) is an endogenous inhibitor of endothelial nitric oxide synthase. Ras is a guanine nucleotide-binding protein that serves as an important second messenger in signaling pathways including that of cellular proliferation. SAM is S-adenosyl methionine, and SAH is S-adenosyl homocysteine, universal cellular metabolites involved in methyl group transfer both for amino acid metabolism and modification of proteins. *(Adapted, with permission, from Lentz, S.R. Mechanisms of thrombosis in hyperhomocysteinemia. Curr. Opinion in Hematol. 5:343-349, 1998.)*

ate blood glucose control without weight gain.

This new finding serves to underscore two points related to this chapter's emphasis on lack of certainty in medicine. First, there is no such thing as a completely benign intervention, even when the benefits of the intervention far outweigh the risks. The risk-to-benefit ratio refers to a population, not an individual patient, who may or may not fit the statistical norm for various reasons (e.g., genes, environment, or chance). Second, often new insights are best applied cautiously rather than by pushing new conclusions to their logical extreme because they may be revised in the future.

11. HOW DOES UNDERSTANDING NORMAL PHYSIOLOGY PROVIDE INSIGHT INTO THE INITIAL CASE PRESENTATION?

Mr. F. A. is a 54-year-old father and office worker who transferred himself to your clinic's primary care area seeking more satisfying care than he had received in the past. His underlying medical problems included ulcerative colitis, chronic obstructive pulmonary disease, hypertension, diabetes mellitus, and depression. He articulated many reasons for his anger and mistrust. He has a long history of unanticipated drug side effects that were rarely fully effective at treating his complaints. Explanations by health care providers as to what they thought was wrong with him were inadequate. The potential limitations of the therapies they prescribed were never clearly presented. Often, the provider's pronouncements came down as inscrutable edicts from above, or when he was involved in decision making he was provided with statistical data on therapeutic efficacy — and expected to choose between clinical approaches whose pros and cons were not obvious. Although he had sought and seen a series of

new health care providers over the years, he was often frustrated because they assumed they understood his illnesses — without listening to his experience of failure with the very therapies they planned to prescribe. His illnesses terrify him and have wreaked havoc in his life.

An extraordinary number of people are disaffected with conventional medicine. Often they turn to alternative therapies from which they may or may not get relief. One interesting problem is that many advocates for alternative therapies make the same epistemological mistakes (e.g., they assume certainty in knowledge and fail to recognize the limitations of their approach), for which allopathic medicine can be criticized. Many disaffected patients are lost to follow-up, drifting from one health care provider to another. Their frustration and anger can contribute greatly to their pain and suffering and interfere with the efforts of providers to treat them. They also often have insight into their illness, which was accumulated through personal experience, that has not been tapped by clinicians who are too harried or busy or dogmatic to listen.

Trying to understand his concerns and to build his trust, you start by taking some time to listen to Mr. A. and by asking questions about his experience with interventions that may have made his symptoms better or worse. Then, following a careful physical examination and inspection of laboratory results, you provide him with a physiological framework in which to view his diseases, including plausible explanations for why previously tried therapies did not work, and why it might be worth trying them, or a variation of them, again.

As part of your approach, you acknowledge that modern medicine's understanding of his diseases is limited and that he may have a disease variant that is uncommon, has been misdiagnosed, or is particularly poorly understood. You assure Mr. A. that, while you cannot guarantee either improvement or cure, you will work with him to come up with a strategy for managing his illnesses that optimizes the quality of his life.

Patients often ignore the recommendations of their health care providers because those recommendations are seen as ephemeral, idealized pronouncements, without rationales that make sense and that are unconnected to the trials and tribulations of day-to-day life. If clinicians more often took the time to hear patients' stories, consider their observations on their illness, and incorporate these insights into things that patients can do to productively affect their care, clinical outcomes would be better, at least for a substantial subset of patients, typified by Mr. A. (see Ref. 16).

Note that this is a powerful use of physiology to facilitate the care of patients that does not rely on the myth of certainty and does not create false hopes or promise more than can be delivered. It synthesizes the art of medicine with the power of science.

First, you make some adjustments to his diabetes and lung disease pharmaceutical regimens. Then you proceed to make recommendations regarding some of his symptomatic complaints. These include nonpharmaceutical measures to address the underlying disturbances of homeostasis whose symptoms will exacerbate any illness (e.g., diet, exercise, and other recommendations to ameliorate his diabetes mellitus and various symptoms such as diarrhea or constipation, difficulty sleeping, and headache). You inform him about likely and possible side effects of any medications you prescribe and ask him to keep a careful log of things that he associates with exacerbations and remissions of his various diseases.

Mr. A. leaves your office more empowered and more confident in you as his new health care provider than he has been with anyone in years. Some of the nonpharmaceutical measures may well make him feel better. In the long run, the relationship he builds with you will likely have a powerful beneficial effect. It remains to be seen how effectively the measures you have initiated, or will institute in the future, will treat his chronic underlying medical conditions. What you are trying may work no better than the therapies instituted by Mr. A.'s previous health care providers. Nevertheless, he is subjectively better already and will almost certainly be no worse than he would be otherwise, as a result of this more accurate, honest, humble, and collaborative approach.

Medicine does not, and probably never will, have all the answers — because the questions will change. The more we learn, the more we rephrase the questions to incorporate a greater sophistication. This patient responded positively to the clinician telling a functional story that provided one reasonable physiological scenario for the patient's medical condition. Thus, quite apart from its other roles, physiological knowledge has been used here in a way that strengthens the patient-health care provider relationship, which currently can use all the strengthening it can get.

SUMMARY AND REVIEW OF KEY CONCEPTS

1. Knowledge is more than just data, it includes or is influenced by: the technology used to collect the data, the interpretation of the data within the conceptual frameworks that are popular at the time, and even political and economic ideology, which influence which conceptual frameworks are taken seriously.
2. Knowledge is also influenced by how questions are posed and the use that is intended for the knowledge. Rather than getting us closer to some absolute truth, it is more helpful to view the explosion

of scientific knowledge as adding more depth to the kind and number of questions we can ask, and nuances to the purposes for which the answers can be used.

3. All experimental sciences, including physiology, pathophysiology, and epidemiology, are based on principles of induction. Thus, lack of certainty is a fundamental characteristic of physiological knowledge in particular and medical knowledge in general.

4. Physiology is the study of organ systems and their interactions over the course of the human life cycle. It can be viewed from the perspective of fundamental physical and chemical principles or from the perspective of biological specializations that allow life to be distinguished from nonliving things. Both approaches are valid and together provide the most coherent and useful view of physiology as it is relevant to medicine.

5. Cells are the smallest living units of the body. They are organized into tissues, organs, and organ systems. Within cells are membrane-delimited organelles, proteins, and other macromolecules. Many proteins are enzymes that are organized into pathways to make chemical reactions proceed in certain directions, at rates and to extents that would not occur in their absence.

6. Biological systems are characterized by feedback, usually negative, but occasionally positive. Feedback can be simple or complex with many layers of specializations.

7. Homeostasis is the tendency of a physiological system to resist deviations from the normal range.

8. Cycles of development are seen in many organ systems, often in conjunction with positive feedback and programmed cell death.

9. The dimension of time is important both in terms of understanding what is going on in the patient at the present time, as a snapshot in the natural history of the disease process, and in terms of understanding when the need for a given therapy will be complete and homeostasis will be restored.

10. The dimension of space: Physiological functions have evolved in a manner that takes into account the anatomic location of organ systems.

11. A mole is 6.0235×10^{23} molecules of any substance, which is equal to the molecular weight of that substance in grams.

12. Complexity and redundancy leads to resilience of biological systems and are a legacy of billions of years of evolution that remains poorly understood.

13. The enormous number of genes that affect any given trait means that it is often difficult to predict the effect of a drug or other treatment on any given individual. The clinician cognizant of physiology is always on the lookout for the unexpected consequences of "biochemical individuality."

14. Physiological knowledge does not provide certainty, but certainty is not necessary for the practice of medicine. What is needed, on any question, is (a) a working hypothesis that we use today, based on currently available technology, data, and concepts; (b) an awareness that these notions are not fixed in stone but rather, are evolving; (c) an appreciation of some of the frontiers that may give rise to the views of the future — and when it is appropriate to call in a specialist to deal with the technical details of which you may not be aware; and (d) a remembrance that the patient is a human being, often in crisis, and that the manner and attentiveness with which you engage the patient can influence the quality and therapeutic effect of the interaction, regardless of the technical issues involved.

A CASE OF PHYSIOLOGICAL MEDICINE

M. D. is a 72-year-old woman who lives alone and works as a writer. She is admitted to the hospital with a possible stroke and a blood pressure of 220/130 (upper limits of normal for her age would be about 160/90). She has a long history of atherosclerotic cardiovascular disease. Her past medical history is most notable for a major thrombotic stroke about two years ago, from which she has largely recovered, with some residual difficulty with speech. Although she may have had hypertension in the distant past, her blood pressure has not been elevated in the last few years. Her cholesterol has been slightly elevated and treated only with dietary modification. On the morning of admission, Ms. D. awoke, felt dizzy and unable to rise from bed, and noticed double vision. After speaking with her primary care provider by phone, she proceeded to call 911 and was taken by ambulance to the emergency room. There her extreme high blood pressure was noted and antihypertensive therapy with sodium nitroprusside, a powerful, intravenous, rapid-acting drug for lowering blood pressure, was initiated. She was transferred to the intensive care unit (ICU) for close monitoring of her medical condition. Prior to going to the ICU, Ms. D. received a computed tomography (CT) scan of the head that revealed signs of ischemia in the left temporal region. A tentative diagnosis of stroke-in-evolution was made, and she was placed on systemic anticoagulation therapy.

A tentative plan to carry out an arteriogram (an x-ray study of the arteries) to identify possible vascular lesions that might be bypassed to avoid further stroke was canceled when Ms. D. refused to consider the possibility of surgery.

Slowly, her double vision and generalized weakness resolved. The nitroprusside was gradually discontinued. Ms. D. was placed on a systemic antihypertensive medication and two cholesterol-lowering agents. Anticoagulation was adjusted to an outpatient regimen, and she was discharged.

One week later she went to her primary care physician, again dizzy, weak, and feeling "lousy," but this time without double vision or other new neurological symptoms. Her blood pressure was noted to be 80/60.

The primary care provider took a careful history and concluded that Ms. D. felt bad because of the effects of the many new drugs she was taking. The high blood pressure medication, the cholesterol-lowering medication, and a sleeping pill were all stopped. Gradually, her blood pressure returned to normal and she returned to her baseline state of well-being.

QUESTIONS

1. After seeing that the patient had dangerously high blood pressure when she had the stroke, the clinicians appropriately initiated antihypertensive therapy. Later, the primary care physician discontinued this treatment, suggesting a difference of opinion. Present the two perspectives and explain the difference.

2. The medical staff felt the angiogram was appropriate and necessary — but the patient disagreed. Assuming that the technical utility and merits of an angiogram and subsequent emergent surgery could prevent further stroke, is there a rationale for the patient's point of view?

3. How might new knowledge change this scenario in the future?

ANSWERS

1. The clinicians in the emergency room appropriately treated Ms. D. for her danger-

ously high blood pressure and then discharged her on medication assuming that the high blood pressure had been a cause of the stroke.

The primary care provider, knowing that she did not have hypertension prior to the stroke but was extremely hypertensive during the stroke, concluded that the high blood pressure was a consequence, not a cause, of the stroke, and thus made the decision to discontinue therapy.

2. Ms. D.'s view might be that the risk of complications outweighs the benefits of potential extension of life. In her view, prolongation of low-quality life might be the most undesirable outcome, in place of which a rapid demise would be preferable. Although we might disagree with the patient, we can only present the case for the alternative position, and must respect the patient's right to make her own decision.

3. New diagnostic modalities will entail less risk of complications than an angiogram. New therapeutic modalities, including thrombolysis, may allow stroke-in-evolution to be terminated effectively or reversed at later and later times after onset of symptoms. These new modalities may carry lower risks of complications.

References and suggested readings

GENERAL REFERENCES

1. Dewey, J. (1923). The quest for certainty.
2. Kuhn, T.S. (1962). *Structure of Scientific Revolutions.* Chicago: University of Chicago Press.
3. Bernard, C. (1927). *An Introduction to the Study of Experimental Medicine.* New York: Dover.
4. Boyd, D.B. (1998). Rational drug design: controlling the size of the haystack. *Mod. Drug Disc.* Nov./Dec. 41-47.
5. Cannon, W.B. *The Wisdom of the Body.* New York: W.W. Norton.
6. Gerhart, J., and Kirschner, M. (1997). *Cells, Embryos, and Evolution.* Malden, MA: Blackwell Science.
7. Gould, S.J. (1982). *The Panda's Thumb.* New York: W.W. Norton.
8. Dawkins, R. (1996). *The Blind Watchmaker.* New York: W.W. Norton.

FRONTIER REFERENCES

9. Hulley, S., et al. (1998). Randomized trial of estrogen plus progestin for secondary prevention of coronary artery disease in postmenopausal women. *JAMA* 280:563-674.
10. Petiti, D. (1998). Hormone replacement therapy and heart disease prevention: Experimentation trumps observation. *JAMA* 280:650-652.
11. Lentz, S.R. (1998). Mechanisms of thrombosis in hyperhomocysteinemia. *Curr. Opinion Hematol.* 5:343-349.
12. Wang, H., et al. (1997). Inhibition of growth and p21(Ras) methylation in vascular endothelial cells by homocysteine but not cysteine. *J. Biol. Chem.* 272:25380-25385.
13. Folsom, A.R., et al. (1998). Prospective study of coronary heart disease incidence in relation to fasting total homocysteine, related genetic polymorphisms, and B vitamins. *Circulation* 98:204-210.
14. Kuller, L.H., and Evans, R.W. (1998). Homocysteine, vitamins, and cardiovascular disease. *Circulation* 98:196-199.
15. Purnell, J.Q. (1998). Effect of excessive weight gain with intensive therapy of type 1 diabetes on lipid levels and blood pressure: results from the DCCT. *JAMA* 280:140-146.
16. Adler, H.M. (1997). The history of the present illness as treatment: Who's listening and why does it matter? *JABFP* 10:28-35.

MOLECULAR FOUNDATIONS OF PHYSIOLOGY

2

1. THE MOLECULAR BASIS OF MODERN PHYSIOLOGY

To understand modern physiology, that is, the current paradigm of physiological knowledge (see Chap. 1), the reader needs some background in biochemistry, cell biology, and genetics. This chapter is intended to provide that background and makes reference to more detailed sources.

Biochemistry, cell biology, and molecular genetics in physiology

Consequences

The ongoing revolution in biochemistry, cell biology, and molecular genetics has had three important consequences for physiology:

1. The level of detail of our currently favored explanations for just about everything has increased enormously. Many drugs, whose actions were discovered empirically, have now had explanations attached to account for their effects. As discussed in the previous chapter, we may be no closer to an ultimate, timeless understanding of "truth," however, we can surely say a lot more about something. As long as that "something" is useful (i.e., facilitates the care of patients or is an engine of economic growth), the value of the scientific enterprise is assured.
2. New concepts have emerged from cellular, molecular, and genetic analysis that require integration into the larger framework of organ system function (i.e., physiology). For example, it has become apparent that cells can die in a programmed fashion, termed *apoptosis*. This process is found to play a crucial role in the physiology of virtually every organ system and the pathophysiology of many complex diseases. These new concepts are only just now being integrated into older ways of thinking about various organ systems. Indeed, much of medicine as currently practiced by most clinicians is oblivious to the current molecular understanding of the underlying physiological phenomena. Then why should we strive to incorporate these insights into clinical thinking? Because these new concepts provide richer explanations for clinicians and their patients, and because these new concepts are setting the stage for the development of new modalities of disease treatment of the future.
3. New tools have been developed that promise to further increase the rate of progress. The phenotypes observed in animal models such as transgenic and "knockout" mice (where specific genes have been deleted through the molecular mechanism of homologous recombination), as well as in the insights from sequence databases of the entire genome of yeast and other organisms, have highlighted ways in which we are similar to, as well as different from, other organisms. Chips containing every single gene in an experimental organism's genome are now used to map the detailed changes in gene expression that occur under different physiological and pathological circumstances (see Ref. 5 and discussion in Frontiers). Within 5 years, the entire 3 billion base pair human genome will be sequenced and DNA array chip technology can be applied directly to human gene expression. These tools will make possible further explanations and new therapies in the future (including many that could not even have been imagined while the current generation of clinicians was receiving their formal medical training.)

Challenges

The molecular revolution in physiology and medicine poses four challenges:

1. For those involved in research, the chal-

lenge is not to let the power of the technology lead to intellectual sloppiness. It is very easy to find what you expect or to interpret high technology-derived data in a boring manner consistent with a well-developed paradigm. More difficult is to make sense of what others might dismiss as "noise" in the data or cobble together a more creative interpretation of the findings and then come up with a way to test it.

2. For clinicians, the challenge is to keep up with modern technical and conceptual advances, knowing when to use them and when not to use them (to minimize risks, costs, etc.) without losing sight of the art of medicine or its ultimate point: the care of patients.

3. As a society, we need to decide to what use we will put the new molecular insights. To sell more drugs, advance disease care (for those who can afford it), and improve profits? Or to heal patients, provide better health care, and improve the quality of people's lives?

4. Finally, all of us, whether students, scientists, clinicians, or patients, need to remember that what we know about biology, physiology, or medicine as a result of these marvelous advances in technology and concepts is still dwarfed by what we do not understand. It will take far longer than any of our lifetimes to unravel the mysteries of billions of years of evolution.

Biochemical form and physiological function in evolution

According to the modern cellular and molecular paradigm, the functions of our organ systems, and of our bodies as a whole, are generally viewed as a consequence of activities carried out by individual cells through chemical reactions facilitated by individual proteins.

Most of our activities, and the organs, cells, organelles, particles and proteins that make them possible, have analogues in activities of other organisms with which we share a common evolutionary heritage. Thus, for example, mice share our use of endogenous heat generation to maintain a constant body temperature at which enzymes work efficiently. This allows us to venture briefly into otherwise forbiddingly cold environments that would stop an organism dependent on ambient heat (e.g., a lizard) in its tracks.

As a general rule, the earlier in evolution that a physiological specialization appeared, the more divergent the subsequent organisms in which that general solution to a particular problem can be found. Thus, both humans and insects use hemoglobin as the primary oxygen-carrying protein. We share homology with even the simplest eukaryotes, such as yeast in the organelle components that make up our individual cells, and the structure of proteins involved in fundamental metabolic pathways and mechanisms of gene expression. Even the most divergent life forms on earth (for example, humans and *Escherichia coli*) use mostly the same building blocks, in terms of precursors to make DNA, RNA, proteins, lipids, and so forth.

Although these similarities usually reflect the fact that we share common ancestors with these organisms, sometimes similarities are a result of convergent evolution — the same good solution to a problem selected independently, more than once, in the course of evolution. Thus, bacteria and humans both have evolved enzymes for protein cleavage (e.g., subtilisin and trypsin, respectively) that function by the same mechanism (i.e., the same amino acid side groups comprise the active site), even though the two proteins as a whole share no significant overall amino acid sequence homology.

Regardless, despite enormous variation in size, external appearance, and other properties, the fundamental conservation of proteins, pathways, and subcellular structures means that we can study physiological processes down to the molecular mechanism in other organisms to understand generally how they work in us. Most of our understanding of human biochemistry, cell biology, and physiology is based on the results of experiments in simpler, more readily studied organisms, such as mice, frogs, fruit flies, worms, yeast, and bacteria. Typically, only a small subset of information is directly known about these processes in humans. But since what little information that is known from studies of human tissues seems consistent with more detailed work from specialized model animal systems, we are inclined to believe that more extensive extrapolations apply as well.

In contrast, while the overall plan is similar between often widely divergent species, sometimes it is the differences, not the similarities, that are most important. In these circumstances, conclusions based on animal studies must be applied to humans with caution. For example, there may be additional levels of regulation or other complexity built into humans that is not apparent in yeast, or mice, or even other primates such as chimpanzees, with whom we share about 98.5% genetic identity. An important unanswered question is: What does the different 1.5% of genetic information between chimpanzees and us encode, and how does it account for the differences between our species?

Even conclusions based on the study of one set of humans are not necessarily applicable to other subsets of humans who may display variations from both other individuals and from the statistical norms for the population as a whole (see Frontiers later). Most likely, this reflects the complex consequences of multiple genes affecting any given trait.

Case Presentation

A. B., a tall, muscular, 56-year-old former restaurateur, whose specialty was sheep brain stew, came to medical attention with a progressive neurodegenerative disease. Mr. B. came to this country from Italy 50 years earlier and worked his way up from waiting tables to owning his own restaurant. He was a charming, cultured, well-read man. With his children grown, he and his wife decided to sell their restaurant and retire to his hometown. There, he got a part-time job as a security guard, mainly to keep himself busy. Then, his dream turned into a nightmare.

Over the space of 6 months, Mr. B. became progressively more forgetful. At first, it provided material for good-natured teasing by his wife and friends. But then he started leaving his gun in places where he should not have. Soon he could not reliably make his way home from work. His speech was slurred. He quit his job. A local physician thought he was depressed and prescribed antidepressant medications. Sometimes his wife would return home to find him standing naked in the front yard. Other times he would fail to recognize family members. In desperation, his wife took him back to the United States. On the flight, he was barely controllable and constantly chased down the aisles by his wife who was trying to give him a sedative by medicine dropper.

Evaluation revealed a man with profound dementia but lacking any focal neurological deficits. Considering the time-course and other features of disease progression, Mr. B. was given the tentative diagnosis of Creutzfeldt-Jacob disease. His family was terrified. They asked the clinicians: What caused this? Is it contagious?

Review Questions

1. What are three consequences of the molecular revolution for physiology?
2. What are four challenges that the molecular tools and concepts pose for students of physiology?

2. PHYSICAL CHEMISTRY OF BIOLOGICAL SYSTEMS

Ways to store and transmit information and energy are necessary conditions of life. The information needs to be encoded in a form that can be passed on from one generation to the next with a high (but not perfect) degree of fidelity. The information also has to be easy to decode and used by the individual. The energy has to be in a form stable enough to be stored but also available to meet the needs of the individual for the work of survival and reproduction.

Energy

Energy is the capacity to do work. It comes in two general forms: kinetic energy, the energy of molecular motion; and potential energy, stored energy of various forms. According to the first law of thermodynamics, barring a nuclear reaction that converts matter into energy, energy can be neither created nor destroyed. However, energy can be transformed from one form to another.

Heat and light are forms of kinetic energy. Sunlight is the original source of most energy in biological systems on earth. It is harnessed by plants through the ability of chlorophyll to absorb the energy in sunlight and convert that form of kinetic energy into various forms of potential energy. One of these forms of potential energy, the energy in chemical bonds, can be passed along the food chain, thereby making animal life possible on earth. Thus, all animals eat either plants or other animals to gain chemical energy that originated from the plants. As potential energy flows along the food chain, some of it is used to do work, but even more of it is dissipated in the environment as heat, as a result of the inefficiency of various kinds of work. When food materials are burned in a fire, all of the energy is released as heat (except for the energy in unburned material, which forms smoke).

Three forms of potential energy are particularly useful for biology, and hence for physiological systems:

1. The energy stored in chemical bonds, such as in glucose, proteins, and fats, as well as in specialized energy transfer molecules such as adenosine triphosphate (ATP). We eat to get this form of energy and our bodies use it to drive many chemical reactions in our bodies.
2. The energy stored in concentration gradients (e.g., across a biological membrane). The potential energy in a concentration gradient can be used to do work, such as driving another molecule "uphill" against its concentration gradient.
3. The energy stored in the separation of electrical charges (manifest as an electrical potential difference, e.g., across a biological membrane).

Of these, only the first, chemical bond energy, can be transferred from one organism to another (by being eaten and assimilated).

The creation of food materials (stored chemical energy) by plants involves reduction of carbon dioxide from the atmosphere to form more complex molecules such as glucose, which are rich in chemical bond energy. Release of that energy, whether suddenly by setting the food on fire or gradually through the action of enzymes in biological systems, is a form of oxidation. In biological systems, oxidation proceeds in a stepwise fashion, sometimes resulting in carbon dioxide and water (the end products of setting the food on fire), in other cases releasing only part of the stored energy. As a result of oxidation, compounds are transformed to a more energetically stable state, with release of potential (chemical) energy.

Information

Biological systems are particularly rich in stored information and in the ability to faithfully copy, transmit, decode, and act upon that information. The macromolecules chosen for this purpose through the course of evolution, such as DNA, RNA, and proteins, have features that are particularly well suited for storage and manipulation of information.

The information that specifies just about every feature that distinguishes us from each other — and from an armadillo or a jellyfish — is encoded in our genes in the form of specific sequences of relatively stable, double-stranded DNA. This information is expressed, first as the more labile and generally single-stranded RNA, and finally as proteins, the molecules that actually do the work that the information makes possible. Thus, in some sense, DNA and RNA act like blueprints to direct the construction of various machines (the proteins). Some proteins play structural roles in holding together parts of our cells, tissues, and organs. Other proteins are used to bind and store specific substances or transfer them from one site to another. Many other proteins are enzymes, biological catalysts that affect the rate and direction of crucial chemical reactions that occur in living systems.

Molecules interact in several sorts of ways that are crucial for the function of biological systems (see Table 2.1 and Figure 2.1). These interactions can be classified according to how much energy it takes to break them. Covalent bonds are interactions in which two atoms within a molecule actually share one or more electrons. Covalent interactions require a relatively large input of energy to be broken. Sometimes the two atoms involved in a covalent chemical bond do not share the electrons evenly, in which case the molecule is said to be polar and different parts of the

TABLE 2.1   COVALENT AND NONCOVALENT CHEMICAL BONDS

Bond type	Strength (in vacuum) kcal/mole	Strength (in water) kcal/mole
Covalent	90	90
Ionic	80	3
Hydrogen	4	1
Van der Waals forces	0.1	0.1

molecule have a relatively + (electron poor) or − (electron rich) charge.

There are several types of noncovalent interactions, which hold atoms together more weakly, taking about twentyfold less energy to break. The major noncovalent interactions are ionic bonds and van der Waals interactions. The hydrogen bond is a special kind of ionic interaction that occurs between various biologically important molecules and water. Polar molecules are more readily able to form ionic bonds and hydrogen bonds compared to uncharged, nonpolar molecules. Hydrophobic interactions are another biologically important kind of noncovalent interaction driven by the inability of nonpolar substances to form hydrogen bonds with water (see Figure 2.1 and later).

The strength of a bond can be measured by the energy required to break it (given in kilocalories per mole or kcal/mole). An aqueous environment, such as exists in cells, greatly weakens ionic and hydrogen bonds between nonwater molecules. Thus, the ionic interactions that hold granite rock together are strong because they are not occurring in an aqueous environment. Ionic interactions are further weakened by salt, which allows counter ions to cluster around the charges. Precisely because ionic interactions are weak in biologically relevant water and salt environments, they, like hydrogen bonds, are crucial for protein-protein interactions. Hy-

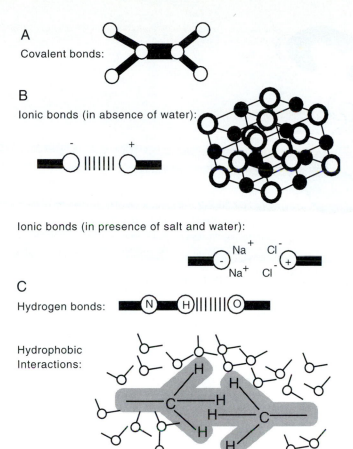

A
Covalent bonds:

B
Ionic bonds (in absence of water):

Ionic bonds (in presence of salt and water):

C
Hydrogen bonds:

Hydrophobic
Interactions:

FIGURE 2.1. Covalent and noncovalent interactions. This figure indicates in schematic form the difference between *A*, a covalent bond and various types of noncovalent interactions including *B*, ionic interactions in the absence and presence of water and salt, and *C*, hydrogen bonds in the absence and presence of hydrophobic molecules. Not shown are another type of noncovalent interaction termed *van der Waals forces*. Open and closed circles represent different atoms. Bold bars (in A, B, C) and solid lines (in A and C) between atoms represent covalent bonds. Na^+, sodium; Cl^-, chloride; N, nitrogen; C, carbon; H, hydrogen. + and − refer to charge, which reflect the relative electron-rich or electron-poor state of the atom, respectively. *(Adapted, with permission, from Alberts, B. et al., (1994). Molecular Biology of the Cell, 3rd ed. New York, Garland, pp. 92-94.)*

drophobic interactions are actually caused by repulsion of hydrophobic groups from hydrogen-bonded water (see Table 2.1).

Without these weak, noncovalent interactions, life could not exist on earth. For example, it is the noncovalent hydrogen bonds between water molecules that allow them to exist in a liquid state. Otherwise, at body temperature, all water would be a gas which would pose a problem for life as we know it, since most living organisms are composed of two-thirds to four-fifths water by weight.

The sum total of many noncovalent interactions is remarkably stable (see Figure 2.2), but can be subject to manipulation in biological systems that render these interactions reversible at a particular time (see Chap. 3). Making and breaking covalent bonds, which involve a large amount of energy, are a useful means of storing energy. Making and breaking noncovalent interactions takes a very small amount of energy, and therefore is a useful way to store information. Characteristic of biological systems are the utilization of certain classes of very large, complex, and information-rich macromolecules, such as DNA, RNA, and proteins, in which

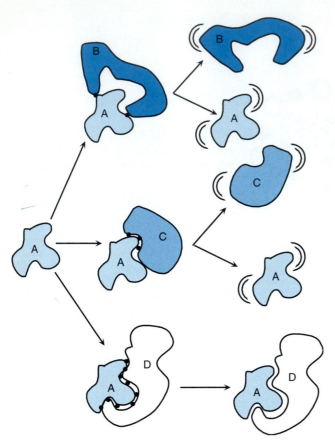

FIGURE 2.2. An indication of how the sum of many noncovalent interactions can serve to hold two complex macromolecules together. Molecule A randomly encounters other molecules (B, C, and D). The surfaces of A and B, and of A and C, are a poor match in terms of forming only a small number of noncovalent bonds (represented by black dots). Thus, random thermal motion (indicted by curved lines), due to the heat generated in the body, is sufficient to disrupt them. The surfaces of A and D, however, match well and form enough weak bonds to withstand the thermal motion occurring at standard biological temperatures. Hence A and D stay bound to each other as a protein complex. *(Adapted, with permission, from Alberts, B. et al. (1994). Molecular Biology of the Cell, 3rd ed. New York, Garland, pp. 91.)*

a large number of noncovalent interactions occur.

Thermodynamics, catalysis, and enzymes

Chemical reactions and equilibrium

The second law of thermodynamics states that the entropy (randomness) of the universe as a whole always increases. While some may find this a depressing thought, it does leave open the possibility that in some local neighborhoods in the universe, entropy may decrease. Thus, even while randomness and disorder are increasing in the universe as a whole, some places in the universe may be more ordered, at least for a while. This is the "loophole" that makes life, a form of local increased order, possible.

Free energy reflects the tendency of chemical reactions to proceed spontaneously (by itself). A general equation that applies to biological systems that reflects the likelihood of a particular reaction occurring is:

$$\Delta G = \Delta H - T \times \Delta S$$

where ΔG is the free energy of the reaction, ΔH is the potential energy in the chemical bonds, T is the temperature, and ΔS the entropy or randomness.

Sometimes the second law of thermodynamics manifests itself in unexpected ways. For example, it turns out that entropy is the driving force behind protein folding, even though a folded protein is more ordered than an unfolded one. The reason is that in the unfolded protein, exposure of hydrophobic amino acid side groups creates a surrounding lattice of water molecules. By burying these groups within a folded protein, need for this ordered structure of water is eliminated and the water molecules can maintain a more disordered structure, thus the total entropy of the universe increases.

There is a relation between the ΔG of a reaction and the concentrations of reactants and products of that reaction at equilibrium (Table 2.2).

Chemical reactions, for example:

$$A + B \rightleftharpoons C$$

proceed in the direction that minimizes the free energy of the system. Thus, those reactions whose ΔG is positive do not occur, to a significant degree, spontaneously. Rather, they require an input of energy, if they are to happen.

The equilibrium between reactants (i.e., A and B) and products (i.e., C) that is reached when the reaction has gone to completion, is determined by the equilibrium constant, K. In mathematical terms, this is equal to the concentration of products over that of the reactants at equilibrium:

$$K = \frac{[C]}{[A][B]}$$

Put another way, equilibrium is reached when the rate of the reaction in one direction is equaled by the rate of the reaction in the opposite direction. Thus, the concentrations of reactants and products influence the direction a chemical reaction will go in order to reach equilibrium. Furthermore, if the distribution of either reactants or products is far from equilibrium, it tends to drive the reaction in the direction that establishes equilibrium, including "backwards" from products to reactants. This is termed *the law of mass action* (see Figure 2.3). Thus, by providing a vast excess of one or more reactants or by removing one or more products as quickly as they are formed, it is possible to get an unfavorable reaction (i.e., one whose ΔG is positive), which would otherwise remain in the form of reactants to proceed to products to some extent.

Activation energy and enzyme action

Free energy and equilibria are two different ways of describing where a reaction will eventually go. However these concepts do not elucidate how the reaction got there or when it will get there. Another way of looking at chemical reactions, which provides insight into these questions, is in terms of the energy involved in bringing reactants together in a productive manner. Whether a chemical reaction will occur quickly or not depends on the size of the activation energy "hump" to be overcome before the reaction occurs (see Figure 2.4A). One way a reaction with a large activation energy can be speeded is to heat the reactants, which increases the energy they

TABLE 2.2 VALUES OF ΔG°′ FOR SOME VALUES OF K_{eq}

K_{eq}	$\Delta G^{\circ\prime}$ (cal/mol)*
0.001	+4086
0.01	+2724
0.1	+1362
1.0	0
10	−1362
100	−2724
1000	−4086

* Calculated from the formula $\Delta G^{\circ\prime} = -2.3\ RT \log K_{eq}$. Adapted, with permission, from Lodish, H.F. et al. (1995). *Molecular Cell Biology,* 3rd ed. New York, W.H. Freeman, p. 37.

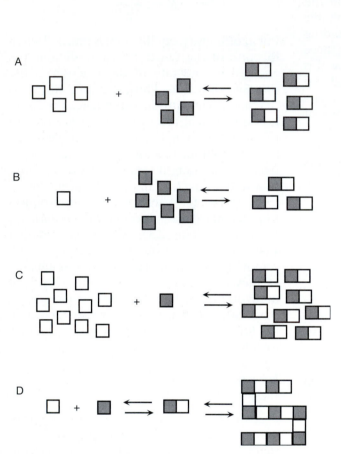

FIGURE 2.3. Various manifestations of the law of mass action. A description of the dependence of chemical reactions on the concentrations of reactants and products, and the consequences of manipulating reactant concentrations on the extent to which the reaction goes to completion. A reaction in which two reactants (white squares and gray squares) combine to make gray-white rectangles is described, in each case, at equilibrium. Equilibrium is reached when the rate of chemical reaction in one direction equals the rate in the other. A indicates the equilibrium reached when equal concentrations of white and gray squares are combined. B and C show what happens when the concentration of one of the reactants (the white squares) is manipulated. When the concentration of white squares is dropped very low in B, less product (fewer gray-white rectangles) will be formed, at equilibrium. Conversely, by raising the concentration of white squares in C, the reaction can be driven such that, at equilibrium, most of the other reactant (gray squares) is consumed to make the product. The reaction can also be driven by consuming the product in a subsequent reaction (here indicated as a polymer of alternating gray and white rectangles). Thus, in D, equilibrium is far to the right, compared to A. Note that the total number of gray squares in reactants and products of all reactions is 10. The distribution of gray squares between reactant and product at equilibrium is thus affected by the concentration of the other reactant (white squares) or the disposition of the product (i.e., in D).

FIGURE 2.4. Enzyme action. A. How catalysts facilitate chemical reactions. The reactants contain substantial chemical energy, but the activation energy "hump" indicated for the uncatalysed reaction forms an energetic barrier that prevents the reaction from proceeding spontaneously. Heating the reactants raises their thermal energy enough to overcome the energetic barrier and allows the reaction to proceed. Alternatively, an enzyme can serve to lower the activation energy to the point where the reaction proceeds without heating. B, How enzymes couple unfavorable reactions to favorable ones such that the ∆G of the combined reaction is favorable. Often high-energy phosphate hydrolysis (e.g., of ATP) is the favorable reaction to which a relatively less favored reaction is coupled. C, How a series of enzymes can make an unfavorable reaction proceed to some extent. The reactions of A to B, B to C, and C to D are all quite unfavorable (∆G positive). Thus, at equilibrium very little will get to D. However, because the final step is so energetically highly favored, at its equilibrium almost all of D will have been converted to E — which will drive more of reactants A, B, and C toward D. This is a variation of the same principle illustrated in Figure 2.3D.

A

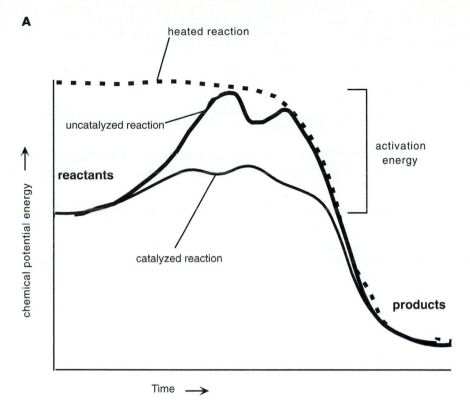

B

$$B + Ap{\approx}p{\approx}p \xrightarrow{\Delta G = -7 \text{ kcal/mol}} B{\approx}p + Ap{\approx}p$$

$$B{\approx}p + C \xrightarrow{\Delta G = +4 \text{ kcal/mol}} D + P_i$$

Coupling the above two reactions gives:

$$B + C + Ap{\approx}p{\approx}p \xrightarrow{\Delta G = -3 \text{ kcal/mol}} D + A{\approx}p{\approx}p + P_i$$

C

$$A \xrightarrow{\Delta G = +2 \text{ kcal/mol}} B \xrightarrow{\Delta G = +4 \text{ kcal/mol}} C \xrightarrow{\Delta G = +5 \text{ kcal/mol}} D \xrightarrow{\Delta G = -14 \text{ kcal/mol}} E$$

contain and decreases the size of the hump, relative to the energy in the reactants (see Figure 2.4A). You can think of the activation energy as reflecting the reactants' need to be positioned correctly, however briefly, for the reaction to occur. The chance of that happening through random motion is increased by heating, which speeds up the motion of the reactants. Since the G for the reaction is negative, all the reactants have to do is bump into each other in just the right way, and the reaction will proceed.

Another way to make a reaction go more quickly without increasing the energy in the reactants (biological systems do not take kindly to being heated too much), is through the action of a biological catalyst, termed *enzyme*. Enzymes are a crucial feature of biological systems that make some remarkable things possible. Enzymes make reactions go more quickly by positioning the reactants properly so that the reaction is more likely to happen (i.e., kinetically more favorable). Thus, enzymes speed up energetically favorable reactions (whose ΔG is negative) by lowering the activation energy (see Figure 2.4A).

Even more remarkable, enzymes can make energetically unfavorable reactions (whose ΔG is positive) happen, by linking them to an energetically highly favorable reaction (see Fig. 2.4B). Thus, when the net ΔG of two linked reactions is negative, being coupled to the favorable reaction drives the unfavorable one. An example of such a favorable reaction is the breaking down or hydrolysis of high-energy molecules such as adenosine triphosphate (ATP) or other nucleoside triphosphates, which can be used to drive the synthesis of biological macromolecules such as DNA, RNA, and proteins. There are many other ways in which energetically unfavorable events can be driven by coupling them to an energetically favorable reaction within biological systems, but hydrolysis of ATP is the most common. The ΔG of various biologically important high-energy phosphate compounds are given in Table 2.3.

TABLE 2.3   VALUES OF $\Delta^{\circ\prime}$ FOR THE HYDROLYSIS OF VARIOUS BIOLOGICALLY IMPORTANT PHOSPHATE COMPOUNDS*

Compound	$\Delta G^{\circ\prime}$ (kcal/mol)
PHOSPHOENOLPYRUVATE	−14.8
CREATINE PHOSPHATE	−10.3
PYROPHOSPHATE	−8.0
ATP (to ADP + P$_i$)	−7.3
ATP (to AMP + PP$_i$)	−7.3
GLUCOSE 1-PHOSPHATE	−5.0
GLUCOSE 6-PHOSPHATE	−3.3
GLYCEROL 3-PHOSPHATE	−2.2

* The bond that is cleaved is indicated by the wavy line.

TABLE 2.4 MAXIMUM TURNOVER NUMBERS OF SOME ENZYMES

Enzyme	Turnover number (per second)
Carbonic anhydrase	600,000
3-Ketosteroid isomerase	280,000
Acetylcholinesterase	25,000
Penicillinase	2,000
Lactate dehydrogenase	1,000
Chymotrypsin	100
DNA polymerase I	15
Tryptophan synthetase	2
Lysozyme	0.5

Adapted, with permission, from Stryer, L. (1995). *Biochemistry*, 4th ed. New York, W.H. Freeman, p. 195.

Sometimes several enzymes acting in sequence can use mass action to drive a reaction that is otherwise unfavorable (see Fig. 2.4C). Consider the situation where the product of one enzyme's action is a reactant for a reaction catalyzed by another enzyme. If activity of the first enzyme generates a large excess of the reactant used by the second enzyme, it will help drive the reaction to a greater extent than would otherwise occur if the concentration of that reactant were lower. Similarly, if a third enzyme uses up as a reactant one of the products of the second enzyme's action, it drives the second enzyme. In both of these cases, the reactions catalyzed by the first and third enzymes serve to move the distribution of reactants and products of the second reaction far from the equilibrium that would have been achieved by the reaction catalyzed by the second enzyme in isolation. The reaction rates catalyzed by enzymes vary tremendously from enzyme to enzyme (see Table 2.4), depending on the kind of reaction being catalyzed, and reflect differences in mechanism from one reaction to another.

Metabolic pathways

The capacity to drive chemical reactions in directions and at rates at which they would not occur otherwise in the physical world are essential features of life and, hence, of physiological systems. Most of the events that occur within the cell are the result of the action of enzymes or are due to other types of protein-protein interactions. Many enzymes are organized into pathways that allow substrates to be rapidly converted into particular products (see Figure 2.5A). Some 500 enzyme activities comprise the core metabolic pathways that occur in most cells that result in substrate production and consumption (see Figure 2.5B). Often these pathways interconnect, allowing the constant flux of materials from those present in excess to those that are deficient. The activity of pathways can be affected either by substrate levels or a change in enzyme activity (e.g., due to hormones that turn on various signaling pathways; see Chap. 3).

The intermediates that move along these pathways can be used for either structural and storage purposes or can be broken down with the release of energy, often harnessed to make ATP. In this regard, not all substrates are alike. Proteins, fats, and carbohydrates each have their own distinctive utility as a building block and also as a source of energy. Proteins can be readily broken down into their component amino acids, which can be used to synthesize other proteins of different amino acid sequence. Those newly synthesized proteins could be enzymes in the cytoplasm, hormones destined to be secreted, or any other polypeptide whose encoding mRNA is available for translation (see later). Fats can be modified and used to build any of the various intracellular biological membranes (see later), each of which have their own unique lipid composition. Fats can also be used to make important signaling molecules, such as steroids, that are involved in intercellular communication (see Chap. 3). Carbohydrates can be used as precursors for synthesis of either fats or amino acids and are used in their own right to covalently modify proteins and lipids.

In addition to these structural, functional, and storage purposes, metabolic intermediates can be used as a source of chemical energy. The most immediate energy source is carbohydrates, in particular glucose. Glucose typically derives either from breakdown of glycogen or from the pathway of gluconeogenesis (see Figure 2.5A).

An intermediate energy source is amino acids, both free and in the form of proteins. However, using proteins as an energy source has two disadvantages. First, since proteins are how genes are expressed, they are necessary for the structural and functional integrity of the organism. Thus, excessive breakdown of protein can compromise survival (e.g., if the organism is too weak to run away or fight a would-be predator). Second, the amino group must be removed before amino acids can feed into the major pathways of energy generation (glycolysis and the tricarboxylic acid cycle, see Figure 2.5A). These free amino groups are highly toxic and must be converted to urea and excreted. Thus, using proteins as a predominant energy source may burden the kidneys, liver, and other organs responsible for detoxification and excretion and may subject them

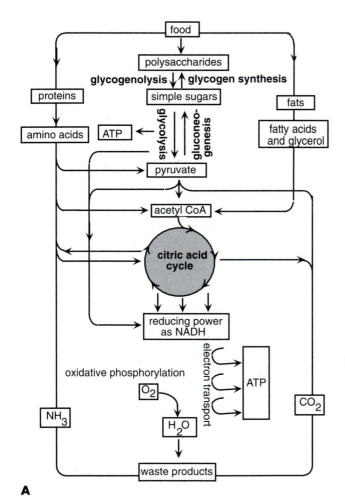

A

FIGURE 2.5. Pathways of intermediary metabolism. *A,* Simplified overview of pathways of substrate generation and utilization highlighting the central role of the citric acid cycle in metabolism. *B,* "Bigger picture" of approximately 500 reactions of intermediary metabolism and focus on specific enzymatic steps of one of them. *(Adapted, with permission, from Alberts, B. et al., (1994). Molecular Biology of the Cell, 3rd ed., New York, Garland, pp. 67, 83.)*

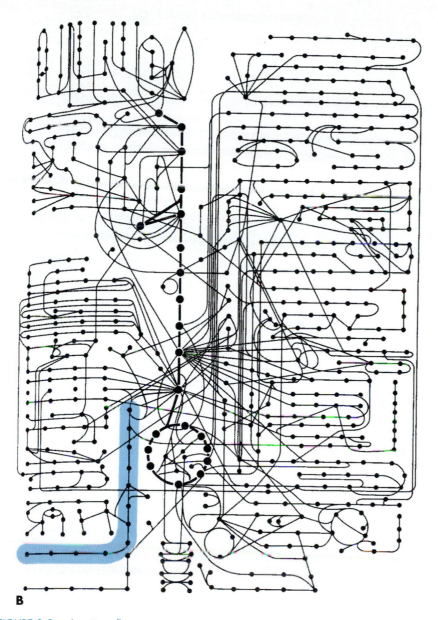

B

FIGURE 2.5 — (*continued*)

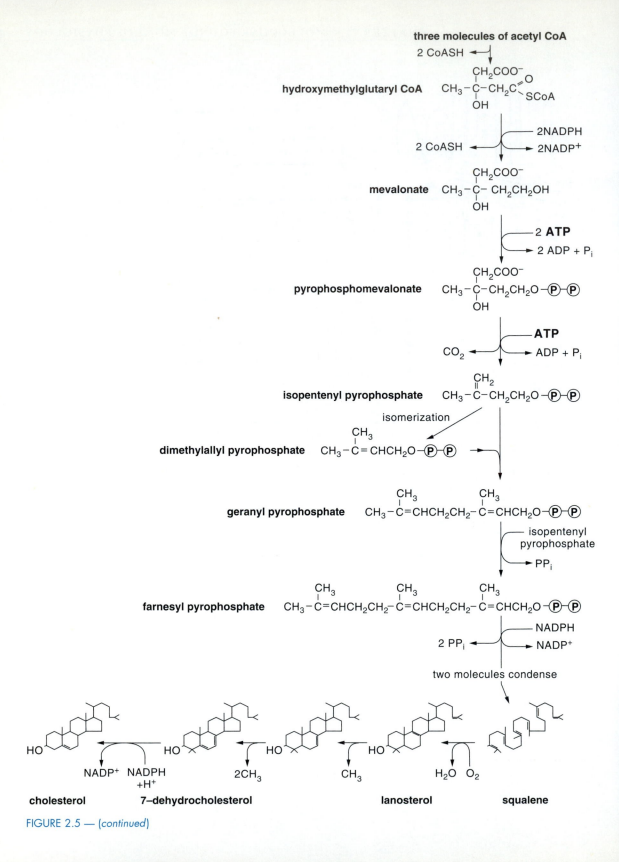

FIGURE 2.5 — (continued)

to more stress and oxidative injury than would occur otherwise.

Long-term energy storage is accomplished by formation of triglycerides (TG) in adipose tissue (fat). This is the physically most compact energy source, releasing 9 calories of energy per gram upon complete oxidation to carbon dioxide and water, where sugars release only 4 Kcal/gram. The basis for this difference is that lipids are much more highly reduced, that is, have more hydrogen-carbon bonds, hence their complete oxidation releases the most energy.

Thus, no one type of food is intrinsically "bad." We could not survive without fats, proteins and carbohydrates. However, above the minimum levels of protein and fat needed to maintain homeostasis, carbohydrates may well be the most versatile energy source. This is because they can be readily used for energy, to make protein or fat, or be stored as glycogen, depending on the needs of the organism, with the least potential long-term toxicity. Perhaps more important than the category of food eaten (e.g., carbohydrate, fat, or protein) is that food intake be characterized by an abundance of variety and fiber. The former provides maximum freedom for absorptive mechanisms of the body to procure minor or trace substances needed, the latter assures rapid transit of undigested materials (and with it numerous toxic products) out of the body in the form of bulky stools (see Chaps. 5 and 20).

Although we have accumulated a lot of useful information about physiological systems through the study of biological chemistry, there are probably fundamental rules that govern such issues as to why enzymes exist at particular levels and degrees of activation in pathways, which we do not currently understand (see Frontiers later). Likewise, for example, it is becoming clear that not all "fat" is the same (adipose tissue stored in the abdomen is associated with more negative long-term consequences compared to adipose tissue in the hips or extremities (see Chap. 6).

Clinical Pearl

○ The therapy for acetaminophen (Tylenol) overdose takes advantage of the law of mass action. As will be discussed in more detail in Chapter 4, deficiency of the reducing reagent glutathione can greatly increase acetaminophen toxicity. This is treated by giving large amounts of acetylcysteine, one of the reactants from which glutathione is made. By increasing the concentration of reactants, more glutathione is made. This facilitates elimination of highly toxic free radicals generated during acetaminophen metabolism.

Review Questions

3. What are some examples of kinetic energy? Of potential energy?
4. In which state are chemical bonds more energy-rich, reduced or oxidized?
5. State the physical principle known as the first law of thermodynamics.
6. What is free energy, and what does it measure?
7. What are enzymes and, in general, how do they work?
8. What are metabolic pathways, and what two general purposes do they serve?
9. What are good short-term, intermediate, and long-term energy sources for humans to eat?

Timescales in biological systems

In our brief consideration of the physical chemistry of biological systems we have mentioned various interactions without regard to their absolute or relative timescales, that is,

A

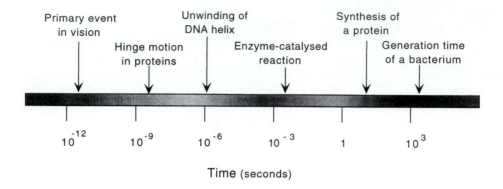

B

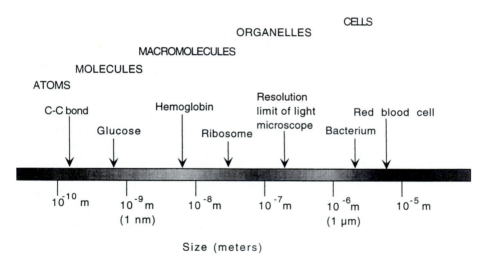

FIGURE 2.6. Biological scales for time and size. *A*, Time. The photochemical basis for vision involves events on a timescale of picoseconds (10^{12}), while doubling of a bacterium takes 20 min. *B*, Size. The difference between atoms, molecules, macromolecules, organelles, and cells is indicated. *(Adapted, with permission, from Stryer, L. (1995). Biochemistry, 4th ed, New York, W.H. Freeman.)*

how long it takes them to happen. Let us consider how long it takes for various physical chemical processes to occur in biological systems.

Light is the fastest thing in our known physical universe. Not surprisingly, therefore, the fastest biological events are those related to light. For example, the primary event in vision, a change in the structure of the light-absorbing group upon being hit by a light particle or photon, occurs in picoseconds (10^{-12} s). This is similar to the timescale of the light-induced electron transfer of photosynthesis, a key step in converting the energy of sunlight into the chemical energy needed to run biological systems.

Noncovalent interactions between proteins are formed and broken a thousand times more slowly, in nanoseconds (10^{-9} s). This is about the time it takes for proteins to change conformation due to rotation around a chemical bond.

The unwinding of DNA, a conformational change, is catalyzed by enzymes, which is a necessary step in its replication (see later), and occurs about a thousand times more slowly than conformational change in proteins, on the order of microseconds (10^{-6} s).

Chemical reactions involving formation and breaking of covalent bonds catalyzed by enzymes typically occur even more slowly, on the order of milliseconds (10^{-3} s). Coordinated biological processes such as protein synthesis take even longer, on the order of seconds to minutes to synthesize a protein, depending on its size. Figure 2.6A compares the timescales of these biophysical events and that of various physiological processes.

3. BIOLOGICAL CHEMISTRY

Structure of macromolecules

Four different kinds of small molecules, carbohydrates, nucleotides, amino acids, and lip-ids are used as building blocks for the macromolecules and biological structures of life (see Figure 2.7). Nucleotides themselves are complex molecules composed of a phosphate group, a five-carbon sugar and a nucleotide base. Four different bases can be used to compose deoxyribonucleotides: adenine (A), guanine (G), cytosine (C), and thymidine (T). In the case of ribonucleotides, the bases used are A, G, C, and uridine (U), which replaces T. Because the sugar phosphate backbone is common to each base, the information encoded in DNA can be stored in a readily "readable" manner.

From two-dimensional drawings on paper it is difficult to appreciate that many of these molecules have an asymmetry in three dimensions, termed *chirality*. This means that, like your left versus right hands, they can occur as mirror images of otherwise identical structures, and by convention are labeled "L" (levo = left) and "D" (dextro = right), that are not interchangeable. For reasons that remain mysterious, life on earth often uses only one of the two mirror images of chiral molecules. Thus, with extremely rare exceptions, only the L but not the D amino acids are used in proteins. Likewise, the D but not L mirror images of sugars such as glucose are made and used in biological systems. Since enzymes work by positioning reactants in the proper manner, chirality is crucial for enzyme action. Perhaps a chance event early during the evolution of life committed all descendents to one form or the other.

Early in evolution, various molecules related to these starting materials were selected for properties that made it possible to use them for particular energetic and informational purposes:

- High-energy phosphates are the most widely used form of immediate energy currency. They were stable enough to allow storage, but sufficiently easily broken down

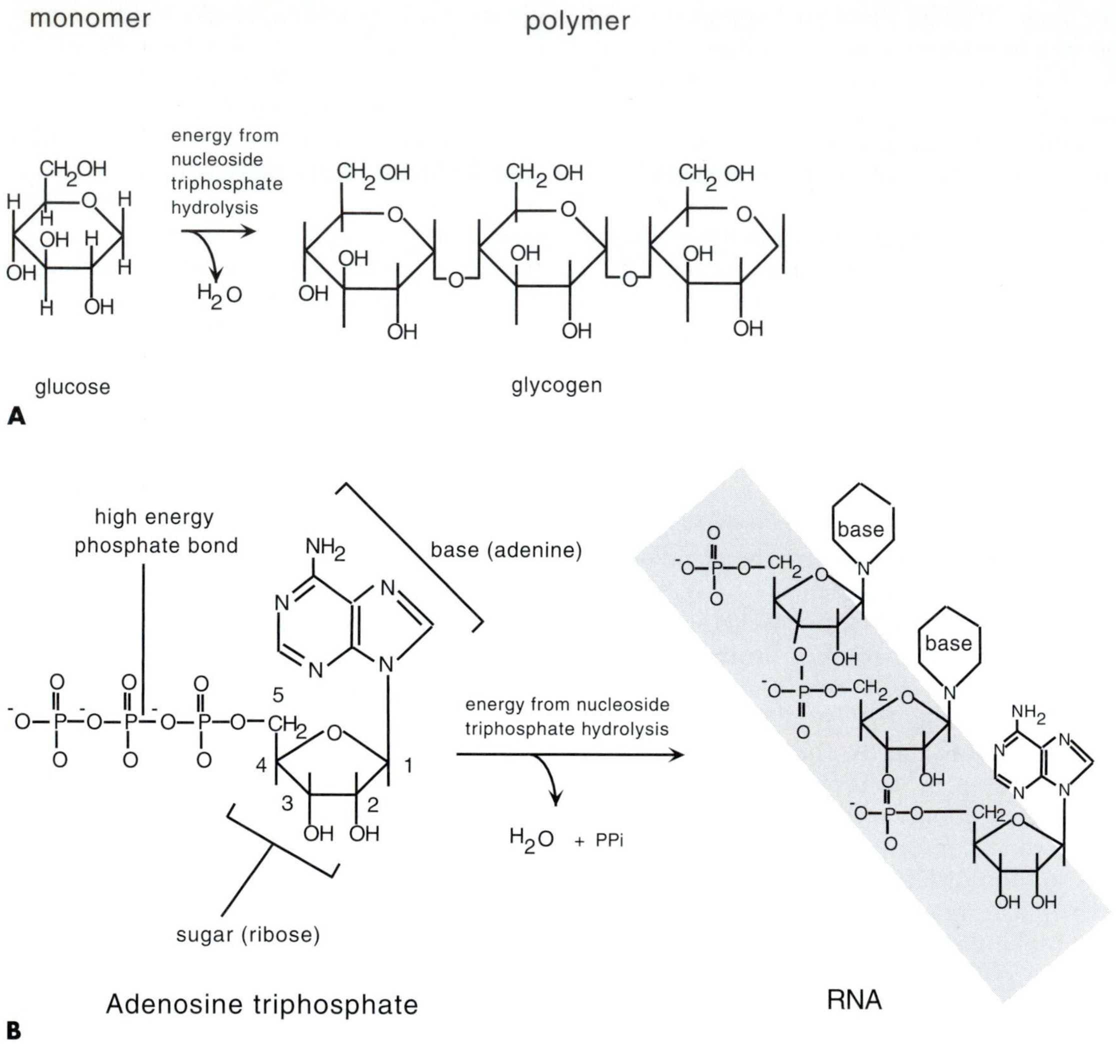

FIGURE 2.7. Monomers and polymers used to build macromolecules. A. Simple sugars assemble into polymers such as glycogen. B. A nucleoside triphosphate, adenosine triphosphate (ATP) is added to a polyribonucleotide (RNA). Gray shading indicates the sugar-phosphate "backbone" onto which the bases are attached. Note that the same ATP molecule that is the major free energy donor in cellular metabolism also is one of the components used to build RNA. Also indicated are one of the two high-energy phosphate bonds whose hydrolysis releases energy that can be used to drive other chemical reactions. Ppi, pyrophosphate, the remaining two phosphate groups released upon incorporation of the adenine nucleotide into the growing RNA molecule. C. Amino acids assemble into polypeptides. D. Acetate is used to make fatty acids of various chain lengths. All of these transformations require an input of energy, usually in the form of nucleotide triphosphate hydrolysis, most commonly that of ATP.

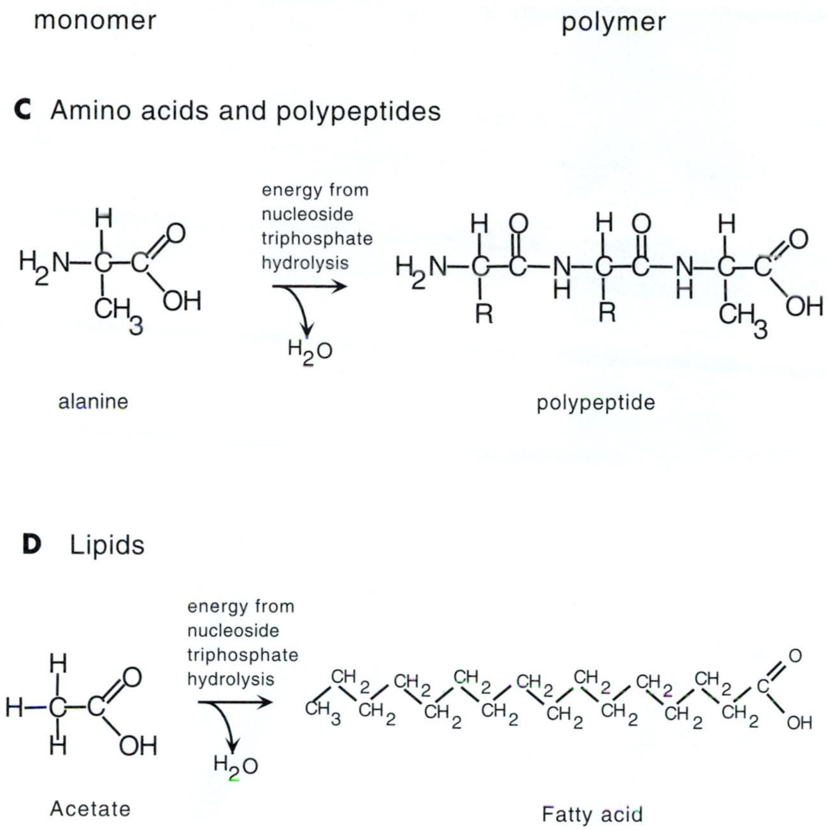
monomer
polymer
C Amino acids and polypeptides
energy from nucleoside triphosphate hydrolysis
H2O
alanine
polypeptide
D Lipids
energy from nucleoside triphosphate hydrolysis
H2O
Acetate
Fatty acid

FIGURE 2.7 — *(continued)*

that they could be used to run many different kinds of protein machines. Adenosine triphosphate (ATP) is the most commonly used high energy phosphate compound (see Figure 2.7B). Usually ATP is broken down to ADP, releasing chemical energy and then rephosphorylated back to ATP. Thus, the body's ATP pool is in a state of flux, constantly being recycled, with food coming in and work, heat, and waste going out. If, instead of being recycled, ATP was used only once, a resting human would consume some 40 kg of ATP per day. During vigorous exercise, ATP consumption would reach levels of half a kilogram per minute. For short-term storage of energy, carbohydrates such as glucose and long polymers of glucose termed *glycogen* (a starch) are generally used.

- Sequences of nucleotides are the most widely used way of encoding information. When joined by phosphodiester bonds, the four different nucleotides could be strung together to make a sequence. A triplet code made possible an extremely large set of possibilities for encoding information in these sequences (see Figure 2.8B and C and Table 2.5). This information could be stored permanently in deoxyribonucleic acid (DNA), a double-stranded sequence of deoxyribonucleotides. Ribonucleic acid (RNA) generally is a single-stranded sequence of ribonu-

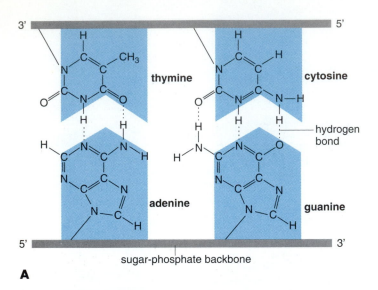

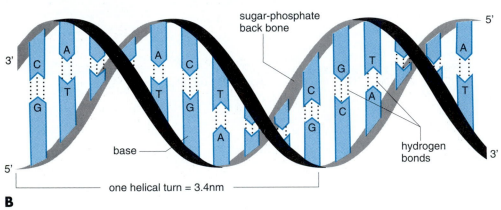

FIGURE 2.8. Nucleotides and nucleic acids involved in information storage, utilization, and transmission. *A.* Structure of bases used to make deoxyribonucleotides. *B.* Structure of a length of DNA indicating the code composed of various permutations of the four bases A, T, G, and C. *(Adapted, with permission, from Alberts, B. et al., (1994). Molecular Biology of the Cell, 3rd ed., New York, Garland, pp. 58, 65, 99, 100.)*

cleotides, which is used to download information encoded in DNA. Although RNA is more flexible, it is less stable than DNA. The sequence of nucleotides in RNA can be translated into a protein, whose amino acids sequence is dictated by the triplet code (see later).

A crucial feature of the use of nucleotides for encoding information in DNA is that the bases adenine and thymidine can interact with each other to form 2 hydrogen bonds per base pair. Guanine and cytosine, in contrast, form 3 base pairs between them (see Figure 2.8A). This recognition and stabilization,

TABLE 2.5 TRIPLET CODE OF NUCLEOTIDES AND AMINO ACIDS

1st position (5′ end) ↓	2nd position				3rd position (3′ end) ↓
	U	**C**	**A**	**G**	
U	Phe	Ser	Tyr	Cys	U
	Phe	Ser	Tyr	Cys	C
	Leu	Ser	STOP	STOP	A
	Leu	Sor	STOP	Trp	G
C	Leu	Pro	His	Arg	U
	Leu	Pro	His	Arg	C
	Leu	Pro	Gln	Arg	A
	Leu	Pro	Gln	Arg	G
A	Ile	Thr	Asn	Ser	U
	Ile	Thr	Asn	Ser	C
	Ile	Thr	Lys	Arg	A
	Met	Thr	Lys	Arg	G
G	Val	Ala	Asp	Gly	U
	Val	Ala	Asp	Gly	C
	Val	Ala	Glu	Gly	A
	Val	Ala	Glu	Gly	G

Amino acids and their symbols

			Codons					
A	Ala	Alanine	GCA	GCC	GCG	GCU		
C	Cys	Cysteine	UGC	UGU				
D	Asp	Aspartic acid	GAC	GAU				
E	Glu	Glutamic acid	GAA	GAG				
F	Phe	Phenylalanine	UUC	UUU				
G	Gly	Glycine	GGA	GGC	GGG	GGU		
H	His	Histidine	CAC	CAU				
I	Ile	Isoleucine	AUA	AUC	AUU			
K	Lys	Lysine	AAA	AAG				
L	Leu	Leucine	UUA	UUG	CUA	CUC	CUG	CUU
M	Met	Methionine	AUG					
N	Asn	Asparagine	AAC	AAU				
P	Pro	Proline	CCA	CCC	CCG	CCU		
Q	Gln	Glutamine	CAA	CAG				
R	Arg	Arginine	AGA	AGG	CCA	CGC	CGG	CGU
S	Ser	Serine	AGC	AGU	UCA	UCC	UCG	UCU
T	Thr	Threonine	ACA	ACC	ACG	ACU		
V	Val	Valine	GUA	GUC	GUG	GUU		
W	Trp	Tryptophan	UGG					
Y	Tyr	Tyrosine	UAC	UAU				

Adapted, with permission, from Alberts, B. et al. (1994). *Molecular Biology of the Cell,* 3rd ed. New York, Garland.

which holds double stranded nucleic acids together, occur when their nucleotide sequences are complementary. Since base-pairing of DNA forms a stable structure termed a *double helix*, it also makes possible the long-term storage of genetic information in chromosomes.

Another fundamental feature of nucleic acid sequences is that they have directionality, that is, one end is not identical to the other. Thus, for any given nucleic acid sequence, the "front" 5′ end and the "back" 3′ end refer to the numbering of the carbon atoms that make up the sugar within the nucleotide, whose hydroxyl group is free. When enzymes add nucleotides to a sequence it is generally done in the 5′ to 3′ direction such that the first nucleotide in the sequence is the 5′ end, and the last nucleotide added is the 3′ end. Furthermore, since the opposite strand (e.g., of a double helix in DNA, or of a newly synthesized strand for either DNA or RNA) is complementary, its 5′ to 3′ orientation is exactly reversed compared with that of the first strand. Thus, when molecular biologists manipulate nucleic acids they are careful to note which strand they want to use. All of these features of nucleic acids have profound implications for their use as a means of storing, copying, decoding, and expressing information.

By convention, unless otherwise specified, a DNA or RNA sequence refers to the coding strand, that is, the strand whose triplet code, when read in the 5′ to 3′ direction, specifies the amino to carboxyl sequence of amino acid residues in the encoded protein.

- Proteins, which are sequences of amino acids, also termed *polypeptides*, are often used by living organisms as tools to carry out work. The 20 amino acids each have a different side group (see Figure 2.9) that confers certain chemical properties to the protein in which they occur. Some side groups are positively charged, some negatively charged, some uncharged but polar, and others, also uncharged, are hydrophobic or nonpolar. The amino acids can be strung together in a near infinite variety of sequences giving rise to an enormous number of shapes and chemical properties. The order of amino acids in the sequence is termed a *protein's primary structure*. The spirals and twists that a given sequence of amino acids takes on due to the angles at which bonds occur in the adjacent amino acid residues is termed the *protein's secondary structure*. When side groups of amino acid residues in different parts of the protein attract one another due to ionic, hydrophobic, or other interactions, the protein's overall shape is further altered. This gives rise to the *protein's tertiary structure*. When individual proteins associate due to multiple noncovalent interactions (see Figure 2.2), the complex is termed the *protein's quaternary structure* (see Figure 2.9). These features that affect a protein's shape are extremely important for biology and medicine, since the shape of a protein determines what roles it can or cannot play, e.g., as a receptor, ligand, enzyme, or machine (see Table 2.6).

By assigning specific nucleic acid sequence triplets to specific amino acids, it was possible to decode a nucleic acid sequence in the form of an amino acid sequence (i.e., making a protein). The sequences of nucleotides that give rise to protein sequences of particular shapes that were most useful were selected in the course of evolution over billions of years. In that way, cells have evolved all manner of enzymes and other protein-based tools that serve as ratchets, levers, pumps, pulleys, wheels, clamps, shears, hammers, cages, glue, springs, corks, pliers, and propellers to carry out work within our cells and between our organs (see Table 2.6). Furthermore, selected side groups of the amino acid residues in a protein can be covalently modified in literally hundreds of different ways (e.g., phosphorylation, glycosylation, acetylation, hydroxylation, etc.), each of which can affect a protein's function or the message it sends in a signaling system. Usually, different enzymes (which are themselves proteins), carry out these modifications. Thus the information content of the human genome, and with it, the functional abilities of its gene products, are greatly amplified.

In order to separate precious biological products from the environment, biological membranes evolved. These barriers mark the boundary between living cells and the outside world. Biological membranes consist of lipids organized into bilayers, into which specialized proteins are embedded (see Figure 2.10C and Table 2.7). Thermodynamically favored hydrophobic interactions between the non-charged, nonpolar surfaces of lipids drive formation of bilayers. Being hydrophobic in their core and hydrophilic on their surface, lipid bilayers provide the environment for a wide range of barrier, carrier, transport, and enzymatic functions on the part of membrane proteins. Different membranes, in different parts of the cell, contain specialized proteins that allow a particular membrane to carry out a particular set of functions. One of the remarkable properties of membranes is that vesicles can pinch off from one membrane and fuse to another. These processes do not occur randomly, but rather are driven in an energy-consuming, directed manner by protein machines that mediate budding, targeting, docking, and fusion of vesicles to membranes (see Chap. 3).

Clinical Pearls

Shape, charge, and modifications of proteins are extremely important for biological function.

○ Different degrees of glycosylation alter the biological properties of the reproductive hormones LH and FSH, most likely by affecting their affinity for receptors.

○ Much of the damage that occurs in patients with the disease diabetes mellitus (see Chap. 6) is probably caused by the fact that, at high glucose concentrations, proteins can be modified nonenzymatically, that is by spontaneous chemical reaction between the amino acid side groups and the sugar. These unintended modifications can change a protein's shape and physical properties so that many proteins no longer work quite right, affecting the efficiency of function in the short term and causing organ failure in the long term.

Review Questions

10. DNA and RNA are synthesized in which direction?

11. In what direction are codons of nucleic acids read to encode amino acids in the amino to carboxyl terminal direction?

12. What are some biologically important properties of lipids?

Gene duplication and expression

Genes are made of the chemical DNA, which encodes the proteins that comprise our bodies and carry out most of our activities at the subcellular level. Our DNA is intricately organized into chromosomes, which are individual double-stranded DNA molecules complexed to specialized scaffolding and other structural proteins. Usually the DNA that makes up chromosomes is in a morphologically indistinct, partially unwound, state. Only during mitosis and meiosis is it suffi-

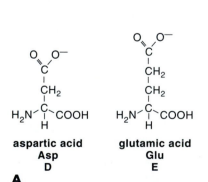

alanine
Ala
A

valine
Val
V

leucine
Leu
L

isoleucine
Ile
I

glycine
Gly
G

cysteine
Cys
C

phenylalanine
Phe
F

tryptophan
Trp
W

methionine
Met
M

proline
Pro
P

uncharged polar amino acids

serine
Ser
S

threonine
Thr
T

tyrosine
Tyr
Y

asparagine
Asn
N

glutamine
Glu
Q

negatively charged (acidic)
polar amino acids

positively charged (basic)
polar amino acids

aspartic acid
Asp
D

glutamic acid
Glu
E

lysine
Lys
K

arginine
Arg
R

histidine
His
H

A

FIGURE 2.9.

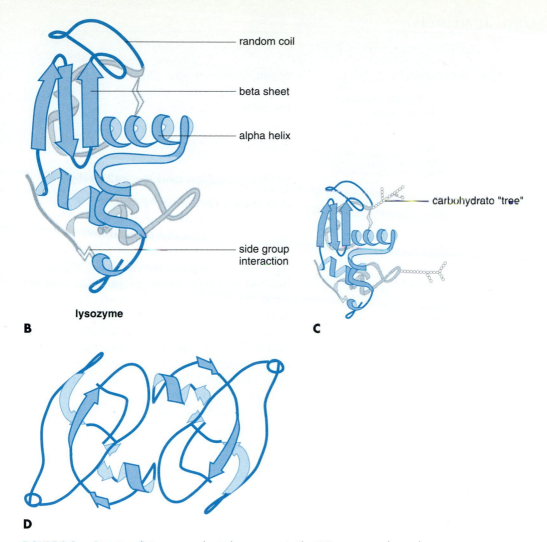

— random coil

— beta sheet

— alpha helix

— side group interaction

lysozyme

B

— carbohydrate "tree"

C

D

FIGURE 2.9 — (*continued*) Amino acids and proteins. *A.* The 20 amino acids used by ribosomes in protein synthesis indicating their side groups, ordered by their chemical properties. *B.* Diagram of the overall structure of a protein (lysozyme) illustrating how the amino acid residues take on secondary structure features such as spirals (termed *α helices*) or zig-zags (termed *β sheets*). Often regions with such ordered structures are connected by less structured loops (termed *random coil*). Note that contacts between side groups of distant regions of the protein can affect its shape (tertiary structure). These conclusions are based on x-ray diffraction studies of protein crystals. *C.* Sometimes proteins can be modified by the addition of carbohydrates or other structures which affect its shape and physical properties including its affinity for other proteins. *D.* Some proteins can form multimeric structures in which several proteins are coassociated (dimer = two, trimer = three, etc.). When two copies of the same protein come together, the structure is termed a *homodimer*. When two different proteins come together, the complex is termed a *heterodimer*. These features of protein structure can be identified by biochemical studies such as susceptibility of a modified protein to enzymes that remove the modification, or biophysical studies that distinguish protein complexes by their size. (*Adapted, with permission, from Lodish, H.F. et al. (1995). Molecular Cell Biology, 3rd ed., New York, W.H. Freeman, pp. 63-65.*)

TABLE 2.6 PROTEIN MACHINES*

Protein	Analogous machine/ common item
G proteins	Timers
Actin	Cables
Kinesin/dynein	Motors
Proteases	Shears, saws, knives and explosives
Glycosyltransferases	Polishing equipment
Tight junctions	Nails and clamps
Signal recognition particle/ receptor	Anchors and docks
TRAM	Adaptor
Protein disulfide isomerase	Monkey wrench for proteins
HSP 70 and other molecular chaperones	Hammers and workbenches
Surface glycolipids	Flags
Various receptors	Magnets
Ribosome	Assembly line for proteins
RNA polymerase	DNA scanner
Membrane vesicles	Container ships loaded with cargo

* A convenient way to think about the structure and function of the cell is in terms of machines we know and use in our lives. These are some examples that should give a ring of familiarity to various cellular mechanisms.

ciently organized for the distinctive morphology of individual chromosomes to be apparent at the light microscopic level. The full human genome comprises 46 chromosomes (see Figure 2.11).

Organisms must be able to do two things with their DNA. First, they have to be able to pass on the information to their offspring, with extremely high fidelity. Copying the DNA through the process of DNA replication does this. Second, organisms have to be able to selectively express subsets of the information encoded in their genomes at different times, in different tissues, and in different amounts. This process is known as gene expression. Only about 1% of the DNA in the human genome encodes expressed genes. The rest are either regulatory sequences or are needed for proper

organization of the chromosomes, or perhaps serve some other as yet unknown function.

DNA replication and the cell cycle

A complex regulatory machinery is involved in assuring that DNA is not only replicated correctly, but that this replication takes place only when it is in the best interest of the multicellular organism as a whole. DNA replication involves a host of proteins that unwind the DNA, unzip the two strands, and faithfully copy each one. Because copying billions and billions of base pairs of DNA will inevitably result in some errors, proofreading mechanisms exist that detect and correct most (but not all) errors that might be accidentally introduced during the process of DNA replication. The intrinsic error rate goes up upon exposure to ionizing radiation, certain environmental insults and the like, which is probably why these exposures are associated with increased risk of developing cancer (see later).

Once the signal for DNA replication has been given and the DNA has been copied, the chromosomes align and pull apart such that each of the two prospective "daughter" cells receives one of the two copies of each chromosome. Thus, upon completion of cell division, each daughter cell has a full complement of human DNA. The process of duplicating nuclear DNA and dividing it between two daughter cells is termed *mitosis* (see Figure 2.12). In meiosis or reduction division (see Chap. 15), haploid germ cells are generated to be used to create a new organism. In this process, the two homologous members of each chromosome pair separate, so that only one of the two genes encoding any given trait ends up in a given germ cell.

The mechanisms for generating diversity

in the gene pool on which selection operates include:

- Random mutations, insertions, deletions in the DNA sequence
- Recombinational events in which chromosomes swap bits of themselves with each other

The cell cycle is the complex set of regulatory events, which lead one cell to become two cells (Figure 2.13). A cell that is going about its business, with no plans for replication, is termed *in the G0 state*. Once a cell has made the decision to divide, it enters the cell cycle, which has four phases termed *G1, S, G2, and M*. G1 corresponds to when the cell is readying itself for cell division, in terms of having enough spare parts, etc., before actually getting started. S phase occurs when the cell duplicates its DNA. G2 is the quiescent period before mitosis (M) when the cell has a chance to "catch its breath" after S and make sure it has everything it needs to consummate M. During embryonic development cells seem to cycle between S and M, spending little or no time in G1 and G2.

Control of the cell cycle is mediated by two families of proteins: the cyclin-dependent protein kinases and the cyclins. The cyclins are proteins that bind the cyclin-dependent protein kinases and by phosphorylation activate their ability to stimulate various downstream events including DNA replication and subsequently, mitosis. The cyclins themselves are regulated by enzymes that break them down to their component amino acids, a process termed *proteolysis.*

RNA synthesis and processing

Transcription is the first step in the process of gene expression. A gene, which is made of a long string of covalently bonded deoxyribonucleotides, is copied by the enzyme RNA polymerase into a complementary copy of RNA. This initial transcript is subject to modifications in which internal regions can be removed, a process termed *splicing*, and a cap and tail are added (see Figure 2.14). Once spliced, the RNA product, termed *messenger RNA (mRNA)*, is exported through the nuclear pores into the cytoplasm. Once in the cytoplasm, mRNA is used to direct the synthesis of proteins (see later).

The process of transcription is extremely complex. In brief, it is regulated by proteins, termed *transcription factors*, that bind to specific regions of DNA to enhance or impede the enzyme, termed *RNA polymerase,* that makes the RNA copy of the DNA sequence from the 5′ to the 3′ direction. Thus, if one transcription factor binds, the rate of formation of a given transcript increases, while binding of another transcription factor will trigger transcription of a different set of genes. Sometimes the production of one transcript can, directly or indirectly, affect transcription of other genes, giving complex patterns of gene expression, which in turn can be influenced by other events in the cell. That is how a cell can be changed from one program of activity to another. Transcription factors can be generated and inactivated by many different mechanisms.

Protein synthesis

Once a molecule of mRNA has entered the cytoplasm, it is bound by proteins. Some mRNA-binding proteins are believed to affect the molecule's localization, while others affect its ability to be utilized to direct protein synthesis. Within the sequence of a mRNA molecule are a number of recognizable regions. First, most eukaryotic mRNA are "capped," meaning they have a structure at the 5′ end that stabilizes them for use. Second, mRNA usually has regions at both ends termed *untranslated* regions, because they are outside the coding sequence. Even though the untranslated region is not expressed, it is

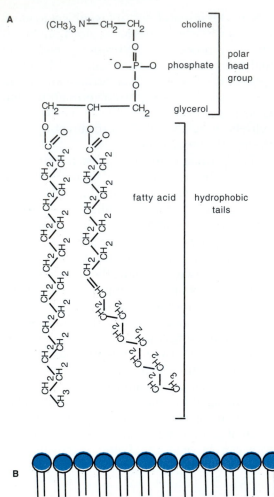

FIGURE 2.10. Lipids, bilayers, and biological membranes. *A.* An individual molecule of phosphatidylcholine (a phospholipid that is an important constituent of biological membranes). *B.* A lipid bilayer. *C.* A biological membrane including both lipids and proteins. *(Adapted, with permission, from Alberts, B. et al. (1994). Molecular Biology of the Cell, 3rd ed. New York, Garland, pp. 479-486.)*

not a waste product. Rather, it plays important roles in regulating when mRNA is to be used and how long-lived it will be. Many regulatory proteins affect the translation of individual mRNA molecules by binding to the untranslated regions. Between the untranslated regions at either end of an mRNA is the coding region. It starts at the initial sequence of three bases that encodes the first amino acid, which, with very few exceptions, is the sequence A-U-G, that is, adenine-uracil-guanine, encoding a methionine residue (see Table 2.5). This also serves to orient the reading frame since, with few exceptions, bases are not skipped in reading the triplet code.

Protein synthesis, the process by which the information encoded in mRNA is translated into a polypeptide chain, consists of three general phases. Initiation is the first phase,

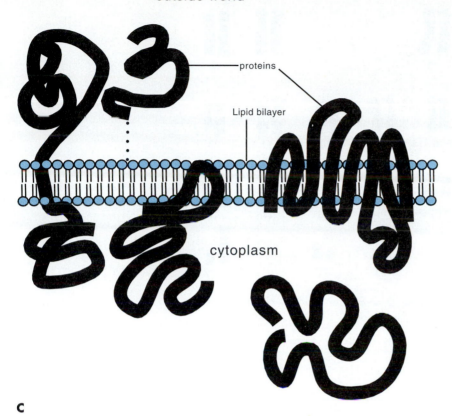

outside world

proteins

Lipid bilayer

cytoplasm

C

FIGURE 2.10 — *(continued)*

TABLE 2.7   FUNCTIONS OF THE ENDOPLASMIC RETICULUM

Protein translocation
Posttranslational covalent modification of proteins
Integration and orientation of proteins in membranes
Assembly and charging of carbohydrate donor lipids
Synthesis and transfer of lipids
Quality control (retention, reverse translocation, refolding of misfolded proteins in the ER lumen)
Protein degradation
Signal transduction to and from other organelles and compartments (e.g., nucleus, plasma membrane, cytosol)

during which an mRNA molecule is chosen to be translated and synthesis of the encoded polypeptide begins. Elongation refers to the repetitive cycles of adding additional amino acid residues beyond the initial methionine. Termination refers to the recognition of the triplet sequence that indicates the end of the protein. The end of the coding sequence is distinct from the end of the mRNA, since the coding sequence is followed by the 3′ untranslated region. The ribosome is a complex of about 100 proteins and several small RNAs that forms a machine which works in conjunction with various initiation, elonga-

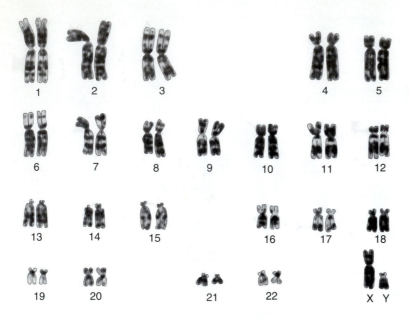

FIGURE 2.11. The human karyotype. A normal set of 46 XY chromosomes of a diploid human cell visualized with Giemsa stain.

FIGURE 2.12. Mitosis. *1*. Prophase. As viewed in the microscope, the transition from the G2 phase to the M phase of the cell cycle is not a sharply defined event. Well-defined chromosomes are slowly formed, containing two copies of the DNA, as a result of duplication in the preceding S phase. Toward the end of prophase, cytoplasmic microtubules that are part of the interphase cytoskeleton disassemble and the main component of the mitotic apparatus, the mitotic spindle, composed of microtubules and associated proteins, begins to form. *2*. Prometaphase starts abruptly with breakdown of the nuclear envelope into membrane vesicles indistinguishable from the endoplasmic reticulum (ER). These vesicles remain visible around the spindle during mitosis. Some of the spindle microtubules enter the nuclear region and attach to structures termed *kinetochores*, while others stay outside. By exerting tension on the chromosomes, the kinetochore-bound microtubules of the spindle set them in motion, while the remaining spindle microtubules keep them from straying off course. *3*. In metaphase, the kinetochore microtubules align the chromosomes in one plane halfway between the spindle poles. Each chromosome is held in tension at the metaphase plate by the paired kinetochores and their associated microtubules, which are attached to opposite poles of the spindle. *4*. In anaphase, the paired kinetochores on each chromosome separate, allowing one set of chromosomes to be pulled toward each spindle pole, at the rate of about 1 μm/min. Anaphase is usually over in a few minutes. *5*. Telophase is when the separated daughter chromosomes arrive at the poles and the kinetochore microtubules disappear. The remaining microtubules of the spindle elongate even further, and the nuclear envelope starts to reassemble around each group of daughter chromosomes. At the same time the chromosomes start to decondense, marking the end of mitosis. *6*. Cytokinesis, the process of separation of the cytoplasm to form two cells is actually initiated during anaphase (see earlier). The connection between the two daughter cells becomes a smaller and smaller ring of cytoplasm until the connection breaks and two cells are formed upon completion of mitosis. *(Adapted, with permission, from Alberts, B. et al. (1994). Molecular Biology of the Cell, 3rd ed. New York, Garland, pp. 916-917.)*

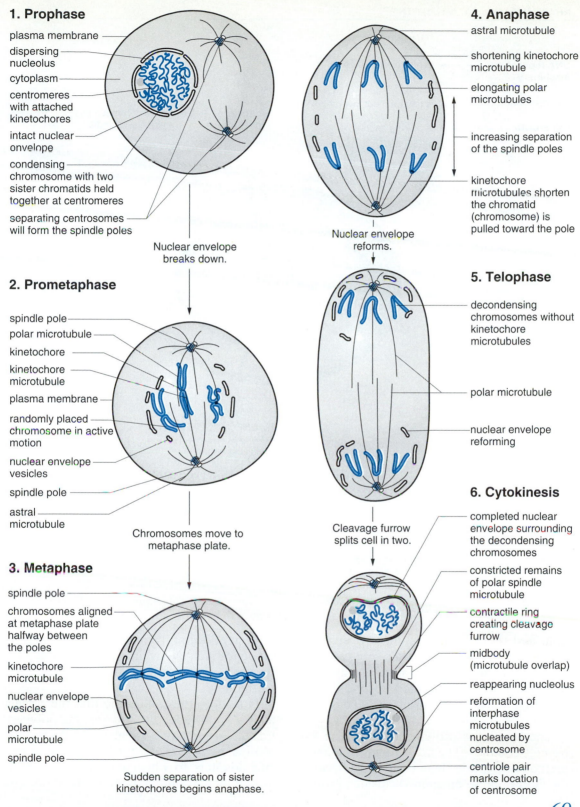

1. Prophase

- plasma membrane
- dispersing nucleolus
- cytoplasm
- centromeres with attached kinetochores
- intact nuclear envelope
- condensing chromosome with two sister chromatids held together at centromeres
- separating centrosomes will form the spindle poles

Nuclear envelope breaks down.

2. Prometaphase

- spindle pole
- polar microtubule
- kinetochore
- kinetochore microtubule
- plasma membrane
- randomly placed chromosome in active motion
- nuclear envelope vesicles
- spindle pole
- astral microtubule

Chromosomes move to metaphase plate.

3. Metaphase

- spindle pole
- chromosomes aligned at metaphase plate halfway between the poles
- kinetochore microtubule
- nuclear envelope vesicles
- polar microtubule
- spindle pole

Sudden separation of sister kinetochores begins anaphase.

4. Anaphase

- astral microtubule
- shortening kinetochore microtubule
- elongating polar microtubules
- increasing separation of the spindle poles
- kinetochore microtubules shorten the chromatid (chromosome) is pulled toward the pole

Nuclear envelope reforms.

5. Telophase

- decondensing chromosomes without kinetochore microtubules
- polar microtubule
- nuclear envelope reforming

Cleavage furrow splits cell in two.

6. Cytokinesis

- completed nuclear envelope surrounding the decondensing chromosomes
- constricted remains of polar spindle microtubule
- contractile ring creating cleavage furrow
- midbody (microtubule overlap)
- reappearing nucleolus
- reformation of interphase microtubules nucleated by centrosome
- centriole pair marks location of centrosome

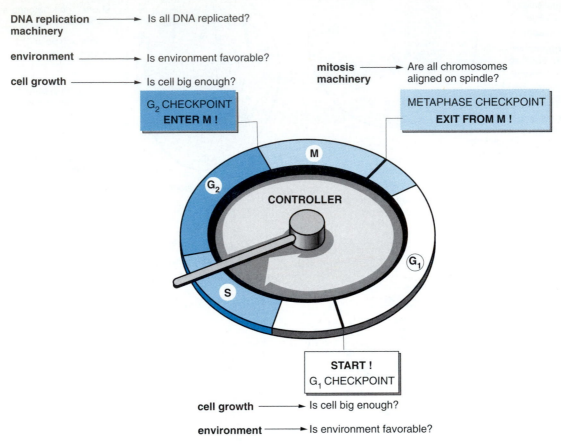

DNA replication machinery ——→ Is all DNA replicated?

environment ——→ Is environment favorable?

cell growth ——→ Is cell big enough?

G₂ CHECKPOINT
ENTER M !

mitosis machinery ——→ Are all chromosomes aligned on spindle?

METAPHASE CHECKPOINT
EXIT FROM M !

M

G₂

CONTROLLER

G₁

S

START !
G₁ CHECKPOINT

cell growth ——→ Is cell big enough?

environment ——→ Is environment favorable?

FIGURE 2.13. Cell cycle. A cell cycle controller, operating in response to feedback from downstream processes and signals from the environment, seems to control transition from G1 to S to G2 to M phases of the cell cycle. A cell in G1 is quiescent; a cell in S phase is engaged in DNA replication, a cell in G2 has completed its replication but has not yet entered mitosis (M). *(Adapted, with permission, from Alberts, B. et al., (1994). Molecular Biology of the Cell, 3rd ed. New York, Garland, p. 868.)*

tion, and termination proteins to carry out protein synthesis. Like people in a cafeteria line, many ribosomes can be engaged in translating an mRNA, lined up one behind the other. Such a structure is called a *polyribosome* or *polysome.*

The events of protein synthesis are extremely complex. The amino acids that make up the polypeptide chain (so termed because the linkage between amino acids in a protein is the peptide bond) correspond to the precise sequence dictated by the triplets of base pairs that follow the A-U-G encoding the initial methionine.

How does the cell ensure that the correct amino acid is added to the growing polypeptide chain? A family of small RNAs termed *transfer ribonucleic acid (tRNA)* serve as specific adapters to which specific amino acids are coupled, resulting in their activation. The

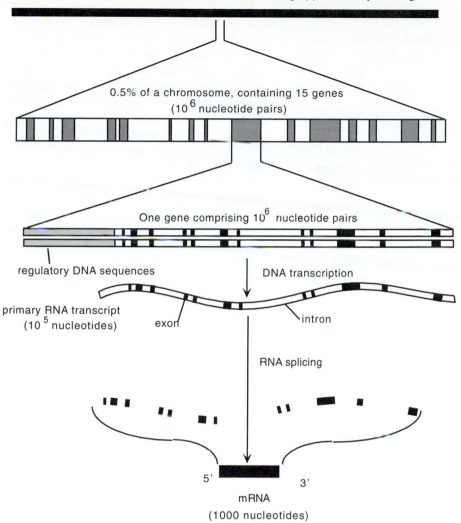

Chromosome of 1.5×10^8 nucleotide pairs containing approximately 3,000 genes

0.5% of a chromosome, containing 15 genes
(10^6 nucleotide pairs)

One gene comprising 10^6 nucleotide pairs

regulatory DNA sequences

DNA transcription

primary RNA transcript
(10^5 nucleotides)

exon

intron

RNA splicing

5'

3'

mRNA
(1000 nucleotides)

FIGURE 2.14. RNA processing. Of the large number of genes on a chromosome (black bar), some smaller number are actually transcribed. The primary transcript is an RNA copy of the gene except for the regulatory information that determined whether or not the gene would be transcribed in that tissue at that time. This is determined by the presence of DNA binding proteins, activated by signaling pathways, that bind to the regulatory regions and initiate transcription (see Chap. 3). The primary RNA transcript is then subjected to splicing, itself a regulated event, wherein defined bits of sequence (exons) are cut out and assembled together to form the coding region of a specific protein. By altering which exons are used, different proteins can be encoded from a single gene. A good example of regulation by alternate splicing is that immunoglobulin genes encode both membrane bound and secreted forms that differ only in which of two possible exons are used to encode the 3' end of the mRNA (corresponding to the carboxyl terminus of the protein, see Chap. 19). *(Adapted, with permission, from Alberts, B. et al. (1994). Molecular Biology of the Cell, 3rd ed. New York, Garland, p. 341.)*

resulting aminoacyl tRNAs can then recognize and hybridize to the next base triplet (codon) in the mRNA, thereby assuring that the correct amino acid is added to the growing polypeptide chain.

Thus, the elongation phase of protein synthesis involves:

1. Selecting the correct aminoacyl tRNA
2. Binding it to the corresponding triplet of base pairs in the mRNA
3. Proofreading to ensure that the correct aminoacyl tRNA is in place
4. Forming a peptide bond
5. Releasing the tRNA adapter to be recycled
6. Advancing the chain to make room for the next aminoacyl tRNA.

Gene expression can be regulated at many different levels. Potential levels of regulation include (a) concentrations and activities of transcription factors and associated regulatory proteins; (b) splicing of mRNAs; (c) transport of mRNAs to the cytoplasm; (d) masking versus selection of mRNA for translation; and (e) changes in the rate of protein synthesis itself, including regulation of initiation, elongation, and termination. Different tissues express different genes and thus contain different proteins, which carry out different functions. Hence physiology, the study of organ systems, involves the study of gene expression in the organ system of interest.

An additional role for RNA in protein synthesis (besides the role of mRNA and tRNA) is seen in ribosomal RNAs, which are structural components of the ribosome itself.

Proofreading in macromolecular synthesis

A challenge faced by biological systems is to devise a system for copying information that has varying levels of accuracy built in. Several strategies for proofreading to correct mistakes have been devised. Thus:

- DNA replication takes advantage of the thermodynamic stability difference between correct and incorrect base pairing. DNA polymerases generally have the ability to remove improperly base-paired nucleotides immediately after they are mistakenly incorporated into the growing DNA strand.
- Protein synthesis uses two proofreading mechanisms. The first operates at the level of formation of aminoacyl tRNAs. The synthetases catalyzing aminoacylation of specific tRNAs have two active sites, one that forms aminoacyl tRNAs and one that will break an incorrect linkage, analogous to the active site of DNA polymerase, which allows excision of a newly incorporated erroneous base. A second mechanism used to further improve accuracy in protein synthesis is termed *kinetic proofreading*. It involves using GTP binding and hydrolysis by an elongation factor to introduce a timed delay in chain elongation. During that delay, an incorrect aminoacyl tRNA is more likely to dissociate and leave the ribosome, hence improving the overall fidelity of protein synthesis.

Clinical Pearls

○ Ribosomes are important sites of antibiotic action. This is possible because the ribosomes of prokaryotes (like bacteria) are sufficiently different from those of eukaryotes (including humans). Thus, many substances that poison bacterial ribosomes do not affect ours. In contrast, the ribosomes of fungi, being eukaryotes, are similar to ours. Thus they are not susceptible to the antibiotics that work against many bacteria, and drugs that would poison their ribosomes are often toxic to humans.
○ Viruses typically use the machinery in cells that they infect (their hosts) to do the work

of replicating their proteins. Thus antibiotics that block prokaryotic ribosomes are not effective against viruses. Hence there are relatively few antiviral drugs currently available, compared to the number of antibiotics used against bacteria and other prokaryotes. The few antiviral products that are available are directed against virus-specific steps, for example, against processes by which viral genes replicate the viral genome (e.g., AZT), or against viral-encoded proteases involved in maturation of viral structure (protease-inhibitors).

Review Questions

13. What are transcription factors, and how do they work?
14. What is the difference between mitosis and meiosis?
15. What are the phases of protein synthesis?
16. What is a ribosome?
17. What are three roles of RNA in protein synthesis?
18. What is the mechanism of proofreading in DNA synthesis? In protein synthesis?

Details of energy generation and storage

Early in the evolution of life, proteins evolved that were able to generate ATP by breakdown of foods such as glucose. Initially this took place under anaerobic conditions, due to the lack of oxygen in the atmosphere by a pathway known as glycolysis (see Fig. 1.6 in Chap. 1). These reactions were relatively energy poor generating a mere net yield of 2 ATP molecules per molecule of glucose, with organic byproducts, such as lactate, being released from the cell. Later, with the appearance of oxygen in the atmosphere,

mechanisms evolved, in the form of the tricarboxylic acid cycle (TCA cycle), that greatly boosted the efficiency of ATP generation to 36 molecules of ATP per molecule of glucose. This involved importing 2 carbon acetyl units into mitochondria where they were subjected to oxidation-reduction reactions in a process termed *oxidative phosphorylation*, with carbon dioxide and water as end products.

In our bodies, both of these approaches to energy generation (i.e., glycolysis and the TCA cycle) continue to be used. We cannot survive without oxygen. The energy needs of the brain, heart, liver, kidneys, and many other organs are simply too great to get by anaerobically, as can many bacteria. However, at certain times and conditions, such as during intense muscular exercise, it is simply not possible to get enough oxygen to run the TCA cycle. In these situations, the tissue that has the greatest need for ATP, exercising muscle, shifts to anaerobic metabolism for a short burst of ATP production (e.g., just enough to get to a tree ahead of a hungry tiger). Soon, however, the accumulation of lactic acid in the bloodstream gives the feeling of fatigue and the inability to continue running.

Clinical Pearl

○ A practical corollary of the 2nd law of thermodynamics is that 90% of the energy consumed by livestock in the form of grain is dissipated as heat or work, and thus is not available to the humans that consume the livestock. By eating a plant-based diet, that "wasted" energy becomes available for use by humans. Thus, plant-based diets conserve energy and make it possible to feed more humans per given amount of resources, including acreage planted, water and fertilizer used, and grain harvested. If, as clinicians, we wish to be more than just technicians, perhaps this is the sort of information we need to be providing our patients, to help motivate their adoption of a more healthy diet and lifestyle (before they get sick).

Review Question

19. What is the difference in ATP yield from one molecule of glucose via the pathway of glycolysis alone versus metabolism through the entire TCA (citric acid) cycle, including oxidative phosphorylation?

4. CELL BIOLOGY: ORGANELLES AND THEIR INTERACTIONS

There are at least 200 different cell types in the human body (see Figure 2.15). Some cells are precursors of others, meaning that changes in the expression of genes normally convert the precursor cell into its differentiated progeny, in response to programmed signals. These signals can change in the course of development, with aging, or in response to changes in the environment. The differences between each of these cell types are a consequence of differences in gene expression as described earlier (see Fig. 2.14).

Each of our cells is surrounded by a plasma membrane, which keeps the "guts" of the cell from spilling all over the place. Within the cell are a number of membrane-bounded structures termed *organelles* that are suspended in the cytoplasm, a gel-like liquid within the cell (see Figure 2.16). Most of the organelles are believed to have evolved either from invaginations of the plasma membrane (e.g., nuclear envelope; ER, endoplasmic reticulum; Golgi; lysosomes), or from bacteria that were somehow engulfed and enslaved by primitive eukaryotes and have given rise to chloroplasts and mitochondria. Figure 2.6B places organelles on a scale of sizes with other structures considered in this chapter.

Cytoplasm

Cytoplasm is the medium within the cell in which the organelles are suspended. It comprises individual proteins, generally in complexes, and particles, sometimes in association with other macromolecules, such as nucleic acids. The cytoplasm has a distinctive ionic composition compared to that of the outside world (see Chap. 10).

Although it is formally an aqueous (water-containing) space, the cytoplasm is extremely crowded (see Ref. 6). Exactly how so many different substances manage to move quickly through such a crowded space is something of a mystery. In part, this crowding may explain why relatively low-affinity interactions can have significant biological consequences. Surely there must be mechanisms, currently unknown, by which the cytoplasm is organized to allow components that need to interact in the crowded environment to be readily accessible to one another.

Among the most important structures and activities that occur in the cytoplasm (as opposed to within other membrane-delimited organelles) are:

- Ribosomes engaged in protein synthesis (translation of mRNA; see earlier).
- Enzymes that comprise metabolic pathways (see later).
- Cytoskeletal proteins that carry out cell and organelle movement. Polymerization of these proteins affects whether the cytoplasm is in a gel or liquid state.

Membranes and organelles

The membranes that surround the cell as a whole and the various organelles within the cytoplasm are all derived from a lipid bilayer. Each type of membrane has a distinctive composition of lipids that make up the bilayer, and of proteins that float in the plane of the membrane. Thus, the different proteins within different organelles and their membranes are responsible for most of the activities of that organelle.

The nucleus

The nucleus is the double-membrane-bounded organelle that houses chromosomal DNA. Specific genes are transcribed and spliced in the nucleus and the resulting mature mRNA is exported via the nuclear pores that traverse the nuclear envelope and lead to the cytoplasm. The space between the inner and outer nuclear membranes (together termed the *nuclear envelope*) is contiguous with the lumen of the endoplasmic reticulum (see later). The nuclear envelope breaks down during mitosis and meiosis to allow chromosome segregation and later reforms after completion of cell division.

Endoplasmic reticulum and secretory pathway

The ER serves as the factory in which proteins are made and assembled, either for eventual export out of the cell, or to meet the cell's own needs (see Table 2.7).

Perhaps the best understood ER function is that of translocation of newly synthesized proteins into the ER lumen, the first step in the secretory pathway by which proteins end up outside the cell (see Figure 2.17). The secretory pathway is central to cell physiology for several reasons. First, almost every cell in the body must secrete some proteins. While protein secretion is almost universal, each cell type displays its own complex variations in terms of proteins expressed, modifications that occur, and regulatory events that govern the secretory process. Some of these distinctive modifications (e.g., glycosylation), occur

initially within the lumen of the ER and are modified in more selective ways in other compartments of the secretory pathway.

A second reason for the importance of the secretory pathway is that a variation of the same mechanism is used by cells to insert membrane proteins into their precise correct transmembrane orientations. Once correctly inserted, membrane proteins are sorted to their correct final compartment for function.

The process of protein secretion is heavily regulated, and there are complex mechanisms currently being unraveled by which the ER and other organelles, such as the nucleus and plasma membrane, appear to talk to one another to stimulate and inhibit various functions. Thus, understanding the secretory pathway is a first step to appreciation of how homeostasis is achieved at cellular and subcellular levels.

The basic plan of the secretory pathway is that nascent proteins destined for either secretion or insertion into membranes must:

1. Target to the ER membrane, where a translocation channel is assembled. This involves recognition of a signal sequence within the nascent protein chain, by a series of receptors in the cytoplasm and in the ER membrane.
2. Then, additional information in the nascent chain is decoded to determine whether the protein is to be translocated (i.e., go all the way into the ER lumen for secretion), or is to stop in the membrane in a particular orientation (i.e., to make a membrane protein). In the case of complex membrane proteins, the translocation channel acts as a special workshop in which proper folding and orientation of the membrane proteins are achieved. During this process of translocation and insertion, many modifications of the nascent chain including addition of carbohydrates occur.
3. Once in the ER lumen (or the bilayer, in the case of membrane proteins), quality

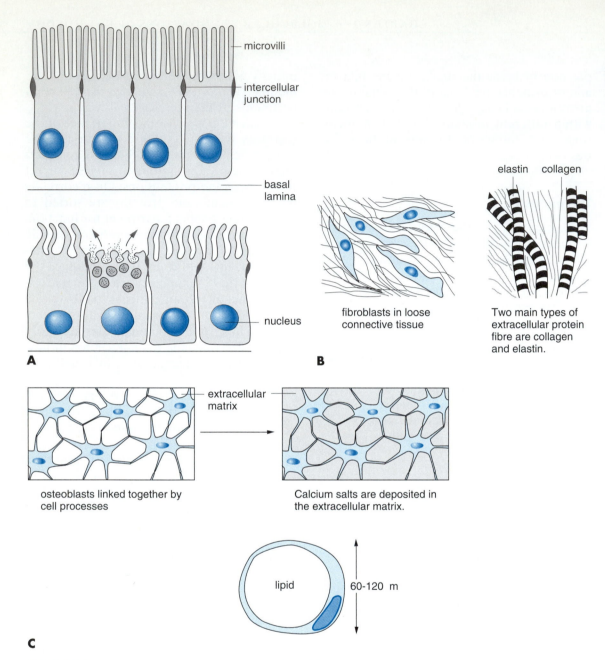

A

microvilli

intercellular junction

basal lamina

nucleus

B

fibroblasts in loose connective tissue

elastin   collagen

Two main types of extracellular protein fibre are collagen and elastin.

C

extracellular matrix

osteoblasts linked together by cell processes

Calcium salts are deposited in the extracellular matrix.

lipid

60–120 m

FIGURE 2.15. Characteristic features of a few of the 200 different cell types in the body *A*. Epithelial cells form sheets that line the inner and outer surfaces of the body and various organ cavities. They are typically connected by tight junctions and have absorptive functions that are facilitated by microvilli projecting from their apical surface. Mucus and other products are secreted from Goblet and other cell types that are often found within an epithelial layer. Some epithelial cells are specialized as receptors (see Chap. 18), others for secretion into the bloodstream (see Chaps. 3 and 6), and others for secretion into the GI tract or other cavities (see Chaps. 5 and 8). *B*. Connective tissue is composed of protein fibers such as elastin and collagen that are secreted, mainly by fibroblasts. Bone is made by osteoblasts that secrete extracellular matrix into which calcium phosphate crystals are later deposited. *C*. Adipose cells produce and store fat, with the nucleus and cytoplasm displaced by a fat droplet that can

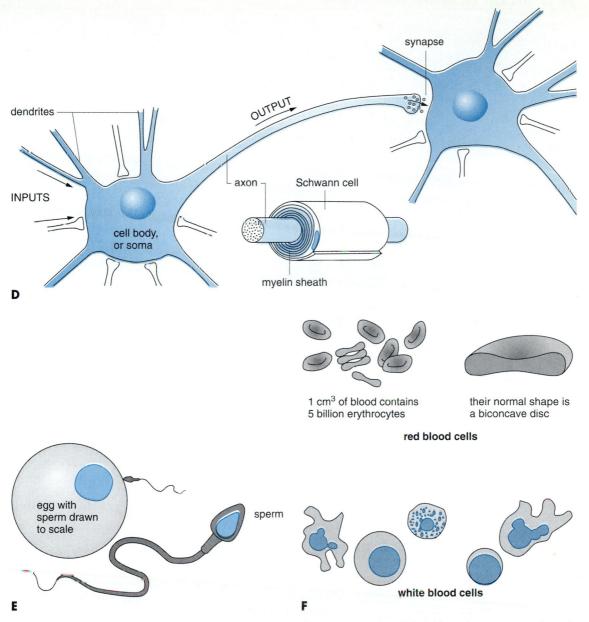

D

synapse

dendrites

OUTPUT

INPUTS

cell body,
or soma

axon

Schwann cell

myelin sheath

E

egg with
sperm drawn
to scale

sperm

1 cm³ of blood contains
5 billion erythrocytes

their normal shape is
a biconcave disc

red blood cells

F

white blood cells

FIGURE 2.15 — (*continued*) reach enormous size. *D.* Nerve cells (neurons) are specialized from communication through the transmission of electrical signals down long processes termed *axons*, followed by release of signaling molecules at specialized junctions termed *synapses* that allow the message to be selectively transmitted to the next cell. Sometimes, specialized cells termed *Schwann cells*, a type of glial cell, wrap the axon for form insulation that greatly increases the speed at which the electrical signals occur (see Chap. 18). *E.* Germ cells have only one set of chromosomes and are specialized for production of a new diploid organism through sexual reproduction (see Chaps. 15 and 16). *F.* Blood cells are generated by maturation of precursors in the bone marrow. Red blood cells are small cells specialized for carrying oxygen by the presence of enormous concentrations of the iron-containing protein hemoglobin. White blood cells are involved in immune defenses (see Chap. 19). (*Adapted, with permission, from Alberts, B. et al. (1994). Molecular Biology of the Cell, 3rd ed. New York, Garland, pp. 36-37.*)

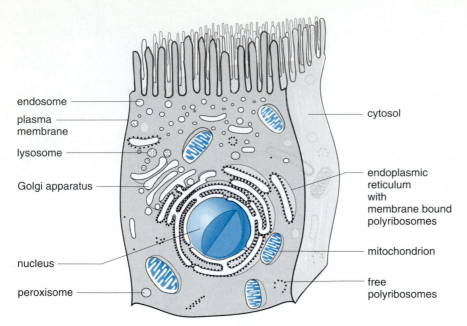

FIGURE 2.16. Internal organization of a typical animal cell, indicating specialized membrane-delimited compartments.

FIGURE 2.17. A. Secretion and endocytosis. Schematic diagram of a typical animal cell depicting the pathway by which newly synthesized proteins leave the cell (secretion) and the pathway by which proteins outside the cell are brought in (endocytosis). Proteins destined for secretion are synthesized on ribosomes bound to the membrane of the ER. After targeting to the ER via the signal sequence (S1) entering the ER lumen via the translocation channel (S2), and maturation/assembly in the ER lumen (S3), as monitored by quality control machinery, these proteins are targeted through a series of compartments by sequential pinching off and fusion of vesicles (S4-S6). From the ER, most vesicle traffic traverses the cis, medial, and trans stacks of the Golgi apparatus, with sorting of vesicles by fate and destination at the trans Golgi network (TGN, S6). There, some vesicles are targeted to some locations (e.g., to the lysosome, see S6a) versus others (e.g., the plasma membrane, see S6b). In each of these pathways, GTP binding proteins serve to provide specificity of targeting, allowing the correct container to dock at the correct compartment of destination. Termed the *rab proteins*, of which at least 10 have been described, these proteins appear to be crucial to intracellular vesicle trafficking. The final step in the secretory pathway is fusion with the plasma membrane (S7), resulting in externalization of secretory product. Not shown is the recycling of membrane, in the form of either vesicles or tubules, from the plasma membrane back to the ER.

Receptor-mediated endocytosis is depicted as starting at the bottom left with receptor-ligand interaction (E1), resulting in multimerization (E2), internalization (E3), and movement or maturation of vesicles to a lower pH compartment in which ligands dissociate from receptors (e.g., due to pH-dependent conformational changes, see E4). In some cases the vesicles, usually containing free ligand, fuse with the lysosome allowing degradation of the ligands (E5). Note that the secretory and endocytic pathways intersect at the lysosome or a related acidic compartment. As with

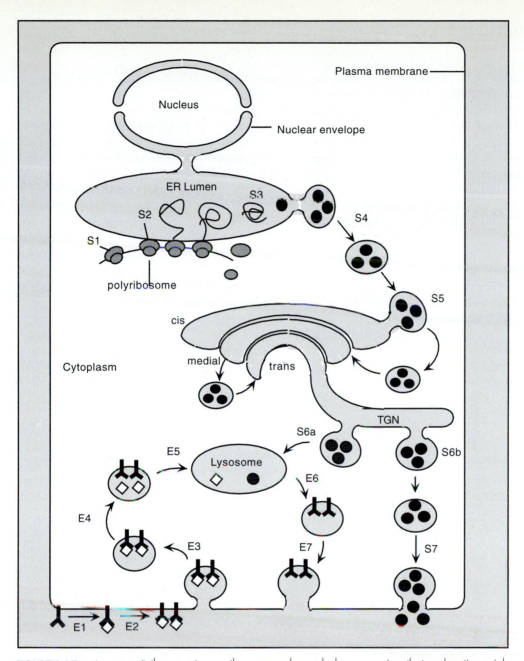

FIGURE 2.17 — (continued) the secretory pathway, membrane balance requires that endocytic vesicles recycle much of the time. In the case of endocytosis, they must recycle back to (see E6) and fuse with, the plasma membrane (E7). Often, the receptors as well as the vesicles themselves are recycled, as indicated in E7.

In both the secretory and endocytic pathways, more than just the destination of the vesicle can be regulated. Particular vesicles loaded with particular cargo are triggered to fuse with the plasma membrane when they receive a specific stimulus. Thus, for example, secretory vesicles containing insulin fuse with the pancreatic β cell plasma membrane only when triggered by a specific signal such as elevated blood glucose. Similarly, glucose uptake in muscle is dependent on insulin to trigger the fusion of endocytic vesicles containing the GLUT-4 transporter (see Chap. 6). However, other cargo in both pathways proceeds in a constitutive fashion, at a particular rate irrespective of hormonal or other triggers.

control machinery carries out and assesses folding and assembly. If either is deemed inadequate, the protein is either retained in the ER to complete the folding and assembly process or, if irreparably misfolded, the protein is returned to the cytoplasm and destroyed.

4. If it passes quality control, the protein is moved to a part of the ER that serves as a dock from which membrane vesicles pinch off. These ER-derived vesicles, loaded with protein cargo, are targeted to other organelles such as the Golgi apparatus, a complex organelle consisting of a stack of membranes. The vesicles dock and fuse in a precise and regulated manner on one side of the Golgi apparatus (called the *cis Golgi*).

5. Other vesicles bud off from the cis Golgi compartment and fuse to the next, medial Golgi compartment, moving protein cargo with them. The different Golgi stacks each contain enzymes to carry out distinctive modifications. Those proteins that are destined to receive a particular modification are recognized and modified. Other proteins are carried on through, without modification. There is growing support for an alternative view in which, within the Golgi complex, transport occurs by maturation of cysteinae. In this view, the major role for vesicular traffic within the Golgi is for the return of "empty" membrane containers.

6. Eventually the cargo gets to a final Golgi-related compartment termed the *trans Golgi network* (TGN) located at the opposite end of the stack, from which sorting takes place. Some vesicles carry proteins destined for the lysosome or lysosomal membrane (see later). Other vesicles carry proteins that are constitutively secreted as well as various plasma membrane proteins targeted to either the apical or basolateral surfaces. Still other vesicles are loaded with regulated secretory cargo. These are secreted only when specific stimuli are received.

7. The final vesicle fusion event is with the compartment of destination. In the case of secretory proteins, the vesicles fuse with the plasma membrane, a process termed *exocytosis*. The flow of membrane from ER to plasma membrane and elsewhere in "professional" secretory cells is so massive that the entire ER membrane would be consumed in a matter of minutes, except that there is an equal and opposite flow of membrane back to the ER. Thus, cells must have a membrane recycling program as massive as that of protein export.

Only once, at the ER, does the chain actually cross a lipid bilayer (via the translocation channel). All other transport is either within a membrane system or from compartment to compartment by fission and fusion of membrane vesicles.

The plasma membrane, endocytosis, and membrane recycling

The heavy traffic of vesicles taking cargo to the plasma membrane, and recycling the empty containers, is but a part of the vesicular traffic of the cell. Independent of, but intersecting with, the secretory pathway, receptors on the cell surface bind hormones and other ligands and are internalized by invagination and pinching off of vesicles, a process termed *endocytosis*. In many ways endocytosis is a simple reversal of exocytosis. However, endocytosis can be either receptor-mediated (in which case it is specific for a particular substance binding to a receptor) or nonspecific (in which case the cell samples whatever is in the fluid bathing the cell). As with secretion, the volume of membranes consumed by endocytosis would exhaust the plasma membrane in minutes were it not for recycling in equal magnitude, which returns membrane containers to the plasma membrane. The speed, extent, and accuracy of membrane-vesicle formation trafficking and fusion in endocytosis and secretion are believed to be of crucial importance in the physiological functioning of organ systems.

Lysosomes

The lysosome is a special organelle that contains digestive enzymes with an extremely acidic pH optimum. The lysosomal membrane has a proton transporter that generates the low pH, which allows these enzymes to work. Lysosomal digestive enzymes are targeted to lysosomes via the secretory pathway. Special targeting machinery recognizes and diverts them to the correct vesicles at the TGN. Upon departure from the TGN, those vesicles are targeted to the lysosome. Endocytic vesicles derived from the plasma membrane are also often targeted to the lysosome, via an intermediate low pH compartment. In this low pH environment the bound ligands dissociate and the "empty" receptors are able to be recycled back to the plasma membrane, while the formerly bound ligand continues on to the lysosome where it is degraded by the low pH-activated digestive enzymes (see Fig. 2.17).

Mitochondria

Eukaryotic cells in general and certain specialized cells in particular (e.g., cells of the renal tubule that do a lot of active transport) have huge ATP requirements. Thus, the development of double-membrane containing organelles called *mitochondria* (see Figure 2.18) that were specialized for energy production, must have been a major step in evolution. It appears that these organelles were derived from primordial bacteria that were somehow engulfed and incorporated as the "power pack" of the early eukaryotic cell. A heritage of their likely origins is that mitochondria have a DNA genome of their own.

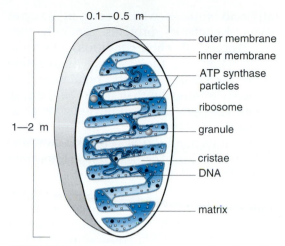

FIGURE 2.18. Mitochondrial structure and function. Cutaway view of a mitochondrion indicating its dimensions and double-membrane structure, and the location of the machinery that carries out the synthesis of ATP through oxidative phosphorylation. (*Adapted, with permission, from Lodish, H.F. et al. (1995). Molecular Cell Biology, 3rd ed. New York, W.H. Freeman, pp. 745-746.*)

Only a handful of the specialized proteins within the mitochondrion are encoded in the mitochondrial genome, however. Most mitochondrial proteins are encoded in chromosomal genes in the nucleus and are made in the cytoplasm. These proteins (including ornithine transcarbamylase, OTC; see Case of Physiological Medicine, later), need to use specialized transport mechanisms to enter the mitochondrion. The mechanisms used are roughly analogous in concept, but different in specific molecular detail, from the mechanism by which secretory proteins enter the ER lumen.

A cascade of enzymes and carrier proteins make possible oxidative phosphorylation, the process by which the energy released from oxidation of pyruvate to carbon dioxide and water is harnessed by generation of ATP, at the inner mitochondrial membrane.

Another valuable use of the mitochondrion is to segregate activities such as fatty acid oxidation from the opposite process, fatty acid synthesis, which occurs in the cytoplasm. Regulatory proteins generally turn one process off when conditions favor the other. However, their spatial segregation allows for greater capacity, regulation, and efficiency of function than might be the case if both activities occurred in the same compartment.

The mitochondrion also plays a key role in the conversion of cholesterol, an important membrane lipid, into steroids such as glucocorticoids, androgens, and estrogens. An enzyme called *side-chain cleavage enzyme* is located in the mitochondrial membrane and is the rate-limiting step in synthesis of most steroids.

Finally, the mitochondria appears to play a central role in carrying out the decision to undergo apoptosis. Like the decision to launch nuclear warheads, the decision to commit suicide is not one that cells take lightly. A series of failsafe mechanisms prevent premature or inappropriate activation of the apoptosis cascade (see later). Release of calcium and specific proteins from the mitochondria are part of this failsafe mechanism that regulates apoptosis.

Review Questions

20. What are the major compartments of eukaryotic cells?
21. For each organelle, name a physiological process that is dependent on that organelle's function. Also name a specific enzyme involved.
22. What are the major compartments of the secretory pathway?
23. How are mitochondria believed to have evolved?

Clinical Pearls

An important role of the endoplasmic reticulum, in addition to actual synthesis and modification of proteins, is the responsibility of ensuring quality control. This can be a double-edged sword. If standards are set too low, proteins that are nonfunctional or poorly functional will be made and decrease the efficiency of the cell. In contrast, if standards are set too high, mutant molecules that would otherwise be functional are prevented from getting to the correct location. The disease of complete deficiency is worse than one of inefficient function.

○ Alpha-1-antitrypsin is an inhibitor that plays a crucial role in protecting individuals from the damaging effects of proteases secreted by cells of the immune system into the lung. Alpha-1-antitrypsin deficiency is a genetic disease where a point mutation in the alpha 1 antitrypsin gene results in accumulation of the protein in the ER. Thus, rather than being allowed to traverse the secretory pathway and exit the cell, the protein is retained and eventually degraded. As a result of the lack of export of this enzyme inhibitor, the person is unable to prevent damage that results in the chronic lung disease emphysema (see Chap. 8). In patients who develop emphysema due to smoking, the same enzyme and inhibitor reactions are involved, but the difference is that in their cases, smoke-triggered hyperactivity of neutrophils results in their secreting more proteases than their normal level of alpha-1-antitrypsin can handle.

○ Another example of a quality control disease is cystic fibrosis. The most common form of this relatively common genetic disease (one in 5000 live Caucasian births are homozygous for the mutation; one in 24 are heterozygous) is a single amino acid change that leaves the protein, termed *cystic fibrosis transmembrane regulator* or *CFTR*, fully functional as a chloride channel. However, the quality control machinery deems the protein misfolded and prevents its exit from the ER, resulting in a far more severe disease phenotype than would otherwise be caused by proper expression of the mutant protein on the plasma membrane (see Chap. 8). In the future, treatment of this disease might be as simple as coaxing the quality control machinery to relax a little, so this protein can escape to the cell surface to do its job.

5. PRINCIPLES OF GENETICS

The science of genetics is based on simple principles of how hereditary traits are transmitted, which were first appreciated in the 1860s by Gregor Mendel, an Austrian monk who studied pea plants. Features of genetics that conform to these principles are known as Mendelian genetics. The subsequent rise of molecular genetics has provided an understanding of the physical basis by which Mendelian rules and principles occur.

Because we are diploid organisms who receive half of our genes from our mother and half from our father, we carry two copies of most genes. When a genetic mutation is said to be dominant, what is meant is that a change in one of the two copies of that gene normally present is manifest as a change in some apparent feature or function of the organism (its phenotype). This is true even though the other copy of the gene (termed the *other allele*) is normal. When a genetic mutation is said to be recessive, what is meant is that the second normal allele, usually 50% of the expressed protein, is able to carry out the normal function sufficiently well enough so that no mutant phenotype is observed.

The only exception is when the mutant gene is carried on the X or Y chromosome and the offspring is a male. In this case, since only one copy of each X and Y chromosome is present, there is no second normal copy to

suppress the phenotype of a recessive mutation.

Most genetic diseases are due to changes in the DNA sequence of a gene and hence alter a single protein. Genotype refers to the genes an individual has. Phenotype refers to how those genes are expressed in any given individual. The point in time at which the mutation arose has important implications for its expression:

- If the mutation was present in the DNA of the germ cell, then every cell in an individual of the next generation will inherit the mutation.
- If the mutation arose during early embryogenesis, then only a subset of cells in the individual will have the mutation.
- If a mutation arises during adulthood, it might increase the risk of malignant transformation into a cancer cell or render the cell dysfunctional in some other way. One theory of aging proposes the accumulation of such somatic mutations in adult cells, resulting in more and more dysfunctional cells over time.

Within the 1% of the human genome that encodes genes are a certain number of differences from one individual to another. On average, 1 in 100 to 200 base pairs within genes are different in different individuals. These differences are due to mutations. Many of them are harmless but some, depending on circumstances, can be a cause of disease or can protect the organism from disease, depending on environment, other genes, etc. When mutations have no obvious phenotype they are termed *allelic polymorphisms* of the human populations. This does not mean that they cannot have a phenotype under different environmental conditions. For example, there are polymorphisms in the gene for the chemokine receptors on T lymphocytes. Prior to the emergence of the AIDS epidemic, these mutations could have been said to have no functional consequence for the individuals displaying them, as their chemokine receptors seemed to work equally well with or without the mutations. However, the human immunodeficiency virus that is the cause of AIDS utilizes these chemokine receptors for its entry into certain immune cells. Individuals with some polymorphisms are protected from HIV infection, because the virus is unable to use the mutant as a coreceptor to enter the immune cell. Such mutations now confer a selective advantage to individuals bearing the mutant coreceptor in areas where HIV infection is widespread. In contrast, the mutation of hemoglobin that causes sickle cell anemia is believed to have conferred some protection from malaria infection to heterozygous individuals, thereby selecting for the presence of the gene in certain human populations. Later, with the advent of antibiotics, this mutation no longer has a selective value and is now viewed as clearly deleterious.

Going from simple observations in pea plants to complex observations in people is a challenging task. The human genome contains some 50,000 to 100,000 genes. Each encodes a different protein. However, about 99% of the DNA in the human genome consists of repetitive sequences that do not code for specific proteins and are of unknown function.

Mutations in DNA are generally characterized in two ways:

First, in molecular terms, mutations can be caused by single base changes (point mutations), deletions, insertions, or substitutions. As a result of the molecular change, the new sequence may encode one or more different amino acids or may terminate in a different place, compared to the nonmutant or wild-type sequence.

Second, mutations can be characterized by their effect on the encoded protein. Some mutations are outside of the coding region for a protein, e.g., in the regulatory regions needed for transcription, splicing, or transla-tion of the gene. Of the mutations that are actually in the coding region, some are functionally neutral and have no effect. Such mutations are allelic polymorphisms (see earlier). Others, termed *amorphic* or *hypomorphic*, result in complete or partial loss of function, respectively. Some are termed *hypermorphic* and result in a gain of function. Those termed *neomorphic* result in acquisition of a new property altogether. Table 2.8 gives some examples of each type of mutation as causes of human disease.

Since it is much more likely that a mutation will interfere with a protein's function rather than improve it, most mutations that are not neutral are amorphic or hypomorphic. These are generally recessive since it would probably require two mutant alleles for the person to have not enough or no functional protein.

The prevalence of phenotypic genetic disease in the population is about 1%. Most mutations are recessive and hence have a phenotype only in individuals in whom both genes are mutant. The spontaneous mutation rate generating new deleterious mutations at any given locus is estimated to be one in 10^{-6} to one in 10^{-5}. Thus it is estimated that each of us carries 4 or 5 highly deleterious mutations. Fortunately, these highly deleterious mutations are recessive, masked by the presence of one normal copy of the gene. As long as our mates are not too closely related to us genetically, the chances of our offspring getting two copies of a bad gene is extremely small.

Clinical Pearl

○ Although genetic diseases are rare, they provide hints as to the proteins that may be involved in the much more common diseases in which environmentally induced organ system dysfunction occurs. This logic has been used to implicate the

TABLE 2.8 EXAMPLES OF VARIOUS PHENOTYPES OF DIFFERENT CLASSES OF GENETIC MUTATIONS IN HUMANS

Disorder	Phenotype	Genetic mechanism	Prevalence
Down's syndrome	Mental and growth retardation, dysmorphic features, internal organ anomalies	Chromosomal imbalance caused by trisomy 21	≈1 : 800; increased risk with advanced maternal age
Fragile X-associated mental retardation	Mental retardation, characteristic facial features, large testes	X-linked; progressive expansion of unstable DNA causes failure to express gene encoding RNA-binding protein	≈1 : 1500 males; can be manifest in females; multistep mechanism
Sickle cell anemia	Recurrent painful crises, increased susceptibility to infections	Autosomal recessive; caused by a single missense mutation in β globin	≈1 : 400 blacks
Cystic fibrosis	Recurrent pulmonary infections, exocrine pancreatic insufficiency, infertility	Autosomal recessive; caused by multiple loss-of-function mutations in a chloride channel	≈1 : 2000 whites; very rare in Asians
Neurofibromatosis	Multiple café au lait spots, neurofibromas, increased tumor susceptibility	Autosomal dominant; caused by multiple loss-of-function mutations in a signaling molecule	≈1 : 3000; about 50% are new mutations
Duchenne's muscular dystrophy	Muscular weakness and degeneration	X-linked recessive; caused by multiple loss-of-function mutations in a muscle protein	≈1 : 3000 males; about 33% are new mutations
Osteogenesis imperfecta	Increased susceptibility to fractures, connective tissue fragility	Phenotypically and genetically heterogeneous	≈1 : 10,000
Phenylketonuria	Mental and growth retardation	Autosomal recessive; caused by multiple loss-of-function mutations in phenylalanine hydroxylase	≈1 : 10,000

Adapted, with permission, from Barsh, G. (1995). Genetic Disease in McPhee, S. et al. eds. *Pathophysiology of Disease*, 2nd ed. Stamford, CT, Appleton & Lange, p. 7.

β-amyloid and presenilin genes in Alzheimer's disease, by virtue of familial forms of this neurodegenerative disorder that occurs in individuals bearing mutations in these genes (see Chap. 18).

Review Questions

24. How many genes encoding different proteins are believed to reside in the human genome?
25. What does it mean to be called a diploid organism?
26. What is the difference between a genotype and a phenotype?
27. What is the difference between a dominant and a recessive trait?
28. What happens if a mutation occurs during embryogenesis?
29. Why might a gene differ in penetrance between two individuals?
30. What is the prevalence of genetic disease in the population?
31. How many deleterious mutations do normal individuals carry, on average? Why aren't these generally a problem?

6. COMPLEX FUNCTIONS OF PROTEINS

Solutions, membranes, and the problem of transport

A substance (termed a *solute*) is dissolved (in solution) in another, more abundant liquid substance (termed the *solvent*), when their molecules are intermixed. It is important to note that molecules in a liquid solution are not as freely intermixed as in a gas due to hydrogen bonding and other noncovalent attractive forces between the molecules.

Substances in solution move from one part of the body to another by several mechanisms. Diffusion is the tendency of a substance to randomly move from a point of high concentration to areas of lower concentration. Osmosis is the result of the effect of a semipermeable membrane on diffusion, impairing the movement of dissolved substances too large to pass through the holes in the membrane. As a result, more of the smaller solvent molecules that can move across the membrane do so. This raises either the volume or the osmotic pressure on the other side (see Figure 2.19). Osmotic pressure is just one of a number of fundamental properties of solutions that form the parameters within which evolution has been free to operate.

Things become more complicated when one of the solutes that is unable to diffuse across a semipermeable membrane is an ion, that is, a molecule with a positive or negative electrical charge. Large, charged molecules such as proteins attract ions to neutralize their charges. But the movement of ions to neutralize these nondiffusible charges in cells (e.g., due to the proteins) creates a concentration gradient of those ions and raises the osmotic pressure. Without an offsetting mechanism, cells would simply swell until they burst. In the course of evolution, a number of ingenious mechanisms have evolved for dealing with the combined effect of charge distribution and concentration gradient, termed *electrochemical potential difference*, between the outside and inside of cells.

- Plant cells have a rigid wall that prevents influx of water. This allows them to passively resist osmotic pressure.

- Some protozoa pump the excess water that enters the cell into a vacuole and periodically dump this back into the medium outside of the cell—the bucket and the leaky boat approach.

- Most animal cells use a remarkable array of transporters and channels to maintain a sufficient membrane potential to just offset the osmotic forces. Thus, the membrane potential is the extent of deviation from electroneutrality (i.e., the charge distribution across the membrane), at which equilibrium with osmotic forces exists.

Transporters and channels

A pure lipid bilayer is freely permeable to gases such as oxygen or carbon dioxide and partly permeable to small uncharged molecules such as water, ethanol, and urea. However, it is almost completely impermeable to small or large charged molecules such as ions, amino acids, sugars, nucleotides, or proteins.

In order to move significant numbers of such molecules across a lipid bilayer, there must be specialized proteins or other structures. Channels are conduits that allow large numbers of specific molecules to flow down the concentration gradient for that substance, through a hole that they create across the membrane. Transporters are molecules that bind the substance to be transported and then undergo a conformational change that allows the molecule to cross to the other side of the membrane (see Figure 2.20). There are two distinctive features of transporters compared to channels:

First, channels move far more molecules per second than do transporters (about 10^8 versus 10^4, respectively). This is because it takes transporters more time to bind the substance, change conformation, release them on the other side, and then change back to the original conformation. In contrast, chan-

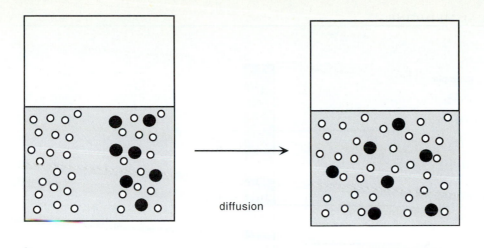

A

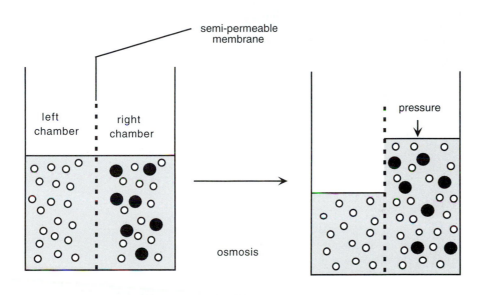

semi-permeable
membrane

B

FIGURE 2.19. *A.* Diffusion. Small white circles are water molecules, large dark circles are solute dissolved in the water. In diffusion, random motion results in both water and solute distributed equally throughout the vessel. *B.* Osmosis. Here, the chamber is divided in two by a semipermeable membrane that allows the passage of water, but not of solute. Equal volumes are placed in each compartment, one with water alone, the other with water and solute. Water moves down its concentration gradient into the chamber containing the solute and, as a result, the volume in the solute-containing chamber increases. Osmotic pressure is the pressure that would have to be applied to prevent movement of water molecules and the resulting change in volume. *(Adapted, with permission, from Ganong, W.F. (1999). Review of Medical Physiology, 18th ed. Stamford, CT, Appleton & Lange, p. 4.)*

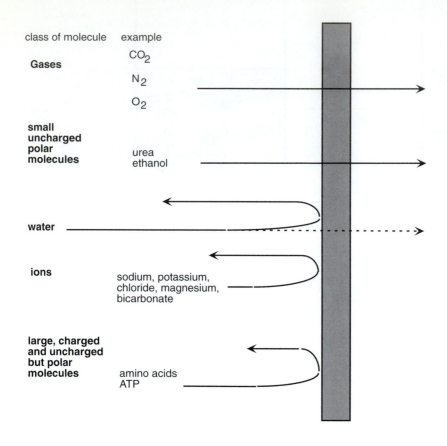

class of molecule   example

Gases CO_2

N_2

O_2

**small
uncharged
polar
molecules**   urea
ethanol

water

ions   sodium, potassium,
chloride, magnesium,
bicarbonate

**large, charged
and uncharged
but polar
molecules**   amino acids
ATP

phospholipid bilayer

A

FIGURE 2.20. Diversity of transporters versus channels. A. Indicates the permeability of a pure phospholipid bilayer in the absence of channels or transporters. It is fully permeable to small hydrophobic molecules and small uncharged but polar molecules, slightly permeable to water, and impermeable to ions and large uncharged polar molecules.

nels let the ions go through constantly and rapidly.

A second difference is that some transporters, also called *pumps*, can move a substance against its concentration gradient, while a channel can allow it only to diffuse down its concentration gradient. Transporters that are pumps must either hydrolyze ATP or link the "uphill" transport against the concentration gradient to transport of another substance

flowing down its concentration gradient. This is highly reminiscent of how enzymes couple unfavorable reactions to favorable ones, and is termed *active transport*. Other transporters (such as most of the glucose transporters) only work in the direction of the concentration substrate gradient.

The electrochemical gradient observed in most animal cells is due to a combination of the Na/K ATPase (a transporter) and potas-

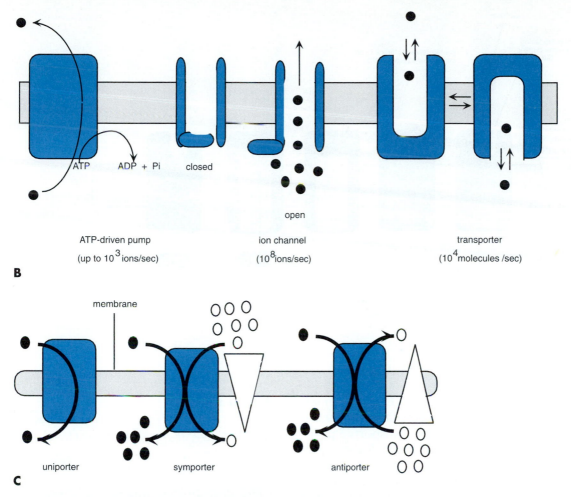

FIGURE 2.20 — (*continued*) *B* and *C*. Schematic diagrams illustrating the action of transport proteins. *B* indicates the three classes of transporters and their relative potential activities. In the case of pumps, the energy of hydrolysis of a phosphoanhydride bond in ATP is used to power the movement of specific ions against their electrochemical gradient. Channels allow the movement of specific ions or water down their electrochemical gradient. Transporters move molecules down their concentration gradients (uniporters), or couple the movement of a molecule down its concentration gradient to transport of another molecule against its concentration gradient (symporters and antiporters). The latter two categories differ in the direction of the transported versus cotransported molecule's concentration gradient, as indicated in *C*. *D* describes in more detail how a transporter (of glucose, in this case) works by shuttling between two different conformational states. In one conformation (a and e), the binding site faces outward. Binding of glucose (b) triggers the conformational change that allows the molecule to leave the transporter only through the other side (c). When the glucose is released (d), it is on the inside, and the transporter returns to its original conformation. Note that the direction of net glucose movement via a transporter is determined by the concentration gradient. Should glucose be higher in concentration within the cell, net movement will be from inside to outside, rather than the other way around. (*Adapted, with permission, from Lodish, H.F. et al. (1995). Molecular Cell Biology, 3rd ed. New York, W.H. Freeman, pp. 639, 654, 659.*)

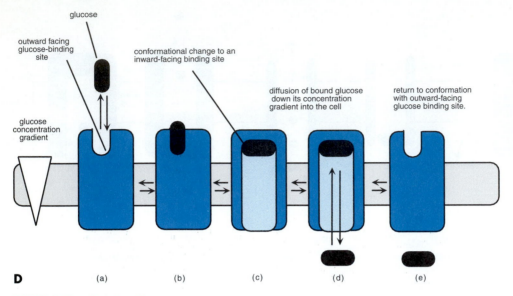

D

(a)   (b)   (c)   (d)   (e)

FIGURE 2.20 — *(continued)*

sium channels. The Na/K/ATPase channel plays a small role in maintenance of membrane potential (because it transports 3 positively charged sodium ions out for every 2 positively charged potassium ions in, leaving a net negative charge on the inside). Its major role, however, is to protect against osmotic damage to cells. The major contribution to maintenance of membrane potential is through the action of voltage-dependent potassium channels.

Physiological organ systems each have their own complement of distinct transporters, ion channels, and receptors to carry out their specialized functions. For example, no less than 6 glucose transporter genes exist. Each has a different set of biophysical and biochemical properties and/or is expressed in different tissues. This diversity makes possible the range of distinctive phenotypes of glucose regulation observed in different organ systems of the body (see Table 2.9).

Clinical Pearls

Osmotic forces are important ones to remember in medicine:

◯ The alert clinician who recognizes signs of excessive brain swelling (termed *cerebral edema*) can save the life of a patient by intravenous infusion of a hyperosmotic solution that pulls water out of the brain and thereby decreases the osmotic pressure that might otherwise result in irreversible brain injury (see Chap. 18).

◯ The patient in profound diabetic ketoacidosis may not seem depleted of potassium ions based on a test for blood potassium concentration.

◯ In acidosis there is a shift of potassium ions from the large intracellular pool to the extracellular space from which it is excreted in the urine. This results in a

TABLE 2.9 PROPERTIES OF GLUCOSE TRANSPORTERS

Name	Major sites of expression	Affinity for glucose	Role in metabolism
GLUT 1	Brain, red blood cells, vasculature, all tissues	High (Km = 1 mM)	Responsible (along with GLUT 3) for basal glucose uptake by all cells; lack of dependence on insulin, means that in the absence of insulin and when blood glucose is low, glucose will go preferentially to those cells that have only GLUT 1 and 3.
GLUT 2	Liver; pancreatic B cell, serosal surfaces of gut and kidney	Low (Km 15-20 mM)	Low affinity for glucose allows GLUT 2 to serve as a monitor of ambient blood glucose concentrations; thus, in response to low blood glucose, hepatic gluconeogenesis is stimulated and in response to a rise in blood glucose, pancreatic β cells secrete more insulin.
GLUT 3	Brain, neurons, all tissues	High (Km < 1 mM)	See GLUT 1.
GLUT 4	Muscle, fat cells	Medium (Km = 2.5-5 mM)	GLUT 4 requires insulin action in order to appear on the cell surface; hence it is used to store glucose in times of plenty and switch from glucose to other substrates such as fatty acids in times of glucose deprivation (e.g., prolonged starvation).
GLUT 5	Jejunum, liver, spermatozoa	Medium (Km = 6 mM)	Na+/glucose symporter brings glucose from gut into intestinal epithelial cells; GLUT 5 moves that glucose from the intestinal epithelial cells into the bloodstream.

Km represents the level of blood glucose at which the transporter has reached one-half of its maximum capacity to transport glucose. −Km is inversely proportional to the affinity.

Reproduced, with permission, from Gardner, D. (1997). Hormone action. In Greenspan, F. and Strewler. G., eds. *Basic and Clinical Endocrinology*, 5th ed. Stamford, CT, Appleton & Lange.

blood potassium concentration close to the normal range, but with substantial depletion of total body potassium stores.

○ Upon correction of the acidosis, the rapid shift of potassium from extracellular fluid back into cells can result in dangerously low blood potassium, which in turn can trigger life-threatening cardiac arrhythmias. By the time this occurs, it may be too late to save the patient. This complication needs to be anticipated and treatment initiated in advance, based on your knowledge of fluid and electrolyte homeostasis (see Chaps. 6 and 10).

○ The patient with rhabdomyolysis has muscle injury with release of myoglobin, an oxygen-binding pigment found in muscle. This can result in precipitation of the myoglobin in the renal tubules and lead to renal failure. Because myoglobin is more soluble in an alkaline environment and is more likely to precipitate in an acidic one, adjustment of body pH slightly in the alkaline direction and expansion of intravascular volume to promote renal tubular flow constitute one effective method of treating this condition. It is especially effective if started early, before precipitation has started to occur. This can be accomplished by expanding the intravascular volume with an isotonic alkaline solution (e.g., of sodium bicarbonate). The resulting large volume flow of alkaline urine keeps the released myoglobin soluble and promotes its excretion (see Chap. 10).

○ A patient can develop life-threatening dehydration due to any one of a number of unrelated conditions such as cholera, diabetes insipidus, hyperglycemia, or failure to drink enough fluids. Recognition of decreased skin turgor, low blood pressure, and rapid heart rate suggests the need for immediate infusion of fluids even before the results of blood studies are available.

Review Questions

32. How do different life forms prevent their cells from exploding in hypotonic solutions?

33. What are the differences between a channel and a transporter?

34. What is the basis for the electrochemical potential difference observed in animal cells?

The cytoskeleton, molecular motors, and muscle contraction

Cell organization and the cytoskeleton

A single human cell expresses about 10,000 out of the 50,000 to 100,000 different genes present in the human genome. The typical human cell also contains about 1 billion protein molecules, representing these 10,000 different coding sequences, in various amounts, all packed in at enormous concentrations (see Ref. 6). One way in which the cell generates order from this potential for chaos is through a tremendous degree of spatial organization. Thus, relatively few proteins float about freely in the cytoplasm. At the level of individual molecules, there are numerous multimeric assemblies of proteins (i.e., groups of proteins physically associated with each other). Some hold together tightly and are known to be multiprotein complexes (e.g., ribosomal subunits); others probably fall apart as soon as an attempt is made to detect them, and thus their ordered association is not easily detected.

The cytoskeleton comprises several families of proteins that polymerize to form structures that can be used to organize the interior of the cell, keeping some proteins together or, at least, nearby, while other proteins are maintained apart. Like workers rearranging the scenery and props between acts of a play, the cytoskeleton can respond to major changes in gene expression by changing the location of various organelles or proteins.

There are three general types of cytoskeletal elements: actin filaments and cables, microtubules, and intermediate filaments (Fig. 2.21). Each has distinctive properties and roles to play in cell biology.

Actin filaments and microtubules are both dynamic polymeric structures in equilibrium with their component monomers, which use nucleotide triphosphate hydrolysis to polymerize the individual monomer proteins into the larger multimeric cytoskeletal structure. GTP hydrolysis is used to assemble microtubules; ATP hydrolysis assembles actin filaments.

A large number of actin filaments are associated with the plasma membrane and play a key role in formation of microvilli and other deformations that are the basis for cell shape and polarity (e.g., apical versus basolateral surfaces). Microtubules emanate from the centrioles, specialized structures that somehow are able to determine and localize to the center of a cell. The so-called "minus end" is at the centriole, and the growing "plus end" is where new monomer subunits are added. Both actin filaments and microtubules contain a number of associated proteins that provide position and cell-type specific information along their lengths.

The intermediate filaments provide a structural scaffolding that contributes to cellular integrity and mechanical stability. Unlike actin filaments and microtubules, intermediate filaments are symmetrical structures and are not in a dynamic state of assembly in equilibrium with monomers. Rather, assembly of intermediate filaments is triggered, often by modifications such as phosphorylation. Thus, in the case of the nuclear lamina,

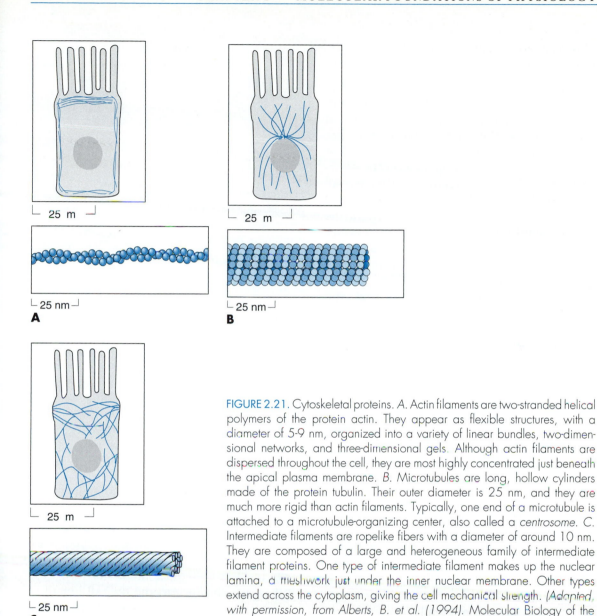

FIGURE 2.21. Cytoskeletal proteins. *A.* Actin filaments are two-stranded helical polymers of the protein actin. They appear as flexible structures, with a diameter of 5-9 nm, organized into a variety of linear bundles, two-dimensional networks, and three-dimensional gels. Although actin filaments are dispersed throughout the cell, they are most highly concentrated just beneath the apical plasma membrane. *B.* Microtubules are long, hollow cylinders made of the protein tubulin. Their outer diameter is 25 nm, and they are much more rigid than actin filaments. Typically, one end of a microtubule is attached to a microtubule-organizing center, also called a *centrosome. C.* Intermediate filaments are ropelike fibers with a diameter of around 10 nm. They are composed of a large and heterogeneous family of intermediate filament proteins. One type of intermediate filament makes up the nuclear lamina, a meshwork just under the inner nuclear membrane. Other types extend across the cytoplasm, giving the cell mechanical strength. *(Adapted, with permission, from Alberts, B. et al. (1994). Molecular Biology of the Cell, 3rd ed. New York, Garland, p. 789.)*

one of the structures made of intermediate filaments, disassembly into component proteins takes place in conjunction with phosphorylation during mitosis. Subsequently, when nuclear membrane reassembly occurs, the same protein is dephosphorylated. Intermediate filaments are comprised of a large number of different proteins. Unlike the actin filaments and microtubules, many of these are cell-type-specific.

Molecular motors and cell movement

In addition to structural and organizational roles in the cell, both actin filaments and microtubules make possible various forms of movement. Various molecular motors are used to position organelles, move cargo, or generate force and movement along these cytoskeletal elements. Members of the myosin gene family in the case of actin filaments, and the kinesin and dynein gene families in the case of microtubules are the motor proteins that make movement via these structures possible. Different motor proteins move specifically toward the "plus" or "minus" end of microtubules, moving various vesicles and other organelles with them.

Changes in the shape and movement of cells are mediated by actin filaments in association with the plasma membrane of the cell. When a cell moves, actin filaments polymerize at the leading edge, generating the force to move the membrane forward.

Muscle contraction

Skeletal muscle is composed of cells packed with a highly specialized form of actin and myosin filaments. By being attached to bones, muscles make possible running, jumping, flying, and other movements. Cardiac muscle is a variant that makes the heart a pump. Smooth muscle in blood vessels and various organs, including the gastrointestinal (GI) tract, make possible less synchronized forms of muscle contraction. Finally, even nonmuscle cells contain actin and myosin and use them to generate various forms of motion at the cellular level.

Muscle is highly specialized in many ways (see Figure 2.22):

- Skeletal muscle is a multinucleate syncytium formed by the fusion of many myocytes during development. However, in cardiac and smooth muscle the cells remain separate.

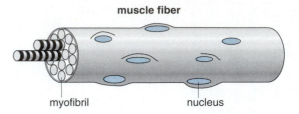

muscle fiber

myofibril   nucleus

FIGURE 2.22. Muscle. Anatomical organization of muscle. In the adult human skeletal muscle exists as huge, multinucleated cells 50 μm in diameter and up to several centimeters long, packed with myofibrils. (Adapted, with permission, from Alberts, B. et al. (1994). Molecular Biology of the Cell, 3rd ed., New York, Garland, p. 848.)

- The cytoplasm of skeletal muscle is entirely filled with bundles of contractile proteins that form myofibrils. Each myofibril is an assembly of contractile proteins that can lead to triggered shortening of the muscle and therefore movement of the bone to which it is attached. The *sarcomere* is the minimum contractile unit that gives skeletal muscle its striated appearance. It consists of overlapping thick (myosin) and thin (actin) filaments. In three dimensions, the thin filaments form a hexagonal array around a thick filament. The Z disks are the morphological boundaries between sarcomeres where the thin filaments are attached. Muscle contraction involves the coordinate sliding of thin and thick filaments past each other, which shortens the overall length of the muscle and generates the tension that makes muscular work possible.
- The process of muscle contraction is highly regulated both by calcium and also by actin-associated proteins. In skeletal and cardiac muscle, calcium regulates binding of the proteins troponin and tropomyosin to actin. In smooth muscle and nonmuscle actin systems, calcium regulates contraction through phosphorylation of a subunit of myosin.

A simplified view of the molecular mechanism of muscle contraction is summarized in Figure 2.23.

Clinical Pearls

○ Epidermolysis bullosa simplex is a human genetic disease caused by mutations in keratin, an intermediate filament component expressed in the basal layer of the epidermis (skin). Individuals with this disease are sensitive to blistering of their skin upon even gentle touch. The mutant phenotype is reproduced in transgenic mice containing these defective genes. This indicates the role of intermediate filaments in protecting cells from mechanical damage.

○ *Listeria monocytogenes* is an invasive bacteria that causes a severe form of food poisoning. Upon gaining entry through the plasma membrane into the cytoplasm of a host cell, these bacteria appear to assemble actin filaments to drive them across the cell to the plasma membrane on the other side of the cell. There, the bacteria appear to mimic the normal actin-based mechanism of cell movement to form a plasma membrane extrusion that is engulfed by a neighboring cell. This allows the bacteria to spread in a manner that cannot be detected by antibodies or other host defenses in the outside world.

Review Questions

35. What are the components of the cytoskeleton?

36. What are some of the roles played by the cytoskeleton in cells?

37. What is the role of actin and myosin in nonmuscle cells?

38. How is muscle contraction regulated?

Apoptosis and cancer

Signal transduction, the act of receiving, recognizing, and responding to a stimulus at the cell surface, is covered in more detail in Chapter 3. Here we will focus on one of the many purposes for which signal transduction is necessary, that of apoptosis and its relation to cancer.

Apoptosis

In multicellular organisms, each cell has a specialized role to play for the benefit of the organism as a whole. In return, each cell is a beneficiary of the efforts of all other cells toward maintaining an optimal internal environment. This "contract of multicellularity" has two key provisions. First, cells must pay attention and respond when called upon (e.g., they must be willing to work overtime in times of need). Second, when certain things go wrong, or at other preordained times built into the genetic code of the cell, each member cell must be willing to sacrifice itself for the good of the organism. This aspect of the contract, calling for programmed cell death or apoptosis, is a central feature in the cell biology and physiology of organ systems in both health and disease.

In its essence, apoptosis involves a large number of signaling pathways (more are being recognized all the time) by which a cascade of protein-protein interactions culminates in activation of proteases and nucleases that destroy cells from within (see Ref. 7). As a result, the apoptosed cell's proteins and nucleic acids are degraded in a distinctive way, and it shrivels up and disappears.

Apoptosis can be distinguished from necrosis, where external insults result in direct death of a cell. In necrosis, the contents of the cell are typically splattered about the neighborhood, with phagocytic cells of the immune system required to come in and clean up the mess. In contrast, apoptosis is often

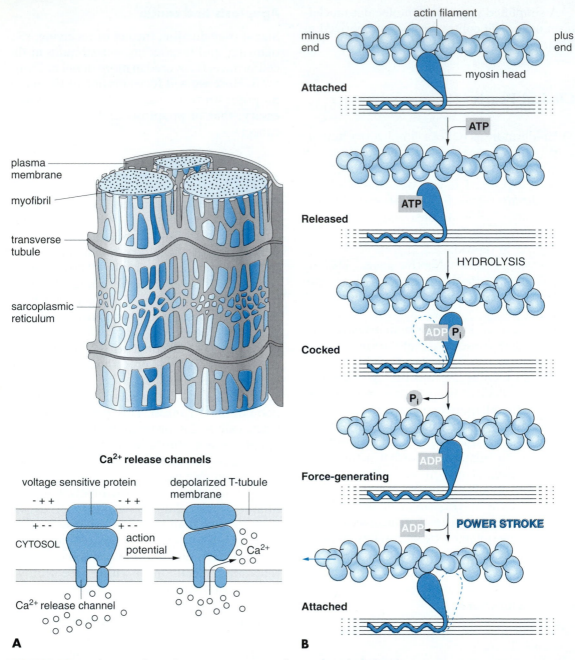

FIGURE 2.23. Mechanism of muscle contraction. *A.* Mechanism by which depolarization of the T-tubule membrane results in calcium flux from sarcoplasmic reticulum to cytosol, triggering muscle contract. *B.* Cycle by which myosin walks along an actin filament. At the start of the cycle, a myosin head is tightly bound to an actin filament in the absence of bound nucleotide. This state is short-lived in vivo,

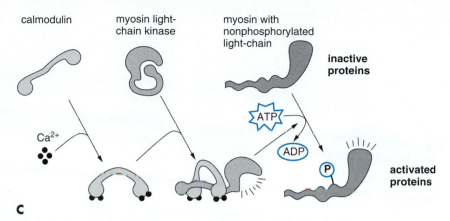

calmodulin

myosin light-
chain kinase

myosin with
nonphosphorylated
light-chain

**inactive
proteins**

ATP

Ca^{2+}

ADP

P

**activated
proteins**

C

FIGURE 2.23 — (continued) due to rapid binding of ATP. However, it is prolonged upon death and is responsible for rigor mortis, the stiffness of a corpse. ATP binding causes a conformational change that decreases affinity for actin, allowing the myosin head to move along the filament. ATP hydrolysis results in a large conformational change of the myosin head that moves about 5 nm along the actin filament. The ADP and Pi remain tightly bound, however. Weak binding to a new site on actin causes release of Pi, which allows tight binding of the myosin head to actin. The release of Pi triggers the power stroke (the force-generating change in shape during which the myosin head returns to its original conformation, concomitant with release of the bound ADP. C. In contrast to the mechanism described in B, regulation of smooth muscle contraction occurs through calcium-dependent phosphorylation of a myosin light chain that is associated with myosin in these cells. (Adapted, with permission, from Alberts, B. et al. (1994). Molecular Biology of the Cell, 3rd ed. New York, Garland, pp. 852-853, 857.)

largely antigenically "silent," leaving no debris behind and activating no inflammatory response.

Part of the complexity of apoptosis is that it does not involve easy decisions. How does the organism know when to give up on a cell versus hoping that it will recover and be a productive member of the multicellular community? The risk in setting the controls too stringently is that too many cells are killed too quickly, impairing survival of the organism. The risk of setting the controls too loosely is that cells that are too impaired to be productive members of the community hang on. As a result, they function inefficiently or are otherwise costly to maintain and are a drag on the functioning of the organism as a whole. Furthermore, such cells are at greater risk of malignant transformation and establishment of a rogue clone gone wild that acts in its own self-interest rather than that of the organism as a whole.

To aid in making the decision of whether or not to trigger apoptosis, a very large family of proteins has evolved that appear to function by adjusting one another's levels in response to various cues so that, ideally, the balance in favor of death is tipped neither too soon nor too late. Apoptosis is not just a response to illness and injury. It is also a key feature of normal development. Thus, for example, apoptosis of intervening cells is what gives rise to fingers and toes of the embryonic limb.

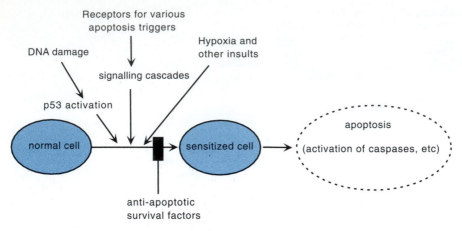

FIGURE 2.24. Pathways of apoptosis (programmed cell death). Description of how many different initial triggers can set off the apoptotic cascade, as data suggest. Whether these triggers (e.g., DNA damage, activation of apoptotic receptors such as that of the cytokine TNF-α, and environmental insults such as low oxygen concentrations termed *hypoxia*) actually push the cell to apoptosis or whether the cell will be arrested or rescued depends on the balance between various pro- and antiapoptotic factors, with the latter blocking the former. Once the cell has been appropriately sensitized, a final common pathway of irreversible events is set in motion (e.g., activation of the caspase proteases), which leads to apoptosis. *(Adapted from Evan, G. and Littlewood, T. (1998). A matter of life and death. Science. 281:1317-1322.)*

Like other signal transduction pathways (see Chap. 3), triggering the apoptotic cascade involves receptors, cytoplasmic effectors, and nuclear effectors (see Figure 2.24). The final common limb initiated by diverse signaling pathways, which defines the apoptotic cascade, includes:

• Families of pro- and antiapoptotic signaling proteins whose association with, and dissociation from, each other, define a wide range of pathways by which apoptosis can be activated. These pathways are often controlled by phosphorylation and dephosphorylation and differ from one cell type to the next. A common feature of the apoptotic cascades is that they can involve either or both the ER and the mitochondria as key weigh stations in the process.

• Cytoplasmic proteases, termed *caspases*, are part of the final common pathway by which apoptosis is carried out.
• Apoptosis culminates in distinctive degradation of nuclear DNA as part of the final common pathway that culminates in cell death.

Cancer

For a single-celled eukaryotic organism, such as a paramecium, the big challenges in life are getting enough food, avoiding bacteria and viruses, and not ending up in some puddle that is going to dry up. The organism has little defense against any of these three terminal situations. Food could be plentiful in the virus-free next puddle over and there is nothing that the paramecium can do about getting there.

An individual cell in a multicellular eukaryote is largely relieved of the worst of these three problems in that a huge amount of effort on the part of the multitrillion-cell organism has gone into the capacity to (1) seek out a food supply, (2) defend against infection, and (3) move to a warm and safe home. However, other obligations come with those solutions. Foremost among these obligations is courtesy to other cells of the organism: no inappropriate dividing, no asking for "more" when the decision has been made to divert meager resources elsewhere. As a member of a multicellular community, you must follow orders even when those orders include self-sacrifice. The logic of multicellularity is that, if everyone goes along, the likelihood of survival of the whole (and therefore of every cell's progeny) is increased.

But what happens if one cell gets the idea to become a freemarketeer, "go it alone" and not fulfill the obligations of multicellularity? That, in essence, is what happens in cancer. Either because of a mutation or for some other reason, the usual apoptotic triggers are disabled, controls on cell division and movement are lost, and a "bad actor" takes over.

Typically, malignant transformation is not an all-or-nothing process, but rather goes through several stages (see Figure 2.25). First, a mutation must occur that disables a key check point which would otherwise prevent the rogue from completing malignant transformation. For example, an apoptotic trigger may be disabled. The mutant cell is not at this point cancerous, but it is particularly susceptible to becoming such. Should another mutation occur which results in out-of-control growth, the failsafe mechanism to trigger apoptosis will not be available. Instead, that cell will divide, forming a tumor. As the tu-

FIGURE 2.25. Stages of progression in the development of cancer of the epithelium of the uterine cervix. (a) Normal epithelium, with dividing cells limited to the basal layer, with full differentiation of the outer layers. (b) Dysplasia in which differentiation is incomplete even far beyond the basal layer. (c) In carcinoma in situ, cells in all layers are proliferating and appear undifferentiated. (d) Malignant carcinoma, begins when cells cross the basal lamina and begin to invade the underlying connective tissue. Several years may elapse from first signs of dysplasia to onset of cancer.

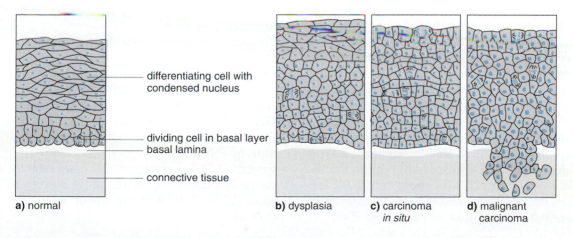

differentiating cell with condensed nucleus

dividing cell in basal layer
basal lamina

connective tissue

a) normal

b) dysplasia

c) carcinoma
in situ

d) malignant
carcinoma

mor grows, there is a chance of more mutations occurring within one of the daughter cells. One of these may further accelerate the loss of control on the part of the organism over the individual cells. For example, loss of genes that make the cell adhesive results in its coming "unglued" from its proper location and start wandering to other locations where it has no business being, a behavior termed *metastasis*. Similarly, expression of a new gene that promotes blood vessel growth and, therefore, preferential access to nutrients would allow a subclone of rogue cells to bypass the needs of the body as a whole. If any of these changes had occurred in isolation, subcellular alarm bells would have gone off, and apoptosis might have been triggered, eliminating the misbehaving cell. But because these changes are occurring in the progeny of a cell that had already lost the capacity to undergo apoptosis, they accumulate and are propagated in the daughter cells. After each mutation, the single mutant cell proliferates into a clone of rogue cells, one of which undergoes the subsequent mutation that moves it further along the pathway of cancer. Some of the mutations occurring in the progression to cancer may be mutations that themselves actually increase the rate of random mutation, making malignant transformation even more likely. It has been estimated that between 3 and 7 such successive mutations are necessary for a cell to go from being entirely normal to being entirely out of control.

The progression from normal cell to cancer may take years to complete. Sometimes the cancer is detected early, when the abnormal cells have not yet left their site of origin. In that case, eradication of all mutant cells (e.g., by surgery) is still a possibility. Unfortunately, by the time a cancer is often detectable by currently available methods, it typically comprises upwards of 1 billion cells. Often, at least a few of those cells have left the site of origin, making the likelihood of complete eradication of the cancer slim.

Protooncogenes are normal genes whose functions, when not properly controlled, can result in inappropriate proliferation of cells. The proteins encoded by protooncogenes include components involved in every level of various signal transduction cascades. Mutations that activate them into oncogenes can be of many different sorts. Thus some oncogenic mutations affect regulation, including level of expression of an otherwise normal protein, while other oncogenic mutations change the protein itself in ways that either boost or impair its signaling in a deleterious way. Some examples of ways in which protooncogenes can become oncogenes include:

- Mutations of genes encoding some receptors result in signals being sent to the nucleus continuously rather than periodically. As a result, DNA synthesis and replication may become a constant preoccupation of the cell, rather than an intermittent event triggered by specific stimuli.
- Mutations of genes encoding some second messenger-generating systems (that normally respond to activation of a surface receptor), when inappropriately activated, can bypass normal controls (e.g., down regulation by endocytosis, or adaptation by phosphorylation) by which a surface receptor would be turned off. As a result, their signaling pathways are inappropriately on, including triggering of growth programs.
- Mutations of genes encoding some transcription factors that result in their constitutive activity can do the same thing, namely bypass the normal controls that prevent a second messenger from being overactive.
- Gene amplification can result in overproduction of a protein normally made in minute quantities.
- Chromosomal rearrangements can result in recombinational events that move a protein from tightly regulated expression to looser control.

Tumor suppressor genes are genes that normally act as triggers of pathways that prevent inappropriate oncogene activation. Many tumor suppressor genes work by activating the apoptotic pathway. When these genes are inappropriately turned off (e.g., by mutations that inactivate their encoded proteins), the rates of malignant transformation are greatly increased. Since we all have two copies of most genes, one from each parent, the loss of one of the two tumor suppressor genes results in a much higher incidence of any particular cancer, since the individual is just one mutation away from losing that particular tumor suppressing line of defense.

The physiology of cancer includes the study of the normal mechanisms by which "bad behavior" is held in check and by which cells are compelled to comply with the "contract of multicellularity." Given that approximately 10^{16} cell divisions occur in a human body over the course of its lifetime and that DNA polymerase has a spontaneous mutation rate of approximately one in 10^6 per gene per cell division, one might expect cancer to be more common than it actually seems to be. An important role of the immune system (see Chap. 19) seems to be to identify cells that have ceased to cooperate with the multicellular contract and kill them before they have a chance to undergo further transformation to the fully malignant cancerous state. At some point during the progression of successive mutations, cells not only develop the ability to ignore instructions and bypass what were intended to be "failsafe" apoptotic controls, but also to evade immune surveillance mechanisms. Once such a mutation occurs, it does not matter that the immune system can still detect and kill all other cells of the tumor. The one evasive mutant cell will proliferate until it comprises billions of cells, all of them resistant to that particular mechanism of host defense.

Further mutations are not the only way in which a mutant cell can progress to cancer.

Tumor promoters include nongenetic ways in which malignant transformation can be favored. Sometimes they can be as simple as injury to tissues that include a mutant cell. The normal healing response is to flood the local injured tissue with growth factors and other substances that stimulate cell division. Although the intent of those growth factors was to support repair of the injury, they may also unwittingly provide a mutant cell the opportunity to proliferate, which increases the likelihood of further mutation and progression down the pathway of malignant transformation, before host defenses arrive on the scene.

Various factors in the environment, from cigarette smoke to drinking burning hot beverages, can serve as either tumor initiators or promoters in the development of cancers. Different populations have different incidences of cancers, reflecting a combination of genetic and environmental factors (see Table 2.10).

Clinical Pearls

○ In 1996 there were an estimated 1.36 million new cases of invasive cancer in the United States alone. Roughly 50% of patients diagnosed with cancer are cured by currently available treatments. This varies tremendously from cancers that are highly curable with treatment (such as basal cell carcinoma of the skin) to others such as pancreatic or esophageal carcinoma whose prognosis today is invariably poor.

The most significant risk factor for cancer, overall, is age: The older you are, the more likely you are to get it. This makes sense in terms of both the occurrence of random tumor initiation events and exposure to environmental tumor promoters. Currently approximately 25% of the population has or will develop some form of cancer in their lifetime.

TABLE 2.10 DIFFERENT INCIDENCES OF CANCER IN DIFFERENT POPULATIONS/ENVIRONMENTS

Site of origin of cancer	High incidence population		Low-incidence population	
	Location	Incidence*	Location	Incidence*
Lung	USA (New Orleans, blacks)	110	India (Madras)	5.8
Breast	Hawaii (Hawaiians)	94	Israel (non-Jews)	14.0
Prostate	USA (Atlanta, blacks)	91	China (Tianjin)	1.3
Uterine cervix	Brazil (Recife)	83	Israel (non-Jews)	3.0
Stomach	Japan (Nagasaki)	82	Kuwait (Kuwaitis)	3.7
Liver	China (Shanghai)	34	Canada (Nova Scotia)	0.7
Colon	USA (Connecticut, whites)	34	India (Madras)	1.8
Melanoma	Australia (Queensland)	31	Japan (Osaka)	0.2
Nasopharynx	Hong Kong	30	UK (southwestern)	0.3
Esophagus	France (Calvados)	30	Romania (urban Cluj)	1.1
Bladder	Switzerland (Basel)	28	India (Nagpur)	1.7
Uterus	USA (San Francisco Bay Area, whites)	26	India (Nagpur)	1.2
Ovary	New Zealand (Polynesian Islanders)	26	Kuwait (Kuwaitis)	3.3
Rectum	Israel (European and USA born)	23	Kuwait (Kuwaitis)	3.0
Larynx	Brazil (São Paulo)	18	Japan (rural Miyagi)	2.1
Pancreas	USA (Los Angeles, Koreans)	16	India (Poona)	1.5
Lip	Canada (Newfoundland)	15	Japan (Osaka)	0.1
Kidney	Canada (NWT and Yukon)	15	India (Poona)	0.7
Oral cavity	France (Bas-Rhin)	14	India (Poona)	0.4
Leukemia	Canada (Ontario)	12	India (Nagpur)	2.2
Testis	Switzerland (urban Vaud)	10	China (Tianjin)	0.6

* Incidence = number of new cases per year per 100,000 population, adjusted for a standardized population age distribution (so as to eliminate effects due merely to differences of population age distribution). Figures for cancers of breast, uterine cervix, uterus, and ovary are for women; other figures are for men.

Adapted, with permission, from Alberts, B. et al., (1994). *Molecular Biology of the Cell,* 3rd ed. New York, Garland, p. 1266.

○ The diagnosis of cancer should never be made without microscopic examination of tissue, e.g., from a biopsy.

○ Prognosis in patients with cancer often correlates with amount of tumor present. This makes sense in that the more tumor there is, the longer the cancer has been present. Similarly, the more the cancer has divided, the greater the chance that further mutations have occurred that make the cancer less responsive to physiological controls.

○ Often the treatments for cancer, such as chemotherapy and radiation, are themselves mutagenic and can result in a secondary cancer, should the patient be cured of the first cancer. The risk is roughly 1% per year of survival in the case of radiation. Also, both radiation and chemotherapy can cause permanent damage to other organs, such as the lung, heart, and gonads.

○ Tumor markers are gene products expressed by cancers as a result of the loss of controls that maintain the normal differentiated phenotype of cells. Often tumor markers are genes that are normally expressed in embryogenesis but are not found in the adult, such as α-fetoprotein (AFP) and carcinoembryonic antigen (CEA). Measurement of the level of these products can often be used to monitor the effectiveness of therapy or the return of a cancer.

○ When cancer recurs after initially success-ful chemotherapy, it is often resistant to further chemotherapy, including other chemotherapeutic agents. There are a number of different mechanisms of che-motherapy resistance. One is that the cells that survive the initial chemotherapy have often been selected because they overex-press p-glycoprotein, a transporter that protects the cancer cell by pumping many different chemotherapeutic drugs out of the cell.

Another mechanism of chemotherapy resistance is the loss of hormone receptors. Often a cancer is dependent on the pres-ence of a particular hormone, for example, to keep it in the cell cycle, etc. Thus, antag-onists of that hormone are often useful forms of chemotherapy to slow down the progression of the cancer. The problem is that, eventually, a clone of the cancer cells is selected (i.e., due to further mutations) that lacks that hormone receptor and is able to proliferate independent of the presence of the hormone. Estrogen recep-tors in breast cancer are an example of this phenomenon.

○ Sometimes cancers make hormones or other products that cause paraneoplastic syndromes (disease states that are due to the biological effects of the hormones or other products made). Cushing's syn-drome due to ACTH excess (see Chap. 13) and hypercalcemia due to parathyroid hormone-related products (see Chap. 14) occur commonly in advanced cancer for this reason.

Review Questions

39. Contrast apoptosis and necrosis as mechanisms of cell death.

40. What are the stages a mutant cell must go through before it becomes a meta-static cancer?

41. Suggest at least 5 mechanisms by which protooncogenes can become func-tional oncogenes.

7. FRONTIERS OF MOLECULAR PHYSIOLOGY

Spontaneous versus protein-mediated events in biology

A recurring debate in modern experimental biological science has been whether various events occur spontaneously or are catalyzed by specific cellular machinery. Folding of polypeptides, translocation of proteins across the membrane of the ER, and assembly of viral capsids are all different examples of events originally believed to be spontaneous, but for which there is growing evidence for nonspontaneous, energy-dependent roles for protein machinery (see Refs 11-16). The no-tion that biological processes might occur spontaneously derives sometimes from theo-retical considerations (see Ref. 9) and some-times from experiments examining the be-havior of purified proteins in solution in a test-tube (see Ref. 10). This view has often been reinforced by the lack of observation of intermediates in these processes in living cells. But perhaps the events in vivo occur too quickly to easily detect such intermedi-ates. That events can occur in purified sys-tems to a small extent does not mean that that is the way they happen in cells where the same events typically occur orders of magnitude faster and to a high degree of com-pletion. Enzymes, after all, deal with the speed, efficiency, and coupling of energeti-cally favorable reactions — they do not make thermodynamically unfavorable reactions occur.

Cell-free extracts that combine at least some of the complexity of living cells with the analytical power of test-tube studies have been one way to address these problems (see

Refs. 11, 15, 16). These systems appear faithful to the in vivo situation by numerous criteria. However, they are slower, thereby allowing intermediates to be detected and mechanism to be dissected in ways that are not possible in living cells. This issue provides good examples of how progress in science is often driven by the development of new technology, which, in turn, leads to new ways of thinking about long-standing observations (see Chap. 1).

Why would the cell have chosen more complex, protein machinery-driven ways of solving problems that might have been solved in simpler, more spontaneous ways? Perhaps because the complex, protein-mediated mechanism provides more avenues for variations on a theme and regulation under different conditions. These are the contingencies that evolution through natural selection can exploit (see Ref. 3).

Biochemical individuality

The concept of biochemical individuality originated from studies of human nutrition that recognized significant differences in the vitamin needs of different individuals (see Ref. 16). Now the notion is broader, reflecting the effects of many different genes on any given trait and the way different individuals can compensate for lack of one with an excess of another (Refs. 17 and 18).

The implications of this concept for physiology and medicine are enormous. First, the huge number of products in the biotechnology pipeline means a major expansion of the potential for drug-induced side-effects in subpopulations of humans, which may not be anticipated from existing studies on a more limited population base.

Second, the utility of so-called evidence-based medicine, derived primarily from clinical epidemiology, is significantly diminished if, for any given question, there are potentially dozens of different subpopulations for whom the answer will be different. The characteristics and identity of these subpopulations and the conditions under which their responses deviate from the studied population remains unknown.

Third, the complex effects of environmental toxins and other biologically active compounds may be difficult to sort out without a better understanding of the relevant interacting gene products. One of the by-products of the human genome project will be the potential to study such interactions in a more comprehensive and streamlined fashion than can be done today (see, for example, current approaches with the yeast genome, Ref. 5). On the other hand, recent studies also suggest the potential for novel protein-protein interactions that cannot be predicted from the simple gene sequence (see Ref. 20).

8. HOW DOES AN UNDERSTANDING OF NORMAL PHYSIOLOGY PROVIDE INSIGHT INTO THE INITIAL CASE PRESENTATION?

Let's revisit the case of Mr. B., the 56-year-old former restaurateur with a progressive neurodegenerative disease, whose specialty was sheep brain stew (see earlier Case Presentation).

Mr. B.'s family was told that "a virus is eating his brain and there is nothing we can do about it."

Sixteen years later, the Nobel Prize was awarded for contributions to the understanding of prion diseases, of which CJD is one. Astounding progress involving cell biology, biochemistry, and molecular genetics has greatly changed our view of CJD and related diseases. This and other prion diseases are no longer viewed as the consequence of infection by a slow virus. They are now viewed by many scientists to be diseases of gene expression encoded entirely in the host, in which an abnormal conformation of a normal protein induces normal copies of that protein to take on the abnormal conformation. By eating scrapie-infected sheep brain (i.e., which contains prion protein in the abnormal conformation), a person plays Russian Roulette with their brain: Should even one molecule of abnormal prion protein appear in the brain (e.g., get absorbed undigested from the gut, escape clearance by the liver, and travel to the brain via the bloodstream), the abnormal conformation may be transmitted to the endogenous prion protein of the host.

A remarkable and still mysterious aspect of these disorders is how an abnormally folded form of a protein encoded in an endogenous gene is able to confer a conformational change in normal copies of the host protein and thereby trigger neurodegeneration. A "knockout" mouse (one lacking both copies of an endogenous normal gene) for the prion protein has been made and is found not to be infectable, confirming an essential feature of the prion hypothesis.

Host factors have been implicated in the progression of these diseases. Bovine spongiform encephalopathy (BSE), also known as Mad Cow disease, is a prion disease that appeared in the 1980s among cattle in Britain, prompting changes in animal feeding practices that were believed to have caused the disease.

More recently, a number of people in Europe have come down with variant CJD, believed to be the human manifestation of BSE from consumption of contaminated beef, gelatin, or other products. The full implication of this outbreak depends on the incubation time of this disorder, which is currently unknown. These may be a few tragic aberrations. In contrast, they may be the harbinger of a much larger cohort of disease with a more delayed time of onset.

Apart from the individual tragic stories of people such as Mr. B., who come down with these rare and devastating diseases, the potential importance of prion disease is three-fold: First, it shares important pathological features with Alzheimer's disease (AD), a much more common dementing disorder of humans. This raises the possibility that an understanding of the prion diseases may provide insight into neurodegeneration as seen in AD (see Ref. 20).

Second, the prion story reminds us that we should not take current hypotheses too seriously, they may be just one astute set of observations away from being exploded.

Finally, prion diseases are the quintessential modern disease. BSE and variant CJD exist, apparently, because modern humans feed ground-up cows (including some that were sick with prion disease) to live cows (who normally consume an entirely plant product-based diet). As a result of this human-introduced aberration in the food chain, herds of cattle, and apparently some of the hamburgers made from them, may have been contaminated with infectious prions. Modern science may give us new information and tools, but if we do not use them in ways that respect evolution and promote homeostasis, our actions are likely to continue to cause unanticipated disasters of this sort.

Although we cannot yet treat these disorders, they can now be studied with the powerful tools of modern molecular physiology, which were not available 16 years ago at the time of this case. Through further study it may some day be possible to pharmacologically interrupt the pathological cascade that gives rise to CJD and other prion diseases. In the meantime, a prudent diet (low on the food chain, high in fiber, and variety), may well be the best means of disease prevention (see Chap. 20).

SUMMARY AND REVIEW OF KEY CONCEPTS

1. In physical-chemical terms, life is about information and energy storage, utiliza-

tion and transmission within the limits imposed by the first (energy cannot be created or destroyed) and second (entropy of the universe always increases) laws of thermodynamics.

2. Enzymes are organized into pathways that interconnect and whose action facilitates chemical reactions with negative free energy (G). Enzymes also couple unfavorable reactions to favorable ones to get them to occur. A series of enzymes can use the law of mass action to drive a reaction that would otherwise be unfavorable.

3. The basic molecular building blocks of life are sugars, nucleotides, amino acids, and simple lipids such as cholesterol and phosphatidyl choline.

4. High-energy phosphates are used to make chemical energy available in an immediately usable form. Sugars and sugar polymers (starches) are the most convenient forms of short-term energy storage. In the intermediate term, energy can be stored in proteins, but with two caveats. First, the organism needs its protein stores for structural purposes and cannot deplete them as a source of energy. Second, ammonia groups derived from amino acid metabolism are quite toxic and must be converted (e.g., into urea). Long-term storage of energy is achieved through the use of fats.

5. Sequences of nucleotides and their capacity to be stabilized by a complementary sequence via hydrogen bonding of base pairs provides the most effective form of information storage and transfer. This information is generally expressed as protein sequences composed of amino acids corresponding to a particular translation of triplets of base pairs, shared by all living organisms.

6. Biological membranes are composed of lipid bilayers with associated proteins. They make possible separation of the intracellular and extracellular worlds and the demarcation of internal organelles devoted to specialized functions within the cell.

7. Complex protein machines mediate various biological processes including DNA replication and cell cycle control, transcription, protein synthesis and secretion, and signal transduction of all sorts.

8. Principles of genetics have emerged to understand how changes in the genetic code occur and are passed on to daughter cells and the next generation of multicellular organisms.

9. Transporters and channels move ions and other substances in and out of cells and organelles and make possible specialization functions such as those that occur in the nervous and muscular systems.

10. The cytoskeleton and associated proteins including molecular motors organize the cytoplasm and make possible various forms of movement of organelles, cells, and organ systems such as muscle.

11. Apoptosis, or programmed cell death, is a complex multipathway means of insuring that eukaryotic cells conform to the multicellular contract of collaboration and self-sacrifice for the good of the whole.

12. Cancer occurs when, as a result of mutations and subsequent selection, a cell breaks away from the controls applied by apoptotic and other pathways.

A CASE OF PHYSIOLOGICAL MEDICINE

A. T. is a 24-year-old man who works at a warehouse. He has OTC deficiency, a genetic disease caused by a mutation in the gene encoding this protein, which results in greatly lowered enzymatic activity. His diagnosis was made when he went to his pediatrician with profound jaundice at age 2. The pediatrician remembered that a few years before the family had had an infant who died with jaundice and liver disease ascribed at the time to Reye's syndrome, a mysterious form of hepatic failure associated with childhood aspirin use during a viral syndrome. Thinking it unusual that one family would have suffered such a rare disease twice, the pediatrician undertook a search for a genetic disease, and uncovered several family members over three generations with similar presentations. Biochemical detective work identified the OTC deficiency (see Figure 2.26A). This enzyme of the urea cycle is needed to convert ammonia into the far-less toxic and more easily excreted by-product urea. Without it, a patient accumulates ammonia, which is believed to be toxic to the brain.

As a child, Mr. T. had two episodes of mild coma, the last one occurring at age 9. During his childhood his parents divorced; he now lives with his mother 500 miles from the academic medical center where his childhood medical records are located.

One day, while at work, Mr. T. had a minor accident, bumping his head. That afternoon he went out drinking with friends, but by evening felt nauseous and was unable to eat. Within 24 hours he was comatose and was brought to the hospital by friends. There, initial puzzlement at his condition was followed by recognition of his unusual history, suggesting that this was not a run-of-the-mill hepatic encephalopathy in a person with underlying liver disease, nor was it coma due to intoxication, trauma, or brain disease. Mr. T. was transferred to the intensive care unit of a university hospital for further evaluation and treatment.

The physicians unearthed his past history and recognized that Mr. T. likely had ammonia toxicity, later confirmed by testing of blood and cerebrospinal fluid. They initiated therapy based on several principles of biochemistry and metabolism. First, using the law of mass action, they gave him large doses of arginine to drive the pathway and thereby consume more ammonia. Second, taking advantage of the interconnection between metabolic pathways, they gave him sodium benzoate and phenylacetate, compounds that drive alternate pathways by which glycine and glutamine (amino acids in which the excess ammonia is trapped) can be converted to more readily excreted compounds (such as hippurate and phenylacetylglutamate). Synthesis of these amino acids normally serves as a relatively minor metabolic sink for excess ammonia. In the absence of OTC, the pathways by which these amino acids are metabolized to products readily eliminated in the urine can serve as substitutes for OTC and the urea cycle as the major pathways of nitrogen excretion (see Figure 2.26B). Finally, using the principle that the level of activity of a pathway is determined by the level of flux of substrates through it, they used classical approaches to minimizing Mr. T.'s ammonia load. These included restricting his intake of protein and giving him lactulose, a nonabsorbable carbohydrate that is metabolized by GI tract bacteria to acid products that trap ammonia in its charged form in the GI lumen and that causes osmotic diarrhea that eliminates the ammonia from the body.

Over the next week Mr. T. gradually recovered and two weeks after admission he was ready for discharge. Once he was awake, Mr. T. was informed that his two-week, $25,000 hospital bill was not covered by his employee insurance since it was due to a "preexisting condition" (his genetic disease). In addition, his insurance did not cover phenylacetate and sodium benzoate administration, the cost of which is substantial (several thousand dollars a year). Even though he seems to acquire ammonia intoxication only during periods of stress, it is essential for Mr. T. to take large doses of these compounds every day, since it is not yet possible to know the amount of

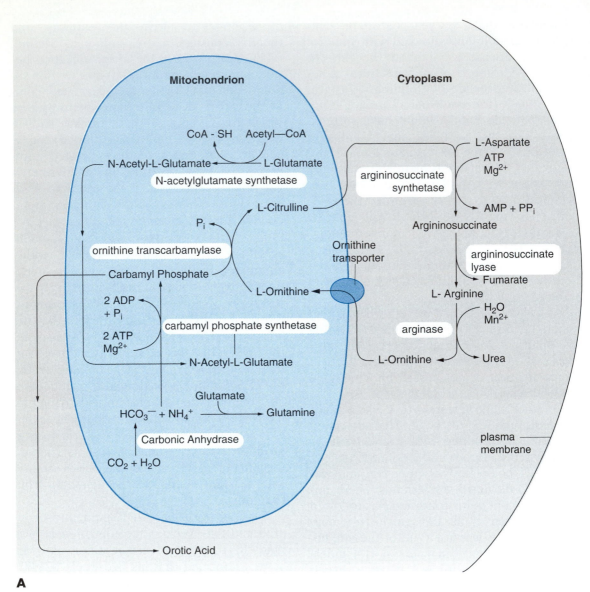

A

FIGURE 2.26. *A.* Schematic representation of the urea cycle showing intra- and extramitochondrial localization of constitutent enzymes. Ornithine transcarbamylase (OTC) is located within the mirochondrion where it is responsible for the condensation of carbamyl phosphate (derived from ammonia and bicarbonate) and ornithine to form citrulline. Congenital OTC deficiency in humans can result in hyperammonemia and severe neurological impairment, but sometimes these patients have symptoms only during times of stress, as in this case. The basis for these differences in manifestation of disease is unknown, but could, for example, be due to subtle defects that render the mechanism of import into mitochondria subject to disruption in times of stress.

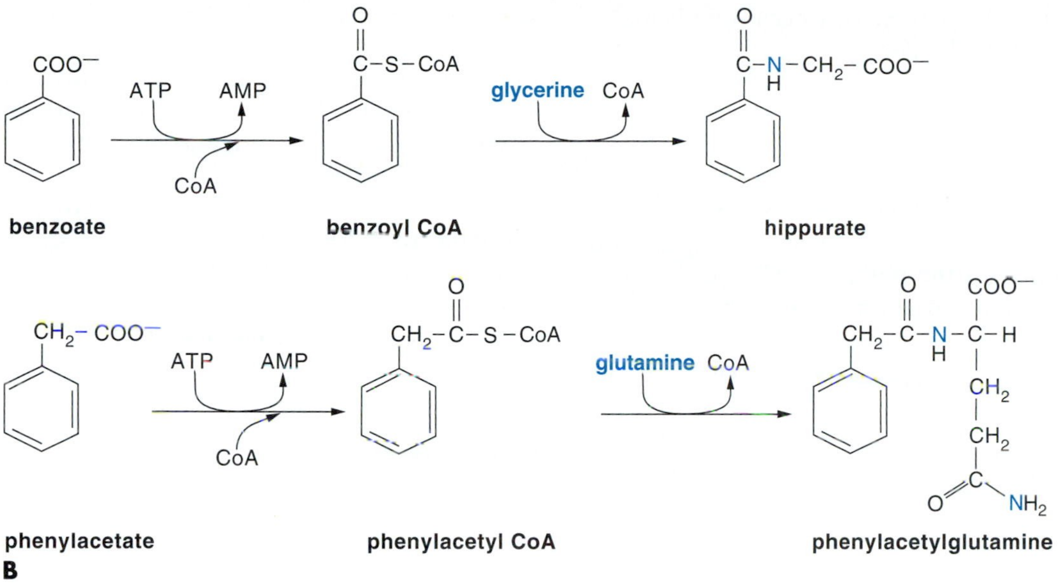

B

FIGURE 2.26 — (continued) B. Ornithine transcarbamylase deficiency can be treated by supplementing the diet with benzoate and phenylacetate. Through the law of mass action, large doses of these agents expand these latent biochemical pathways to bypass the genetic defect. In effect, hippurate and phenylacetylgluta- mate substitute for urea, allowing the body to dispose of excess nitrogen. (A, Adapted, with permission, from Brusilow, S.W. (1997). Inborn errors of urea synthesis, in Glew, R.H. and Ninomiya, Y. eds. Clinical Studies in Medical Bio- chemistry, 2nd ed. Oxford,. B, Adapted, with permission, from Stryer, L. (1995). Biochemistry, 4th ed. New York, W.H. Freeman, p. 637.)

stress necessary to trigger manifestation of OTC deficiency in Mr. T.

QUESTIONS

1. Why is OTC deficiency only a problem for individuals homozygous for the mutation?
2. How does Mr. T.'s OTC deficiency disease relate to that of individuals with alcohol-induced liver disease who develop hepatic encephalopathy in response to an ammonia load?
3. Explain the law of mass action and how it was used in this case to compensate for a lack of OTC.

4. "Simple" genetic diseases such as OTC de- ficiency often, on close inspection, have annoying complications and mysteries that suggest that either they are not so simple or our understanding of the underlying simple biochemistry is incomplete. For example, this patient is able to go for years, by report even eating protein, (and, therefore, am- monia) loads such as cheeseburgers some- times without a problem, but then occa- sionally get into trouble during times of stress. Based on the survey of modern biol- ogy presented in this chapter, and knowing that OTC is a mitochondrial matrix enzyme encoded in the nucleus and subsequently transported from cytoplasm to mitochon- dria, suggest some possible explanations

for why the patient only occasionally manifests OTC deficiency.

ANSWERS

1. If an individual also has a normal gene (in the normal location), it will be expressed and half of the person's OTC protein will be normal. Therefore, since a normal individual has a vast excess of enzyme activity capacity, the urea cycle should function normally even with only half of the usual level of OTC protein and enzyme capacity.
2. In Mr. T.'s case, he does not have enough OTC enzyme activity in his liver to handle a normal ammonia load during certain times of stress. In the case of patients with hepatic encephalopathy due to alcohol-induced destruction of the liver, the problem is one of inadequate numbers of functional liver cells and inadequacy of all of the enzymes of the urea cycle, rather than a selective defect in one enzyme.
3. The law of mass action states that the levels of reactants and products will affect the direction in which a chemical reaction will go. Thus, manipulations that elevate nontoxic reactions will help eliminate toxic coreactants, and manipulations that consume products (e.g., down side pathways) will tend to increase conversion of reactants to products.

   If the level of one (nontoxic) reactant (arginine) is extremely high, it can be used to drive the next step in the reaction generating ornithine. When ornithine levels are high, they tend to drive what little OTC activity the patient may have, which will increase consumption of the toxic reactant (ammonia). Phenylacetate and sodium benzoate drive the side reaction consuming glycine and glutamine, thereby driving the ammonia-consuming pathways by which they are formed (see Figure 2.26B).

4. Molecular chaperones play multiple roles in protecting cells from injury — and have also been implicated in uptake of proteins such as OTC into mitochondria. Perhaps Mr. T.'s molecular chaperones were too busy performing other duties during stressful situations when he became ill and were unable to mediate import into mitochondria of his low level of OTC, resulting in a loss of activity and making him acutely susceptible to ammonia toxicity.

COMMENTS

Complex genetic diseases are not suffered by rich people only. However, the poor, who have less access to care and to expensive evaluations are less often diagnosed. Thus Mr. T.'s deceased brother, who never had a genetic evaluation, almost certainly had OTC deficiency, not Reye's syndrome.

Although biochemical physiology is important in treating patients with complex diseases, nonscientific, nonmedical issues can intrude into the care of the patient, as in the health insurance dilemma indicated here. It is interesting to consider the argument that, although Mr. T. has a genetic disease, the primary genetic aspect does not account for the exacerbation at some times and not others. What does account for exacerbation is not understood, but likely goes beyond simple genetics and suggests an environmental component. Hence, a case could be made that his insurance should cover his illness.

References and suggested readings

GENERAL REFERENCES

1. Alberts, B. et al. (1994). *Molecular Biology of the Cell*, 3rd ed. New York. Garland.
2. Stryer, L. (1995). *Biochemistry*, 4th ed.: New York, W.H. Freeman.

3. Gerhart, J., and Kirschner, M. (1997). *Cells, Embryos, and Evolution*. Malden, MA., Blackwell.
4. McPhee, S. et al. (1996). *Pathophysiology of Disease*. Stamford, CT, Appleton & Lange.
5. Derisi, J.L. et al. (1998). Exploring the metabolic and genetic control of gene expression on a genomic scale. *Science* 278: 680-686.
6. Fulton, A. (1982). How crowded is the cytoplasm? *Cell* 30:345-347.
7. Ashkenazi, A., and Dixit, V. (1998). Death receptors: Signaling and modulation. *Science* 281:1305-1308.

FRONTIER REFERENCES

8. Alberts, B.M. (1998). The cell as a collection of protein machines. *Cell* 92:291-294.
9. Steitz, T., and Engleman, D. (1982). The spontaneous insertion of proteins into and across membranes: The helical hairpin hypothesis. *Cell* 23:411-416.
10. Ganser, B.K. et al. (1999). Assembly and analysis of conical models for the HIV-1 core. *Science* 283:80-83.
11. Blobel, G., and Dobberstein, B. (1975). Transfer of proteins across membranes I and II. *J. Cell Biol.* 67:371-377.
12. Simon, S., and Blobel. G. (1991). A protein-conducting channel in the endoplasmic reticulum. *Cell* 65:371-377.
13. Buchner, J. (1996). Supervising the fold: Functional principles of molecular chaperones. *FASEB J.* 10:10-19.
14. Lingappa, J. et al. (1997). A multistep, ATP-dependent pathway for assembly of human immunodeficiency virus capsids in a cell-free system. *J. Cell Biol.* 136:567-581.
15. Hegde, R.S., and Lingappa, V.R. (1999). Regulation of protein biogenesis at the endoplasmic reticulum. (perspectives) *Trends Cell Biol.* 9:132-137.
16. Williams, R.J. (1956). *Biochemical Individuality*. New York, Wiley.
17. Kadlubar, F.F. (1994). Biochemical individuality and its implications for drug and carcinogen metabolism. *Drug Metab. Rev.* 26:37-46.
18. Calabrese, E.J. (1996). Biochemical individuality: The next generation. *Regulatory Tox. Pharm.* 24:S58-67.
19. Michalak, A., and Butterworth, R.F. (1997). Ornithine transcarbamylase deficiency: Pathogenesis of the cerebral disorder and new prospects for therapy. *Metab. Brain Dis.* 12:171-180.
20. Hegde, R.S. et al. (1999). Transmissible and genetic prion diseases share a common pathway of neurodegeneration. *Nature* 402: 822–826.

COMMAND AND CONTROL OF ORGAN SYSTEMS

3

1. INTRODUCTION TO ENDOCRINOLOGY

Foundations of intercellular commmunication

Over 1 billion years ago, in the course of evolution, a selective advantage was achieved in a certain set of environmental niches by cells coming together to form multicellular organisms. A key benefit of multicellularity was the potential for specialization. That is, by becoming expert at a subset of activities, a cell could enhance its survival, and that of the organism as a whole. Eventually, controls evolved that skewed in favor of survival of the organism as a whole, at the sacrifice of individual cells (e.g., apoptosis). Indeed, "suicidal" cell types evolved that sacrifice themselves in a programmed fashion for the benefit of the organism (e.g., red and white blood cells).

Exploitation of the full potential of multicellular specialization required novel modes and increased sophistication of communication between cells. Specialized cells in multicellular organisms had to communicate in two particular ways. First, they had to be able to coordinate their actions with the actions of all other cells needed for a particular function, including other cell types. This form of communication makes it possible for cells to work together as organs (groups of cells that perform a particular function for the organism as a whole), rather than as unconnected component tissues (cells of a particular type). For example, the **exocrine** pancreas consists of both enzyme-secreting acinar cells, as well as duct cells that secrete bicarbonate and serve as a conduit to the gastrointestinal (GI) tract. The bicarbonate neutralizes stomach acid as it enters the small intestine, which is necessary if the enzymes secreted by the acinar cells are to work. The entry of food into the GI tract is communicated to both types of exocrine pancreatic cells so that both pancreatic enzymes and bicarbonate can be secreted in concert.

Second, specialized cells of a particular type must have ways to inform other classes of specialized cells on whom they depend, when their needs change. For example, when exercising, much ATP must be generated to drive muscle contraction. This need can quickly outstrip the available oxygen, requiring the muscle to switch to anaerobic metabolism (which does not use oxygen). However anaerobic metabolism uses up glucose faster, since it generates far less ATP per molecule of glucose, than aerobic metabolism. The lactic acid end product of anaerobic metabolism of glucose spills into the bloodstream where it has several effects, including:

- Driving the liver to produce more glucose
- Increasing the respiratory rate to bring in more oxygen
- Increasing muscle blood flow to take the oxygen and glucose to where they are needed, the exercising muscle
- Promoting the unloading of oxygen from red blood cells; this allows the generation of more ATP, which allows the muscle to continue contracting and, therefore, has tremendous survival value.

Multicellular animals have evolved a number of modes of communication. The nervous system and the endocrine system are the best studied. Both of these systems release substances that bind to specific receptors on specific target cells, often far away, to trigger responses. However, each of these systems has features that make them better suited to integrate certain specific organ system functions over others.

The fundamental feature of the nervous system is the transmission of electrical signals termed *action potentials* by individual cells called *neurons*, which deliver chemical messages known as **neurotransmitters** to special structures termed *synapses* and *neuromuscu-*

lar junctions (see Chap. 18). This mode of communication is notable for its speed and precise localization. Generally, a message transmitted by the nervous system needs to be repeated after a short time, and only those cells with direct neural inputs through synapses can "hear" the message.

The fundamental feature of the endocrine system is the secretion of substances called *hormones* into the bloodstream. Hormones are distributed throughout the body, but have no effect on cells unless the cells have receptors to which the hormones can bind. Such receptor-bearing target cells may all be found in a single organ or may be scattered throughout the body. Upon reaching a target cell, the hormone binds and activates the receptor. The activated receptor then triggers concerted changes in the activity of sets of enzymes within the target cell, termed *signaling pathways*, that serve a particular biochemical purpose (e.g., to produce more glucose, in the example of the exercising muscle). This process of converting a neural or hormone-mediated message into an activated signaling pathway within a receptor-bearing target cell, culminating in a biochemical response, is termed *signal transduction*.

Generally, the time course over which a message is transmitted, carried out, and terminated in the endocrine system is much slower than in the nervous system. While relatively slow and diffuse compared to that of the nervous system, hormonal communication in the endocrine system has the advantage that the message generally does not need to be repeated anywhere near as often. An additional advantage is that even a very low concentration of hormone reaching a distant site is able to convey the message. Table 3.1 summarizes the key features that distinguish the classical nervous and endocrine systems of communication. There are, however, ambiguities that make a distinction between these two systems of

TABLE 3.1   CHARACTERISTICS OF THE NERVOUS AND ENDOCRINE SYSTEMS

Nervous system	Endocrine system
• Speed	• Distance
• Precise localization	• Diffuse recipients
• Short action	• Longer action
• Low affinity	• High affinity
• High concentration	• Low concentration

Adapted with permission from Funder, J.W. (1987). Receptors, hummingbirds and refrigerators. *News Physiol. Sci.* 2: 231-232.

communication less clear cut, as will be discussed later.

What is endocrinology?

Classically, endocrinology is the subspecialty of medicine that deals with the physiology and pathophysiology of the **endocrine glands**. These are the organs of the body that are specialized for the secretion of hormones.

For example, insulin is a hormone made by the **islets of Langerhans** in the pancreas, an endocrine organ. Insulin is released into the bloodstream in response to an increase in blood glucose. After release from the islets, insulin travels first to the liver (via the portal vein) where it binds to insulin receptors, which tells the liver to stop exporting glucose (because there is enough already in the blood). After leaving the liver, insulin enters the systemic circulation and travels throughout the body triggering the uptake and storage of glucose by muscle and fat cells (which also have insulin receptors). Thus, different cells (e.g., liver, muscle, and fat) can respond to the same hormone (e.g., insulin) because they all have insulin receptors. However, because the insulin receptors in different cell types are hooked up to different signaling pathways, the effect of insulin on liver cells is different from the effect on muscle or fat cells (see Chap. 6).

Receptor-mediated signal transduction is involved in far more than just the classical actions of the traditional endocrine hormones. There are a variety of ways in which cells communicate with one another that have at least some features in common with the classical endocrine system, but are distinctive in other ways.

For example, sometimes cells release hormone-like substances in such tiny amounts that they achieve sufficient concentrations to have effects only on the cells in the immediate neighborhood of the secreting cell. These would-be hormones work just like classical hormones in that they bind receptors and activate signal transduction mechanisms. However, they either are degraded before they can travel long distances or are too low in concentration and thus do not have effects at long distances, even if there are distant cells that have receptors. This kind of locally, but not systemically, effective secretion is termed *paracrine* *secretion*, and such hormone-like substances are termed *local mediators* or *biological response modifiers*. The **eicosanoids**, including **prostaglandins**, are examples of local mediators, as are the **cytokines** and **chemokines**.

Sometimes cells release local mediators for which they themselves have receptors. Thus the secreting cell is able to stimulate itself, a process termed *autocrine* *secretion*. Local mediators include some of the same peptides that serve as neurotransmitters or blood-borne hormones when released in large amounts by specialized cells of the nervous or endocrine systems, respectively. In other cases, completely novel substances serve as local mediators. These can be by-products of enzyme action on membrane lipids, or even gases such as nitric oxide (generated by metabolism of the amino acid arginine). Finally, in some cell types, signaling pathways are triggered by activation of receptors that de-

tect physical forces (e.g., stretch, pressure, photons, and sound waves, see Figure 3.1).

Given the ambiguities discussed, a broader definition of endocrinology would be the study of **receptor-mediated actions** within and between cells, tissues, and organ systems. By this definition, endocrinology is *not* just another medical subspecialty, such as cardiology (study of the heart), nephrology (study of the kidneys), or gastroenterology (study of the GI tract). Rather, endocrinology is the study of cell and organ system integration applicable in principle to all organ systems of the body.

Why is endocrinology important for medical practice?

Defined as the study of the molecular basis for organ system integration, endocrinology is essential for proper care of all patients, not just patients with disorders of the classical endocrine glands. Classical concepts of "the heart as a pump," "the kidney as a filter," and "the brain as a computer," are being replaced with a view that emphasizes the unique variations on the common theme of receptor-mediated signal transduction that make possible each organ's specialized function. Thus, every organ can be understood in terms of its signal transduction pathways in response to special stimuli. To be a good cardiologist, nephrologist, neurologist, urologist, or orthopedist one needs to be able to think in endocrinological terms as they relate to a particular field of specialization. Likewise, to be a good generalist one needs to appreciate the common themes of cellular signaling that interconnect different organ systems.

Modern medicine often involves pharmaceutical interventions directed at one organ system, which have direct and indirect inadvertent consequences (including adverse side effects) on other organ systems. This reflects the delicate interplay between organ systems.

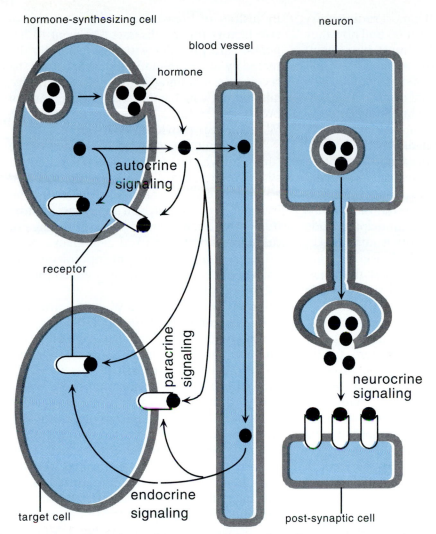

FIGURE 3.1. Different forms of receptor-mediated cell-to-cell communication: endocrine (effects occurring at a distance via the bloodstream to diffuse receptors), neurocrine (effects at a distance to a specific location such as a synapse, as typically occurs via the nervous system), paracrine (local effects on neighboring cells), autocrine (when the same cell that sends the message responds to it). (Adapted, with permission, from Baxter, J.D. (1997). Introduction to endocrinology. In Greenspan, F.S. and Strewler, G.J. Basic and Clinical Endocrinology, 5th ed. Stamford, CT, Appleton & Lange, p. 2.)

We currently have only the most rudimentary understanding of organ systems and how they are integrated, a fact that must be remembered in approaching the treatment of patients. An appreciation of the complexities of receptor-mediated signal transduction (endocrinology) should be a humbling force to counter our exuberance at applying the latest, greatest, just-approved agent to the care of patients. A good "rule of thumb" might be to limit the use of new and specialized drugs and other therapies to those cases where existing therapies are unsuccessful. In this way, the risk to the patient of unanticipated side effects with the newer agents is minimized.

As medicine becomes increasingly complex, and with the advent of new therapies, one will be limited as a clinician unless one is a good practitioner of signaling medicine — an endocrinologist. A walk through any intensive care unit will demonstrate the disaster that unfolds in multiorgan system failure where the best treatment for one problem exacerbates another, in effect, due to the "**cross-talk**" between signaling pathways. Likewise "**spillover**" of hormones onto receptors for which they have lower affinity, is a mechanism by which unintended side effects can occur. Whether these variations occur in any given individual can be affected by genetic differences and the set point of other hormone systems. Ultimately, an appreciation of endocrinology as organ system integration will allow us to better care for these patients. Perhaps in the future it will be possible to prevent disease through diet, lifestyle, and other nonmedical interventions, based on better understanding of their effect on signaling pathways in various organ systems of the body.

Case Presentation

M. W. is a 42-year-old hard-working, stressed teacher and single mother of two, with a fam-ily history of breast cancer and a variety of risk factors for the disease. She went to her health care provider with a breast lump detected by self-examination. In short order she received a mammography, ultrasonography, and biopsy, which confirmed the diagnosis of breast cancer. Initially in a state of shock, Ms. W. asked her provider, "Why me?"

Ms. W. underwent surgical excision of the tumor, at which time evidence was found for systemic spread of the disease. She received an intensive regiment of chemotherapy and was placed on an estrogen antagonist, tamoxifen. Subsequently she developed a range of side effects that mimicked menopause. Nevertheless, in the hope of optimizing her chance of "beating the odds," she continued the therapy.

Four years later, Ms. W. noted arm and back pain, and made an appointment to see her health care provider. The day before the appointment, while shopping at a downtown department store, she fell to the floor in a tonic-clonic seizure. Evaluation in the emergency room of a local hospital revealed a brain mass and other signs of metastatic disease. Further studies revealed that her tumor was no longer responsive to antiestrogen therapy and that she had metastases to bone, accounting for her pain and elevated blood calcium. Ms. W. wondered why her cancer would no longer respond to the therapy that was previously effective. As her HMO will not pay for "experimental" therapies, she was frustrated and angry at the apparent lack of alternatives.

After consultation with her health care provider, Ms. W. opted to receive nothing more than a course of **palliative** radiation therapy for her bone metastases. She became profoundly discouraged. After a short disease-free period, she developed signs of liver failure. She was admitted to the hospital and noted to have liver metastases. A difficult discussion with her family and her health care provider resulted in her being transferred home with care focused on keeping her pain free. Ms. W.'s final question to her health care provider is: "What can my daughter do to avoid this disease?"

Review Questions

1. How are the classical neural and endocrine modes of communication different?
2. How are endocrine, paracrine, and autocrine modes of communication different?

2. CLASSICAL CONCEPTS OF ENDOCRINOLOGY

Hormone structure

It has become clear that just about any product released from a cell can, in principle, be a hormone. All that is required is:

- A way for cells to produce and export the substance.
- **Specificity** of binding of the substance to a receptor.
- A means of delivery of the substance, typically via the bloodstream or, in the case of local mediators, via extracellular fluid. This feature distinguishes the nervous system (where neurotransmitters are delivered via synapses) from the endocrine system (where hormones are delivered via the bloodstream) and from the large group of local mediators (which are delivered via extracellular fluid).

Classical hormones can be categorized structurally into several general types (to be discussed in subsequent chapters):

- Peptides and proteins
- Steroids
- Modified amines and amino acids

In many cases some of the effects ascribed to classical hormones are actually carried out by local mediators whose synthesis and release is triggered by classical hormones.

Nitric oxide gas (NO) has been recognized to be an important signaling molecule, both in its own right and in response to neural and classical endocrine signals. The smooth muscle relaxation induced by acetylcholine released from autonomic nerves in blood vessel walls, for example, is an indirect effect of NO. The acetylcholine triggers endothelial cells to make NO by action of the enzyme NO synthase. NO is also produced as a signaling molecule by many neurons, including those involved in vasodilation of blood vessels that mediate processes as diverse as renal perfusion and penile erection. Independent of its role in smooth muscle tone, NO is also an important intermediate in the pathway of action of glutamate, acting in the CNS as a neurotransmitter.

Our ability to pharmaceutically manipulate enzymes involved in the synthesis and metabolism of local mediators (e.g., with drugs such as aspirin, ibuprofen, and prednisone) has outstripped our understanding of the subtleties of their role in overall homeostasis. The result is that, in addition to many profound benefits, we have created a substantial burden of **iatrogenic disease** (disease caused by the treatment prescribed by the health care provider). This is likely to be a dark side of the overexuberant application of the fruits of the biotechnology revolution that is currently under way. However, the development of more selective drugs can also ameliorate this problem (for example, as seen in the development of drugs that selectively inhibit COX-2, thereby decreasing the risk of the GI side effects of nonsteroidal anti-inflammatory drugs [NSAIDs], see Clinical Pearls). Figure 3.2 summarizes the structures

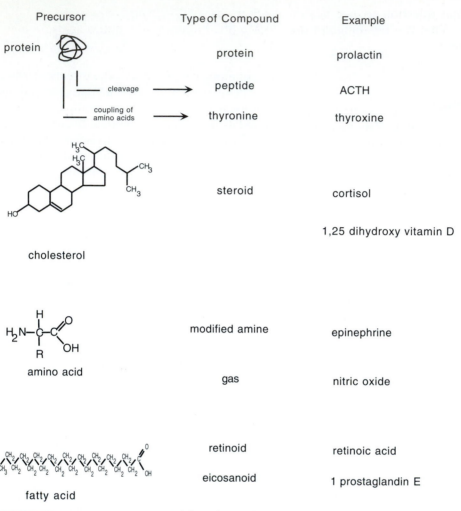

Precursor	Type of Compound	Example
protein	protein	prolactin
cleavage →	peptide	ACTH
coupling of amino acids →	thyronine	thyroxine
cholesterol	steroid	cortisol
		1,25 dihydroxy vitamin D
amino acid	modified amine	epinephrine
	gas	nitric oxide
	retinoid	retinoic acid
fatty acid	eicosanoid	1 prostaglandin E

FIGURE 3.2. Hormone structures. At left is shown the schematic structure of the precursors from which are derived various biochemical classes of hormones (listed in the middle column). The far right column gives a specific example of each class of hormones. (Modified, with permission, from Baxter, J.D. (1997). Introduction to endocrinology. In Greenspan, F.S. and Strewler, G.J. Basic and Clinical Endocrinology, 5th ed. Stamford, CT, Appleton & Lange.)

of various classes of conventional and unconventional hormones.

Receptors and receptor affinity

The classical, best studied, actions of neurotransmitters, hormones, and local mediators are receptor-mediated. The term **ligand** refers to anything that binds a receptor, including neurotransmitters, hormones, local mediators, and even antibodies that mimic or block the actions of any of the previously mentioned.

Once released from the synthesizing cell,

hormones must reach and bind with specific, high-affinity proteins called **receptors**. These may be located on the surface of the target cell, or inside, either in the cytoplasm or within a subcellular compartment (see Chap. 2). If a hormone binds a receptor in a manner that "activates" the receptor, a signal (whose nature will generally depend on the "class" of receptor we are talking about; see later) is transmitted. This signal ultimately alters one or more fundamental cellular processes (e.g., enzyme activities, mRNA transcription, protein synthesis, or intracellular vesicle trafficking) and, thereby, leads to the target tissue's characteristic response to the hormone.

If a cell has no receptors for a hormone, no hormone-mediated actions can occur, because the cell is, in effect, oblivious to the hormone's presence. However, having an appropriate receptor is not sufficient to guarantee all (or even any) of the possible biologic responses to the hormone by a cell. The number of receptors, their intracellular location, and modifications that increase or decrease their sensitivity each affect the consequence of hormone-receptor interaction.

Ligand-receptor interaction can be viewed in two different ways, first in terms of how quickly the ligand goes on and comes off the receptor (reaction rates), and second, at equilibrium. The initial binding of a ligand such as a hormone (H) to a receptor (R) is described by the equation:

$$[H] + [R] \xrightarrow{k_{on}} [HR]$$

where k_{on} is a measure of the rate at which hormone binds to the receptor.

Because hormone-receptor complexes are not held together by covalent interactions (see Chap. 2), a bound hormone will also readily dissociate from the receptor, as described by the equation:

$$[H] + [R] \xleftarrow{k_{off}} [HR]$$

where k_{off} is a measure of the rate at which bound hormone comes off the receptor. In this view, the higher the **affinity** of the hormone for the receptor, the greater the **on rate** compared to the **off rate**.

Alternatively, ligand-receptor interaction can be viewed at **equilibrium**, the steady state reached when the hormone comes off the receptor as often as the hormone goes on, with the distribution of hormone between free and receptor-bound forms reflecting the difference between on and off rates. In this formulation, affinity reflects the distribution of hormone between the free and receptor-bound states, as measured by the **equilibrium constant**, K. Thus, at equilibrium:

$$[H] + [R] \underset{k_{off}}{\overset{k_{on}}{\rightleftarrows}} [HR]$$

and

$$[HR]/[H]\,[R] = k_{on}/k_{off} = K$$

The physical chemical basis for the differences in properties between the nervous, classical endocrine, and local mediator systems can be traced to the differences in affinity of these ligands for the receptors to which they bind, and has two important implications:

1. For binding to low affinity receptors to occur, the ligand must be present at relatively high concentrations. This best described events at a synapse, and thus most neurotransmitters work via low-affinity receptors.
2. Because affinity is low, the rate at which the neurotransmitter comes off its receptor is high, hence the actions triggered can be very transient.

Conversely, for classical hormones, exactly the opposite is true. Affinity for receptors is relatively high. Thus, even low concentrations of hormone reaching a distant site via the bloodstream can be sufficient to occupy enough receptors to trigger an action. But this same property (high affinity binding to its receptor) means that the hormone will dissociate from its receptor relatively slowly and hence will signal actions for a longer time. Indeed, endocrine cells have special mechanisms to terminate long-lived hormone-receptor interactions (see later).

Thus, because the classical endocrine hormones must act at a great distance and at relatively low concentration, they must have high affinity for their receptors. Otherwise, the hormone concentration achieved in the peripheral blood would be too low to bind a sufficient number of receptors to cause an effect.

Clinical Pearl

○ Anatomy plays an important role in determining hormone concentration and, therefore, the spectrum of receptor-mediated actions that occur. Peptides made in the hypothalamus of the brain flow via a special blood supply to the anterior pituitary gland allowing them to have effects not possible had their concentrations been lowered by dilution into the systemic circulation. For the same reason, many of these peptides can serve as local mediators in various peripheral tissues without affecting the pituitary gland.

Review Questions

3. What are the three major structural classes of classical hormones?
4. What is an equilibrium constant, and what does it tell you about hormone receptor interaction?

5. What are the implications of low (versus high) affinity of a hormone for its receptor, with respect to (a) hormone concentrations needed for an effect, and (b) frequency with which the hormone needs to be provided?

Signal transduction: amplification, memory, and contingency

Once a receptor has been activated, there are a number of distinct mechanisms by which it can trigger signaling cascades within the cell. Generally cell surface receptors are coupled to one or more **second messengers**. These are small molecules, often the product of enzymes, that bring about consequences of hormone binding to the inside of the cell (see later). Figure 3.3 indicates some of the classes of second messengers that are used to control signaling, and how they are part of **signal transduction pathways**.

Regulatory proteins (called *G proteins*) that bind the nucleotide guanosine triphosphate (GTP) are used by many different cell types to couple cell surface receptor activation to generation of second messengers. Classical G proteins have three subunits that are inactive when together. When the nucleotide GTP binds to the G protein, it induces dissociation of the α from the β and γ subunits. The GTP-bound free α subunit then binds to and activates an enzyme such as adenylate cyclase that makes cyclic adenosine monophosphate (cAMP, cyclic AMP) from ATP. The cyclic AMP in turn stimulates phosphorylation of other enzymes. The phosphorylated enzymes are activated (or inactivated), which increases (or decreases) the activity of the biochemical pathways in which these enzymes occur, thereby carrying out the effects of the hormone.

The α subunit is available to activate adenylate cyclase only for the brief window of time during which it is not bound to the β and

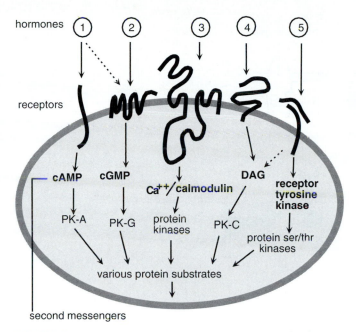

FIGURE 3.3. Some signal transduction pathways involved in hormone action. Indicated are examples of five different hypothetical cell surface receptors for five different hypothetical hormones. Note the wide range of structures of the receptors in the plasma membrane. In some cases, one hormone may have significant affinity for more than one receptor (see dotted line for hormone #1). In these cases, the different receptors may cause different effects and, therefore, which receptor a given cell has will determine the effects of the hormone on that cell. Furthermore, at high hormone concentrations "spillover" onto the lower affinity receptor may cause actions not seen at low hormone concentrations. Each receptor activates one (and often more than one) second messenger for different signaling pathways (see for example dotted line from receptor of hormone #5). These pathways manifest as phosphorylation or other modification of diverse protein substrates, affecting enzymatic activities, protein synthesis, transcription of mRNA, and, potentially, a multitude of other steps in gene expression. Because different tissues have different subsets of genes expressed, a given hormone, acting via a given receptor, can have different effects in different tissues due to differences in downstream mediators. Not shown are G proteins and other mechanisms of regulation of pathways. PK-A = A kinase; PK-C = C kinase; PK-G = cyclic GMP-dependent protein kinase; cAMP = cyclic adenosine monophosphate; cGMP = cyclic guanosine monophosphate; DAG = diacylglycerol. *(Adapted, with permission, from Berne, R.M. and Levy, M.N. Physiology, 4th ed. St. Louis, Mosby, p. 61.)*

γ subunits. This corresponds to the lifespan of the bound GTP-molecule. The "timer" that determines the length of this window of time is a GTP degrading activity within the α subunit that converts the GTP to GDP. Once the GTP is hydrolysed to GDP, the α subunit once again binds to the β and γ subunits, which makes it unavailable to activate adenylate cyclase. Without the G protein α subunit, adenylate cyclase activity shuts off and hormone action is terminated as various phosphodiesterase enzymes inactivate cyclic AMP and dephosphorylate activated enzymes (see Figure 3.4).

Evolution has built tremendous complexity into this system. In addition to its intrinsic **GTPase activity**, GTP binding proteins often recognize so-called **GTPase activating proteins** (GAPs) that increase the intrinsic rate of GTPase activity in the G protein α subunit, thereby shortening the time available for signaling. These negative regulators of signaling

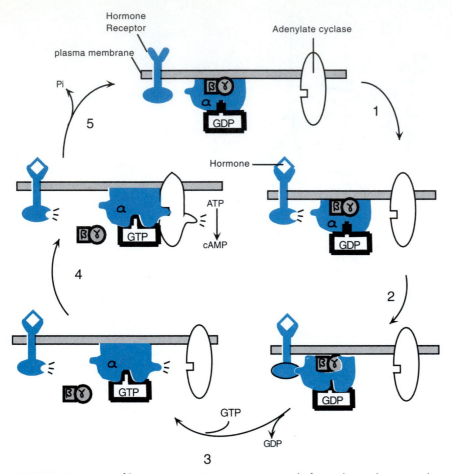

FIGURE 3.4. Function of heterotrimeric G proteins in control of signal transduction pathways. Example of how G α couples receptor activation to adenylyl cyclase activation. In the absence of hormone, receptor is inactive, G protein is in inactive GDP-bound state and adenylate cyclase is inactive (top). Upon hormone binding, receptor is activated (1). Binding of G α subunit to the receptor causes GDP to leave and GTP to bind (2). GTP binding causes dissociation of β and γ subunits, exposing the binding site for adenylate cyclase (3). G α binding activates adenylate cyclase resulting in more cyclic adenosine monophosphate (cAMP) production (4). Cyclic AMP, in turn, activates various protein kinases that are the effectors of particular signal transduction pathways. Hydrolysis of GTP causes G α to dissociate from adenylate cyclase and reassociate with β-γ complex, with GDP remaining bound (5). As long as the extracellular hormone remains bound, the receptor continues to activate more G α. As long as GTP is bound but not hydrolysed, free G α continues to activate adenylate cyclase, which generates the second messenger cyclic AMP. When GTP is hydrolysed and continued activation of adenylate cyclase ceases, the balance is shifted in favor of other enzymes that destroy cyclic AMP, thereby turning off further signaling. Many variations on this scheme have been discovered (see Table 3.2). *(Adapted, with permission, from Alberts, B. et al. (1994). Molecular Biology of the Cell, 3rd ed., New York, Garland, pp. 736 and 739.)*

TABLE 3.2   THE MAJOR FAMILIES OF TRIMERIC G PROTEINS*

Some family members	α Subunits	Functions	Modified by bacterial toxin
Gs	α_s	activates adenylyl cyclase; activates Ca^{2+} channels	cholera activates
Golf	α_{olf}	activates adenylyl cyclase in olfactory sensory neurons	cholera activates
Gi	α_i	inhibits adenylyl cyclase; activates K^+ channels	pertussis inhibits
Go	α_o	activates K^+ channels; inactivates Ca^{2+} channels; activates phospholipase C-β	pertussis inhibits
Gt (transducin)	α_t	activates cyclic GMP phosphodiesterase in vertebrate rod photoreceptors	cholera activates and pertussis inhibits
Gq	α_q	activates phospholipase C-β	no effect

* Families are determined by amino acid sequence relatedness of the α subunits. Only selected examples are shown. About 20 α subunits and at least 4 β subunits and 7 γ subunits have been described in mammals.
Adapted, with permission, from Alberts, B. et al., (1994). *Molecular Biology of the Cell,* 3rd ed. New York, Garland, p. 755.

may themselves be regulated by phosphorylation and probably also by features such as location (bound to membranes versus free in the cytosol).

In some systems, it is the β and γ subunit pair rather than the α subunit which is the active mediator of second messenger formation. In other systems, rather than activating an enzyme, the G protein is inhibitory and turns off an enzyme system. Table 3.2 indicates some of the major families of G proteins.

Thus, hormone action involves diverse pathways of receptors, some of which activate G proteins, which activate an array of second messengers, which affect different **kinases** or **phosphatases** (enzymes that phosphorylate or dephosphorylate various proteins). Some of these protein **substrates** of kinases and phosphatases are transcription factors, and therefore their phosphorylation or dephosphorylation affects which genes are expressed directly. Other protein substrates of kinases and phosphatases affect protein synthesis. Still others are enzymes involved in any of the hundreds of enzymatic steps of metabolism, and, as a result of phosphorylation or dephosphorylation, the enzyme is more or less active. Why did hormone action in eukaryotic cells evolve such complex mechanisms? Three important reasons are:

1. These pathways provide a means of **amplification** of a signal. For example, a single molecule of a hormone bound to a G protein-coupled receptor is able to generate hundreds of G protein molecules which generate thousands of molecules of second messenger (e.g., cyclic adenosine monophosphate) and thereby affect the many copies of responsive enzymes in the cell. Figure 3.5 gives another example of receptor-mediated signal transduction and amplification involving G proteins.

2. These pathways provide cells with a **memory** of signaling events. Once activated, a G protein stays active for a certain period

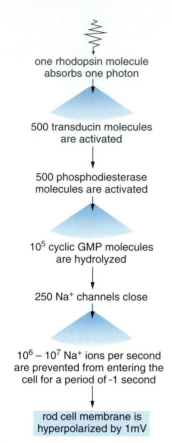

one rhodopsin molecule
absorbs one photon

500 transducin molecules
are activated

500 phosphodiesterase
molecules are activated

10^5 cyclic GMP molecules
are hydrolyzed

250 Na$^+$ channels close

$10^6 - 10^7$ Na$^+$ ions per second
are prevented from entering the
cell for a period of ~1 second

rod cell membrane is
hyperpolarized by 1mV

FIGURE 3.5. An example of amplification of signaling through GTP binding proteins: the light-induced catalytic cascade of phototransduction in vision. *(Adapted, with permission, from Alberts, B. et al. (1994). Molecular Biology of the Cell, 3rd ed., New York, Garland, p. 755.)*

Clinical Pearl

○ The ubiquitous nature of signal transduction is seen in the fact that G protein activation is at the heart of otherwise completely unrelated disease processes. Somatic mutations in the G protein α subunit can render it unable to hydrolyse GTP and, hence, be constitutively and irreversibly "on." In some cells, for example, in the pituitary gland, this activates signaling pathways that control cell growth and proliferation. Thus the pathway of signal transduction involved in growth spirals out of control resulting in a pituitary tumor.

The cholera bacterium uses a toxin to covalently modify the G protein α subunit in epithelial cells of the GI tract. As a result of this modification, the G protein α subunit is permanently "on," until it is degraded and replaced by a new copy of the G protein without the toxin-mediated modification. In the case of GI tract epithelial cells, G protein signaling stimulates ion channels and the resulting flow of ions and water into the GI tract lumen causes profuse diarrhea. Without treatment, the patient may succumb from dehydration before the modified G protein can be eliminated and replaced with a new functional copy.

of time (until the bound GTP is hydrolysed to GDP, perhaps in seconds to minutes), even if the surface receptor, whose activation initiated signaling, becomes inactive (e.g., because of dissociation of the hormone). This is another way of thinking about the amplification of the signaling event in the dimension of time rather than quantity.

3. These pathways allow more complex regulation choices than would be possible without these options or contingencies.

Feedback

The purpose of a system of integration, coordination, and control is generally to maintain **homeostasis** (constancy of the internal environment). Thus, in addition to being able to sense the need to secrete a hormone (i.e., when a particular effect is desired by the body), hormone-secreting cells need to know when to stop.

Thus, hormonal systems are typically governed by **negative feedback** control: One of the effects triggered by a hormone on a target tissue is that, directly or indirectly through its actions, the target cell notifies the hormone-releasing cell that the message was received. When sufficient hormone-mediated action has been triggered in the target cells, the hormone-secreting cell is notified that further hormone release should cease. For example, hyperglycemia is a potent trigger for the release of the hormone insulin. Secreted in response to hyperglycemia, insulin's actions on target tissues lowers blood glucose, which alleviates the initial stimulus (hyperglycemia) for insulin secretion. As a result, further insulin secretion is halted until blood glucose levels rise again.

Negative feedback control on a hormonal system can occur at any of several different levels:

• The substrates whose levels are affected by hormone action can provide feedback to the secreting organ directly; for example, the interrelation of glucose level and insulin secretion just mentioned.

• Direct input from the autonomic or central nervous systems. For example, when there is a major fall in blood pressure, sympathetic stimulation of the renal nerves is one of several events that triggers renin secretion. Renin initiates a hormonal cascade that elevates blood pressure. The return of normal blood pressure turns off the neural stimulus for renin release.

• Feedback inhibition by one hormone affecting the secretion of another hormone. Sometimes hormones are placed "in series." That is, the consequence of secretion of one hormone is to trigger secretion of a second hormone, the consequence of which secretion is release of a third hormone. This is sometimes termed *feed-forward* control. Typically, in those cases, the third hormone has negative feedback effects on secretion of the first and second hormones. For example, growth, reproduction, and stress responses are all controlled by such cascades

of hormones. A signal to the brain can trigger release of the first hormone (from the hypothalamus), which triggers release of a second hormone (from the pituitary), which travels to a target organ to trigger release of a third hormone. This third hormone not only triggers effects in target tissues but also travels back to both the hypothalamus and the pituitary to inhibit further secretion of hormones one and two.

• The signaling pathways activated by a hormone can include upregulation of transcription for the GAP protein that shortens the life of the activated G protein second messenger, thereby diminishing the memory and amplification of the system.

Rarely, hormonal systems display **positive feedback** control. Typically, positive feedback occurs when **maturation** rather than homeostasis is the goal of the signaling pathway. Chapter 16 will describe positive feedback as it occurs in the female reproductive system.

Receptor subtypes and agonists versus antagonists

It is simplest to think of each hormone as having its own specific receptor. However, reality is far more complex. Often multiple, distinct receptor types exist for a given hormone. Sometimes several different hormones may share recognition of a given receptor, but with different relative affinities. When blood levels of one of these hormones rises, that hormone can "spill over" and bind, in addition to its highest affinity receptor, to other receptors besides that for which it has the highest affinity. This causes effects via those lower affinity receptors that would not normally have been activated at normal blood concentration of the hormone (see Figure 3.3). For example, the structurally related catecholamines epinephrine and norepinephrine each recognizes the multiple subtypes of adrenergic receptors (e.g., α_1 and α_2, β_1 and

β_2 receptors, see Chap. 13). However, the affinity of epinephrine is lower for α receptors than it is for β receptors, while that of norepinephrine is higher for α than it is for β receptors.

Analogues of a hormone, which are capable of binding to that hormone's receptor and induce action that mimics the effects of the natural hormone, are termed **agonists**. Analogues that block hormone action, either because they prevent hormone binding or because they bind but do not activate the receptor, are termed **antagonists**.

Clinical Pearl

○ Agonists and antagonists of hormones have proved to be of significant clinical utility. Table 3.3 indicates some of these uses.

Review Questions

6. Describe the levels at which negative feedback can occur in an endocrine system.

7. When is positive feedback of hormones generally observed?

8. What is the difference between an agonist and an antagonist?

Receptor number, tissue effects, and time course of action

Another feature of hormone action is the relation of receptor number to tissue effect. For some hormones, cells have significant numbers of "spare" receptors, meaning that hormone binding of only a small percentage of the total number of receptors displayed on the surface will give the maximum biological response. However, this does not mean that the extra receptors serve no purpose.

These so-called spare receptors render the target cell more sensitive to the hormone.

TABLE 3.3   EXAMPLES OF HORMONE ANTAGONISTS USED IN THERAPY

Antagonist to	Use
Progesterone receptor	Contraception, abortion
Glucocorticoid receptor	Spontaneous Cushing's syndrome
Mineralocorticoid receptor	Primary and secondary mineralocorticoid excess
Androgen receptor	Prostate cancer
Estrogen receptor	Breast cancer
GnRH receptor	Prostate cancer
β-adrenergic receptor	Hypertension, hyperthyroidism

Adapted, with permission, from Greenspan, F.S. and Strewler, G.S. (1997). *Basic and Clinical Endocrinology,* 5th ed. Stamford, CT, Appleton & Lange, p. 22.

Biological effects of the hormone occur in the target tissue at a lower hormone concentration than would have been required for effects if the cell had fewer receptors (see Figure 3.6).

Since any given hormone can have a variety of biological effects, one biological effect may occur upon occupation of a smaller number of receptors than is necessary to achieve a second biological effect. Thus, receptors that need not be occupied for one response, may need to be occupied to trigger another. This reflects the fact that not all responses to a hormone are necessarily elicited at a given hormone concentration or on the same time scale. For example, we mentioned earlier that insulin promotes decreases in blood glucose concentration. It does so by triggering certain tissues to take up glucose, an action that occurs within minutes. At higher concentrations and over several days insulin can trigger growth and proliferation of these same tissues.

These growth-promoting effects of insulin have many possible explanations, including that they are:

• A direct result of growth triggered by occupancy of a large number of insulin re-

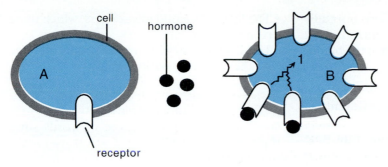

Low hormone concentration

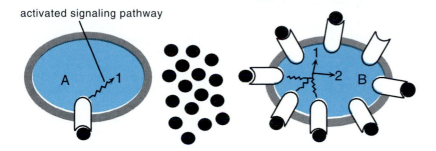

High hormone concentration

FIGURE 3.6. Implications of "spare receptors." Cell A has only a few copies of a particular hormone receptor, while cell B has many copies of that same hormone receptor. At low hormone concentration (top panel), no receptors on cell A may be occupied, where a few receptors are occupied on cell B, activating signaling pathway 1. Thus the "spare" receptors on cell B made it more sensitive to low hormone concentrations. At high hormone concentration (bottom panel), activation of many receptors on cell B may allow additional signaling pathways (e.g., both 1 and 2) to be activated. In cell A with a low concentration of receptors, the threshold of signaling for activation of the second signal transduction pathway may never be achieved. For both of these reasons, increased sensitivity and increased effects, additional receptors are not really "spare." (Adapted, with permission, from Alberts, B. et al. (1994). Molecular Biology of the Cell, 3rd ed., New York, Garland.)

ceptors (the specific scenario envisioned earlier).
• The result of occupying a small number of insulin receptors for a long time (perhaps having more receptors occupied is irrele-vant, it may just take longer for those effects to be manifest).
• Due to "spillover" binding of insulin to other receptors (e.g., the receptors for the insulin-like growth factors), for which insu-

lin has low affinity and therefore normally does not interact at the concentrations at which insulin is normally found in the bloodstream.

Whether some or all of these different explanations are involved in accounting for the different effects of insulin on different time scales is not completely clear. The point is that one can envision each of these variables affecting hormone action on different time scales.

The effects of hormones can be influenced in complicated ways by other hormones. Sometimes, one hormone can have the effect of making the body, or a particular tissue, more sensitive or less sensitive to the actions of another hormone. When one hormone makes another more effective, it is said to potentiate the actions of the second hormone or be permissive for its action. When a hormone makes another hormone less effective, it is said to counter the actions of the second hormone. For example, thyroid hormone induces the transcription and synthesis of catecholamine receptors and consequently is necessary for catecholamines to have their normal effects on heart rate and blood pressure, even though thyroid hormone itself has very different actions from the catecholamine (see Chaps. 10 and 13). Thus, the action of thyroid hormone is termed *permissive* for catecholamine action. Conversely, glucagon, which inactivates many of the enzymes activated by insulin, is termed *counter-regulatory* to insulin (see Chap. 5).

In principle, permissive or counter-regulatory effects of one hormone on the effects of another hormone can occur due to any number of reasons, including effects on the following:

• The number and distribution of various receptors, including the receptors of these hormones themselves

• The level of second messengers, which these receptors activate

• The level of enzymes or substrates affected by the signaling pathways

From a physiological perspective, "permissive" may be a poor choice of words since the potentiating effects are necessary for the optimal function of the other hormone-target tissue system.

Clinical Pearls

○ In certain cancer-related syndromes, massive overproduction of a hormone spills over onto receptors for which it normally has too low an affinity to be clinically significant. With the cancer-induced overproduction, hormone levels can be high enough to activate a significant number of the other receptors and thereby cause inappropriate hormonal effects.

○ Sometimes spillover of one hormone onto the pathway of another is prevented by other means. For example, glucocorticoids have a roughly tenfold lower affinity for mineralocorticoid receptors than they do for their own receptor. Glucocorticoids, however, are present in the bloodstream at 1000 times the concentration of mineralocorticoids. To prevent spillover of glucocorticoids onto mineralocorticoid receptors, cells with mineralocorticoid receptors have an enzyme to inactivate glucocorticoids. Licorice contains an inhibitor of this enzyme, and sometimes patients who consume too much licorice can develop a syndrome of high blood pressure due to glucocorticoid spillover onto mineralocorticoid pathways (see Chaps. 10 and 13).

Review Questions

9. What is the role of receptors in excess of the number needed for maximum response to a given hormone?
10. Explain how a given hormone might have different actions on different time scales?
11. What is meant by permissive actions of a hormone?

Adaptation

Another level of control of target tissue effects is that of **adaptation** or **desensitization**. There are five general mechanisms by which target tissues diminish their degree of response in the face of persistent elevation of a hormone:

1. Receptor down-regulation through sequestration. In some cases, particularly for certain cell-surface receptors (see later in Figure 3.7), the hormone-receptor complex is not degraded but is moved to an intracellular compartment whose conditions (e.g., pH) favor dissociation from the hormone and hence termination of cell signaling. Until this receptor is recycled back to the cell surface, it is not available for hormone binding, regardless of the concentration of hormone present in the bloodstream.
2. Receptor down-regulation through degradation. As a result of hormone-receptor interaction, the occupied receptors can be degraded.
3. Receptor desensitization through phosphorylation. Sometimes the receptor remains at the cell surface and may even stay bound to a hormone, but modification of the receptor protein by a specific protein kinase renders it ineffective at signaling. Alternatively, receptor affinity for the hormone might decrease.
4. Receptor desensitization through G protein inactivation. Even though a receptor may be activated, if the G protein that mediates its action cannot be fully activated, signaling and hence action of this hormone will be blunted. Enzymes exist in cells to phosphorylate G proteins and thereby partially or completely inactivate them in this manner. This may serve as a sort of "safety valve" to prevent the cell from getting too "exhausted" when hormone levels in the bloodstream are very high.
5. Regulation of timing of GTPase activity. Another way to decrease the activity of G proteins is to shorten the time that it takes for them to hydrolyse GTP, which is the window during which they are active. A large family of **GTPase activating proteins** called *GAPs* serve that function and are themselves regulated by phosphorylation events.

Review Questions

12. What are some mechanisms of adaptation by which the response of a cell to a hormone can be changed?
13. What are five mechanisms by which the sensitivity of a target cell to a hormone can be diminished without a change in hormone concentration?

3. SIGNALING PATHWAYS IN HORMONE ACTION

There are three broad classes of mechanisms of hormone action:

1. Proteins, peptides, and modified amines bind to cell-surface receptors triggering the production of second messengers that have many effects altering transcription, translation, and posttranslational events such as protein modifications, sorting, degradation, and so on.
2. Steroid and thyroid hormones can form

complexes with receptor proteins inside the cell that directly regulate transcription. Thus, steroid hormone receptors can be thought of as ligand-dependent transcription factors, where the steroid hormone serves as the ligand needed to activate them, much as a key fits into a lock to open a door (see later in Figure 3.9).

3. Nitric oxide (NO) and other molecules can directly modify enzymes that produce second messengers.

The physical properties of different classes of hormones are also reflected in the fundamental features of their cognate receptors and their mechanisms of action. Because of their smaller size and greater hydrophobicity, steroids and thyroid hormone diffuse into cells directly and bind intracellular receptor proteins in the cytosol or nucleus. In contrast, proteins, peptides, and some amine-related hormones cannot enter cells by diffusion. Instead, they must bind to cell-surface receptor proteins through which they indirectly trigger intracellular signals within the target cells.

Cell surface receptor-mediated hormone action

After a polypeptide hormone binds to its cell-surface receptor, the receptor is activated. This may involve a conformational change (change of shape) in the receptor protein itself. In some cases, upon hormone binding, two copies of receptors bind to each other, forming a protein dimer in the plane of the plasma membrane. The activated receptor is now able to carry out signaling. Unlike the activated steroid hormone-receptor complex, activated cell-surface receptors do not themselves leave the membrane. Instead, they work through second messengers. They are, however, typically endocytosed to an internal compartment from which signaling is eventually terminated (see Figure 3.7).

Many subtypes of cell-surface receptor-mediated signaling have been discovered.

• Some surface receptors are (or are linked directly to) gated ion channels. The effect of receptor activation is therefore to open a specific ion channel, which results in a change in intracellular conditions.
• Other surface receptors have protein kinase domains that phosphorylate protein substrates inside the cell, which in turn change intracellular enzyme action and ultimately gene transcription.
• Still other surface receptors are linked to G proteins. A whole array of distinct G protein subtypes serve as adaptors to couple numerous hormone receptors to particular effector systems within cells. Some of the most important G proteins are those whose action results in changes in the level of various small molecules, which serve as second messengers of hormone action (see Figure 3.8).

Steroid hormone action

After diffusing across the plasma membrane, steroids bind to receptor proteins in the cytosol or nucleus. An activated hormone-receptor complex is thus formed. In this state, the hormone-receptor complex is able to bind DNA and induce or repress the transcription of certain genes (primary response). Some of the products of the primary response may then lead to an induction or repression of the transcription of other genes (secondary response). Cell types that respond differently to a given steroid often have the same intracellular receptor for that particular steroid. The basis for the different responses by different cell types in these cases is that the cells express different combinations of other gene-regulating proteins (e.g., transcription factors) that are capable of modifying in different ways the pattern of gene expression in response to a common activated steroid hormone-receptor complex (see Figure 3.9).

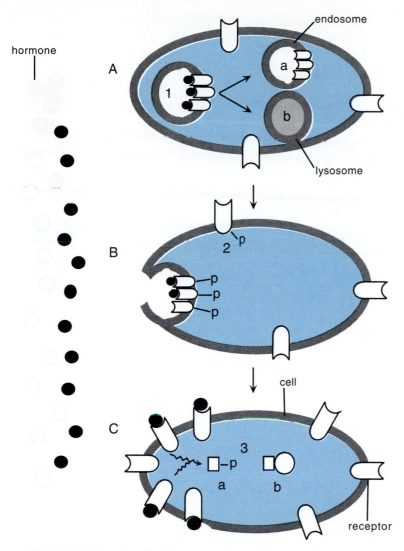

FIGURE 3.7. Mechanisms of adaptation and desensitization in hormone action. Signaling by a hormone can be decreased by a number of different mechanisms. In *A*, the receptor is (a) sequestered or (b) degraded. In *B*, the receptor is phosphorylated or otherwise modified so that it does not transduce a signal. Some receptors must dimerize before they can signal and thus signaling can be blocked by preventing dimerization. In *C*, signaling is attenuated by modifying an adaptor such as a GTP-binding protein (small white square). This can occur either through inactivation, such as modifications that maintain it in its inactive GDP bound state (3a), or through the action of GAP proteins (3b), which increase GTP-binding protein GTPase activity, so that GTP is hydrolyzed more quickly, thereby shortening the window of time during which the GTP-binding protein is active. *(Adapted, with permission, from Alberts, B. et al. (1994). Molecular Biology of the Cell, 3rd ed., New York, Garland, p. 772.)*

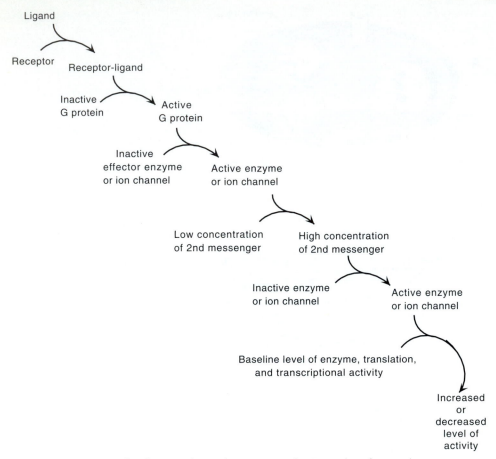

Ligand

Receptor   Receptor-ligand

Inactive   Active
G protein   G protein

Inactive
effector enzyme   Active enzyme
or ion channel   or ion channel

Low concentration   High concentration
of 2nd messenger   of 2nd messenger

Inactive enzyme   Active enzyme
or ion channel   or ion channel

Baseline level of enzyme, translation,
and transcriptional activity

Increased
or
decreased
level of
activity

FIGURE 3.8. An example of a signal transduction cascade. Examples of second messengers whose level increases as a result of signaling include cyclic adenosine monophosphate (cAMP), cyclic GMP (cGMP), inositol triphosphate (IP_3), diacylglycerol (DAG), and calcium ions. Each of these steps are, in principle, subject to many kinds of regulation including modifications that inactivate the protein that carries out that step, changes in the localization of that protein from one part of the cell to another, or bound to a membrane versus free. These differences can affect the rate at which an enzyme finds its substrate. Finally, a particular step might be regulated by other signal transduction cascades that are the domain of other hormones. The cross-talk between hormones can be influenced by hormone concentration, receptor density and dynamics (the time a hormone receptor spends inside the cell versus on the surface; see Figs. 3.6 and 3.7). Typically the final effects of such a cascade include multiple reinforcing effects such as transcription of new mRNA, enhanced translation of certain preexisting mRNAs, and activation of preexisting copies of specific enzymes. (*Adapted, with permission, from Berne, R.M. and Levy, M.N. (1998). Physiology, 4th ed. St. Louis, Mosby, p. 63.*)

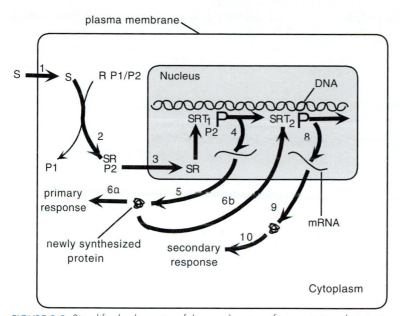

FIGURE 3.9. Simplified schematic of the mechanism of transcriptional activation in reponse to a steroid hormone. Steroid (S) enters the cell by diffusion across the plasma membrane (1). Once in the cytoplasm, S binds the receptor (R) displacing some of the proteins (P1 but not P2) to which the receptor is bound (2). For some steroids binding to receptor occurs first in the nucleus (not shown), while for others, receptor binding occurs in the cytoplasm, with subsequent transport into the nucleus (3). The steroid-receptor complex, in conjunction with various transcription factors (T_1), activates transcription by binding to specific regions of DNA and allowing RNA polymerase (large P) to transcribe the adjacent gene (4). The transcripts are processed and the resulting mRNA exported to the cytoplasm (5), where they are translated into proteins. The proteins encoded by the first set of genes expressed in response to S are termed the *primary response*. Some of these have various enzymatic or other effects (6a). Other primary response proteins return to the nucleus (6b), and serve, sometimes in conjunction with other transcription factors, to induce transcription of another set of genes (8). Processing, export, and translation of these mRNAs (9) results in secondary response proteins (10). Some secondary response proteins may return to the nucleus to serve as negative feedback regulators that shut off the primary response genes to maintain homeostasis. In reality the mechanism of steroid-induced gene expression is far more complex, with regulation at many levels. Possible levels of regulation include (a) which proteins bind the steroid, (b) whether those proteins are active or inactive, (c) if active, whether they inhibit binding of other proteins, (d) whether the proteins bound facilitate or impair transport to the nucleus, and (e) whether the complex binds to all possible regions of DNA with potential binding sites for the steroid-receptor complex, or just to a subset. This decision is, in turn, dependent upon which other proteins (not shown) are bound to the active steroid-receptor complex, modifying its transcriptional activation properties. (Modified, with permission, from Griffin, J.E. and Ojeda, S.R. (1996). Textbook of Endocrine Physiology, 3rd ed. New York, Oxford, p. 52.)

Mechanism of action of nitric oxide

NO is produced by an enzyme, NO synthase (NOS) by deamidation of the amino acid arginine, which is thereby converted to citrulline. NOS comes in three forms. Two of these, nNOS and eNOS, so named because they were first discovered in neurons and endothelial cells, respectively, are **constitutive**, and new protein synthesis is not needed for their activation. However both of these constitutive forms of NOS are exquisitely calcium sensitive and are probably highly regulated by calcium-mediated pathways. Thus, G protein coupled receptors activate **phospholipase C** with subsequent generation of the lipid **phosphatidyl inositol**, which is released from the membrane. One of the effects of phosphatidyl inositol is elevation of cytosolic calcium. Among its many effects on intracellular signaling, calcium ions trigger increased activity of nNOS and eNOS pathways. The third form, iNOS, is induced primarily in response to cytokines. One way NO works is by binding to the iron in the active site of guanylyl cyclase, stimulating the production

of cGMP, a second messenger (see later). Both NO and cGMP have a short half-life, which is a crucial characteristic that allows them to fulfill their regulatory functions.

Second messengers in signal transduction

Both hormones that bind to cell surface receptors and local mediators such as NO can work through second messengers. Here we discuss several examples of second messengers.

Cyclic adenosine monophosphate as a second messenger

Cyclic adenosine monophosphate (cyclic AMP; see Figure 3.10 and Table 3.4) was one of the first second messengers discovered. Its level is controlled by the enzyme that synthesizes it, adenylate cyclase, and the enzyme that degrades it, cyclic AMP phosphodiesterase. Adenylate cyclase activity is increased by different stimulatory G proteins or decreased

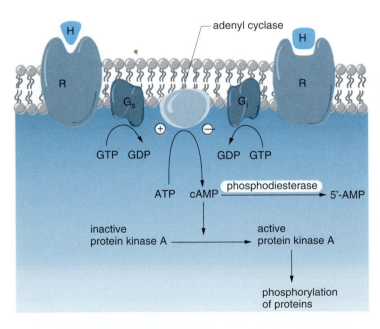

FIGURE 3.10. The adenylate cyclase signaling system. Hormone (H) binds receptor (R), which interacts with either stimulatory (G_s) or inhibitory (G_i) G proteins. Association with G_s activates adenylyl cyclase, which increases cyclic AMP production and hence activates protein kinase A. Association with G_i decreases cyclic AMP production. GTP = guanosine triphosphate; GDP = guanosine diphosphate; ATP = adenosine triphosphate; cAMP = cyclic adenosine monophosphate; 5'-AMP = adenosine monophosphate. *(Modified, with permission, from Porterfield, S. (1997). Introduction to the endocrine system. In Endocrine Physiology. St. Louis, Mosby, p. 8.)*

TABLE 3.4   SOME HORMONE RESPONSES MEDIATED BY CYCLIC ADENOSINE MONOPHOSPHATE

Target tissue	Hormone	Major response
Thyroid	Thyroid-stimulating hormone (TSH)	Thyroid hormone synthesis
Adrenal cortex	Adrenocorticotropic hormone (ACTH)	Cortisol secretion
Ovary	Luteinizing hormone (LH)	Progesterone secretion
Muscle, liver	Epinephrine	Glycogen breakdown
Bone	Parathyroid hormone	Bone resorption
Heart	Epinephrine	Increase in heart rate and contractility
Kidney	Vasopressin (ADH)	Water resorption
Fat	Epinephrine, ACTH, glucagon, TSH	Triglyceride breakdown

Modified, with permission, from Porterfield, S. (1997). *Endocrine Physiology*. St. Louis, Mosby, p. 15.

by different inhibitory G proteins. These G proteins respond to activation of cell surface hormone receptors. Cyclic AMP works as a second messenger by **allosterically** activating a number of cyclic AMP-dependent protein kinases (so-called **A kinases**), which participate in a cascade of protein phosphorylation. As a result of such protein phosphorylation events, both specific enzyme activities as well as the transcription of specific genes are altered. Thus, a common second messenger such as cyclic AMP may affect different processes in different cell types. This occurs because each cell type has its own characteristic set of responding proteins whose actions are affected by A kinase-mediated phosphorylation in response to changes in levels of cyclic AMP.

Calcium and phosphatidyl-inositol derivatives as second messengers

Another important second messenger of hormone action is intracellular free calcium ion. Changes in calcium ion (Ca^{2+}) concentration appear to be generated by a distinct G protein-linked signaling pathway, termed the *phosphatidyl-inositol pathway* (see Figure 3.11 and Table 3.5). In this pathway, G protein activation by cell surface receptors results in an alteration of the activity of an enzyme that cleaves a specific phospholipid termed *phosphatidyl-inositol bisphosphate* (PIP_2, which is found as a minor constituent of the plasma membrane). When this lipid is cleaved, it generates two products that have profound effects on cell signaling: **inositol 1,4,5 triphosphate** (IP_3, also sometimes called *ITP*) and **diacylglycerol** (DAG).

IP_3 mediates the release of calcium from a specialized intracellular compartment. The increase in cytoplasmic free calcium activates a protein called *calmodulin*. Unlike A kinase, which is activated by cyclic AMP, calmodulin is not itself an enzyme. Rather, calmodulin is a regulatory protein that binds to, and alters the activity of, various enzymes. It does this only in response to the presence of high-cytoplasmic free calcium ion concentration. These calmodulin-sensitive enzymes include (but are not limited to) another set of specific protein kinases. IP_3 itself is also a substrate for conversion to other second messengers.

DAG, the other cleavage product besides IP_3 generated from PIP_2 in response to sur-

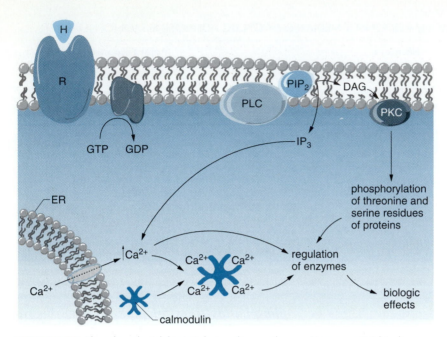

FIGURE 3.11. The phosphatidyl-inositol signaling pathway. Hormone (H) binding to the receptor (R) activates phospholipase C (PLC) via Gi or other similar G proteins. This results in phosphatidyl-inositol biphosphate (PIP$_2$) hydrolysis to produce inositol 1,4,5 triphosphate (IP$_3$) and diacylglycerol (DAG). IP$_3$ releases calcium from the endoplasmic reticulum. DAG activates C kinase (PKC). *(Modified, with permission, from Porterfield, S. (1997). Endocrine Physiology. St. Louis, Mosby, p. 9.)*

TABLE 3.5   SOME HORMONE RESPONSES MEDIATED BY PHOSPHATIDYL INOSITOL

Target tissue	Signaling molecule	Major response
Liver	Vasopressin (ADH)	Glycogen breakdown
Pancreas	Acetylcholine	Amylase secretion
Smooth muscle	Acetylcholine	Contraction
Pancreatic β cell	Acetylcholine	Insulin secretion
Mast cell	Antigen	Histamine secretion
Blood platelets	Thrombin	Serotonin and PDGF secretion

Modified, with permission, from Porterfield, S. (1997). *Endocrine Physiology*. St. Louis, Mosby.

face receptor activation, is itself a second messenger. DAG activates another kinase known as **C kinase** (also called *protein kinase C*). Like A kinase, C kinase activation results in a cascade of phosphorylation that affects enzyme activities and, ultimately, gene transcription in a cell-type-specific fashion. DAG is probably also a second messenger whose generation activates other signaling pathways.

Protein kinases and phosphatases

Different hormone receptors often utilize distinct pathways of signaling. An important class of signaling pathways are mediated by direct phosphorylation of a tyrosine residue on the receptor itself. Such tyrosine kinase activity can, in turn, trigger various other protein kinases or activate other pathways of signal transduction. The "ripple effects" from these cascades of signaling pathways ultimately generate the characteristic effects on a cell that we associate with a particular hormone. Although these various pathways of protein kinase activation (e.g., cyclic AMP and Ca^{2+}-mediated) are distinct, they are not entirely independent of one another. Some of the substrate proteins that are phosphorylated by one protein kinase may also serve as direct substrates for other protein kinases or act as important regulators within other pathways. In this "combinatorial" manner, different hormones can either reinforce or counteract one another's effects in very complex ways.

Review Questions

14. What are some differences between the mechanisms of steroid and polypeptide hormone action?
15. What is calmodulin, and how does it work?
16. Name three second messenger systems.

4. HORMONE BIOGENESIS

Polypeptide hormones

Polypeptide hormones are, generally, secretory proteins, made on membrane bound ribosomes of the rough endoplasmic reticulum (ER). The **secretory pathway** refers to the complex movement of newly synthesized secretory and membrane proteins from their site of synthesis to their final destination. In the case of secretory proteins such as hormones, the ultimate destination is typically outside of the cell. In the case of membrane proteins such as receptors for polypeptide hormones the destination is typically the plasma membrane. Other classes of proteins, such as lysosomal enzymes, follow this pathway part of the way, before being diverted to another destination, such as the lysosome (see Figure 2.17).

Steroid hormones

Unlike the polypeptide hormones, the steroids are not presynthesized and stored for secretion on demand. Rather, they are made as they are needed and are generally believed to diffuse out of the cell (see Figure 3.12).

The precursor of all steroid synthesis is the lipid **cholesterol**, a vital constituent of cellular membranes. Steroid synthesis involves a complex shuttle from mitochondria, where the first step, carried out by **side chain cleavage enzyme** occurs. Subsequent steps vary from tissue to tissue and are carried out by a series of enzymes distributed between the mitochondria and the ER.

Amines

Catecholamines are derived from modified amino acids. Like proteins, catecholamines are stored in secretory granules and released upon demand. Unlike proteins, they are not made via the ER, but rather are directly taken up into the granular containers from the cytoplasm.

Prostaglandins

Arachidonic acid is a 20-carbon polyunsaturated fatty acid that is a component of membrane phospholipids, and which gives rise to several classes of local mediators, including the **leukotrienes**, **prostaglandins**, **prostacyclins**, and **thromboxanes** (see Figure 3.13). Specific phospholipases (e.g., phospholipase A_2) release arachidonic acid from membrane phospholipids, which constitutes the rate-

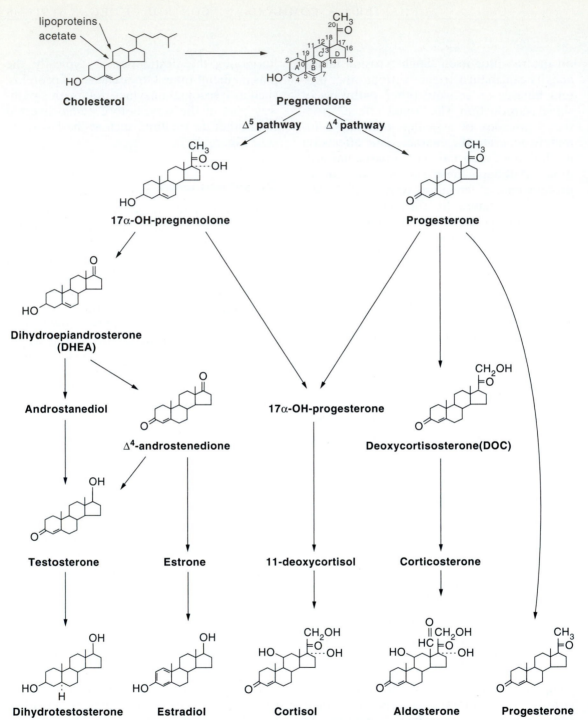

FIGURE 3.12. Pathways of synthesis of the major classes of steroid hormones. Cholesterol, the precursor for steroid synthesis, can either by synthesized by the cell from acetate (see pathway in Figure 2.5b), or is derived from breakdown of lipoprotein particles taken up from the bloodstream (see Chap. 4). The numbering of the steroid molecule is shown for pregnenolone. The major pathways thought to be used are shown. (Adapted, with permission, from Mellon, S. and Lingappa, V. Hormone synthesis and release, in Greenspan, F.S. and Strewler, G.S. (1997). Basic and Clinical Endocrinology, 5th ed. Stamford, CT, Appleton & Lange, p. 50.)

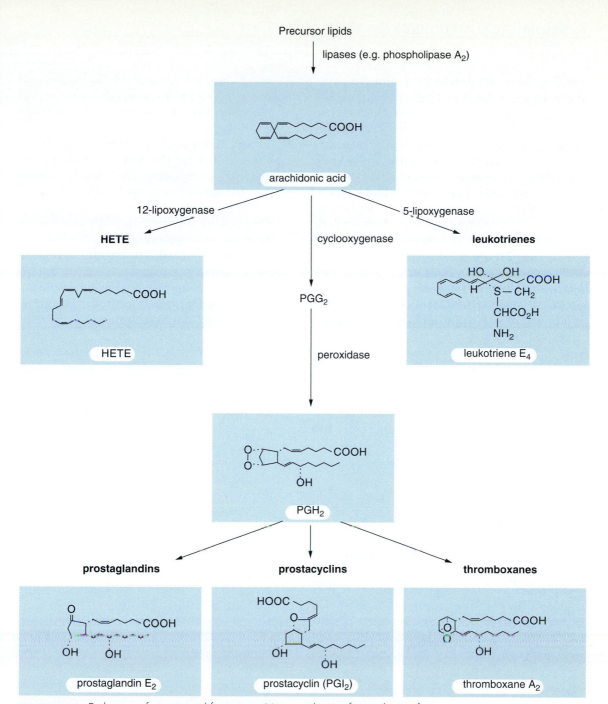

FIGURE 3.13. Pathways of eicosanoid formation. Major pathways for synthesis of the major classes of eicosanoids: prostaglandins, prostacyclins, thromboxanes, and leukotrienes. All steps in the pathways are not shown. Below each pathway enclosed by boxes is a representative compound of the class. HETE = hydroxyeicosantetraenoic acid; PGG_2 = prostaglandin G_2; PGH_2 = prostaglandin H_2.

limiting (slowest) step in the pathway of synthesis of these local mediators.

The free arachidonic acid is subject to two general pathways. The first is the **cyclooxygenase pathway**, which results in prostaglandins, prostacyclins, and thromboxanes. Cyclooxygenase is an enzyme that converts arachidonic acid into prostaglandin H, an unstable intermediate that gives rise to thromboxanes, prostaglandins and prostacyclins through the action of specific synthetic enzymes (see Figure 3.13).

The second pathway of arachidonate metabolism is the **lipoxygenase pathway**, whose products include the leukotrienes. These products are important immune modulators.

Nitric oxide

NO synthase is a calcium and calmodulin-dependent enzyme that generates NO while converting the amino acid arginine into citrulline. NO is rapidly oxidized and therefore has a lifetime lasting seconds.

Clinical Pearls

○ There are two forms of cyclooxygenase. Cyclooxygenase 1 (COX-1) is present in all cells and is the target of aspirin and other NSAIDs. Aspirin acetylates COX enzymes and thereby permanently inactivates them, while most other NSAIDs such as ibuprofen inhibit the enzyme but do not permanently inactivate it. COX-2 is another form of this enzyme that is believed to be responsible for the development of certain cancers and is selectively expressed in certain tissues. Consistent with this notion, some epidemiological studies suggest that aspirin, which inactivates both COX-1 and COX-2, can prevent colon cancer. New COX-2 selective inhibitors (e.g., Celebrex) may have the potential to provide cancer prevention and pain relief comparable to aspirin and other NSAIDs without the risk of GI bleeding that is due to inhibition of COX-1.

○ The cardioprotective value of aspirin includes blocking the formation of thromboxanes, compounds that are important for formation of platelet thrombi and which may contribute to occlusion of coronary arteries in patients with atherosclerotic coronary artery disease.

○ The chemical nature of hormones reflects their pathways of synthesis and secretion and indicates the steps at which clinically relevant defects may occur. For example, the different steroid hormones are synthesized from a common precursor (cholesterol) by various interconnected enzymatic pathways. A genetic defect, which cripples an enzyme in one pathway, results in a backup of precursors that flow down unaffected pathways. As a result, the affected individual will not only suffer the consequences of deficiency of the hormone whose synthesis could not be completed, but also may display pathologic effects from excessive secretion of the alternate steroid products. An example is adrenogenital syndrome in patients with 21 hydroxylase deficiency who cannot produce cortisol. Lack of negative feedback results in excessive stimulation of the adrenal gland. Since it is defective in the enzyme for cortisol synthesis, the precursors spill into the pathway leading to androgens, resulting in virilization and precocious puberty (see Chap. 13).

In contrast, peptide hormones are often synthesized initially as large polypeptide precursors that are proteolytically converted to the mature hormone. In general, polypeptide hormones are stored in **secretory granules** from which they may be secreted on demand. Defects in the ability of cells to sense and respond appropriately to signals that would normally result in secretion of stored hormone may be involved in subsets of patients with the most common form of diabetes mellitus (non-insulin-dependent diabetes mellitus). Others may have processing errors that occur during the cleavage of precursor forms of the protein hormone insulin. The resulting products do not fit the insulin receptor correctly, thereby contributing to insulin resistance (see Chap. 6).

Review Questions

17. Describe the major steps in the secretory pathway for polypeptide hormones.
18. From what chemical substance are steroid hormones derived?

5. HORMONE TRANSPORT, METABOLISM, AND CLEARANCE

Some hormones travel entirely unbound in the bloodstream (e.g., many, but not all, peptide hormones). Other hormones travel bound to carrier proteins, either tightly or weakly, in equilibrium with the unbound fraction.

It is useful to think of protein binding as a way for the body to achieve the following:

1. Alter the amount of hormone seen by the tissues. Carrier protein-bound hormone is not available to bind the receptor until it has dissociated.
2. Alter the clearance rate (removal of a hormone from the circulation, generally by the liver or kidney). Hormones bound to carrier proteins are often poorly filtered by the kidney and therefore circulate in the bloodstream for a longer period of time.
3. Provide a reservoir of circulating hormone, which can be constantly mobilized (by dissociation to equilibrium) to maintain a basal level of free hormone. Carrier proteins are nature's "slow-release patch" to provide a steady supply of hormone over time.

Clinical Pearls

○ Most hormones are inactivated in the liver or kidney. One consequence of diseases of the liver or kidneys is a significant increase in effect of action of the many hormones, by changing the half-life and hence effective concentration.
○ Liver disease can also affect synthesis of many hormone-binding proteins since many of them are made by the liver. Hence, the decreased clearance of various hormones due to liver disease is often exacerbated by a shift in equilibrium in favor of free hormone, due to binding protein deficiency.
○ Some hormones require kidney or liver function for their production or activity and hence their effects are strikingly lacking in patients with severe liver or kidney disease. Erythropoietin, a hormone that stimulates red blood cell production, is made by the kidney and so patients with kidney failure typically also have low red blood cell counts. The precursor to angiotensin II, a blood pressure regulating hormone, is made in the liver. Its deficiency contributes to the low peripheral vascular resistance and blood pressure observed in patients with liver disease (see Chap. 9).

6. MEASUREMENT OF HORMONES

Methods of hormone measurement and their pitfalls

Hormones are measured either directly or indirectly. Consider the following different

A. Starting Materials

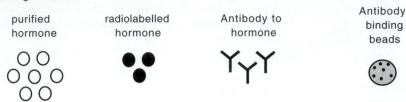

B. Procedure

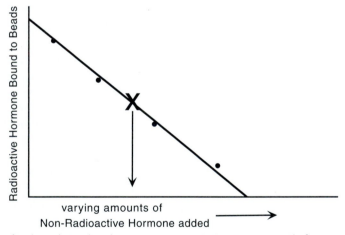

C. Determination of Hormone Concentration in Patient's plasma from standard curve.

FIGURE 3.14. Workings of a hypothetical radioimmunoassay. A. Starting materials for a radioimmunoassay are purified hormone, some of which has been made radioactive, to allow its use as a tracer; antibody to the hormone and antibody-binding beads that allow antibody to be removed easily (e.g., by centrifugation). B. The procedure is to first generate a standard curve that characterizes the hormone-antibody interaction. This is done by mixing various amounts of pure, nonradioactive hormone with constant amounts of radioactive hormone, antibody, and antibody-binding beads. The reaction is allowed to go to completion (an hour should be sufficient), and the beads are removed, taking with them a fraction of the hormone, both radioactive and not. The amount of radioactive hormone bound by the antibody will vary as the amount of nonradioactive hormone is varied. This allows the amount of pure hormone a given amount of the antibody binds to be determined, as monitored by the amount of radioactive hormone bound (which is easily measured by removing the beads and putting them in a radioactivity-measuring

ways of determining how much hormone is in a given blood sample:

- The sample could be subjected to a separation system such as a **high-pressure liquid chromatography** (HPLC) column. "Peaks" corresponding to the hormone can be identified in the material coming off the column, which can be directly identified and quantified by **mass spectrometry**.
- An antibody that recognizes the hormone could be used to quantify the total "immunoreactive" material in the sample by **radioimmunoassay** (see Figure 3.14).
- The amount of biological activity of the hormone can be measured by applying the sample to living cells (e.g., in culture or injected into mice) and then quantifying an effect (e.g., amount of DNA, RNA, or protein synthesis in response).

Each of these approaches has different drawbacks:

- The HPLC/mass spectrometry approach is typically expensive, because the machines to carry out this analysis are expensive and their cost usually has to be amortized by charging for each sample so analyzed.
- The radioimmunoassay is indirect and does not distinguish between multiple forms of the hormone that may or may not be active. Conversely, forms of the hormone may exist that do have biological activity but are not measured by the radioimmunoassay because they are not recognized by the particular antibody available. These assays also generally measure total hormone rather than just the active fraction not bound to proteins.
- Biological assays are extremely slow, extremely expensive, and often not easily reproducible from one testing site to another.

Clinical utility requires the best compromise between these various advantages and drawbacks. In practice, the most common tests are the indirect assessment of hormone levels by radioimmunoassay: determining the ability of the unknown sample (e.g., of serum) to compete with a radioactive sample of purified hormone of known concentration, for binding to an antibody. These tests are rapid, quantitative, inexpensive, and relatively reproducible from day to day and laboratory to laboratory (given the same antibody). For these reasons, radioimmunoassays are commonly used in clinical practice. You should understand how they are done and their limitations.

Radioimmunoassay

To carry out a radioimmunoassay to determine the amount of a given hormone in a sample (e.g., of blood or urine) you need the following (see Figure 3.14):

- A sample of purified radioactive hormone
- A sample of purified nonradioactive hormone
- An antibody that recognizes the hormone
- A way of separating antibody from everything else without disrupting antibody-

---

FIGURE 3.14 — *(continued)* machine called a *scintillation counter*). C. Once a standard curve has been generated, it is a simple matter to mix the unknown sample (e.g., the patient's blood plasma or serum) with the same amount of antibody and radioactive hormone used to generate the standard curve, determine how much radioactive hormone it displaced from the antibody, and plot that amount on the standard curve. A crucial requirement is that the hormone-binding capacity of the antibody not exceed the amount of hormone present in generating the standard curve. Advantages and pitfalls of radioimmunoassays are indicated in Table 3.6.

TABLE 3.6 ADVANTAGES AND PITFALLS OF RADIOIMMUNOASSAY

Advantages (compared to alternatives)	Pitfalls (if results are not interpreted cautiously)
Fast (hours)	Interfering substances (e.g., autoantibodies)
Reproducible	Aberrant hormone processing alters or abolishes antibody recognition
Quantitative	
Inexpensive	Degradation of hormone during sample collection and assay procedure
Adaptable to large-scale use	
Comparison between institutions using the same reagents possible	Cross-reaction of antibody with other substances that are not active hormone
Uses standard laboratory equipment; no large investment in new technology required	Failure of antibody to distinguish molecular forms of hormone with different activity (e.g., glycosylation differences)
Adaptable in concept to a huge variety of clinically relevant questions	Human error (such as mislabeling which sample came from which patient)
	Insufficient sensitivity to detect clinically significant differences
	Inaccessibility of receptor (the problem is not with the hormone)
	Altered signal transduction mechanisms (the problem is not with the hormone)

hormone binding (e.g., beads containing a protein that binds to antibodies are often used; see Figure 3.14)

First, a "standard curve" is generated. This indicates how much of the known radioactive hormone the antibody will bind in the presence of different amounts of purified unlabeled hormone of defined concentration.

Then, the ability of the mystery sample (whose hormone content you wish to know) to compete with the radioactive hormone for binding to the antibody is determined. By plotting how much radioactive hormone binds to antibody in the presence of the mystery sample and by comparing that value with the standard curve, an approximate hormone concentration in the mystery sample can be determined.

Always remember that when you order a laboratory test in clinical practice, you are usually getting this sort of indirect measure. When the test result does not fit your clinical judgment about what is going on with a patient, always consider the possibility that the test result may be in error. Table 3.6 summarizes some of the potential advantages and disadvantages of radioimmunoassays.

Review Questions

19. What are some roles of hormone binding to proteins in the bloodstream in hormone physiology?
20. Why is it important to know what kind of assay is used when you request determination of a hormone level in a patient's bloodstream?
21. How is a radioimmunoassay done?
22. What are some advantages and shortcomings of radioimmunoassays?

7. CLINICAL ENDOCRINOLOGY

In contrast to the broad definition of endocrinology described at the outset of this chapter, clinical endocrinology is typically defined more narrowly. Clinical endocrinologists are

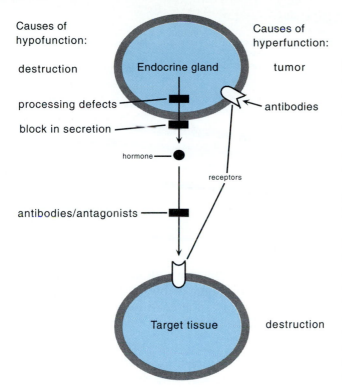

Causes of hypofunction:

Causes of hyperfunction:

destruction — Endocrine gland — tumor

processing defects — antibodies

block in secretion

hormone

receptors

antibodies/antagonists

Target tissue — destruction

FIGURE 3.15. Causes of endocrine gland hyper- and hypofunction. Endocrine disorders can be caused by hypofunction, hyperfunction, or disregulation of the endocrine glands. Indicated are some of the common mechanisms by which dysregulation through hyper- or hypofunction occur. Antibodies can either fool the hormone-producing cell into thinking the organism needs more hormone (agonist antibodies), or can block hormone action either at the level of the signal for hormone secretion or the target for hormone action (antagonistic antibodies). Besides generating antibodies, the immune system can target endocrine cells or their targets for destruction through immune attack on receptors or other antigens that characterize these cell types. More subtle forms of dysregulation can involve processing and secretory mechanisms for either hormones or their receptors. Examples include released hormone that is not as active as it should be, or impairment in the sensing of signals that govern the kinetics of hormone storage or release.

subspecialists who are consulted in a narrow spectrum of clinical situations, usually for dysfunction of specific endocrine glands (e.g., thyroid, adrenal, or pituitary).

Any endocrine gland can have simple disorders of excessive function or insufficient function or more complex aberrations in sensing, timing, or response that can look like disorders of hormone excess or insufficiency (see Figure 3.15).

There can be aberrations related to hormone metabolism (i.e., transport and clearance) and dysfunction due to abnormal tissue effects (e.g., change in receptor number, distribution, and sensitivity of action). These will be mentioned in the discussion of each endocrine system (see Chaps. 11-16).

Finally, since endocrine systems exist to integrate the other organ systems, a primary disturbance in any major organ system will have its manifestations in the endocrine system responsible for its control. Table 3.7 summarizes some of the classical disorders of endocrine systems.

8. FRONTIERS IN ENDOCRINOLOGY

Cross-talk between classes of hormones, receptors, and signaling pathways

A hormone can activate a number of different second messenger signal transduction pathways. Some of these pathways may intersect with other ligand-activated receptor pathways, reinforcing them in some cases, canceling each other out in other cases.

There is growing evidence that an even more profound level of cross-talk occurs between pathways of signal transduction. It has been discovered that different steroid hormone receptors can form homo- and hetero-

TABLE 3.7   SOME CLASSICAL ENDOCRINE DISORDERS

Endocrine gland	Disorder of hormone excess	Disorder of hormone lack	Miscellaneous
Pituitary	Prolactin, GH or ACTH secreting adenomas	Panhypopituitarism	
Adrenal	Cushing's disease; Cushing's syndrome; Adrenal adenoma	Addison's disease	Precocious puberty
Thyroid	Hyperthyroidism	Hypothyroidism	
Islets of Langerhans	Insulinoma	Diabetes mellitus	Diabetes mellitus
Parathyroid glands	Hyperparathyroidism	Hypoparathyroidism	

Greenspan, F.S. and Strewler, G.S. (1997). *Basic and Clinical Endocrinology*, 5th ed. Stamford, CT, Appleton & Lange, p. 29.

dimers to give hybrid molecules with unique transcriptional activation characteristics. Furthermore, phosphorylation events induced by ligands, such as peptide hormones, acting via a cell-surface receptor, may be able to alter the activity of these hybrid steroid hormone receptors inside the cell and, possibly, even activate them so that they can turn on transcription in the absence of binding by a ligand!

"Orphan" receptors and the human genome project

The massive outpouring of DNA sequence data in recent years has led to the recognition that there are numerous variants of genes for many classes and families of hormone receptors. It was initially presumed that they differed from the prototypic member of the family in that they bound a different ligand (e.g., insulin-like growth factor 1 versus insulin) or that they activated a different pathway of signal transduction in response to binding the same ligand as did the "classical" receptor. In many cases, however, the reason for the existence of these other family members remains unknown; that is, no other ligands that might bind to these receptors preferentially have yet been identified. Some of these recep-

tors may function without ligands, when activated by other pathways of signal transduction, such as the cross-talk described earlier (see Refs. 5 and 6).

Dioxin receptor: the endocrinology of environmental pollution

Dioxin is a byproduct of polychlorinated biphenyl compounds (PCBs) that were once widely used as insulators. It is now recognized that dioxin and related molecules are extremely toxic and their use has been largely discontinued. Unfortunately, massive amounts of this and related toxins are found in waste dumps around this country and throughout the world. Quite unexpectedly, the study of dioxin biology has yielded a fascinating insight into the endocrine system, and a terrifying realization of the implications of environmental pollutants as endocrine disruptors (see Refs. 7-9).

Dioxin binds to a receptor termed the **aromatic hydrocarbon** (AH) receptor (so named because it can bind other aromatic hydrocarbons besides dioxin). Animal studies suggest that the AH receptor acts like a steroid hormone receptor. When occupied, it travels to the nucleus where it activates transcription of a subset of the genes that would normally be activated by thyroid hormone, androgens, estrogens, and some growth factors. Thus, the presence of such compounds in the environment can serve to scramble homeostatic mechanisms in many ways, with different effects occurring in different individuals depending on the levels of hormones, transcription factors, and patterns of gene expression going on in that person at that time. The endogenous ligand, if any, for the AH receptor remains unknown.

Protease-activated receptors: more variations on receptor-ligand interaction

We have seen how many different classes of compounds can serve as hormones and how a hormone can activate many different forms of receptors that can, in turn, activate many different signaling pathways. While the combinatorial possibilities for complexity may be dizzying to us, it apparently is not too much for cells, which have evolved even more complex mechanisms of receptor ligand activation. Consider the thrombin receptors on platelets, whose activation results in the platelet-dependent phase of blood clotting (see Refs. 10-13). These receptors are activated by proteolytic cleavage, which generates a new free amino terminus of the receptor. The new amino terminus acts as what has been termed a *tethered ligand*, it is both part of the receptor as well as what binds to, and activates, the receptor. However, this unusual mechanism has other implications. Since such a receptor is now permanently on (you can not uncleave a protein, the thermodynamics of the reaction make it irreversible, for all practical purposes), how do you turn off its signaling? In addition to mechanisms such as receptor phosphorylation, it appears that alternate pathways of trafficking have evolved by which the thrombin receptor is targeted to the lysosome for degradation rather than being simply recycled to the surface. Mutations and other analysis at the cellular level suggest that there may be a number of points of regulation at which cells can affect various aspects of the functioning of receptor systems. One of the features that can be regulated is the distribution between surface and internalized receptors. Furthermore, there are a number of different thrombin receptors that are activated by different mechanisms that play important roles in development, blood clotting, and, pathologically, atherogenesis. Different individual members of this receptor system appear to have been selected to be the primary thrombin receptor in mouse versus humans.

9. HOW DOES UNDERSTANDING NORMAL PHYSIOLOGY PROVIDE INSIGHT INTO THE INITIAL CASE?

We will reconsider the initial case of M. W., the 42-year-old hardworking, stressed teacher and single mother of two, with a family history of breast cancer and a variety of risk factors for the disease. She went to her health care provider with a breast lump detected by self-examination. In short order she received mammography, ultrasonography, and biopsy, which confirmed the diagnosis of breast cancer. Initially in a state of shock, Ms. W. asked her provider, "Why me?"

Why breast cancer develops in one individual and not another remains unknown. Overall, women in the U.S. have a 1 in 8 lifetime risk of developing breast cancer. Known risk factors include family history and genetics, early onset of periods and late onset of menopause, late or no childbearing and breastfeeding, and exogenous estrogen and radiation exposure. Suspected risk factors include high-fat diets and environmental toxin exposure.

A patient wondering "why me," as most do, whether or not she asks a health care provider about this, usually has a number of related questions: Why now? What caused this? How does it work? How long will it last? Individuals often view an illness as a consequence of something they did or did not do. Exploring these questions with patients and providing physiological explanations at a level of simplicity or sophistication that is appropriate for the individual patient are an important part of clinical medicine. Likewise, exploring fears about the illness and the problems caused by the illness can be highly therapeutic.

Ms. W. had undergone surgical excision of the tumor, at which time evidence was found for systemic spread of the disease. She then received an intensive regiment of chemotherapy and was placed on an estrogen antagonist, tamoxifen. Subsequently, she developed a range of side effects that mimicked menopause, but chose to continue the therapy.

It has been observed that growth of breast cancers that have estrogen and progesterone receptors is inhibited by treatment with estrogen antagonists such as tamoxifen, or elimination of endogenous sources of estrogen by removal of the ovaries, adrenals, and/or pituitary gland. Eventually, however, this treatment selects for tumor cells whose growth is independent of estrogen and is generally not a cure. It is not known why some tumors respond better than do others.

A problem with estrogen antagonist treatment is that it can mimic menopause, causing acute and chronic complications including dizziness, hot flashes, vaginal inflammation (see Chap. 16), and bone loss (see Chap. 14).

Four years later, studies revealed that Ms. W.'s tumor was no longer responsive to antiestrogen therapy and that she had metastases to bone.

Commonly breast cancer metastasizes to the brain, causing seizures and confusion, or to bone, causing pain, fractures, and elevated blood calcium. Our lack of understanding of numerous features of the endocrine system impair our ability to treat this and many other disorders.

There is a fine line between experimental and nonexperimental therapy. A patient who is desperate often turns to experimental therapies. A real problem in modern medicine is that the rise of for-profit health care greatly complicates the issue of what a patient should be offered in the way of "experimental" therapy. The resulting conflict of interest undermines both clinical judgment and the patient's trust.

Ms. W. opted to receive nothing more than a course of palliative radiation therapy for her bone metastases. She later developed liver metastases as well. Ms. W.'s final question to her health care provider was: "What can my daughter do to avoid this disease?"

Approximately 5 to 10% of breast cancers are due to specific mutations in the recently discovered $BRCA_1$ and $BRCA_2$ genes. The risk of breast cancer by age 70 is as high as 60 to 80% in individuals who are carriers of these mutations. It is not currently known whether hormones affect the risk associated with these or other genes. Cancers associated with BRCA genes seldom have estrogen receptors. Since Ms. W.'s tumor did have estrogen receptors, she can be reassured, without genetic testing, that she and her daughter are unlikely to carry these genes and that her daughter's risk is unlikely to differ much from that of the general population. Ms. W.'s daughter can attempt to reduce her own risk through a prudent diet, early childbearing and breast feeding, and avoidance of carcinogens, radiation, and exogenous estrogens. She might also consider early detection through screening mammography and breast exams.

Should prophylactic mastectomy be offered to patients identified as having BRCA genes? Will any insurance company want to cover a patient known to be at high risk of breast cancer? Will determining your genotype result in you or your children not being able to get health insurance because you are a "bad risk"? These are just a few of the difficult questions clinicians and patients face today, and currently there are no satisfying answers.

Breast cancer is a terrifying modern epidemic that has many endocrinological features. Even while new research promises to clarify long-obscure features of this disorder, the complexity of the underlying mechanisms should remind us to have great respect for the meaning of the term *organ system integration*.

SUMMARY AND REVIEW OF KEY CONCEPTS

1. Receptor-mediated signaling systems are specialized for particular purposes. For example, the endocrine system is best used when signaling needs to occur over large distances, to diffuse recipients for long-lived actions. The ligands that are best suited for these characteristics are generally those with high affinity for their receptors, since this allows low concentrations of hormones to work.

2. Feedback is a nearly universal theme in endocrinology. Negative feedback comprises various means of limiting the extent of a hormone's action once it has accomplished its primary purpose. In systems with more than one hormone in series, the final hormone's actions include feedback inhibition of secretion of the earlier hormones. Rarely, usually in the context of a change in gene expression as a consequence of development, hormones participate in positive rather than negative feedback loops.

3. The major classes of hormones are proteins and peptides, steroids, amines and thyronines, eicosanoids, and certain gases such as NO. Classically, receptors are ei-

ther on the cell surface (for protein hormones) or intracellular (for steroids). A given hormone can have more than one receptor, each of which can have different affinities for the hormone and can activate different signaling pathways.

4. A typical signaling pathway involves a hormone whose binding activates a receptor, which then activates a G protein which results in an increased level of a second messenger which activates enzymes which phosphorylate or dephosphorylate other proteins that either serve as transcription factors or regulate protein synthesis or regulate enzyme activities, or all of the above.

5. Cyclic AMP and Phosphatidyl-inositol/calcium are some of the most common signaling pathways that operate in hormone-responsive systems. Different effects of second messengers occur in different cells even when they have the same receptors, due to the differences in transcription factors and enzymes that are present in one cell versus another.

6. Chemical compounds that mimic hormone-receptor interactions are termed *agonists*. Those that block hormone-receptor actions are termed *antagonists*. The number of receptors present on a cell determines the sensitivity of that cell to a particular hormone.

7. There are differences in the time course of receptor-mediated actions. A hormone can have a variety of actions that occur over different time courses depending on variables such as whether the actions are via the highest affinity receptor versus another lower affinity receptor, or due to the primary versus secondary transcriptional response, or due to more or less complex second messenger interactions in the signaling pathways.

8. There are five general mechanisms of adaptation or desensitization by which a cell can diminish the extent of signaling in re-

sponse to a hormone. These are receptor sequestration with or without degradation, receptor phosphorylation, G protein inactivation, and GAP action.

9. Signal transduction pathways allow amplification and memory of hormone action by altering the number of molecules carrying the message and affecting the duration of time for which the message is carried.

10. Hormones are often transported in the blood stream bound to other proteins. The extent to which protein binding occurs is itself often reguated and can affect the half-life, and therefore concentration and actions, of various hormones.

11. Hormones can be measured a number of ways. One of the most common is through radioimmunoassays, where the concentration of hormone (e.g., in a blood sample) is determined indirectly by its ability to displace radioactive pure hormone from binding sites, and correlation of that displacement with a standard curve.

A CASE OF PHYSIOLOGICAL MEDICINE

R. V. is a 48-year-old-man with coronary artery disease and diabetes mellitus. Recently he moved to another state to take a new job at a small software firm. The move was quite stressful, and during the transition his weight went up and his diet switched almost exclusively to junk food, which he had previously avoided. He began to see a new health care provider who did not have time to elicit his diet and lifestyle history. The physician did note, however, that Mr. V.'s blood glucose was too high and that his angina (pain due to insufficient blood flow to the coronary arteries) episodes were more frequent. The new physician chose to increase the dosages of Mr. V.'s medicines.

Unfortunately, Mr. V. was already being treated with fairly high doses of long-acting agents. Soon after the dosages were further increased, the medicines seemed to be having even less effect. Mr. V.'s blood sugar was higher than ever and his angina was even more frequent. After one particularly severe episode of angina, he was admitted to the cardiac care unit as a precautionary measure (he did not have a heart attack, although he did have significant coronary artery disease), and he saw a new clinician.

Taking a careful history and noting the adjustment in dosage of medicines, the new clinician suggested that down-regulation of receptors might have contributed to the lack of response to the diabetes and heart medicines.

On the previous regimens, Mr. V. was taking nitrates (medicines whose effects include increasing blood flow to the coronary arteries) around the clock. On the new regimen, he does not take them at night allowing his body an opportunity to recover from high dose therapy during the day.

On the previous regimens, Mr. V. was taking high doses of a long-acting medicine to stimulate insulin secretion. On the new regimen, he was switched to a shorter-acting drug. The thinking was that both of these maneuvers should allow the relevant cells to up-regulate their receptors during the drug-free period.

Furthermore, the important role of his weight gain in decreasing the sensitivity of his cells to the glucose-lowering effect of insulin was considered, and he was put back on a good weight-loss diet and a gentle exercise program.

Over the following two weeks Mr. V. notes the disappearance of his angina, allowing him to walk pain free. The additional exercise, together with a more careful diet and the diabetes medicine adjustments, results in gradually improved blood glucose control over the next several months.

QUESTIONS

1. Describe how hormones in general work and how signal transduction is likely to be an important part of the patient's medical problems at a molecular level.
2. Explain what is meant by down-regulation and desensitization of receptors, and how too much of a medicine can paradoxically make the medicine lose its effectiveness.
3. What are some mechanisms by which down-regulation and desensitization might be reversed?

ANSWERS

1. Hormones bind to receptors, activating them and thereby triggering changes in protein function and gene expression. Signalling is how cells respond to their environment in both health and disease and in response to therapy that may affect more signalling pathways and more cell types than we might like.
2. Down-regulation and desensitization refer to mechanisms of adaptation by which cells respond less well to particular stimuli. Many drug actions are receptor-mediated. Hence receptor adaptation makes cells less sensitive to the action of that particular drug, especially if taken at high dose over the long term.
3. Physiological manipulation (e.g., exercise to increase insulin sensitivity, see Chap. 6), and decreased dose or increased dosing interval of a drug.

References and suggested readings

1. Alberts, B. et al. (1994). *Molecular Biology of the Cell*, 3rd ed. New York, Garland.
2. Greenspan, F.S., and Strewler, G.S. eds. (1997). *Basic and Clinical Endocrinology*, 5th ed. Stamford, CT, Appleton & Lange.
3. McPhee, S. et al. eds. (1996). *Pathophysiology of Disease*. 3rd ed. Stamford, CT, Appleton & Lange.
4. Funder, J.W. (1987). Receptors, hummingbirds and refrigerators. *News Physiol. Sci.* 2:231-232.
5. Turgeon, J.L. and Waring, D.W. (1992). Functional cross-talk between receptors for peptide and steroid hormones. *Trends Endocrinol. Metab*. 3:360-363.
6. Hammer, G. et al. (1999). Phosphorylation of the nuclear receptor SF-1 modulates co-factor recruitment: integration of hormone signaling in reproduction and stress. *Mol Cell* 3:521-526.
7. Whitlock, J.P. (1994). The aromatic hydrocarbon receptor, dioxin action and endocrine homeostasis. *Trends Endocrinol. Metab*. 5:183-186.
8. Cheek, A.O. et al. (1998). Environmental signaling: a biological context for endocrine disruption. *Environ. Health Perspect*. 106:5-10.
9. Zacharewski, T. (1998). Identification and assessment of endocrine disruptors: limitations of in vivo and in vitro assays. *Environ. Health Perspect*. 106:S2 577-582.
10. Coughlin S.R. (1998). Sol Sherry lecture in thrombosis: how thrombin 'talks' to cells: molecular mechanisms and roles in vivo. *Arteriosclerosis, Thromb., Vasc. Biol*. Apr, 18(4): 514-518.
11. Kahn M.L.; Zheng Y.W.; Huang W. et al. (1998). A dual thrombin receptor system for platelet activation. *Nature* Aug 13, 394(6694): 690-694.
12. Trejo J., and Coughlin S.R. (1999).The cytoplasmic tails of protease-activated receptor-1 and substance P receptor specify sorting to lysosomes versus recycling. *J. Biol. Chem*. Jan 22, 274(4):2216-2224.
13. Shapiro M.J., and Coughlin S.R. (1998). Separate signals for agonist-independent and agonist-triggered trafficking of protease-activated receptor 1. *J. Biol. Chem*. Oct 30, 273(44): 29009-29014.
14. Liri, T. et al. (1998). G protein diseases furnish a model for the turn-on switch. *Nature* 394: 35-38.

LIVER PHYSIOLOGY

4

1. INTRODUCTION TO THE LIVER

Why is the liver medically important?

- The liver is involved in the normal function of just about every organ system in the body. Proteins made by the liver participate directly in an extremely wide range of functions. Many products are either cleared from the bloodstream by the liver, or are bound to a protein made by the liver, and thus metabolism is broadly affected in liver disease.

- Liver disease has diverse manifestations. In some patients liver disease may present primarily with mental confusion (termed *hepatic encephalopathy*); in others it is bleeding (for any of several different reasons) that brings them to medical attention; some may have intractable itching or fat malabsorption; still others may have ascites, edema, or infections as their major symptom. Some patients may have all of these signs and symptoms, while others manifest only one or two. Therefore, you must understand the liver well to recognize what is wrong with your patient and why, among such a kaleidoscope of clinical presentations.

- Liver disease has consequences that affect other aspects of a patient's health care. For example, patients with liver disease are much more sensitive to some drugs. These patients are also at greater risk of certain infections and have a much higher incidence of liver cancer (see Mechanisms of Hepatic Carcinogenesis, in Sec. 12). Thus you have to be particularly careful of drug dosage and vigilant about noticing early warning signs (e.g., of infection or cancer), when treating a patient with liver disease.

- Liver cells are a model system for many different areas of medical research. This includes both the study of basic questions, such as gene expression, apoptosis, protein trafficking, and intracellular signaling, and the development of practical applications for new technology, such as strategies for gene therapy. Insights from liver cells have advanced our understanding of phenomena of diseases of many other organ systems.

- Liver disease is extremely common: It is one of the 10 leading causes of death in the United States today. Consider the following case:

Case Presentation

J. S. is a 46-year-old patient with alcoholic cirrhosis, who stopped drinking alcohol 2 years ago and has just been brought to the outpatient clinic for evaluation of altered mental status. His mother, with whom he has lived for the past month, noted that he stopped taking one of his medications earlier in the week because it gave him diarrhea. Shortly thereafter, she noted that her son was somewhat more absent-minded than usual. Yesterday he succumbed to temptation and had a double cheeseburger for dinner. This morning she found him in bed barely able to wake up, and called the paramedics. After taking a history from the mother and performing a careful physical examination, some blood tests are ordered. The results reveal a clotting abnormality, high glucose, and abnormally high white blood cell count with low hematocrit (red blood cell count). On the physical exam it is noted that he has a significantly increased abdominal girth compared to his last clinic visit 2 weeks ago and that he has 2+ edema in both feet. His lungs, however, are clear, and there is blood in his stool. A distinct, intermittent jerking motion (termed *asterixis*) occurs when he is asked to stick out his tongue or to "hold up traffic" with his hands extended. He knows his name and who the physician is, but has no idea where he is, what time or day it is, or his address. None of these abnormalities of mental status was present at his last clinic visit. His mother is anxious about his condition and wants to know why each of these abnormalities have occurred, what they might mean, and what she can do to prevent them in the future. What are you going to tell her? What can be done for Mr. S. and his mother?

Mr. S. demonstrates a number of acute (new onset) complications of chronic, long-standing liver disease. After evaluating him, you may conclude that he needs to be admitted to the hospital. Suppose (as is often the case) his health maintenance organization (HMO) tries to deny payment for the hospital admission. How will you justify your decision?

A knowledge of normal liver physiology will help you understand what is going on with Mr. S., decide whether he needs to be hospitalized, justify your decision, and anticipate the likely causes and best treatments of his current altered condition, without having to remember an arcane constellation of seemingly unconnected clinical findings.

Review Question

1. Give five general reasons why the liver is medically important.

2. ANATOMY, HISTOLOGY, AND CELL BIOLOGY OF THE NORMAL LIVER

The liver is located in the right upper quadrant of the abdomen, in the **peritoneal space** just below the right diaphragm and under the rib cage (Figure 4.1A). It weighs approximately 1400 g (about 2.5% of total body weight) in the adult and is covered by a fibrous capsule. It receives nearly 25% of the cardiac output, approximately 1500 mL of blood flow per minute, via two sources of blood supply, the **portal vein** and the **hepatic artery**.

- The **portal vein** carries venous blood from the gut, rich in freshly absorbed nutrients, directly to the liver (Figure 4.1B).
- The portal venous blood is also notable for high concentrations of toxins and drugs absorbed from the gastrointestinal (GI) tract.
- Being venous, portal blood is relatively poor in oxygen. Yet, because of the liver's dual blood supply, complete blockage of flow in liver disease is unusual.
- Also, flowing into the portal vein, prior to its entry into the liver, is the pancreatic venous drainage, rich in pancreatic hormones (e.g., insulin, glucagon, and somatostatin, see Chap. 6).
- The portal vein forms a special capillary bed that allows individual hepatocytes to be bathed directly in portal blood.

Clinical Pearl

○ Because of its portal blood supply, the liver is a prime site for the spread of neoplasms from elsewhere in the body, especially from the GI tract, breast, and lung (see Figure 4.1B).

The hepatic artery carries arterial blood and is important for liver oxygenation and for supplying the **biliary system** (see later). The separate portal venous and hepatic arterial blood supplies converge within the liver and exit together via the **central veins** that drain into the **hepatic vein** and, ultimately, the **inferior vena cava**.

Concepts of liver organization: lobule versus acinus

Viewed under the microscope at low power magnification, liver architecture has been traditionally described in terms of the **lobule**

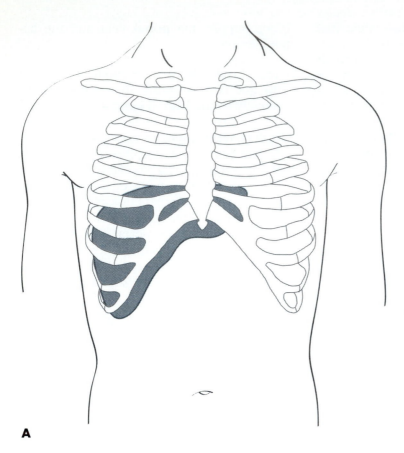

A

FIGURE 4.1. *A.* Location of the liver in the right upper quadrant of the abdomen. *B.* Venous drainage to the liver. Note that venous drainage from the pancreas, stomach, small and large intestine, gallbladder, and spleen flow into the liver via the portal vein. (*A. Modified, with permission, from Wolf, D.C. in Walker et al., eds.,* Clinical Methods, *3rd ed. Butterworths, 1990, p. 478. B. Modified, with permission, from Mackenna, B.R. and Callander, R.* Illustrated Physiology, *5th ed. New York, Churchill Livingstone, 1990, p. 84.)*

(see Figure 4.2A). This view derives from the neat arrays of hepatocytes that are organized in plates around individual central veins. Sinusoids are the endothelial cell-lined spaces in which blood flows past the basolateral surfaces of a plate of hepatocytes. Thus each cell in a plate of hepatocytes is in contact with two sinusoids (which separate one plate of hepatocytes from another).

The bile canaliculi comprise a completely separate system of vessels originating at the hepatocyte apical plasma membrane. In three dimensions, the bile canalicular membrane forms a ring around the individual hepatocyte. This canaliculus leads to vessels that take bile flow in the opposite direction as blood, that is, from the vicinity of the central vein to that of the portal triad, which contains the larger bile vessels leading eventually out of the liver (see Figure 4.2B).

The set of plates that radiate from a given central vein make up a hexagon with **portal triads** (sheathlike structures containing a portal venule, hepatic arteriole, and bile canaliculus) at the corners (Figure 4.2A).

However, it is more physiologically revealing to think of liver architecture in terms of the portal-to-central direction of blood flow. Blood entering the sinusoids from a terminal portal venule or hepatic arteriole first flows past hepatocytes closest to those vessels (termed *zone 1 hepatocytes*). The blood then percolates past zone 2 hepatocytes (so called because they are not the first hepatocytes passed by blood entering the hepatic parenchyma). The last hepatocytes passed by the

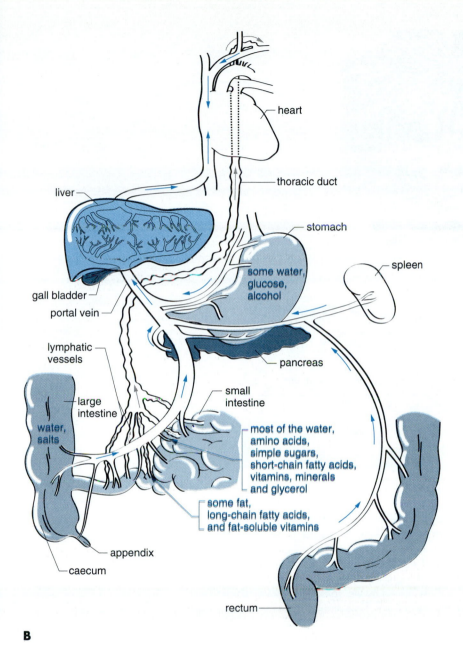

heart

thoracic duct

liver

stomach

spleen

some water,
glucose,
alcohol

gall bladder

portal vein

lymphatic
vessels

pancreas

large
intestine

small
intestine

water,
salts

most of the water,
amino acids,
simple sugars,
short-chain fatty acids,
vitamins, minerals
and glycerol

some fat,
long-chain fatty acids,
and fat-soluble vitamins

appendix

caecum

rectum

B

FIGURE 4.1 — *(continued)*

blood before it enters the central vein on its way out of the liver are termed *zone 3 hepatocytes*. In this way of viewing the microscopic organization of the liver, a liver **acinus** is defined as the unit of liver tissue centered around the portal venule and hepatic arteri-

ole whose hepatocytes can be imagined to form concentric rings of cells ordered by which ones "see" fresh portal blood, first to last (Figure 4.2C).

Hepatocytes at either extremes of the acinus (i.e., zones 1 and 3) appear to differ in

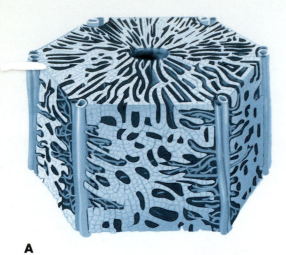

A

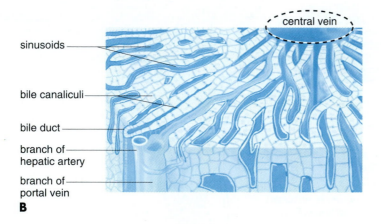

central vein

sinusoids

bile canaliculi

bile duct

branch of
hepatic artery

branch of
portal vein

B

FIGURE 4.2. Histology of the liver. *A.* Lobule concept of liver histology. At the center of the liver lobule lies the central vein from which radiates plates of hepatocytes. Around the edges that define the hexagonal liver lobule are the portal triads containing branches of the portal vein, hepatic artery, and bile duct. *B.* Relation of blood and bile flow in the liver. Magnification of part of a liver lobule indicating the flow of bile from the canaliculi formed by the apical hepatocyte plasma membrane into larger vessels in the portal triad. Note that the direction of flow of bile is from the center of the lobule to the periphery, exactly opposite that of blood. Note also how the branches of the hepatic artery and portal vein join at the sinusoids and drain together into the central vein. *C.* Liver acinus concept of liver histology. Illustrating the functional unit of the liver and the relationship of zones 1 to 3 to morphological landmarks. *(A. Adapted, with permission, from Jones, A. The liver and gallbladder. in Weiss, L., ed. Cell and Tissue Biology, 6th ed. Urban and Schwartzenberg, 1988, p. 687. B. and C. Adapted, with permission, from Fawcett, D. A Textbook of Histology, 11th ed. Saunders, 1986, pp. 682-683.)*

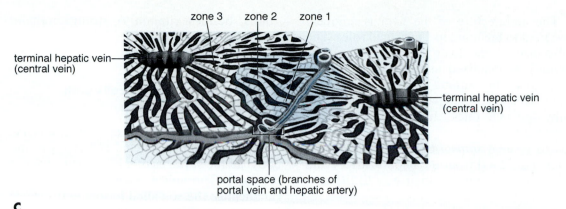

zone 3   zone 2   zone 1

terminal hepatic vein
(central vein)

terminal hepatic vein
(central vein)

portal space (branches of
portal vein and hepatic artery)

C

FIGURE 4.2 — *(continued)*

both enzymatic activity and physiological functions, having been tailored for (perhaps by) their environment. Thus, zone 1 hepatocytes, exposed to the highest oxygen concentrations, are particularly active in gluconeogenesis and oxidative energy metabolism. They are also the major site of urea synthesis (since freely diffusible substances, such as ammonia absorbed from protein breakdown in the gut, will be largely extracted in zone 1). Conversely, zone 3 hepatocytes are more active in glycolysis and lipogenesis (i.e., processes requiring less oxygen).

Clinical Pearl

○ Because zone 3 cells are most susceptible to hypoxia, metabolism of substrates that consume oxygen (e.g., alcohol) may lead to more pronounced cell injury in this region.

This **functional zonation** applies only to processes that are driven by the presence of diffusible substances. However, the liver is involved in many pathways involving **receptor-mediated uptake** and active transport of substances unable to diffuse freely into cells. These substances will enter whichever hepatocytes have the appropriate transporters, regardless of their zone. Similarly, substances that are tightly bound to carrier proteins likely will not be free to enter cells in any of the three zones, unless a cell has receptors allowing endocytosis of these substances.

Review Questions

2. What are the components of the portal triad?

3. What is the difference between the lobule and acinus concepts of liver subarchitecture?

4. What is the significance of functional zonation in the liver?

5. What activities are found in zone 1 hepatocytes? zone 3 hepatocytes?

6. Given your knowledge of functional zonation, which hepatocytes are most at risk for injury in times of oxygen deprivation?

7. What are four characteristics of portal venous blood?

8. Why is the liver a prime site for metastasis of malignant neoplasms from other parts of the body? For which neoplasms in particular?

The architecture of the liver is uniquely designed to facilitate its functional roles. The substance of the liver (termed the *parenchyma*) is organized into plates of hepatocytes that lie among various other cell types. The plates of hepatocytes are generally only one cell thick. Individual plates are separated from each other by vascular spaces termed *sinusoids*. It is in these sinusoids that blood from the hepatic artery and the portal vein mix on their way to the central vein.

Approximately 30% of all cells in the liver are **nonhepatocytes**, including phagocytic **reticuloendothelial cells**. Because they are smaller than hepatocytes, the reticuloendothelial system constitutes only about 2 to 10% of the total protein in the liver. The nonhepatocytes perform specific functions and communicate with each other as well as with hepatocytes. These cells include the following:

- Endothelial cells, which make up the walls of the sinusoids and secrete powerful vasoactive peptides such as **endothelins** in response to mediators such as **nitric oxide**.
- **Kupffer cells** (resident liver macrophages), which live in the sinusoidal space and make up about one-third of all reticuloendothelial cells. They are a crucial dimension of host defense. Kupffer cells can engulf bacteria directly, secrete powerful **cytokines** that can modulate other cellular elements of the immune system, and make other products that affect the liver, and perhaps even the body as a whole.
- **Stellate cells** (or lipocytes), which are nestled between the hepatocytes and the endothelial cells (Figure 4.3). Stellate cells normally store small amounts of fat and contain vitamin A within cytoplasmic droplets. They are now recognized to be extremely important in the pathophysiology of liver disease (see later), even though their normal func-

tions, besides vitamin A storage, remain quite mysterious.

Hepatocytes: polarized cells with segregation of functions

Hepatocytes are modified epithelial cells. As with many other epithelial cell types in the body, all the surfaces of a hepatocyte are not the same. The **apical surface** forms the **bile canaliculus**; the so-called **basolateral** surface is in contact with the bloodstream via the sinusoids. Most other epithelia are comprised of cells that have a single apical surface (e.g., those facing the lumen of the GI tract or the pancreatic acinus; see Chap. 5).

However, each hepatocyte has two small apical regions, one on each side, making up the bile canalicular wall. Each apical surface is surrounded by basolateral surface. Very different activities take place at these different regions of the hepatocyte plasma membrane, with tight junctions between hepatocytes serving to maintain segregation (see Figures 4.4A, B). Processes related to bile transport and excretion occur at the apical plasma membrane. Uptake from, and secretion into, the bloodstream occur across the basolateral membrane.

Mild hepatocyte dysfunction can sometimes involve disruption of bile flow (cholestasis) with relative preservation of other functions. There is, however, no absolute separation between the consequences of disturbed apical and basolateral functions: Cholestasis ultimately manifests at the basolateral surface where, for example, bilirubin and other substances to be excreted apically into the bile must be taken up from the bloodstream. Similarly, disruptions of energy metabolism or protein synthesis, while initially impinging on the secretory and metabolic processes of the hepatocyte, ultimately affect the bile transport machinery in the apical plasma membrane, because it too is com-

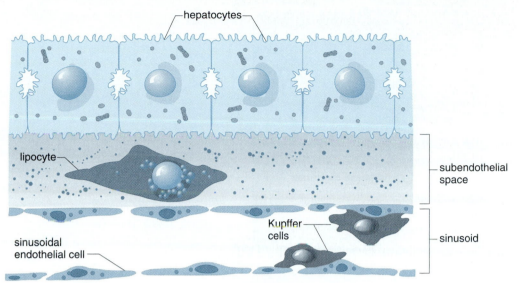

FIGURE 4.3. Relation of hepatocytes and endothelial cells. Shown are the hepatocytes and their relation to three types of reticuloendothelial cells, the endothelial cells (that make up the walls of the sinusoid, separating the space of Disse from the bloodstream), the Kupffer cell (a tissue macrophage), and a stellate cell, also called a lipocyte, within the space of Disse. *(Modified, with permission, from Friedman, S.L. (1993). The cellular basis of hepatic fibrosis. N. Engl. J. Med. 328: 1828.)*

posed of proteins that eventually need to be synthesized and replaced.

The liver: a remarkable capacity for regeneration

The normal liver has very few cells engaged in mitosis. However, when hepatocytes are lost, proliferation of the remaining hepatocytes is stimulated by mechanisms that are not well understood (see Prospects for Human Gene Therapy, in Sec. 12). Thus, in most cases of fulminant hepatitis with massive hepatocellular death, if the patient survives the initial period of inadequate liver function, recovery will be complete with no residual evidence of liver disease, because regenerated liver cells replace those that died with no disruption of hepatic architecture. Similarly, surgical resection of liver tissue is followed by rapid and architecturally precise hypertrophy and proliferation of the remaining hepatocytes. However, under certain conditions of chronic or repetitive injury associated with inflammation, regeneration is limited and complicated by scarring. This results in a condition known as cirrhosis (see later).

Review Questions

9. From which vascular sources do the hepatic central veins derive their blood flow?

10. What functions are associated with the apical plasma membrane of hepatocytes?

11. What cell types make up the liver? What are their distinguishing characteristics?

12. What happens to the remaining hepatocytes when part of the liver is surgically resected?

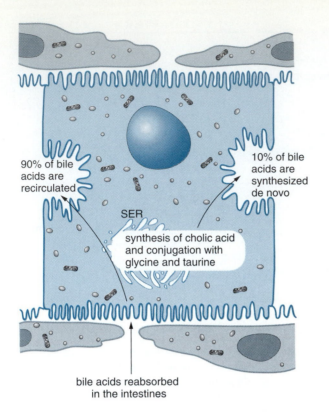

90% of bile acids are recirculated

10% of bile acids are synthesized de novo

SER

synthesis of cholic acid and conjugation with glycine and taurine

bile acids reabsorbed in the intestines

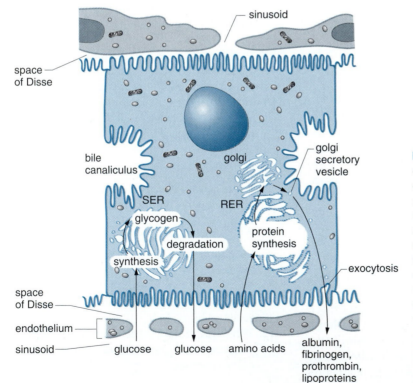

sinusoid

space of Disse

bile canaliculus

golgi

golgi secretory vesicle

SER

RER

glycogen

degradation

protein synthesis

synthesis

exocytosis

space of Disse

endothelium

sinusoid

glucose

glucose

amino acids

albumin, fibrinogen, prothrombin, lipoproteins

FIGURE 4.4. *A*. Mechanism of secretion of bile acids by hepatocytes. About 90% of bile acids derive from enterohepatic circulation (recycling), with about 10% derived from hepatocyte synthesis of cholic acid followed by conjugation with the amino acids glycine or taurine in the smooth endothelial reticulum (SER). *B*. Protein synthesis and carbohydrate storage in hepatocytes. *(Modified, with permission, from Junquiera, L.C. et al. (1995). Basic Histology, 8th ed. Stamford, CT, Appleton & Lange, pp. 328-329.)*

3. LIVER HEMODYNAMICS

The portal blood flow, being venous in nature, is normally under low hydrostatic pressure, about 10 mm of mercury. Accordingly there must be little resistance to its flow within the liver, allowing it to percolate through the sinusoids achieving maximal contact with hepatocytes. A number of unique features make this possible. Loss of these unique features contributes to the cellular basis of some of the cardinal manifestations of liver disease.

The endothelium of the hepatic sinusoid is fenestrated

Between the endothelial cells that make up the walls of the portal capillary system are spaces termed *fenestrations* that allow plasma and its proteins, but not red blood cells, free and direct access to the surface of the hepatocytes. This feature is crucial to the liver's function of uptake from, and secretion of, substances into the bloodstream. Most of the other capillary beds in the body lack such fenestrations, which are believed to contribute to the efficiency of the liver as a low-pressure filter of portal blood.

Hepatic sinusoids lack a typical basement membrane

In the liver, unlike most other organs, very little basement membrane exists between the capillary endothelial cell and the functional cells of the organ (i.e., the hepatocytes). This feature further enhances the exchange of dissolved substances between liver and portal blood.

If these specializations that allow blood to percolate through the liver under low pressure are lost, it would take higher pressures to force the portal blood to flow through the liver. But as portal pressure increases, a greater and greater proportion of portal blood flow will be diverted to other venous channels that return blood to the systemic circulation without going through the liver. Over time, these initially tiny vessels become engorged with blood, forming **varices**. Such channels have two very bad consequences. First, they defeat the purpose of having the liver as the first site for absorbed substances from the GI tract, and they allow substances into the systemic circulation that the liver would normally remove (see Loss of Protective Functions, in Sec. 8). Second, varices greatly increase the risk of bleeding. Since these thin vessels were never intended to carry so much blood, they are relatively fragile and their location (e.g., around the lumenal aspect of the esophagus) makes it impossible to control their bleeding by application of external pressure.

Review Questions

13. Why is it important for the liver to be a low-pressure circuit for blood flow?
14. What cell biological specializations normally make this possible?

4. PHYSIOLOGICAL FUNCTIONS OF THE NORMAL LIVER

The remarkably diverse functions of the liver fall into several broad categories (see Table 4.1). Although there is considerable overlap between these categories, a systematic consideration of each one is a useful way to approach the patient with liver disease.

Energy generation and substrate interconversion

Much of the body's carbohydrate, lipid, and protein is synthesized, metabolized, and interconverted in the liver. Many of the prod-

TABLE 4.1   SUMMARY OF NORMAL FUNCTIONS OF THE LIVER

Energy metabolism and substrate interconversion

Glucose production through gluconeogenesis and glycogenolysis
Glucose consumption by pathways of glycogen synthesis, glycolysis, tricarboxylic acid cycle, and fatty acid synthesis
Cholesterol synthesis from acetate, triglyceride synthesis from fatty acids, and secretion of both in very low density lipoprotein (VLDL) particles
Cholesterol and triglyceride uptake by endocytosis of high density lipoprotein (HDL) and low density lipoprotein (LDL) particles with excretion of cholesterol in bile, β oxidation of fatty acids and conversion of excess acetyl CoA to ketones
Deamination of amino acids and conversion of ammonia to urea via urea cycle
Transamination and synthesis de novo of nonessential amino acids

Solubilization, transport, and storage functions

Drug and toxin detoxification through phase I and phase II biotransformation reactions and excretion in bile
Solubilization of fats and fat soluble vitamins in bile for uptake by enterocytes
Synthesis and secretion of VLDL and pre-HDL lipoprotein particles and clearance of HDL, LDL, and chylomicron remnants
Synthesis and secretion of various binding proteins including transferin, steroid hormone binding globulin, thyroid hormone binding globulin, ceruloplasmin, and metallothionein
Uptake and storage of vitamin A and D, B12, and folate

Protein synthetic functions

Synthesis of various plasma proteins including albumin, clotting factors, binding proteins and apolipoproteins, angiotensinogen, and insulin-like growth factor I

Protective and clearance functions

Detoxification of ammonia through the urea cycle
Detoxification of drugs through microsomal oxidases and conjugation systems
Synthesis and export of glutathione
Clearance of damaged cells and proteins, hormones, drugs, and activated clotting factors from the portal circulation
Clearance of bacteria and antigens from the portal circulation

---

ucts of this metabolism are removed from, and/or released into, the bloodstream in response to the energy and substrate needs of the body (see Figure 4.5A). **Anabolic pathways** are those biochemical reactions involved in making carbohydrates, proteins, and lipids. **Catabolic pathways** are those biochemical reactions involved in the breakdown of carbohydrates, proteins, and lipids.

Carbohydrate metabolism

After a meal, the liver takes up glucose and uses it for glycogen synthesis and/or generation of metabolic intermediates via glycolysis and the tricarboxylic acid cycle. Up to 10%

of the weight of the normal liver is glycogen. The stimulus for glucose uptake occurs due to the increase in the concentration of glucose in the portal vein together with changes in the concentration of hormones (e.g., increase in insulin and decrease in glucagon, see Chap. 5). The liver responds to these changes by a corresponding change in the levels of enzymes that control pathways of glucose utilization and production (see Sec. 5) in the hepatocyte.

During fasting or stress, changes in hormone and substrate levels in the bloodstream drive metabolic pathways of the liver in the opposite direction and are responsible for net glucose production and release into the bloodstream by the liver (e.g., the pathways of glycogenolysis and gluconeogenesis). Although glycogen is stored in both liver and muscle, only liver glycogen can be used to provide glucose to the bloodstream. This is because the end-product of glycogenolysis (glycogen breakdown) is glucose-6-phosphate, which cannot leave the cell unless it is dephosphorylated by the enzyme glucose-6-phosphatase. This enzyme is present in the liver, but not in muscle.

The net effect of hepatic glucose consumption and production under different substrate and hormonal conditions is to maintain the peripheral blood glucose concentration in the normal range in spite of wide and sudden changes in the rate of blood glucose input and output.

An overnight fast substantially depletes hepatic glycogen reserves. Upon subsequent eating of a meal, direct and indirect pathways contribute about equally to hepatic glycogen storage, as the body attempts to replenish those reserves. The direct pathway is glucose to glycogen. The indirect pathway involves first metabolizing glucose to lactate via glycolysis in both the liver and in peripheral tissues (e.g., exercising muscle). Lactate is then converted into glucose-6-phosphate via gluconeogenesis in the liver, and finally, incorporated into glycogen. The prominence of the indirect pathway might be to make sure the liver has a plentiful supply of intermediates that connect different pathways of carbohydrate, lipid, and protein metabolism. It is also a way of interconnecting the liver with muscle and adipose tissue, from which gluconeogenic precursors will flow in times of fasting, exercise, and so on.

Clinical Pearl

○ In liver disease, either the ability to store glucose as glycogen or the ability to produce glucose from glycogen breakdown or by gluconeogenesis may be impaired.

Thus, a patient with liver disease could manifest either hyperglycemia or hypoglycemia (see Sec. 8). Generally, hyperglycemia is an earlier but mild manifestation as a consequence of blood bypassing the liver in portal hypertension. Hypoglycemia is typically an end-stage occurrence in chronic liver disease and is a grave prognostic sign.

Protein metabolism

The liver is also a major site for processes of the urea cycle, oxidative deamination, and transamination:

- The urea cycle allows nitrogen to be excreted in the form of urea, which is much less toxic than free amino groups in the form of ammonium ions (see Figure 4.5B).
- Oxidative deamination and transamination allow amino groups to be shuffled among molecules in order to generate substrates for both carbohydrate metabolism and amino acid synthesis. A key reaction in these pathways is the amidation of the tricarboxylic acid cycle intermediate α-ketoglutarate to form glutamate. This allows nitrogen to be spared from the waste generation pathway and to be recycled instead.

Amino acids may play additional regulatory roles in the liver. It appears that, after a meal, branched chain amino acids (leucine, isoleucine, and valine) preferentially enter the systemic circulation, perhaps as a signal to stimulate protein synthesis (e.g., in muscle).

Clinical Pearl

○ In liver disease, the ability to handle an ammonia load from protein metabolism is compromised. Thus hepatic encephalopa-

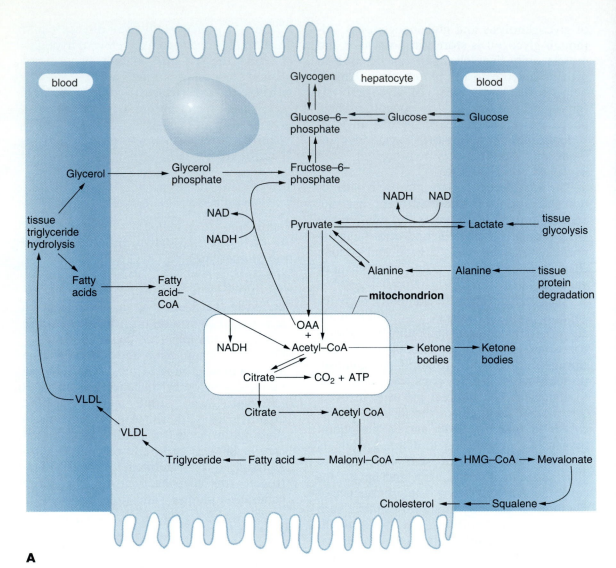

A

FIGURE 4.5. *A. Pathways of carbohydrate and lipid metabolism in hepatocytes. B. Pathway of urea detoxification in the liver. Dashed lines signify pathways whose extent of involvement varies from patient to patient, depending on genetic, dietary, and other factors. (A. Modified, with permission, from Schwartz, C.C. (1989). in Kelley, W.N., ed. Textbook of Internal Medicine, New York, Lippincott. B. Modified, with permission, from Powers-Lee, S.G. and Meister, A. (1988). in Arias, I.M. et al., eds. The Liver: Biology and Pathology, 2nd ed. New York, Raven Press.)*

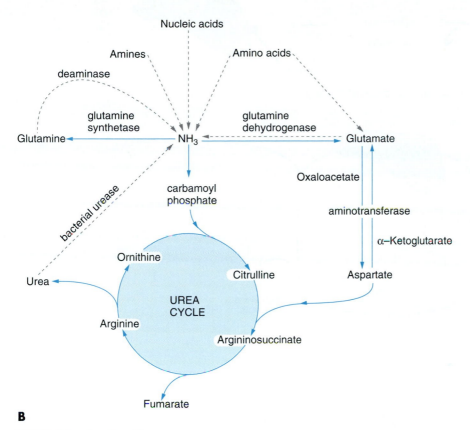

B

FIGURE 4.5 — (continued)

thy (manifest as altered mental status) may be the first sign of (a) infection (associated with increased endogenous protein breakdown), (b) gastrointestinal bleeding (blood is a protein load dumped into the gut), or (c) an increased dietary protein load (such as in Mr. S. who ate the double cheeseburger).

Lipid metabolism

Nearly 80% of the cholesterol synthesized in the body is made in the liver from acetyl coenzyme A via a pathway that connects carbohydrates with anabolic lipid metabolism (see Figure 4.5A).

The liver can also synthesize fatty acids, primarily palmitate, through biochemical reactions that occur in the cytoplasm. The other fatty acids of the body are derived largely by modification (shortening, lengthening, or desaturating) of palmitate. Fatty acids are stored and exported in the form of triglycerides. In order to manipulate the body's cholesterol and triglyceride stores, the liver assembles, secretes, and takes up various lipoprotein particles (see Figure 4.6).

Triglyceride-rich lipoprotein particles (termed ***very-low-density lipoproteins*** or ***VLDL***) are assembled in the liver at the endoplasmic reticulum during synthesis of the protein **apolipoprotein B**. VLDL serves to distribute lipid to adipose tissue for storage as fat, and to other tissues for immediate use.

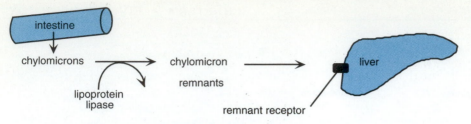

A. Exogenous Fat Transport Pathway

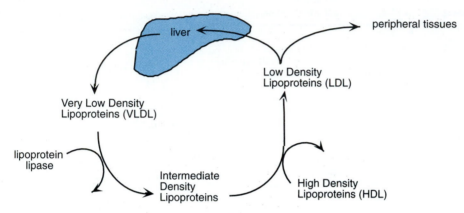

B. Endogenous Fat Transport Pathway

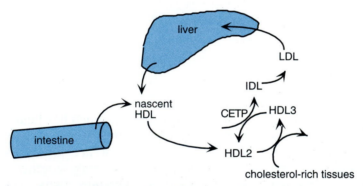

C. Reverse Cholesterol Transport Pathway

FIGURE 4.6. Lipoprotein metabolism involving the liver. In each of these three pathways lipoprotein particles are used to solubilize cholesterol esters (and triglyceride), either for the purpose of import from the GI tract (A), distribution to various tissues (B), or transport to the liver for excretion in bile (C). During their circulation, specific lipoprotein particles are transformed by addition and removal of apoproteins and by the action of enzymes in plasma or in tissues. (Lipoprotein lipase = LPL; cholesterol ester transfer protein = CTEP). Intermediate density lipoproteins (IDL) are intermediates in the conversion of VLDL to LDL. High Density Lipoproteins = HDL; HDL2 and HDL3 refer to modified forms of HDL due to removal of cholesterol from tissues to IDL and LDL. (Low Density Lipoproteins = LDL) *(Modified, with permission, from Breslow, J.L. (1989). Genetic basis of lipoprotein disorders. J. Clin. Invest. 84:373.)*

During these processes, the structure of a VLDL particle is modified by loss of lipid and protein components.

Cholesterol-rich **low-density lipoprotein** particles (**LDL**) result from metabolism of VLDL. The LDL particles are then returned to the liver, or to peripheral tissues, by virtue of their affinity for a specific hepatocyte surface receptor, the LDL receptor.

Other lipoprotein particles (termed **high-density lipoproteins** or **HDL**) are synthesized and secreted from the liver and the intestine, in order to scavenge excess cholesterol and triglycerides from other tissues and from the bloodstream. Cholesterol taken up by HDL is then transferred to LDL (by cholesterol ester transfer protein, CETP) for subsequent removal from the plasma via the liver. This process is called **reverse cholesterol transport**. Thus secretion of HDL and removal of LDL are both mechanisms by which cholesterol in excess of that needed by various tissues is removed from the circulation. Once returned to the liver in the form of LDL, cholesterol can be excreted from the body in bile, both directly and by conversion to bile acids.

In addition to its role in reverse cholesterol transport, HDL plays a role as an antioxidant serving to prevent conversion of LDL to oxidized LDL, the actual cause of atherosclerosis. Both the reverse cholesterol transport pathway and the antioxidant functions of HDL can be thought of as one of the liver's protective functions (see later).

The one class of newly synthesized lipoprotein particles *not* made in the liver are the triglyceride-rich chylomycrons (see Chap. 5). However, the liver is responsible for removing chylomicron remnants, the term used to describe what is left of the chylomicron (including most of the cholesterol) after these particles have served up much of their triglyceride to adipose and other tissues and exchanged various component proteins.

We have focused on the liver's role in lipid metabolism from an anabolic perspective.

But the liver also plays a crucial role in lipid catabolism as a primary site of fatty acid oxidation. Besides carbon dioxide, water, and ATP, the end products of fatty acid oxidation are β-hydroxy butyrate and acetoacetate, commonly termed **ketones**. This pathway is physiologically very important. It is the basis for the transition from a carbohydrate- to a lipid-based fuel economy (e.g., in times of starvation, see Chap. 6).

Normally, ketones are only generated at relatively low levels during fasting and are metabolized by brain, heart, and renal cortex. However, in patients with out-of-control diabetes mellitus, ketones can be overproduced to the point that they lower blood pH, resulting in the life-threatening syndrome of diabetic ketoacidosis (see Chap. 6). While the liver is an efficient producer of ketones, it cannot itself metabolize them, because it lacks the necessary enzyme (ketoacid CoA transferase).

Solubilization, transport, and storage functions

The liver plays an important role in solubilization, transport, and storage of a variety of very different substances that would otherwise be difficult for other tissues in the body to obtain or move in and out of cells. Specific cells in the liver perform these functions by making specialized proteins. The broad categories of solubilization, transport, and storage functions can be divided into those involving the following:

1. Metabolism and detoxification of various substances including drugs and toxins in the hepatocyte
2. Excretion and absorption of various substances in **bile**
3. Packaging, circulation, and recycling of lipoprotein particles in the bloodstream (as previously discussed)

4. Storage and transport of various other lipophilic substances

Drug detoxification

Most of the enzymes that carry out metabolism necessary for the detoxification and excretion of drugs and other substances are located in the endoplasmic reticulum of hepatocytes. These pathways of drug detoxification are used not only for metabolism of exogenous drugs but also for many endogenous substances that would otherwise be difficult for cells to excrete (e.g., including both bilirubin and cholesterol previously described). In most cases this metabolism involves the conversion of **lipophilic** (lipid-loving) substances which are difficult to excrete from cells because they like to stay in cellular membranes, into more **hydrophilic** (water-loving) substances. This involves catalysis of chemical modifications to make the substance more charged so that it will partition more favorably into an aqueous medium or at least be solubilized sufficiently in bile. As a result of these processes, collectively termed **biotransformations**, some substances are modified in ways that allow them to be excreted directly in the urine. Other substances are modified in ways that allow them to be transported into the bile for excretion in feces.

Biotransformation generally occurs in two phases. **Phase I reactions** involve oxidation-reduction reactions in which an oxygen-containing functional group is added to a lipophilic substance (e.g., a drug) that diffuses into a hepatocyte from the bloodstream. Although oxidation itself often has only a small effect on water solubility, it usually introduces a reactive group into the drug to serve as a "handle" that makes possible other enzymatic reactions to render the modified substance highly water soluble. These subsequent **phase II reactions** usually involve covalent attachment of the drug to a water-soluble carrier molecule such as sugar glucuronic acid or peptide glutathione. The biochemical reactions by which these sugar molecules are added is termed **conjugation**. The resulting drug-carrier conjugate can be excreted either in bile (and therefore feces) or urine. Not only drugs, but bile salts themselves undergo conjugation.

Unfortunately, phase I oxidation reactions often convert mildly toxic drugs into much more toxic reactive intermediates in order to facilitate their conjugation by phase II enzymes. This feature of drug detoxification has important clinical implications (see later).

Clinical Pearl

○ The major phase I metabolite of Tylenol is a highly toxic reactive intermediate that is normally conjugated to glutathione to render it water soluble and harmless. In a setting of nutritional deprivation resulting in cysteine deficiency (needed for glutathione synthesis) and enzyme induction (e.g., from alcohol intake, see Sec. 5), and underlying chronic liver disease, even very small doses of Tylenol are sufficient to cause substantial liver injury and result in hepatic failure (e.g., manifest as hepatic encephalopathy). Thus, a careful drug history and urine "tox screen" are mandatory to rule out this reversible cause of worsened liver function in such a patient (see A Case of Physiological Medicine at the end of the chapter).

Functions of bile

Many of the components of **bile** are synthesized, exported, and recycled in hepatocytes. This detergent-like substance allows a variety of otherwise insoluble substances to be dissolved in an aqueous environment for transport into or export out of the body. Bile acids undergo an **enterohepatic circulation** that starts with their synthesis from cholesterol, conjugation to the amino acids glycine or taurine, and secretion at the apical plasma membrane of the hepatocyte into the bile canaliculus.

One role of bile is to solubilize and eliminate hydrophobic substances including drugs and toxins. Bile acids and their salts and the substances whose excretion they promote are collected via the biliary tract, and are sometimes stored in the gall bladder prior to excretion via the common bile duct into the duodenum.

From the duodenum, bile acids and salts travel down the GI tract (see Chap. 3). During this transit, bile performs a second function, which is to solubilize and promote the absorption of fats and fat-soluble vitamins. Both conjugated and deconjugated bile salts are absorbed from the lumen of the terminal ileum into the portal blood through the action of specific sodium-dependent active transporters (see Figure 4.7). In the colon, bacterial action on primary bile salts results in their deconjugation and modification to so-called secondary bile salts.

Portal blood flow takes the bile salts that were absorbed in the terminal ileum back to the liver where they are taken up by hepatocytes and transported back into bile, bound to various bile salt-binding proteins present in the hepatocyte cytoplasm. Normally, about 75% of the bile acids in the liver are destined to be recycled each day, so only about a quarter of the 2 g of bile acids in the enterohepatic circulation are a result of new synthesis.

Miscellaneous binding, transport, and storage functions

Cells in the liver synthesize proteins that bind particular substances (e.g., certain vitamins, minerals, and hormones) very tightly. In some cases these proteins are secreted out of the liver into the bloodstream. There they allow substances to be transported in the bloodstream that otherwise would not be soluble (e.g., steroids bound to steroid-binding globulin which is synthesized and secreted by hepatocytes).

In other cases, proteins secreted by the liver allow substances to be cleared from the bloodstream (e.g., binding of free heme by hemopexin or binding of free iron by transferrin), often involving uptake of the bound complex by specific cells in the liver. This is an important line of host defense because many pathogens are critically dependent on a source of specific nutritive substances, such as free iron. By binding all the free iron in the bloodstream, proteins such as hemopexin and transferrin make it more difficult for a pathogen to gain a foothold in the body.

In still other cases, tight binding proteins made by the liver are retained in the cytoplasm where they allow accumulation of specific substances to high concentration in particular cells, serving as a reservoir for future needs in times of scarcity (e.g., vitamin A binding proteins in the stellate cell).

Clinical Pearls

○ Obstructive jaundice presents initially with predominantly conjugated hyperbilirubinemia, but metabolites eventually back up enough to elevate unconjugated bilirubin as well.

Thus, examination of the urine gives you an idea of whether new onset jaundice is likely to be obstructive or not. Conversely, if you know a patient has an obstructive lesion (e.g., indicated by ultrasound of the biliary tract showing dilated bile ducts behind a mass), whether the elevated bilirubin is largely conjugated (also called direct bilirubin) or unconjugated (termed indirect bilirubin) tells you if the

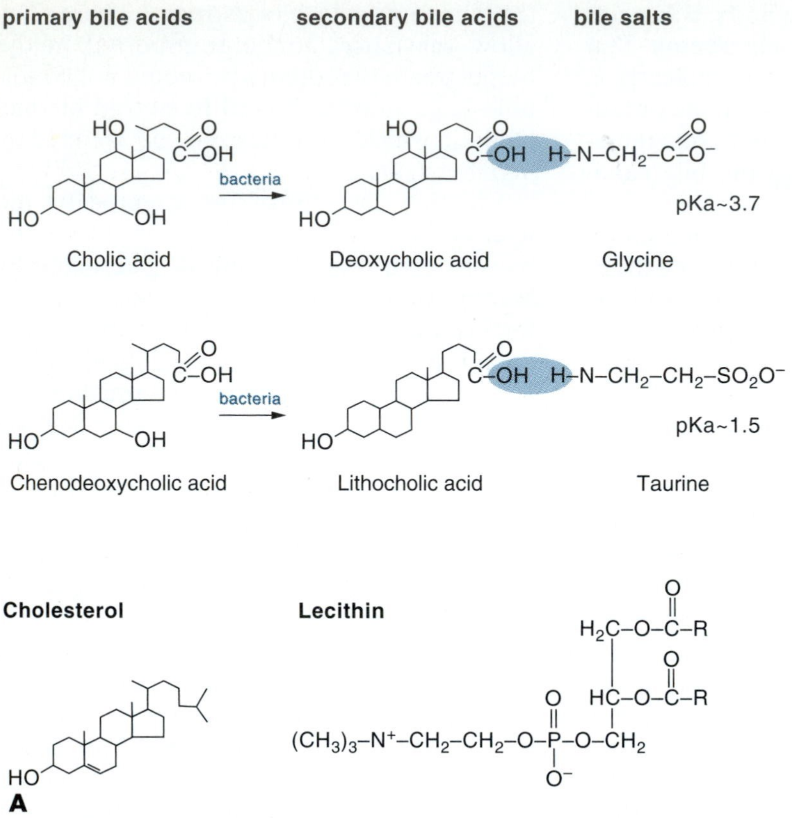

primary bile acids **secondary bile acids** **bile salts**

Cholic acid

Deoxycholic acid

Glycine

pKa~3.7

Chenodeoxycholic acid

Lithocholic acid

Taurine

pKa~1.5

Cholesterol **Lecithin**

A

FIGURE 4.7. *A.* Principal organic constitutents of bile. The two primary bile acids may be converted into secondary bile acids in the intestine through bacterial action. Each of these four bile acids may be conjugated to either glycine or taurine. *B.* Lecithins are phospholipids that are found in association with bile salts in aggregates termed *micelles* that act as a detergent to disperse and eliminate via bile substances (such as cholesterol) that are too hydrophobic to be excreted efficiently any other way. *(A. Modified, with permission, from Johnson, L.R. (1992). in* Essential Medical Physiology. *New York, Raven Press. B. Modified, with permission, from Sleisenger, M.H., and Fordtran, J.S., eds.* Gastrointestinal Disease, *3rd ed. Philadelphia, Saunders.)*

obstruction is recent or has been building for some time.

○ Jaundice (yellow discoloration of the "whites" of the eyes) occurs from buildup in tissues of metabolites of bilirubin (by products of hemoglobin degradation as a result of clearance of old red blood cells) that are normally eliminated from the body via bile (giving feces its normal brown color). These disorders can be distinguished into three categories:

1. Hemolysis (rupture of large numbers of red blood cells), which can result in transient jaundice in the absence of any liver disease simply by exceeding, for a time, the capacity of the liver to clear the released heme metabolites

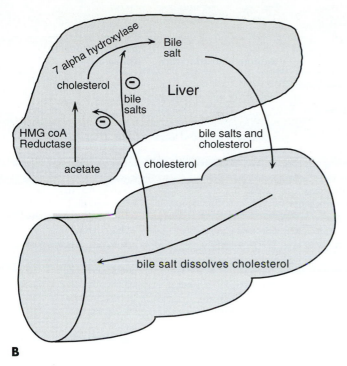

B

FIGURE 4.7 — (continued)

2. A hepatocellular defect that results in increase in unconjugated bilirubin
3. Obstruction of bile flow (e.g., by a gallstone or tumor), resulting in backup of, initially, largely conjugated bilirubin into the bloodstream. Light, chalky-colored feces and the GI consequences of lack of bile flow (steatorrhea, fat-soluble vitamin deficiencies) are seen in categories 2 and 3, but not category 1.

○ Conjugated bilirubin (e.g., in category 3) is more water soluble than unconjugated bilirubin and can be filtered into urine, which becomes dark in color as a result. Unconjugated bilirubin is more lipophilic and partitions to a greater extent into tissues than does conjugated bilirubin.

Synthesis and secretion of plasma proteins

The liver has a tremendous protein-synthetic capacity. It is the site of synthesis and secretion of many of the proteins found in plasma. These include albumin, the vitamin K-dependent clotting factors (II, VII, IX, and X), a number of binding proteins (including those for steroids, thyroid hormone, copper, and iron), and even certain hormones and hormone precursors (angiotensinogen and IGF-1). By virtue of the actions of these proteins, the liver has important roles in maintaining plasma oncotic pressure (serum albumin), coagulation (clotting-factor synthesis and modification), blood pressure (angiotensinogen), growth (insulin-like growth factor I), metabolism (steroid and thyroid hormone binding proteins) and so on. Table 4.2 lists

TABLE 4.2 PROTEINS OF THE LIVER

Name	Principal function	Binding characteristics	Serum or plasma concentration
Albumin	Binding and carrier protein; osmotic regulator	Hormones, amino acids, steroids, vitamins, fatty acids	4500-5000 mg/dL
Orosomucoid	Uncertain; may have a role in inflammation		Trace; rises in inflammation
α_1-Antiprotease	Trypsin and general protease inhibitor	Proteases in serum and tissue secretions	1.3-1.4 mg/dL
α-Fetoprotein	Osmotic regulation; binding and carrier protein*	Hormones, amino acids	Found normally in fetal blood
α_2-Macroglobulin	Inhibitor of serum endoproteases	Proteases	150-420 mg/dL
Antithrombin-III	Protease inhibitor of intrinsic coagulation system	1 : 1 binding to proteases	17-30 mg/dL
Ceruloplasmin	Transport of copper	Six atoms copper/mol	15-60 mg/dL
C-reactive protein	Uncertain; has role in tissue inflammation	Complement C1q	<1 mg/dL; rises in inflammation
Fibrinogen	Precursor to fibrin in hemostasis		200-450 mg/dL
Haptoglobin	Binding, transport of cell-free hemoglobin	Hemoglobin 1 : 1 binding	40-180 mg/dL
Hemopexin	Binds to porphyrins, particularly heme for heme recycling	1 : 1 with heme	50-100 mg/dL
Transferrin	Transport of iron	2 atoms of iron per molecule	3.0-6.5 mg/dL
Apolipoprotein B	Assembly of lipprotein particles	Lipid carrier	
Angiotensinogen	Precursor to pressor peptide angiotensin II		
Proteins, coagulation factors II, VII, IX, X	Blood clotting		20 mg/dL
Antithrombin III, protein C	Inhibition of blood clotting		
Insulin-like growth factor I	Mediator of anabolic effects of growth hormone	IGF-I receptor	
Steroid hormone-binding globulin	Carrier protein for steroids in bloodstream	Steroid hormones	3.3 mg/dL
Thyroid-binding globulin	Carrier protein for thyroid hormone in bloodstream	Thyroid hormones	1.5 mg/dL
Transthyretin (thyroid-binding prealbumin)	Carrier protein for thyroid hormone in bloodstream	Thyroid hormones	25 mg/dL

*The function of fetoprotein is uncertain, but because of the structural homology to albumin it is often assigned these functions.

Modified, with permission, from Donohue, T.M. et al. (1990). in Zakim, D. and Boyer, T., eds. *Hepatology: a Textbook of Liver Disease,* Philadelphia, Saunders.

the proteins synthesized by the liver and their physiological functions, many of which will be discussed specifically in subsequent chapters.

Protective and clearance functions

The final broad category of normal liver functions are those that can be viewed as "protective" functions. These include the following:

1. Phagocytic and endocytic functions of Kupffer cells, such as the removal of bacteria and antigens that breach the defenses of the gut to enter the portal blood, as well as clearance of endogenously generated

cellular debris. Kupffer cells appear to have various receptors (such as the Fc receptor that binds material coated with immunoglobulin, and the C3 receptor that binds activated complement proteins). Using these receptors, Kupffer cells are able to clear damaged plasma proteins, activated clotting factors, immune complexes, senescent blood cells, and the like from the circulation. Impaired function of Kupffer cells may account for the increased risk of blood-borne infection in patients with severe liver disease.

2. Endocytic functions of hepatocytes. Hepatocytes have a number of specific receptors (e.g., the asialoglycoprotein receptor) for damaged plasma proteins, distinct from the receptors present on Kupffer cells.

3. Ammonia metabolism. Ammonia generated from deamination of amino acids is metabolized by hepatocytes into the much less toxic substance urea. Loss of this function results in altered mental status, a common manifestation of severe or end-stage liver disease.

4. Hepatocyte synthesis of **glutathione**. Glutathione is the major intracellular (cytoplasmic) reducing reagent and, thus, is crucial for preventing oxidative damage to cellular proteins. This interesting molecule is a nonribosomally synthesized tripeptide (γ-glutamyl-cysteinyl-glycine), which is also a substrate for many phase II drug detoxification conjugation reactions. The liver is also believed to export glutathione for use by other tissues.

Many of the liver functions already discussed under other categories of functions can also be considered "protective." These include drug detoxification, lipoprotein particle dynamics (especially HDL), and biliary excretion. Despite this overlap, it is useful to conceptualize protective functions as a separate category because of their tremendous

importance in the care of patients with liver disease (see later).

Review Questions

15. Summarize the role of the liver in carbohydrate, protein, and lipid metabolism.
16. Why is liver rather than muscle glycogen a source of blood glucose?
17. What are two physiological mechanisms by which the body moves cholesterol?
18. Explain phase I and phase II reactions in drug detoxification.
19. Name and explain four clearance/protective functions of the liver.
20. What is conjugation, where does it occur, and for what is it used? Name some substances that are conjugated.

5. CONTROL OF LIVER FUNCTION

Perhaps because so much of what the liver does is essential for the basic, minute-to-minute functioning of the organism (e.g., maintaining blood glucose and removing toxins from the bloodstream), the liver has evolved to be particularly attentive to the state of affairs in the rest of the body. Thus, the liver normally is able to monitor substrate concentrations in the bloodstream and respond to changes in a way that promotes homeostasis.

Control by substrates

Unlike many other tissues such as muscle and adipose tissue, the liver is freely permeable to glucose. This is because the specific form of the glucose transporter found in the liver (termed *GLUT II*) always resides in the plasma membrane. Thus the liver takes up glucose in direct proportion to its concentration in the bloodstream. In contrast, the glucose transporter (termed *GLUT IV*) found in muscle and adipose tissue is inserted into the plasma membrane only in response to the hormone insulin, returning to an endosome compartment in insulin's absence. Thus, unlike the liver, muscle and adipose tissue take up glucose only when insulin is present. By this mechanism, the liver "sees" the glucose concentration in the blood whether or not there is insulin around, allowing it to "decide" whether to store glucose as glycogen or produce glucose from other substrates.

Consider the fate of blood glucose. As discussed earlier, glucose can freely enter hepatocytes. Once in the hepatocyte cytoplasm, glucose can be phosphorylated by specific enzymes. The phosphorylated glucose molecule is unable to leave the hepatocyte freely. Thus phosphorylation serves as a trap, creating a gradient by which the liver extracts glucose from the bloodstream in response to hormonal dictates. Furthermore, phosphorylation of glucose is the first step to either glycogen synthesis or pathways of glucose metabolism leading to fat or protein synthesis.

The key question for understanding hepatic control of blood glucose concentration is, what controls the activity of the enzyme that phosphorylates glucose (termed *glucokinase*)? Glucokinase has a much higher K_m (lower affinity) for glucose than the isoform (termed *hexokinase*) that occurs in most other tissues. Thus, the activity of the enzyme (i.e., the rate of glucose phosphorylation in hepatocytes) goes up dramatically as blood glucose (in the portal vein) rises above about 100 mg/dL. Of course, this is precisely when the body would want the liver to extract glucose from the bloodstream. Conversely, when blood glucose falls below about 60 mg/dL, activity of glucokinase drops, in part because its affinity for glucose is not sufficient to maintain the high rate of enzyme activity displayed when blood glucose concentrations were higher. Similar principles govern other pathways. For example, the levels of glycerol and free fatty acids available in the bloodstream

are determinants of how much VLDL the liver produces in order to maintain lipid homeostasis.

Control by hormones

Control of liver function by substrate concentration is only part of the story. The enzymes of the liver are tremendously dependent on hormones, which turn on (or off) signal transduction pathways that can enormously increase (or decrease) activity of various liver enzymes.

Even though glucose uptake in the liver is independent of insulin, many other liver functions are under the control of this or other hormones. Some of these hormonal effects on the liver are very rapid. For example, the effects of glucagon and of epinephrine, released in response to hypoglycemia to stimulate glycogen breakdown and, thereby, raise blood glucose, occur in *minutes*.

Some hormonal effects are manifested on a somewhat more delayed timescale. Thus, insulin, released from the endocrine pancreas (see Chap. 6) in response to the high blood glucose, stimulates an increase in synthesis of the enzymes involved in glucose metabolism in the liver, manifest over a timescale of *hours*.

Finally, other hormones have delayed effects on the liver, which occur over *days*. Estrogens and androgens, for example, change the patterns of protein synthesis in the liver, allowing more of some proteins to be made relative to other proteins.

In addition, the action of insulin greatly increases the glucokinase activity in the hepatocyte. Insulin does this by triggering signaling pathways that activate the following:

1. Dephosphorylation of the glucokinase protein itself, thereby increasing its activity directly
2. Dephosphorylation of ribosomal proteins to increase translation of glucokinase and other mRNAs

3. Activation of transcription of the glucokinase gene to make more glucokinase mRNA, which upon translation results in more glucokinase protein
4. Decrease in synthesis and activity of a variety of enzymes that oppose the action of glucokinase, such as glucose-6-phosphatase
5. Degradation of enzymes involved in opposing pathways

In these ways, the intrinsic control by substrate concentration discussed earlier is synergistically amplified by the hormonal milieu. Exactly the opposite changes happen in response to glucagon, a hormone that opposes the action of insulin and promotes breakdown of glycogen by the liver and release of free glucose into the bloodstream.

The effects of hormones on the liver are, of course, mediated by **receptors** on the surface of hepatocytes or, in the case of the steroid hormone receptors, inside the cell. Through these receptors hepatocytes monitor a wide range of activities and trigger increases in synthesis of specific proteins in order to maintain homeostasis.

Receptor-mediated regulation of cellular homeostasis in the liver

Regulation by receptors can occur in many complex ways. Consider, for example, iron homeostasis, which we understand perhaps better than most regulatory pathways (see Figure 4.8).

The transmembrane **transferrin receptor**, the iron-binding secretory protein **transferrin**, and the cytoplasmic iron-binding protein **ferritin** are all made in the hepatocyte and work together to regulate iron storage. In iron deficiency, synthesis and secretion (into blood) of apotransferrin (the transferrin polypeptide chain without bound iron) is greatly increased in order to augment the body's ability to scavenge free iron in the bloodstream (absorbed from the GI tract).

At the normal pH of the bloodstream (pH 7.4), the apo form of transferrin has low affinity for the transferrin receptor. However, upon binding iron, its conformation changes and its affinity for the transferrin receptor increases greatly. Once bound to the transferrin receptor, transferrin is internalized by endocytosis and is localized to an intracellular vesicle termed an *endosome*. In the endosome, the pH is substantially lower than that in either the cytoplasm or the bloodstream. In this low pH environment, transferrin again changes its conformation, resulting in dissociation of the bound iron. However, at low pH, it is the apotransferrin that has high affinity for the transferrin receptor, in contrast to the situation in the bloodstream at a more neutral pH. Thus, when the transferrin receptor cycles back to the cell surface, it brings with it the apotransferrin, which is released in the neutral pH of the bloodstream. Meanwhile, back in the acidic endosome, the iron is transported to the cytosol where it is bound to ferritin. This system is set up to yield a net uptake of iron, but only when it is needed.

This is just one of many ways in which iron homeostasis is likely to be controlled at the molecular level. For example, in another form of regulation, binding proteins stimulate or inhibit translation of ferritin and transferrin mRNA in an inverse relationship: When ferritin levels are high, apotransferrin synthesis is low, and vice versa. Somehow, under normal circumstances the cell is able to integrate all of these mechanisms such that homeostasis is achieved.

Disordered iron metabolism can result in a condition known as **hemachromatosis** in which excessive iron accumulation leads to inexorable liver destruction.

Clinical Pearl

○ Some clinical conditions are characterized by lysis of red blood cells in the circulation (termed *hemolysis*). Frequent blood trans-

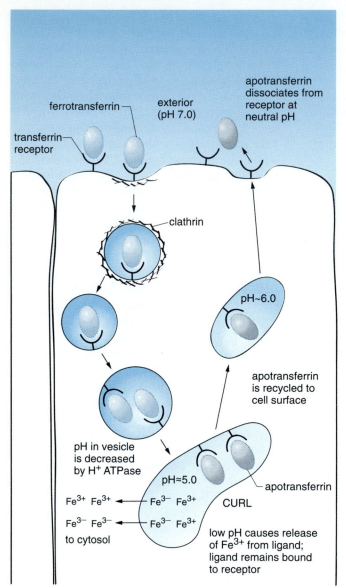

transferrin receptor

ferrotransferrin

exterior (pH 7.0)

apotransferrin dissociates from receptor at neutral pH

clathrin

pH~6.0

apotransferrin is recycled to cell surface

pH in vesicle is decreased by H^+ ATPase

$pH \approx 5.0$

CURL

apotransferrin

Fe^{3+} Fe^{3+} ← Fe^{3-} Fe^{3+}

Fe^{3-} Fe^{3-} ← Fe^{3-} Fe^{3+}

to cytosol

low pH causes release of Fe^{3+} from ligand; ligand remains bound to receptor

FIGURE 4.8. Iron homeostasis. Recycling of transferrin and its receptor upon unloading of iron in a low pH endocytic compartment (see Chap. 2). *(Modified, with permission, from Lodish, H. et al. (1995). Synthesis and sorting of plasma membrane, secretory, and lysosomal proteins, in Lodish, H., Baltimore, D., Berk, A. et al., eds. Molecular Cell Biology, 3rd ed. New York, Scientific American Books, p. 728.)*

fusions to treat these conditions can result in excessive free iron in the blood that, probably by the law of mass action, can drive excessive iron uptake into the liver by the transferrin-transferrin receptor pathway described earlier. One complication of many years of such transfusion therapy is iron accumulation and toxicity, a condition known as transfusional hemochromatosis or hemosiderosis. The problem, it seems, is that the iron homeostatic mechanisms were not designed to deal with the concept of a blood transfusion.

Enzyme induction and changes in gene expression

In addition to immediate control by substrate concentrations and receptor binding, internalization, and dissociation, there is regulation of liver function by changes in gene expression termed **enzyme induction**.

Enzyme induction is the increase in transcription and/or translation and/or activity of a particular enzyme in response to the presence of the substrate on which that enzyme acts. The cytochrome P450 enzymes that mediate phase I oxidation-reduction reactions are a good example of inducible enzymes. What happens when a patient who is on a drug that induces these enzymes is subsequently put on another drug that is metabolized in the same manner? A higher dose of the second drug is generally needed to get the same blood level that would have been achieved had the patient not been chronically on the first drug. This phenomenon is due to enzyme induction.

Review Questions

21. Why is the liver, but not muscle, freely permeable to glucose?
22. What are some short-, medium-, and long-term effects of the hormone insulin on the liver?
23. How does the body regulate iron stores?
24. Define enzyme induction and give an example of where it occurs.

More generally, gene expression in any cell can be affected by exogenous compounds. For poorly understood reasons, "unphysiological" compounds can inadvertently turn on or off transcription of various genes, and activate or inactivate pathways of signal transduction, or "cross-talk" between one pathway or another (see Chap. 1). Presumably, these effects reflect some normal pathway that was unintentionally activated by the unphysiological compound. The liver provides great examples of this, since the blood flow from the portal vein makes the liver the organ that "sees" orally ingested compounds first, after they have been absorbed into the bloodstream. Alcohol is a good example of a toxin that often is ingested in liberal quantities resulting in hepatic oxidative enzyme induction.

6. PRESENTATIONS AND CONSEQUENCES OF LIVER DISEASE

Presentations of liver disease

Although there are many different kinds of disease-causing agents and processes that can affect the intrinsic functions of the liver, they generally manifest in the patient as one of five common presentations (see Table 4.3):

1. In some cases liver disease is so mild that only a subset of functions are affected, as seen for example in certain forms of drug-induced impairment of bile formation by the liver (termed **cholestasis**).
2. In other cases moderate degrees of liver injury result in transient effects on the entire range of liver functions. This is termed **acute hepatitis** and is typical of clinically symptomatic viral infection of the liver.
3. Occasionally viral and other causes of acute liver injury present in an overwhelming manner with massive liver cell death and destruction. Termed **fulminant hepatic failure**, this syndrome carries a high mortality. However, if the patient survives, liver function will return to normal and there will be no residual evidence of liver disease.
4. Sometimes liver injury continues beyond the initial acute episode or is recurrent. Such processes are termed **chronic hepati-**

TABLE 4.3 DIVERSE CAUSES OF THE BROAD CATEGORIES OF LIVER DISEASE

Cholestasis

Direct causes (intrahepatic biliary atresia, cholangiocarcinoma, viral hepatitis, alcoholic hepatitis, primary biliary cirrhosis, pericholangitis)

Reactions to certain classes of drugs (including anabolic steroids, oral contraceptives, phenothiazines, erythromycins, oral hypoglycemics, and antithyroidals)

Secondary causes (postoperative, endotoxin, total parenteral nutrition, sickle cell crisis, hypophysectomy, some porphyrias)

Acute hepatitis

Viral (including hepatitis viruses A, B, C, D; Epstein-Barr virus; Herpes Simplex virus; and cytomegalovirus) and bacterial (Brucellosis, Leptospirosis) infections

Reactions to certain classes of drugs (anesthetics such as halothane, anticonvulsants such as phenytoin, antihypertensives such as methyldopa, chemotherapeutic agents such as isoniazid, thiazide, diuretics, and laxatives such as oxyphenisatin)

Toxins (such as ethanol)

Fulminant hepatic failure

Infections (viral hepatitis A, B, D; yellow fever; cytomegalovirus; Herpes viruses; *Coxiella burnetii*)

Poisons, chemicals, and drugs (Amanita phalloides toxin, phosphorus, ethanol, solvents including carbontetrachloride and dimethylformamide, anesthetics including halothane, analgesics including acetaminophen and pirprofen, antimicrobials including tetracycline and isoniazid, and other drugs including methyldopa, monoamine oxidase inhibitors, valproate)

Ischemia and hypoxia (vascular occlusion, circulatory failure, heat stroke, gram-negative sepsis with shock, congestive heart failure, pericardial tamponade)

Miscellaneous metabolic anomalies (acute fatty liver of pregnancy, Reye's syndrome, Wilson's disease, Galactosemia)

Chronic hepatitis

Viral hepatitis (types B, C, and D)

Primary autoimmune disorders (idiopathic autoimmune chronic active hepatitis, primary biliary cirrhosis, and sclerosing cholangitis)

Therapeutic drug-induced (methyldopa, nitrofurantoin, oxyphenisatin containing laxatives)

Genetic diseases (Wilson's disease, α-1 antitrypsin deficiency)

Infiltrative disorders (Sarcoidosis, amyloidosis, hemachromatosis)

Cirrhosis

Infectious (viral hepatitis B, C, D; cytomegalovirus; toxoplasmosis; schistosomiasis)

Genetic diseases (Wilson's disease, hemochromatosis, α-1 antitrypsin deficiency, glycogen storage diseases, Fanconi syndrome, cystic fibrosis)

Drugs and toxins (ethanol and methotrexate)

Miscellaneous (sarcoid, graft versus host disease, inflammatory bowel disease, jejunoileal bypass, diabetes mellitus)

Focal or extrinsic diseases with variable manifestations on liver

Vascular (hepatic vein thrombosis, occlusion by parasites such as echinococcus or schistosomiasis)

Biliary (duct obstruction due to stones or tumor or bacterial infection)

Infectious (systemic sepsis, bacterial, fungal, or parasitic abscesses)

Granulomatous diseases (sarcoidosis, tuberculosis)

Infiltrative diseases (hemochromatosis, amyloidosis, Gaucher's and other lysosomal storage diseases, lymphoma)

---

* Note that liver disease of a given cause (e.g., drug-induced) may be manifest differently in different patients.

Modified from Chapter 261, Isselbacher, K.J., and Podolsky, D.K., in Isselbacher, K. et al. eds. (1994). *Harrison's Principles of Internal Medicine*, 13th ed. New York, McGraw-Hill, p. 1439.

tis. In some cases liver function remains stable or the process ultimately resolves altogether, while in other cases progressive deterioration of liver function occurs.

5. **Cirrhosis** of the liver is the ultimate consequence of progressive liver injury that occurs in a subset of cases of chronic hepatitis. It is characterized by irreversible scarring of the liver (see Mechanisms of Hepatic Fibrosis in Sec. 12) and sets the stage for devastating complications to be discussed below.

This categorization into five presentations of liver disease is not absolute, but rather forms a continuum that differs not only from one agent of liver injury to another but also from patient to patient. The differences between patients in their response to the same agent of liver injury are presumably due to a variety of poorly understood genetic, immunologic, nutritional, and other factors.

In addition, features of the structure and location of the liver render it susceptible to focal or systemic disease processes (e.g., cancer), which can alter the relation of the liver to other organs of the body. Even without causing direct liver injury such extrinsic processes can have profound consequences.

Consequences of liver disease

The consequences of liver disease can be divided into two groups. One group includes those that arise from direct damage to **hepatocytes**, as occurs in inflammation of the liver (hepatitis). Like many organs of the body, the normal liver has a huge excess capacity, with many times the number of hepatocytes that are actually needed to carry out its roles. Thus, the abnormalities arising from loss of hepatocyte function are generally mild in the early stages, and patients present with complaints that are relatively nonspecific, such as malaise, nausea, mild abdominal pain, and lack of appetite. The health care provider needs to be vigilant about the possibility that such complaints are a sign of liver disease rather than just "the flu." Only in extremely severe (e.g., fulminant) cases of acute hepatitis, or after many years of gradual loss of hepatocytes (e.g., due to alcoholic liver injury or other chronic inflammatory disorders) are sufficient hepatocytes lost to compromise the ability of the liver to carry out its daily functions.

A second group of consequences of liver disease includes those that are due to alteration in liver hemodynamics, that is, the physics of liver blood flow. These alterations result in diversion of blood around, rather than through, the liver. This is termed ***portal-to-systemic shunting*** and is of prime importance in the pathophysiology of many of the complications of cirrhosis.

Studies suggest that the reason for altered hemodynamics is abnormal collagen production by the stellate cell of the reticuloendothelial system. This creates a "basement membrane" in the liver sinusoids which normally do not have such a structure. This "scar tissue" disrupts both the low-pressure flow and the efficient extraction of substrates that characterize the normal liver parenchyma.

Review Questions

25. What are the five broad categories of liver disease? Describe the defining features of each.
26. How can a given agent of liver injury (e.g., drugs or viruses) have profoundly different manifestations in different individuals?
27. The clinical consequences of liver disease can be divided into those related to hepatocyte dysfunction and which other category?

7. CLINICAL ASSESSMENT OF DISORDERED LIVER FUNCTION BY COMPARISON TO NORMAL VALUES

Liver disease can be assessed by laboratory tests in two very different ways that are used clinically in different circumstances:

1. The level of certain enzymes in serum can be monitored as a direct indicator of hepatocyte death. These are often called "liver function tests," but, in fact, have nothing to do with liver function. Rather, they are enzymes that are normally present in the cytoplasm of hepatocytes. Their presence in the bloodstream indicates recent liver injury and hepatocyte necrosis. Examples are aspartate aminotransferase (abbreviated SGOT or AST), alanine aminotransferase (abbreviated SGPT or ALT), lactate dehydrogenase (abbreviated LDH), and alkaline phosphatase (Alk Phos).

2. Failure of the liver to carry out some of its functions is a sensitive indicator not only of the presence of liver disease, but also, in some cases, of the precise nature of the disorder. Thus a patient with an elevated level of conjugated bilirubin in the bloodstream may have an obstructive disorder (e.g., a gallstone or tumor blocking the hepatic duct, preventing excretion of conjugated bile). However, a patient with an elevated unconjugated bilirubin may have a hepatocellular problem (preventing bilirubin uptake and conjugation in the first place). Likewise the differences between the half-life of albumin (1-2 weeks) and clotting factors (a few hours in some cases) can sometimes allow an assessment of whether the liver disease is of very recent onset or is more likely to have been long-standing.

8. EFFECTS OF LIVER DISEASE ON HOMEOSTASIS

Liver capacity for energy metabolism

Loss of liver capacity for energy metabolism due to insufficient viable hepatocytes manifests as hypoglycemia (due to an inability to maintain an adequate level of glycogen or capacity for gluconeogenesis to maintain blood glucose). This is an end-stage event in liver disease and such patients are usually moribund. However, aberration in liver energy metabolism due to portal hypertension can occur much earlier in the course of liver disease, because of inability of the liver to efficiently clear portal blood of absorbed glucose after a meal (from blood bypassing the liver via collateral veins). This usually manifests as mild to moderate postprandial hyperglycemia.

Defects in biliary function as indicators of liver disease

Defective biliary tract function can often be a sensitive indicator of liver disease. One readily detectable way this can manifest is **jaundice** (a yellow discoloration of the eyes and mucous membranes). This occurs as a result of rising bilirubin, a pigment generated in the breakdown of heme released from old red blood cells, which is normally removed from the bloodstream via the biliary system.

Patients in whom jaundice is due to a disruption of bile flow may present with steatorrhea (fat loss in stool) and with deficiency in fat-soluble vitamins, because bile salts are necessary for absorption of these nutrients from the bowel (see Chap. 5). Of the fat-soluble vitamins, vitamin K is distinctive because its deficiency results in formation of inactive clotting factors by the liver. As a result, patients with vitamin K deficiency are at increased risk of bleeding.

It is important to recognize the distinction between a patient with liver disease bleeding because of a defect in solubilization and one bleeding because of insufficient synthesis of clotting-factor protein. The former condition is common, often occurring early in the course of end-stage liver disease (especially if the patient is somewhat malnourished), and can be corrected by injection of vitamin K (thereby bypassing the defective biliary flow in the GI tract). However, bleeding because of insufficient synthesis of clotting-factor protein, is rare except for patients with fulminant hepatic failure or the very end stages of cirrhosis. The only way to correct bleeding from lack of sufficient hepatic factor synthesis is by infusion of functional clotting factors. This is quite expensive and only done if the patient is experiencing active, life-threatening bleeding.

Patients with biliary tract disease can develop intense itching due to accumulation in the bloodstream of bile acids and other substances normally removed in bile. These patients can also have abnormal deposition of fat in tissues (xanthomas), reflecting defective fat solubilization and transport.

Loss of protective functions

Long before patients have an insufficient number of functioning hepatocytes to carry out specific biochemical functions, they may develop loss of the protective functions (described in Sec. 4), as a consequence of portal hypertension. As portal pressure rises (e.g., due to repeated cycles of hepatocyte inflammation and necrosis, leading eventually to stellate cell activation and scar formation), the portal blood returns to the systemic circulation via varices. Besides the increased risk of bleeding (see Sec. 3), these pathologic changes in the plumbing result in the liver's failure to adequately carry out its protective functions (e.g., removal of ammonia and other toxins, activated clotting factors, and bacteria), not because the liver does not have the capacity to, but rather because blood simply no longer gets into the liver efficiently.

Thus, patients may have altered mental status from the toxic effect on the brain of ammonia and other compounds normally cleared by the liver. A telltale sign of such a metabolic cause of altered mental status (encephalopathy) is asterixis. This refers to the rhythmic, intermittent, jerking motion that occurs when the patient is asked to "hold up traffic" with hands extended. It can often also be seen when the patient sticks out his or her tongue. This is believed to be due to impairment in nerve conduction caused by the uncleared toxins.

The treatment for this condition makes physiological sense: First, the patient should avoid high levels of dietary protein, particularly protein from animal sources, because this may increase the ammonia load that the compromised liver must detoxify through the urea cycle.

Second, the patient should be put on lactulose, a nonabsorbable carbohydrate. Bacterial action on lactulose in the gut creates an acid environment, which keeps ammonia and other toxins in charged forms (e.g., NH^{4+} rather than NH^3) that do not cross the mucosal barrier as readily, thereby trapping them in the gut. Furthermore, lactulose breakdown by the colonic bacteria greatly increases its osmolarity, thereby drawing water into the colonic lumen and causing an osmotic diarrhea, which shortens transit time and speeds elimination of toxins and substrates from which toxins might otherwise be generated. Diarrhea is no fun, but it sure beats coma.

Third, patients with liver disease and portal hypertension are at high risk for the accumulation of fluid into the peritoneal cavity (termed *ascites*), which can be uncomfortable and can increase their risk of infection and other complications.

Loss of synthetic functions

An important question in the evaluation of a patient with liver disease is to determine whether the condition is acute or chronic. How can you tell? You can take advantage of the fact that the liver makes some proteins with a very short half-life (e.g., some of the clotting factors have a half-life of a few hours) and others with a relatively long half-life (e.g., albumin with a half-life of 1 to 2 weeks). If albumin is relatively normal but clotting parameters are abnormal, you will have a strong suspicion that the liver failure is relatively acute. If both are abnormal, it is likely to be a relatively chronic disease. The suspicion of chronic disease might be corroborated by changes on physical exam (e.g., vascular "spiders" or testicular atrophy in the male patient).

Review Questions

28. What do the "liver function tests" really tell you?
29. For each of the four broad categories of liver functions, describe how a patient with a disorder of those functions might be expected to present.

9. EFFECTS OF SYSTEMIC DISEASE ON THE LIVER

An assessment of the effects of systemic disease on the liver can provide the clinician with insight into the nature of the patient's disorder.

Effects on liver energy metabolism: alcoholism

In moderation, the direct effects of ethanol on the central nervous system can be pleasing. In contrast, in excess it is also a terrible toxin that harms essentially every organ in the body, especially the liver. The pathophysiological basis for liver injury in response to alcohol is still, fundamentally, a mystery. However, there are a lot of interesting hypotheses that make sense and that are supported by one line of evidence or another. Most likely, all of these contribute to alcoholic liver disease, depending on the genetic makeup of the individual, exposure to other toxins, and probably aspects of normal liver physiology that we are not aware of today.

Alcohol is a protein denaturant. It also alters membrane fluidity and, hence, membrane properties and functions. This may account for short-term effects.

Alcohol is metabolized by phase I enzymes into the far more reactive and dangerous compound **acetaldehyde**. This is believed to cause peroxidation of lipids, permanently altering their function, and covalent modification of proteins that render them not only dysfunctional but "foreign" by the immune system. The resultant inflammatory response results in acute alcoholic hepatitis, that is, liver inflammation. Repeated episodes of such acute inflammation result in a change in the pattern of gene expression in the liver, with increased collagen production, much like what occurs upon scar formation. This is probably the result of both inflammatory cytokines and direct effects of ethanol to induce collagen gene expression, resulting in hepatic fibrosis. Fibrosis, in turn, alters the physics of blood flow through the liver, with its resultant metabolic consequences.

Alcohol metabolism generates a lot of calories compared to carbohydrate (7 versus 4 kcal/g, respectively), almost as much as fat (9 kcal/g). This means that massive alcohol ingestion will tremendously distort hepatic intermediary metabolism. For example, the NAD^+ will be tied up as NADH, as alcohol dehydrogenase tries desperately to metabolize acetaldehyde to acetate. Because of such alterations and consequent changes in the levels of ATP in the cell, the normal setpoints that govern intracellular metabolism do not respond properly, resulting in chaos. The excess calories are converted into fat, but the liver's ability to export that fat as lipoproteins seems to be impaired, causing so-called alcoholic "fatty liver." The full extent to which signal transduction is altered in response to these metabolic derangements is only beginning to be discovered.

Finally, as if that were not enough, the increased oxygen consumption needed to oxidize ethanol may lead to hypoxia of zone 3 hepatocytes (see Concepts of Liver Organization in Sec. 2), further exacerbating liver injury.

Effects on the synthetic function: starvation

A patient with profound protein-calorie malnutrition may develop hypoalbuminemia or fatty liver even without a specific liver disorder. This is because the synthetic capacity of the liver depends not only on adequate energy generation, but on sufficient amounts of amino acids as well. In the absence of enough amino acids to make lipoproteins, the fat cannot be mobilized out of the liver, even in a person who is starving.

Effects on the protective functions: sepsis

Cytokines (polypeptide mediators of immune system functions) released by the reticuloendothelial cells of the liver may result in damage of nearby hepatocytes. This has been proposed as an explanation for the jaundice and hyperbilirubinemia often observed during overwhelming systemic infections (a syndrome termed *sepsis*), even when they do not involve infection in the liver.

Effects on biliary functions of the liver: autoimmune disease

Primary biliary cirrhosis is an autoimmune disease in which immune attack on bile ducts results in progressive loss of hepatocytes, scarring, regeneration, portal hypertension, and ultimately liver failure. Thus, in primary biliary cirrhosis, a systemic autoimmune disorder manifests as liver disease.

10. SIGNS AND SYMPTOMS IN LIVER DISEASE

Each of the disease manifestations discussed previously can be detected by the physical exam of patients with severe or chronic liver disease, although rarely will all findings manifest prominently in any one patient. Typically, different individuals will display prominence of one or two findings but not of others. Presumably this reflects features of the natural history of their particular disease process, or different genetic susceptibility to failure of one liver function versus another (see Table 4.4).

However, it is important to realize that early in the course of liver disease, there may be few or no specific physical findings and nothing that allows you to distinguish liver disease from the flu. The examining clinician often has to "ride a hunch" in ordering the test that makes the diagnosis. This involves the use of true clinical judgment, the art of medicine at its finest, identifying risk factors by taking a careful history. Ultimately, the most important role of normal physiological understanding of the liver is sometimes the simple recognition that there is no certain way to be sure whether a patient has early liver disease without blood studies for liver injury. The decision to order those tests depends on judgment that may not be readily

TABLE 4.4   PATHOPHYSIOLOGY OF SYNDROMES IN LIVER DISEASE

Syndromes of aberrant function in liver disease	Hepatocellular dysfunction	Portal-to-systemic shunting
Energy metabolism and substrate conversion		
Alcoholic hypoglycemia	✓	
Alcoholic ketoacidosis	✓	
Hyperglycemia		✓
Familial hypercholesterolemia	✓	
Hepatic encephalopathy	✓	✓
Fatty liver	✓	
Solubilization, transport, and storage function		
Reactions to drugs	✓	
Drug sensitivity	✓	✓
Steatorrhea	✓	✓
Fat-soluble vitamin deficiency	✓	✓
Hemochromatosis	✓	✓
Coagulopathy	✓	✓
Protein synthetic function		
Edema due to hypoalbuminemia	✓	
Protective and clearance functions		
Hypergammaglobulinemia		✓
Hypogonadism and hyperestrogenism	✓	✓
Renal dysfunction		
Sodium retention		✓
Impaired water excretion		✓
Impaired renal concentrating ability		✓
Deranged potassium metabolism		✓
Prerenal azotemia		✓
Acute renal failure		✓
Glomerulopathies		✓
Impaired renal acidification		✓
Hepatorenal syndrome		✓

From Lingappa, V. (1999). Liver disease. in McPhee, S. et al. eds. *Pathophysiology of Disease*, 3rd ed. New York, McGraw-Hill, p. 338.

determined by an algorithm, as is so trendy today.

11. PATHOPHYSIOLOGY OF ASCITES FORMATION IN LIVER DISEASE

Sometimes pathophysiological manifestations, such as ascites, provide insight into normal functions of the liver that we might not otherwise appreciate. So it is with ascites and the role of the liver in fluid homeostasis and renal function (see Chap. 8).

Liver disease with ascites formation occurs on a wide clinical spectrum. At one end is mild portal hypertension with no ascites present. Here the volume of ascites generated is less than the approximately 800 to 1200 mL daily capacity of the peritoneal lymphatic drainage, so the disorder is fully compensated by homeostatic mechanisms. At the other extreme is the so-called **hepatorenal syndrome**. This typically fatal condition, which occurs in patients with liver disease who usually have massive ascites, is one in which the patient succumbs to rapidly progressing acute renal failure. The hepatorenal syndrome seems to be precipitated by intense and inappropriate renal vasoconstriction. This syndrome is characterized by extreme sodium retention, as if the kidneys "thought" the body was severely volume depleted, in the absence of true volume depletion. Its pathophysiology remains poorly understood. Some of the following discussion of the pathophysiology of ascites formation may make more sense after you read Chapter 10 on fluid, electrolyte, and blood pressure regulation.

Over the years various mechanisms have been proposed to explain ascites formation (see Figure 4.9). Some hypotheses have proposed intravascular volume depletion, either real or "imagined" by the kidney, as a common theme in the pathophysiology of ascites. In this view, it is the underlying hemodynamic disorder that triggers reflex renal sodium re-

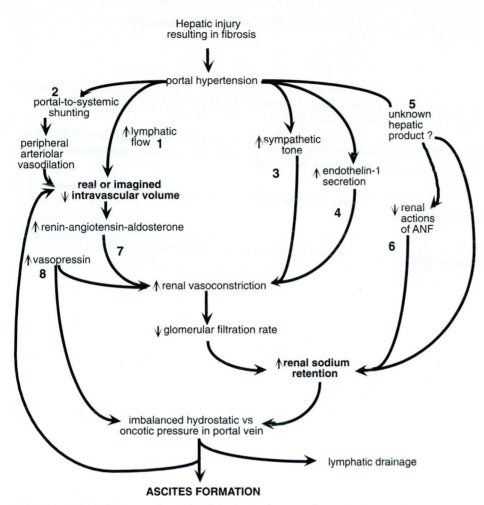

ASCITES FORMATION

FIGURE 4.9. Hypotheses on the pathophysiology of ascites formation in patients with liver disease. Hypotheses involving real or imagined intravascular volume depletion in triggering ascites formation. 1. "Underfilling" hypothesis; 2, peripheral vasodilation hypothesis. Hypotheses involving inappropriate increased renal sodium retention: 3, increased sympathetic tone; 4, increased endothelin-1 secretion; 5, unknown hepatic product working directly; 6, indirectly via antagonism of ANF, or mechanisms 3 or 4, to trigger renal sodium retention. Regardless of initiating mechanism, once ascites has formed, response to real or imagined intravascular volume depletion triggers 7 and 8. (*Adapted, with permission, from Lingappa, V.R. (1999). Liver disease. in McPhee, S. J. et al. eds.* Pathophysiology of Disease, *3rd ed. New York, McGraw-Hill, p. 358.*)

tention. Thus, elevated hepatic sinusoidal pressure results in "underfilling" of the central vein with diversion of intravascular volume to the hepatic lymphatics, which, like the central vein, drains the space of Disse. When this excess fluid exceeds the capacity of lymphatic drainage, **hydrostatic pressure** (the pressure of the fluid in the vessel) increases. The fluid can then be seen to visibly "weep" from the lymphatics and pool in the abdominal cavity as ascites.

Another hemodynamic hypothesis involves portal-to-systemic shunting in liver disease. With shunting, vasodilatory products (e.g., nitric oxide) that are normally cleared by the liver are instead delivered to the systemic circulation. There they cause peripheral arteriolar vasodilation, decreased renal arterial perfusion and reflex renal arterial vasoconstriction, and increased renal tubular sodium resorption. Retention of sodium expands the intravascular volume, which exacerbates portal venous hypertension. The imbalance between hydrostatic versus **oncotic pressure** (the tendency of proteins in plasma to hold fluid in the vessel) in the portal vein results in ascites formation, as described earlier.

In contrast to these views, others have proposed that inappropriate renal sodium retention, rather than a hemodynamic disorder, is the crucial early event in the development of ascites. In this view, ascites is the consequence of "overflow" from the intravascular volume expanded portal system. But what triggers the inappropriate renal sodium retention in the first place?

One possibility is that there may exist a hepatorenal reflex by which elevated sinusoidal pressure triggers increased sympathetic tone or secretion of the hormone **endothelin-1**. Either of these pathways could cause an inappropriate degree of renal vasoconstriction, a fall in glomerular filtration rate and, by tubuloglomerular feedback, sodium retention. Note that **endothelin-1** is both a renal vasoconstrictor and a stimulant of epinephrine secretion. Epinephrine, in turn, stimulates more endothelin-1 secretion.

Alternatively, it is possible that an as yet unidentified product from the diseased liver interferes with atrial naturetic factor action at the kidney or in some other way is responsible for an inappropriate increase in renal sodium retention. Regardless of the initial inciting event, once ascites formation has occurred, intravascular volume depletion will develop and trigger activation of both the renin-angiotensin-aldosterone system and vasopressin as mechanisms of compensation through sodium and water retention, respectively.

No single hypothesis of pathogenesis easily explains all findings, at all points in time, during the natural history of portal hypertension. Most likely, multiple mechanisms can contribute to the development of ascites and to its perpetuation, worsening, or improvement in diverse clinical situations. In any patient, depending on genetic, environmental, and other factors, including where the patient is at in the natural history of liver disease, one mechanism may dominate over others.

An important development has been the use of TIPS (transhepatic intrajugular portal to systemic shunting) as a means of decompressing the portal vein in patients with ascites. Although encephalopathy can be a problem in some, most patients have a remarkable improvement in the degree of accumulation of ascites. As a result of the procedure, peripheral arteriolar vasodilation appears to increase (perhaps due to shunting of vasodilators such as nitric oxide that are normally cleared by the liver), yet ascites is generally dramatically improved. This finding suggests that arteriolar vasodilation is not the primary precipitant of ascites formation, although it may nevertheless be a contributor. Other studies suggest a role for a sympathetic neural reflex as a trigger of renal sodium retention in response to elevated portal sinusoidal pressure, which would be relieved by TIPS. Regardless of the initial events, once fully established, many if not all of the mechanisms described in Figure 4.9 are likely to contribute to ascites formation.

Review Questions

30. Why do alcoholics often develop "fatty liver"?
31. Describe the mechanism of ascites formation.

12. FRONTIERS IN THE STUDY OF LIVER DISEASE

Our understanding of the normal and the diseased liver is in flux. We are constantly learning new things. Here are some areas in which research on the liver is advancing in ways that promise to affect our understanding of liver physiology, pathophysiology, and treatment of disease.

Mechanisms of hepatic fibrosis

Fibrosis is one of the hallmarks of chronic liver injury culminating in cirrhosis. It is useful to think of this process as similar to the development of a scar: an excessive deposition of extracellular matrix proteins, compared to what used to be there before the injury. Evidence strongly suggests that the **stellate cell** is the main source of extracellular matrix in liver injury.

Normally, stellate cells store vitamin A, although their normal function is not well understood. They reside in the subendothelial space, which normally contains a low density of extracellular matrix proteins. In chronic liver injury stellate cells are **activated**. Once activated, perhaps in part through communication with Kupffer cells, a stellate cell loses its vitamin A and starts to secrete high concentrations of extracellular matrix proteins. At the same time, other changes characteristic of cirrhosis occur (loss of hepatocyte microvilli and sinusoidal fenestrations). Together, these changes lead to increased resistance to portal blood flow resulting in portal hypertension. Studies are underway to better understand the process of stellate cell activation, the key early event in hepatic fibrosis. Such an understanding may make possible new prevention and treatment strategies for patients with chronic liver disease (see Refs. 2 and 10).

Mechanisms of hepatic carcinogenesis

All forms of liver disease, but especially chronic hepatitis B and C infection, are associated with increased risk of developing hepatocellular carcinoma. Epidemiological studies suggest that patients with chronic hepatitis B or C and cirrhosis have a 1000 times greater incidence of hepatocellular carcinoma than those in the same population without chronic hepatitis B or C. It has been estimated that up to 80% of cases of this malignancy, the eighth most common cancer in the world, occur in patients with chronic hepatitis B infection. Patients with chronic hepatitis B infection typically express a variety of gene products including the protein encoded by the "X" gene, a viral gene. Studies have suggested the possibility that, in at least a subset of patients, coding sequences of the "X" gene product may bind to, and interfere with, the functioning of p53, a tumor suppressor gene product. Inactivation of p53 is known to be a cause of many human cancers. Moreover, an increased incidence in mutations in p53, which inactivates the tumor suppressor, is seen in patients with chronic hepatitis B and in patients exposed to the potent hepatic carcinogen aflatoxin. These mechanisms may provide an explanation for the association between hepatitis B and liver cancer. Eventually, these insights, if proved correct, may result in developing a means of preventing liver cancer in patients with chronic hepatitis B and C infection (see Refs. 4 and 5).

New insights into hepatic regeneration

One of the remarkable features of the liver is its ability, after either extensive damage (e.g., fulminant hepatitis A) or actual removal (partial hepatectomy), to regenerate itself with normal histology and architecture. In recent years the roles of various products from hepatocytes, nonparenchymal cells of the liver, and products delivered to the liver via the bloodstream have been recognized as important contributors to hepatic regeneration. Included in this list of hepatic growth regulators are complete mitogens, comitogens, and growth inhibitors. Complete mitogens are products such as cytokines (including hepatocyte growth factor) that are by themselves capable of stimulating DNA synthesis and mitosis of otherwise quiescent hepatocytes. Comitogens enhance the effect of complete mitogens or diminish the effect of growth inhibitors, but alone are not capable of stimulating DNA synthesis and mitosis. They include various hormones, neurotransmitters, and nutrients. Growth inhibitors that can prevent DNA synthesis and mitosis include transforming growth factor β (see Table 4.5). An area of intensive investigation is to understand how these various classes of growth factors interact with parenchymal and nonparenchymal cells of the liver, with the extracellular matrix and with other agents to initiate and control the

TABLE 4.5 GROWTH REGULATORS OF HEPATIC REGENERATION

Growth stimulatory factors
  Hepatocyte growth factor
  Transforming growth factor-α
  α Fibroblast growth factor
  Epidermal growth factor
  Hepatocyte stimulating substance
  Insulin-like growth factors
  Tumor necrosis factor

Hormones, neurotransmitters, nutrients, immunosuppressive drugs
  Insulin
  Glucagon
  Catecholamines
  Steroids
  Calcium
  Vitamin D
  Parathyroid hormone
  Triiodothyronine
  Vasopressin
  Angiotensin
  Prolactin
  Estradiol
  Ions
  Cyclosporine
  FK-506
  Azathioprine (in selected cases)
  FKBP (receptor for FK-506 and Rapamycin)
  15-Deoxyspergualin
  Prostaglandins

Growth inhibitory factors
  Transforming growth factor β
  Regenerating liver inhibitory factor-1
  Rapamycin
  Interleukins 1, 2, and 6

Adapted from Hoffman, A.L. et al. (1994). Hepatic regeneration: current concepts. *Sem. Liver Dis*. 14:190.

process of regeneration (see Figure 4.10). Such an understanding may eventually make it possible to regenerate a normal liver in many conditions currently remedied only by hepatic transplantation. Studies using a "knockout" mouse lacking the gene for the cytokine interleukin 6 has demonstrated its crucial role in hepatic regeneration and its

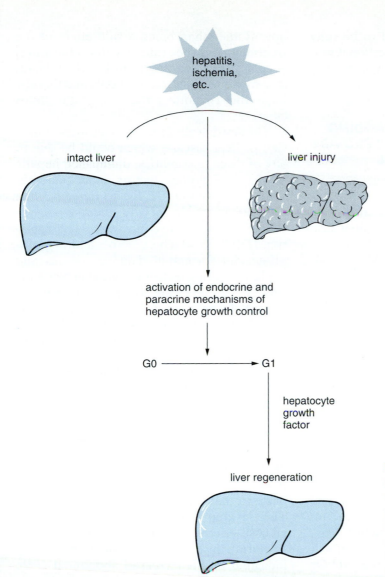

FIGURE 4.10. Events in hepatic regeneration. Actue liver injury triggers proliferation of hepatocytes through endocrine and paracrine mechanisms involving transition from resting G0 state to G1. *(Adapted, with permission, from Hoffman, A.L. et al. (1994). Hepatic regeneration: current concepts. Sem. Liver Dis. 14:190.)*

potential for therapeutic use (see Refs. 7 and 8).

Prospects for human gene therapy

By using recombinant DNA methods, it is now possible, in the laboratory, to take hepatocytes from an animal, introduce various new genes into those cells in culture by any of several methods of transfection, and then inject the transfected hepatocytes into the portal vein from which they can colonize the liver. In this way, defective liver genes in individual patients can, in principle, be corrected or replaced. Before these strategies are generally applied to human disease, however, a number of technical improvements need to be made and concerns regarding risks of the procedure need to be fully addressed (e.g., potential for insertional mutagenesis when using retroviral vectors; see Refs. 9 to 11.

13. HOW DOES AN UNDERSTANDING OF NORMAL PHYSIOLOGY PROVIDE INSIGHT INTO THE INITIAL CASE PRESENTATION?

Let us now look at J. S., the 46-year-old patient with alcoholic cirrhosis (see initial case presentation in Sec. 1).

You should now realize that Mr. S.'s altered mental status is most likely due to loss of a key protective function of the liver, namely, filtering toxins from portal blood, resulting in hepatic encephalopathy. The observation of asterixis strongly supports this explanation over the myriad of other causes of altered mental status (e.g., Might he have been hit on the head? Might he be drunk or on drugs?).

The bigger problem is the cause of the increased toxins: It probably was a protein load greater than his liver could handle, given portal to systemic shunting and diminished hepatocyte reserve. However, which of several possible protein loads? That double cheeseburger (these patients need to be on strict low-protein diets)? GI bleeding (e.g., from esophageal varices), which in itself will drop a protein load (blood) into the gut? Or infection (which will create a catabolic state with increased protein breakdown in various organs including muscle)? Mr. S. needs to be admitted to the hospital for several reasons. First, because he is in a coma, a condition requiring close monitoring and the cause of which needs to be determined, but also because if he is in hepatic coma it could be due to life-threatening bleeding or infection, not just dietary protein intoxication.

The diarrhea he had had earlier in the week was probably due to his lactulose ther-

apy. Rather than being a side effect of the treatment, diarrhea (along with acidification) is central to the mechanism by which lactulose works to eliminate ammonia and thereby keep the cirrhotic patient's mental status clear.

The clotting abnormality is another telltale sign of liver disease, which could be due to any of three possibilities: diminished hepatic synthesis of clotting factors, inadequate absorption of vitamin K due to defective bile production, or the poorly understood syndrome of disseminated intravascular coagulation (DIC), in which excessive and inappropriate clot formation damages organs and depletes clotting factors resulting in bleeding. This grave situation develops more frequently in patients with liver disease, perhaps because the normal role of the liver in clearing activated clotting factors is impaired and because patients with liver disease are at greater risk of systemic infection (sepsis), of which DIC is a dreaded complication.

The abnormal white blood cell count is a further sign that the patient may have a systemic infection brewing, for which he is likely to be at increased risk, since he has lost the protective function of the liver in clearing bacteria that breach the GI mucosal barrier. The elevated blood glucose reflects impaired glucose clearance from the portal vein due to portal hypertension, as does the ascites indicated by his increased abdominal girth. The edema suggests that the patient's synthetic functions are also affected with a low albumin and diminished plasma oncotic pressure.

What are you going to do for this patient? He would most likely be admitted to the hospital. In view of his altered mental status and your concerns about systemic infection, you will want to take a sample of his blood, cerebral spinal fluid, and ascites fluid for examination and culture (to be sure he does not have a bacterial infection). Perhaps you may even put him on antibiotics right away, stopping them when you are sure he is not infected. Knowing the other risks associated with portal hypertension (besides encephalopathy), you will monitor him closely for GI bleeding, determine whether his clotting abnormality responds to vitamin K, and treat his ascites and edema with mild diuretics. Once you are sure he does not have active GI bleeding, you would restart him on a low-protein diet and on lactulose therapy, which will resolve his encephalopathy over the next day (and will give him diarrhea).

You should now understand how each of these issues is related to the normal physiology of the liver in a patient with liver disease.

SUMMARY AND REVIEW OF KEY CONCEPTS

1. Implications of liver anatomy and histology, functional zonation; cell biology (fenestrations, polarized plasma membrane) for function and pathophysiology
2. The liver is involved in four broad categories of functions:

- Intermediary metabolism of carbohydrates, proteins, and fats (know the broad outlines of the pathways and how they are controlled)
- Synthesis of a wide range of serum proteins involved in many different endocrine and homeostatic pathways (know the main ones)
- Solubilization of various substances needed to be brought into or exported out of the body (know the main ones)
- Protection of the body from various toxins (know the broad categories of protection)

3. Important principles of normal liver function include the following:

- Functional zonation of hepatocytes

- Oxidation and conjugation steps of drug detoxification
- Functional differences between the apical and basolateral hepatocyte surfaces
- Capacity of hepatocytes to undergo regeneration
- Differences between liver sinusoids and capillaries in most other tissues (lack of a basement membrane; fenestrations allowing low-pressure blood percolation)
- Regulation of hepatic function by substrate concentration (thanks to the K_m of key liver enzymes such as glucokinase versus the isoforms found in other tissues)
- Regulation of hepatic function by hormones (such as insulin and glucagon) that affect transcription, translation, modification, activity, and degradation of enzymes
- Regulation of hepatic function by receptors (such as transferrin-transferrin-receptor interaction in iron homeostasis);
- Regulation of hepatic function by enzyme induction (e.g., in drug detoxification).

4. Liver disease generally results from the combination of consequences of the following:

- "Plumbing abnormalities" (i.e., bypass of blood around rather than through the liver) due to portal hypertension and intrahepatic scar formation
- Diminished hepatic function due to hepatocyte injury, inflammation, and necrosis.

A CASE OF PHYSIOLOGICAL MEDICINE

The patient is a 52-year-old man with a long history of alcohol abuse complicated by numerous prior bouts of alcoholic hepatitis and acute pancreatitis, until 8 years ago when he stopped all alcohol consumption. Since then, he was largely symptom free, although physical examination revealed evidence of chronic liver disease, and blood clotting studies demonstrated a mildly prolonged prothrombin time. For the latter reason he has been advised not to use aspirin for pain relief because it might exacerbate his tendency to bleed. Instead, he has always used small amounts of acetaminophen (Tylenol) for pain control. One year ago, he was mugged and Tylenol, in larger doses, effectively controlled the pain from his bruises and contusions.

Last month, he was laid off from work. Despondent, he returned to abusing alcohol. Two days ago, after a one-week drinking binge, he was again mugged as he staggered home from a bar. Since Tylenol so effectively treated his injuries one year ago, he self-instituted the same therapy again. Twenty-four hours later he was brought to the emergency room with altered mental status. Complete evaluation revealed evidence of fulminant hepatic necrosis with massive transaminase elevation and markedly worsened clotting parameters. His physicians assumed that the acute hepatic failure was a consequence of alcoholic liver disease and instituted supportive measures only. Luckily for the patient, he was seen by an astute third-year medical student who took a careful history from both the patient and his friends and discovered the recent acetaminophen use. The student sent a blood sample for Tylenol level, and suggested an appropriate therapy for acetaminophen toxicity. The patient rapidly improved on this therapy.

QUESTIONS

1a. What is the normal mechanism of drug detoxification by the liver?

1b. What aspects of the normal mechanism are altered in this case?

2. Explain why the patient had no adverse response one year ago to the same amount of acetaminophen, which this time re-

sulted in fulminant liver failure. Describe the mechanism at work.

3a. What mechanisms (involving functions of the liver) can you think of that would account for the mildly abnormal blood clotting parameters the patient demonstrated one year ago?

3b. How might you distinguish between these mechanisms of clotting abnormality in patients with mild blood clotting abnormalities associated with liver disease, as in this case?

4. Knowing the normal functions of the liver, what supportive measures would you institute while you waited for the patient to recover from his acute episode of hepatic necrosis?

5. Suppose that instead of going on a drinking binge, the patient developed a seizure disorder and was placed on the antiseizure medicine phenytoin, which is metabolized by the liver. Why might that have resulted in the same bad response to acetaminophen?

ANSWERS

1a. The normal mechanism of drug detoxification is phase I oxidation, which makes compounds more reactive (and often more toxic), followed by phase II modification, in which bulky, hydrophilic groups are attached to the reactive products to make them water soluble (and less toxic). The hydrophilic groups attached include glucuronic acid and glutathione, with different compounds being a substrate for different modifications, depending on their recognition by specific transferase enzymes.

1b. The patient has liver disease, so many functional hepatocytes are replaced by fibrotic scar tissue, hence there is a lower net capacity for drug detoxification and the patient is more sensitive to the loss or dysfunction of even a relatively small number of hepatocytes. The patient has been drinking acutely, which has induced the phase I enzymes. He is nutritionally deprived, so his stores of glutathione (made of amino acids) are likely to be depleted.

2. Acetaminophen is converted to a more toxic metabolite by phase I oxidation reactions carried out by cytochrome P450 enzymes, induced by ethanol ingestion. Thus, the patient's ability to activate acetaminophen to a more dangerous metabolite was out of proportion to his ability to complete its metabolism by conjugation to glutathione (due to the combination of progression of his underlying liver disease, enzyme induction, and possibly nutritional deprivation).

3a. Vitamin K deficiency due to either lack of bile or nutritional deprivation combined with liver disease; reduced levels of clotting factor protein synthesis due to liver disease (less likely).

3b. Improved clotting parameters after a few days of oral vitamin K suggests nutritional deprivation; response to parenteral vitamin K only suggests inadequate bile production; lack of response to either suggests a liver protein synthesis problem.

4. The supportive measures that should be instituted include the following:

- IV hydration with glucose containing solutions;
- lactulose to decrease ammonia absorption from the GI tract;
- parenteral vitamin K to correct the worsened bleeding parameters or clotting factor;
- transfusions if the patient has significant bleeding; and
- a close watch on the patient for early signs of sepsis, which would be treated with IV antibiotics.

5. The phenytoin will also induce phase I enzymes. The nutritional deprivation need not be due solely to his drinking binge. He could be not eating well due to poverty (remember he recently lost his job) or depression.

COMMENTS

A crucial aspect of good medical practice is meticulous attention to detail. A doctor who makes assumptions (e.g., once an alcoholic, always an alcoholic) or who neglects the possibility of a disorder (e.g., liver failure) in a susceptible individual that may be due to something other than or in addition to the obvious (e.g., Tylenol in addition to alcohol) is being careless and may do the patient grave harm (in this case, by not recognizing the need for instituting therapy for acetaminophen toxicity).

When you look at a patient, you need to simultaneously see the person from several perspectives: First, you need to objectively assess the evidence from the history, physical exam, and laboratory studies. Second, you need to put yourself in the patient's shoes and hear the person sympathetically and nonjudgmentally. This is the only way you can appreciate the person's pain and suffering. Finally, you need to step back and ask: Is my judgment being distorted by unconscious prejudices about the patient (e.g., because they are poor or smell or look bad)?

In this case, despite the fact that the third-year medical student was the least experienced, it was her meticulous attention to detail that was crucial in management of this patient's medical condition.

References and suggested readings

GENERAL REFERENCES

1. Achord, J.L. (1995). Alcohol and the liver. *Sci. Am. Sci. Med* March/April.

2. Friedman, S.L. (1993). The cellular basis of hepatic fibrosis. *N. Engl. J. Med.* 328:1828.

3. Michalopoulos, G.K., and DeFrances, M.C. (1997). Liver regeneration. *Sci.* 276:60-66.

4. Chang, A.G.Y., and Wu, G.Y. (1994) Gene therapy: Applications to the treatment of GI and liver diseases. *Gastro.* 106:1076.

5. Greenblatt, M.S. et al. (1997). Integrity of p53 in Hepatitis B X antigen-positive and negative hepatocellar carcinomas. *Cancer Res.* 57: 426-432.

6. Kim, S.-O. et al. (1996). Increased expression of IGF-1 receptor gene in hepatocellular carcinoma cell lines: Implications of IGF-1 receptor gene activation by HBV $\times$ gene product. *Cancer Res.* 56: 3831-3836.

7. Cressman, D.E. et al. (1996). Liver failure and defective hepatocyte regeneration in interleukin-6 deficient mice. *Sci.* 274:1379-1381.

8. Bautista, A.P. (1997). Chronic alcohol intoxication induces hepatic injury through enhanced macrophage inflammatory protein-2 production and intercellular adhesion molecule-1 expression in the liver. *Hepatol.* 25: 335-342.

9. Chowdhury, J.R. et al. (1991). Long-term improvement of hypercholesterolemia after ex vivo gene therapy in LDLR-deficient rabbits. *Sci.* 253:1802.

10. Ilan, Y. et al. (1997). Insertion of the adenoviral E3 region into a recombinant viral vector prevents antiviral humoral and cellular immune responses and permits long-term gene expression. *Proc. Natl. Acad. Sci. USA* 94: 2587-2592.

11. Nakamura J. et al. (1997). Treatment of surgically induced acute liver failure by transplantation of conditionally immortalized hepatocytes. *Transplantation* 63:1541-1547.

GASTROINTESTINAL PHYSIOLOGY

5

1. INTRODUCTION TO THE GASTROINTESTINAL TRACT

Why is understanding gastrointestinal physiology important for medical practice?

Gastrointestinal (GI) tract complaints, including abdominal pain, nausea and vomiting, difficulty swallowing, lack of appetite, diarrhea or constipation and weight loss (or gain), are among the most common reasons that patients seek medical attention. Some patients with these problems end up being highly unsatisfied with their health care provider. In a substantial number of these cases, a better appreciation of GI physiology (by both provider and patient) might have resulted in a more satisfactory medical encounter.

Serious illnesses of other organs can present as a GI problem (e.g., constipation in a patient with hypothyroidism, or bloody diarrhea due to ischemic colitis in a patient with cardiomyopathy and congestive heart failure). Conversely, GI disorders may be the true cause of symptoms initially assumed to reside elsewhere (e.g., chest pain due to esophageal disease rather than angina). The better your understanding of GI physiology, the less likely you are to be fooled in these and other situations.

The GI tract is more complex than many people realize (did you know there are more neurons in the GI tract than in the entire spinal cord?). An important frontier for future study is the way the GI tract interacts with other systems including the nervous system to produce so-called "functional" bowel disorders whereby patients (often with depression or other psychiatric disorders) may have GI symptoms in the absence of any apparent structural lesion.

Dietary modification is an important dimension of preventive health care. If followed by the population as a whole, this alone would greatly reduce the incidence of some of the current leading causes of morbidity and mortality, including cardiovascular disease, diverticular disease, and colon cancer. Perhaps if health care providers understood what is currently known — and not known —

about the GI tract, they would pay more attention to this "environmental influence" on patients' well-being.

Clinical scenarios illustrating the importance of gastrointestinal physiology

A common problem in medicine is that sometimes things just happen too fast — and you can never recall the list you once memorized when you really need it. An alternative to memorizing lists you are going to forget anyway is based on the fact that it is often a lot easier to figure out what might be wrong when you understand how something is supposed to work. The GI tract is a great example, because the symptoms that bring patients to medical attention (pain, diarrhea or constipation, nausea/vomiting/difficulty swallowing, and bleeding) can have very different causes that can either take a long time to sort out or be quickly distinguished by the right questions and observations, based on an understanding of normal physiology. Consider the following:

You are just starting your shift as the sole physician in a busy emergency room. Usually, following standard etiquette, the preceding physician leaves a clean slate: no backup of patients waiting to be seen. Unfortunately, your shift today follows that of a doctor notorious for being slow, scattered, and inefficient — and for treating symptoms without adequate consideration for the pathophysiological cause. The result: The waiting room is overflowing with patients, some who have waited many hours, some who were treated for symptoms earlier and now are back because the underlying problem is getting worse, some who are potentially seriously ill, and all are very, very angry — and this is before the usual after-dinner surge of new patients. Acutely aware of the situation, the administrative staff starts panicking

at the increasing likelihood of a night from hell. All eyes are upon you. Calmly, you bid farewell to your fleeing colleague and survey the patients' complaints. It is quickly apparent that the preceding physician's problem is a lack of a systematic, physiological approach to GI disorders. Moving quickly from patient to patient, your knowledge of GI physiology leads you to ask questions your predecessor neglected and direct therapy to the underlying cause of the patients' symptoms.

For example, a history of prior ulcer surgery suggests to you the dumping syndrome in one patient with diarrhea, for whom you quickly prescribe dietary changes — and tear up the prescription for opiates given by the previous M.D. A patient with chest pain is rescued from admission to the cardiac care unit by a successful therapeutic swig of antacids — cured and out the door with a diagnosis of reflux esophagitis and a number of dietary and other recommendations. Another patient who has abdominal pain and was awaiting a consult from the surgeons is diagnosed as having failed prior treatment for ulcer disease, most likely because antibiotics weren't prescribed to eradicate *Helicobacter pylori* infection. His medical regimen is revised (and the expensive specialist consultation for which he had been referred is canceled). Three more patients with diarrhea are quickly sorted into likely infectious, osmotic and neuropathic causes and treated appropriately. Even more importantly, you identify two patients who have been more seriously misdiagnosed. The first has severe constipation, which turns out to be due to profound hypothyroidism. She needs thyroid hormone replacement — not just the regimen of enemas prescribed by the previous M.D. The second misdiagnosed patient is one with a metabolic acidosis who appears to have early signs of a life-threatening bowel obstruction. He needs an emergency consultation with a surgeon — not bicarbonate tablets as your colleague prescribed. Soon, all has been set right, and the emergency room is quiet. Less drugs have been sold, but more patients are satisfied, all thanks to your ability to put physiology into action.

Case Presentation

C. W., a 42-year-old administrative assistant, arrived at the hospital with dizziness. She told of a three-year history of intermittent burning pain in the upper abdomen, which was somewhat relieved by food. During this time she used antacids intermittently, with some relief. She frequently took nonsteroidal anti-inflammatory drugs such as ibuprofen both for dysmenorrhea and for tension headaches. She also said she drinks heavily on occasion, has smoked a pack of cigarettes per day for the last 10 years, and has a particular fondness for fancy chocolates ("I start on them right after breakfast"). She was a thin woman with mild upper abdominal tenderness. Tarry guaiac positive stool was found during the rectal exam. Routine laboratory studies were normal except for a complete blood count revealing a hematocrit of 30% (normal is 35 to 45%). Upper GI x-ray series showed normal stomach folds and upper small intestine, with a possible ulcer in the area of the pylorus, a finding confirmed subsequently on upper GI endoscopy, which also revealed scarring of the distal esophagus and moderate gastritis. Cultures of the stomach at that time were positive for *H. pylori*. Ms. W. was advised to change some of her habits and was placed on aggressive medical therapy for duodenal ulcer, with documented healing of the ulcer on repeat endoscopy 1 year later, at which time cultures were negative for *H. pylori*. Her therapeutic regimen was then changed to maintenance therapy with a single bedtime dose of a proton pump inhibitor.

2. OVERVIEW OF STRUCTURE AND FUNCTION IN THE GASTROINTESTINAL TRACT

The most obvious function of the GI tract is to: (a) separate ingested food into needed nutrients and wastes, and (b) absorb the former while getting rid of the latter. To successfully carry out these tasks, the GI tract has evolved a number of elaborate mechanisms involving four functions: motility, secretion, digestion, and absorption. Each of these functions manifests slightly differently in different portions of the GI tract, starting from the mouth and oropharynx and progressing through the esophagus, stomach, small intestine, and large intestine (see Figure 5.1). In some of these regions one of these functions takes on a prominence that is not seen in the other regions.

We will first consider the structure and function of the GI tract as a whole, establishing certain concepts that are recurrent themes, and then consider the nuances that distinguish one part of the GI tract from the other.

Structure

The GI tract is a long tube with a continuous lumen from mouth to anus (see Figure 5.1). The various parts of the GI tract display unique structural features in one or more of these layers, which allow them to carry out specialized functions under neural and hormonal control. In addition, the liver, gallbladder, and pancreas provide secretions that feed via specialized ducts into the GI lumen, and thus can be considered accessory organs of the GI tract.

Histologically the wall of the GI tract is comprised of four layers. From the lumen outward these are the mucosa, the submucosa, the muscularis, and the serosa (see Figure 5.2).

The mucosa is the innermost layer of the

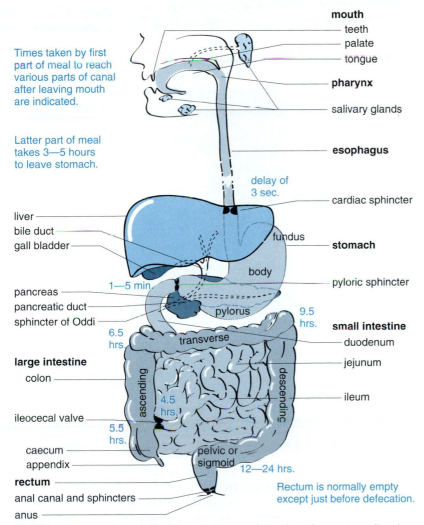

Times taken by first part of meal to reach various parts of canal after leaving mouth are indicated.

Latter part of meal takes 3—5 hours to leave stomach.

mouth
teeth
palate
tongue
pharynx
salivary glands

esophagus

delay of 3 sec.
cardiac sphincter

liver
bile duct
gall bladder
fundus
stomach
body
pyloric sphincter

1—5 min.
pancreas
pancreatic duct
sphincter of Oddi
pylorus
9.5 hrs.
small intestine
duodenum
6.5 hrs.
transverse
jejunum

large intestine
colon
ascending
descending
ileum

ileocecal valve
4.5 hrs.
5.5 hrs.
caecum
appendix
pelvic or sigmoid
12—24 hrs.
rectum
anal canal and sphincters
Rectum is normally empty except just before defecation.
anus

FIGURE 5.1. Transit through the GI tract. Times indicate how long it typically takes food to pass the indicated point after ingestion. *(Adapted, with permission, from Mackenna B.R., and Callander R. (1990). Illustrated Physiology, 5th ed. New York, Churchill Livingstone, p. 65.)*

GI tract, in contact with the contents of the lumen. The mucosa is the direct site of secretion, absorption, and even some digestion.

The submucosa contains connective tissue that supports the mucosa structurally. The submucosa also contains other cells, as well as glands, which provide valuable secretions that maintain, assist, and otherwise influence the functions of the mucosa.

The muscularis contains an inner circular muscle layer that upon contraction makes the cross-section of the lumen smaller, and an outer longitudinal muscle layer whose contraction shortens the length of the GI tract. Together these muscle layers make possible the various motility programs of the GI tract.

The serosa is the outer covering of the GI

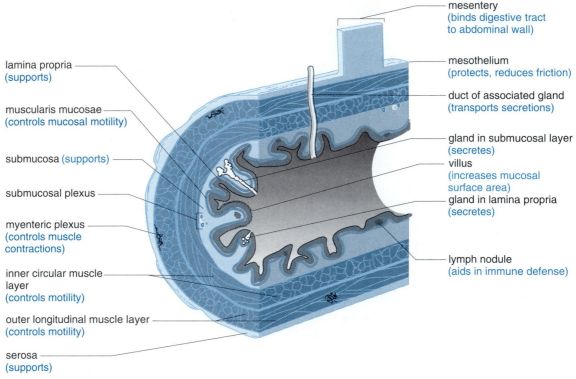

lamina propria
(supports)

muscularis mucosae
(controls mucosal motility)

submucosa (supports)

submucosal plexus

myenteric plexus
(controls muscle
contractions)

inner circular muscle
layer
(controls motility)

outer longitudinal muscle layer
(controls motility)

serosa
(supports)

mesentery
(binds digestive tract
to abdominal wall)

mesothelium
(protects, reduces friction)

duct of associated gland
(transports secretions)

gland in submucosal layer
(secretes)

villus
(increases mucosal
surface area)

gland in lamina propria
(secretes)

lymph nodule
(aids in immune defense)

FIGURE 5.2. Schematic of a cross-section of the GI tract, indicating some typical components.

tract. At the intestines, the serosa is continuous with the peritoneum.

Motility

Motility in the GI tract is achieved as a result of the intrinsic contractility of its smooth muscle under the influence of neural input and hormonal control. The result is a series of programmed responses (e.g., peristalsis) that allow delivery of material from one part of the GI tract to another and (generally) not in the opposite direction. The frequency, direction, and distance of propagation of muscle contraction, as well as the determination of when a contraction can occur, are controlled by an oscillating sodium pump in GI tract smooth muscle. The action of this pump results in the intrinsic contractility of the smooth muscle in the GI tract and is characterized by what is called *slow wave* electrical activity.

Certain smooth muscle cells serve as **pacemakers** in the proximal part of the distal stomach, proximal duodenum, and midcolon. By their spontaneous electrical activity, these cells determine the intrinsic frequency of slow waves in these regions (see Disorders of Motility in Sec. 11). The actual initiation of contraction is caused by a second form of electrical activity: spike action potentials in response to either stretch, neural, or hormonal impulses (see Figure 5.3). Long bursts of spikes (depolarization due to increased membrane conductance of calcium) cause tonic muscle contraction. **Sphincters** are specialized regions of the GI tract where such protracted bursts of spike action potentials

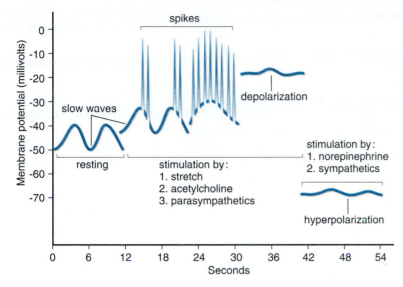

FIGURE 5.3. Membrane potentials in intestinal smooth muscle. Slow waves are intrinsic to the GI tract smooth muscle. Superimposed on the slow waves are spikes that exceed the threshold for depolarization (indicated to the right), in response to stretch, acetylcholine and parasympathetic stimulation, and result in muscle contraction. In contrast, physiological sympathetic nervous system stimulation results in hyperpolarization and inhibition of GI tract motility. *(Adapted, with permission, from Guyton A.C. and Hall J.E. (1996). Textbook of Medical Physiology, 9th ed. Philadelphia, W.B. Saunders, p. 794.)*

occur. As a result, sphincters are usually contracted (closed), but relax (open) from time to time, usually in a highly regulated fashion. This is in contrast to most of the rest of the tube that makes up the GI tract, between sphincters, where short bursts of spikes cause transient contraction resulting in phasic motor activity.

The degree of **central nervous system** (CNS) control over gut motility also varies from region to region of the GI tract:

- Striated muscle seen in the mouth, pharynx, and proximal esophagus is under direct CNS control.
- The small intestine is almost totally independent of the CNS.
- The stomach, colon, and distal esophagus are under partial CNS control.

Regardless of the extent of CNS versus hormonal control, neurons in the GI tract that are part of the enteric nervous system (ENS) are the final common pathway by which instructions are given to the muscular and glandular structures of the gut.

The ENS is composed of two **plexuses** (groups) of nerves, one of which, termed the **myenteric plexus**, directs gut motility. The other, termed the **submucosal plexus**, is involved in the control of intestinal secretion (see later). The myenteric plexus has two programmed responses, **segmented** and **peristaltic**. The segmented program, involving to-and-fro mixing, predominates in the postprandial period. The peristaltic program dominates during fasting. Program selection is determined by hormonal, neural, and other factors and manifests in different ways in the various parts of the GI tract.

Secretion

Secretion in the GI tract involves the diverse processes by which water, ions, and proteins are exported out of cells. It is remarkable for both its magnitude and diversity: In a typical day, the human body makes over 1.5 liters of saliva, 2.5 liters of gastric juice, 0.5 liter of bile, 1.5 liters of pancreatic juice, and 1.0 liter of intestinal secretions. The fluid produced in different parts of the GI tract displays tremendous variation in both ionic and macromolecular composition. Moreover, while some GI secretions are directed into the lumen of the GI tract, others are secreted into the bloodstream.

Certain epithelial cells lining the GI tract lumen, or comprising ducts that are contiguous with and draining into the lumen, are specialized to secrete large volumes of fluid. Depending on the region of the GI tract, this fluid may contain acid or base, digestive enzymes or binding proteins. Normally these processes are set to maintain homeostasis. At one extreme of GI tract secretory dysfunction, a patient with cholera can have a volume of as much as 30 L or more of stool water daily. In this case, secretions from the small intestine are far in excess of the absorptive capacity of the colon, resulting in life-threatening diarrhea and dehydration. At the other extreme, a patient with hypothyroidism may present with profound constipation, not having had a bowel movement in weeks, due to the combination of defective motility and secretion, in the absence of thyroid hormone (see Chap. 12).

Transport

Several mechanisms can be used to transport substances in the GI tract. Ions as well as small charged molecules such as amino acids, small peptides, and sugars are moved directly across the epithelial plasma membrane via **transporters**. These transport processes may be driven by diffusion, facilitated diffusion, and active transport.

Only active transport requires metabolic energy, by which it is able (e.g., such as ATP hydrolysis), to move substances against a concentration gradient. Active transport can be of two sorts, either **primary** (where energy from ATP hydrolysis is used to transport a specific molecule directly across the membrane) or **secondary** (where transport of one substance is coupled to that of another).

An example of primary active transport is the role of H^+/K^+ ATPase in secreting acid in the stomach. An example of secondary active transport is the coupling of monosaccharide and amino acid uptake to the Na^+ gradient established by Na^+/K^+ ATPase in the small intestine.

For large molecules such as proteins, transport is via pinching-off/fusion of membrane vesicles from/with the plasma membrane. These processes are termed **endocytosis** (uptake into) and **exocytosis** (export out of) epithelial cells.

Generally, structures in the first part of the GI tract (e.g., mouth, stomach, and pancreas) are more involved in secretion (e.g., of saliva, acid and mucus, bicarbonate and digestive enzymes, respectively). Conversely, structures in the latter part of the GI tract (e.g., small and large intestine) are more involved in absorption (e.g., of products of digestion and of water, respectively). In the small intestine, epithelial cells of the vilus tip are prominently involved in absorption while those of the crypts are involved in secretion.

The submucosal plexus of nerves of the ENS serve to tonically inhibit fluid and electrolyte secretion and limit the absorptive capacity of the intestines. These effects are mediated by neurotransmitters released by the motor neurons, which interact with receptors on intestinal epithelial cells to influence the functional state of the ion channels through which electrolytes pass.

Digestion

Digestion is a potentially dangerous process because it involves breakdown of substances very similar to what the body is made of. As you might expect, the GI tract has multiple lines of defense against autodigestion (see later). Moreover, since the amount and composition of meals vary, there are reflex mechanisms to modify digestion to accommodate the composition of a particular meal.

The underlying mechanism of most digestion is hydrolysis, the breaking up of large molecules of carbohydrate, lipid, and protein into their components by insertion of H^+ and OH^- ions derived from water. Because their structures are distinct, different types of carbohydrates, lipids, and proteins use different enzymes as catalysts of this fundamental chemical reaction. Some of the enzymes to carry out hydrolysis are located in the GI tract lumen, secreted by the pancreas (see Pancreas and Gallbladder in Sec. 5), while other digestive enzymes are part of the plasma membrane of **enterocytes**, the epithelial cells that make up the mucosal surface of the GI tract. Most digestion occurs in the small intestine.

Absorption

Absorption as it occurs in the GI tract solves two remarkable problems:

- How to reclaim the enormous volume of fluid, approximately 9 L, entering or secreted into the lumen of the GI tract each day. From this daily input of fluid, approximately 100 mL ends up in stool daily, with the balance recycled back to the body.
- How to recognize specific nutrients, some of them present in only trace quantities, and to absorb them selectively and efficiently. The molecular mechanisms by which this is carried out are multifaceted, involving active, passive, and coupled transport.

Review Questions

1. What are the layers of the GI tract viewed in cross-section?
2. Name some landmarks along the length of the GI tract.
3. What are the four broad processes through which the GI tract carries out its primary functions?
4. What determines the intrinsic frequency of slow waves in GI tract smooth muscle?
5. To what extent does the CNS exert control over the GI tract?
6. What classes of products does the GI tract secrete? Where do these secretions come from and go to? What are their approximate volumes from each source?
7. What two problems does the GI tract solve in the course of its absorptive functions?

3. OROPHARYNX AND ESOPHAGUS

Anatomic organization and histologic characteristics

The **oropharynx** is the place where several orifices intersect, providing entry to either the GI or respiratory tracts, depending on whether swallowing or breathing is the desired activity. It also includes the vocal cords, which serve a crucial role in the separation of respiratory and ingestion-related activity and provide the structural basis for speech. Much of the oropharynx is lined with a respiratory-type ciliated pseudocolumnar epithelium.

The **esophagus** is a hollow muscular tube that connects the pharynx to the stomach. Lined with a stratified squamous epithelium, its muscular wall is notable for the transition from striated (first one-third of the length starting from the pharynx) to smooth muscle (latter two-thirds of the length from pharynx to stomach). A key functional feature is the lower esophageal sphincter (LES) at the transition from low-pressure (intrathoracic) to high-pressure (intraabdominal) sections of the GI tract. The LES remains closed due to tonic contractions intrinsic to its smooth muscle, thereby keeping acidic stomach contents out of the esophagus. Specialized neural control governs relaxation of the LES to allow passage of food into the stomach during swallowing.

Physiological role of the oropharynx: swallowing

The major role of the oropharynx is swallowing: to get food into the esophagus without some of it ending up in the lungs or coming back out the nose. After mixing of food is initiated in the oropharynx (i.e., chewing), swallowing involves the following set of events:

1. A bolus of material is directed posteriorly by the tongue and muscles of the mouth, under voluntary control.
2. Involuntary peristaltic contractions of the pharyngeal muscles take over. The upper esophageal sphincter opens and the bolus of food is propelled into the esophagus.
3. Simultaneously, the larynx is protected from food entry by involuntary forward and upward movement of the cricoid cartilage and approximation of the vocal cords. All of the involuntary events are coordinated by an interplay of CNS and ENS.
4. Entry of the bolus of food into the esophagus is accompanied by a primary peristaltic wave and, if necessary to move the bolus, a secondary peristaltic wave.

Clinical Pearl

○ The importance of oropharyngeal motility is seen when it is lost, as in patients who have suffered a stroke or are demented. Aspiration pneumonia is a polymicrobial lung infection as a result of inhaling food or secretions (including vomited material). This common consequence of failure to properly coordinate breathing and swallowing is due to impaired oropharyngeal motility. This is a final common pathway of death in many elderly and chronically ill patients. Proper positioning (i.e., sitting the patient up or on the side), so that gravity does not favor aspiration, is a crucial nursing measure in the care of these patients.

Esophageal motility

Peristalsis is the dominant motor program of the esophagus. Primary peristalsis in the esophagus is initiated by the act of swallowing with a reflexly relaxed upper esophageal sphincter. Esophageal peristalsis involves a progressive wave of ringlike smooth muscle contractions that propels food down to the LES. Once triggered by swallowing, esophageal peristalsis will occur whether or not food is present, although the presence of food will intensify the peristaltic contractions. If the primary peristaltic wave fails to move food into the stomach, the persistence of the food bolus in the esophagus will set off secondary peristaltic waves to complete the job.

The upper esophageal sphincter is under acetylcholine-mediated CNS control.

The LES, like most sphincters, is tonically contracted. However, this tonic contraction can be influenced either to relax or to contract further, by hormonal and neural input (e.g., release of the neurotransmitters nitric oxide and vasoactive intestinal peptide, VIP, in response to the events triggered by swallowing).

A complex coordination between the ENS and the CNS swallowing center in the brainstem, via the vagus nerve, normally mediates reflex relaxation of the LES to allow passage of ingested food into the stomach. Various foods can increase (e.g., protein) or decrease (e.g., fat, ethanol, or chocolate) LES pressure (see Table 5.1). Presumably, foods that decrease LES are (directly or indirectly) triggering receptors that coincidentally connect

TABLE 5.1   FACTORS INFLUENCING LES PRESSURE

	Increase	**Decrease**

Hormones	Gastrin
	Motilin
	Substance P
		Secretin
		Cholecystokinin
		Glucagon
		Somatostatin
		Gastric inhibitory poly-
		  peptide (GIP)
		Vasoactive intestinal
		  polypeptide (VIP)
		Progesterone

Neural agents	α-adrenergic
	  agonists
	β-adrenergic
	  antagonists
	Cholinergic agonists
		β-adrenergic agonists
		α-adrenergic antagonists
		Anticholinergic agents

Foods	Protein meals	Fat Chocolate Ethanol Peppermint

Other	Histamine
	Antacids
	Metoclopramide
	Domperidone
	Prostaglandin $F_{2\alpha}$
	Migrating motor
	  complex
	Raised intraab-
	  dominal pressure
		Theophylline
		Caffeine
		Gastric acidification
		Smoking
		Pregnancy
		Prostaglandins E_2, I_2
		Serotonin
		Meperidine, morphine
		Dopamine
		Calcium channel-
		  blocking agents
		Diazepam
		Barbiturates

Modified, with permission, from Diamant, N.E. (1993). *Physiology of the Esophagus*, in Sleisenger, M.H. and Fordtran, J.S. eds. *Gastrointestinal Disease*, 5th ed. Philadelphia, Saunders, p. 322.

to the normal pathway of LES relaxation in response to an esophageal peristaltic wave, since there is no obvious other reason for a decrease in LES pressure.

Even though motility is the most important function of the oropharynx and esophagus, their secretory, digestive, and even absorptive capacities are evident.

Salivary secretion

Salivary gland secretions aid in lubrication and digestion of food, and enhance speech, taste, and swallowing. Moreover, patients who cannot produce saliva (a condition known as xerostomia) suffer from dental caries, dry mouth, and inflammation of the buccal mucosa.

These secretions initially resemble plasma in composition: high in sodium and chloride and low in potassium. However, the salivary gland duct epithelium is impermeable to water, but allows reabsorption of sodium, chloride, and bicarbonate and secretes potassium into the fluid. Thus, by the time secretions actually leave the salivary gland they are generally hypotonic. Parasympathetic and sympathetic neural pathways (e.g., via acetylcholine and norepinephrine) control the volume of fluid. The more fluid secreted, the less time it spends in the ducts and, therefore, the more similar to plasma it is in composition.

Salivary secretion is entirely under autonomic nervous system (ANS) control. An unusual feature of salivary secretion is that both sympathetic and parasympathetic nerve stimulation result in the same effects: increased secretion, vasodilation, myoepithelial cell contraction, metabolism, and tissue growth.

In addition to basal secretion, various conditioned reflexes involving smell, taste, pressure, and nausea stimulate salivary secretion, generally by parasympathetic-mediated pathways. Conversely, fatigue, sleep, fear, and dehydration are inhibitory influences on these pathways. Both inhibitory and stimulatory influences act on the **salivary nucleus of the medulla**, which affects the parasympathetic output of acetylcholine through cranial nerves IX and X.

Salivary digestion

The complex process of nutrient assimilation actually starts in the mouth through the action of salivary amylase, lingual lipase, and the act of chewing, although the most important digestive processes occur in the small intestine (see Sec. 6).

Review Questions

8. The oropharynx is crucial for the proper fulfillment of what three functions?
9. What are the steps involved in swallowing and how are they controlled?
10. What are some factors influencing LES tone?
11. How is salivary secretion controlled and under what conditions is it stimulated?

Clinical Pearls

○ In Chagas' disease, common in certain parts of South America, the parasite *Trypanosoma cruzi* destroys ganglion cells of the ENS in the esophageal wall, resulting in a permanently contracted LES that causes difficulty in swallowing (**dysphagia**). How might you treat this condition? It could be treated with anything that relaxes or stretches the smooth muscle that makes up the LES. Thus, calcium channel blockers, which are smooth muscle relaxants, can help, as can mechanical dilation or surgery to cut the muscle fibers rendering the sphincter at least partially incompetent.

○ An even more common problem is loss of LES tone resulting in acid from the stomach splashing back up the esophagus, termed **esophageal reflux** and manifest as "heartburn." Clinical management of this common problem involves a combination of lifestyle changes and pharmacologic intervention that makes physiological sense (i.e., have the patient elevate the head of the bed at night, take antacids and blockers of acid secretion, avoid chocolate and ethanol, and take "prokinetic" drugs such as bethanechol and metachlopramide that increase peristalsis). Complications of this condition if left untreated include strictures (causing dysphagia), aspiration (resulting in pneumonia), and epithelial cell irritation predisposing to cancerous changes (termed **Barrett's esophagus**).

4. STOMACH

In the **stomach** (see Figure 5.4) ingested food is subjected to thorough mixing and attack by hydrochloric acid and the proteolytic enzyme pepsin.

Anatomic organization and histologic characteristics

The mucosal surface of the stomach is a simple columnar epithelium of mucus-secreting cells interrupted occasionally by various types of glands in the form of surface invaginations. Within these glands the surface epithelial cells are replaced by specialized secretory cells. Some of these specialized secretory cells are **exocrine cells** (their secretions enter the GI tract lumen); others are **endocrine cells** (their secretions enter the bloodstream).

The exocrine cells secrete various substances from their apical surface (e.g., acid from **parietal cells** and pepsin from **chief cells** of the **oxyntic glands** in the fundus and body of the stomach) into the GI tract lumen.

The endocrine cells secrete hormones from their basolateral surface. Perhaps the best understood of these hormones is **gastrin**, secreted from so-called **G cells** in the **antral glands** of the antral mucosa into the adjacent capillary bloodstream (see Gastrin/Cholecystokinin Family in Sec. 9).

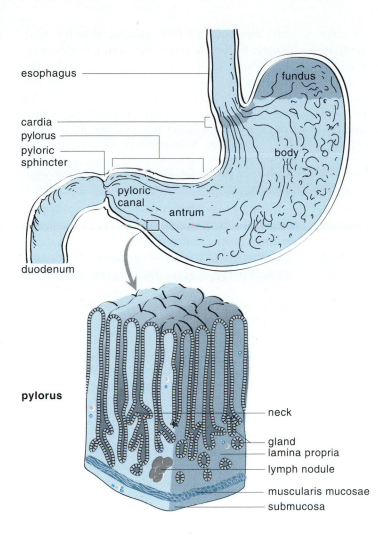

esophagus

cardia
pylorus
pyloric
sphincter

fundus

body

pyloric
canal

antrum

duodenum

pylorus

neck

gland
lamina propria
lymph nodule

muscularis mucosae
submucosa

FIGURE 5.4. Structure and histology of different regions of the stomach. *(Adapted, with permission, from Junqueira L.C., et al. (1992). Basic Histology, 7th ed. Norwalk, CT, Appleton & Lange, p. 291.)*

Physiology

The stomach performs the following functions:

1. Acts as a temporary storage depot for both ingested liquids and solids.
2. Secretes gastric juice, which has various components, most notably **acid**.
3. Facilitates digestion by vigorously mixing ingested liquids and solids. As a result, the particle size of solids is reduced and, together with the liquid, forms a slurry.
4. Delivers this slurry to the proximal small intestine in small spurts. The rate of movement of slurry from stomach to small intestine is modified by characteristics of food composition.

Stomach motility

From the perspective of motility, the stomach is two organs in one. The proximal stomach handles liquids; the distal stomach is more important for solids. Both parts of the stomach are involved in mixing ingested materials. In addition, the proximal stomach prevents reflux and the distal stomach promotes transit to the duodenum.

During and after a meal the proximal stomach displays tonic contraction with **receptive relaxation**. This term refers to the tendency of distension in one part of the GI tract (e.g., by food) to induce relaxation of muscle in the upcoming part of the tract, followed by muscle contraction in the first part when the distension is relieved. At maximum relaxation, the stomach can accommodate about 2 L of both solids and liquids.

The distal stomach has a pacemaker, which generates a wave of peristalsis with simultaneous contraction of the pyloric sphincter. Thus only a small amount of ingested substances get through before the pyloric sphincter closes. Most of the material in the stomach smashes up against the closed pylorus and is churned backwards, creating a motion that pulverizes particles. Both the small particle size and the controlled release of small spurts of food suspension are critical for subsequent absorption. This process is under control of fibers of the vagus nerve. Its importance is seen in the high rate of complications of "dumping syndrome" characterized by nausea and diarrhea in patients with partial gastrectomy or vagotomy.

The force of stomach contractions is influenced by hormonal and neural input. Stomach smooth muscle contraction is stimulated by acetylcholine (vagus nerve), the hormone **motilin** and possibly the hormone **gastrin**, and is inhibited by the hormone **secretin** (see Secretin in Sec. 9). Although the strength of stomach contractions will decrease without CNS input (e.g., after vagotomy), they are not abolished.

Gastric emptying and satiety

Gastric emptying occurs by coordinated contraction of muscle in the wall of the stomach and relaxation of the pyloric sphincter. The rate of gastric emptying is controlled by several factors. The most important is volume, but pH, osmolarity, caloric content, chemical composition, and liquidity also significantly influence this rate with neutral, isotonic, non-caloric liquids leaving the stomach most rapidly. The rate of emptying slows with increasing acidity, caloric content, amino acid, and fat content. These effects on gastric emptying are a consequence of the effects of activating (poorly understood) stimulatory and inhibitory receptors. These receptors act either directly on the gastric smooth muscle or indirectly through neural or hormonal signals (see Figure 5.5).

During fasting, a very different motor program occurs in the stomach. Termed the **migrating motor complex** (MMC), it is a cyclic (once every 80 to 100 min) pattern of peristalsis featuring no resistance on the part of the pyloris, allowing indigestible matter to be swept out of the stomach and down through the intestine. Loss of MMC occurs in a variety of diseases, including diabetes mellitus, and can result in retention of indigestibles and the formation of bezoars (concretions of hair and indigestible foul-smelling debris) which can cause symptoms ranging from nausea, bloating, and bad breath to life-threatening intestinal obstruction.

These "motor programs" depend on both intrinsic muscular activity as well as neural and hormonal modification. In addition to control via the vagus nerve, hormones are also likely to be involved in control of gut motility, albeit in less well-defined ways. For example, the hormones cholecystokinin (CCK, which increases proximal stomach relaxation and pyloric contraction) and motilin (which increases gastric emptying) have been suspected to play such a role.

Disorders of gastric motility can occur as a result of alteration in a number of normal gastric functions, including the stomach's role as the following:

- Reservoir for ingested solids and liquids (e.g., due to resection of the stomach)
- Mixer and homogenizer of ingested food
- Barrier that only allows small spurts of well-mixed chyme beyond the pyloric sphincter

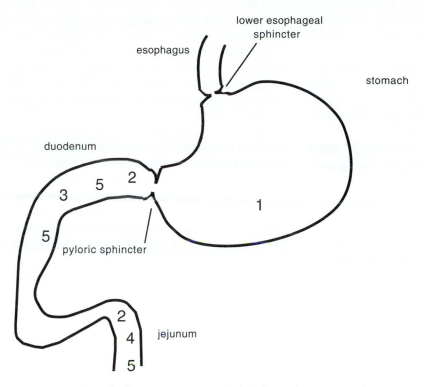

FIGURE 5.5. Control of gastric emptying. 1. Mechanical receptor in the gastric musculature, which triggers gastric emptying upon stimulation. 2. Acid receptor in proximal duodenum and jejunum, which inhibits gastric emptying upon stimulation. 3. Osmotic receptor in duodenum sensitive to electrolytes, carbohydrates, and amino acids (except L-tryptophan), which inhibits gastric emptying upon stimulation. 4. Fat receptor in the jejunum, which inhibits gastric emptying upon stimulation. 5. L-tryptophan receptor in all portions of the duodenum and in jejunum, which inhibits gastric emptying upon stimulation. Note: 2 to 5 are all inhibitory receptors whose action is likely mediated by neural and/or hormonal pathways. Hormonal candidates include gastrin, CCK, secretin, GIP, glucagon, VIP, and somatostatin. *(Adapted, with permission, from Trier, J. (1989). Sleisenger, M.H., and Fordtran, J.S., eds. Gastrointestinal Diseases, 4th ed. Philadelphia, W.B. Saunders.)*

The resulting diseases span the gamut from gastric outlet obstruction to excessively rapid emptying, and may result from interference with the normal mechanisms by which these functions are controlled, including the following:

1. The intrinsic contractility of gastric smooth muscle

2. The ENS

3. The autonomic nervous system's control over ENS function

4. Gut hormones

The pyloric sphincter, like all sphincters, is usually contracted, but undergoes intermittent transient relaxation. Loss of vagal control typically results in excessive contraction, even fewer periods of relaxation, and therefore, symptoms of various degrees of gastric outlet obstruction.

Disorders that affect the ENS, such as the neuropathy of diabetes mellitus and surgical cutting of the stomach wall or vagal trunk, typically cause delayed emptying. However, in some cases delayed emptying can result in symptoms expected from excessively rapid emptying. For example, an excessively contracted pylorus that can open completely, but which does so infrequently, will result in too large a bolus of chyme entering the duodenum from the excessively distended stomach when the sphincter does relax. Such a bolus may be too large to be digested efficiently in the small intestine, resulting in poor absorption and diarrheal symptoms characteristic of the dumping syndrome.

Hormones play a poorly defined, but clearly important role in regulation of GI motility in health and disease.

Because different patients may well have different relative contributions of intrinsic smooth muscle, ENS, ANS, higher centers of the CNS, and hormones over control of their GI tract motility, various treatments for gastroparesis work to different extents in different patients, even when they all have the same initial complaints.

Satiety is a complex sense of fullness after consuming a meal that is due to the interplay of peripheral and central factors. The peripheral factors regulating satiety are numerous. Some are oral (the taste of food). Other are gastric in origin (mechanical distension and release of hormones such as bombesin). Still others are intestinal [digestion of food resulting in activation of receptors facing the intestinal lumen that affect gastric emptying (see Figure 5.6) and absorption of food resulting in elevation of blood glucose, amino acids, and fatty acids]. Finally, some satiety factors are pancreatic in origin (hormones such as pancreatic polypeptide). These factors are interrelated. For example, when a high fat meal slows gastric emptying, continued eating automatically causes gastric distention. Similarly, hormones can work directly on the brain or indirectly, such as on peripheral blood glucose and other nutrient concentrations, which are monitored by the brain.

Central regions in the brain, in particular the ventromedial hypothalamus (satiety center) and lateral hypothalamus (feeding center), integrate the peripheral input with central input from the frontal cortex, the amygdala, and elsewhere, to come to a decision as to the urge for additional feeding versus satiety (see Chap. 11). Gastric emptying is a crucial part, but only one part, of this complex story.

Vomiting

When the GI tract is excessively distended, irritated, or excited, it can respond by sending ingested materials back out the way they came in, a process termed **vomiting**. Any part of the GI tract can initiate this reflex, although it is most often initiated by distention or irritation of the duodenum. Usually vomiting is a normal physiological response to some other disorder, rather than a disorder in itself. However, on occasion, violent vomiting or retching can induce upper GI mucosal lacerations and substantial bleeding.

Vagal and sympathetic nerve afferent fibers transmit a signal to the vomiting center of the medulla near the tractus solitarus at the level of the dorsal motor nucleus of the vagus. This results in automatic motor responses from the vomiting center via the V, VII, IX, X and XII cranial nerves to the upper GI tract and via the spinal nerves to the diaphragm and abdominal muscles to trigger the vomiting act, which involves the following:

1. A deep inspiration
2. Raising the hyoid bone and larynx to open the upper esophageal sphincter

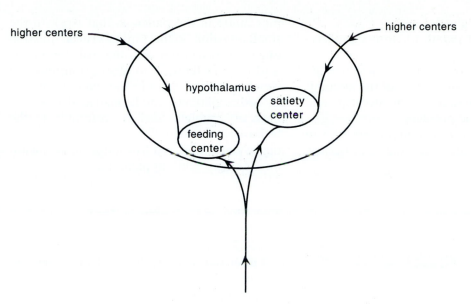

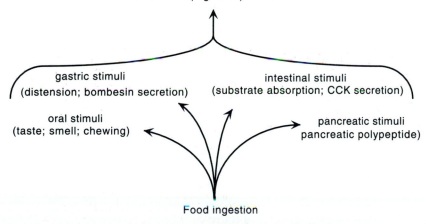

substrates (glucose, amino acids, fatty acids) via blood

neural pathways (vagus nerve)

hormones (e.g. CCK) via blood

FIGURE 5.6. Control of satiety. Food ingestion (bottom) triggers oral, gastric, intestinal, and pancreatic responses that comprise the peripheral components of the mechanism of satiety. These peripheral triggers act via nerves, or through substrates or hormones released into the bloodstream, to stimulate or inhibit the lateral hypothalamic feeding center or ventromedial hypothalamic satiety center. These hypothalamic centers integrate the various peripheral inputs with inputs from higher centers, especially frontal cortex and amygdala, to come to a final decision regarding satiety and hunger, at any given point in time. Only one of the two pairs of hypothalamic feeding and satiety centers is shown (looking down on the hypothalamus from above).

3. Closure of the glottis
4. Lifting the soft palate to close the posterior nares
5. Simultaneous downward contraction of the diaphragm and contraction of the abdominal muscles to squeeze the stomach and raise intragastric pressure
6. Sudden transient relaxation of the LES in response to the elevated intragastric pressure

Clinical Pearl

○ The antibiotic erythromycin has been discovered to be a motilin analogue, that is, it binds and activates the receptor for the GI peptide hormone motilin. As a result, unrelated to the mechanism of its antibiotic effect, erythromycin stimulates GI motility. In many patients who take erythromycin, this manifests as the unpleasant "side effect" of diarrhea. However, in some patients with disorders of GI hypomotility such as diabetic gastroparesis, substantial improvement is observed with erythromycin or its nonantibiotic analogues. This is especially true when the patient's complaints are suggestive of partial gastric outlet obstruction, such as bloating, nausea, and constipation.

Secretion by the stomach

Roles of gastric acid

Gastric acid secretion was probably much more important as a normal physiological function in the days before refrigeration, basic concepts of hygiene, and antibiotics when a fiery barrier to undesirables entering the GI tract (e.g., pathogenic microorganisms) was imperative for survival. Gastric acid also activates the proteolytic enzyme pepsin in the stomach, but there are plenty of other proteases made in the pancreas that work in the small intestine, so this is not a crucial function of gastric acid either. Another role for gastric acid is to facilitate iron absorption, most of which actually occurs in the duodenum.

Today, patients who lack all acid secretion have no problems directly referable to the lack of gastric acid. That is, they are able to digest their food and live a normal life without taking "acid supplements" or the like. They often need regular vitamin B_{12} shots, but that is because the same cells that make acid also make **intrinsic factor**, a protein needed to absorb vitamin B_{12}, and not because of a lack of acid secretion per se.

Other indirect effects of a lack of acid secretion include a small increased risk of infection and perhaps a small increased risk of stomach cancer. This increased cancer risk has been suggested to be due to either overproduction of hormones (e.g., gastrin), which are trying to stimulate acid secretion, or associated with chronic *H. pylori* infection.

The major clinical significance of gastric acid secretion, however, is not the consequences of its lack, but rather the consequences of its relative or absolute excess.

Mechanism of gastric acid secretion

Acid secretion by the stomach is a receptor-mediated process stimulated by **histamine**, **gastrin**, and **acetylcholine** working via both the cyclic AMP and inositol phosphate pathways and inhibited by prostaglandins (see Figure 5.7).

Hydrochloric acid is secreted by parietal cells of the gastric mucosa. The molecular mechanism of acid secretion is complex (see Figure 5.8). What follows is a reasonable current model:

1. A large negative potential difference (40 to 70 mV) is generated by active transport of chloride ions (Cl^-) from parietal cell

cytoplasm to stomach lumen. Potassium follows passively.

2. Water dissociates into H^+ and OH^- ions in parietal cell cytoplasm and H^+/K^+ ATPase drives the exchange of cytoplasmic H^+ for lumenal K^+, generating concentrated hydrochloric acid in the stomach lumen.

3. OH^- ions combine with CO_2 from the bloodstream to form HCO_3, which is exported across the basolateral surface into the bloodstream in exchange for chloride ions.

This process is regulated at the cellular level where H^+/K^+ ATPase is stored in internal (endocytic) vesicles in the parietal cell cytoplasm. In reponse to stimuli for acid secretion (e.g., acetylcholine, histamine, or gastrin binding to their receptors), signaling pathways are activated that trigger fusion of these H^+/K^+ ATPase containing vesicles with the plasma membrane. Once in the plasma membrane, H^+/K^+ ATPase is able to function — perhaps because it now has access to the potassium in the stomach lumen (due to active Cl^- transport, as indicated earlier).

A concentration of up to 100 mM HCl (pH = 1) can be achieved by this mechanism. Tight junctions keep the H^+ in the lumen. The net effect is to maintain **electroneutrality** in the parietal cell, with low pH in the stomach lumen and an elevated pH in the blood downstream of the parietal cell. This local, blood-borne "alkaline tide" may protect against damage from acid backleak in the event of mucosal damage.

Secretion of acid occurs in a basal diurnal pattern, but it can be stimulated by such diverse factors as the thought of food, distention of the stomach, protein ingestion, and acidification.

Basal acid secretion is normally about 10% of maximum.

Acetylcholine released from the vagus mediates the so-called cephalic phase (acid secretion in response to the thought of food)

as well as the so-called gastric phase (acid secretion in response to gastric distention). Gastrin is secreted in the intestinal phase (in response to the amino acid and peptide composition of a meal).

Histamine has a **paracrine** effect to stimulate acid secretion. That is, it is released by cells in the neighborhood of the parietal cells and reaches them by local diffusion rather than via the bloodstream.

The various stimuli of acid secretion act in an additive fashion: Blocking one but not the others decreases, but does not entirely stop, all acid secretion.

Acid secretion can be inhibited as well as stimulated. Thus, **prostaglandins** act in a paracrine fashion to inhibit acid secretion.

The importance of control of acid secretion is seen in the pathogenesis and therapy of acid-mediated injury to the GI tract: Exacerbations are often traced to the use of drugs that inhibit prostaglandin synthesis (e.g., aspirin, Motrin, and so forth). Likewise, infection of the mucosa by the bacterium *H. pylori* results in inflammation and diminution of mucosal defenses, thereby increasing the risk of gastritis and ulcer disease.

Other stomach products secreted into the gut lumen

Intrinsic factor is a vitamin B_{12} binding protein. It is synthesized and secreted constitutively by parietal cells of the gastric mucosa, the same cells that generate gastric acid. Thus, autoimmune destruction of parietal cells produces not only impaired acidification but also **pernicious anemia** due to vitamin B_{12} deficiency.

Secreted into the lumen of the stomach, intrinsic factor travels to the small intestine, where it binds vitamin B_{12}. The vitamin B_{12}-intrinsic factor complex is then taken up by receptor-mediated endocytosis by enterocytes of the **terminal ileum**, from which

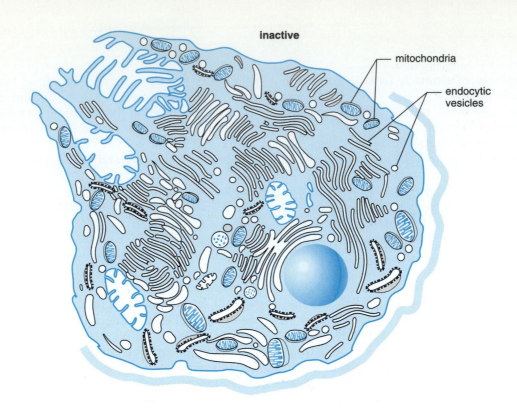

inactive

mitochondria

endocytic
vesicles

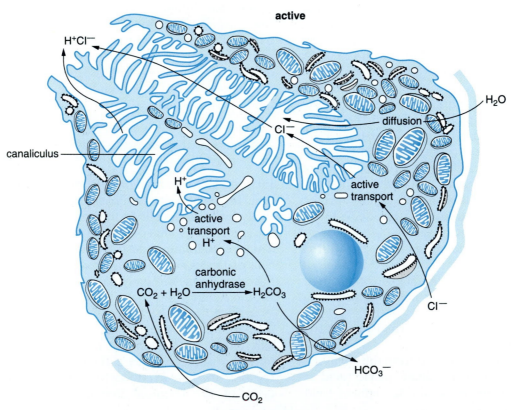

active

H^+Cl^-

H_2O

Cl^-

diffusion

canaliculus

H^+

active
transport

active
transport
H^+

carbonic
anhydrase

$CO_2 + H_2O \longrightarrow H_2CO_3$

Cl^-

HCO_3^-

CO_2

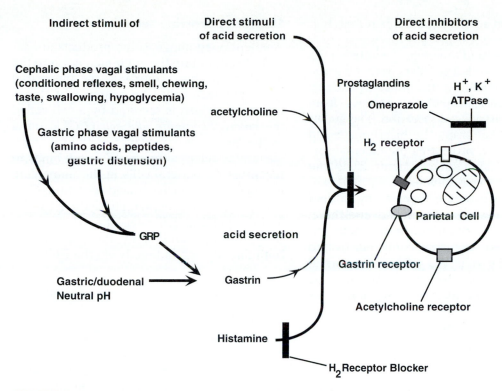

FIGURE 5.8. Regulation of acid secretion. Various indirect and direct stimuli result in acid secretion. Acid secretion can be blocked either by omeprazole, which works directly on the H⁺/K⁺ ATPase that generates the acid, or by prostaglandins or H₂ receptor blockers that work by blocking stimuli to acid secretion. Indicated are the H₂ receptor, acetylcholine receptor and gastrin receptor on the parietal cell surface, by which those agents stimulate acid secretion. Note that prostaglandins have many protective roles, including enhancement of mucus and bicarbonate production as well as inhibition of acid secretion. *(Adapted, with permission, from Lingappa, V.R. (1999). in McPhee S.J. et al.,* Pathophysiology of Disease, *eds. 3rd ed. New York, McGraw-Hill, p. 304.)*

FIGURE 5.7. Mechanism of acid secretion by the parietal cell. Schematic of a parietal cell showing numerous mitochondria (which generate ATP) and the apical canalicular membrane to which endocytic vesicles bearing H⁺/K⁺ ATPase fuse. As a result of the combination of carbonic anhydrase and H⁺/K⁺ ATPase activity, H⁺ ions are pumped into the intestinal lumen and bicarbonate into the bloodstream (see text). Note the remarkable canalicular system of tubules and vesicles bearing H⁺/K⁺ ATPase that fuse to the plasma membrane or undergo endocytosis, depending on whether more or less acid secretion is required, respectively.

it is delivered to the bloodstream (see Figure 5.9).

Bicarbonate and mucus are secreted in the stomach by so-called goblet cells that line the glands that punctuate the mucosal surface. These products protect the mucosa from damage by gastric acid secretion. The mucus forms a gel that traps the bicarbonate and holds it in place, protecting the mucosal surface without immediately neutralizing the acid in the stomach lumen.

Pepsin is a protease secreted by distinct cells in the gastric antrum and elsewhere, which initiate proteolysis in the acid environment and are irreversibly inactivated at neutral pH. It is not critical for normal digestion and has never been proved to be involved in peptic ulcer disease, despite its name.

Stomach products secreted into the bloodstream

Gastrin is the primary hormonal effector of acid secretion by the parietal cells. It is synthesized as a precursor polypeptide, processed and secreted by distinct endocrine cells in the antral and duodenal mucosa under negative feedback control by acid. Gastrin also has a trophic effect on gastric mucosa.

Somatostatin is another polypeptide product derived from a larger precursor. Somatostatin is produced in various other locations of the body as well, including the endocrine pancreas (delta cells), brain, and gut. It appears to be a general inhibitor of secretion of various other hormones perhaps acting in both paracrine (locally by diffusion through interstitial fluid) and endocrine (into the bloodstream) fashion.

Various neurotransmitters of the gastric division of the ENS are also secreted across the basal surface, including vasoactive intestinal polypeptide (VIP), enkephalins, substance P, and neuropeptide Y (NPY).

Stomach paracrine secretion

As mentioned above, some products are secreted neither into the gut lumen nor into the bloodstream, but rather into the interstitial space between cells. An example of this is histamine, which is secreted by a cell called the *enterochromaffin-like cell* (*ECL*) found in the lamina propria layer of the GI tract. Histamine released by the ECL cell binds to receptors on parietal cells in the immediate neighborhood to trigger acid secretion. Gastrin receptors are found on both the ECL cell and the parietal cell, suggesting that gastrin triggers acid secretion by the parietal cell both directly and indirectly via the ECL cell.

Clinical Pearls

○ Based on this discussion what would you expect to be a rational initial treatment for acid-mediated injury? That depends on its type and severity.

For abdominal pain after or between meals without other complications, you might start with recommendations for dietary/lifestyle changes. Treatment should include avoiding stimulants of gastrin secretion such as protein-rich meals, stress, coffee, Motrin, and other nonsteroidal anti-inflammatory drugs (NSAIDs) that are known to potentiate acid secretion and/or diminish host defenses. Treatment with antacids, which neutralize secreted acid, should follow.

If antacids alone are ineffective, you might switch the patient to histamine receptor blocking drugs (e.g., cimetidine, ranitidine, famotidine, etc.).

If pain persists, you might test the patient for *H. pylori* infection (serum antibody titer) and refer him or her for endoscopy (direct visualization of the gastric mucosa through a flexible scope) to see if

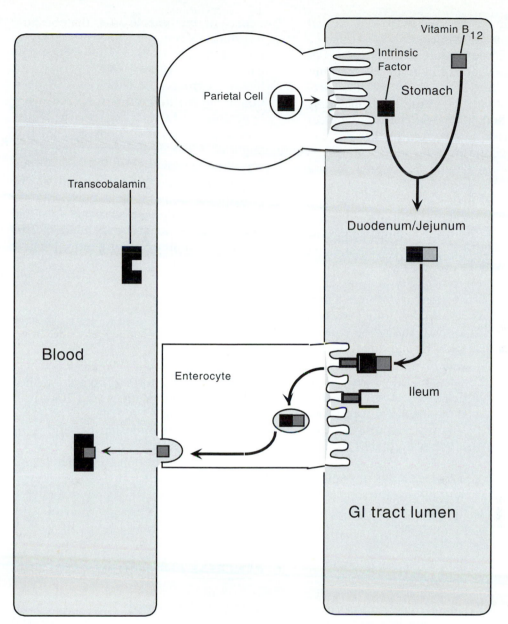

FIGURE 5.9. Intestinal absorption of vitamin B_{12}. Parietal cells in the stomach secrete intrinsic factor into the GI tract lumen. In the duodenum and jejunum, Intrinsic Factor binds to vitamin B_{12}. The complex is taken up into intestinal enterocytes by receptor-mediated endocytosis in the terminal illeum. Vitamin B_{12} is subsequently released into the bloodstream. Once released in the bloodstream, vitamin B_{12} is bound to a serum protein, transcobalamin, that serves as a vitamin B_{12} carrying protein. *(Adapted, with permission, from Rhoades, R.A. and Tanner, G.A. (1992). Digestion and Absorption, in Medical Physiology. Boston, Little, Brown, p. 564.)*

there is an ulcer and, if so, to be sure that the ulcer is not associated with a cancer.

If this study reveals an ulcer that needs to be healed, one or more of several drugs besides the H_2 blockers already prescribed, should be considered, including the drug sucralfate, which coats the ulcer crater, protecting it from further damage and allowing it to heal.

The patient should also be treated with an antibiotic regimen demonstrated to eradicate *H. pylori* infection, if present, since in many patients with ulcer disease, the cause of the ulcer is diminished host defenses due to *H. pylori* infection.

If the patient did not have signs of *H. pylori* infection or a history of using drugs that inhibit prostaglandin synthesis (such as steroids or NSAIDs), other (rarer) causes of ulcer disease should be considered, such as a gastrin-secreting tumor.

An elderly patient or one whom for other reasons you think may have diminished mucosal defenses could be treated with a prostaglandin agent (misoprostol), especially if the patient has disabling arthritis and therefore really needs to take NSAIDs.

If you do not consider the physiology of ulcer disease and address the root cause (e.g., *H. pylori* or NSAIDs), the patient is likely to have a recurrence.

○ Severe disease and cases resistant to simpler therapy might call for bigger guns: somatostatin analogues or the K^+/H^+ ATPase antagonists such as omeprazole.

A life-threatening complication (massive gastrointestinal bleeding or perforation) would short-circuit this progression of therapy and bring the patient to surgery.

○ Omeprazole is a nearly complete inhibitor of the final common pathway of acid secretion. Then why do we bother to use drugs such as H_2 receptor blockers that are incomplete in their action? One conse-

quence of omeprazole use is that, because it results in a complete block of acid secretion, it results in extremely high serum gastrin levels. Although the short-term effect of gastrin is stimulation of acid secretion, it has the long-term effect of causing hypertrophy of the gastric mucosa. Hence someone on chronic omeprazole therapy might be at risk of increased stomach cancer, although this theoretical concern has not yet been proved. Nevertheless, the principle of using the least powerful drug that has the desired effect seems a prudent one to follow, in order to minimize the chance of unintended long-term negative consequences of drug therapy.

Review Questions

12. What does the stomach do and how does it do it?
13. Describe the vomiting reflex.
14. What are the motor programs of the stomach and intestines and how are they controlled?
15. What is the relationship of satiety to gastric emptying?
16. How is acid secretion controlled?
17. Name some endocrine, exocrine, and paracrine products secreted by the stomach.

5. PANCREAS AND GALLBLADDER

Anatomy and histology

Gallbladder

The **gallbladder** is a muscular sac lined with a columnar epithelium that lies on the inferior surface of the liver (see Figure 5.10). It has a resting volume of about 50 mL and is connected to the hepatic biliary system by the cystic duct which also connects to the common bile duct. The opening of the biliary system into the proximal duodenum is controlled by the sphincter of Oddi, where the common bile duct and the pancreatic duct usually join.

Pancreas

The **pancreas** is a solid secretory tissue that lies transversely across the posterior abdominal wall deep within the upper abdomen (see Figure 5.10). It is firmly fixed in the retroperitoneal space in front of the abdominal aorta and the first and second lumbar vertebrac. It is 15 cm long and weighs about 100 g. The pancreas is covered by a thin capsule of connective tissue that sends septa into the organ, separating it into lobules. The exocrine tissue of the pancreas is organized into acini that open into ducts, which come together to form the pancreatic duct (see Figure 5.11).

Physiological roles of the gallbladder and pancreas

Gallbladder

The gallbladder stores and modifies bile, the detergent produced by the liver that facili-

FIGURE 5.10. Anatomic location of the gallbladder and pancreas. *(Adapted, with permission, from Lindnar, H.H. (1989). Clinical Anatomy, Norwalk, CT, Appleton & Lange.)*

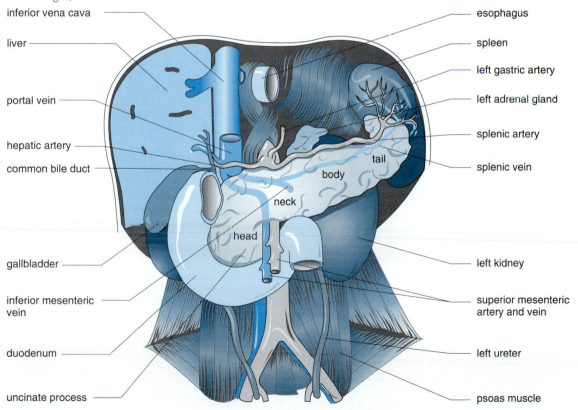

inferior vena cava

liver

portal vein

hepatic artery

common bile duct

gallbladder

inferior mesenteric vein

duodenum

uncinate process

esophagus

spleen

left gastric artery

left adrenal gland

splenic artery

splenic vein

tail

body

neck

head

left kidney

superior mesenteric artery and vein

left ureter

psoas muscle

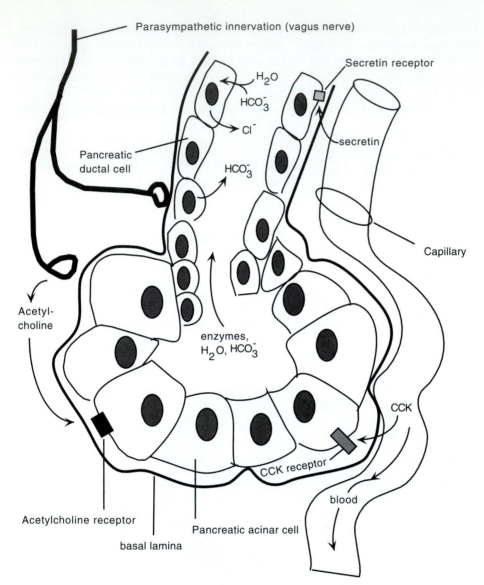

Parasympathetic innervation (vagus nerve)

Secretin receptor

H_2O

HCO_3^-

Cl^-

Pancreatic
ductal cell

HCO_3^-

secretin

Capillary

Acetyl-
choline

enzymes,
H_2O, HCO_3^-

CCK

CCK receptor

blood

Acetylcholine receptor

basal lamina

Pancreatic acinar cell

FIGURE 5.11. Diagram of pancreatic acini indicating water, bicarbonate and enzyme secretion, and the ability of ductal cell transport activity to modify the ionic composition, especially in low flow states. The relation between flow rate and bicarbonate concentration is described in the text. Also indicated is the ability of hormones traveling via the bloodstream to stimulate secretion of enzymes (by CCK) and bicarbonate (by secretin), from the acinar and ductal cells, respectively. Also shown is control of pancreatic secretion through parasympathetic innervation with release of acetylcholine. (Adapted, with permission, from Kelley, W. N. ed. (1989). Textbook of Internal Medicine, Philadelphia, Lippincott.)

tates excretion and absorption of lipophilic substances. Bile is secreted by hepatocytes into the bile canaliculus, from which it flows down the hepatic duct and into the gallbladder via the cystic duct. There it is stored until stimulation of gallbladder contraction expels the bile back through the cystic duct into the common bile duct and, via the sphincter of Oddi, into the duodenum. Stimuli for gallbladder contraction and sphincter of Oddi relaxation necessary for proper bile flow include both hormones, such as **cholecystokinin** (CCK), and neural inputs, in response to fat-rich meals.

During its time in the gallbladder, bile normally undergoes a substantial degree of concentration. Bile composition is further modified in the gallbladder by mucin production under the control of prostaglandins, and saturation of bile cholesterol controlled in part by estrogen.

Pancreas

The pancreas serves three general functions:

1. The pancreas is the source of key hormones that control carbohydrate metabolism (insulin, glucagon, and somatostatin; see Chap. 6).
2. The pancreas is the source of bicarbonate to neutralize gastric acid. This is produced by the cells lining the ducts and enters the duodenum along with the digestive enzymes. This establishes an environment with a pH greater than 6 at which pepsin is inactive and in which pancreatic digestive enzymes, once activated, are functional.
3. The pancreas is the source of digestive enzymes, secreted by the **acinar tissue** that composes the bulk of the pancreas. These pancreatic digestive enzymes (actually in the form of larger polypeptide precursors that normally are not activated until they enter the small intestine) are secreted in a small volume into a system of ducts. These

ducts converge to form the pancreatic duct that leads to the duodenum of the small intestine. The pancreatic enzymes are activated in the small intestine and play a crucial role in digestion.

Control of pancreatic secretion

Let us consider a simple framework for understanding pancreatic bicarbonate and enzyme secretion, and then add some complications.

The hormone secretin is released into the bloodstream from endocrine cells in the duodenal mucosa, in response to acid entering the duodenum. Secretin travels through the blood and binds to receptors in the pancreas, triggering secretion of bicarbonate, which neutralizes the acid and thereby turns off the initial stimulus for secretin secretion (see Figure 5.12). Cholecystokinin (CCK) is another hormone secreted from endocrine cells of the duodenal mucosa. It stimulates digestive enzyme secretion from the pancreas in response to a protein-rich meal (see Figure 5.12). Thus, together these two hormones contribute to regulation of the composition of pancreatic "juice" (see Table 5.2). The presence of either CCK or acetylcholine increases the amount of bicarbonate secreted in response to a given amount of secretin.

Bicarbonate secretion from the pancreas differs from that of the salivary gland in that its duct epithelium is permeable to water, and thus pancreatic juice is always isotonic with plasma. However its composition changes with flow rate. As flow rate increases, bicarbonate concentration increases and chloride concentration decreases (see Figure 5.11). Thus, in response to secretin, the flow rate of pancreatic ductal cell secretion increases, which leaves less time for exchange with chloride and therefore results in an increase in the bicarbonate concentration in pancreatic juice, which facilitates neutralization of acid. Remember your GI-ography: Acid is on

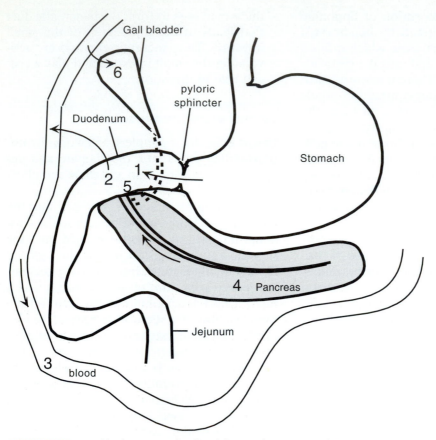

FIGURE 5.12. Simplified negative feedback loops of secretin and CCK secretion. For secretin: acidic chyme enters the duodenum (1), and is sensed by secretin-secreting cells in the duodenal mucosa (2), which respond by releasing secretin into the bloodstream (3). Secretin travels to the pancreas where it stimulates increased bicarbonate secretion from pancreatic ductal cells (4), which enters the duodenum via the pancreatic duct and neutralizes the acid that was the initial stimulus for secretin secretion (5). For CCK: entry of food into the duodenum (1), triggers release of a CCK-stimulating peptide (2), which causes release of CCK, from endocrine cells in the duodenal mucosa, into the bloodstream (3), which stimulates increased pancreatic enzyme secretion from acinar cells (4). Once the pancreatic enzyme trypsin is through digesting dietary protein in the small intestine, it is free to digest the CCK-stimulating peptide, thereby relieving the initial stimulus for CCK secretion. In addition, CCK travels to the gallbladder [6] where it stimulates contraction of the gallbladder and relaxation of the sphincter of Oddi, to further facilitate digestion of the meal. Additional neural and hormonal pathways contribute to stimulation of secretin and CCK secretion, but are not shown here for simplicity.

TABLE 5.2 CONTROL OF PANCREATIC SECRETION

Stimulant	Mediator	Action
Sight, smell, taste of food	Vagus nerves (acetylcholine)	Stimulation of enzyme secretion
Gastric distention	Vagal reflex (acetylcholine)	Stimulation of enzyme secretion
Digestion products of protein or fat in intestine	CCK, vagal reflex (acetylcholine)	Stimulation of enzyme secretion, potentiate bicarbonate secretion
Gastric H^+, fatty acids in intestinal lumen	Secretin, VIPergic reflexes?	Stimulation of bicarbonate secretion
Not known	Somatostatin, pancreatic polypeptide	Inhibit release or effects of CCK, acetylcholine, secretin.

Modified, with permission, from Kelley, W.N. ed. (1989). *Textbook of Internal Medicine*. Philadelphia, Lippincott.

the gut lumenal side; it triggers secretin secretion into the bloodstream, which triggers bicarbonate secretion into the pancreatic ductal lumen that connects to the GI lumen.

In humans, the hormone CCK and neurogenic pathways (e.g., acetylcholine) appear to be equally important effectors of pancreatic enzyme secretion. However, this view may be somewhat oversimplified because there is reason to believe that many other peptide and neurotransmitters may also be involved in potentiation of pancreatic secretion.

The pancreatic digestive enzymes are stored and secreted as inactive precursors. A protease among them (trypsinogen) is activated by a membrane-bound enzyme of the brush border, enterokinase, which cleaves trypsinogen to trypsin. Trypsin in turn can activate the other precursors generating active digestive enzymes exclusively in the small intestine lumen. This and other features of the system are designed to protect the pancreas and gut wall from autodigestion.

A feedback loop involving CCK secretion involves release of a specific peptide (called **CCK-releasing factor**) that stimulates intestinal CCK secretion. CCK, in turn, stimulates pancreatic enzymes secretion. Upon activation, trypsin (and other pancreatic proteases) is initially occupied digesting protein in the intestinal lumen. Once protein digestion is largely complete, trypsin turns its attention to digestion and inactivation of the stimulating peptide, thereby removing the initial stimulus for CCK release and therefore, for further pancreatic enzyme secretion.

The feedback loops described earlier are not the only ones involved in secretin and CCK regulation. A host of other hormones and factors are likely to contribute in currently obscure ways. The complex regulation of pancreatic secretion (both bicarbonate and enzymes) can be distinguished into four specific phases.

1. Basal secretion (the unstimulated state) represents 10% of the **maximal secretory output** and is synchronized with the interdigestive myoelectrical complex under vagal control. This is actually enough pancreatic secretion to digest most meals, even though it is a small fraction of the maximal response to stimulation. Perhaps the vast excess of digestive enzyme secretory capacity is a vestige from our evolutionary origins in the pre-cooking era? In contrast, this is close to the degree of excess capacity we start off with for most vital functions.
2. The thought of eating also stimulates an increase in pancreatic secretion (termed the **cephalic phase**).
3. Vagal reflexes in response to distention of the stomach stimulate pancreatic secretion (termed the **gastric phase**).

4. Finally, the **intestinal phase**, strongest of them all, occurs in response to acid and nutrients.

Clinical Pearls

○ Acute pancreatitis is an attack of abdominal pain associated with nausea, vomiting, and signs of pancreatic inflammation. It is believed to be inappropriate activation of pancreatic enzymes before their export to the duodenum, and is most commonly due to alcohol or gallstones. Amylase levels in the blood are typically dramatically elevated, which is how this condition can be distinguished from other causes of abdominal pain. Presumably this is because activation of enzymes in the pancreas results in tissue damage and release of cellular contents, which are absorbed into the blood stream. Complications of acute pancreatitis can be extremely severe due to either infection or production of powerful cytokines (secreted proteins that regulate host immune defense systems).

○ Chronic pancreatitis is an attack of abdominal pain in a patient whose pancreas is badly scarred from prior episodes of acute pancreatitis. In these patients, often no acute inciting event (e.g., alcohol or gallstone) is needed to set off an attack, and the serum amylase is often minimally elevated if at all. A possible explanation is that small amounts of enzymes can leak out of the pancreatic scar tissue to initiate low-level inflammation and pain. As a result of the underlying degree of pancreatic damage and scar tissue, these patients often do not produce sufficient pancreatic enzymes for normal digestion and, therefore, have signs and symptoms of pancreatic insufficiency (e.g., fat malabsorption resulting in steatorrhea and weight loss).

Steatorrheal symptoms typically improve with pancreatic enzyme replacement (pills taken orally at meals).

Biliary motility

The smooth muscle in the gallbladder wall can be stimulated to contract by the hormone CCK, resulting in augmentation of bile secretion necessary to assimilate the digestion products of a fat-rich meal.

Clinical Pearl

○ Patients with gallbladder disease (e.g., stones in the common bile duct) develop pain upon eating fatty foods as a consequence of CCK-stimulated gallbladder contraction against a partially occluded duct lumen.

Review Questions

18. What are the functions of the gallbladder and the pancreas?
19. How is pancreatic secretion regulated?
20. How is gallbladder contraction regulated?

6. SMALL INTESTINE AND COLON

Anatomic organization and histologic characteristics

Three regions can be distinguished along the 6 to 7 m linear length of the small intestine. The pyloric sphincter marks the beginning of the **duodenum**, which is largely retroperitoneal and fixed in its location. Thanks to this sphincter, stomach contents normally enter the duodenum in small spurts of tiny suspended particles. The mechanism by which this happens will be discussed later. A characteristic feature of the duodenum is the presence within the submucosa of numerous **Brunner's glands** (which contain cells secreting both mucus and other products), and a relative paucity of mucus-secreting **goblet cells**. In the duodenum, gastric contents are mixed with that of the common bile duct and pancreatic ducts.

Beyond the duodenum, the small intestine is mobile and suspended in the peritoneal cavity by a mesentery. The proximal two-fifths is called the **jejunum**; while the distal three-fifths is termed the **ileum**, ending with the ileocecal valve at the start of the large intestine. Each region has its characteristic gross and microscopic structural features. The jejunum is notable for the presence of submucosal folds (termed **plicae circulares**)

and the ileum has numerous goblet cells and mucosal lymphoid cell collections called **Peyer's patches**. However, it is more useful to consider the functional distinctions (see later).

The most striking gross structural feature of the small intestine are the numerous villi (small, approximately 1-mm height projections of the mucosa) that confer the apt name of "brush border" to its lumenal surface and greatly increase its surface absorptive area (Figure 5.13A). Each villus contains a single terminal branch of the arterial, venous, and lymphatic trees, with the villus surface composed of epithelial cells termed **enterocytes**. Enterocytes, particularly those at the villus tip, carry out the efficient absorption of specific substances from the gut lumen, and their

FIGURE 5.13. *A and B. Structure of the small intestine. (B. Adapted, with permission, from Sleisenger, M.H., and Fordtran, J.S. eds. (1986). Gastrointestinal Disease, 3rd ed. Philadelphia, Saunders.)*

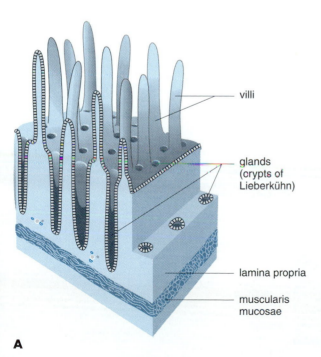

villi

glands (crypts of Lieberkühn)

lamina propria

muscularis mucosae

A

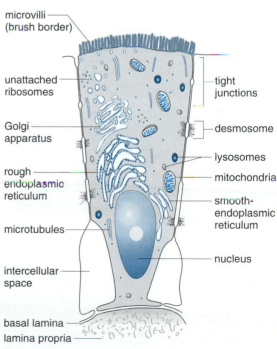

microvilli (brush border)

unattached ribosomes

Golgi apparatus

rough endoplasmic reticulum

microtubules

intercellular space

basal lamina

lamina propria

tight junctions

desmosome

lysosomes

mitochondria

smooth-endoplasmic reticulum

nucleus

B

subsequent transfer to the circulatory system. The **crypts of Lieberkuhn** between villi are the site of cell proliferation and are involved in fluid and electrolyte transport into the intestinal lumen. The cells differentiate as they ascend the villus to be rapidly shed from the tip (average lifespan about 3 to 5 days).

At the electron microscopic level, each enterocyte displays numerous microvilli, plasma membrane evaginations that further increase the absorptive surface area (Figure 5.13B). The magnitude of the surface area expansion due to villi and microvilli is enormous, as indicated in Figure 5.14.

Beneath the enterocytes, but still within the mucosa, is a layer termed the **lamina propria** — loose connective tissue in which travel immune cells involved in defense

FIGURE 5.14. Expansion of intestinal surface area by folds, villi, and microvilli. *(Adapted, with permission, from Schmidt, R.E. and Thews, G. (1993). Human Physiology. New York, Springer-Verlag.)*

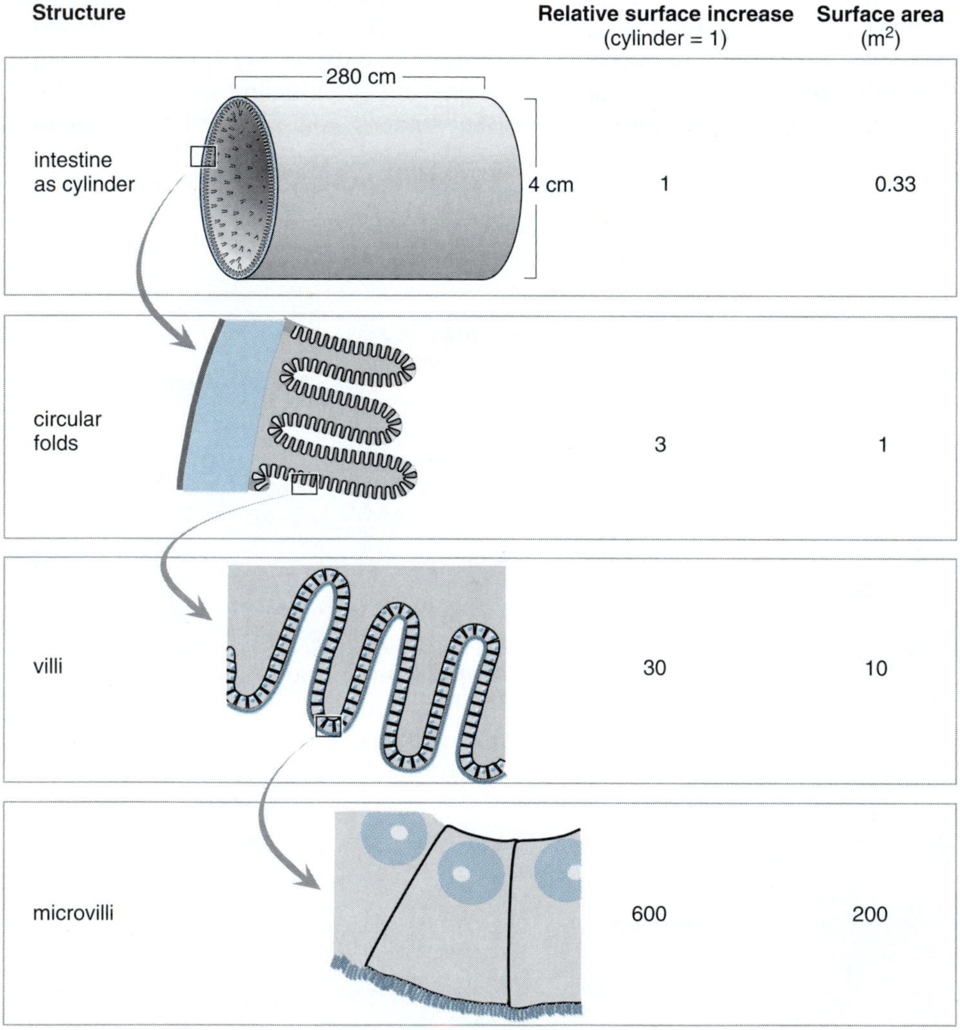

Structure		Relative surface increase (cylinder = 1)	Surface area (m^2)
intestine as cylinder		1	0.33
circular folds		3	1
villi		30	10
microvilli		600	200

against pathogens and potential pathogens of the gut lumen. In addition to this layer within the mucosa, numerous collections of lymphocytes (e.g., Peyer's patches and lymph nodes) are also found in the submucosa.

Small intestinal motility

As with other regions of the GI tract, the small intestine has two programs of activity, one during feeding and another during fasting. During feeding the intestinal program, termed **segmentation**, displays a predominance of (to and fro) motion designed to promote optimal mixing. Because the rate of segmentation is greater proximally than distally, this program is also responsible for most of the net forward movement of chyme along the intestine. Every now and then there is a peristaltic wave that also moves chyme along the intestine. The force of intestinal smooth muscle contractions is increased by CCK, gastrin, and insulin and decreased by secretin.

During fasting, a program termed the *migrating motor complex* (*MMC*) occurs. The MMC consists of a repetitive (every 80 to 100 min) three-phase cycle of peristaltic activity that keeps the GI tract clear of debris (bacteria, undigested material, desquamated cells, secretions) as part of "housekeeping" functions. Phase I is quiescent, phase II consists of spontaneous irregular activity, and phase III displays a burst of rhythmic propagated contraction. The MMC appears to be at least partly under the control of the gut hormone motilin.

Clinical Pearls

○ Some of the most common GI tract disorders involve aberrant small intestine motility. For example, many individuals complain of complex sets of symptoms including alternating constipation, diarrhea, and abdominal pain. A full medical investigation often turns up no apparent structural problem or underlying disease. These individuals may have a disorder of function in the absence of any gross structural abnormality. They are often classified as having "irritable bowel syndrome," probably from disordered small intestinal motility of unknown etiology.

○ Disordered small intestine motility (in which the MMC is altered or lacking) can be seen in diseases such as diabetes mellitus, familial pseudoobstruction, and scleroderma. Complications can include bezoar formation, intestinal bacterial overgrowth, excessively rapid small bowel transit time associated with diarrheal states, symptoms of nausea and vomiting, abdominal distention, and constipation.

Small intestinal secretion and transport

The intestinal mucosa is armed with an array of transporters for electrolytes that allow it to absorb a tremendous volume of fluids and electrolytes in the course of a normal day. Much of the fluid and electrolyte transport in the intestine can be compared to the same processes in the kidney beyond the proximal tubule (except that the tube from which the fluid is being absorbed in the former case is bigger and contains the products of food digestion). In both organs, facilitated diffusion, cotransport, and the like operate to absorb both fluid and electrolytes.

Fluid and electrolyte secretion and absorption vary along the villus. The tip is involved in all sorts of absorptive functions, including both nutrients and electrolytes, with water passively following the electrolytes (sodium and chloride). Transporters in the crypts of Lieberkuhn actively secrete chloride and bicarbonate ions into the small intestinal lumen, with passive movement of water and sodium.

Enterocytes are able to absorb sodium because the basolaterally located Na^+/K^+ ATPase establishes an electrochemical gradient. They use this gradient to drive sodium absorption from the lumen in three ways (see Figure 5.15):

1. Cotransporters localized to the villus tip selectively absorb nutrients such as glucose, galactose, amino acids, vitamin C, and small peptides along with sodium. Water follows the sodium passively in these cases. These cotransporters are lacking in the colon, one reason why its maximum absorptive capacity (5 L/day) is considerably less than that of the small intestine (12 L/day).

2. Neutral cotransport systems move sodium and chloride or sodium for hydrogen. In the jejunum, sodium for hydrogen exchange allows neutralization of excess pancreatic bicarbonate, forming carbon dioxide and water. The carbon dioxide diffuses into blood for excretion via the lungs.

3. Sodium and chloride are passively absorbed down the electrochemical gradient. In addition, some sodium is absorbed by following water through the junctions between enterocytes, a phenomenon termed **solvent drag**. This only occurs in "leaky" parts of the GI tract such as the proximal small intestine and not in the "tight" epithelium of the distal small bowel and colon.

A disturbance in gut fluid homeostasis resulting in diarrhea can be either malabsorptive, osmotic, or secretory in nature:

1. Malabsorptive diarrhea can result from damage to the intestinal epithelial surface (for example, due to excessive alcohol ingestion), or impairment of the ability of the intestinal epithelial cells to function in nutrient absorption (for example, due to pancreatic enzyme insufficiency or congenital disaccharidase deficiency).

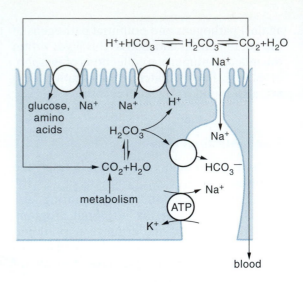

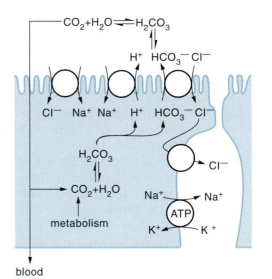

FIGURE 5.15. Mechanism of small intestinal sodium absorption. *(Adapted, with permission, from Rhoades, R.A., and Tanner, G.A. (1995). Boston, Little, Brown, p. 565.)*

2. Osmotic diarrhea is typically caused by malabsorbed nutrients or poorly absorbed electrolytes, which retain water in the lumen. In this case, enzyme action on foodstuffs actually makes matters worse because food breakdown increases their

osmolarity and therefore pulls more water into the intestinal lumen.

3. Secretory diarrhea is the result of secretagogues (substances that stimulate secretion) maintaining elevated rates of fluid transport out of intestinal epithelial cells (i.e., in the crypts). Secretagogues can include such substances as hormones (such as vasoactive intestinal peptide acting from the bloodstream), bacterial toxins (acting within the enterocytes themselves), or bile acids (acting from the lumen).

In its capacity to transport fluid, the small intestine far exceeds the colon (in part because of the enormous surface area of the small intestinal brush border). Thus conditions that result in maximal efflux of fluid out of the small intestinal epithelial cells (e.g., the presence of bacterial toxins) will overwhelm the ability of the colon to compensate by increased fluid absorption.

Clinical Pearl

○ Under certain circumstances the physiological mechanism of sodium and glucose cotransport can be put to valuable therapeutic use. A simple view of the pathophysiology of the diarrheal disease cholera is that G protein modification by a bacterial toxin results in uncontrolled chloride channel activation in the small intestinal villus crypts (see Frontiers in Sec. 12 for a more complex view of cholera toxin action). Loss of huge amounts of chloride, and with it sodium and water (10-20 L/day), can rapidly cause dehydration and death. An effective treatment is oral rehydration with glucose-containing solutions. The glucose drives the sodium-glucose cotransporter to transport both molecules into enterocytes, and with them goes chloride and water. This offsets the fluid efflux mediated by the bacterial toxin. This approach is much less expensive than intravenous hydration, which requires sterile equipment that is often not available "in the field," especially in a poor country and with epidemic numbers of cases. This "low tech" intervention has probably saved more lives worldwide than all interventions to date for heart disease or cancer combined!

Digestion and absorption in the small intestine

In the small intestine the processes of digestion and absorption can be resolved into four phases:

1. Hydrolysis in the intestinal lumen
2. Hydrolysis at the enterocyte brush border
3. Transport into the enterocyte
4. Processing within and export from the enterocyte into the portal or lymphatic circulation

Carbohydrate digestion and absorption

Dietary carbohydrates include simple sugars, **complex carbohydrates** (such as starches), and indigestible carbohydrates, termed **dietary fiber**. Complex carbohydrates are particularly valuable because they are a source of energy, dietary fiber, and essential vitamins and minerals.

Mechanism of carbohydrate absorption

Most carbohydrate absorption occurs in the jejunum. Salivary and pancreatic amylases start the process of carbohydrate digestion by hydrolysing α 1-4 linkages (but not α 1-6 or β 1-4 linkages such as occur in cellulose) between sugar residues. The resultant oligosaccharides are further digested to simple sugars by enterocyte brush border enzymes (see Figure 5.16A).

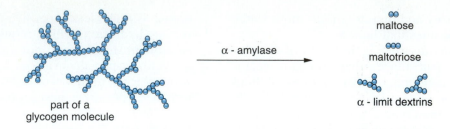

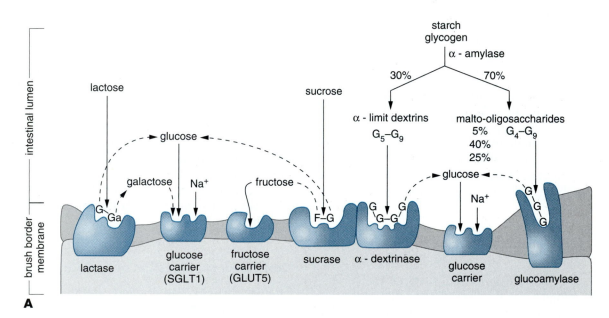

A

FIGURE 5.16. Dietary carbohydrate, protein, and fat breakdown and absorption. *A.* Carbohydrate digestion and absorption. Schematic diagram (upper half) indicates the structure of a glycogen molecule and its breakdown products, while (lower half) shows the functions of most brush border oligosaccharidases. The glucose, galactose, and fructose molecules released by enzymatic hydrolysis are then moved into the epithelial cell by the specific transporters indicated. *B.* Protein digestion and absorption. Schematic diagram shows major features of protein digestion and uptake into enterocytes. Approximately 40% of ingested amino acids are absorbed as free amino acids or as di and tripeptides following lumenal digestion. The remaining 60% are absorbed after being broken down further by membrane-bound peptidases. Free amino acids leave the cell by both facilitated and simple diffusion. *C.* Fat digestion and absorption. Schematic diagram of three major classes of fats and their digestion products. *(A. Adapted, with permission, from Berne R.M., and Levy, M.N., eds. (1998). Physiology, 4th ed., p. 648. B. and C. Adapted, with permission, from Johnson, L.R. (1992). Essential Medical Physiology. New York, Raven Press, pp. 514, 515.)*

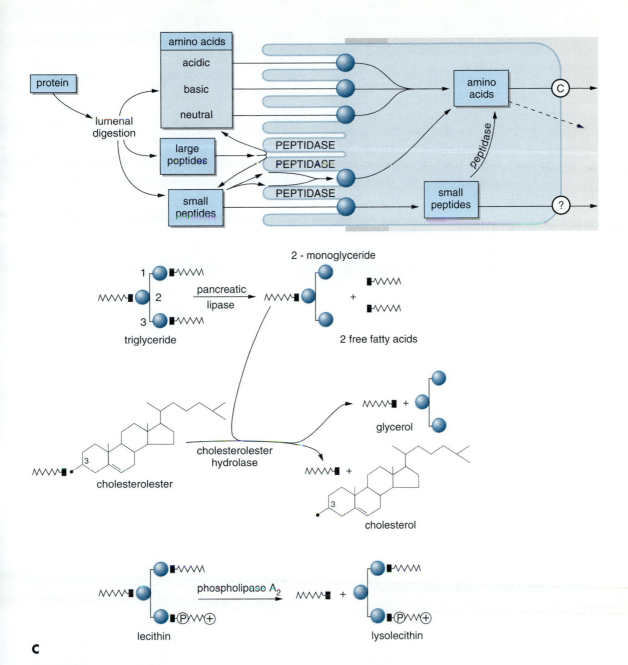

C

FIGURE 5.16 — (*continued*)

Whereas glucose and galactose are taken up by a Na$^+$ dependent active glucose transport system (GLUT1, see Figure 5.16A), fructose is absorbed by carrier-mediated facilitated diffusion (GLUT5). From the enterocyte, various sugars are transported into the blood stream by yet another glucose transporter isoform (GLUT2). The venous drainage from the GI tract flows into the portal vein. Thus simple sugars are transported to the liver and converted into glycogen.

Value of dietary fiber

Even though it is not digested, dietary fiber is an extremely valuable component of the diet because its ingestion:

- Prevents constipation
- Provides a food source for the normal, beneficial human colonic microbes
- May assist in removal of dietary toxins by tight binding and rapid excretion
- May help establish an optimal time course of absorption of simple sugars through lower affinity binding
- Contributes to satiety without providing excess calories
- Is epidemiologically associated with lower rates of cardiovascular diseases and digestive diseases including cancer, probably for reasons related to the previous points.

Protein digestion and absorption

The recommended daily intake of protein in the diet recommended by the U.S. National Academy of Sciences is currently 45 g/d for women and 56 g/d for men. However, this is likely to be a substantial overestimate, given that the average male placed on a protein-free diet loses an amount of nitrogen equivalent to about 24 g of protein a day.

The quality of protein ingested depends on its amino acid composition. Nine amino

TABLE 5.3   ESSENTIAL AND NONESSENTIAL AMINO ACIDS

Essential	Nonessential
Histidine	Alanine
Isoleucine	Arginine
Leucine	Aspartic acid
Lysine	Glutamic acid
Methionine	Glycine
Phenylalanine	Proline
Threonine	Serine
Tryptophan	Tyrosine
Valine	Cystiene
	Glutamine
	Asparagine

acids are termed *essential* because they cannot be synthesized via intermediary metabolism, and therefore, must be ingested (see Table 5.3). High-quality protein sources are those that provide balanced amounts of the essential amino acids.

Protein digestion, termed *proteolysis*, is initiated in the acid environment of the stomach (pepsin). Proteolysis continues in the neutralized environment of the small intestine, where pancreatic endoproteases (trypsin, chymotrypsin, elastase) generate small peptides. These peptides are further acted upon by both pancreatic enzymes (carboxypeptidases) and brush border membrane-bound enzymes (e.g., aminopeptidases) to generate free amino acids, dipeptides, and tripeptides.

Free amino acids and small peptides can be taken up across the enterocyte plasma membrane by specific transporters in the apical enterocyte plasma membrane. In the enterocyte cytosol, an additional set of proteases converts the transported peptides to free amino acids. Transporters on the basolateral surface of the enterocyte move free amino acids into the portal vein, where they travel in the bloodstream to the liver and are taken up by hepatocytes and subject to further metabolism.

Fat digestion and absorption

Fat is the most concentrated energy source. Oxidation of 1 g of fat generates 9 kcal, while 1 g of carbohydrate or protein generates 4 kcal each. Diets with as little as 10% fat are generally considered safe. The average American diet contains more than 50% fat. High-fat diets are epidemiologically associated with higher rates of obesity and cardiovascular disease. Therefore, a decrease in dietary fat to 30% of total calories is generally recommended, although there are reasons to believe that a diet of 15 to 20% of total calories from fat could be even more beneficial (see Ref. 13). Table 5.4 gives the nutritional composition of some common foods.

The major components of dietary fat are fatty acids, mostly in the form of **triglycerides** and **cholesterol**. Dietary fat is also necessary to provide the essential fatty acid **linoleic acid**. The fatty acids derived from animal sources are largely saturated (contain 2 extra hydrogen atoms instead of carbon-to-carbon double bonds), while those from plant sources are mono- or polyunsaturated (con-

TABLE 5.4 NUTRITIONAL CONTENT OF SOME COMMON FOODS

Food	% Protein	% Fat	% Carbohydrate	Fuel value per 100 grams, calories
Apples	0.3	0.4	14.9	64
Asparagus	2.2	0.2	3.9	26
Bacon, fat	6.2	76.0	0.7	712
broiled	25.0	55.0	1.0	599
Beef, medium	17.5	22.0	1.0	268
Beets, fresh	1.6	0.1	9.6	46
Bread, white	9.0	3.6	49.8	268
Butter	0.6	81.0	0.4	733
Cabbage	1.4	0.2	5.3	29
Carrots	1.2	0.3	9.3	45
Cashew nuts	19.6	47.2	26.4	609
Cheese, Cheddar, American	23.9	32.3	1.7	393
Chicken, total edible	21.6	2.7	1.0	111
Chocolate	(5.5)	52.9	(18.0)	570
Corn (maize), entire	10.0	4.3	73.4	372
Haddock	17.2	0.3	0.5	72
Lamb, leg, intermediate	18.0	17.5	1.0	230
Milk, fresh whole	3.5	3.9	4.9	69
Molasses, medium	0.0	0.0	(60.0)	240
Oatmeal, dry, uncooked	14.2	7.4	68.2	396
Oranges	0.9	0.2	11.2	50
Peanuts	26.9	44.2	23.6	600
Peas, fresh	6.7	0.4	17.7	101
Pork, ham, medium	15.2	31.0	1.0	340
Potatoes	2.0	0.1	19.1	85
Spinach	2.3	0.3	3.2	25
Strawberries	0.8	0.6	8.1	41
Tomatoes	1.0	0.3	4.0	23
Tuna, canned	24.2	10.8	0.5	194
Walnuts, English	15.0	64.4	15.6	702

Reproduced, with permission, from Guyton, A.C., and Hall, J.E. (1996). *Textbook of Medical Physiology*, 9th ed. Philadelphia, Saunders, p. 890.

TABLE 5.5 WATER-SOLUBLE AND FAT-SOLUBLE VITAMINS

Water-Soluble Vitamins

Vitamin	RDA	Sources	Site and mode of absorption	Role
C	60 mg/day	Fruits, vegetables, organ (liver and kidney) meat	Active transport by the ileum	Coenzyme or cofactor in many oxidative processes
B_1 (thiamine)	1 mg/day	Yeast, liver, cereal grains	At low lumenal concentrations, by active, carrier-mediated process; at high lumenal concentrations, by passive diffusion	Carbohydrate metabolism
B_2 (riboflavin)	1.7 mg/day	Dairy products	Active transport in the proximal small intestine	Metabolism
Niacin	19 mg/day	Brewers' yeast, meat	At low lumenal concentrations, by a Na^+-dependent, carrier-mediated, facilitated transport	A component of the coenzymes NAD(H) and NADP(H); metabolism of carbohydrates, fats, and proteins; synthesis of fatty acid and steroid
B_6 (pyridoxine)	2.2 mg/day	Brewer's yeast, wheat germ, meat, whole grain cereals, dairy products	By passive diffusion in small intestine	Amino acid and carbohydrate metabolism
Biotin	200 μg/day	Brewer's yeast, milk, liver, egg yolk	At low lumenal concentrations, by active transport; at high lumenal concentrations, by simple diffusion	Coenzyme for carboxylase, transcarboxylase, and decarboxylase enzymes; metabolism of lipids, glucose, and amino acids
Folic acid	0.5 mg/day	Liver, beans, dark green leafy vegetables	By Na^+-dependent facilitated transport	Nucleic acid biosynthesis, maturation of red blood cells, and promotion of growth
B_{12}	3 μg/day	Liver, kidney, dairy products, eggs, fish	Absorbed in terminal ileum. By active transport involving binding to intrinsic factor	Normal cell division; bone marrow and intestinal mucosa most affected in deficiency state, characterized by pernicious anemia

Fat-Soluble Vitamins

Vitamin	RDA	Sources	Site and mode of absorption	Role
A	1000 RE	Liver, kidney, butter, whole milk, cheese, β-carotene (yields 2 molecules of retinol)	Small intestine; passive	Vision, bone development, epithelial development, reproduction
D	200 IU	Liver, butter, cream, vitamin D-fortified milk, conversion from 7-dehydrocholesterol by ultraviolet light	Small intestine; passive	Growth and development, formation of bones and teeth, stimulation of intestinal Ca^{2+} and phosphate absorption, mobilization of Ca^{2+} ions from bones
E	10 mg	Wheat germ, green plants, egg yolk, milk, butter, meat	Small intestine; passive	Antioxidant
K	70-100 μg	Green vegetables and intestinal gut flora	Phylloquinones from green vegetables are absorbed actively from the proximal small intestine; menaquinones from gut flora are absorbed passively	Blood clotting

RE, retinol equivalent; IU, international unit; 1 IU = 0.025 μg.

Reproduced, with permission, from Johnson, L.R. (1992). in *Essential Medical Physiology*, New York, Raven Press.

tain 1 or more double bonds). Unsaturated fatty acids are associated with lower serum cholesterol and lower cardiovascular risk. Daily cholesterol intake is recommended to be less than 300 mg/day. The average American diet contains about 450 mg/day of cholesterol.

Fat absorption occurs in the proximal small intestine (duodenum and jejunum). Most ingested fats are long-chain triglycerides, either saturated (animal fats) or unsaturated (plant products).

The action of bile acids is to solubilize fats; that is, convert them from large globs to small micelles so that the enzymes can have access to their constituents and digest them, and the digestion products in the micelles can be absorbed.

Once hydrolyzed by digestive enzymes, micelles containing the digestion products (including triglycerides, phospholipids, and cholesterol, see Figure 5.16), diffuse across what is called the **unstirred layer** of liquid between the intestinal epithelial cell brush border and the gut lumen. Upon reaching the enterocyte plasma membrane, the hydrophobic digestion products either enter the membrane directly or, more likely, are transported in.

On the cytosolic side, special binding proteins (e.g., fatty acid binding protein) transport specific components to sites where they are re-esterified to form triglycerides and assembled with nascent lipoproteins in the endoplasmic reticulum to form chylomicrons. The resulting lipoprotein particles traverse the secretory pathway and enter the lymphatic drainage, from which, eventually, they rejoin the systemic circulation.

Essentially the same process, resulting in incorporation into chylomicrons, also occurs for less abundant fats such as lecithin (from which arachidonic acid is synthesized) and the hydrophobic "fat soluble" vitamins A, D, E, and K. These hydrophobic substances are transported in lipoprotein particles and thus are made available to various tissues. Ulti-

mately, they are transported to the liver for storage or disposal (see Chap. 4).

Specialized absorptive mechanisms

Specialized mechanisms exist in the ileum for absorption of Vitamin B_{12} and bile acids. The vitamin B_{12}-intrinsic factor complex is bound to the enterocyte cell surface at the terminal ileum and internalized by receptor-mediated endocytosis (see Figure 5.8). Other vitamins and their mechanism of absorption are indicated in Table 5.5.

Bile acids are absorbed efficiently in the terminal ileum, probably by uptake from the lumen by sodium-dependent transporters in the apical enterocyte plasma membrane. From the enterocyte they enter the portal circulation, from which they are extracted by the liver to complete the cycle of enterohepatic bile circulation.

Iron is absorbed in two places. Heme-bound iron is absorbed to some extent by the gastric mucosa, however, most of both heme-bound and free iron is largely absorbed in the duodenum and proximal jejunum. The degree of saturation of enterocyte ferritin determines the degree to which iron is absorbed from the GI tract lumen (see Figure 5.17).

Review Questions

21. What are the programs of small intestinal motility and how are they regulated?
22. What is dietary fiber and what is its role?
23. Where is protein digestion initiated? Where does the bulk of protein digestion occur?
24. What are the major classes of dietary fats? What is the mechanism of their digestion and absorption?
25. How is vitamin B_{12} absorbed?

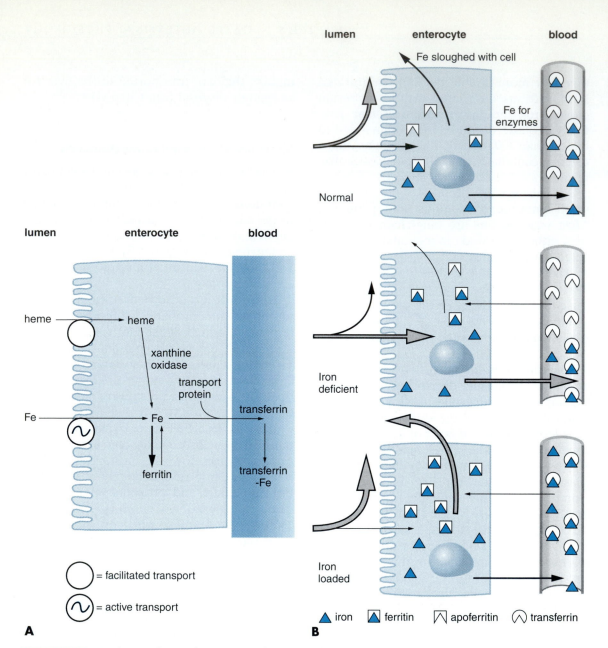

FIGURE 5.17. Regulation of iron absorption in the intestinal mucosa. A. Iron is absorbed from the intestine by facilitated transport of heme, from which free iron is released in the enterocyte cytoplasm, and by active transport of iron. Iron released in the cytosol is bound to ferritin and transported into the bloodstream where it binds transferrin for transport to other tissues. B. Regulation of iron absorption by the intestinal mucosa. The degree to which iron binding proteins (such as ferritin in the enterocyte and transferrin in the bloodstream) are saturated determines the extent to which dietary iron is absorbed or eliminated, either by not being absorbed in the first place, or by sloughing of the enterocyte. Somehow, the intestine receives a signal to increase iron absorption under conditions of hypoxia, iron deficiency or increased erythropoesis. (Adapted, with permission, from Rhoades, R.A. and Tanner, G.A. (1995). Medical Physiology. Boston, Little, Brown, p. 568.)

240

7. COLON

Anatomic organization and histologic characteristics

The colon is the section of the GI tract that follows the small intestine. It is approximately 1.5 m in length and can be divided into various segments: cecum, ascending, transverse, descending and sigmoid colon, rectum and anal canal, and anal sphincter (see Figure 5.1).

The colon has distinctive anatomic features:

The outer longitudinal smooth muscle of the bowel wall is organized in the form of three bands termed the **taeniae coli**.

Between the taeniae are outpouchings called **haustra**, which are separated by folds. The size and shape of the haustra change with the contraction state of the taeniae.

On a plain x-ray film of the abdomen the distinction between the small and large intestine can often be made on the basis of the distinctive presence of gas in the colon.

Microscopically the colon is similar to the small intestine in organization (i.e., its lining columnar epithelium displays microvilli and a glycocalyx); however, there are no villi and the microvilli are far less abundant. Biochemically, it lacks many of the channels present in the small intestine (e.g., there are no nutrient-coupled active sodium cotransporters). Unlike the proximal small intestine, there are tight junctions that prevent water from leaking in between enterocytes.

Physiological functions of the colon

The major functions of the colon are:

- Propulsion/storage of unabsorbed material
- Provision of a niche for normal resident microbes
- Absorption of water and electrolytes

Colonic motility

Unlike the stomach and small intestine, which have quiet periods, the colon is rarely without activity. However, activity is less easily characterized than that of the stomach (e.g., receptive relaxation versus MMC) or the small intestine (segmental peristalsis versus MMC). Some patterns of activity in the colon are discernible, however, such as the **gastrocolic reflex**. This is the phenomenon of colonic mass peristalsis following a meal.

Colonic secretion

Normally, the colonic epithelial cells are involved largely in mucus secretion. However, the colon also is involved in either absorption or secretion of K^+, depending on the lumenal K^+ concentration. The colon is normally responsible for approximately 10% of daily K^+ excretion when dietary K^+ is plentiful (the rest leaves via the kidney). Upon irritating stimuli, fluid and electrolyte secretion can be stimulated in the colon, providing another mechanism for diarrhea.

Clinical Pearl

○ The colon's potential for K^+ secretion can be put to good use in a patient with moderately elevated serum potassium. Potassium-binding resins are administered together with nonabsorbable carbohydrates (e.g., sorbitol), in the form of an enema. Lumenal potassium is bound by the resin, triggering K^+ secretion while the nonabsorbable carbohydrate triggers osmotic diarrhea. The net effect is substantially increased colonic K^+ loss and, ultimately, lowering of serum potassium. However, this process takes up to several hours to be fully effective, so if serum potassium elevation is life-threatening (e.g., above 6.0 eq/L), other interventions should be made in addition (see Chap. 10).

Colonic absorption

The cells of the colonic epithelium do not have the digestive enzymes found on the brush border enterocytes of the small bowel. However, unlike the small bowel which is normally free of bacteria, the colon is host to a large resident bacterial population whose health and well-being is crucial for normal GI tract function. Colonic microbes digest dietary fiber generating short chain free fatty acids (SCFAs) that are readily absorbed by colonic enterocytes, providing most of the nourishment for the colon.

These SCFAs are more than just a major source of nutrition in that they appear to affect signaling pathways within the colonic enterocytes quite profoundly. Normal colonic enterocytes appear to be stimulated to proliferate under the influence of the SCFAs produced by colonic microbe. In contrast, colonic epithelial cells that have undergone malignant transformation are forced to undergo apoptosis by SCFAs. Thus, SCFAs are protective in more ways than one, indicative of a true symbiosis between the colon and its resident bacterial flora.

A major function of the colonic enterocytes is the absorption of fluid and electrolytes. The colon has an absorptive capacity of up to 5 L of water per day, although normally less than 1 L is actually absorbed there. Furthermore, the colonic epithelium can also take sodium up against a considerable concentration gradient. Aldosterone, a hormone involved in fluid and electrolyte homeostasis, increases the colonic sodium conductance in response to volume depletion, thus playing an important role in maintaining the body's fluid and electrolyte balance similar to its role in the kidney. Fluid conservation by the colon is critically important, despite that it accounts for only a very small percentage of total absorption that occurs in the GI tract, because of the following reasons:

- Although small as a percentage of total fluid absorbed, it is a large enough amount that uncorrected, its loss would rapidly result in serious dehydration.
- Being the last step before exit from the body, there is no further opportunity for downstream regulation to compensate for lack of colonic absorption.

Review Questions

26. What are the structural differences between the small and large intestine? What are the physiological functions of the colon and the unique features of colonic motility, secretion, and absorption?
27. What are some histologic and functional differences between the regions of the small intestine?

8. GASTROINTESTINAL BLOOD FLOW

Nearly a quarter of the cardiac output goes to the GI tract, and up to one-third of blood volume can reside there at any given time. Collectively, the vasculature and blood flow of the GI tract and spleen is termed the **splanchnic circulation**.

Splanchnic blood flow is highly regulated, with ingestion of food serving as a major stimulus to increase GI blood flow, particularly to the mucosa. The magnitude of this effect, which accounts for as much as an eightfold difference in blood flow between active and quiescent states, depends on many factors, including the following:

- The caloric and nutritional composition of food

• Paracrine vasodilators such as the kinin peptides released by various GI tract glands at the same time as they secrete substances into the GI lumen.

• The fall in oxygen concentration that accompanies increased metabolic activity which in turn results in release of **adenosine**, a powerful local vasodilator.

• Nervous system regulation of GI blood flow. Parasympathetic input is believed to contribute to vasodilation indirectly, by triggering some of the other factors previously named. Sympathetic activity directly results in intense constriction of arteriolar smooth muscle, thereby decreasing and redirecting blood flow away from the GI tract. This sympathetic nervous system effect is transitory, however, because of a phenomenon called **autoregulatory escape**. Probably this reflects the dominance of a vasodilatory factor (such as adenosine) over sympathetic vasoconstriction under conditions of hypoxia.

In addition to affecting blood flow, many of the paracrine mediators that increase GI blood flow also increase capillary permeability. Physiologically, this is part of the normal inflammatory response that defends the GI tract from invasion by pathogens. However, under certain circumstances, that response proceeds in excess of what is beneficial to the patient, resulting in bowel edema and/or intestinal ischemia. In extreme cases this can be life-threatening, resulting in hypotension and even multiorgan system failure.

Clinical Pearl

○ The complaint of blood in the stool without a history of vomiting is, by itself, a poor basis for localizing the site of bleeding. Very brisk bleeding from an upper GI source (e.g., gastritis or a gastric or peptic ulcer) may, fortuitously, present as blood per rectum without vomiting. A tip-off is that the presence of melena (black tarry stools from mixing fresh blood with stomach acid) is suggestive of an upper source while bright red blood from the rectum suggests a lower source. All patients with substantial GI bleeding should initially have a nasogastric (NG) tube placed, at least temporarily, to help localize the source of the bleeding. If flushing out the stomach with saline through the NG tube does not demonstrate blood, then colonoscopy (looking up a flexible tube inserted from the anus) rather than upper endoscopy (looking down into the stomach from the mouth) is the appropriate first study.

Review Questions

28. What is autoregulatory escape? What is believed to be its molecular basis?

29. What additional action is associated with many paracrine effectors that increase GI blood flow?

9. CONTROL OF GASTROINTESTINAL TRACT FUNCTION

Together, neural and hormonal factors regulate the processes of motility, secretion, digestion, and absorption (see Figure 5.18) and, as just described, GI blood flow.

Neural

GI tract functions are controlled by both the ENS and the CNS, working through autonomic components of the peripheral nervous system (Figure 5.19). The ENS receives sensory input from neurons specialized to detect chemical, osmotic, or thermal changes in the lumen or mechanical activity involving the gut wall. This information is integrated with and modified by input from the CNS via the

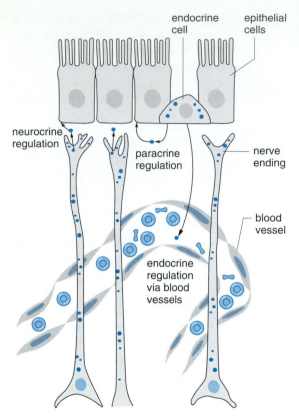

FIGURE 5.18. Neural and hormonal control of the intestine. Indicates the role of paracrine, endocrine, and neural factors in regulation of intestinal function. *(Adapted, with permission, from Dharmsathaphorn (1989). in Kelley, W.N. ed.* Textbook of Internal Medicine, *Philadelphia, Lippincott.)*

sympathetic and parasympathetic neurons, which synapse with intramural neurons and provide the program for motor neurons. In this way, otherwise uncontrolled and random motor and secretory activity of the gut becomes purposeful and coordinated (e.g., as manifested by characteristic gut activities such as peristalsis, migrating motor complex, and sphincter control, to name a few).

Motor neurons in the ENS do not release their neurotransmitters at a single site as occurs at the motor endplates in skeletal muscle. Instead, a neurotransmitter is released

from small bulges along the length of the axon called *varicosities*. Also, the spacing between motor axon and muscle cell is larger than occurs in skeletal muscle. Thus, ENS-mediated neural responses in the GI tract are generally slower and more diffuse than those mediated by skeletal neuromuscular junctions.

Recall (from earlier in this chapter) that the ENS consists primarily of two major networks of neurons and their processes, termed the *myenteric (Auerbach's) plexus* and the *submucosal (Meissner's) plexus*. The myenteric plexus is largely involved with muscular contraction while the submucosal plexus tonically suppresses fluid and electrolyte transport and limits the absorptive capacity of the intestine. These effects are mediated by neurotransmitters released by the motor neurons. The neurotransmitters work by triggering signaling via receptors on intestinal epithelial cells. Signaling from the receptor alters the activation state of ion channels.

The dependence of the ENS on CNS control varies with the embryologic origin of gut structures. The characteristic functions of structures derived from the embryonic foregut (proximal to the ampulla of Vater) are more dependent on CNS control (e.g., esophageal peristalsis, relaxation of the lower esophageal sphincter, gastric accommodation and peristalsis, pyloric sphincter function). However, mid- and hindgut-derived structures (e.g., small and large intestine) function relatively well when their connections to the CNS are disrupted.

The importance of the ENS itself is seen in diseases where its function is lost, which can occur at any of the several levels of the GI tract. For example, in achalasia (in the esophagus) loss of ENS function results in an esophagus that is quiet and a lower esophageal sphincter that is tonically contracted. As a result, ingestion of food is difficult or impossible. Similarly, loss of ENS function in pseudoobstruction of the small bowel or Hirschsprung's disease in the colon have severe clinical consequences, including abdominal pain, distension, and risk of catastrophic intestinal perforation.

Hormonal

Unlike the other endocrine glands, the gut endocrine system is a diffuse collection of individual cells distributed throughout the mucosa of the GI tract. Armed with apical microvilli and crammed with basal secretory granules, they are ideally situated to respond to a change in the lumenal environment by releasing their secretory products into the bloodstream.

Some gut peptides are true hormones, meaning they are released into the bloodstream, and it is difficult to sort out which gut peptides are local mediators, hormones, or neurotransmitters. Many are likely to play more than one of those roles under particular circumstances. Regardless of mechanism, gut peptides have a range of effects on their target tissues in the GI tract, including the following:

• Stimulation or inhibition of water, electrolyte, or enzyme secretion
• Stimulation or inhibition of gut motility
• Stimulation or inhibition of release of other gastrointestinal peptides
• Stimulation or inhibition of blood flow
• Stimulation of growth of the GI tract (different hormones affect different regions)

Many GI peptides have effects at high concentrations that are unrelated to the effects that occur at the concentrations that are actually achieved in the bloodstream. Distinguishing pharmacologic systemic effects (effects that occur at doses that are higher than would normally be seen in the body) from the physiological effects at particular target sites is one of the challenges for modern gastrointestinal endocrinology.

Five gut peptides have been shown unequivocally to serve as hormones (mediators of signal transduction that are transported to their target cells via the bloodstream): secretin, gastrin, CCK, GIP, and motilin. The data implicating others remain controversial (see Table 5.6).

Gastrin/cholecystokinin family

Gastrin is the 34 amino acid peptide generated from a much larger precursor that is secreted by endocrine cells of the antral and duodenal mucosa. It is released in response to protein-rich meals (i.e., to the presence of amino acids and peptides in the gut lumen). Gastrin also responds to increased calcium, various neurotransmitters, catecholamines, and other GI hormones, especially when the pH is elevated.

• The major action of gastrin is to stimulate acid secretion by the parietal cells of the gastric mucosa. Acid serves as a "brake" to close the negative feedback loop by neutralizing the elevated pH that was a powerful stimulant of gastrin release in the first place.
• Gastrin also inhibits gastric and intestinal smooth muscle contraction.
• On a delayed timescale of days, gastrin is trophic to gastric mucosa, promoting DNA synthesis and cell proliferation. In excess it will result in hyperplasia.

CCK is a 33 amino acid peptide secreted from endocrine cells of the small intestine. An 8 amino acid form is found in the brain. CCK has the same carboxy terminal 5 amino acid residues as does gastrin, and this region is required for both hormones' biological activities. Sulfation of a tyrosine residue 7 amino acids in from the carboxy terminus is specific for CCK and critical for its biological activity by causing a major change in both receptor affinity and selectivity.

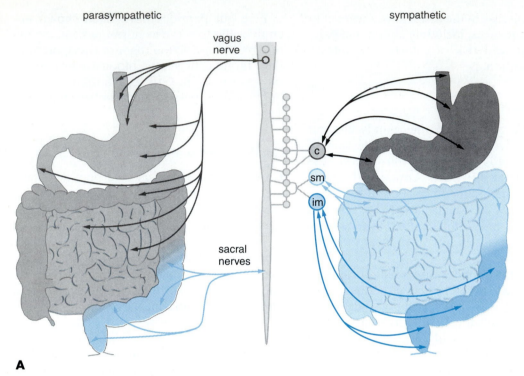

parasympathetic

sympathetic

vagus
nerve

sacral
nerves

A

FIGURE 5.19. ENS and its control by the ANS. *A.* The extrinsic branches of the autonomic nervous system. Parasympathetic (left hand panel). Dashed lines indicate cholinergic innervation of the striated muscle in the esophagus and external anal sphincter. Solid lines indicate afferent and preganglionic innervation of the remaining GI tract. Sympathetic (right hand panel). The afferent and preganglionic efferent pathways between the spinal cord and the prevertebral ganglia (c, celiac; sm, superior mesenteric; im, inferior mesenteric) are indicated on the left hand side; the afferent and postganglionic efferent innervation are indicated on the right hand side. *B.* Parasympathetic input to the ENS. Upper panel shows the preganglionic fibers of the parasympathetic system synapsing with ganglion cells located in the myenteric and submucosal plexuses of the ENS. Their cell bodies in turn send signals to smooth muscle, secretory, and endocrine cells. Lower panel shows a vagovagal reflex where information from receptors in the smooth muscle or mucosa is relayed through the ENS to higher centers via vagal afferents. This may trigger a response carried by vagal efferent resulting in alteration of motility, secretion, or hormone release. *C.* Efferent sympathetic innervation. Postganglionic fibers from the sympathetic ganglia innervate the elements of the ENS. However, they may also innervate blood vessels and cells of the smooth muscle layers and mucosa directly. *(B and C. Adapted, with permission, from Johnson, L.R. (1992). in* Essential Medical Physiology. *New York, Raven Press, pp. 451–452.).*

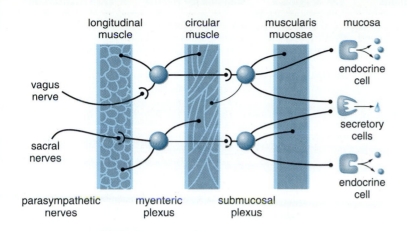

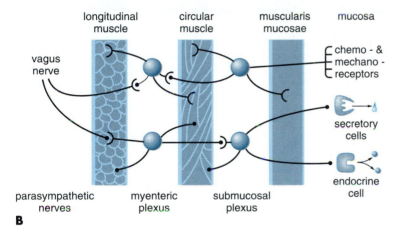

B

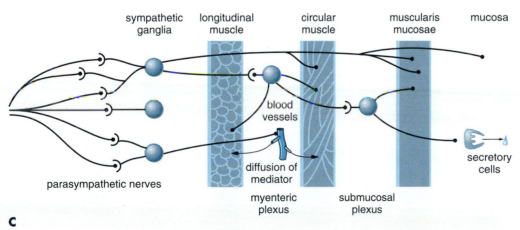

C

FIGURE 5.19 — (*continued*)

TABLE 5.6 SECRETORY PRODUCTS OF THE GI TRACT

Products	Physiologic actions	Site of release	Stimulus for release	Disease association
True hormones				
Gastrin	Stimulates acid secretion and growth of gastric oxyntic gland mucosa	Gastric antrum (and duodenum)*	Peptides, amino acids, distention, vagal stimulation	Zollinger-Ellison syndrome, peptic ulcer disease
CCK	Stimulates gallbladder contraction, pancreatic enzyme and bicarbonate secretion, and growth of exocrine pancreas	Duodenum and jejunum	Peptides, amino acids, long chain fatty acids, (acid)	
Secretin	Stimulates pancreatic bicarbonate secretion, biliary bicarbonate secretion, growth of exocrine pancreas, pepsin secretion; inhibits gastric acid secretion, trophic effects of gastrin	Duodenum	Acid (fat)	
GIP	Stimulates insulin release (inhibits gastric acid secretion)	Duodenum, jejunum	Glucose, amino acids, fatty acids	
Candidate hormones				
Motilin	Stimulates gastric and duodenal motility	Duodenum and jejunum	Unknown	Irritable bowel syndrome; diabetic gastroparesis
Pancreatic polypeptide	Inhibits pancreatic bicarbonate and enzyme secretion	Pancreatic islets of Langerhans	Protein (fat and glucose)	
Enteroglucagon	Elevates blood glucose?	Ileum	Glucose and fat	
Paracrines				
Somatostatin	Inhibits release of most other peptide hormones	Gastrointestinal tract mucosa, pancreatic islets of Langerhans	Acid stimulates, vagus inhibits release	Gallstones
Histamine	Stimulates gastric acid secretion	Oxyntic gland mucosa	Unknown	
Neurocrines				
VIP	Relaxes sphincters and gut circular muscle; stimulates intestinal and pancreatic secretion	Mucosa and smooth muscle of gastrointestinal tract	Enteric nervous system	Secretory diarrhea
Bombesin	Stimulates gastrin release	Gastric mucosa	Enteric nervous system	
Enkephalins	Stimulate smooth muscle contraction; inhibit intestinal secretion	Mucosa and smooth muscle of gastrointestinal tract	Enteric nervous system	
Other products				
Intrinsic factor	Binds vitamin B_{12} to facilitate its absorption	Parietal cells of the stomach	Constitutive secretion	Autoimmune destruction resulting in pernicious anemia
Mucin	Lubrication and protection	Goblet cells along entire gastrointestinal tract mucosa	Gastrointestinal tract irritation	Viscid mucus in cystic fibrosis. Attenuation in some cases of peptic ulcer
Acid	Initiates digestion of food; prevents infection	Parietal cells of the stomach	Gastrin, histamine, acetylcholine, NSAIDs (indirectly)	Acid-peptic disease

*Parentheses indicate minor components and effects.
NSAIDs, nonsteroidal anti-inflammatory drugs.

CCK does the following:

- Causes gallbladder contraction and sphincter of Oddi relaxation
- Is a powerful stimulant of pancreatic enzyme secretion (by acinar cells)
- Is a weak stimulant of bicarbonate and water secretion by pancreatic duct cells
- Exerts important long-term trophic effects on the growth of pancreatic acini
- May be a major hormonal signal of satiety, thereby limiting the size of meals
- Increases gastric and intestinal smooth muscle contraction (opposite the effects of secretin)

CCK release is stimulated directly by amino acids (especially phenylalanine), fatty acids, and monoglycerides, and indirectly by HCl, which lowers the pH of chyme entering the duodenum and triggers secretin secretion. Bile acids have no influence on CCK release.

Secretin family

The secretin family of gut peptides includes secretin, glucose-dependent insulinotropic peptide (GIP), glucagon, and vasoactive intestinal polypeptide (VIP).

- **Secretin** is a 27 amino acid polypeptide structurally related to glucagon, vasoactive intestinal polypeptide (VIP), and glucose-dependent insulinotrophic peptide (GIP), which are all secreted from endocrine cells of the intestine. Acid (pH < 4.5) is the major stimulant for secretion of secretin. The endocrine cells from which secretin is released are found in the mucosa of the duodenum and upper jejunum. Secretin's major action is to stimulate pancreatic ductal cells to increase their volume of bicarbonate and water secretion (which neutralizes acid and thereby shuts off the stimulus for further secretion of secretin).

- **GIP** (gastric inhibitory peptide) is released in response to a carbohydrate- and fat-rich meal. Its major role probably is to potentiate insulin release, although it may have a minor action as an inhibitor of acid secretion. GIP may be responsible for the observation that a greater amount of insulin is released in response to an oral glucose load than to an identical load infused intravenously.
- **Glucagon** is made not only from the α cells of the islets of Langerhans in the pancreas, but also from endocrine cells in the mucosa of the terminal ileum and colon. Islet cell glucagon is processed to a 29-residue peptide whose major effect is to stimulate hepatic glucose production and release. However, the predominant form of glucagon in the gut is a larger, less fully processed polypeptide termed **glycentin**, whose major effects are believed to be on the GI tract rather than the liver. Glycentin's role may be largely that of a trophic hormone stimulating growth of the small intestine (e.g., in response to malabsorption). Glycentin may also slow gastric emptying and intestinal motility — effects that, interestingly, would result in more glucose absorption from the gut and thereby reinforce the glucose-mobilizing effects of islet cell glucagon.
- **VIP** has secretin-like effects on the pancreas, dramatically increasing the volume of water and bicarbonate output. It may also affect GI blood flow and gut motility, both as a hormone and a neurotransmitter. VIP may also stimulate intestinal secretion in a manner similar to cholera toxin (i.e., by increasing cyclic adenosine monophosphate).

Secretin and CCK potentiate each other's effects on the pancreas. Thus, a protein-rich meal stimulates acid secretion. The protein also stimulates CCK release, and the acid stimulates secretin release. The combination of secretin and CCK stimulates more pancreatic enzymes than would have been released in response to that amount of CCK alone, and more bicarbonate than would have been released in response to that amount of secretin alone. Secretin also decreases the force of contraction of smooth muscle in the wall of the stomach and the intestine.

Other gastrointestinal hormones

Of the many other GI hormones and candidate hormones, the most prominent include the pancreatic polypeptide family, the opioid peptides, motilin, somatostatin, and epidermal growth factor. Their physiological roles are under active investigation.

At present, **somatostatin** is probably the best understood of these molecules. It has a broad range of inhibitory effects, mainly by inhibiting secretion of various peptides from endocrine cells throughout the body that, in turn, have diverse effects on tissues throughout the body. The effects of somatostatin on the GI tract include the following:

- Inhibition of secretion in the stomach, small intestine, pancreas, and liver
- Diminution of GI motility
- Reduction of splanchnic blood flow

Clinical Pearl

○ An analogue of somatostatin called *octreotide*, which is notable for a longer half-life, has been developed and found to be useful in a variety of clinical situations including:

- Zollinger-Ellison syndrome, where massive gastrin hypersecretion by a tumor results in intractable peptic ulcer disease.
- Carcinoid/VIPoma syndromes, where a variety of peptides secreted from GI endocrine tumors result in profuse secre-

tory diarrhea and/or disabling symptoms of flushing.
- Acromegaly, where octreotide is able to inhibit growth hormone hypersecretion.
- Detection and imaging of a variety of tumors that display somatostatin receptors, including some lung cancers and some malignant lymphomas.
- Control of certain forms of upper GI bleeding, including esophageal varices (presumably by reducing splanchnic blood flow).
- Control of secretory diarrhea due to infectious causes, including cryptosporidium and cytomegalovirus (e.g., in patients with AIDS).
- Treatment of GI motility disorders such as dumping syndrome.

Review Questions

30. How do motor neurons of the ENS differ from those of skeletal muscle elsewhere in the body?
31. Describe the major actions and regulators of gastrin, CCK, and secretin.
32. Name four other GI tract hormones and their actions.

10. SPECIAL TOPICS

Gastrointestinal immunology

In the course of carrying out its primary mission — the separation of food into nutrients to be assimilated and wastes to be eliminated — the intestinal mucosa inevitably is in close contact with all manner of undesirables, including pathogenic microbes. Thus, a crucial accessory function of the GI tract is defense against pathogenic microbial invasion across the intestinal epithelial barrier. This defense is organized at several levels:

- The intestinal epithelium defends nonspecifically against invasion by having tight junctions between cells, as well as by its continuous secretion of mucus and its glyco-calyx coat.

- The intestinal epithelial defense has a second component that is more specific: the GI tract immune system. This system needs to be powerful and multifaceted, and yet flexible, specific, and selective. The potential for invasion once the epithelial cell barrier has been breached is great, the variety of pathogens can be equally enormous, yet only a small subset of all antigens seen by the GI tract will be pathogenic. Thus, to attack all of them equally would be not only wasteful but dangerous — if any of those antigens are related to self-components, autoimmune disease might be triggered. The GI immune system is well suited for this responsibility. The prominent role afforded the GI tract in host defense often is not fully appreciated: by weight, the GI tract has as much lymphoid tissue (the anatomical equivalent of a police station) as does the spleen.
- Additional lines of immune defense, should pathogens breach the intestinal epithelium, are provided by mesenteric lymph nodes and the reticuloendothelial cells of the liver.

Subpopulations of gastrointestinal tract immune cells

GI tract associated lymphoid tissue can be divided into Peyer's patches, lamina propria lymphoid cells (LPLCs), and intraepithelial lymphocytes (IELs).

- The Peyer's patches are small lymphoid follicles of the small intestine that play a role in initiation of the immune response. Thus they contain many precursor cells, which subsequently migrate to become part of immune cell populations at other locations.
- The LPLCs consist of B lymphocytes secreting IgA, T lymphocytes serving helper/inducer functions, macrophages involved in

antigen presentation and phagocytosis, and eosinophils and mast cells involved in controlling vascular permeability and recruitment of additional immune cells (see Figure 5.20A).

- The IELs play a less well-defined role. Notably, they are separated from the GI lumen by the tight junctions of the surface intestinal epithelium.

Functions of gastrointestinal tract associated lymphoid tissue

A primary function of B lymphocytes in the gut is to synthesize IgA and IgM — but not IgG. This IgA and IgM is transported across the intestinal epithelium by a specialized form of endocytosis termed **transcytosis**: The immunoglobulins are bound by an immunoglobulin receptor on the basal surface of the epithelium (the side facing the bloodstream). They are then internalized into a vesicle that travels to the apical surface (the side facing the GI lumen). During transport to the apical surface, the receptor that bound the immunoglobulin is cleaved, which allows the immunoglobulin, together with the bound fragment of its cleaved receptor, to be released into the GI tract lumen upon fusion of the vesicle to the apical plasma membrane. In this way, specific Ig directed against various pathogens defends the epithelium.

In addition to their role in the GI tract immune system, specific lymphocytes from Peyer's patches migrate to other mucosal sites including the mammary gland, cervix, vagina, uterus, and bronchus comprising a systemic mucosal immune system (see Figure 5.20B).

Unlike other classes of Ig, IgA (the major Ig of mucosal immunity) does not participate in all of the inflammatory responses mediated by the complement system. This feature may provide one basis for the flexibility and selectivity of the GI tract immune system. In addition to its role in secretory immunity, the GI

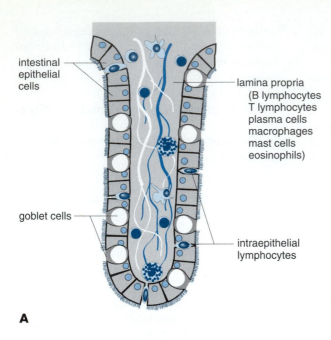

intestinal epithelial cells

lamina propria
(B lymphocytes
T lymphocytes
plasma cells
macrophages
mast cells
eosinophils)

goblet cells

intraepithelial lymphocytes

A

FIGURE 5.20. Immunology of the gastrointestinal tract. A. Schematic description of a villus indicating presence of immune cells. B. Circulation of immune cells from intestine via regional lymph nodes to the systemic circulation, other tissues, and back to the intestine again. (B. Adapted, with permission, from Kagnoff, M. (1989). Immunology and inflammation of the GI tract, in Sleisenger, M.H. and Fordtran, J.S., eds. Gastrointestinal Disease, 4th ed. Philadelphia, Saunders, p. 58.)

tract immune system carries out cell-mediated immune functions as well. These and many other features of the GI tract immune system are poorly understood and constitute an important frontier of investigation, which is likely to provide insight into a wide range of human disease.

Gastrointestinal microflora

The distal GI tract is home to a complex family of bacteria, which play important roles in the maintenance of health and the development of disease. These roles include:

- Fermentation of undigestible dietary fiber to generate short-chain fatty acids (SCFAs). These SCFAs are a major nutritional source for the colon and have trophic effects to promote normal mucosal growth and development. They also promote apoptosis (programmed cell death) of damaged colonic cells that might otherwise undergo malignant transformation.

- Creation of an environment that is inhospitable to pathogenic microorganisms and thereby preventing their colonization of the GI tract. The mechanisms by which this occurs include simple crowding — if there are a million of the "good guys" present, it is hard for one "bad guy" to take over — furthermore, many of the normal flora have a low pH optimum, whereas many pathogens favor a neutral or more alkaline environment.

- Metabolism of various compounds including bile salts, drugs, and nutrients, some of which are made available to the host.

Understanding the full implications of these interactions represents an important future frontier for medical science.

Review Questions

33. What are the lines of defense that prevent pathogen invasion via the GI tract?

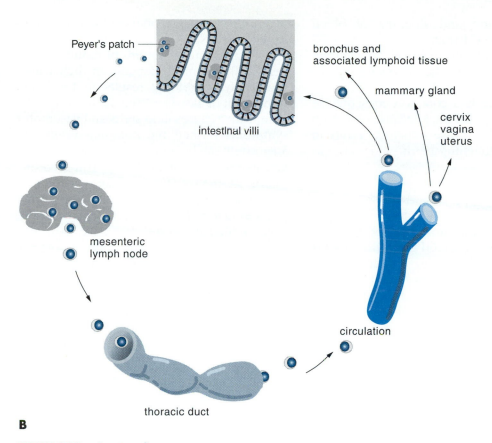

Peyer's patch

intestinal villi

bronchus and
associated lymphoid tissue

mammary gland

cervix
vagina
uterus

mesenteric
lymph node

circulation

thoracic duct

B

FIGURE 5.20 — (*continued*)

34. What are IELs and LPLCs and what do they do?
35. What are some likely roles of the normal GI tract microbial flora?

11. AN OVERVIEW OF GASTROINTESTINAL PATHOPHYSIOLOGY

Disorders of each of the physiological functions discussed previously (motility, secretion, digestion, and absorption) are prominent causes of GI disease in one part or another of the GI tract (see later).

GI bleeding and intestinal ischemia are important GI consequences of disease in the GI tract or other organ systems. Damage to the GI tract can be conceptualized as occurring due to the following reasons:

• The primary disease process (e.g., trauma)
• Subsequent hypotension
• Reactive oxygen metabolites produced upon reperfusion (so-called reperfusion injury)

Intestinal ischemia can occur through many pathophysiological mechanisms including the following:

• A "watershed" effect of hypoperfusion due to fall in blood pressure

- Vasoconstriction and shunting of blood away from the GI tract
- Clot formation resulting in ischemia, infarction, and necrosis of the GI tract

Bloody diarrhea is a common consequence of ischemia in the GI tract because of its high vascularity and because ischemia results in necrosis and sloughing of the mucosal epithelium.

Disorders of motility

Disorders of motility are observed to affect all major regions of the GI tract. Because GI tract motility is a complex consequence of smooth muscle contraction under the influence of neural and hormonal controls, abnormal motility of the GI tract can occur through either damage to GI smooth muscle or to the neural and hormonal mechanisms by which it is controlled.

Esophagus

An example of muscle damage leading to abnormal motility is seen in **esophageal stricture** as a result of caustic ingestions or acid reflux.

Abnormal neural control of motility is seen in the esophageal disorder termed **achalasia**, in which degeneration of the nerves controlling esophageal smooth muscle results in disordered muscular contraction.

All esophageal motility disorders are characterized by **dysphagia** (difficulty swallowing) and **odynophagia** (painful swallowing).

Stomach

Motility disorders of the stomach include **gastroparesis**, a complication of diabetes mellitus (see Sec. 11) and dysmotility as a consequence of stomach surgery, either due to resection of part of the stomach or **vagotomy** (surgical transection of the vagus nerve to interrupt vagal-stimulated acid secretion, but which also cuts vagal fibers influencing motility via the ENS).

The signs and symptoms of motility disorders in the stomach depend on their cause. Classically, vagotomy results in too rapid movement of gastric contents into the duodenum, which causes fluid shifts and vasomotor symptoms termed the *dumping syndrome*. Vagotomy can be done to treat some cases of acid hypersecretion due to a gastrin-secreting tumor (termed *Zollinger-Ellison syndrome*) and in severe peptic ulcer disease. Over the years surgeons have learned how to do so-called selective and superselective vagotomy procedures by which transection of some of the motility-controlling vagal fibers can be avoided.

In contrast to vagotomy, intrinsic neuropathy (e.g., in diabetes mellitus) results in delayed gastric emptying, nausea, vomiting, and constipation, rather than the classical dumping syndrome. The pathophysiological basis for these differences is not known.

Small intestine and colon

In the small intestine and colon disordered motility is believed to be responsible for some cases of "irritable bowel syndrome," a condition characterized by recurrent episodes of abdominal pain, bloating, and diarrhea alternating with constipation. Although the pathophysiology of this disorder is poorly understood, altered levels of GI tract hormones such as motilin have been suggested as a cause, perhaps influenced by emotional and psychological factors.

Disorders of secretion

The major defined disorders of secretion in the GI tract are those involving production of the following:

- Acid or intrinsic factor by the stomach (acid peptic disease)

- Digestive enzymes by the pancreas (pancreatitis)
- Bile by the liver (cholestasis)
- Water and electrolytes by the small intestine in response to inflammation of the mucosa, blood-borne secretagogues, or lumenal-derived toxins (diarrhea)

As mentioned earlier, irritable bowel syndrome may be quite heterogeneous in etiology and some cases may be due in part to disordered secretion of GI hormones.

Stomach

Either elevated gastric acid secretion or diminished mucosal defense can predispose to development of **ulcers**, discrete, circumscribed regions of erosion through the mucosa that are surrounded by apparently normal tissue. Acid-induced damage may occur in the form of an ulcer either in the stomach (**gastric ulcer**) or in the first part of the small intestine (**duodenal ulcer**). Acid-induced injury may also occur in the form of more diffuse and less clearly demarcated inflammation anywhere along the length of the GI tract from the lower esophagus through the duodenum. It appears that elevated acid secretion is relatively more important in the development of duodenal ulcer while diminished mucosal defense (perhaps due to diminished mucus secretion in some cases), is the crucial factor in development of gastric ulcer.

Helicobacter pylori and ulcer disease

An extremely important advance in understanding the pathophysiology of acid peptic disease has been the recognition that infection by the bacteria *H. pylori* appears to be the cause of most cases of gastric and duodenal ulcers. *H. pylori* is an extremely common infection, found in 50 percent of the world's population, with rates of infection even higher in the poorest countries where sanitation and hygiene are particularly deficient. The most likely route of spread from person to person is fecal-oral contamination. As many as 90% of infected individuals show signs of inflammation (gastritis and/or duodenitis) on endoscopy, although typically many of these individuals are clinically asymptomatic.

Despite this high rate of association of inflammation with *H. pylori* infection, the important role of other factors is indicated by the fact that only about 15% of infected individuals develop a clinically significant ulcer during the course of their lifetime. Thus, other factors (both genetic and environmental) must account for the individual variations observed and are pathophysiologically important.

Treatment for ulcer disease that does not eradicate *H. pylori* is associated with a high rate of ulcer recurrence. Studies have also associated different strains of *H. pylori* with different forms and degrees of acid-peptic disease and implicated *H. pylori* infection in development of GI tract cancers.

These observations suggest the importance of altered local production of cytokines by the host immune system in the pathophysiology of *H. pylori*-induced disease. The details of these relations remain to be clarified by further investigation.

Disorders of digestion and absorption

Physiologically significant digestion and absorption can occur throughout the GI tract. Thus, amylase in salivary secretions initiates carbohydrate digestion and the effectiveness of sublingual nitroglycerin therapy for patients with angina is a testimonial to the efficacy of that mode of absorption. Nevertheless, the clinically prominent disorders of digestion and absorption focus on the small intestine and colon and the accessory organs (pancreas and liver) whose secretions (digestive enzymes and bicarbonate versus bile, respectively) are necessary for proper digestion and absorption in the small intestine.

Thus pain and disordered digestion and absorption are common complaints of patients with chronic pancreatitis and inability to secrete appropriate amounts of pancreatic enzymes into the duodenum. Capsules containing pancreatic enzymes can be taken orally by these patients at mealtime to improve their ability to digest and absorb a meal.

Common causes of gastrointestinal bleeding

The most common sites of bleeding along the course of the GI tract are as follows:

- Esophagus: varices (in a patient with portal hypertension, e.g., due to liver disease)
- Stomach: gastritis (superficial inflammation, e.g., due to NSAID use), gastric ulcer (a circumscribed erosion, sometimes associated with cancer), or gastric laceration (seen in some patients after intense retching)
- Small intestine: duodenal ulcer, inflammatory bowel disease, infectious gastroenteritis
- Colon: cancer, diverticular disease, polyps, amoebas and other parasites, hemorrhoids (in the rectum)

Clinical Pearls

As is apparent from the vignette at the beginning of this chapter, diarrhea is a symptom of many different pathophysiological entities. A number of powerful antidiarrhea drugs are available, their use without an understanding of the underlying cause can limit therapeutic effectiveness — or even cause more harm than good, thanks to side effects and complications.

One useful approach is to recognize that disorders of each of the major GI tract activities (motility, secretion, digestion, and absorption) can result in diarrhea. Thus:

○ Diarrhea that persists even when a patient is taking in nothing by mouth (with dehydration prevented by intravenous feedings) cannot be osmotic, but rather must be secretory or inflammatory.
○ Inflammatory causes of diarrhea can be distinguished by the presence of white blood cells in the stool, by classical appearance on biopsy of involved epithelium, and by stool culture, which identifies infectious causes.
○ A patient with longstanding diabetes mellitus is at high risk for development of diarrhea, alternating with constipation as a consequence of dysmotility due to autonomic neuropathy. These patients are probably also at increased risk of infection, especially if their diabetes is poorly controlled.
○ Secretory diarrheas can result from either blood-borne products (e.g., hormones produced by a tumor) or products in the GI lumen (bacterial products such as cholera toxin; bile acids), which damage the secretory or absorptive apparatus of gut epithelial cells, respectively.
○ Patients with chronic pancreatitis and liver cirrhosis can develop fat malabsorption (steatorrhea and/or diarrhea) and fat-soluble vitamin deficiencies, due to lack of digestive enzyme and bile, respectively. Analysis of the stool for fat, together with therapeutic trial of pancreatic enzyme replacement, typically clinches the diagnosis in these cases.

Review Questions

36. What are the major motility, secretory, and digestion/absorption disorders of the GI tract?

37. What is the role of *H. pylori* in GI disease?
38. What are the common sites of bleeding along the GI tract and their causes?

12. FRONTIERS OF GASTROENTEROLOGY

Molecular basis of gastrointestinal motility

What is the origin of the slow waves that are responsible for the intrinsic contractility of the GI tract smooth muscle? Cells of mesenchymal origin, termed the *interstitial cells of Cajal (ICC)*, have been implicated as the pacemakers from which the slow waves originate. Isolated ICCs display slow wave activity. ICCs are located within the muscle layers of the GI tract and have a distribution consistent with the extent of slow-wave activity in different regions of the GI tract. ICCs express a protooncogene termed *c-kit*, which is a receptor with endogenous tyrosine kinase activity. When mutant mice are examined that lack either a normal functioning c-kit gene, or lack the gene for the protein with which the c-kit gene product interacts, the number of ICCs in the small intestine is greatly diminished and electrical activity is absent.

Other work demonstrates severe abnormalities of GI motility and abolition of slow waves when monoclonal antibodies to c-kit are used to block development of ICCs in otherwise normal mice. Together, these studies suggest ways in which the integration of intrinsic, hormonal, and neural input to GI motility can be studied, understood, and eventually modulated in order to treat currently intractable GI motility disorders, such as irritable bowel syndrome (see Refs. 1–6).

Pathogenesis of infantile pyloric stenosis

Nitric oxide is an important signaling molecule in the nervous system. A surprising observation was that the targeted disruption of the neuronal nitric oxide synthase gene resulted in viable, fertile mice with no obvious CNS defect — but with profound abnormalities of the gastrointestinal tract, in particular grossly distended stomachs, hypertrophied circular muscle layer, and pyloric stenosis. Indeed, the common disorder of infantile pyloric stenosis is often due to a comparable genetic lesion in humans (see Refs. 7 and 8).

Trefoil peptides: a newly appreciated line of gastrointestinal defense

The trefoil peptides are a group of small proteins that constitute an important newly appreciated line of GI defense. In the absence of acute injury, they are made by mucous secreting cells and are believed to play a role in stabilization of mucus. Upon acute injury, trefoil peptides are also made by enterocytes in the neighborhood of the lesion(s) (e.g., in peptic ulcer disease and inflammatory bowel disease) and are believed to aid in repair at the site of injury. Experimentally, trefoil peptides given systemically — but not intragastrically — appear to protect against NSAID-mediated GI tract injury, when given in pharmacologic doses. Similarly, transgenic mice overexpressing a trefoil peptide in the jejunum were protected from NSAID injury. A "knockout" mouse lacking the gene for a trefoil peptide makes no gastric mucus — and develops gastric adenomas. However, the mechanism by which the trefoil peptides act remains unknown (see Refs. 9 and 10).

What is the real mechanism of cholera toxin action?

Cholera is a dread diarrheal disease that continues to take thousands of lives around the world every year. It is caused by infection of the GI tract by the bacterium *Vibrio cholerae*. This organism actually is not invasive and does not erode the GI tract mucosa as do

Salmonella, Shigella, E. coli, and other causes of bacterial gastroenteritis. Instead, *V. cholerae* produces a protein toxin, a cholera toxin, which causes uncontrolled fluid secretion into the small intestinal lumen. Distal absorptive mechanisms are overwhelmed, and unless quickly treated (e.g., by oral rehydration; see Clinical Pearl in Sec. 6), the patient quickly succumbs to dehydration. Although it is known that cholera toxin can inactivate a G protein that controls chloride channels and therefore fluid egress from the small intestine, it has never been proved that this is actually the cause of diarrhea in cholera.

Data suggest that the pathogenesis of diarrhea in cholera may be more complex. It appears that nerves of the ENS are part of a secretory reflex of the GI tract. If the ENS is interrupted, cholera toxin has no effect on fluid and electrolyte transport. This and other data have been interpreted to suggest that cholera toxin triggers a unique form of electrical activity in GI smooth muscle (a kind of action potential), and that the resulting motor activity triggers an intestinal mechano-receptor to induce fluid secretion. Further experiments are needed to determine whether this motor activity is the actual cause of the fluid secretion, or is an independent effect of cholera toxin (see Ref. 11).

Are gallstones an infectious disease?

Why do gallstones form? Some years ago an appealing hypothesis was that supersaturation of particular substances (e.g., cholesterol) in bile, together with impaired gallbladder motility, were an important cause of gallstones. Later it was recognized that mucous secretion and fluid and electrolyte absorption and secretion served to modify bile composition and therefore solubility of substances in bile. It was also recognized that there were various proteins in bile that could promote or retard nucleation and precipitation of supersaturated substances, thereby influencing the tendency for gallstone formation.

Data suggest a further wrinkle. It appears that colonization of the gallbladder with *Propionibacterium acnes*, a bacteria found in dental plaque, may tip the balance of forces in favor of gallstone formation in many patients. As with the revolution in thinking about peptic ulcer disease brought about by recognition of the role of *H. pylori* infection, these observations may ultimately result in new ways to effectively prevent or treat gallstones (see Ref. 12).

13. HOW DOES AN UNDERSTANDING OF NORMAL PHYSIOLOGY PROVIDE INSIGHT INTO THE INITIAL CASE PRESENTATION?

Recall the case of C.W., the 42-year-old accountant who presented to the hospital with dizziness.

Her history includes a number of factors that might help explain her symptoms. First, her chocolate and ethanol consumption will decrease her lower esophageal sphincter tone, resulting in acid reflux and injury. Furthermore, both smoking and drinking predispose the patient to development of gastritis and ulcer disease. Her use of NSAIDs, which diminishes protective prostaglandins, also substantially increases the risk of acid-induced GI tract injury. Acid-mediated injury is normally avoided by mucus and bicarbonate secretion by the stomach; the presence of tight junctions between epithelial cells lining the stomach normally prevents acid from leaking back. Also, an "alkaline tide" in the gastric mucosal blood flow due to bicarbonate-for-chloride exchange on the basolateral surface of parietal cells defends against acid. Finally, there are negative feedback controls over hormones such as gastrin, which stimulate acid secretion.

Antibiotics eradicate chronic *H. pylori* infection, thereby removing a major cause of mucosal inflammation, which weakens host defenses and potentiates acid-mediated injury. Antacids neturalize gastric acid directly. Cytoprotectants (such as sucralfate) bind to areas of denuded mucosa and prevent it from coming into direct contact with acid, allowing reformation of the mucus-bicarbonate defense. Histamine receptor antagonists diminish acid secretion by blocking one (of the several) stimuli to acid secretion.

Acid secretion can also be blocked by antagonists of other pathways, such as somatostatin, which inhibits gastrin secretion, and vagotomy to remove cholingeric neural input to the stomach. Proton pump inhibitors, such as omeprazole, directly block the H^+/K^+ ATPase that is the final common pathway for acid secretion by all stimuli. Prostaglandin analogues prevent ulcer formation (e.g., in patients on NSAIDs) by stimulating mucus and bicarbonate secretion and perhaps by promoting mucosal blood flow and the resulting protective alkaline tide.

H. pylori causes ulcer disease in only a small minority of infected individuals because the risk of acid-mediated injury is the result of an imbalance between protective forces (mucus, bicarbonate, feedback inhibition, etc.) and injurious forces (acid production, changes in gene expression induced by *H. pylori* infection, etc.). Thus, patients most likely to develop ulcer disease are those with *H. pylori* infection (as a result of genetics or environment, including stress), or those who have some predisposing genetic or environmental basis for excessive acid production or diminished mucosal defenses, either with or without *H. pylori* infection. In infected patients, *H. pylori* infection is sometimes enough to tip the balance of factors in favor of acid-mediated injury. In others, while the

margin of safety may be diminished, the balance is not yet tipped, and injury does not occur.

Ms. W. was advised to change some of her habits and was placed on aggressive medical therapy for duodenal ulcer, with documented healing of the ulcer on repeat endoscopy 1 year later, at which time cultures were negative for *H. pylori*. Her therapeutic regimen was then changed to maintenance therapy with a single bedtime dose of a proton pump inhibitor.

If she is cured, why put her on maintenance therapy with a proton pump inhibitor? She has a chronic scarring of the distal esophagus that will not go away. Thus, the proton pump inhibitor therapy will not only decrease influx pain by decreasing acid secretion, but will also break the cycle of further scarring of the esophagus due to acid reflux, which is worse at night in the recumbent position.

SUMMARY AND REVIEW OF KEY CONCEPTS

1. Oropharynx: Swallowing is a complex set of events initiated voluntarily but completed involuntarily, which includes contributions from both the CNS and the ENS. Major disorder: aspiration of food due to defective swallowing/gag reflexes.

2. Esophagus: Has a peristaltic motor program initiated upon swallowing, which culminates in transient lower esophageal sphincter relaxation. Major disorders: reflux esophagitis and esophageal spasm (achalasia).

3. Stomach: Displays receptive relaxation in response to food entry, and mixing function during and after meals that is programmed to allow only small spurts of well-homogenized chyme past the pylorus. Between meals, the stomach displays a different motor program, the "housekeeping"

migrating motor complex. The stomach secretes hormones into the blood, and mucus, bicarbonate, acid, and vitamin B_{12}-binding intrinsic factor into the stomach lumen. Motility and secretion are controlled by hormones (gastrin stimulates acid secretion), CNS (vagus nerve), ENS, and paracrine mediators (e.g., histamine). Major disorders: acid-mediated injury (gastritis/ulcer), motor dysfunction in diabetes mellitus, cancer, and bleeding from ulcers and gastritis.

4. Pancreas: Secretes digestive enzyme precursors (in response to hormone CCK) and bicarbonate (in response to secretin) into the proximal duodenum to neutralize acid in chyme and start digestion. Also has endocrine islets of Langerhans that secrete insulin and glucagon into the bloodstream. Major disorder: acute and chronic pancreatitis (usually due to gallstones or alcohol).

5. Gallbladder: Stores bile, modifies bile, contracts in response to CCK to eject bile into ducts leading to the small intestine. Major disorder: gallstones.

6. Small intestine: Motor functions include segmentation, peristalsis, and housekeeping migrating motor complex. Secretory functions include fluid and electrolyte transport in response to blood-borne or lumenal secretagogues. Digestive functions include brush border enzymes. General absorptive functions include most carbohydrate, fat, and protein (amino acid) absorption. Specialized absorptive mechanisms in the terminal ileum for bile acids and vitamin B_{12}-intrinsic factor complex. Major disorder: diarrhea (secretory, osmotic, malabsorptive, infectious, and inflammatory causes).

7. Colon: Major functions are water and electrolyte absorption, storage of feces, housing normal microbial flora. Major disorders: diverticular disease, infectious gastroenteritis, irritable bowel syndrome and inflammatory bowel disease, and cancer.

A CASE OF PHYSIOLOGICAL MEDICINE

Gastrointestinal bleeding

MP is a 68 year old woman in general good health whose only complaint had been knee pain occurring after extended periods of gardening, for which she took an occasional Tylenol. Last month at a social gathering, a friend said that high-dose ibuprofen, 800 mg 3 times a day, had dramatically improved his similar knee symptoms. Assuming that they would never sell something over the counter if it was not "safe," Ms. P self-initiated this regimen for control of her knee symptoms.

At first, she noted substantial improvement. However within a few weeks, she noted a strange sense of abdominal discomfort that seemed to get significantly worse when she took the ibuprofen on an empty stomach. These symptoms were present, off and on, for nearly two months.

One day the patient had a sudden urge to defecate and noted black, tarry stools, quite different in character from usual. She also felt profoundly dizzy upon rising from the toilet seat, and noted her pulse racing. She mentioned these signs and symptoms to her son who immediately made arrangements for her to be taken to a local emergency room.

In the ER, her blood pressure was 60/40 with a heart rate of 120. Hematocrit was noted to be 18 before hydration. The patient was admitted to the hospital and transfused four units of blood. A gastroenterologist was consulted, and several recommendations were made.

QUESTIONS

1. What kinds of GI pathology might the gastroenterologist see on endoscopy in this patient to account for her symptoms?
2. Interference in what normal, protective

physiological mechanisms may have contributed to the patient's gastrointestinal bleeding?

3. What determines whether a GI bleed presents with bright red blood from the rectum versus dark, tarry stools?

4. What recommendations would you make regarding medications, if you were the GI physician, based on the likely physiology of acid-mediated injury in this case?

5. With appropriate therapy, what would a follow up endoscopy likely show?

ANSWERS

1. Endoscopy might reveal reflux esophagitis, gastritis, and gastric or duodenal ulcer.

2. NSAIDs diminish mucosal defenses by impairing prostaglandin production.

3. (a) Location of the site of bleed (blood from an upper GI source more likely to mix with acid and become "tarry," while blood from the colon is likely to still be red when it appears); (b) Briskness and volume of bleeding. Thus a large, fast, arterial source of bleeding, even from an upper GI source, may appear bright red.

4. The GI physician should recommend the patient stop taking NSAIDs or, if absolutely necessary, take them with oral prostaglandin preparations that are believed to give some protection from the negative effects of NSAIDs alone, or take newer agents that are selective COX-2 inhibitors believed less likely to cause GI-side effects of NSAID use (e.g., Celebrex).

5. An endoscopy would likely show healing of the lesions.

Diarrhea

A homeless woman is admitted to the hospital with fever, altered mental status, and electrolyte abnormalities. She is noted to have a high serum ethanol level and is reported to have had profuse diarrhea for the last 24 h. As best you can piece the facts together, given her somewhat incoherent history, she is a chronic alcoholic with diabetes mellitus secondary to pancreatic insufficiency. She has also been on an ethanol binge for the last two weeks. She says this all started after eating some food that she found in a garbage can outside of a posh restaurant yesterday. On physical exam, you note findings of chronic liver disease. Cultures of blood, cerebrospinal fluid, urine, and stool are all negative for pathogens. The patient's hospital course is complicated by signs of alcohol withdrawal, including seizures.

You approach work up of her diarrhea in a physiological manner.

QUESTIONS

1. What are the major categories of physiological dysfunction that can result in diarrhea?

2. What are some prominent causes that are suggested by this patient's history and physical findings?

3. How would you go about distinguishing these possibilities?

4. What recommendations based on your understanding of GI physiology, would you give to the patient for each of the broad categories of causes of diarrhea you suggested earlier?

5. If the diarrhea were grossly bloody and persisted, why might you consider (or decide not) to do upper or lower GI endoscopy?

ANSWERS

1. Diarrhea can be caused by disorders of motility, digestion, secretion or absorption, as well as by mucosal destruction due to infection or inflammation.

If motility is disordered, the bolus of material leaving the stomach or moving down the small intestine may be (intermittently) too large for efficient mixing, digestion, or absorption, resulting in malabsorption and diarrhea.

If digestion is altered (e.g., lack of pancreatic digestive enzymes in a patient with chronic pancreatitis), obviously absorption is altered resulting in malabsorption and diarrhea.

If secretion in the small intestine is excessive (e.g., as in an endocrine tumor or cholera infection, where a vibrio bacterial toxin results in covalent modification of the G protein subunit controlling various ion channels into the "on" position), the absorptive capacity of the colon will be exceeded, resulting in diarrhea.

If absorption is abnormal due to a genetic, immunological, or inflammatory disorder, or an infection, the patient may develop diarrhea. Digestion will increase the number of moles of solute in the lumen. In the absence of a functioning absorptive mechanism to pull solute into cells, the solute will pull water out of cells and thereby provide an additional osmotic cause of diarrhea.

Both infections and immunological disorders with or without infection can damage the integrity of the mucosal barrier, resulting in excessive sloughing of cells, bleeding, loss of absorptive capacity, which are all manifest as diarrhea.

2. The following are some prominent causes that are suggested by this patient's history and physical findings:

- Fever: infectious or inflammatory disorder
- Acute alcohol use: direct damage to enterocytes
- Pancreatitis: enzyme deficiency
- Eating out of a garbage can: infection or toxin-mediated altered secretion
- Chronic liver disease: malabsorption due to biliary tract dysfunction

- Homelessness: stress-mediated gastritis and GI tract dysfunction.

3. Culture and examination of stool for white blood cells should be done to rule out infection and inflammation (sigmoidoscopy or colonoscopy would reveal the nature of the mucosal injury, infectious versus inflammatory, if this was suspected). This does not, however, rule out diarrhea caused by a toxin produced by a noninvasive organism (e.g., as in the case of cholera), where diarrhea occurs through toxin-mediated secretion rather than inflammatory erosion of the GI mucosa.

Analysis of stool (e.g., for fat) will reveal malabsorption. Measurement of blood levels of gut hormones (e.g., VIP) might indicate presence of such a secretogogue (e.g., due to a hormone-secreting tumor) and the patient's symptoms would be expected to respond to treatment with a somatostatin analogue.

Withholding food (giving the patient intravenous feedings only) will diminish the volume or resolve a malabsorptive or osmotic diarrhea due to any cause. However, a secretory diarrhea would continue.

Drugs that manipulate motility, acidity, or replace enzymes would reveal those bases for motility and digestive disorders.

4. The recommendations would include antibiotics for non-self-limited infections; enzyme replacement for pancreatic enzyme deficiency; good control of diabetes mellitus for diabetic neuropathy; drugs that alter motility; and changes in diet, timing, and volume of meals.

5. You might want to localize the source of the bleeding and characterize the nature of the lesions. While a lower source seems likely from this history, formally you could not rule out an upper source with rapid transit. Lavage of the stomach with a nasogastric tube is a quick and easy (for the doctor) way to make an upper source far

less likely, at which point endoscopy from below might be indicated first. It can sometimes be difficult to distinguish infectious causes from inflammatory bowel disorders (autoimmune causes). The histology on biopsy of the lesions sometimes helps, as can the response to antibiotics versus steroids and bowel rest.

References and suggested readings

REVIEWS

1. Sleisenger, M. and Fordtran, J. (1993). *Gastrointestinal Disease*, 4th ed. Philadelphia: Saunders.

2. Geoghegan, J., and Pappas, T.N. (1997). Clinical uses of gut peptides. *Ann. Surg.* 225:145-154.

3. Hagger, R. et al., (1997). Role of the interstitial cells of Cajal in the control of gut motility. *Br. J Surg.* 84:445-450.

4. Bueno, L. et al. (1997). Mediators and pharmacology of visceral sensitivity: From basic to clinical investigations. *Gastroenterology* 112:1714-1743.

5. Maeda, H. et al. (1992). Requirement of c-kit for development of intestinal pacemaker system. *Development* 116:369-375.

6. Torihashi, S. et al. (1995). c-kit-dependent development of interstitial cells and electrical activity in the murine GI tract. *Cell Tissue Res.* 280:97-111.

7. Huang, P.L. et al. (1993). Targeted disruption of the neuronal nitric oxide synthase gene. *Cell* 75:1273-1286.

8. Milla, P.J. (1992). Gastric-outlet obstruction in children. *N. Eng. J. Med.* 327: 558-560.

9. Playford, R.J., et al. (1996). Transgenic mice that overexpress the human trefoil peptide pS2 have an increased resistance to intestinal damage. *Proc. Natl. Acad. Sci. USA* 93:2137-2142.

10. Mashimo, H. et al. (1996). Impaired defense of intestinal mucosa in mice lacking intestinal trefoil factor. *Science* 274:262-265.

11. Nocerino, A. et al. (1995). Cholera toxin-induced small intestinal secretion has a secretory effect on the colon of the rat. *Gastroenterology* 108:34-39.

12. Swidsinski, A. et al. (1995). Molecular genetic evidence of bacterial colonization of cholesterol gallstones. *Gastroenterology* 108:860-864.

13. Ornish, D. et al. Intensive lifestyle changes for reversal of coronary heart disease. *JAMA*, 1998 Dec 16, 280:2001-2007.

PHYSIOLOGY OF THE ENDOCRINE PANCREAS AND FUEL HOMEOSTASIS

6

1. SIGNIFICANCE OF DISORDERS OF THE ENDOCRINE PANCREAS

Why is the endocrine pancreas medically important?

- Obesity (see Chap. 11), due in most cases to excess fuel substrate intake and storage, is a modern epidemic, afflicting one-third of the adult American population. It is associated with substantially increased rates of many diseases including cardiovascular disease, the number one cause of death in the United States today. The hormones of the endocrine pancreas can play a crucial role in the development of obesity.
- Ten million Americans have a disorder of fuel storage regulation termed **diabetes mellitus**. Many of these patients are also obese, but some are not. Diabetes mellitus is the third leading cause of death in the United States and is associated with long-term complications including kidney failure, amputations, blindness, neuropathy, and immune dysfunction. Much of the morbidity (suffering) and mortality (death) caused by cardiovascular disease is actually a secondary complication of coexisting diabetes mellitus.
- Acute syndromes, such as diabetic ketoacidosis, which occur in subsets of patients with diabetes mellitus, continue to have a high mortality even in the best of medical facilities — especially when precious time is lost by not anticipating complications in a physiologically rational manner.
- Treatment of diabetes mellitus involves walking a therapeutic tightrope: undertreatment accelerates devastating complications, but overtreatment can be rapidly and directly lethal, by causing hypoglycemia. And even appropriate treatment may sometimes worsen complications. An understanding of the physiology is crucial to caring for patients in a way that maximizes therapeutic potential without doing harm. We must humbly remember that medical management is, at best, a feeble attempt to replicate the exquisite normal homeostatic mechanisms that have been fine-tuned through a billion years of metazoan evolution in ways that we far from fully understand.

Case Presentation

A. R. is a 65-year-old Russian immigrant and homemaker with a 10-year history of non-insulin-dependent diabetes mellitus. The diagnosis was made by blood and urine testing after several weeks of frequent urination, thirst, weight loss, hunger, and blurry vision. Initially treated adequately with pills, she required higher and higher doses of these medicines over time. Eventually, the pills were ineffective. For the last 5 years, she has been taking injections of the fuel storage hormone insulin, twice a day. During this time her weight increased by nearly 30 kg (66 lb).

Recently, she developed chest pains on exertion. She also noted a general sense of fatigue, puffiness in her face and legs, and dizziness on sudden standing.

She came to your clinic for the first time concerned about symptoms of bloating, nausea, alternating diarrhea and constipation. She notes some sores that were healing poorly on her toes. Her vision has started to deteriorate again.

On further questioning, Ms. R. reported that her sugars have often been high in recent years despite insulin injections. Blood tests corroborated her report.

She wants an explanation as to why she is developing these new symptoms, how they are related to diabetes, and what she can do to prevent them from getting worse. She also does not understand why her diabetes mellitus is getting worse, why she was told she has non-insulin-dependent diabetes but is now on insulin, and why the insulin injections seem to be inadequate. She has observed that the more insulin she takes at bedtime, the higher rather than lower her blood sugar is in the morning, which doesn't make any sense to her. She wants to understand how to better treat her diabetes and decrease the unpleasant and worrisome symptoms she is experiencing.

2. THE LOGIC OF FUEL HOMEOSTASIS

Why do we need to eat food?

We need to eat food to:

1. Generate the energy to carry out current activities.
2. Acquire the fuel substrates for storage from which we generate energy between meals.
3. Provide the raw materials to synthesize and repair our cells and tissues.

The major classes of ingested nutrients that serve as both fuel substrates and building materials are termed *carbohydrates*, *fats*, and *proteins*. The tissues of the body contain enzymes to break down and to synthesize each of these classes of fuel substrates, and in many cases, to convert them from one to another to better meet the metabolic needs of the body.

A molecular perspective on fuel homeostasis

Energy is obtained in immediately usable form by oxidizing fuel substrates in food (ultimately to carbon dioxide and water), with the generation of adenosine triphosphate (ATP). This occurs primarily through the pathways of glycolysis and the citric cycle. ATP is a small molecule that contains a high-energy phosphodiester bond. When this bond is broken, energy is released that allows otherwise energetically unfavorable chemical reactions to occur. Thus, ATP serves as an energy "cur-rency" within cells, allowing the energy released from a thermodynamically favorable reaction to be captured and used to drive a less-favorable reaction.

In the absence of oxygen, a relatively small amount of ATP is generated through glycolysis (the breakdown of the 6-carbon glucose molecules into three carbon pyruvate molecules, with a net yield of 2 mol of ATP per mol of glucose).

In the presence of oxygen, we make a net of 30 mol of ATP per mol of glucose, largely because of the **citric acid cycle** (also called the **tricarboxylic acid cycle**, **TCA cycle**, or **Krebs cycle**), in which the two molecules of pyruvate produced per molecule of glucose are, in effect, oxidized to carbon dioxide and water.

Glucose can be stored as long polymers termed *glycogen*. Like money in your checking account, glycogen is readily accessible to generate energy on a minute-to-minute basis (by reconversion back to glucose, which in turn can be oxidized to make ATP).

When far more fuel substrates are taken in than are needed for short-term needs, the excess fuel substrates are stored as fat. This can take place either directly or by conversion of glucose to fat.

When blood glucose levels fall below the normal range, hormonal changes convert the liver from a consumer of glucose into a producer of glucose. Those same hormonal changes induce alterations in the metabolism of other tissues that reinforce the effects on the liver (see later).

Physiology of fuel substrate utilization

Glucose is a fuel substrate that is "as good as cash" for short-term needs. Essentially every living cell is able to generate ATP from glucose. For some organs, such as the brain, glucose is the preferred energy source. For other tissues, such as muscle, glucose is used only under certain circumstances and when other fuels are unavailable or insufficient for metabolic needs (see later).

Amino acids, the constituents that make up proteins, are primarily a building material. However, when necessary, they can be converted into fuel substrates and used for energy generation. Thus, the pathways of carbohydrate, protein, and lipid metabolism interconnect allowing many but not all substrates to be interconverted. Although amino acids can be converted into citric acid cycle intermediates, no mechanism exists in animals to convert acetate directly into citric acid cycle intermediates.

Free fatty acids are a fuel substrate ideal for storage of energy in that they can be used to form triglycerides that are deposited in cells as fat. Not all triglyceride deposits are the same. Fat deposited in some locations is more metabolically active than in others. Excess fat in some locations is more strongly associated with diseases (e.g., cardiovascular disease and diabetes mellitus) than the same amount of fat in other locations (see Visceral versus Subcutaneous Fat in Pathogenesis of Diabetes Mellitus in Frontiers, Sec. 9).

Fuel substrate regulation is extremely complex, with different responses to various situations in which the body might find itself. In clinical practice we tend to simplify the pathways of intermediary metabolism and their regulation in order to focus on those aspects that are most relevant to therapeutics.

As a species, we evolved under conditions in which getting enough food was a constant problem. Thus, the mechanisms that evolved to allow us to survive in periods of relative food scarcity are generally more powerful than the mechanisms to curtail our food intake in times of plenty.

In Western societies today we eat too many calories for the amount of physical activity we do, a situation against which there has been relatively little evolutionary defense. Thus obesity has become a major cause of morbidity and mortality.

Review Questions

1. Give three fundamental reasons why we need food.
2. What is the difference in net ATP yield per molecule of glucose via glycolysis versus the TCA cycle?

3. CONTROL OF INTERMEDIARY METABOLISM

Perhaps the greatest challenge faced by the body in regulating the assimilation of nutrients from food is in dealing with requirements that can change under a variety of different circumstances:

- We are not always eating and thus must shift from storage of fuel substrates to utilization of stored fuels several times during the course of a day (i.e., during versus between meals).
- Sometimes we have to change activities extremely rapidly (such as suddenly recognizing danger and either running away or fighting). Under these circumstances, the rate of energy utilization changes even more rapidly than would otherwise occur in the transition from feeding to fasting states during the course of the day.
- Sometimes we have to adapt to long-term changes: A bad harvest meant that our ancestors might face starvation in the winter. Under such circumstances, survival meant living off of stored energy substrates such as fat, for a long time. The average nonobese adult has enough fat to meet all of the body's energy needs for one to two months. Somehow, regulation must be tailored to allow access to the fat reserve while "sparing" protein. Otherwise, breakdown of structural protein would render the individual too weak to survive even in the presence of a substantial fat reserve.

To accommodate these varied circumstances, we have evolved sets of biochemical reactions to store fuels (termed **anabolic** *pathways*), and sets of biochemical reactions to break down stored materials to generate energy (termed **catabolic** *pathways*). We use hormones to rapidly switch from having predominantly anabolic pathways active to having predominantly catabolic pathways active. **Insulin** is the primary hormone that promotes anabolic pathways. It does this by promoting glucose transport into many tissues, by activating the enzymes that make up the anabolic pathways and by stimulating the transcription and translation of mRNAs for those enzymes. Insulin also has the effect of inactivating the enzymes that promote catabolic pathways. **Glucagon** and **epinephrine** are the primary hormones that promote catabolic pathways, although a host of other hormones (see Counterregulatory Hormones, in Sec. 6) contribute to countering the actions of insulin. These hormones, to one degree or another, impair the pathways that insulin promotes, and promote the pathways that insulin impairs. They do this by different effects on different tissues, as will be discussed later.

Thus, anabolic states (situations in which fuel substrates are being stored) are characterized by a relative increase in the insulin-to-glucagon ratio in the bloodstream. They are also characterized by the use of diet rather than already stored materials as the primary fuel source, and predominance of the processes of glycogen synthesis, glycolysis, triglyceride, and protein synthesis. This results in a net flow of the energy stored in glucose in the bloodstream to tissues, where it is stored in the form of glycogen, protein, or fat (largely triglycerides) for later use (see Figure 6.1A).

Catabolic states (situations in which fuel stores are being broken down) are notable for a decrease in the insulin-to-glucagon ratio in the bloodstream. Catabolic states are also characterized by the use of stored sources of fuel. Thus in a catabolic state intermediary metabolism is geared toward glycogenolysis, lipolysis (breakdown of triglycerides into fatty acids and glycerol), proteolysis (breakdown of protein), gluconeogenesis (production of glucose from other substrates), and ketogenesis (the production of ketones, which is a measure of fatty acid oxidation and provides the brain with a crucial alternate food source should glucose be lacking). This results in a net flow of energy from stored glycogen, protein, and triglycerides in tissues into glucose, amino acids, and free fatty acids that can be readily oxidized to provide energy (see Figure 6.1B).

Differences in the mix of hormones released are one way the body is able to achieve an optimal response to particular metabolic situations. For example, running fast for 5 min triggers a different catabolic hormonal mix than starving for a week (see Fasting and Starvation, in Sec. 7).

Despite these changes from fuel substrate storage to utilization and back again, most individuals maintain relatively constant body weight over long periods of time (months to years). This suggests that the biochemical pathways of anabolism and catabolism are integrated with neural pathways that relate to feeding, fasting, satiety, and other behaviors, a subject that will be considered in more detail in Chapter 11.

Since, at rest, the brain consumes approximately 6 g of glucose per hour, and other tissues some 4 g of glucose per hour, at least 240 g of glucose (or its equivalent of some other substrate for energy generation, e.g., free fatty acids) are required for daily basal activity.

The effects of insulin and other hormones of fuel storage and mobilization are best conceptualized in terms of their effects on the liver versus the **periphery**, of which fat and muscle tissue are most prominent. Thus, in the liver, which has receptors for both insulin and glucagon, it is the balance of the two

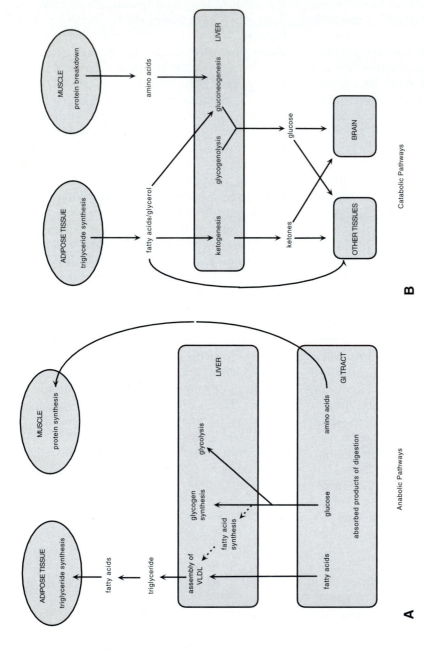

A Anabolic Pathways

B Catabolic Pathways

FIGURE 6.1. Intermediary metabolic pathways of (A) anabolism and (B) catabolism. In A, the fed state, absorbed glucose is extracted by the liver for storage as glycogen and generation of metabolic intermediates for other synthetic reactions (e.g., fatty acid or amino acid synthesis). The liver converts absorbed fatty acids and newly synthesized fatty acids into very low density lipoprotein (VLDL) particles that are exported to peripheral tissues. Under anabolic conditions, absorbed amino acids flow primarily to muscle for use in protein synthesis. In B, the fasted state, the liver is a net producer of glucose using its own supply of glycogen and, when that is exhausted, substrates from fat and protein breakdown in adipose tissue and muscle, respectively. The liver also converts from fatty acid synthesis and lipoprotein particle production to fatty acid oxidation, releasing ketones that are usable by the brain as an alternate energy source in the absence of glucose. Dotted line in A refers to the fact that the degree of activity of some pathways, such as that of fatty acid synthesis, will depend on the composition (e.g., in this case, fatty acid content) of the diet.

hormones (i.e., their ratio) that is a major determinant of metabolic status. When the ratio is shifted in favor of insulin, the liver removes glucose from the bloodstream and forms glycogen, lipoproteins, and so on. When the ratio is shifted in favor of glucagon, metabolism in the liver is dominated by glycogenolysis and gluconeogenesis, with net release of glucose into the bloodstream. In the periphery, glucagon generally has no direct effect. Instead, insulin action, or its lack, determines whether glucose is taken up and protein and fat synthesized, or whether protein and fat are being broken down (to provide substrates that flow to the liver to support gluconeogenesis).

In addition, we must consider the needs of "special" tissues, including the brain, red blood cells, and the renal medulla. The brain directs and coordinates the activities of all the other organs of the body. You cannot really survive very long on "autopilot" without conscious brain function, therefore providing the brain a steady supply of glucose is a priority. Red blood cells have no mitochondria and, therefore, cannot carry out the citric acid cycle. Instead, they must generate energy through low-yield glycolysis and thus have ready access to glucose. The renal medulla functions under conditions of very low oxygen tension often inadequate for aerobic metabolism; therefore, it, too, is particularly dependent on glycolysis. The best way to afford priority in glucose distribution to these special tissues is to have them take up glucose independently of insulin. Thus, in the absence of insulin, uptake by other tissues goes down, and glucose is preferentially made available to the insulin-independent tissues.

Review Questions

3. What are the anabolic pathways of intermediary metabolism and their key steps?

4. What are the catabolic pathways of intermediary metabolism, their key steps, and their connections to anabolic pathways?
5. What are three fundamentally different circumstances in which fuel requirements change?
6. What are some tissues that have priority for glucose and why?
7. How many grams of glucose does the body use at rest, per 24 hours?
8. How does the liver differ from the periphery, in terms of fuel substrate metabolism and control?

4. ANATOMY AND HISTOLOGY OF THE ENDOCRINE PANCREAS

Insulin and glucagon are synthesized in and secreted from specific cells of the **islets of Langerhans** that make up the endocrine pancreas. A healthy human has about a million of these islets, small clumps of cells distributed throughout the pancreas, interspersed among the far more predominant acinar tissue and ducts that make up the exocrine pancreas. Each islet contains but a few hundred endocrine cells each.

The islets have a peculiar structure in which the glucagon-secreting α cells (approximately 20% of the endocrine cells in an islet) form a rim with insulin-secreting β cells (approximately 65% of the cells) in the center, and **somatostatin**-secreting δ cells (10% of the cells) scattered between them (see Figure 6.2). Perhaps this histologic organization reflects paracrine interactions between these different cell types. These cells are also connected by gap junctions to form a functional **syncytium** (meaning that small signaling molecules can pass directly from cell to cell without being diluted by the surrounding environment).

The β cells of the islets of Langerhans are

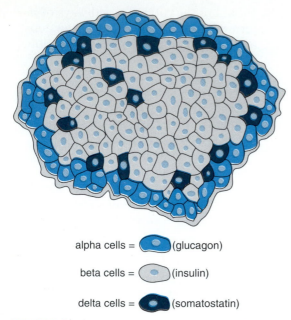

alpha cells = (glucagon)

beta cells = (insulin)

delta cells = (somatostatin)

FIGURE 6.2. Cellular organization of the islets of Langerhans. Illustrates the distinctive organization of endocrine cells in the typical islet of Langerhans (see text). alpha (α) cells, beta (β) cells, delta (δ) cells.

the sole source of insulin in the body. However, glucagon is not only made by the α cells of the islets, it is also synthesized by endocrine cells in the gut. Somatostatin is synthesized in the δ cells of the islets and also in both the gut and various sites in the brain. Most likely these hormones are involved in both paracrine and endocrine actions, in different places at different times.

A few cells in the endocrine pancreas make other secretory products whose function and significance are not well understood.

The hormones of the endocrine pancreas are secreted into the portal vein, which flows directly to the liver before entering the systemic circulation. In the liver, these hormones have receptor-mediated effects. A substantial amount of these hormones are removed from the blood in the liver before circulating to the rest of the body. Thus, the peripheral tissues will see lower concentrations of these hormones than did the liver.

Clinical Pearls

○ One of the reasons insulin injections are a poor replacement for β cells of the islets of Langerhans is that exogenous injections deposit the hormone peripherally, whereas endogenous secretion directs it into the portal vein. Thus, endogenous insulin is seen first by the liver, where much of it is cleared, resulting in a lower concentration of insulin seen by the periphery. Subcutaneous insulin injections thus provide a higher peripheral insulin concentration than would normally occur and alter the normal balance of insulin action between the liver and periphery. The higher peripheral insulin concentration may contribute to the development of hypertension, atherosclerosis, and ultimately coronary artery disease.

○ Another deficiency of injected insulin is that it is generally given as a bolus. Endogenous insulin is released by β cells in coordination with input from α and δ cells of the islet of Langerhans. Hence the fine-tuning made possible by paracrine interactions and the gap junction-mediated communication within the islet do not occur with injected insulin.

5. INSULIN

Biosynthesis

The primary hormone of fuel substrate storage, insulin, is initially synthesized as a larger precursor (preproinsulin), which is cleaved during **translocation** across the membrane of the endoplasmic reticulum (ER) during its synthesis to generate proinsulin. **Disulfide bonds** are also formed in the ER lumen at this time. During subsequent intracellular traffic through the secretory pathway, proinsulin is subject to further proteolytic cleavage, which removes the so-called connecting (C) peptide. This occurs after the protein has left the Golgi apparatus and continues in the secretory granules. The resulting mature insulin consists of two chains termed *A and B chains*. Since the C peptide remains in the secretory granule, it is secreted from the β cells in parallel with mature insulin (see Figure 6.3). Insulin is cleared from the bloodstream by both hepatic and renal metabolism.

Clinical Pearl

○ C peptide, the fragment of proinsulin generated upon processing of insulin in β cells, has no known function. However, because it is released in parallel with insulin from the β cell and has a longer half-life of clearance than insulin, its measurement by radioimmunoassay can be useful, under certain circumstances. In particular, it allows straightforward diagnosis of whether severe hypoglycemia with no other explanation is likely due to an insulin-secreting tumor or due to surreptitious insulin injection (e.g., by a patient with a psychiatric disorder). Injected insulin is purified free of any remaining C peptide, whereas endogenous insulin secretion (either normal or from a tumor) will result in circulating C peptide in the bloodstream.

Actions of insulin

Insulin's actions can be categorized by the following:

- Their time of onset (rapid, intermediate, and late-onset actions)
- The fuel substrate metabolic pathways affected (carbohydrate versus protein versus lipid metabolism)
- The primary site of action (liver versus adipose tissue versus muscle)

Categorization of insulin action by time of onset

Some actions of insulin are extremely rapid, occurring within seconds to minutes after the insulin binds to its receptors on the cell surface. These are effects on proteins already present in the cell that simply need a change in location or a chemical modification (e.g., phosphorylation) in order to be active.

Other actions affect transcription or translation of messenger RNA (mRNA) to increase or decrease the rate at which new copies of specific proteins (e.g., those phosphorylated previously) are made. It can take up to several hours for these effects of insulin to be fully manifest.

Finally, some effects of insulin are delayed, occurring on a time scale of days. This delay could be for several reasons:

- The effect being measured may require many steps and pathways, only some of which are directly under the control of insulin. The other steps may take place under another control that takes its own time.
- Some effects may require occupancy of more insulin receptors than other effects. This is another way of saying that insulin turns on multiple signaling pathways, some of which are more sensitive to insulin than others. It may simply take more time to reach the threshold level of a particular signaling molecule needed to send the message.
- Some delayed effects of insulin may be a result of "spillover" of insulin onto other receptors (e.g., those for insulin-like growth factors) that are, in effect, low-sensitivity insulin receptors. Only when insulin is at very high concentrations or is around for a very long time will these lower affinity receptors be occupied sufficiently to trigger signaling.

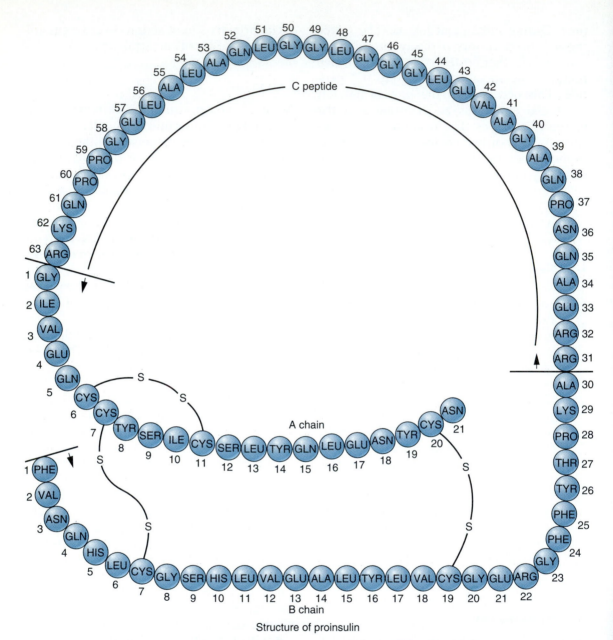

FIGURE 6.3. Structure of proinsulin. Indicating the sequence of proinsulin, including the disulfide bonded A and B chains that make up mature insulin and the connecting C peptide that are removed during maturation in the Golgi and post-Golgi compartments. The signal peptide, removed during synthesis, is not shown. *(Adapted, with permission, from Shaw, W.N. and Chance, R.R. (1968). Diabetes 17:737.)*

It should be noted that this distinction between the time courses of different insulin actions is in some ways more theoretical than practical because, for many of its effects, insulin actions reinforce each other on different time scales. That is, the effects on prexisting proteins occurring in minutes is generally reinforced by the effect on new enzyme synthesis occurring in hours (see Figure 6.4). Thus, the longer insulin is present (or absent), the more entrenched are the consequent changes in overall body metabolism due to changes in the amounts of various enzymes, as well as in their state of activation. Insulin activates anabolic pathways (an effect that is usually reinforced by the lack of glucagon and epinephrine). The lack of insulin activates catabolic pathways (which are usually further reinforced by the presence of elevated concentrations of glucagon or epinephrine).

That high concentrations of insulin for long periods of time should cause growth is not surprising. The same phenomena of long-term or delayed actions that promote tissue growth occur for many other hormones (see Chap. 3).

Categorization of insulin action by effects on different pathways

Insulin is the consummate fuel storage hormone, affecting pathways of carbohydrate, lipid, and protein metabolism (see Figures 6.1, 6.4). For carbohydrates, insulin promotes glycogen synthesis and glycolysis and inhibits the opposing pathways of **glycogenolysis** and **gluconeogenesis** (see Figure 6.4). The reason for the effects on glycogen synthesis and glycogenolysis is obvious — insulin promotes fuel storage. But why should insulin promote glycolysis? Because an increase in the amount of substrates fluxing down the glycolytic cycle expands the supply of intermediary metabolites that ultimately will be used for fatty acid, triglyceride, and VLDL synthesis. Thus by revving up the glycolytic pathway, insulin is

enlarging the pipeline for the production of lipoprotein particles needed to offer excess storage fuels to other tissues.

For protein storage, insulin promotes amino acid uptake and protein synthesis, especially in muscle.

For lipid storage, insulin not only promotes fatty acid, triglyceride, and VLDL synthesis, it also inhibits pathways of fatty acid oxidation and the so-called **hormone-sensitive lipase** in adipose tissue. This enzyme normally displays a baseline level of activity, constantly hydrolyzing stored triglycerides in adipose tissue into free fatty acids and glycerol. In the absence of insulin, the activity of this enzyme is elevated. This provides substrates that flow to the liver and fuel gluconeogenesis. In the presence of insulin, the activity of hormone-sensitive lipase is inhibited, thus turning off a pathway that would otherwise push metabolism in a direction that would counter the action of insulin.

In addition to turning off hormone-sensitive lipase, insulin stimulates **lipoprotein lipase**. This enzyme, located on the cell surface of vascular endothelium, releases free fatty acids from lipoprotein particles and thereby promotes storage of fat in the periphery (i.e., in adipose tissue). Thus, lipoprotein lipase promotes the metabolic pathway that is opposite that which is enhanced by hormone-sensitive lipase (see Figure 6.4).

Categorization of insulin action by effects on different tissues

Insulin has different effects on different tissues. Uptake of glucose is a classical response to insulin and occurs prominently in muscle and adipose tissue. However, some tissues lack receptors for insulin. These insulin-independent tissues include organs whose function is of critical importance for survival of the organism (e.g., brain), those which operate under low oxygen tension (e.g., renal tu-

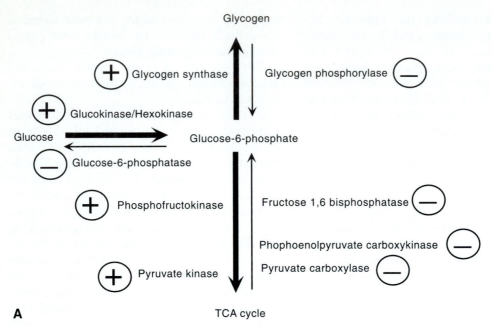

A

FIGURE 6.4. Effects of insulin on anabolic and catabolic pathways of intermediary metabolism. *A.* Indicates specific steps of glucose utilization and production pathways that are enhanced (thick arrows) or diminished (thin arrows) by insulin. Enzymes activated by insulin action are indicated with +, those inactivated by insulin action are indicated with −. Activation involves either phosphorylation of an activating kinase or dephosphorylation of an inactivating phosphatase. The effects of phosphorylation or dephosphorylation on enzymes flowing in one direction are generally the opposite of the effects on a pathway flowing in the other direction, allowing a change in metabolic program to be doubly reinforced by concerted effects on pathways in both directions. *B.* Indicates the key steps of lipid utilization and production pathways that are affected by insulin. Insulin stimulates lipoprotein lipase enhancing VLDL breakdown, which makes triglycerides available for storage in adipocytes. Insulin also inhibits hormone-sensitive lipase that would break down stored fat in the adipocyte. Thus, in the presence of insulin, the net flow of triglyceride is into storage (to the right), while in the absence of insulin, the net flow reverts to the left. In the absence of insulin more free fatty acids and glycerol enter the bloodstream and flow to the liver where they fuel gluconeogenesis and fatty acid oxidation, pathways whose enzymes are enhanced by the lack of insulin. Note that in both *A* and *B*, the effect of insulin is initially on the enzymes themselves, but a delayed reinforcing effect on transcription and translation of messenger RNA for the stimulated or inhibited enzymes is also observed. *(A. Adapted, with permission, from Rhoads, R.A. and Tanner, G.A. (1995). Medical Physiology. Boston, Little, Brown, p. 713. B. Adapted, with permission, from Foster, D. and McGarry, J.D. (1996), in Griffin, J.E. and Ojeda, S.R., eds. Textbook of Endocrine Physiology, 3rd ed. New York, Oxford, p. 367.)*

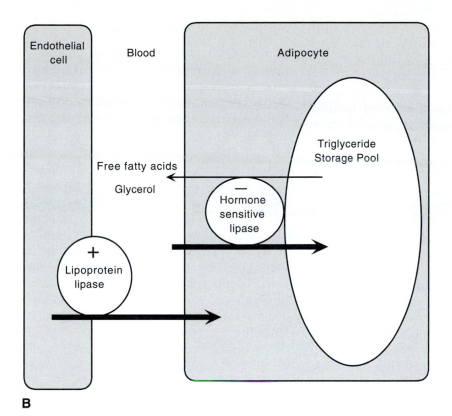

B

FIGURE 6.4 — (continued)

bule) or those lacking mitochondria (e.g., red blood cells).

In some organs, most notably the liver, even though there are insulin receptors, glucose uptake is not dependent on insulin. This is because there are several different members of the glucose-transporter gene family. Activity of the glucose transporter expressed in liver is not dependent on insulin action for its activity (see later).

It is most useful clinically to view insulin action on different tissues from several perspectives: that of the liver versus that of muscle and adipose tissue (the so-called periphery). Generally, insulin's effects on the periphery reinforce its action on the liver.

In the presence of insulin, fuel storage is promoted in both the liver and in the periphery (see Figure 6.1A):

• The most prominent effects in the liver are glycogen and lipoprotein particle formation.
• The most prominent effects in muscle are glycogen and protein synthesis.
• The most prominent effect in adipose tissue is triglyceride synthesis.

In the absence of insulin, the liver becomes a producer of glucose because of the following events (see Figure 6.1B):

• The pathways of glycogenolysis and gluconeogenesis are activated in the liver.

• Fatty acid and lipoprotein synthesis within the liver cease, and pathways of fatty acid oxidation and ketone formation are promoted.
• In the periphery, hormone-sensitive lipase becomes active in the absence of insulin, breaking down triglycerides to generate free fatty acids and glycerol, which flow to the liver to fuel the pathways of gluconeogenesis and fatty acid oxidation, the enzymes for which are being activated there.
• The breakdown of protein in muscle releases amino acids into the bloodstream that flow to the liver and provide further substrate for gluconeogenesis.

Note that the program of metabolism activated by insulin is the anabolic program described in Figure 6.1A, while that in the absence of insulin (or the relatively insulin-deficient, glucagon-excess state), the catabolic program described in Figure 6.1B is activated.

Mechanism of insulin action

Fundamental aspects of the mechanism of insulin action remain a mystery. The insulin receptor consists of a heterodimer of 2 α and 2 β subunits of 135,000 **Daltons** and 95,000 Daltons each, respectively (see Figure 6.5). It is known that binding of insulin to the α subunit activates an intrinsic tyrosine kinase activity, which is resident in the cytoplasmic domain of the β subunit. When activated by binding of insulin, the receptor phosphorylates itself on a tyrosine residue of the β subunit, which allows it to bind to, and phosphorylate, other proteins in the cytoplasm that are themselves kinases. These kinases are activated by phosphorylation and, when active, phosphorylate other enzymes. Some of these enzymes are phosphatases that dephosphorylate other enzymes, and so on. This cascade of phosphorylation and dephosphorylation events activates various second messengers

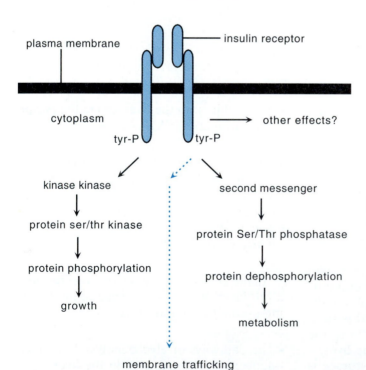

FIGURE 6.5. Signal transduction in insulin action. Indicates the structure of the insulin receptor, the key role of tyrosine phosphorylation in activation of the receptor, and some of the many signaling pathways that are activated in response, affecting membrane trafficking, metabolism, and growth through cascades of phosphorylation and dephosphorylation. (Adapted, with permission, from Saltiel, A. (1994). The paradoxical regulation of protein phosphorylation in insulin action. FASEB J. 8:1034-1040.)

in a host of intracellular metabolic pathways and inactivates others. Activation and inactivation of various second messengers lead to the molecular events of insulin action on different pathways and time scales including as follows:

• Vesicle trafficking (see later)
• Enzyme (i.e., metabolic pathway) activation and inhibition
• Changes in transcription and translation
• DNA synthesis

The net effect of these molecular events is to reinforce the physiological roles of insulin as a hormone of fuel storage and to antagonize the actions of hormones that work to push cellular metabolism in the opposite direction (see Sec. 6).

The differences in insulin's actions in different tissues are caused either by the activation of different pathways of second messengers or by differences in gene expression in different tissues. For example, as already mentioned, expression of a different glucose transporter allows for insulin-dependent glucose uptake in muscle but not liver despite that both liver and muscle have insulin receptors.

Molecular mechanism of increased glucose uptake in response to insulin

At the cellular level, insulin's ability to increase glucose transport in adipose and muscle tissue in minutes is not primarily due to a change in transporter affinity for glucose, but rather due to an increase in the number of glucose transporters on the cell surface. This increase in glucose transporter number on the cell surface is a consequence of fusion to the plasma membrane of endosomal vesicles enriched in glucose transporters. Later, when insulin action is terminated, patches of membrane enriched in glucose transporters will be endocytosed, returning the cell back to the baseline state in which it does not take up glucose in the absence of insulin.

The glucose transporter found in muscle and adipose tissue is termed **GLUT 4**. Specific amino acid sequences present in GLUT 4, but not in the coding region of other glucose transporter genes, are believed to be responsible for trafficking of GLUT 4 into the endosomal vesicles whose fusion to the plasma membrane is regulated by insulin. Since GLUT 4 is not expressed in liver, this organ does not display insulin-sensitive glucose uptake (see Figure 6.6).

Clinical Pearl

○ Another rapid action of insulin is uptake of potassium from the bloodstream into the same cells that respond to insulin with glucose uptake (e.g., adipose and muscle tissue). Although this observation has little impact on our thinking about carbohydrate metabolism, it has important practical implications: If you have a patient with a life-threatening elevation in blood potassium concentration, treatment with insulin and glucose will transport K^+ intracellularly in minutes and can thus be a life-saving maneuver. Of course, you need to give glucose along with the insulin since otherwise hypoglycemia would accompany the lowering of blood potassium that occurs in response to insulin action. Also remember that this does not treat the underlying cause of the elevated potassium—but at least buys you some time to do that!

Regulation of insulin secretion

The secretion of insulin is under several forms of control (see Table 6.1). The primary control is by glucose. When the plasma glucose level falls to within the normal range (approx-

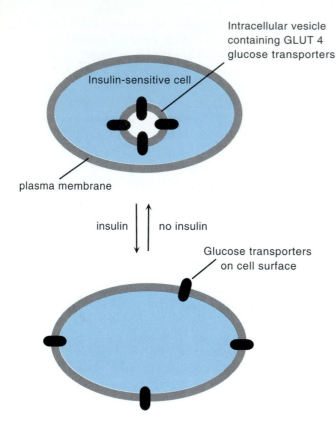

Intracellular vesicle
containing GLUT 4
glucose transporters

Insulin-sensitive cell

plasma membrane

insulin | no insulin

Glucose transporters
on cell surface

FIGURE 6.6. Translocation of GLUT 4 containing vesicles in response to insulin. In the absence of insulin, the GLUT 4 glucose transporter resides in intracellular endocytic vesicles and does not see glucose in the bloodstream. Upon activation of the insulin receptor by insulin, signaling pathways trigger fusion of these vesicles to the plasma membrane allowing the glucose transporter to sense the blood glucose concentration and transport glucose into the cell. When insulin-mediated signaling is terminated, the GLUT 4 is once again collected into patches of membrane that reendocytose, terminating their uptake of glucose.

imately 80 mg per 100 mL), insulin secretion declines to very low levels even in the presence of other stimuli for its secretion. When plasma glucose levels rise, insulin secretion is initiated and the insulin response to any other stimulus for its secretion is magnified. The proposed molecular mechanism for this is that glucose metabolism raises ATP levels in the β cell, which closes channels for potassium efflux out of the cell. As a result, the β cell is **depolarized**, which opens voltage-dependent channels for calcium influx. This effect is reinforced by elevated cyclic adenosine monophosphate- (cyclic AMP) stimulated calcium release from intracellular compartments. The rise in intracellular calcium stimulates the microtubule-dependent secretion of insulin secretory granules (see Figure 6.7).

Other important stimuli for insulin secretion are other fuel substrates such as amino acids as well as some gut hormones (such as glucose-dependent insulinotropic peptide, GIP), which are secreted in response to carbohydrate-rich meals that allow the body to anticipate impending substrate influx. Glucagon also stimulates insulin secretion directly via glucagon receptors on β cells. Of course, direct hyperglycemia is a far greater stimulus to insulin secretion than is glucagon.

In contrast to such direct effects on insulin secretion, anything that serves to raise blood glucose indirectly results in increased insulin secretion (as part of a homeostatic mechanism to maintain constancy of blood glucose). Thus glucagon also stimulates insulin secretion indirectly, i.e., by raising blood glucose (see Table 6.1).

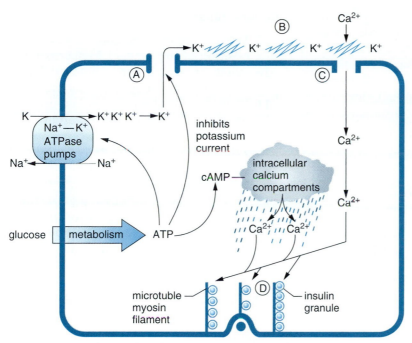

FIGURE 6.7. Regulation of insulin secretion in the β cell. Schematic diagram of glucose-stimulated insulin release from β cell. Potassium (K+) efflux (A), polarizes the β-cell membrane and prevents calcium entry by closing a voltage-dependent calcium channel (B). When glucose is taken up by β cells, its metabolism is believed to inhibit potassium efflux, thus depolarizing the cell and allowing calcium (Ca^{2+}) entry (C). Calcium stimulates the secretion of insulin-containing vesicles (D). *(Adapted, with permission, from Greenspan, F. and Baxter, J.D. eds. (1994). Basic and Clinical Endocrinology, 4th ed. Stamford, CT, Appleton & Lange, p. 623.)*

Together, these direct and indirect controls are a key part of the feedback mechanism by which homeostasis is normally maintained without "overshooting" in reaction to hypoglycemia. Normal pancreatic islets usually do a better job of controlling blood glucose than do people injecting insulin with a syringe, because of these reinforcing features of feedback.

Catecholamines (epinephrine and norepinephrine secreted from the adrenal medulla) play a secondary role in regulation of insulin secretion. β cells have different types of receptors for catecholamines. Some, called α_2 receptors, are direct inhibitors of insulin secretion. Others, termed, confusingly enough, β *receptors*, directly stimulate insulin secretion. Normally, α receptor activity dominates, and thus the net effect of catecholamines is generally inhibitory of insulin secretion.

Clinical Pearls

○ The observation that the inhibitory effects of catecholamines on insulin secretion (via α-**adrenergic receptors**) normally outweigh the stimulatory effects of catecholamines on insulin secretion (via β-adrenergic receptors) may explain why β-adrenergic receptor blockers (e.g., used as a treatment for hypertension) do not generally worsen diabetes mellitus.

○ Despite the practical clinical insignificance of β-adrenergic blockers as inhibitors of insulin secretion (see earlier), these drugs should still be avoided in patients being treated with insulin. This is because some of the most prominent signs and symptoms of hypoglycemia are mediated by β-adrenergic receptors (e.g., **tachycardia** and palpitations). In the event of an insulin overdose, a patient on a β-adrenergic receptor blocker (e.g., propranolol) may not be aware of the telltale symptoms, and the first sign of profound hypoglycemia may be loss of consciousness.

Review Questions

9. What is the location and cellular composition of the islets of Langerhans?
10. What are some rapid, intermediate, and long-term actions of insulin?
11. How does insulin cause an almost immediate increase in glucose uptake by most insulin-sensitive tissues?
12. What is the difference between "hormone sensitive lipase" and "lipoprotein lipase"?
13. What are the major physiological stimuli and inhibitors of insulin secretion?
14. What is known about the molecular mechanisms of insulin action?

TABLE 6.1   REGULATION OF ISLET CELL HORMONE SECRETION

	β cell insulin release	γ cell somatostatin release	α cell glucagon release
Nutrients			
Glucose	↑	↑	↓
Amino acids	↑	↑	↑
Fatty acids	—	—	↓
Ketones	—	—	↓
Hormones			
Enteric hormones	↑	↑	↑
Insulin	↓	↓ ?	↓
GABA	—	—	↓
Somatostatin	↓	↓	↓
Glucagon	↑	↑	—
Cortisol	—	—	↑
Catecholamines	↓	—	↑
	(α-adrenergic)		(β-adrenergic)
Neural			
Vagal	↑	—	↑
β-adrenergic	↑	—	↑
α-adrenergic	↓	—	↓

↑ = increased; ↓ = decreased; — = no effect or no known effect.

Reproduced, with permission, from Funk, J.L. and Feingold, K.R. (1999), in McPhee et al., eds. *Pathophysiology of Disease: An Introduction to Clinical Medicine,* 3rd ed. New York, McGraw-Hill, p. 434.

6. COUNTERREGULATORY HORMONES

Inasmuch as insulin is the sole hormone promoting storage of glucose and other fuels during periods of glucose abundance, an array of hormones defends the body against hypoglycemia, the so-called counterregulatory hormones. Teleologically this makes sense in that hyperglycemia causes problems in the long run while hypoglycemia can be deadly in minutes and therefore needs to be prevented at all costs. Of these counterregulatory hormones, some studies have implicated **glucagon** and **epinephrine** as the primary lines of defense against hypoglycemia, with **growth hormone** and **cortisol** playing a secondary role, and **placental lactogen** being specialized for protecting the fetus (see Chap. 17). It appears that, as a person becomes progressively more hypoglycemic, secretion of all four of these counterregulatory hormones are elicited at blood glucose levels below the high 60s, fully 10 mg/dL before onset of autonomic symptoms of hypoglycemia (anxiety, sweating, palpitations, tremor). Blood glucose must drop another 10 mg/dL before normal individuals start to demonstrate effects of glucose deprivation on the brain (dizziness, blurred vision, difficulty thinking). Thus, under normal conditions defense mechanisms are activated well before the occurrence of dangerous hypoglycemia. Indeed, the autonomic symptoms serve as a line of defense to normally prevent the development of **neuroglycopenic** symptoms.

In some cases of diabetes mellitus, in addition to the defect in insulin secretion, the counterregulatory mechanisms may also be impaired. Perhaps this is because, in the absence of β cells, paracrine interactions needed for proper α cell function are also disrupted. In some patients, counterregulatory responses may be excessive, while in others the responses are inadequate.

Glucagon

Actions of glucagon

The primary role of glucagon is to antagonize insulin's actions on the liver. Thus, it promotes glycogenolysis, gluconeogenesis, and fatty acid oxidation while inhibiting glycolysis, and glycogen and fatty acid synthesis (Figure 6.8). Glucagon's actions are mediated by a rise in intracellular cyclic AMP with its resultant corresponding effect on protein kinases, transcription, and so on, which in turn activate or inactivate the relevant enzymes. Glucagon has no role in the metabolism of peripheral tissues (e.g., fat and muscle). Instead, these peripheral tissues respond to the lack of insulin. As described in Sec. 5, their response is to convert from a substrate-storing to a substrate-generating economy.

Regulation of glucagon secretion

Glucagon is the major hormone involved in redirecting the liver toward glucose production and its release into the bloodstream, rather than storage (as glycogen) or use in intrahepatic intermediary metabolism. The primary stimulus for glucagon secretion is glucose, with the controls operating in the reverse direction as compared to insulin: As glucose concentration falls, glucagon secretion is stimulated. As glucose concentration rises above normal, further glucagon secretion is halted. Another milder stimulus for glucagon secretion is a protein-rich meal, which makes sense in an anticipatory way in that it prevents a transient hypoglycemia due to concurrent insulin secretion, stimulated by a protein-rich but glucose poor meal.

Likewise, catecholamines act through β-adrenergic receptors to trigger an increase in glucagon secretion over and above that expected for any given level of hypoglycemia. In this way, adequate supplies of fuel are maintained in the event of a "fight or flight" decision.

Insulin serves to inhibit glucagon secretion directly, as a paracrine effect, within the islets. Note that this is in contrast to the indirect effect of insulin to stimulate glucagon secretion as a consequence of lowering the blood glucose mentioned previously.

Other counterregulatory hormones

In addition to the major counterregulatory hormones, a number of other hormones can affect insulin's actions to a lesser degree, indirectly, and often in unpredictable ways, depending on other factors. These include thyroid hormone, estrogen, and progesterone.

Also, somatostatin secreted by the δ cells of the islets of Langerhans, as well as from other sources in the gut and brain, likely plays various endocrine and paracrine roles in fuel homeostasis. Its concentration in portal blood is too high for islet somatostatin to be solely a paracrine mediator, but its precise role and significance are not clear at this time.

Somatostatin is a direct inhibitor of secretion of insulin, glucagon, and growth hormone, among others. Somatostatin also decreases intestinal glucose absorption and hepatic glucose production, probably through inhibition of secretion of various hormones.

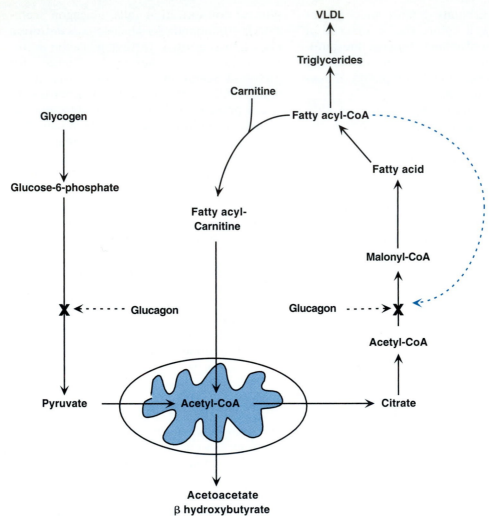

FIGURE 6.8. Actions of glucagon in regulation of glucose and lipid metabolism. Glucagon counters the action of insulin primarily in the liver through effects on both glucose and lipid metabolism (indicated by X). Its effects on glucose metabolism are largely the opposite of those shown for insulin in Figure 6.4A. However, whereas an important effect of insulin on lipid metabolism occurs peripherally through effects on lipoprotein lipase and hormone-sensitive lipase, the effects of glucagon are different. Glucagon inhibits enzymes involved in synthesis of malonyl CoA. This key intermediate normally inhibits carnitine acyl transferase, the enzyme involved in fatty acylcarnitine formation, without which fatty acids cannot be imported into mitochondria for fatty acid oxidation. As malonyl CoA levels fall, fatty acid uptake into mitochondria, and subsequent oxidation, is enhanced. At the same time, the block in malonyl CoA formation induced by glucagon diminishes the substrates needed for fatty acid synthesis and, therefore, VLDL production ceases. (Adapted, with permission, from Foster, D.W. and McGarry, J.D. (1983). The metabolic derangements and treatment of diabetic ketoacidosis, in N. Engl. J. Med. 309:160, 162.)

7. HORMONAL CONTROL OF METABOLIC STATES

Figure 6.9 indicates the major programs of metabolism for which insulin and glucagon secretion are coordinated under particular circumstances.

Basal

Under basal conditions glucose utilization by the brain and body is equal to glucose production by the liver, a balance maintained by the insulin-to-glucagon ratio. It has been estimated that up to 75% of this basal glucose production is driven by glucagon's signaling effects.

Fight or flight

In these situations there is a huge increase in glucose utilization by muscle. Muscle may be working so hard that it is not able to get enough oxygen to drive the citric acid cycle. In this circumstance, ATP production occurs anaerobically (i.e., via glycolysis with a low yield of ATP per mole of glucose), with pyruvate converted to lactate which is released into the bloodstream. In these circumstances, available glucose in the bloodstream would be quickly depleted, causing hypoglycemia and resulting in impaired brain function except that the increased glucose utilization by muscle is matched precisely by a rise in hepatic glucose production.

How does the liver "know" to increase its glucose output to meet this sudden demand from muscle? This effect is largely due to adrenergically mediated glucagon and epinephrine secretion. Both glucagon and catecholamines affect the liver directly, stimulating glycogenolysis, gluconeogenesis, and fatty acid oxidation.

Catecholamines have the additional reinforcing effect of inhibiting insulin secretion via α_2-adrenergic receptors on β cells of the islets. These effects of catecholamines are in large part responsible for the greater magnitude of hepatic glucose production in the fight or flight response, as compared with the more modest response to an overnight fast.

Furthermore, the flood of lactate back to the liver from muscle provides additional substrate for gluconeogenesis in the case of extreme exercise.

Fasting and starvation

Initially, the fall in insulin and rise in glucagon that accompanies fasting promotes glycogenolysis and gluconeogenesis in the liver. However, even at maximum rates of gluconeogenesis, the liver cannot provide adequate fuel substrates to meet the long-term needs of all tissues in the body. Thus, after a few hours of fasting, breakdown of muscle protein and lipolysis of stored triglycerides occurs, releasing amino acids and free fatty acids into the bloodstream. Not only does this provide more substrate for hepatic gluconeogenesis, it allows many tissues to use free fatty acids rather than glucose, which is, by default, preferentially allocated to the brain. Indeed, given a choice, muscle cells will preferentially use free fatty acids rather than glucose when aerobic metabolism is possible.

After about 1 week of fasting, there is a shift in brain fuel utilization from exclusive dependence on glucose to consumption of ketones. Ketones are a product of fatty acid oxidation in the liver and can be utilized by most tissues. Thus the onset of lipolysis spares further breakdown of muscle. The more delayed shift from glucose to ketone utilization on the part of the brain completes the transition of the entire body to a lipid-based fuel economy for survival during long-term starvation.

Transition to a lipid-fuel substrate economy requires not only the provision of free

a) Resting state

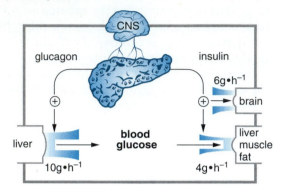

b) "Fight or flight" (acute stress)

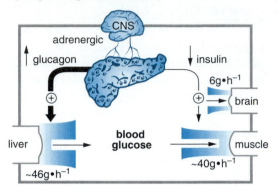

c) Famine (chronic stress)

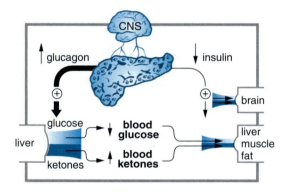

d) Severe injury

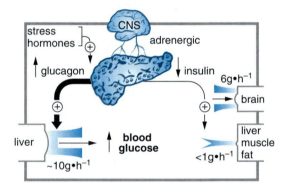

e) Alimentary glucoregulation

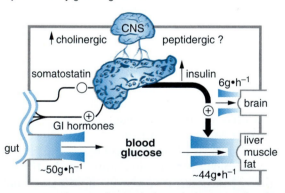

f) Diabetes (Type II)

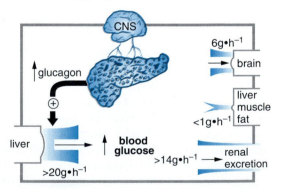

FIGURE 6.9. Hormonal control of metabolic states. The islet of Langerhans is depicted with neural connections to the CNS. The extracellular space is depicted as a box (heavy border) into which glucose flows from the liver or gut and from which it flows, independently of insulin action, to the brain, and, under insulin mediation,

fatty acid substrate to the liver, but also induction of enzymes of fatty acid catabolism and ketone production. Conversely, once a lipid-driven economy has been established, simply diminishing the level of free fatty acids generated in the periphery is not enough to return to baseline. The body must also inactivate and degrade the excess catabolic enzymes that are present in the liver. The change in insulin and glucagon levels helps orchestrate these alterations.

Severe injury

Under conditions of severe injury, glucagon secretion is increased by all of the counterregulatory hormones (glucagon, epinephrine, cortisol, and growth hormone) working together.

Fed

Signals in the form of GI hormones and **cholinergic** and **peptidergic** neurotransmitters reach the islets of Langerhans immediately upon a person eating. They elicit an anticipatory response of insulin and glucagon secretion tailored in magnitude to the protein versus carbohydrate content of the meal. This prevents even transient hyperglycemia (from a large amount of ingested glucose) or hypoglycemia (during the delay time needed to convert absorbed amino acids into glucose) following a meal. It is notable that dietary protein (i.e., amino acids) is the only simultaneous stimulus for both insulin and glucagon secretion.

Review Questions

15. What are the major counterregulatory hormones? What does this term mean?
16. Name the major (and some minor) stimuli and inhibitors of glucagon secretion.
17. How do insulin and glucagon levels change from baseline in the fasted, prolonged starvation, flight or fight, and injured states?

FIGURE 6.9 — (continued) into other tissues. Values given for rates of glucose utilization and production are estimates not based on true data. a. In the resting state, insulin and glucagon maintain equality between the rate of glucose utilization and hepatic glucose production. b. In fight or flight situations, the huge increase in glucose utilization by muscle would cause hypoglycemia if the liver did not replace this glucose precisely, largely through adrenergically mediated increase in glucagon and a decrease in insulin. The latter minimizes the uptake of endogenously produced glucose by tissues other than the exercising muscles and the brain. c. In famine, the rise in glucagon, coupled with a decline in insulin, promotes glycogenolysis and gluconeogenesis and, within one week, induces a shift to ketones required for continuation of survival. d. In severe injury, an adrenergically mediated increase in glucagon and a decrease in insulin stimulate hepatic glucose production and minimize glucose utilization by insulin-responsive tissues. The other stress hormones (growth hormone, epinephrine, and cortisol) all trigger an increase in glucagon secretion. e. In regulation after feeding, signals arising in the gastrointestinal tract immediately after a meal (GI hormones and various neurotransmitters of the ENS and autonomic nervous system) reach the islets and elicit an anticipatory response of insulin secretion, thereby avoiding even a transient rise above normal in peripheral blood glucose concentration. The magnitude of the insulin response to these signals is determined by the blood glucose concentration. When at the low end of normal, insulin response is less, when on the high side of normal, the response is greater. f. In insulin-dependent diabetes, the islets contain no β cells and therefore make no insulin. Without exogenous insulin injections, glucagon is unrestrained, unopposed, and unbuffered in its actions. Under these conditions, glucose rise is limited only by peripheral utilization by insulin-independent tissues and renal excretion. If glucagon, as well as insulin, were absent, massive overproduction of ketones and glucose would not occur. (Adapted, with permission, from Unger, R.H. and Orci, L. (1981). Glucagon and the A cell, in N. Engl. J. Med. 304:1519.)

8. DISORDERS OF FUEL HOMEOSTASIS

Insulin resistance and its consequences

Insulin resistance is the inability of a given amount of insulin to have its usual blood glucose-lowering effect. This could be either a general failure of insulin action, a tissue-selective insulin resistance, or both.

Any of a number of factors and mechanisms can result in such an abnormality in insulin action. For example, the following may occur:

- Counterregulatory hormone levels can be elevated. This could be a normal physiological response (e.g., to stress), a complication of pharmacological therapy (e.g., with glucocorticoids), or a pathologically excessive counterregulatory response.
- Specific tissues can become insulin-resistant. Obesity can cause a defect in the responsiveness of fat cells to insulin. The mechanism of this defect has not yet been fully elucidated, but it is likely to be a postreceptor defect, meaning one that interferes in the signaling pathway downstream of insulin binding to its receptor.
- Antibodies (either to insulin or to the insulin receptor) that interfere with insulin binding can develop.

Recent data suggest the role of obesity in insulin resistance is even more complicated than previously imagined: different "types" of obesity and fat in different locations (visceral versus subcutaneous) can influence the degree of insulin resistance tremendously (see Visceral versus Subcutaneous Fat in Pathogenesis of Diabetes Mellitus, in Frontiers, in Sec. 9).

Regardless of whether the initial insulin resistance is due to elevated counterregulatory hormones, diminished receptor activation, interfering antibodies, or for some other reason, this situation can set in motion several

vicious cycles. Because of this insulin resistance, less glucose is taken up and the blood glucose level rises. Initially, an elevated blood glucose level results in increased insulin secretion, achieving glucose homeostasis at a higher blood insulin level. However, the increased insulin level has effects on other tissues (remember the different effects of insulin on different timescales). Thus, the resultant hypertrophy and proliferation of vascular smooth muscle may contribute to **hypertension** and **arteriosclerosis**.

Increased insulin secretion in response to hyperglycemia (a consequence of insulin resistance) can eventually lead to a form of "β-cell exhaustion" where the islets can no longer maintain the required high level of insulin secretion. Either because of accumulation of **amyloid** deposits (proteinaceous garbage precipitated around individual islet cells) or for other reasons, islets may display more and more significant defects in either the regulation or processing of the insulin that they secrete. These defects in turn manifest as increased insulin resistance, requiring further increase in insulin secretion. Eventually, the ability to further increase insulin secretion is exhausted and blood glucose rises to a new steady state.

Faced with high blood glucose concentrations, other tissues (e.g., muscle) may downregulate their glucose transporters. Thus a major source of glucose disposal (i.e., uptake by muscle) is lost, further worsening the tendency to hyperglycemia.

Rising steady state blood glucose is toxic not only to the β cell (via β-cell exhaustion and amyloid deposition, as already discussed), but also to cells in the periphery. At least two mechanisms have been proposed to explain this effect.

One mechanism is that many proteins can be covalently modified by addition of glucose residues by a chemical reaction dependent only on high glucose concentrations (see Figure 6.10). This nonenzymatic glycosylation of

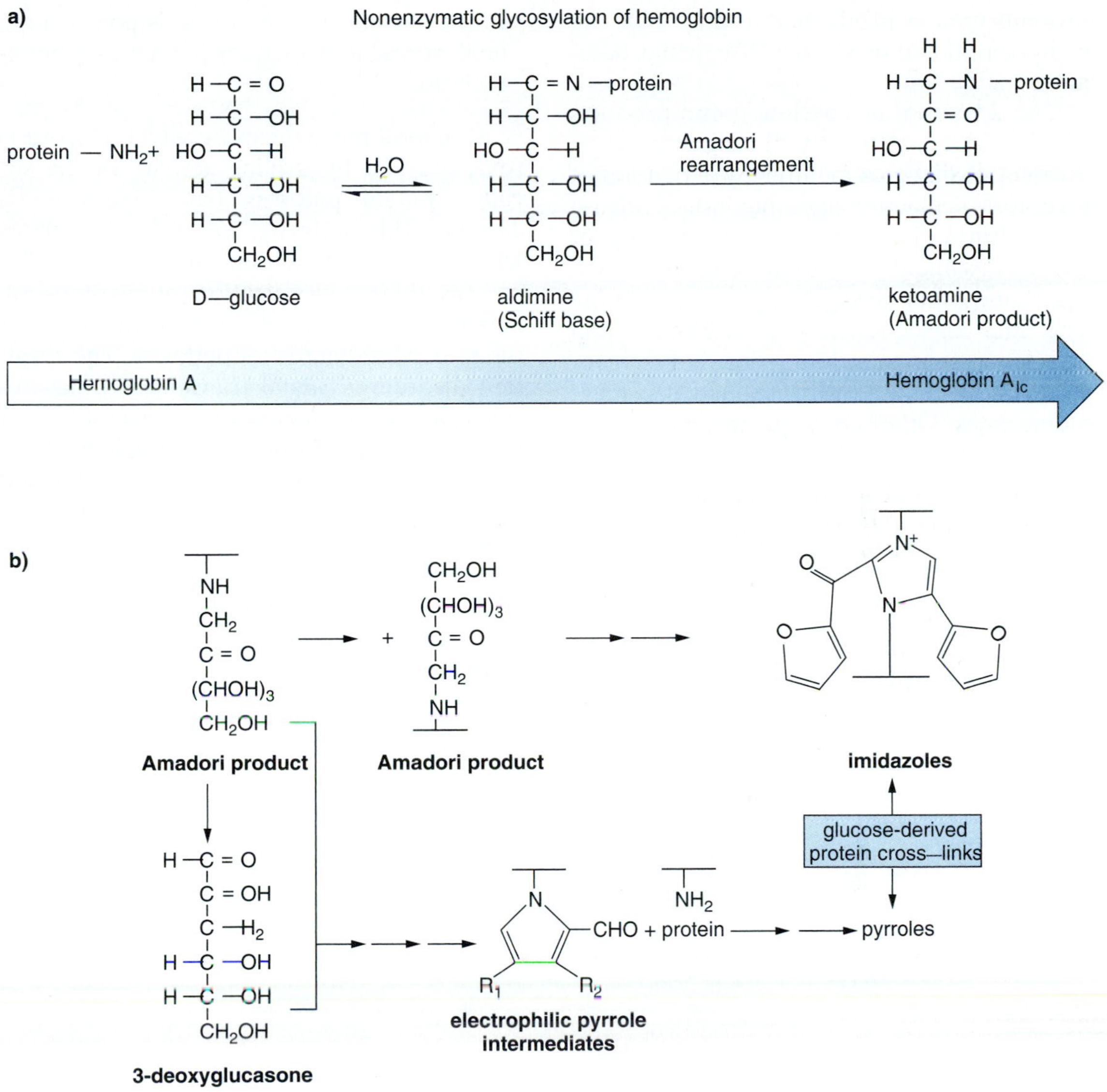

a)

Nonenzymatic glycosylation of hemoglobin

Hemoglobin A → Hemoglobin A$_{Ic}$

b)

FIGURE 6.10. Complications of hyperglycemia: Formation of Amadori and advanced glycosylation end products. *a.* Indicates the nonenzymatic reaction by which high blood glucose concentration results in covalently modified, dysfunctional proteins. *b.* The Amadori products can go on to form various imidazoles and pyrroles that cross-link proteins and contribute to basement membrane thickening and other aspects of organ system dysfunction as key steps in diabetes-associated complications. *(a. Adapted, with permission, from Wyngaarden et al., eds. (1992). Cecil's Textbook of Medicine. 19th ed. Philadelphia, PA, W.B. Saunders. b. Adapted, with permission, from Kohler, P.O., Jordan, R.M., eds. (1986). Clinical Endocrinology. New York, Wiley.)*

proteins creates products that may alter the composition and properties of vascular basement membranes.

The advanced glycosylation end products (AGEs) also contribute to the chronic consequences of diabetes mellitus by activation of receptors on macrophages that induce release of cytokines. The cytokines in turn trigger altered basement membrane component synthesis and other changes in gene expression. The final consequence is small blood vessel disease, with impaired nutrition and oxygenation of tissues due to thickened basement membranes. Other consequences are:

- In the eye, the result is proliferation of fragile new blood vessels with a propensity to rupture and bleed, ultimately causing blindness.
- In the kidney, the result is dysfunction and, eventually, death of nephrons.
- In the autonomic nervous system, the result is dysfunction and, eventually, death of neurons, causing autonomic neuropathy.

- In the extremities, the result is poor wound healing and a propensity for developing infections.

A second mechanism by which glucose is toxic may be by driving activity of the so-called **polyol pathway** (see Figure 6.11). Through this pathway, sorbitol accumulates within cells, changes their osmolarity, and decreases their concentration of myoinositol, an important signal transduction precursor of the phosphatidylinositol pathway. The resultant disordered signal transduction may result in a cascade of abnormalities in different tissues. Cataract formation in the lens of the eye, for example, is associated with elevated sorbitol levels. Altered nerve conduction, believed to be one of the bases for diabetic neuropathy, is another consequence associated with this biochemical pathway.

Diabetes mellitus

Perhaps because fuel storage is controlled by a single hormone (insulin) synthesized in a

FIGURE 6.11. Complications of hyperglycemia: The sorbitol pathway. Hyperglycemia increases intracellular sorbitol, which in turn is associated with depletion of intracellular myoinositol levels. Hyperglycemia may also decrease myoinositol by inhibiting its uptake from the blood. *(Adapted, with permission, from Wyngaarden et al., eds. (1992). Cecil's Textbook of Medicine. 19th ed. Philadelphia, PA, W.B. Saunders.)*

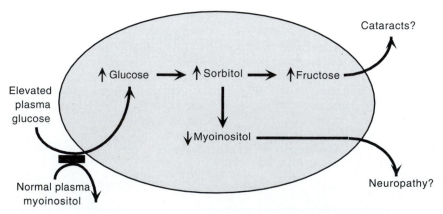

single cell type, the disease of aberrant insulin production and action, diabetes mellitus, is extremely common. The unifying feature of different causes of diabetes mellitus is hyperglycemia. As we have seen, this can result from various combinations of abnormalities including total or relative insulin lack, relative resistance of peripheral tissues to insulin action, excess of counterregulatory hormones, and genetic defects in insulin receptors or signal transduction pathways, just to name a few. Some degree of β-cell dysfunction, either genetic or acquired, must generally be involved, because the normal endocrine pancreas of a young person has enough β-cell secretory reserve to overcome most insulin resistance and maintain normal blood glucose.

A total lack of insulin is only one of several subtypes of diabetes and accounts for approximately 10% of patients with diabetes. This form of diabetes (termed *type 1*) does not have as strong a genetic basis as the other major category of diabetes. Type 1 diabetes mellitus tends to occur in a young age group and is believed to be due to autoimmune attack on the islets. These patients eventually become devoid of β cells as a consequence of the autoimmune attack and thus have a severe disease. Their long-term survival is absolutely dependent on insulin injections. Without insulin therapy, those with type 1 diabetes are at great risk of developing severe hyperglycemia (due to the unopposed action of glucagon in activating gluconeogenesis in the liver and the lack of insulin-activating peripheral substrate production) and elevated blood ketone levels (due to the unopposed action of glucagon on the liver activating fatty acid oxidation, the end products of which are ketones). These abnormalities rapidly cause profound dehydration (due to an osmotic diuresis induced by the high blood glucose) and acidosis (due to both dehydration and the accumulation of ketones), which

untreated result in coma and death. This syndrome is termed **diabetic ketoacidosis**.

The much more common so-called type 2 diabetes mellitus results from a heterogeneous group of disorders in which insulin secretion is defective or inadequate to some degree, and in which there is also resistance to the effects of insulin. These patients have a strong family history of the disease, tend to develop diabetes after the age of 40, tend to be obese, and often have normal or even high blood levels of immunoreactive insulin, which appears inadequate to properly control their fuel metabolism. These patients also have acute hyperglycemia, but rarely develop ketoacidosis because their endogenous circulating blood insulin levels are sufficient to prevent excessive fatty oxidation and ketone production by the liver.

The intrinsic heterogeneity of type 2 diabetes mellitus from patient to patient makes it difficult for clinicians to treat. This difficulty is probably further exacerbated by evolution of the disorder in any given patient over time. Thus, a patient whose initial presentation is out-of-control diabetes may be driven largely by insulin resistance (as might be brought on by obesity, for example) and may go on to develop other abnormalities that independently contribute to, or maintain, diabetes mellitus even if the insulin-resistance precipitant is brought under control.

Suggested pathophysiological mechanisms responsible for such abnormalities include the following:

- **β-cell exhaustion** from elevated insulin secretion rates in response to insulin resistance. The β cell is driven to secrete more and more insulin in an effort to achieve the effect normally seen in the absence of insulin resistance. Somehow, the resulting secretory overactivity can result in either impaired insulin secretion or secretion of defective insulin (e.g., due to acquired trafficking or processing errors during insulin biosynthesis).

- **Glucose toxicity** due to deleterious effects of elevated glucose concentration (e.g., on function of glucose transporters in the periphery). This occurs as the β cell "falls behind" despite elevated insulin secretion (see earlier). It is likely that this effect is distinct from the mechanisms discussed earlier (β-cell exhaustion, amyloid, AGE products, and sorbitol accumulation). However, the precise mechanisms have not been delineated.

Like someone struggling to keep up with payments on a high-interest rate card balance, these mechanisms set up a vicious cycle of worsening insulin resistance and rising glucose concentration, which causes further glucose transporter downregulation and glucose toxicity, making it impossible to maintain homeostasis.

Regardless of its type or mechanism, as diabetes mellitus gets further and further out of control, the patient will experience worsened symptoms. Initially, mild polyuria (increased volume and frequency of urination) will occur from the **osmotic diuresis** induced by the uncleared blood glucose. Then blurry vision may develop, as the high glucose drives production and accumulation of sorbital and other sugars in the lens of the eye. Symptoms of neuropathy may develop or worsen acutely due to deposition of such products in peripheral nerves. Risk of infection is increased. Infection triggers even more release of counterregulatory hormones in response to stress, further worsening glucose control.

At some point the acute complications may go into a potentially lethal spiral. For the person with type 1 diabetes, it may be the development of ketoacidosis with the accumulation of **ketones** exceeding the metabolic and respiratory buffering capacity of the body and causing a fall in blood pH (see

Chap. 10). For others with type 2 diabetes, the osmotic diuresis driven by high blood glucose filtered in the kidney and pulling water with it may exceed the patient's ability to keep up with oral fluid intake. As a result, progressive dehydration and intravascular volume contraction can occur, culminating in renal failure and hyperosmolar coma (see Figure 6.12).

Chronically, both those with type 1 and type 2 diabetes develop devastating complications. Some of the complications are due to small blood vessel disease (from basement membrane changes). The ultimate result can be blindness, kidney failure, neuropathy, a tendency to develop infections, and poor wound healing. The poor wound healing and infections often require amputation of extremities. Other complications of diabetes mellitus are a consequence of large blood vessel disease (arteriosclerosis). This is a result of **hyperinsulinemia** and **hyperlipidemia** (due to increased activity of hormone-sensitive lipase in adipose tissue), as a consequence of insulin resistance.

The Diabetes Control and Complications Trial (see Ref. 4a) was an important study that demonstrated slowing of the development of these complications in patients whose blood glucose was kept as close to normal as possible through intensive insulin injection therapy. However, there remains substantial controversy over when the benefits of tight control are offset by the risks of hypoglycemia.

Clinical Pearls

○ Besides insulin, how might you treat diabetes mellitus? Since insulin resistance is the major problem, at least initially, in most people with diabetes with type 2 disease, drugs that either increase insulin secretion or decrease peripheral resistance to insulin action should improve blood

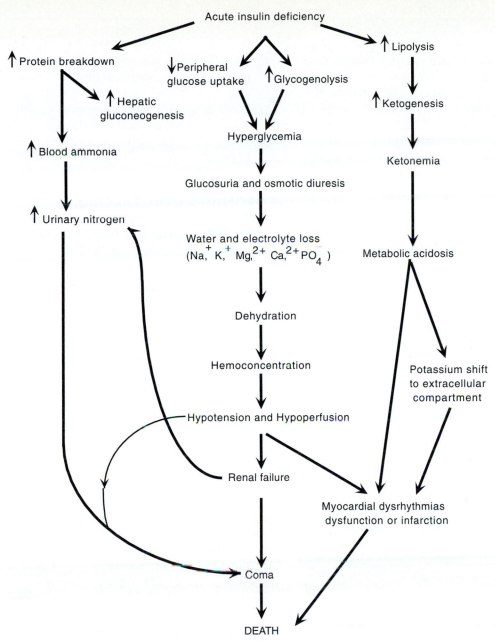

FIGURE 6.12. Pathophysiology of acute complications of diabetes mellitus. Acute insulin deficiency and the consequent change in insulin to glucagon ratio result in the metabolic abnormalities indicated. Once metabolic acidosis and dehydration induced hypotension have developed, the patient is at risk for multiple forms of organ system failure and even death, by multiple mechanisms whose relative prominence will vary from patient to patient. (Adapted, with permission, from Tepperman, J. and Tepperman, H.M. (1987). Metabolic and Endocrine Physiology. 5th ed. St. Louis, YearBook Medical Publishers.)

glucose control. An example of the former is the sulfonylureas, such as the drug glyburide. An example of the latter is the drug troglitizone.

○ Since glucose overproduction by the liver, as a result of a relative imbalance in the glucagon versus insulin effect, is an important contribution to high blood glucose in diabetes mellitus, a third class of drugs are those that block hepatic gluconeogenesis. Metformin is a drug that works by this mechanism.

○ Importantly, none of these drugs work in patients with type 1 diabetes, for whom insulin injections are mandatory.

○ The "see-saw" of insulin and glucagon can confuse the interpretation of blood glucose levels in patients. Injection of too much insulin (e.g., at bedtime) can result in hypoglycemia at night when the patient is not aware of the usual symptoms of tachycardia, sweating, and confusion. Instead, hypoglycemia at night is often manifest as nightmares and vivid dreams. The hypoglycemia in turn triggers release of counterregulatory hormones that drive blood glucose very high by morning. Noting the high morning glucose, patients may think they took too *little* insulin the previous night, when in fact they took too much. But increasing the insulin dose only makes the nocturnal hypoglycemia, and subsequent morning hyperglycemia, worse. The physician needs to recognize this so-called **Somogyi phenomenon** and recommend a *decrease* instead of an increase in the evening insulin dose.

Review Questions

18. Name three mechanisms of insulin resistance.
19. Name two mechanisms of glucose toxicity.
20. Explain the concept of β-cell exhaustion in insulin-resistant diabetes mellitus.
21. What are some acute complications of out-of-control diabetes mellitus?
22. What are some chronic complications of poorly controlled diabetes mellitus?

9. FRONTIERS IN RESEARCH ON HORMONES OF THE ENDOCRINE PANCREAS AND THE CONTROL OF INTERMEDIARY METABOLISM

Etiology and prevention of type 1 diabetes mellitus

A large body of evidence supports the notion that type 1 diabetes is an autoimmune disorder involving attack on the β cell. But what sets off this autoimmune attack and how might it be prevented? Studies have found that an early antigen against which autoimmune attack is directed in type 1 diabetes is glutamic acid decarboxylase (GAD). It appears that this enzyme is more than just an "innocent bystander" in the autoimmune process, because induction of immune tolerance to GAD in a mouse model of type 1 diabetes prevents development of diabetes. Induction of tolerance to other autoantigens observed in type 1 diabetes did not prevent the development of diabetes, suggesting a special role for GAD. Other work has observed a sequence identity between some part of the coding region for viral genes and GAD and suggests that the immune response mounted against certain viral infections by patients with certain **major histocompatibility complex** (MHC) genes may be a trigger of the autoimmune process against GAD in the first place (see Ref. 5).

Molecular mechanism of insulin action

A tyrosine phosphoprotein termed *insulin receptor substrate-1* (IRS-1) has been identified to be an apparent central regulator of the many pathways of signaling activated by insulin. When investigators generated mice in which the IRS-1 gene was disrupted, they found that the animals were insulin resistant and growth retarded but still displayed a substantial amount of insulin action with appearance of a new insulin receptor substrate (IRS-2), representing an IRS-1 independent pathway of insulin action. One explanation for this result may be that organisms have evolved a certain degree of redundancy in their control of important metabolic pathways such as those of insulin action, so that loss of one gene product does not abolish all regulatory control. In this way there would be fewer genetic "weak links" at which mutations would be rapidly lethal. Those aspects of a system for which redundancy has not been developed may be precisely the ones that are more likely to be involved in a genetic disease (see Refs. 6 and 7). These results suggest that the molecular mechanisms of insulin action will be even more complex than would have otherwise been expected (see Ref. 14 for a review of the current view of the mechanism of insulin action).

Visceral versus subcutaneous fat in pathogensis of diabetes mellitus

Although obesity has long been strongly implicated as a cause of insulin resistance, studies suggest that not all obesity is the same. Rather, obesity that is a result of adipose tissue in the abdominal organs is associated with more complications of diabetes mellitus than obesity that is subcutaneous. It appears that individuals who exercise a lot (e.g., Sumo wrestlers) and who are fat (because they eat many-thousand-calorie diets) deposit fat subcutaneously rather than into the abdominal viscera. Such individuals do not develop the complications of diabetes to the extent observed for equally obese sedentary individuals (see Ref. 8). As with most physiological

variables, both genetics and environment (e.g., diet and exercise) are likely to contribute to the extent of visceral fat accumulation in any given individual.

Molecular mechanism of insulin resistance

It is generally acknowledged that most cases of type 2 diabetes involve an insulin-resistant state, but the molecular mechanism of insulin resistance remains unclear. Evidence has been presented that, in at least some cases, a membrane glycoprotein, termed *PC-1*, is induced in the muscle of patients with type 2 diabetes mellitus. When studied in cell culture systems, this protein is found to interfere with the action of insulin receptor kinase. When expressed in cells that do not normally make this protein, PC-1 results in a decrease in at least some of insulin's actions. Further work needs to be done to determine whether this potential mechanism is indeed a major one in the pathogenesis of type 2 diabetes (see Ref. 9).

Understanding the logic of metabolic states

The flight or fight physiology described earlier (see Sec. 7) seems to present a pleasing teleology. But here is a problem: During exercise, insulin levels fall and glucagon levels rise to trigger hepatic gluconeogenesis. How, then, does muscle (an insulin-dependent tissue) maintain its ability to take up glucose in the face of falling insulin levels? It has been determined that muscle contraction stimulates translocation of glucose transporters to the plasma membrane in skeletal muscle by a mechanism distinct from the response to insulin, providing a potentially simple physiological solution to this dilemma (see Ref. 10).

How do obesity and diabetes mellitus cause cardiovascular disease?

A study has directly demonstrated defective endothelial vasodilation in response to the high blood insulin levels that occur during insulin resistance. Since defective vasodilation might be expected to result in a tendency toward development of hypertension, this observation may provide a potential pathophysiological mechanism for cardiovascular complications associated with diabetes (see Ref. 11).

Is diabetic neuropathy an autoimmune disease?

The conventional hypotheses for the pathogenesis of chronic complications of diabetes mellitus, including neuropathy, have been either (a) blood vessel basement membrane thickening and consequent poor nutrition of cells, (b) a consequence of accumulation of advanced glycosylation end products, or (c), defective signal transduction (e.g., due to altered myoinositol levels). However, a remarkable set of observations raise the possibility that an autoimmune syndrome may contribute to at least some forms of chronic diabetic complications (see Ref. 12). It appears that serum from diabetic patients with neuropathy causes apoptosis of cultured neuronal cells, a finding that was not observed with serum from diabetic patients without neuropathy, or in normal controls. Other experiments suggest that the effect is due to an immunoglobulin and that the mechanism involved is elevation of intracellular calcium, a known common step in a number of other forms of apoptosis. If reproduced and extended, these findings would have significant implications both for pathogenesis and therapy of these disabling consequences of diabetes. They also provide appreciation of a potentially new and unanticipated dimension of heterogeneity in patients who are lumped together as having a single disease (see Ref. 13).

10. HOW DOES AN UNDERSTANDING OF NORMAL PHYSIOLOGY PROVIDE INSIGHT INTO THE INITIAL CASE PRESENTATION?

Let's look back on A. R., the 65-year-old Russian immigrant and homemaker with a 10-year history of non-insulin-dependent diabetes mellitus.

Frequent urination reflected the osmotic diuresis induced by hyperglycemia, as did the thirst. Weight loss and hunger occurred because she was losing the calories that she consumed, in the form of glucose in her urine.

Blurry vision was due to the acute effects of hyperglycemia on the eye, perhaps aggravated by sorbitol accumulation and, eventually, cataract formation. Retinopathy due to leakage from fragile blood vessels in the eye may also contribute to her visual impairment.

Ineffectiveness of the oral hypoglycemic agents may have been due to "β cell exhaustion," as her pancreas worked to lower blood glucose in the face of an increasingly insulin-resistant periphery. The action of insulin injection to promote fuel storage contributed to the weight gain, which further worsened the insulin-resistance of the periphery.

In addition, exertional chest pains may be the first sign of myocardial ischemia due to atherosclerosis of the coronary arteries. Puffiness of the face and legs may reflect fluid overload, either because of her heart disease, or more likely, because of diabetic kidney disease, resulting in loss of albumin in the urine, and/or renal failure.

Her new gastrointestinal and neurological symptoms may reflect diabetic neuropathy, resulting in gastroparesis and autonomic vascular dysfunction. Diabetic retinopathy may account for her vision changes.

Measurement of glycohemoglobin (hemoglobin A$_{1c}$), an AGE product (see Disorders of Fuel Homeostasis, Sec. 8), will indicate whether the blood sugar observed is reflective of her average blood sugars over recent weeks.

It is important for Ms. R. to understand how diabetes causes her symptoms and what she can do about it. She is asking for explanations and deserves them, in her language, from you or a member of your health care team. Good health education is an essential part of good diabetes care and helps decrease symptoms and complications caused by end-organ damage.

You might explain to Ms. R. that when her blood sugar is too high for too long, the blood vessels are damaged, especially the smallest ones that nourish the eyes, kidneys, feet, heart, and the nerves that help her stomach and intestines function. The symptoms of bloating, nausea, diarrhea, and constipation may be caused by this nerve damage. Likewise, the changes in her vision may be related to blood vessel and nerve damage in her eyes. Sores are not healing on her feet because the damaged blood vessels cannot carry the cells and materials needed for healing and defense against infection.

She can slow the progress of this damage by lowering her blood sugar. This may be accomplished with exercise (which in her case may be limited by her heart disease), diet, weight loss, and/or medication. She can also decrease the damage to her kidneys by keeping her blood pressure in a normal range, especially by using angiotensin-converting enzyme inhibitors, which have protective effects on the kidneys.

She may relieve some of her symptoms related to digestion through use of a high fiber diet and medications that stimulate nerve activity to compensate for the nerve function damaged by the diabetes. She may improve her vision through laser treatment of damaged and bleeding blood vessels in the retinas of her eyes.

Ms. R. has non-insulin-dependent diabetes, meaning she does produce some insulin, but her body's ability to respond to the amount of insulin she can make is inadequate. The β cells in the pancreas that produce it can be impaired or lost through exhaustion, glucose toxicity, or amyloid deposits. If insulin doses are causing hypoglycemia, she may need to adjust the type, time, frequency, and/or quantity of insulin she is using.

Ms. R. should know that with adjustment to her insulin treatment and changes in diet and activity, she would probably be able to significantly reduce her average blood sugars without frequent hypoglycemia. It is important also for her to understand that if she does not do this, she is at significantly increased risk of blindness, kidney failure, heart attacks, infections, amputation, strokes, and, ultimately, an early death.

SUMMARY AND REVIEW OF KEY CONCEPTS

1. Insulin is the primary hormone of fuel substrate storage.
2. Glucagon is the primary counterregulatory hormone opposing insulin's action on the liver.
3. Epinephrine, cortisol, and growth hormone are the major additional counterregulatory hormones opposing insulin's action both at the liver and the periphery.
4. The primary stimulus for insulin release is higher-than-normal blood glucose. The primary stimulus to glucagon secretion is lower-than-normal blood glucose.
5. Glucagon and other fuel substrates (amino acids, free fatty acids) are minor stimuli to insulin secretion. Insulin directly inhibits glucagon secretion.
6. Insulin action occurs on various time-scales, with rapid, intermediate, and long-term effects.

7. Insulin has various effects on carbohydrate, lipid, and protein metabolism that reinforce the anabolic state by promoting glycogen and protein synthesis, glycolysis, and deposition of triglycerides in adipose tissue.

8. Glucagon and other counterregulatory hormones promote glycogenolysis, fatty acid oxidation, ketone production, and protein breakdown, as part of various catabolic states.

9. The mechanism of insulin action involves binding a cell-surface receptor that is itself a tyrosine kinase. Activation of various pathways of signal transduction, often involving protein phosphorylation, is likely to be the molecular basis for specific insulin effects.

10. The effects of insulin and glucagon on the liver are coordinated with insulin's effects on muscle and adipose tissue to give tight control of blood glucose.

11. Insulin resistance occurs when a given amount of insulin that used to be adequate to maintain blood glucose is no longer sufficient. There are many molecular mechanisms by which insulin resistance might occur in different patients including insufficient insulin receptors, interfering antibodies, excessive counterregulatory hormones, poor quality insulin (e.g., due to defective processing in the β cell), defective receptors, and glucose toxicity).

12. Type 1 diabetes mellitus is an autoimmune disorder of β-cell destruction.

13. Type 2 diabetes mellitus is a heterogeneous collection of disorders of insulin resistance, defective insulin synthesis, or secretion.

14. The concepts of β-cell exhaustion and glucose toxicity are relevant for understanding the progression of diabetes mellitus.

15. Acute complications of diabetes mellitus are a consequence of changes in physiology of the liver and the periphery in the absence of insulin resulting in hyperglycemia with or without ketoacidosis. Dehydration caused by hyperglycemia-induced osmotic diuresis leads to renal failure. Acidosis from ketone accumulation leads to cardiac arrhythmias, respiratory failure, and, rapidly thereafter, death.

16. Chronic complications of diabetes mellitus are due to hyperglycemia-related alteration in basement membrane function leading to disease of small blood vessels and ultimately, retinopathy, nephropathy, and neuropathy. Metabolic abnormalities related to insulin resistance and hyperlipidemia in diabetes mellitus also causes atherosclerotic disease of large vessels, which are a major cause of heart attacks and stroke.

A CASE OF PHYSIOLOGICAL MEDICINE

T.D. is a thin, 38-year-old health care worker with insulin-dependent diabetes mellitus. She first came to medical attention at age 16 with polyuria, polydipsia, and weight loss and was found to be in ketoacidosis. Her sister is quite healthy, with normal fasting blood glucose and no evidence of diabetes to date. Ms. D. in contrast, started taking insulin injections at age 16 and has had multiple medical problems over the subsequent 22 years. Her medical problems include elevated blood sugars (usually), hypothyroidism, autoimmune ovarian failure, and Addison's disease (for which she is taking thyroid hormone, estrogen, and cortisol replacement). For many years she has had extremely high insulin requirements, needing as much as 80 U of insulin daily (those of us without any insulin resistance may secrete about 20 U a day). In addition she has had numerous infections, ranging from superficial cellulitis to bacterial pneumonia. Recently she had new complaints that were diagnosed as due to autonomic neuropathy. She is also seen frequently in the opthalmology clinic for severe retinopathy. Now she notes total body puffiness and wonders if something new is happening. Despite 2 and sometimes 3 injections of insulin per day, her glycosylated hemoglobin values have been greater than 10 mg/dL (upper limits of normal = 6 mg/dL). Surprisingly (at least to her), her insulin requirements have decreased substantially in the last month, although her blood glucose remains high.

QUESTIONS

1. Why didn't Ms. D. develop overt diabetes until age 16? Why has her sister not developed diabetes at all?
2. Is there a relation between diabetes mellitus in this patient and the thyroid, adrenal, and ovarian failure she has subsequently developed?
3. Decrease in the effectiveness of a given amount of insulin is termed *insulin resistance* and may be due to many different causes. Suggest some potential causes of insulin resistance in Ms. D.
4. Suppose Ms. D. were, instead, an overweight 45-year-old with adult-onset disease. Suggest some other causes of insulin resistance that would be more likely in this case.
5. How might you relate the patient's symptoms of total body puffiness to the recent decrease in her insulin requirements without invoking an unrelated disease process?
6. Is oral hypoglycemic agent therapy appropriate for Ms. D. or not?

ANSWERS

1. Most insulin-dependent diabetes mellitus is believed to be due to autoimmune destruction of β cells triggered by events such as a particular viral infection. Presumably, Ms D's immune system was triggered to attack her islets by such an event occurring around age 16, while her sibling has been fortunate not to have such an inciting event (as yet).
2. They may all be manifestations of a genetic predisposition to autoimmune disease.
3. Some potential causes of insulin resistance are high antibody titers (that either block binding of insulin or occupy the insulin receptor without activating it), glucose toxicity, excessive cortisol replacement, or inadequate thyroid hormone replacement.
4. More likely causes of insulin resistance in this case would be obesity or poor quality endogenous insulin (processing and secretion timing defects) perhaps related to β-cell exhaustion.
5. Insulin is substantially metabolized in the kidneys, so worsening of renal function may be associated with *increased* insulin half-life and, therefore, more hypoglycemic effect per unit insulin. The patient's puffiness is consistent with a possible decrease in renal function.
6. No, she is lacking β cells and therefore needs insulin therapy.

References and suggested readings

GENERAL REFERENCES

1. Karam, J. (1997). Pancreatic hormones and diabetes mellitus. Chapter 18, in Greenspan, F.S. and Strewler, G.S., eds. *Basic and Clinical Endocrinology*, 5th ed. Stamford, CT, Appleton & Lange, pp. 595-663.
2. Foster, D.W. and McGarry, J.D. (1983). The metabolic derangements and treatment of diabetic ketoacidosis. *N. Eng. J. Med.* 309:159-169.
3. Mitrakou, A. et al. (1991). Hierarchy of glycemic thresholds for counterregulatory hormone secretion, symptoms and cerebral dysfunction. *Endocrinol. Metab.* 23:E67-E74.

4. Saltiel, A. (1994). The paradoxical regulation of protein phosphorylation in insulin action. *FASEB J.* 8:1034-1040.

4a. The Diabetes Control and Complications Trial Research Group. (1993). The effect of intensive treatment of diabetes on the development and progression of long-term complications in insulin-dependent diabetes mellitus. *N. Eng. J. Med.* 329:973.

FRONTIERS REFERENCES

5. Solimena, M. and DeCamilli, P. (1993). Spotlight on a neuronal enzyme. *Nature* 366:15-17.

6. Tamemoto, H. et al. (1994) Insulin resistance and growth retardation in mice lacking insulin receptor substrate-1. *Nature* 372:182-186.

7. Araki, E. et al. (1994). Alternative pathway of insulin signaling in mice with targeted disruption of the IRS-1 gene. *Nature* 372:186-189.

8. Matsuzawa, Y. et al. Pathophysiology and pathogenesis of visceral fat obesity, in Sakamoto et al., eds. *Pathogenesis and Treatment of NIDDM*. New York, Elsevier.

9. Maddux, B.A. et al. (1995). Membrane glyco-protein PC-1 and insulin resistance in non-insulin-dependent diabetes mellitus. *Nature* 373:448-451.

10. Lund, S. et al. (1995). Contraction stimulates translocation of glucose transporter Glut IV in skeletal muscle through a mechanism distinct from that of insulin. *Proc. Natl. Acad. Sci. USA* 92:5817-5821.

11. Steinberg, H.O. et al. (1996). Obesity/insulin resistance is associated with endothelial cell dysfunction: implications for the syndrome of insulin resistance. *J. Clin. Invest.* 97:2601-2610.

12. Srinivasan, S. et al. Serum from patients with type 2 diabetes with neuropathy induces complement-independent, calcium-dependent apoptosis in cultured neuronal cells. *J. Clin. Invest.* 102:1454-1462.

13. Nathan, D.M. (1996). The pathophysiology of diabetic complications: How much does the glucose hypothesis explain? *Ann. Int. Med.* 124:86-89.

14. Virkamaki, A. et al. (1999). Protein-protein interactions in insulin signaling and the molecular mechanisms of insulin resistance. *J. Clin. Invest.* 103:931-943.

THE CARDIOVASCULAR SYSTEM

7

1. INTRODUCTION TO THE CARDIOVASCULAR SYSTEM

The cardiovascular system consists of the heart and various vessels by which blood circulates through the body (see Figure 7.1). **Arteries** carry blood from the heart to either the lungs or the peripheral tissues. **Veins** carry blood from the lungs or the peripheral tissues back to the heart. **Capillaries** connect the smallest arteries with the smallest veins and allow efficient exchange of substances between tissues and blood. **Lymphatic vessels** drain extracellular fluid that escapes from the vessels back into the circulation.

The role of the cardiovascular system is the pumping and distribution of blood. The blood it carries allows every cell in the body to benefit from the ultimate in franchising: a constant internal environmental pipeline with which to exchange information (e.g., hormones and their regulators), from which to obtain nutrients, and into which to send wastes to be eliminated.

Why is understanding cardiovascular physiology important for medical practice?

- Cardiovascular disorders, including hypertension and atherosclerosis that predispose to heart attacks and stroke, are the leading cause of morbidity and mortality in the developed world.
- Much of current thinking about the pathophysiology of heart disease follows directly from an understanding of simple physiological principles regarding the heart as a mechanical pump under electrical control, which is critically dependent on adequate blood supply for its nourishment.
- Greater attention to simple preventive physiological principles involving diet and lifestyle could greatly diminish the burden of cardiovascular disease on our society.

- Treatment of heart disease is profitable for almost everyone involved. However, expensive cardiac procedures are likely to benefit some, but not all, of the patients who receive them. Some patients who need these procedures may not get them for reasons of cost. At least in some cases, a consideration of physiological principles can help distinguish between patients who will benefit from such interventions and those who will not.
- Important breakthroughs in molecular biology, cell biology, genetics, and the pathophysiology of cardiovascular disease may contribute to vastly improved prognosis for subsets of patients with currently poorly treatable cardiovascular disorders.

Case Presentation

N.P., a vigorous 74-year-old retired legal secretary, came to medical attention for the first time with a syncopal episode. On her evaluation in the emergency room, a loud systolic murmur was heard, and carotid upstroke was felt to be prolonged. Echocardiogram confirmed the diagnosis of nearly critical **aortic stenosis**, probably due to age-related calcification of the aortic valve. Further evaluation revealed an intermittent cardiac dysrhythmia, a conduction system disorder, and left ventricular hypertrophy with possible ischemic changes on the electrocardiogram (ECG). By history, she probably also has exertional angina.

Ms. P.'s HMO was reluctant to authorize an expensive aortic valve replacement procedure. They said that the combination of her age, cardiac rhythm disturbance, ischemic heart disease, and new onset syncope of unclear etiology all suggested that she would not be a good candidate to undergo this invasive (and expensive) procedure. At first, her primary care physician was swayed by their argument. But after reviewing cardiac physiology and pathophysiology, she changed her mind and made a compelling argument for the procedure. Faced with her logic, the bureaucrats eventually backed down (after 6 months of foot-dragging), but required a second opinion. The second examining physician noted worsening of the syncope, angina, and arrhythmia, but found the aortic stenosis murmur to have become softer. At first, the HMO tried to argue that the second physician's assessment supported their view against surgery, arguing that the aortic stenosis was not the patient's most severe problem, and therefore valve replacement was not appropriate. Luckily, the patient's primary care physician was able to identify the physiologically evident logical flaws in their argument and successfully obtained coverage for the surgery, which Ms. P. subsequently underwent.

Ms. P. came through valve replacement surgery with flying colors and had a protracted but uncomplicated postoperative course followed by many years of high quality, independent life. She eventually died peacefully, at home, at the age of 96, surrounded by five generations of her family.

How did an understanding of the physiology of the heart assist the physician in arguing on behalf of Ms. P.'s best interests in this case?

2. THE HEART

The heart consists largely of muscle organized into a highly specialized set of four pumps. Two of the pumps (called the **right side of the heart**) deliver blood to the lungs for oxygenation and elimination of carbon dioxide, while the other two (called the **left side of the heart**) pump oxygenated blood to the rest of the body. Contraction of cardiac muscle generates the force to run the pumps,

while relaxation of the muscle allows filling of the pumps (with blood), between cycles of contraction. Each side of the heart consists of a low-pressure pump, termed the **atrium**, and a high-pressure pump, termed the **ventricle.**

Oxygen-depleted blood returns to the heart from the rest of the body via veins that drain into the **vena cava**, which empties into the **right atrium**. Blood then enters the **right ventricle**, from which it is pumped to the lungs. Oxygenated blood from the lungs returns to the heart via the **pulmonary veins** and fills the **left atrium**. From there, blood enters the **left ventricle** whose contraction sends the oxygenated blood out to the rest of the body via the arteries (see Figures 7.1 and 7.2). On both sides of the heart, approximately 80% of ventricular filling is passive. However, contraction of the atria serves the priming function of delivering the final 20% of blood to the corresponding ventricle. Because the left ventricle must pump blood to all of the organs of the body except the lungs, it contains more muscle and generates higher pressures than the right ventricle.

Clinical Pearls

○ The extra 20% of ventricular filling that is due to atrial contraction (also termed the *atrial "kick"*) normally is not needed at rest because a healthy heart has the capacity to pump about 4 times more blood than necessary. Thus, loss of atrial function only becomes apparent with extreme exercise or in individuals whose ventricular function is substantially diminished (e.g., because of various kinds of heart disease and/or drugs that impair the heart's ability to increase its output to compensate for loss of the atrial kick).

○ Another condition in which atrial kick is important for ventricular filling is in mitral

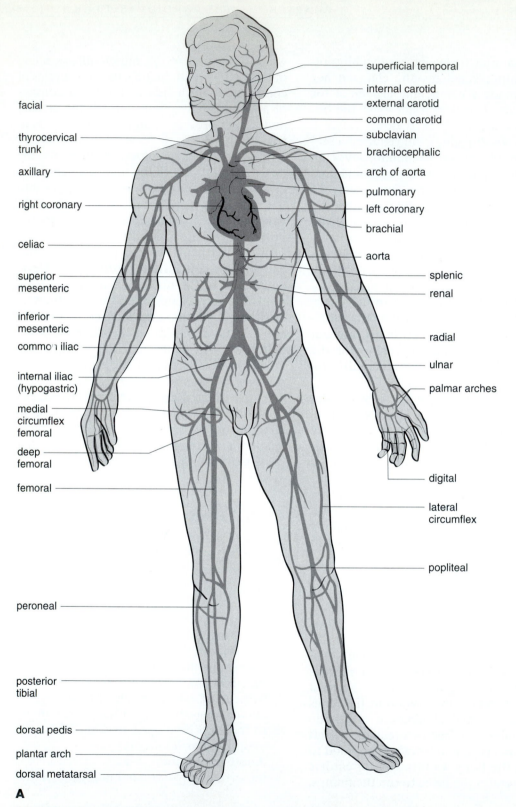

superficial temporal

internal carotid

external carotid

common carotid

subclavian

brachiocephalic

arch of aorta

pulmonary

left coronary

brachial

aorta

splenic

renal

radial

ulnar

palmar arches

digital

lateral circumflex

popliteal

facial

thyrocervical trunk

axillary

right coronary

celiac

superior mesenteric

inferior mesenteric

common iliac

internal iliac (hypogastric)

medial circumflex femoral

deep femoral

femoral

peroneal

posterior tibial

dorsal pedis

plantar arch

dorsal metatarsal

A

FIGURE 7.1. Overview of the circulatory system. A. Schematic diagram of the heart and major blood vessels, with arteries indicated in gray (left) and veins indicated in turquoise (right)

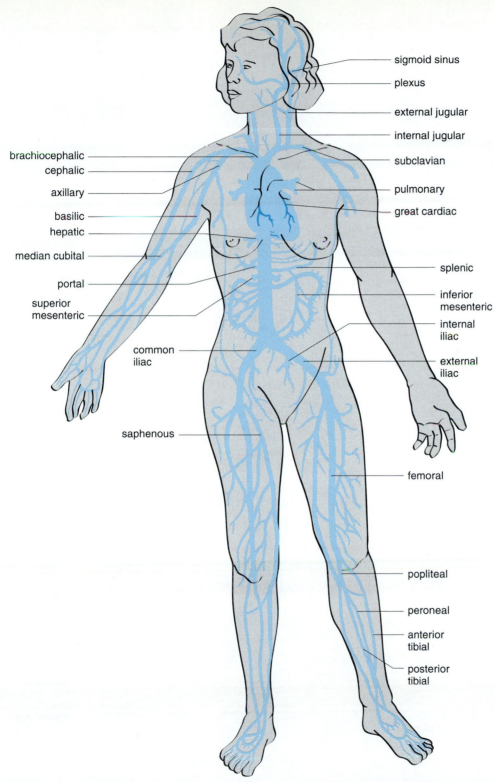

sigmoid sinus

plexus

external jugular

internal jugular

brachiocephalic

cephalic

subclavian

axillary

pulmonary

basilic

great cardiac

hepatic

median cubital

splenic

portal

inferior mesenteric

superior mesenteric

internal iliac

common iliac

external iliac

saphenous

femoral

popliteal

peroneal

anterior tibial

posterior tibial

FIGURE 7.1 — (continued)

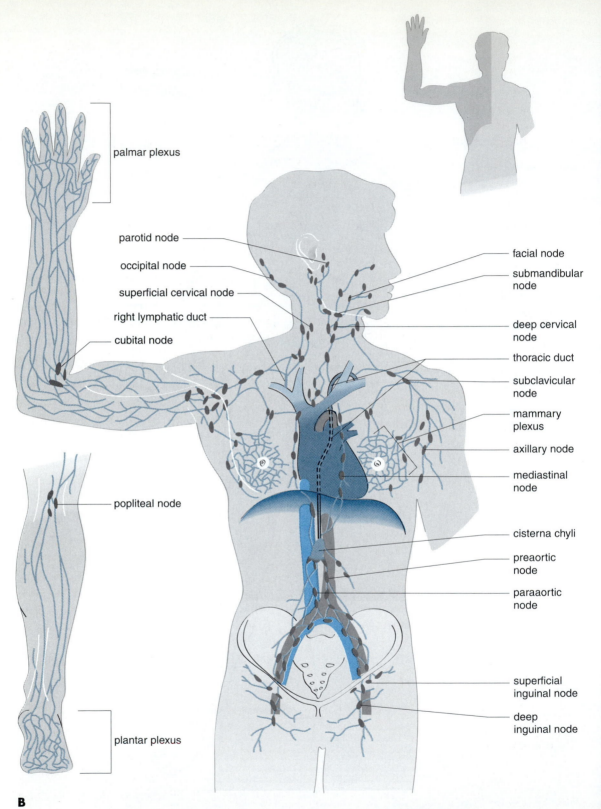

palmar plexus

parotid node

occipital node

superficial cervical node

right lymphatic duct

cubital node

facial node

submandibular node

deep cervical node

thoracic duct

subclavicular node

mammary plexus

axillary node

mediastinal node

cisterna chyli

preaortic node

paraaortic node

popliteal node

superficial inguinal node

deep inguinal node

plantar plexus

B

FIGURE 7.1 — (*continued*) *B*. Schematic diagram of the major lymphatic vessels of the body and lymph nodes to which they drain.

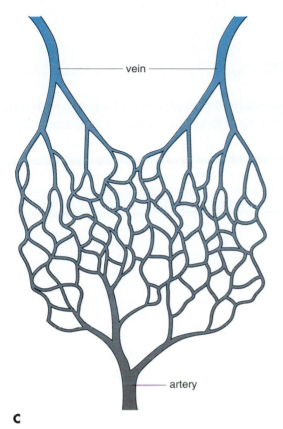

C

FIGURE 7.1 — (continued) C. Schematic diagram of how capillaries derive from the smallest arteries and feed into the smallest veins. (A. and B. Adapted, with permission, from Luciano, D.S., Vander, A.J., and Sherman, J.H. (1978). Human Function and Structure. New York, McGraw-Hill.)

The labels in the figure read, top: "vein"; bottom: "artery".

threatening than one involving just the right side of the heart.

Cardiac valves

Between each atrium and ventricle, and after each ventricle, lies a valve (see Figures 7.2A and B). Closure of the **tricuspid valve** between the atrium and ventricle on the right, and the **mitral valve** between the atrium and ventricle on the left, allows ventricular contraction to drive blood forward, but not backward into the atrium. This greatly increases the efficiency of cardiac function. The mitral and tricuspid valves have attached structures, termed **chordae tendineae** and **papillary muscles,** which prevent the valve from bulging too far into the atrium upon ventricular contraction, which would also dissipate the energy that would otherwise maintain forward flow at high pressure.

Upon onset of relaxation, after each ventricle has emptied, the **pulmonic valve** on the right, and **aortic valve** on the left, close. This maintains the unidirectional flow of blood to the lungs and body, respectively. These valves are smaller than the mitral and tricuspid valves. This allows much higher pressures to be generated in the ventricular outflow tracts, which is necessary because the ventricles have to pump blood farther than the atria. However, these higher pressures also subject the valves to greater physical trauma and result in their closure with greater force. Hence the aortic and pulmonic valves are much sturdier than the mitral and tricuspid valves.

Clinical Pearl

○ One consequence of a heart attack may be rupture of the chordae tendineae or paralysis of a papillary muscle, resulting in excessive bulging and severe leaking of

or tricuspid valve (see Sec. 5) **stenosis** in which the valves do not open properly, creating a mechanical obstruction to passive filling.
○ One consequence of the larger size (and workload) of left ventricular muscle is that its oxygen needs are greater. Another consequence of the difference in ventricular size is that a heart attack (death of cardiac tissue due to lack of oxygen) involving the left side of the heart is more often life-

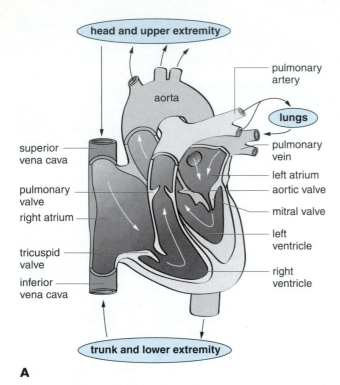

head and upper extremity

pulmonary artery

aorta

lungs

superior vena cava

pulmonary vein

left atrium
aortic valve
mitral valve

pulmonary valve

right atrium

tricuspid valve

left ventricle

inferior vena cava

right ventricle

trunk and lower extremity

A

FIGURE 7.2. Structure of the heart. *A. Course of blood flow through the heart chambers. B. Structure of the heart valves. C. Coronary blood vessels and their principal branches. (A. Adapted, with permission, from Guyton, A.C. and Hall, J.E. (1997). Human Physiology and Mechanisms of Disease, 6th ed. Philadelphia, Saunders, p. 86.)*

the mitral or tricuspid valve. The resulting loss of efficiency of ventricular contraction can result in sudden, life-threatening heart failure and is a significant cause of morbidity and mortality in patients during the first 24 h after a heart attack.

The entire heart is encased in a thin, double-layer of connective tissue termed the **pericardium**. Usually there is only a tiny, lubricating amount of fluid between the layers of the pericardium, serving to minimize friction during motion of the heart. However, in some pathological conditions, large amounts of fluid can accumulate there (called **pericardial effusions**). In extreme cases, especially when it accumulates rapidly, the fluid can form a kind of "straightjacket" around the heart, preventing proper filling with blood. This life-threatening condition is called **cardiac tamponade**.

Clinical Pearls

○ Cardiac tamponade due to fluid between the layers of the pericardium (termed a *pericardial effusion*) can occur in diseases as diverse as infections (such as tuberculosis) or kidney failure.
○ The common signs that raise the concern of cardiac tamponade include (a) the presence of a sound heard by a stethoscope, termed a *pericardial friction rub*, that is caused by fluid sloshing around the beating heart; (b) prominently engorged neck veins, due to blood difficulty draining from the head because of the restriction on filling of the heart caused by a large pericardial effusion; and (c) loss of variation in the intensity of heart sounds and blood pressure with breathing. Usually during inhalation, left ventricular cardiac output, blood pressure, and intensity of heart

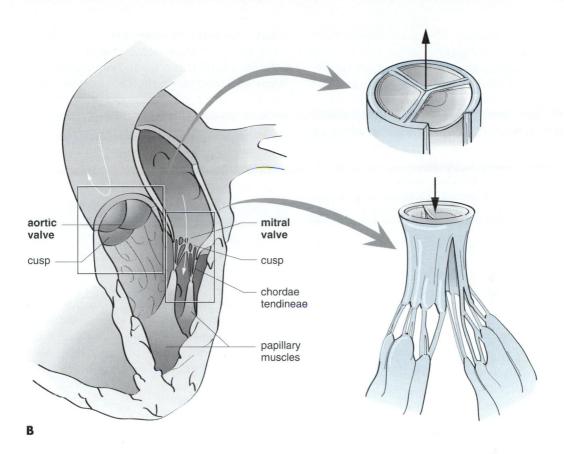

B

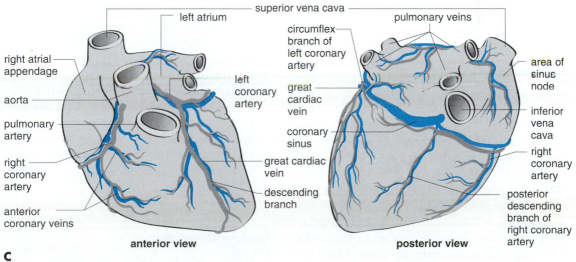

anterior view

posterior view

C

FIGURE 7.2 — *(continued)*

sounds diminishes. The physiological basis for this observation is that the fall in intra-thoracic pressure during inhalation results in more blood being returned to the right side of the heart, which causes bulging of the interventricular septum that impairs left ventricular filling. Also, pooling of blood in the lungs decreases pulmonary venous return to the left side of the heart. When filling of the entire heart is restricted, as occurs in cardiac tamponade, the drop in cardiac output, blood pressure, and heart sound intensity with inspiration is further enhanced. In patients in intensive care units in whom special monitors have been floated into the right side of the heart, cardiac tamponade can manifest as an equalization of the pressures between the normally low-pressure right and high-pressure left sides.

○ Because it starts to impair the movement of the heart, a pericardial friction rub can, paradoxically, get softer as an effusion enlarges. Treatment of cardiac tamponade requires emergency drainage of the pericardial space by insertion of a needle directly into the pericardium (don't try this one at home, kids!).

Cardiac blood supply

Another crucial anatomical feature of the heart is its blood supply (see Figure 7.2C). The heart must contract without fail approximately 100,000 times per day or more, resting for milliseconds between cycles of contraction, for the duration of an entire lifetime. Thus it is imperative that the heart have an efficient circulation for obtaining energy and eliminating wastes. The left and right **coronary arteries** arise from the root of the aorta. The large **left main coronary artery** branches into the **left anterior descending** and **circumflex** coronary arteries, which generally supply the left ventricle, the largest muscle of the heart. The **right coronary artery** usually supplies the right ventricle. From the coronary arteries, blood traverses the capillaries of the heart and returns via the cardiac veins to the coronary sinus, which empties into the right atrium.

Clinical Pearls

○ The coronary circulation is somewhat variable from individual to individual. For example, a branch of the right coronary artery, the posterior descending artery, supplies the posterior left ventricular wall in 80% of people (right dominant circulation). In the remaining 20%, this supply is provided from the circumflex artery (left dominant circulation). These variations are important because they determine whether sudden occlusion of one or another coronary artery branch (e.g., as typically occurs in a heart attack) will have a major effect on left ventricular function.

○ When occlusion of a coronary artery occurs gradually over months or years, there is time for **collateral circulation** to develop, allowing adequate blood supply from a separate, nonoccluded vessel. In contrast, since atherosclerosis is typically a diffuse process, occlusion of other vessels will eventually occur. When that happens, the result is a devastating and often lethal loss of myocardial function because a disproportionately large amount of cardiac blood flow was dependent on a single collateral branch.

Review Questions

1. What are the chambers and valves of the heart, and what are their roles in overall cardiac function?

2. Describe the branches of the coronary arteries and the territory to which they usually supply blood.

Cardiac muscle and the cardiac conduction system

Heart muscle has features that are both different from and similar to skeletal and smooth muscle. Like skeletal muscle, cardiac muscle is striated, which allows it to contract in a rapid, repetitive, and forceful way. However, like smooth muscle, cardiac muscle is largely under involuntary control, regulated by autonomic innervation.

Like other muscle cells, cardiac myocytes are electrically excitable (see Chap. 2). Upon depolarization, an action potential is generated and propagated along the plasma membrane of the muscle fiber, from cell to cell. In the wake of the action potential, a flood of calcium ions brings about a corresponding wave of contraction of the actin and myosin filaments within the muscle fiber.

The heart also has specialized features that make its electrical activity distinct from that of skeletal muscle:

First, the heart has **pacemaker cells** that normally initiate action potentials automatically. These electrical impulses originate at a location where the superior vena cava meets the right atrium, termed the *sinoatrial (SA) node*, whose intrinsic rate of impulse generation is approximately 60 per minute.

Second, the heart has a specialized **conduction system** that propagates action potentials generated at the SA node in such a way that the muscle in different parts of the heart contract in a coordinated manner (see Figure 7.3). Thus, impulses generated at the SA node travel quickly to the **atrioventricular (AV) node** and from there to the **His bundle** and **Purkinje fibers**. The cells that make up this impulse conduction system have little or no contractile function. Their normal role is sim-

ply to propagate action potentials quickly throughout the heart.

Third, the action potential generated in cardiac muscle is quite distinct from that of other muscles, lasting 3 to 15 times longer (see Figure 7.3), as a result of an array of specialized sodium, potassium, and calcium channels. Serious abnormalities of cardiac function can occur when cardiac ion channel function is disordered (see Sec. 6).

Electrical activity of the functioning heart

From its spontaneous origin in the pacemaker cells of the SA node, an action potential is propagated through the atria and, simultaneously, down the rest of the conduction system, and from there to ventricular muscle (see Figure 7.3). Conduction slows down through the AV node, which allows the atria to contract about one-sixth of a second before the ventricle, facilitating their role as priming pumps in loading the ventricles. Once through the AV node, conduction speeds up through the His Bundle and Purkinje systems, so that the entire ventricle can contract simultaneously.

At rest, all myocytes, including those of the heart, have a voltage potential difference across their plasma membrane of approximately -90 mV. Under these resting conditions, many potassium channels, but only a few sodium channels, are open. The resting voltage potential difference is where the chemical potential energy of the potassium gradient across the plasma membrane is equal to the electrical potential energy difference resulting from protein anions being too big to accompany potassium leaking through those channels out of the cell.

There is also a slow leak of sodium into the myocyte, due to the few open sodium channels present, and driven by the large sodium gradient in the opposite direction of the potassium gradient. Eventually this sodium

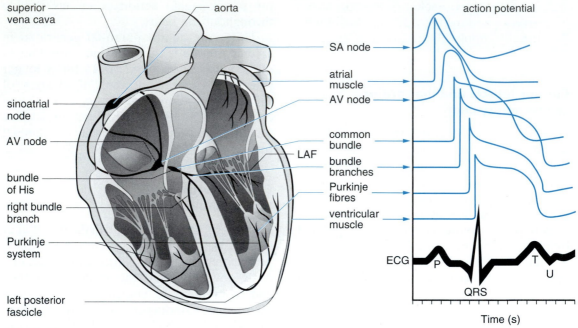

FIGURE 7.3. Conducting system of the heart and its correlation to the cardiac action potential. Typical transmembrane action potentials for the sinoatrial (SA) and atrioventricular (AV) nodes, other parts of the conduction system, and the atrial and ventricular muscles are shown along with the correlation to extracellularly recorded electrical activity (the electrocardiogram, ECG). The action potential and ECG are plotted on the same time axis, but with different zero points on the vertical scale. LAF is the left anterior fascicle of the cardiac conduction system. *(Adapted, with permission, from Ganong, W.F. (1997). Review of Medical Physiology, 18th ed. Stamford, CT, Appleton & Lange.)*

leak would dissipate the resting equilibrium voltage potential difference, if it were not for the activity of sodium and potassium adenosine triphophatase (Na^+/K^+ ATPase). This enzyme uses metabolic energy, generated through ATP hydrolysis, to pump 3 sodium atoms out of the cell for every 2 potassium atoms that are pumped in and, thereby, serves to maintain the resting potential difference.

This description of life in the resting cardiac myocyte changes when, in response to an action potential, depolarization occurs, which transiently throws ion fluxes topsy-turvy for a period of about 0.1 to 0.2 s. A flurry of ion transport, in conjunction with various chan-nel openings and closings reestablishes the resting potential, but not before setting in motion two important events. First, the depolarization propagates the ion flux down the plasma membrane of the muscle fiber. Second, depolarization triggers the molecular events of muscle contraction within the cardiac muscle fiber.

Cardiac muscle action potential

The distinctive features of the cardiac muscle action potential results from the function of various ion channels (see Figure 7.4). Phase 0, rapid depolarization, like the corresponding

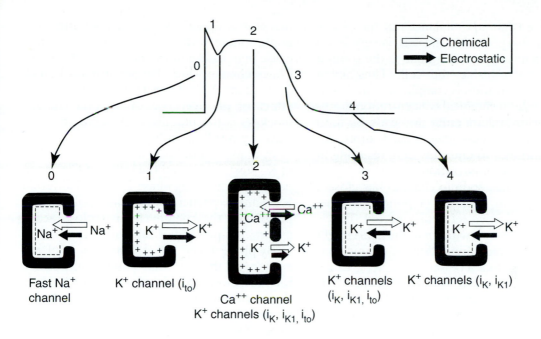

FIGURE 7.4. Principal ionic currents and channels involved in generation of the cardiac muscle action potential. During phase 0 both the chemical and electrostatic forces normally favor sodium entry into the cell through fast Na^+ channels which generates the rapid upstroke. During phase 1, both chemical and electrostatic forces favor efflux of K^+ through the so-called i_{to} K^+ channel. This generates early partial repolarization. During phase 2, the plateau, the net influx of Ca^{++} through Ca^{++} channels is balanced by the efflux of K^+ through i_k, i_{k1}, and i_{to} types of potassium channels. During phase 3, the chemical forces favoring efflux of K^+ through the i_k, i_{k1}, and i_{to} types of potassium channels dominate over the electrostatic forces favoring K^+ influx through the same channels. Finally, during phase 4, chemical forces favoring K^+ efflux through i_k and i_{k1} channels exceeds very slightly the electrostatic forces that favor influx of K^+ through these same channels. See text for details. (Adapted, with permission, from Berne, R.M. and Levy, M.N. (1997). Cardiovascular Physiology, 7th ed. St. Louis, Mosby, p. 17.)

feature of action potentials in nerves and skeletal muscle, results from opening of fast sodium channels in response to an initial depolarizing stimulus. As more and more fast sodium channels open, they let in more and more sodium, which further depolarizes the cell. Depolarization is both responsible for propagation of the impulse (by causing more fast sodium channels to open further down the plasma membrane) and also for closing the fast sodium channels when depolarization proceeds beyond a certain extent.

Despite that individual fast sodium channels close "automatically" as depolarization proceeds, in the cell as a whole they tend to "overshoot" slightly. This lets more sodium into the cell than is needed to completely dissipate the electrical potential. Why does this happen? The number of sodium ions needed to dissipate the electrical potential difference (that is, to balance out the excess negative charges inside the cell) is very small and does not appreciably change the sodium concentration inside the cell. Thus, even when depolarization is complete, there is still a large sodium chemical concentration gradient favoring sodium entry into cells. So until all sodium channels have closed, more sodium continues to enter the cell, resulting in transient hyperpolarization.

Once the fast sodium channel has closed, it is unable to open for a period of time, called the **effective refractory period**. This is important because, without it, the heart might respond to rapid stimulation by tetanic contraction (e.g., like a closed sphincter), which would not allow time for filling of the heart with blood. Subsequent to depolarization, a myocyte must repolarize, during which time it is relatively refractory to another depolarization.

In phase 1, partial repolarization occurs, as special potassium channels open in response to hyperpolarization. This is because, during the brief period that the cell is hyperpolarized due to sodium influx, there is no electrical potential to offset the chemical gradient that provides a driving force for potassium efflux. During hyperpolarization, both the chemical and the electrical gradients favor potassium efflux.

Subsequently, the plateau phase (phase 2) is reached, where calcium influx through voltage-regulated Ca^{2+} channels is balanced by the efflux of K^+ through various types of potassium channels. These calcium channels activate and inactivate far more slowly than the fast sodium channels that give rise to phase 0. The calcium that enters during phase 2 of the cardiac action potential is responsible for activation of cardiac muscle contraction.

Several different types of calcium channels are involved. One type, called L-type calcium channels, is particularly important because its opening is enhanced by catecholamines (see Chap. 12), which work via the β-adrenergic receptor and increased cyclic adenosine monophosphate (cyclic AMP) production, and cause increased contractility of heart muscle. These channels are also acted upon by calcium channel blocking drugs. Thus, one side effect of an overdose of calcium channel blockers is the potential for decreased contractility resulting in heart failure.

In phase 3, final repolarization, the efflux of K^+ starts to exceed the influx of Ca^{2+} compared to that during phase 2. Several different K^+ channels participate and, as repolarization progresses, the calcium channels close, accelerating the process of repolarization.

By phase 4, Na^+/K^+ ATPase has, in effect, exchanged the Na^+ that entered in phase 0 for the K^+ that left in phase 2 and 3. Thus, the resting membrane potential, mainly determined by plasma membrane conductance of K^+, has been reestablished. Similarly, the excess Ca^{2+} influx during phase 2 is compensated for by the activity of both a 3:1 Na/Ca^{2+} exchanger and a K^+/Ca^{2+} pump (see Figure 7.5). This description of the cardiac muscle action potential applies not only to myocytes, but also to the cells of His bundle and Purkinje fibers.

However the action potential generated in the cells of the SA and AV nodes is substantially different (see Figure 7.3). Initial depolarization in these regions is slower and is initiated by Ca^{2+} channels rather than fast Na^+ channels. There is no phase 1 and very little phase 2 that blend together with the repolarization phase. The final voltage potential difference in pacemaker cells and other slow action potential cells is approximately -70 mV.

Impulses normally begin in the SA node for two reasons. First, all cells in the conduction system have a property called *automaticity* that allows them to depolarize spontaneously. The basis for automaticity is simply that these cells are not able to maintain their resting membrane potential. There is a slow leak of sodium ions that results in a steady

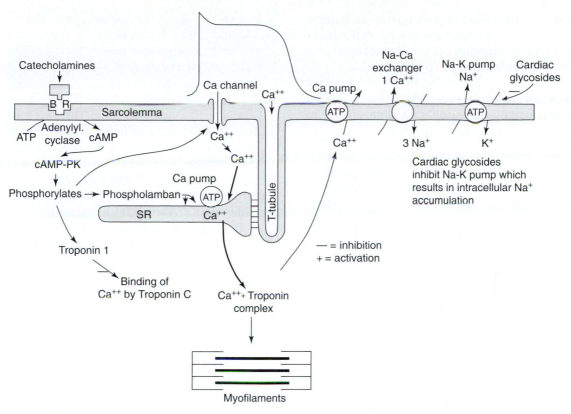

FIGURE 7.5. Mechanism of excitation-contraction coupling. Schematic diagram of the movements of calcium in excitation-contraction coupling in cardiac muscle. The influx of Ca^{++} from the interstitial fluid during excitation raises cytosolic free calcium and also triggers the release of even more calcium from intracellular stores, mainly from a calcium-rich membrane compartment related to the endoplasmic reticulum, termed the *sarcoplasmic reticulum* (SR). The free cytosolic Ca^{++} activates contraction of the myofilaments, which brings about systole. Relaxation (diastole) occurs as a result of uptake of Ca^{++} by the SR due to extrusion of intracellular Ca^{++} by Na^{+}/Ca^{++} exchange, and to a limited degree by the Ca pump. BR = β-adrenergic receptor; cAMP = cyclic adenosine monophosphate; cAMP-PK, cyclic AMP-dependent protein kinase. (*Adapted, with permission, from Berne, R.M. and Levy, M.N. (1997). Cardiovascular Physiology, 7th ed. St. Louis, Mosby, p. 62.*)

depolarization, until the threshold for triggering an action potential (approximately -40 mV) is reached. This leak is greatest in the cells of the SA node and is less pronounced the further along the conduction system you go, which translates into slower and slower spontaneous impulse generation (e.g., SA node versus AV node versus His bundle versus Purkinje fibers). Indeed, even isolated cardiac myocytes display a very slow rate of spontaneous impulse generation.

The second reason for dominance of the SA node in impulse generation is the relative refractory period. This property of the cardiac muscle action potential ensures that once a cell with a slower rate of spontaneous depolarization has been depolarized by an impulse from the SA node, it cannot be depolarized again (spontaneously or otherwise) until after the SA node is ready to refire.

Despite having an intrinsic rate at which they depolarize, SA node pacemaker cells are controlled by the autonomic nervous system, which can affect the following:

- The magnitude of the resting potential achieved
- The rate of spontaneous depolarization from the resting potential and hence the time it takes to reach the threshold for triggering an action potential
- The threshold potential at which depolarization triggers an action potential

The autonomic nervous system also affects the rate at which impulses are conducted through the AV node to the ventricles.

Dysfunction of the sodium, calcium, and potassium channels that generate the cardiac muscle and conducting system action potentials are the basis for most cardiac dysrhythmias and for the action of many cardiac drugs (see later).

known as atrial fibrillation, (see Figure 7.7f and later), it can often be controlled by the drug **digoxin,** whose effects include a slowing of conduction through the AV node.

In contrast, some dysrhythmias due to a congenital defect in the conduction system (e.g., the Wolf-Parkinson-White syndrome) can actually be made worse by this drug. This is because these patients have so-called "bypass tracts" that can usurp the normal conducting role of the AV node. Slowing the AV node further only accentuates the takeover of impulse propagation by the bypass tract. Careful inspection of the ECG in these (typically young) patients will often detect a characteristic electronic signature of the bypass tract (termed a δ *wave*; see Figure 7.7G and later). Recognition of these and other features of the ECG may be crucial to avoiding an otherwise fatal diagnostic and therapeutic error.

When the dysrhythmia is due to an irritable (e.g., ischemic) focus in the ventricle (i.e., below the AV node), it is often best suppressed by a drug such as **amiodarone,** which prolongs refractoriness of ventricular muscle.

Clinical Pearl

○ Patients with dysrythmias can have either genetic or acquired aberrations in impulse generation and/or conduction that result in rates of impulse propagation faster than can be generated in the SA node. At these rapid rates, ventricular filling is impaired and myocardial oxygen demand is greatly increased. As a result, these dysrythmias can be life-threatening. When the dysrythmia is due to excessive impulse generation prior to the AV node (e.g., somewhere in the atria, as in the case of the dysrythmia

Clinical Pearls

○ Regardless of the specific cause of a dysrythmia, a pacemaker placed to deliver impulses to the heart at faster than the dysrythmia rate for a few seconds will typically terminate a rapid abnormal rhythm, allowing the SA node and normal conduction to reestablish control. This technique, termed "overdrive pacing," or a cruder but often effective version in the form of delivery of an external shock to the chest, is often the last chance to save the life of an individual unable to perfuse vital organs at the elevated dysrythmic heart rate.

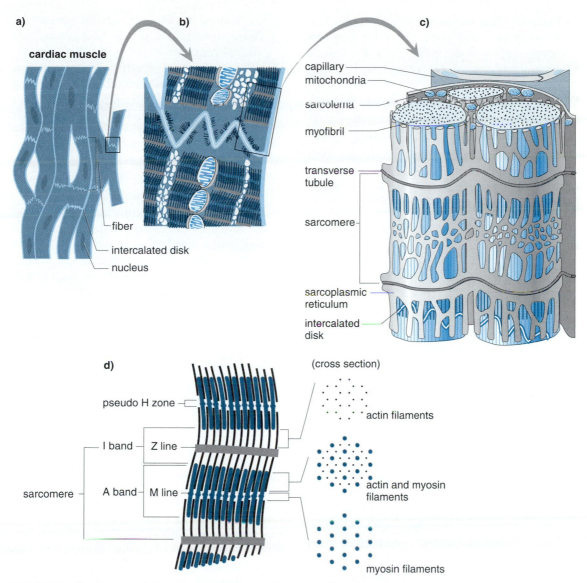

a)

cardiac muscle

fiber

intercalated disk

nucleus

b)

c)

capillary
mitochondria
sarcolemma
myofibril

transverse
tubule

sarcomere

sarcoplasmic
reticulum

intercalated
disk

d)

pseudo H zone

I band — Z line

A band — M line

sarcomere

(cross section)

actin filaments

actin and myosin
filaments

myosin filaments

FIGURE 7.6. Cardiac muscle histology and structure. Drawing of cardiac muscle at low (*a*), high (*b*), and higher (*c*) resolution. (*d*) Diagram of a sarcomere along the length of the muscle (left) and in cross-section (right).

○ Despite their negative effect on cardiac contractility and their potential (e.g., in overdose) to cause heart failure, calcium channel blockers are often used in the treatment of patients with heart failure. This is because calcium channels are also involved in control of constriction of vascular smooth muscle. By causing relaxation of arterial smooth muscle, calcium channel blockers can decrease the work the heart must do in order to pump blood. Fortunately, the calcium channels in the blood vessels are more sensitive to these drugs than those in the heart. Thus, the beneficial effect on heart failure usually occurs at doses of calcium channel blockers that do not affect the contractility of the heart significantly.

○ Sympathetic nervous system activity, primarily through norepinephrine, increases heart rate by increasing the slope at which spontaneous depolarization occurs, allowing the threshold for depolarization to be achieved more quickly. This is how exercise, fever, and anxiety all increase the heart rate.

○ Vagal activity slows heart rate by hyperpolarizing the pacemaker cells (further lowering the resting potential) and decreasing the slope of the pacemaker potential so it takes longer to reach threshold. The Valsalva manuever (bearing down as if to have a bowel movement) and carotid sinus massage (first make sure the patient does not have a bruit upon auscultation of the neck, to avoid an increased risk of stroke!), are two ways to increase vagal tone. Such manuevers can sometimes slow a rapid cardiac dysrhythmia (e.g., atrial fibrillation or paroxysmal atrial tachycardia) or convert back to normal sinus rhythm.

○ In certain forms of heart disease, the atria themselves, other regions of the conduction system, or even the ventricles can be the source of origin of action potentials. These dysrhythmias are dangerous for several reasons:

First, they can result in either too fast or too slow a heart rate. Too rapid a rate does not allow enough time for ventricular filling. Too slow a rate (e.g., as might occur in complete conduction system failure where the ventricles spontaneously depolarize on their own at a rate of about 40 impulses per minute) does not generate enough cardiac output.

Second, these rhythms tend to be unstable and are more likely to degenerate into **ventricular fibrillation** in which individual muscle cells contract chaotically rather than in a synchronized fashion. As a result, there is no cardiac output—a lethal situation.

Finally, some dysrhythmias (such as atrial fibrillation) can result in abnormal pooling of blood within regions of the heart, with formation of blood clots and risk of stroke (see Chap. 18) or pulmonary embolism (see Chap. 8).

Excitation-contraction coupling

As a result of specialized features of cardiac muscle structure, calcium is able to play a key role in coupling the cardiac action potential with the events of cardiac muscle contraction. The action potential that excites a cardiac myocyte gets propagated internally along membrane invaginations termed **T tubules**. The T tubules allow interstitial fluid (and with it, calcium) to have access to the interior of a cardiac muscle fiber (see Figure 7.6). The **sarcoplasmic reticulum** is a distinct, entirely internal membrane network related to the endoplasmic reticulum (see Chap. 2) that serves as another subcellular storehouse of calcium ions. The sarcoplasmic reticulum of cardiac muscle is less well developed than that of skeletal muscle, but its T tubules have twenty-five-fold greater volume and are filled with calcium-binding mucopolysaccharides. Due to the T tubules, which open to the extracellular space, extracellular calcium ions can greatly affect the strength of contraction of cardiac muscle. In contrast, contraction of skeletal muscle is largely independent of extracellular calcium concentration, relying instead on a well-developed sarcoplasmic reticulum and internal calcium stores.

At the end of the plateau phase of the cardiac action potential, the influx of calcium ions is cut off and calcium is pumped back into the lumen of the sarcoplasmic reticulum and T tubules, terminating muscle contraction until the time of the next action potential. Thus, the duration of the time of cardiac muscle contraction is roughly equal to the duration of time of the cardiac muscle action potential, about 0.2 s in the atria and 0.3 s in the ventricle.

Cardiac muscle contraction

The heart uses the same machinery (actin and myosin filaments, regulated by tropomyosin and the calcium-binding protein troponin) and the same mechanism (sliding of the filaments mediated by ATP hydrolysis-driven conformational change in the myosin head group) to generate force as does skeletal muscle (see Chap. 2). Like skeletal muscle cells, cardiac myocytes are filled with bundles of actin (thin) and myosin (thick) filaments termed *myofibrils*. Transient release and uptake of free calcium ions in the cytosol regulate these interactions.

However, unlike skeletal muscle, cardiac myocytes must pump, without a break, for an entire lifetime (several billion beats). Transient anaerobic metabolism, followed by periods of rest and recovery, as occurs in vigorously exercising skeletal muscle, is not an option for the heart. Thus, cardiac myocytes

depend on oxygen and are packed with mitochondria to provide a constant source of ATP.

Like other muscles, the heart is a **functional syncytium**, meaning that even though individual myocytes are, in fact, separate cells, the presence of gap junctions connecting one cardiac myocyte with another allows them to act, electrically, as if they were all connected (see Figure 7.6). Thus the flow of ions from one cell to the next allows impulses to be rapidly propagated and actions to be highly coordinated. Electrical resistance through the gap junctions is about 1/400 of that across the plasma membrane. In cardiac muscle, the arrangement of the syncytium is a bit different from that of skeletal muscle. Individual cells are connected only at their ends, at so-called **intercalated disks** (see Figure 7.6). In effect, the heart comprises two syncytia, one for the atria and the other for the ventricles, joined via the AV node. This underscores the importance of AV conduction and the seriousness of the clinical condition known as complete heart block (see later).

The ECG as a monitor of cardiac electrical activity

Electrical leads placed on the surface of the body can detect characteristic signatures of the phases of electrical activity of the heart, in the form of the surface ECG (see Figure 7.3). The key features of the normal ECG are the P wave, QRS complex and T wave. The P wave reflects the spread of depolarization through the atria. The QRS complex reflects ventricular depolarization and occurs just before ventricular contraction. The T wave represents ventricular repolarization and occurs slightly before the end of ventricular contraction. Figure 7.7 shows some abnormalities of the ECG and their clinical correlation.

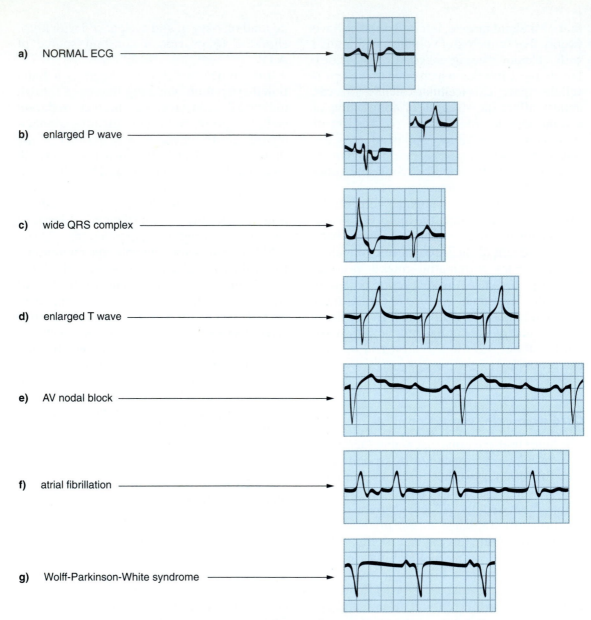

a) NORMAL ECG

b) enlarged P wave

c) wide QRS complex

d) enlarged T wave

e) AV nodal block

f) atrial fibrillation

g) Wolff-Parkinson-White syndrome

FIGURE 7.7. The normal and pathological electrocardiogram (ECG). *a.* Normal ECG. *b* to *f*. Illustrated abnormalities of (b) P wave, (c) QRS complex, and (d) T wave, as well as (e) conduction system abnormality (heart block), (f) rhythm disturbance (atrial fibrillation), and (g) Wolff-Parkinson-White syndrome.

Clinical Pearls

The ECG is a most valuable noninvasive means of assessing the cardiac conduction system and detecting features of heart disease that manifests as conduction system abnormalities. Besides determination of the rate and basic cardiac rhythm, specific components of the ECG have physiological and pathophysiological diagnostic importance:

○ P waves: Large P waves suggests atrial enlargement, as might occur with pulmonary hypertension or pulmonary embolism, on the right side of the heart and mitral stenosis on the left side of the heart. A P-to-P rate that is out of synch with the QRS-to-QRS rate indicates dissociation of the atria from the ventricles. This can be due either to complete heart block (total failure of normal conduction beyond the AV node), or to the presence of a dysrhythmia such as ventricular tachycardia (in which the ventricles are independently activated by abnormal mechanisms).

○ QRS complex: Widened QRS complex indicates that it is taking the electrical impulse longer than normal to travel down the conduction pathway. This suggests a conduction system defect, such as a block in conduction through the bundle branches that synchronize activation of the ventricles. Widened QRS is also seen in certain atrial and ventricular dysrhythmias that bypass the normal conduction system. Some of these may be life-threatening.

○ T wave: Peaked T waves are seen with hyperkalemia and myocardial infarction (death of myocardial tissue, usually due to inadequate blood flow). Prolonged QT interval reflects prolonged ventricular repolarization and is a risk factor for ventricular arrhythmias. Sometimes this is due to a genetic lesion in ion channels. Other times it is a result of ischemia or due to the effect of drugs that poison cardiac ion channels or their normal mechanisms of regulation. Inverted T waves are seen with hypokalemia, hypocalcemia, or ischemia.

○ Various disorders of electrical conduction and cardiac rhythm can be apparent by inspection of the ECG, as seen in the following example.

In complete heart block, a failure of conduction through the AV node results in impulses from the SA node being unable to reach the ventricles. As a result, there is either no ventricular contraction, or it results from spontaneous contraction of the ventricles, often at a rate inadequate to maintain blood pressure. Sometimes complete heart block occurs transiently and is manifest as a sudden loss of consciousness. This condition is typically due to ischemic or degenerative disease of the conduction system, sometimes exacerbated by increased activity of the parasympathetic nervous system.

In atrial fibrillation, which can be triggered by such insults as hypoxia, alcohol, thyrotoxicosis, or simple distention, ectopic pacemakers can result in rapid bombardment of the AV node with hundreds of impulses per second. Not only is the atrial kick for ventricular filling lost, but often, conduction through the AV node occurs at a rate too high to allow adequate time for ventricular filling. Without adequate filling, cardiac output falls and blood pressure is insufficient to perfuse vital organs. The drug digitalis slows conduction through the AV node by poisoning sodium channels, thereby slowing the ventricular response and resulting in adequate time for ventricular filling, which maintain an adequate cardiac output.

Physiology of the heart as a pump

A period of ventricular contraction is termed **systole**. That of ventricular relaxation (and refilling with blood) is termed **diastole**. As the empty ventricles relax, the tricuspid and mitral valves open to allow refilling for another cycle of pumping. As the full ventricle contracts, the aortic and pulmonic valves open.

Although the opening of the valves is a slower, essentially silent process, the valves close rather suddenly with changes in intracardiac pressures, resulting in the noises we call **heart sounds**, the "lub-dub" that is heard through the stethoscope. The first heart sound (lub), termed S_1, is the closely spaced closure of tricuspid and mitral valves. The second heart sound (dub), termed S_2, is the closely spaced closure of the aortic and pulmonic valves. Thus systole is the time between S_1 and S_2, and diastole is the time between S_2 and the next S_1. Together, systole and diastole make up the cardiac cycle, the events occurring from one heart beat to the next.

Preload is the venous pressure that results in filling of the heart in diastole. Without adequate preload, even an otherwise healthy heart cannot fill sufficiently and, therefore, may not be able to pump enough blood to meet the needs of the body. Preload can be affected by many variables including intravascular volume, vascular smooth muscle tone, and even the activity of the immune system (which makes powerful cytokines, see Chap. 19, that affect vascular smooth muscle tone).

Afterload is the pressure against which the heart must work to pump blood. High (diastolic) blood pressure substantially increases the amount of work the heart must do, since the heart must exceed that pressure to achieve any output of blood.

Since the role of the heart is to pump blood, a central relation for understanding the physiology of the heart is as follows:

> **Cardiac Output** (L/min)
> = **Heart Rate** (beats per minute)
> × **Stroke Volume** (mL of blood ejected from the left ventricle with each cycle of contraction)

Thus, both time and volume are important parameters of ventricular muscle function. The cardiac cycle describes the pressures generated within the ventricles as a function of time (see Figure 7.8). The **ejection fraction** refers to the percentage of blood in the heart at the end of systole compared to what was there at the end of diastole. This is an important indicator of contractility and therefore is an important contributor to having a normal cardiac output (see discussion of ischemic cardiomyopathy later). Pressure-volume analysis (see Figure 7.9) describes the changes in the pressure generated by the ventricle (work performed) as a function of the volume of blood in the ventricle at the onset of systole (due to stretch of myocardial fibers). Each of these ways of thinking about the function of the heart are important for understanding how the heart is supposed to work normally and what can go wrong in various disease states.

Events of the cardiac cycle (pressure-time analysis)

The events of the right side of the heart parallel that of the left side of the heart. The volume of blood pumped is normally the same, however, the pressures generated in the right side of heart are only about one-sixth as great as that of the left. Consider the events of the cardiac cycle of the left side of the heart (see Figure 7.8):

1. At the beginning of the cardiac cycle, right after S_2, the aortic valve is closed, the mitral valve is open, and the atrium is a passive conduit for blood flowing into the ventricle.
2. As the atrium contracts, an "a wave" is reflected back into the venous circuit.
3. Closure of the mitral valve at the end of atrial contraction generates S_1 and initiates the period of isovolumic contraction of the ventricle, in which both mitral and aortic

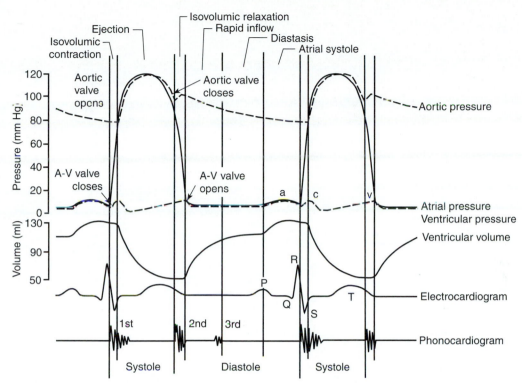

FIGURE 7.8. Events of the cardiac cycle for left ventricular function. Shown are changes in left atrial pressure, left ventricular pressure, aortic pressure, ventricular volume, the ECG, and the sounds heard by stethoscope. (Adapted, with permission, from Guyton, A.C. and Hall, J.E. (1997). Human Physiology and Mechanisms of Disease, 6th ed. Philadelphia, Saunders, p. 88.)

valves are closed and contraction of ventricular muscle raises the pressure in the closed ventricle.

4. The pressure increases with further ventricular contraction and when it exceeds that in the aorta (the diastolic blood pressure), the aortic valve opens and blood flows out of the ventricle into the aorta.

5. At the end of ventricular contraction, with onset of ventricular relaxation, the pressure within the ventricle falls below that of the aorta, resulting in closure of the aortic valve (S_2).

The effect of a change in the left ventricular pressure-time curve under different physi-ological and pathophysiological conditions can be seen in Figure 7.10.

Intrinsic regulation of cardiac pump function (pressure-volume analysis)

During systole, the heart normally pumps out almost all of the blood that entered during diastole. If it did not, there would be a "back up" of blood into the left atrium, which would be reflected as an increased hydrostatic pressure in the pulmonary veins and capillaries from which blood normally flows to the left side of the heart. When the hydrostatic pressure in the pulmonary vessels gets sufficiently high, fluid moves from the capillary lumen to

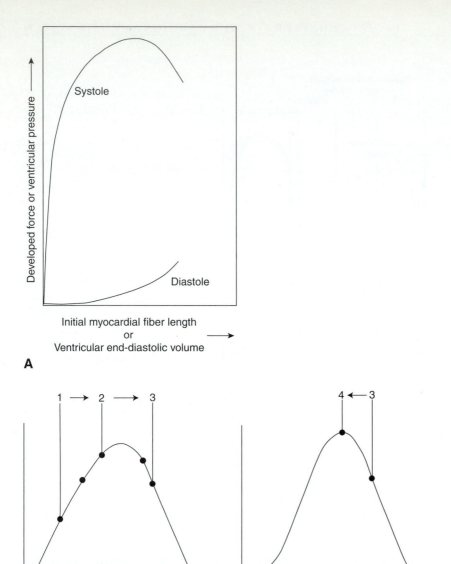

FIGURE 7.9. *A.* Relation of myocardial resting fiber length (sarcomere length) or end-diastolic volume to developed force or peak systolic ventricular pressure during ventricular contraction in the heart (Frank-Starling curve). Increased end-diastolic volume, as occurs for example in heart failure, distends the heart, changing the resting myocardial fiber length and, therefore, affecting the efficiency of subsequent ventricular contraction (i.e., in systole). Another way of thinking of this relation is to recognize that more energy is required for the distended heart to eject the same volume of blood per beat compared to that of the normal, nondilated heart due to the increase in wall tension as a consequence of increased end-diastolic volume. *B.* Shift in position on the Frank-Starling curve from rest (1) with vigorous exercise (2), and in heart failure (3). *C.* Effect of preload and afterload reduction (4) to decrease myocardial fiber length and thereby improve the efficiency of cardiac muscle contraction from that seen in heart failure (3). *(Adapted, with permission, from Patterson et al. (1914). J. Physiol. 48:465.)*

the alveolar space, which impairs gas exchange (see Chap. 8). A patient with this condition is said to have **pulmonary edema** due to **congestive heart failure.**

Failure of the heart to empty the ventricles during systole does not normally happen because of several coordinated mechanisms. One of the mechanisms by which the heart matches work done with need is termed the **Frank-Starling mechanism** and is intrinsic to cardiac muscle function (see Figure 7.9). Normal cardiac muscle contraction, at rest, functions slightly inefficiently. At the molecular level, this means that actin and myosin cross-bridge formation in the sarcomere is not maximal. Thus, when normal cardiac muscle gets stretched because of increased venous blood return to the heart (e.g., as might occur in going from rest to sudden intense exercise), the efficiency of actin and myosin interaction actually improves. As a result, within the normal physiological range, the force of contraction (contractility) increases with stretch of cardiac muscle fibers, allowing the ventricle to pump a greater amount of blood for the same amount of work. This relation between myocardial fiber length and force of contraction is also known as **Starling's law of the heart**. Other factors, such as catecholamines, improve cardiac contractility in a similar manner.

However, if myocardial fibers are stretched too much, their contraction starts becoming less and less efficient (see Figure 7.9B). Thus, the patient with uncompensated congestive heart failure faces a vicious cycle: beyond a certain point: as more and more blood is left unpumped in the ventricle at the end of systole, it results in more and more stretch which makes the next contraction even less efficient, which leaves even more blood in the ventricle leading to even more stretch, etc. Such a patient is highly unstable and may rapidly progress to pulmonary edema, myocardial infarction, and death (see later).

The Frank-Starling mechanism is coordinated with other changes that increase heart rate and venous return, so that when the body needs more cardiac output that need is met through a combination of increased work and increased efficiency of work, all paid for through chemical energy in the form of ATP hydrolysis. Largely because of the Frank-Starling mechanism, cardiac output will normally adjust to whatever is needed to accommodate venous return. Additional neural and hormonal control over heart rate and contractility serve as a secondary mechanism (see Sec. 4).

Clinical Pearls

○ An increased end-systolic volume is a typical finding in heart failure. In such a heart, rapid filling of the ventricle early in diastole results in an audible third heart sound, termed S_3, which occurs after S_2. This can be heard in patients with systolic dysfunction.

○ The final filling of the ventricle that occurs with atrial contraction is normally silent. However, in patients with diastolic dysfunction (see Diastolic Dysfunction, in Sec. 4), this end-diastolic blood flow against a stiff, noncompliant ventricle results in an audible fourth heart sound, termed S_4, which occurs just before S_1.

Review Questions

3. What are the components of the cardiac conduction system?
4. What are the relative rates of automaticity of different regions of the heart?
5. Why do cardiac action potentials normally arise in the SA node?
6. How is cardiac muscle contraction similar to and different from that of skeletal or smooth muscle?

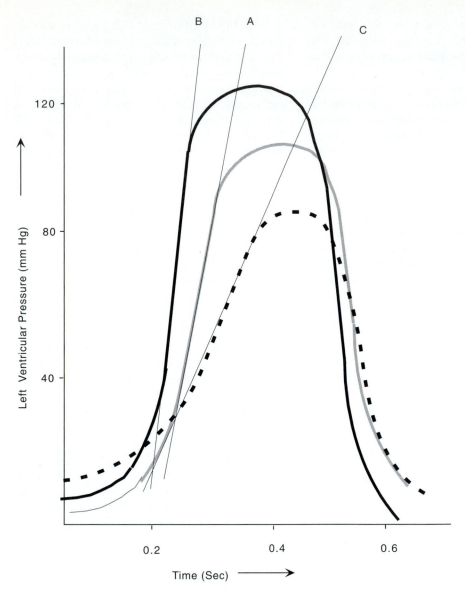

FIGURE 7.10. Changes in the left ventricular systolic pressure curves as a function of time, under different physiological and pathophysiological circumstances. The normal heart at rest is represented by the gray line, whose slope is A. Norepinephrine (e.g., as a result of sympathetic nervous system activation) causes physiological increase in contractility (shown by the solid black line) so that more force is generated more quickly, as indicated by the steeper slope (B as compared to A). The increase in contractility, together with the decreased cycle time (shown on the x axis) and the increased heart rate (not shown), translates into an increased cardiac output, under such conditions. Ventricular end-diastolic volume (not shown) need not change going from A to B, because of increased venous return to the hyperdynamic heart. Heart failure due to systolic dysfunction is shown by the dashed line.

7. What is the physiological basis for the heart sounds?
8. What is preload and afterload?
9. Describe the events of the cardiac cycle.
10. What is the Frank-Starling mechanism? Why does it normally result in cardiac output being determined by preload?

3. THE VASCULATURE AND INTERSTITIAL SPACE

The vasculature comprises a series of conduits of various diameter and structure by which three crucial functions are achieved:

• Distribution and flow of blood and its components pumped by the heart, throughout the body
• Exchange of substances between blood and tissues
• Maintenance of a reservoir of blood to be called upon instantly in times of need

The interstitial space is the space outside of blood vessels and between cells. It constitutes about one-sixth of the entire volume of the body. It is a hydrated matrix of collagen fibers and hyaluronic acid that has gel-like properties (see Figure 7.11), but which also allows, in some cases, free flow of fluid, which is drained by another set of vessels termed *lymphatics*.

The total volume in the intravascular space is approximately 4 to 5 L. The volume in the interstitial space is about 4 times this, nearly 20 L, though much of this is in the form of a hydrated gel that is not free flowing.

Clinical Pearls

○ Under certain pathological conditions, the volume of the interstitial space can expand enormously:
○ In response to certain cytokines produced during infection and inflammation (see Chap. 19), specific subsets of blood vessels can become suddenly more "leaky" and lose fluid to the interstitial space. This results in intravascular volume depletion and low blood pressure, which can set in motion a cascade of events leading to kidney failure in some patients, heart attack or stroke in others, etc. Sometimes this phenomenon, also called "third spacing," can occur selectively in organs such as the gastrointestinal tract in which edema is not as easily assessed as it is peripherally (e.g., in the feet).
○ Chronically, an imbalance between hydrostatic and oncotic pressure can result in a new equilibrium in which more fluid is in the interstitial space, resulting in pedal edema (see later).

FIGURE 7.10 — (*continued*) In this condition, the underlying pathology (e.g., ischemia) may result in a diminished capacity for contraction. Thus, the slope of the increase in left ventricular pressure during systole is less steep (see C), and the peak pressures achieved are lower. Not shown in this analysis of pressure over time is that end-diastolic volume increases in the change from B to C. At first, the increased end-diastolic volume actually improves the efficiency of myocardial contraction by moving to a more efficient part of the Frank-Starling curve (more overlap of actin and myosin to form cross-bridges in the sarcomeres, see Figure 7.9). However, with further increase in end-diastolic volume the left ventricle becomes excessively stretched which further impairs left ventricular contractility and cardiac output, resulting in the condition described in C.

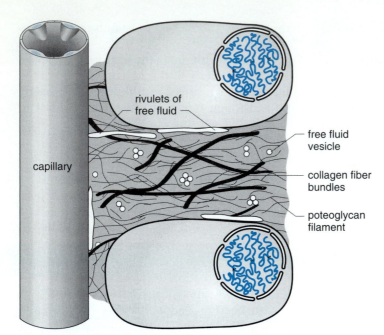

rivulets of
free fluid

capillary

free fluid
vesicle

collagen fiber
bundles

poteoglycan
filament

FIGURE 7.11. Structure of the interstitial space. Proteoglycans fill the spaces between collagen fibers in the interstitium. Excess free fluid (above that needed to hydrate the proteins of the interstitial space) is drained by the lymphatic vessels.

Anatomy of the vasculature

The arteries take blood from the heart via smaller and smaller vessels down to the level of arterioles and metarterioles. The primary functions of the arterial vessels are to get oxygenated blood to the tissues and to regulate the flow of blood into tissue capillaries by constriction and relaxation of the precapillary sphincters. Out of 4 L of blood only about 600 cc, approximately 13% of total blood volume, resides in the arteries at any given time at rest.

The precapillary sphincter is a muscular structure of the smallest arterioles beyond which the vessels are termed capillaries (see Figure 7.12A). These are the vessels through which exchange of substances between blood and tissues occurs (see Figure. 7.12B). At any given point in time only, about 300 mL of blood (7% of total blood volume) reside in the capillaries.

Beyond the capillaries, vessel diameter increases, forming the venous tree and culminating in the large veins that return blood to the heart. The large veins are the capacitance vessels in which most of the blood is stored: at any given time at rest about 2600 mL of blood (64% of total blood volume) reside in the veins (see Figure 7.13).

The lymphatic vessels that drain interstitial fluid empty into the venous system (see Figure 7.14). Lymph from the lower extremities and the left side of the body returns via the **thoracic duct** which joins the junction of the internal jugular and subclavian veins. Much of the rest of the body drains to the **right lymph duct** that empties into the junction of the right subclavian and internal jugular veins. When leakage of fluid out of capillaries exceeds the capacity of the lymphatic vessels, for any of a variety of reasons (see later), edema occurs.

Histology and cell biology of the vasculature

The structures of the arteries, capillaries, and veins differ, because each is specialized for

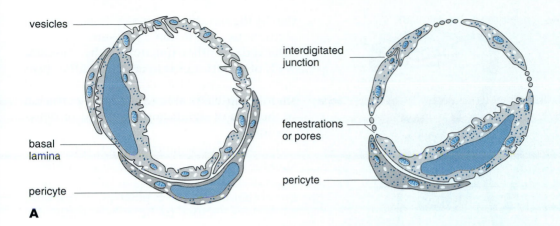

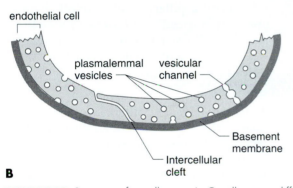

FIGURE 7.12. Structure of capillaries. *A.* Capillaries in different parts of the body have different degrees of "leakiness." This is because some are fenestrated (see right), while others are continuous, meaning that they have no fenestrations (see left), despite the fact that the circumference of the capillary at any given level may be composed of several different cells (note the intercellular junctions or clefts). Still others, as in most of the brain, for example, have tight junctions between their component cells. This further limits the exchange of substances between blood and the tissues through which the capillaries pass. *B.* Schematic drawing indicating that transport across the capillary can occur either through the intercellular clefts, through pinocytosis of vesicles, or through the actions of transporters (not shown here, see Chap. 2). In reality, the vesicles involved in pinocytosis would be too small to be seen at this degree of magnification. *(Adapted, with permission, from Fawcett, D.W. Bloom and Fawcett Textbook of Histology, 11 ed. Philadelphia, Saunders, 1986. B. Adapted, with permission, from Guyton, A.C. and Hall, J.E. (1997). Human Physiology and Mechanisms of Disease, 6th ed. Philadelphia, Saunders, p. 131.)*

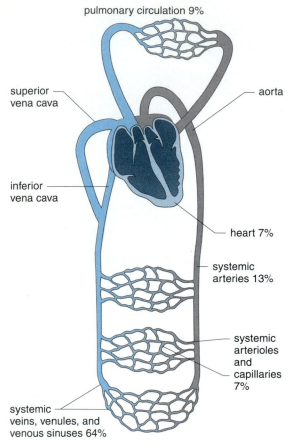

pulmonary circulation 9%

superior
vena cava

aorta

inferior
vena cava

heart 7%

systemic
arteries 13%

systemic
arterioles
and
capillaries
7%

systemic
veins, venules, and
venous sinuses 64%

FIGURE 7.13. Distribution of blood volumes in different portions of the circulatory system. *(Adapted, with permission, from Guyton, A.C. and Hall, J.E. (1997). Human Physiology and Mechanisms of Disease, 6th ed. Philadelphia, Saunders, p. 116.)*

its respective perfusion, exchange, and capacitance functions (see Figure 7.15). The inner wall (in contact with blood) of all blood vessels is composed of a single layer of endothelial cells.

Arteries have a substantial layer of smooth muscle in their walls beneath the endothelial cell layer. In the large arteries this allows them to be highly compliant, dampening out the swings in blood pressure that would otherwise occur between systole and diastole, so

that by the time blood reaches tissues a nearly continuous perfusion pressure can be achieved. Another function of the muscular walls of the arteries is to adjust to differences in blood volume. Thus, constriction of arterial smooth muscle is able to maintain perfusion in the face of significant blood loss or dehydration.

In the smallest metarterioles, the ring of smooth muscle is discontinuous, but allows regulation of tissue perfusion (the amount of blood that enters the capillaries) in response to various factors to be subsequently discussed.

In most capillaries, the endothelial cell layer is reinforced by a **basement membrane** (see Figure 7.12). Exchange of substances between blood and tissues occurs by three routes (Figure 7.12B):

- Between each endothelial cell is a small space, the so-called **intercellular cleft**. In different tissues these spaces are relatively more or relatively less accessible. Thus, in the brain, tight junctions between vascular endothelial cells allows only the smallest substances to traverse between cells. This comprises the **blood-brain barrier**.
- A second slower means of exchange between blood and tissues is **via pinocytic vesicles** of the endothelium that take up substances nonspecifically from the blood plasma and transport them across the endothelial cells for exocytosis on the tissue side.
- Finally, all cells in the body, including endothelial cells have transporters that can be used to take up and move specific substances from the blood stream to the tissues or vice versa.

The veins that receive the blood after it traverses the capillaries (see Figure 7.1C) also have a smooth muscle coat, but it is less pronounced than that of the arteries, because it does not have to serve the dampening func-

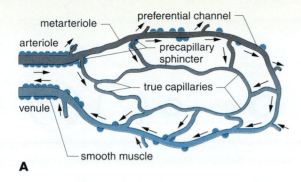

A

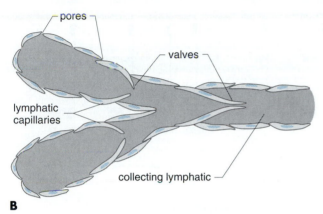

B

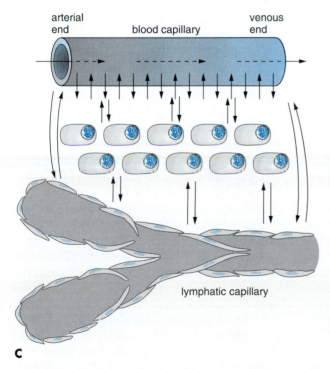

C

FIGURE 7.14. *A*. Structure of the mesenteric capillary bed. *B*. Structure of lympahatic capillaries and a collecting lymphatic, also showing the lymphatic valves. *C*. Hydrostatic and oncotic forces at work moving fluid in and out of the capillary and in and out of the interstitial space. Lymphatic vessels are the "safety valve" that normally balances out any net difference between these forces. *(A. Adapted, with permission, from Zweifach. Factors Regulating Blood Pressure. New York, Josiah Macy Jr. Foundation, 1950. B. and C. Adapted, with permission, from Guyton, A.C. and Hall, J.E. (1997). Human Physiology and Mechanisms of Disease, 6th ed. Philadelphia, Saunders, p. 131.)*

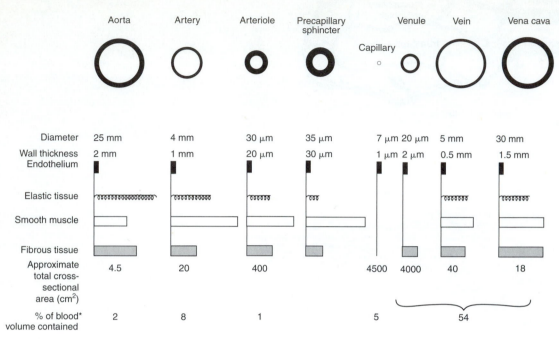

	Aorta	Artery	Arteriole	Precapillary sphincter	Capillary	Venule	Vein	Vena cava
Diameter	25 mm	4 mm	30 μm	35 μm	7 μm	20 μm	5 mm	30 mm
Wall thickness Endothelium	2 mm	1 mm	20 μm	30 μm	1 μm	2 μm	0.5 mm	1.5 mm
Elastic tissue								
Smooth muscle								
Fibrous tissue								
Approximate total cross-sectional area (cm²)	4.5	20	400		4500	4000	40	18
% of blood* volume contained	2	8	1		5		54	

* In systemic vessels. There is an additional 12% in the heart and 18% in the pulmonary circulation.

FIGURE 7.15. Structure of the blood vessel wall. Characteristics of systemic blood vessels. Note that the cross-sections are not to scale since the range of sizes would be too huge to depict comprehensibly. *(Adapted, with permission, from Burton, A.C. (1954). Relation of structure to function of the tissues of the wall of blood vessels. Physiol. Rev. 34:619.)*

tion on blood pressure as does the arterial wall. Instead, venous smooth muscle contributes to the capacitance function of veins. Upon its constriction, a large reservoir of venous blood can be returned to the heart. Figure 7.13 indicates the amounts of blood that reside in various venous beds that can be released to circulation by constriction. Because the veins are larger and more distensible than the arteries and are under much lower pressure, the small amount of smooth muscle in their wall is sufficient to compress them and regulate their function as a reservoir of blood.

The lymphatic vessels have a unique structure that facilitates their role of collecting extravasated fluid and plasma proteins for return to the systemic circulation (see Figures 7.14A and B). **Anchoring filaments** attached to the connective tissue of the interstitial space create a valve effect between the edges of the endothelial cells that comprise lymphatic capillaries, allowing unimpeded access of interstitial fluid to the capillary lumen, but preventing backflow. Together with valves along the length of the larger lymphatic vessels, these specializations in effect comprise a "pump" that propels returning interstitial fluid to the locations where it empties directly into the venous circulation. Lymph in the upper right quadrant of the body drains via the right lymphatic duct (while that from most of the rest of the body drains via the thoracic duct, see Figure 7.1B).

Physiology of the vasculature

Clearly the role of the heart as a pump is a crucial determinant of blood flow. However other factors play an important role in determining where the blood pumped by the heart actually goes. Thus:

$$\text{Blood flow} = \frac{\text{Difference in Pressure between Ends of a Vessel}}{\text{Resistance}}$$

The determinants of resistance to blood flow are as follows:

- Viscosity of blood. The greater the viscosity, the less the flow. Blood is about three times more viscous than water, due to the effect of frictional drag of cells against each other and against the vessel wall.
- Vessel diameter. Flow is proportional to the fourth power of the diameter. Thus a four-fold increase in vessel diameter results in a 256-fold increase in flow. This is because most of the resistance to flow occurs near the vessel wall. Therefore, resistance at the level of arterioles of the body is tremendous, while that in the large arteries is almost nothing. From this it follows that, normally, blood flow is controlled largely at the level of changes in arteriolar vasoconstriction. Vasoconstriction and vasodilation are important means by which blood flow to different organs is regulated, as will be discussed later.

Clinical Pearls

○ Since flow is proportional to viscosity of blood, any process that increases the **hematocrit** (the percentage of blood volume made up of cells) above normal impairs flow and requires a higher blood pressure to achieve tissue perfusion, all other factors being equal. Increased hematocrit can occur in patients with lung disease, as the body compensates for poor oxygenation by increasing the amount of oxygen carrying capacity (i.e., red blood cells) in the blood. However, by increasing the viscosity of blood, the increased hematocrit places the patients at greater risk of failure to perfuse an organ (e.g., the brain or the kidneys). Thus increased viscosity compounds the risk of nonperfusion posed by occlusion of vessels with atherosclerotic plaques and clot formation. Such events can last long enough to result in death of nonperfused tissue. When this occurs in the brain, a patient is said to have had a stroke. When this occurs in the heart, the patient is said to have had a myocardial infarction or heart attack.

○ Often in clinical practice, a "ticking time bomb" (such as high hematocrit in a patient with lung disease and atherosclerosis) is set off by an event that would be otherwise entirely benign. For example, the mild dehydration that might accompany the "flu" could result in tachycardia (increased heart rate) and a slight further increase in blood viscosity which might be just enough to trigger a stroke or myocardial infarction at a partially occluded blood vessel in the brain or heart, respectively.

The **pulse pressure** is the difference between the peak arterial pressure of systole and the arterial pressure at the end of diastole. Over the course of the arterial tree, this difference is dampened due to (a) compliance of the arterial vessel walls and (b) resistance to flow as vessel diameters become smaller (see Figure 7.16). This is important for maintaining tissue perfusion throughout the cardiac cycle. In effect, the compliance of the large arteries stores some of the ejected blood so that flow through the capillaries will be continuous throughout the cardiac cy-

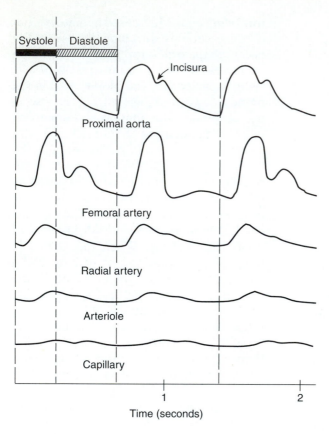

FIGURE 7.16. Changes in pulse pressure contour as the pulse wave travels toward the smaller vessels. Note how the compliance of arteries allows dampening of the pressure variation of the cardiac cycle such that the capillary sees a relatively constant perfusion pressure. *(Adapted, with permission, from Guyton, A.C. and Hall, J.E. (1997). Human Physiology and Mechanisms of Disease, 6th ed. Philadelphia, Saunders, p. 123.)*

cle. Another result of arterial compliance is that by the time the blood reaches the capillaries, flow is nonpulsatile. With age, compliance in the arteries decreases. The less compliant the arteries are, the more work the heart must do to maintain a given cardiac output.

Clinical Pearls

○ **Essential hypertension** is the term used to describe cases of hypertension for which we cannot point to a simple primary cause, in contrast to so-called secondary hypertension that occurs, for example, in response to a specific problem, such as a catecholamine-secreting tumor, or renal artery stenosis resulting in excessive renal production of renin.

○ Systolic hypertension with normal diastolic pressure is common, especially in the elderly. It is believed to be due to atherosclerosis with loss of part of the normal contribution of arterial compliance to the dampening of systolic pressure.

○ Essential hypertension is typically diastolic, with or without a systolic component. Despite these differences in etiology and presentation, both systolic and diastolic hypertension result in increased perfusion pressure and carry a potential for end-organ injury (especially stroke) over the long term, and therefore should be aggressively treated — but not just pharmacologically:

Weight loss, abstinence from alcohol, stress reduction, and gentle exercise (e.g., walking) are likely to improve blood pressure control in the long-term.

Hydrostatic pressure is the pressure contributed by the weight of the blood in the vessels. In an individual standing still, the pressure at the level of the heart is 0, while that in the feet would be 90 mmHg. However, because the veins have valves, once blood flows past the valve its pressure is lowered to that of the valve. In this way, venous hydrostatic pressures are lowered substantially, to an average of 25 mmHg.

Clinical Pearls

The act of walking normally results in muscle contraction that forces blood up the veins of the lower extremities, augmenting venous return to the heart.

❍ Individuals who spend excessive periods "standing around" (e.g., a homeless person in line at a soup kitchen with nowhere to sit) have increased venous pressures that contribute to the development of varicose veins with damaged venous valves. Especially in combination with poor hygiene, these individuals have an increased risk of venous stasis disease. This is manifest as painful, edematous feet with poorly healing skin infections.

❍ Individuals who spend excessive periods sitting (e.g., a business executive who spends large amounts of time on airplane flights), which results in increased pooling and stagnation of blood in the veins, are at increased risk for development of blood clots (thrombophlebitis), particularly in the calves or thighs.

❍ One way to help maintain healthy vasculature is to regularly intersperse mixed activity to break up periods of prolonged sitting or standing.

Capillary-fluid exchange

Another variable of cardiovascular function is the extent to which fluid is localized to the intravascular space versus the extravascular extracellular space (see Chap. 10).

Intercellular clefts comprise 1/1000 of the area of the vascular endothelium, yet rates of diffusion through them are great. Water molecules diffuse across the intracellular clefts 80 times faster than the time it takes for plasma to traverse from the arterial to the venous end of a single capillary. Thus there is plenty of time for exchange of oxygen to, and carbon dioxide from, tissues.

The dimensions of the intracellular cleft in most tissues are such that a molecule of albumin is slightly too big to fit through the space. Thus, the fluid that bathes most tissues is an ultrafiltrate of plasma that is depleted of both cells and most proteins. Some protein does get through, but the protein concentration in tissue fluid is only about one-third of that in plasma. Table 7.1 indicates the relative

TABLE 7.1   VASCULAR PERMEABILITY TO VARIOUS SIZED MOLECULES

Substance	Molecular weight	Permeability
Water	18	1.00
NaCl	58.5	0.96
Urea	60	0.8
Glucose	180	0.6
Sucrose	342	0.4
Insulin	5000	0.2
Myoglobin	17,600	0.03
Hemoglobin	68,000	0.01
Albumin	69,000	0.001

Reproduced, with permission, from Guyton, A.C. and Hall, J.E. (1997). *Human Physiology and Mechanisms of Disease*, 6th ed. Philadelphia, Saunders, p 132. Based mainly on data from Papperheimer. (1953). *Physiol. Rev.* 33:389.

permeability of capillaries to differently sized molecules.

Four different forces, collectively termed **Starling forces**, contribute to fluid movement through a capillary membrane:

1. Capillary pressure, which forces fluid out of the capillary
2. Interstitial fluid pressure, which can be either positive or negative, and which forces fluid into the capillary when it is positive
3. Plasma colloid oncotic pressure, the osmotic activity of plasma proteins within the capillary, which will tend to hold fluid in the capillary
4. Interstitial fluid colloid osmotic pressure, which is usually substantially lower than its plasma counterpart

These Starling forces are not to be confused with the Frank-Starling curve and mechanism and Starling's law of the heart, discussed in in Sec. 2. They are named after the same person, but they deal with an entirely different physiological concept.

Normally there is a gradient of these forces along the length of a capillary. Forces tending to push fluid out of the capillary predominate at the arterial end, forces returning fluid to the capillary predominate at the venous end. About 90% of filtered fluid is returned to the intravascular space by the time blood reaches the veins. There is, however, a slight excess of forces pushing fluid out of the capillaries over those tending to keep it in, resulting in a small net production of interstitial fluid over time, under normal circumstances. The **lymphatic system** collects this small amount of extravasated fluid from the interstitial space and returns it to the circulation.

Lymph reenters the venous circulation at the rate of about 120 mL/h, resulting in a total daily flow of approximately 2 to 3 L.

Lymph from the liver is distinctive in that the lack of a basement membrane results in lymph whose protein concentration is essentially the same as that of plasma. Since up to two-thirds of total body lymph is derived from the liver, the average protein concentration in lymph is 3 to 5 g/L, compared to about 2 g/L for lymph derived from most tissues of the body, and compared to plasma, whose protein concentration is about 6 g/L.

Clinical Pearl

○ Ascites occurs when, due to an imbalance of Starling forces, the fluid extravasation from the vasculature of the liver is greater than the capacity of the lymphatic system. The excess lymph pools in the peritoneal space. Common causes of this phenomenon are portal hypertension from alcoholic liver disease in industrialized countries and hypoalbuminemia from protein-calorie malnutrition in developing countries.

Review Questions

11. What are the functions of the vasculature?
12. What are the four major types of vessels that comprise the vasculature?
13. What are two mechanisms of exchange of solutes between blood and tissues?
14. What are the determinants of blood flow and resistance to blood flow?
15. What are the four Starling forces that contribute to fluid movement across the capillary membrane?
16. What is the daily volume of lymph returned to the intravascular system and its average protein concentration?

4. CARDIOVASCULAR REGULATION

In order to function normally, the heart muscle and its ability to contract and relax, the conduction system, chamber size, valves, and ionized free calcium and potassium concentrations must be within normal limits. Assuming these features are intact, there are a number of mechanisms by which cardiac output can be controlled to give the range (approximately 3 to 10 L/min) observed in different physiological states.

Control of cardiac output

The pump function of the heart has been described earlier by the equation:

Cardiac Output
= Heart Rate × Stroke Volume

Regulation of the heart involves intrinsic features of cardiac muscle contractility already discussed (Frank-Starling mechanism) and its response to changes in venous return, as well as neural and hormonal control.

Neural control is via the autonomic nervous system. The sympathetic nervous system stimulates both heart rate and contractility. The parasympathetic nervous system primarily inhibits heart rate, with a smaller effect on contractility. The effects on contractility are largely due to changes in the activity of adenylate cyclase, with the resulting change in cyclic AMP altering calcium conductance. Neural control of the heart includes various reflexes that respond instantaneously to monitored parameters including changes in blood pressure and blood concentration of O_2, CO_2, and H^+.

Hormonal control of cardiac output is mediated primarily by catecholamines, which are released by the adrenal medulla and function to increase both heart rate and contractility. But other hormones, including glucocorticoids, thyroid hormone, insulin, glucagon, and anterior pituitary hormones, also affect myocardial contractility.

Atrial natruietic factor (ANF) is a small peptide released from the atria upon stretch (as would occur in the setting of excess intravascular volume). It serves to induce sodium and water loss from the kidney, thereby decreasing intravascular volume and relieving the stimulus (stretch) that triggers its release in the first place.

Finally, both gravity and respiration affect cardiac output, through their effect on pooling of blood in the veins. When an individual inhales, intrathoracic pressure falls, increasing the volume of blood in the pulmonary vessels, which will augment preload. When an individual exhales, intrathracic pressure increases, less blood is held in the pulmonary vessels and preload will subsequently fall.

Control of blood flow and distribution

There are many factors that contribute to the regulation of blood pressure, flow, and distribution:

• Local tissue perfusion. This is maintained largely by the ability of arterioles, or more precisely, the precapillary sphincter, to contract or dilate in response to oxygen deprivation, accumulation of vasodilatory metabolites, or both. Adenosine has been suggested as a key vasodilatory metabolite. At any given instant, flow through one capillary may have ceased while it continues through another, in response to the presence or absence of such local factors. The average perfusion of a tissue is the sum of flow through the individual capillaries over time.

• Regional blood flow regulation, largely via the autonomic nervous system. All vessels except for metarterioles, precapillary sphincters, and capillaries have autonomic innervation. Normally the smooth muscle surrounding the vascular endothelium is in a state of partial contraction called **vasomotor tone**, which plays a major role in control of blood pressure (see Figure 7.17).

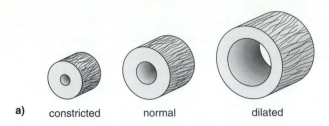

a)   constricted   normal   dilated

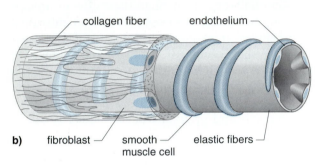

b)   fibroblast   smooth muscle cell   elastic fibers

collagen fiber   endothelium

FIGURE 7.17. Change in the lumen diameter and wall thickness of an arteriole in response to factors resulting in either dilation or constriction compared to normal. Note that the partial state of contraction resulting from normal "vasomotor tone" makes possible regulation in either direction, with resultant changes in both perfusion pressure and volume of blood flow to a given tissue. *(Adapted, with permission, from Luciano, D.S., Vander, A. J., and Sherman, J.H. (1978). Human Function and Structure. New York, McGraw-Hill, p. 426.)*

- Hormones that function as vasoconstrictive or vasodilatory agents. Often the same hormone has other functions on the heart or the kidney that reinforce its vascular effects in particular physiological circumstances. Some vasoactive substances such as endothelins may function under specific circumstances such as injury. Table 7.2 indicates the most important of these vasoactive substances and summarizes their key features.
- Long-term regulation of blood flow through induction of new blood vessels. A large number of peptide growth factors can cause new vessels to sprout from venules or capillaries. Some of these so-called **angiogenic factors** are indicated in Table 7.3.

Effect of cardiac blood flow on cardiac function

The principles that govern local short- and long-term regulation of blood flow throughout the body are especially important for tissues such as cardiac muscle, whose oxygen demand is high and constant. This is apparent by considering the response of cardiac muscle to ischemia, the inadequacy of blood flow despite compensatory local regulation. When ischemia is severe and prolonged, the result is rapid death of cardiac muscle cells through necrosis and their replacement with scar tissue. However, when a brief period of ischemia is followed by reperfusion, cardiac muscle may appear to be **stunned** for a time, failing to contract properly, which may manifest in patients as heart failure. If good perfusion is maintained, proper function may return. Conversely, if subjected to mild ischemia, cardiac muscle reflexly diminishes its metabolism and function, a process termed **hibernation**. These patients also may present with signs of heart failure. Later, if perfusion improves (e.g., due to bypass surgery), proper function may return. If perfusion remains poor, but sufficient to avoid necrosis in the short term, excessively stretched cardiac myocytes may undergo death through apoptosis, resulting in a largely irreversible disorder termed **dilated cardiomyopathy**.

TABLE 7.2   KEY FEATURES AND ROLES OF VARIOUS VASOACTIVE SUBSTANCES

Constriction
  Local factors
    Decreased local temperature
    Autoregulation
    Locally released platelet serotonin
  Endothelial cell products
    Endothelin-1
  Hormones
    Norepinephrine
    Epinephrine (except in skeletal muscle and liver)
    Arginine vasopressin
    Angiotensin II
    Circulating Na^+-K^+ ATPase inhibitor
    Neuropeptide Y
  Neural control
    Increased discharge of noradrenergic vasomotor nerves
Dilation
  Local factors
    Increased CO_2, K^+, adenosine, lactate
    Decreased O_2
    Decreased local pH
    Increased local temperature
  Endothelial cell products
    Nitric oxide
  Hormones
    Vasoactive intestinal peptide
    CGRPα (calcitonin gene-related peptide, the α form)
    Substance P
    Histamine
    Kinins
    Atrial natriuretic peptide
    Epinephrine in skeletal muscle and liver
  Neural control
    Activation of cholinergic dilator fibers to skeletal muscle
    Decreased discharge of noradrenergic vasomotor nerves

Reproduced, with permission, from McPhee S. et al. (eds.) *Pathophysiology of Disease* (1997). 2nd ed. Stamford, CT, Appleton & Lange, p. 263.

Clinical Pearls

○ Patients with myocardial ischemia manifest as angina are often treated with a combination of vasodilators and β-adrenergic receptor blockers. The vasodilators serve to both decrease preload and afterload and to increase coronary circulation. The β blockers slow heart rate and thereby decrease the work of the heart. In treating angina, it is important to remember to use both modalities together since vasodilators alone can cause a reflex tachycardia, which, by increasing oxygen utilization, may exacerbate the ischemia.

○ Treatment of such patients with these drugs involves walking a fine line: Judicious doses of vasodilators and β blockers may improve perfusion or decrease workload, respectively. However, excessive treatment can have exactly the opposite effect. Too much vasodilator can result in hypotension and impaired myocardial perfusion, due to inadequate venous return and cardiac output. Conversely, excessive β-adrenergic receptor blockade can decrease the work performed by the heart to the point of causing congestive heart failure. Thus, never forget to examine the patient in order to assess the effectiveness and balance of therapy.

Blood pressure regulation

By convention, blood pressure is usually measured in terms of millimeters of mercury (mmHg) at sea level, reflecting the development of the mercury manometer, which measures the degree to which a given pressure displaces a column of mercury, which is about 13.6 times as dense as water.

Blood pressure
  = Cardiac Output × Peripheral Resistance

Regulation of blood pressure is a complex integration of function of the following components:

• Organs (heart, vessels, kidneys)
• Systems of control (peripheral autonomic nervous system, central nervous system, hormones)
• Timescales (instantaneous, seconds, minutes, hours, days)

TABLE 7.3 ANGIOGENIC FACTORS

Growth factors	Endothelial cell receptors	Growth factor tissue distribution	Target tissues other than EC
FGF-1 (acidic)	FGFR-1, 2, 3, 4	Brain, bone, matrix, kidney, EC, retina, heart, others	Multiple
FGF-2 (basic)	FGFR-1, 2	Brain, retina, pituitary, kidney, placenta, testes, monocytes, corpus luteum, heart, many others	Multiple
FGF-4	FGFR-1, 2	Embryonic tissue	Megakaryocytes, multiple others
FGF-5	Unknown	Neonatal brain, CNS	CNS, hair follicles
VEGF-A	VEGFR-1 (flt-1)(fms) VEGFR-2 kdr/flk-1	Pituitary cells, monocytes (macrophages), smooth muscle, heart, lung, skeletal muscle, prostate	Monocytes, coagulation system, hematopoeitic stem cells
VEGF-B	Unknown	Heart, skeletal muscle, pancreas, prostate, many others	Unknown
VEGF-C	fit-4 (VEGFR-3)/VEGFR-2	Heart, placenta, ovary, small intestine, others	Unknown
HGE (scatter factor)	c-met	Lung, liver, skin, blood, many others	Multiple
PDGF-BB	PDGFR β	Platelets, malignant cells, macrophages, EC, fibroblasts, VSMC, glial cells, astrocytes, myoblasts, kidney cells	Connective tissue, smooth muscle, neutrophils
EGF	EGFR (c-erbB)	Ectodermal cells, monocytes, kidney, duodenal glands	Epithelial cells, gastric glands
TGF-α	EGFR (c-erbB)	Monocytes, keratinocytes, many normal tissues, neoplastic cells	Epithelial cells, gastric glands
1L-B	1L-B receptor (2)	Monocytes, lymphocytes, granulocytes, fibroblasts, EC, bronchial epithelial cells, keratinocytes, hepatocytes, mesangial cells, and chondrocytes	Neutrophils, lymphocytes, basophils, monocytes
Proliferin	MRP/PLF receptor	Placenta, fibroblasts, muscle	Uterus, muscle, numerous other tissues

Reproduced, with permission, from Ware, A. and Simons, M. (1997). Angiogenesis in ischemic heart disease. *Nat. Med.* 3:159.

- Purposes (changes in posture, activity, fluid status)

Let us consider examples of some different types of situations demanding regulation of blood pressure and perfusion. An example of a short-term blood pressure decision is when you decide to stand up after lying down for a time. Suddenly perfusion of your head and upper body would fall, all else being equal. A baroreceptor system operates on the seconds-to-minutes timescale to ensure that the vasomotor center has the information it needs to determine exactly how much to increase vasomotor tone. Another short-term blood pressure regulatory decision occurs when you run 50 yards, as fast as you can. Here, a sudden increased need for perfusion of muscle mandates an increased cardiac output, which requires increased venous return (see Figure 7.18).

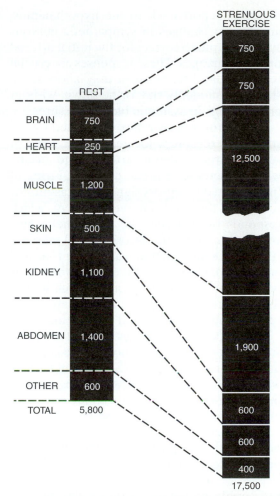

FIGURE 7.18. Distribution of blood flow to the various organs and tissues of the body at rest and during strenuous exercise. The numbers show blood flow in milliliters per minute. *(Adapted, with permission, from Luciano, D.S., Vander, A. J., and Sherman, J.H. (1978). Human Function and Structure. New York, McGraw-Hill, p. 425.)*

Clinical Pearl

○ Most cases of hypertension are essential hypertension, with no known specific remediable cause. About two-thirds of these

patients will be treated with drugs for the rest of their life. However, as many as 1 in 10 cases of hypertension is secondary to a specific endocrine or structural cause. Given the millions of individuals with hypertension and the long course of therapy otherwise entailed, it is crucial that all newly diagnosed cases of hypertension be evaluated for such secondary causes. Such an evaluation includes auscultation of the femoral arteries for bruits (renal artery stenosis), measurement of serum potassium (if low, a sign of mineralocorticoid excess, see Chap. 13), and careful history and physical exam for thyroid, adrenal, and other endocrine causes of hypertension.

Review Questions

17. Define cardiac output.
18. What are the mechanisms by which blood flow and distribution are regulated?
19. Define blood pressure.
20. What organs, systems of control, timescales, and purposes are utilized to control blood pressure?

Neural control of vasomotor tone

Baroreceptors send input from the carotid sinus, aortic arch, heart, and elsewhere to the vasomotor centers of the medulla and brainstem. These in turn stimulate or inhibit the autonomic nervous system. In addition, the vasomotor centers communicate with the hypothalamus, which integrates input from the cerebral cortex, the reticular activating system, and other centers to provide both short- and long-term alterations of vascular tone.

The vasoconstrictor and cardioaccelerator functions of the sympathetic nervous system are stimulated as a unit for the purposes of rapid control of blood pressure, resulting in vasoconstriction of all arterioles and large veins, and up to threefold increase in heart rate. These changes allow blood pressure to either be maintained with sudden changes in posture or to be changed substantially (as much as doubled or halved) in the space of 5 to 30 s, in response to changes in activity.

For example, consider strenuous exercise, during which the metabolic activity of muscles can increase up to sixtyfold and blood flow can increase up to twentyfold to meet these needs. To achieve this increased blood flow, several factors come into play:

• Local vasodilation, as discussed earlier;
• Thirty to 40% increase in blood pressure resulting in a twofold increase in muscle blood flow. Special features of neural regulation are triggered at the same time that the motor pathways of the nervous system initiate exercise. This neural regulation is mediated by the reticular-activating system and the sympathetic nervous system. This results in an increase in heart rate and increased systemic vasoconstriction. As a result, blood pressure and cardiac output increase, helping to meet the increased perfusion needs of exercising muscle.

Other kinds of stress besides strenuous exercise result in increased sympathetic activity and blood pressure, as typified by the **fright reaction**. Teleologically, this serves to anticipate the imminent need for the increased muscle blood flow of a response to danger. A number of involuntary, neurally mediated reflex arcs serve to maintain blood pressure (e.g., upon changes in posture; see Figure 7.19).

Baroreceptor mechanisms

Various reflex neural arcs exist whereby specialized receptors sense changes in arterial pressure, report back to the hypothalamus, and trigger changes in sympathetic nervous system output to correct for the initial arterial pressure changes. These responses are crucial for everyday life, because they allow us to stand up, suddenly run, or lie down, without gross swings in systemic blood pressures.

The **baroreceptor reflex** is initiated by the stretch of receptors located in the walls of several large systemic arteries and occurs with an increase in blood pressure. Firing of the activated receptors signals the vasomotor centers of the central nervous system, which responds by ordering the sympathetic nervous system to reduce arterial blood pressure (through changes in both vasomotor tone and heart rate). One type of baroreceptor is particularly abundant in the aortic arch and in the **carotid sinus**, the area of the carotid artery just above the carotid bifurcation.

This reflex system serves as a sort of "pressure buffer," offsetting both increases and decreases in blood pressure that would otherwise occur (e.g., with postural changes) on a minute-by-minute basis, to about one-third of what they would otherwise be.

However, the baroreceptor system is not believed to be important for long-term blood pressure regulation:

• It rapidly acclimates within a day or two, such that whatever pressure the body has had recently is the new baseline from which postural and other pressure-based changes occur.
• From animal experiments it appears that the average blood pressure over a long period (e.g., days) is the same, with or without a functioning baroreceptor system. In the absence of this system, there are simply wider swings in blood pressure in both directions.

A second form of baroreceptors is found in the atrial and pulmonary arteries. These are called **low-pressure receptors** and are believed to be important determinants of blood

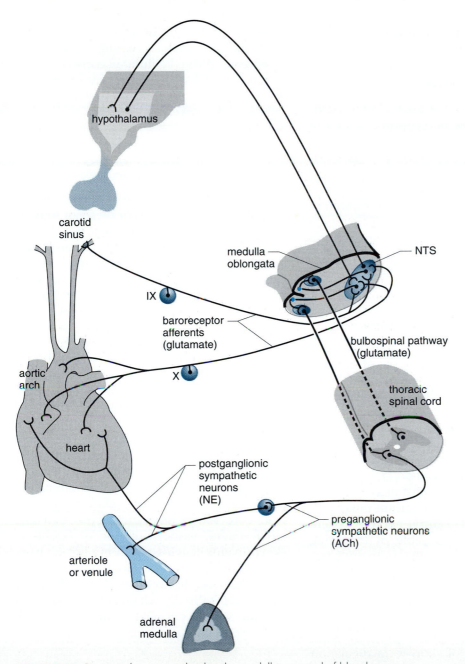

FIGURE 7.19. Basic pathways involved in the medullary control of blood pressure. The vagal efferent pathways to the heart are not shown. The probable neurotransmitters in the pathways are indicated in parentheses. ACh, acetylcholine; NE, norepinephrine; IX, glossopharyngeal nerve (cranial nerve IX); NTS, nucleus tractus solitarius; X, vagus nerve (cranial nerve X).

pressure changes in response to change in overall volume status.

Chemoreceptor mechanism

In close proximity to the arterial baroreceptors are a set of **chemoreceptors** located in the **carotid and aortic bodies**. Instead of responding to stretch, these receptors are sensitive to oxygen lack, carbon dioxide excess, or hydrogen ion excess. They respond by triggering increased rate and depth of respiration and peripheral vasoconstriction. This receptor system will be discussed in more detail in Chapter 8, because arterial baroreceptors play a more important role in control of respiration than they do in blood pressure.

Central nervous system response to ischemia

Normally, the vasomotor centers of the central nervous system are triggered only in response to appropriate stimuli from the baroreceptor or chemoreceptor systems discussed earlier. When arterial hypotension is sufficiently severe or prolonged to result in cerebral ischemia, the vasomotor centers will fire independently of the peripheral receptor systems. Under these circumstances, perhaps in response to the rise in carbon dioxide in ischemic tissues, this **central nervous system ischemic response** is capable of triggering sympathetic nervous stimulation to drive tremendous increases in arterial pressure.

Clinical Pearl

○ The importance of short-term regulation of vascular tone is seen in patients with autonomic neuropathy due to diabetes mellitus who often have disabling symptoms of dizziness upon standing, because of damage to the system that normally carries out instantaneous correction of postural blood pressure changes. Avoiding

dehydration, adjusting antihypertensive therapy, or even increasing intravascular volume through mineralocorticoid therapy (see Chap. 13), are ways of helping patients for whom these symptoms are unacceptably severe.

Capillary leak and inflammation

The movement of fluid from intravascular to extravascular spaces is governed not only by the forces discussed previously, but also by parameters such as the inflammatory response. The release of powerful mediators by cells of the immune system can have a major effect on the permeability of vascular endothelium and is extremely important in the pathophysiology of disease. This will be discussed in more detail in Chapter 19.

The net effect of the various neural, hormonal, and local metabolic factors regulating overall blood flow is to constantly redistribute blood to the most active tissues. The local metabolic factors appear to be the most important of these mechanisms.

Blood flow through the skin is regulated somewhat differently from the other organs. It is regulated primarily by temperature, responding as needed to minimize variation from core body temperature. Thus, in a cold environment, vasoconstriction of vessels in skin prevents heat loss, while in a hot environment vasodilation of vessels in skin dissipates excess heat. As discussed in Chapter 11, fever works centrally by changing the setpoint around which peripheral vasoconstriction and vasodilation operate.

Review Questions

21. How is the sympathetic nervous system controlled?
22. What factors account for the increased blood flow to muscle during exercise?

23. Where are the two types of barorecep-tors located and what are their roles?

24. To what do the chemoreceptors that control blood pressure respond?

5. PATHOPHYSIOLOGY OF SELECTED CARDIOVASCULAR SYSTEM DISORDERS

As with many other organs, understanding the disorders of the cardiovascular system is complicated by two recurrent themes of pathophysiology: (a) a given pathological process can manifest differently in different patients and conversely, and (b) multiple mechanisms can contribute to the development of any given disease, with the precise mix of contributors varying from patient to patient. Consider, for example, atherosclerosis, a common pathophysiological entity of the cardiovascular system. Certain lifestyles (that promote hypertension) can contribute to atherosclerosis, as can certain dietary practices (e.g., high fat and cholesterol intake), and genetic backgrounds (e.g., LDL receptor defects). It has been recognized that, as a further complication, certain infections may accelerate atherosclerosis as well (see Frontiers, in Sec. 6).

Likewise, the consequences of atherosclerosis can range from myocardial infarction and stroke to dysrhythmias, heart failure, kidney failure, and peripheral vascular disease. Why different manifestations are more prominent in one individual versus another is not well understood, but presumably has an explanation rooted in either genetics environment/lifestyle, and/or chance.

We will briefly consider some of the most prominent pathophysiological processes in cardiovascular disease, hypertension, and atherosclerosis, by placing them in a physiological context. Then we will consider the consequences of myocardial ischemia and its diverse manifestations (e.g., angina and myo-cardial infarction, heart failure, and dys-rythmias).

Atherosclerosis

Given the incessant work the heart must perform, provision of adequate nutrition and removal of wastes is essential. Occlusion of cardiac vessels interferes with these essential physiological functions. Blood vessels are commonly occluded because of **atherosclerotic plaques** or **blood clots** or a mixture of both. Plaques form in arterial vessels that are under high pressure; clots can form in either arteries or veins. In the arterial system, clots often occur in areas that have plaques, which appear to serve as a nidus for clot formation.

Formation of atherosclerotic plaques involve aberrations of normal physiological functions related to the stress response (see Chap. 19). Two key contributors are as follows:

- The response to **shear stress** (the force of turbulent blood rushing by) on the endothelium
- High concentrations of **oxidized LDL** in the bloodstream

As a result of abnormally elevated sheer stress, as occurs in the arterial system with **hypertension**, vascular endothelial cells change their expression of adhesion molecules. The new adhesion molecules whose expression is induced are ones that promote migration of monocytes to the subendothelial (intimal) space. There, under the influence of cytokines derived from either (or both) the endothelium and T-cells, the monocytes differentiate into macrophages.

Macrophages express **scavenger receptors** and hence they endocytose oxidized LDL and are converted into **foam cells**, which constitute the **fatty streak** of an early atherosclerotic plaque seen even in childhood. Macrophages also secrete cytokines and other products that (a) induce certain cells to migrate toward them, and (b) change the pattern of gene expression in the attracted cells.

Thus, subsequent to foam-cell formation, smooth muscle cells migrate toward the foam cells and are induced to proliferate and accumulate calcium. This results, somehow, in inflammatory ulceration of the fatty streak to form an atherosclerotic plaque. The higher the concentration of LDL in the blood, the longer any given LDL molecule circulates before its removal. Blood is an oxidizing environment; hence the longer LDL circulates, the greater the fraction with which it will be oxidized.

Although the initial changes in adhesion-molecule expression and subsequent cellular migration somehow may be adaptive for hypertension in the short run, in the long run they set in motion formation of plaques, which are in turn associated with serious disease processes such as clot formation, vessel occlusion, and ischemia.

Thus, atherosclerotic plaques cause disease in two ways:

- They can narrow and eventually occlude the vessel lumen directly.
- They can serve as a nidus for blood clot formation.

In addition to hypercholesterolemia and hypertension, a number of other conditions can accelerate the progression of atherosclerosis including the following:

- Smoking, which increases the rate of LDL oxidation that would otherwise occur at any given serum LDL concentration and may also injure the endothelium through carbon monoxide exposure, thereby triggering the adhesion protein changes that initiate atherosclerosis.
- Diabetes mellitus (both insulin-dependent and non-insulin-dependent disease) results in insulin resistance, elevated serum insulin

levels in the periphery, and the undesired side effects of long-term insulin action: endothelial cell hypertrophy resulting in increased vasoconstriction; worsening of the patient's serum lipid profile, which results in more LDL oxidation, etc.
- Low estrogen states. Estrogens have a serum LDL-lowering effect, possibly by increasing the number of LDL receptors in the liver. This mechanism probably accounts for the increased severity of atherosclerosis in relatively low estrogen states such as occur in men and in postmenopausal women.
- Hypothyroidism, which elevates serum LDL, probably by decreasing LDL receptors in the liver.
- Lipoprotein (a) (see the following Clinical Pearl).
- Nephrotic syndrome, which is associated with increased hepatic lipid output including lipoprotein (a).
- Obesity, partly an independent risk factor and partly due to its association with hypercholesterolemia, hypertriglyceridemia, diabetes, and hypertension; each of which are all independent risk factors for atherosclerosis.
- Family history, reflecting the presence of genes that predispose to development of atherosclerosis.

The hypothesized mechanism of atherosclerosis is summarized in Figure 7.20.

Hypertension

Hypertension is extremely common. It is defined as an elevation of the baseline systolic or diastolic blood pressure at rest. Although there are a few well-defined genetic, hormonal, and mechanical causes of hypertension (so-called **secondary hypertension**, see Table 7.4), in most cases hypertension occurs for currently unknown reasons. This is termed **essential hypertension**.

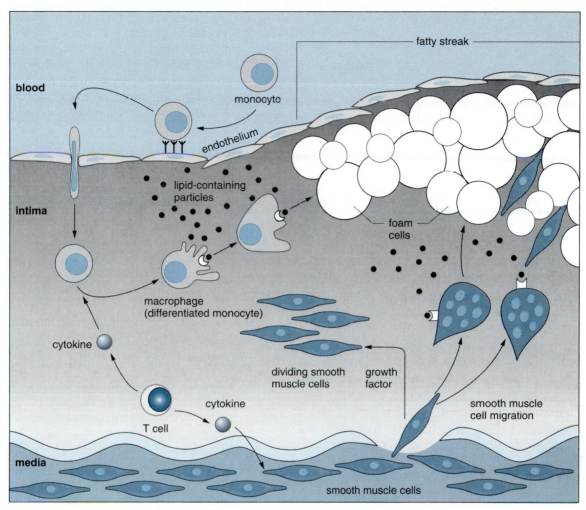

FIGURE 7.20. Formation of a fatty streak in an artery. Following vascular injury, monocytes bind to the endothelium, cross to the subendothelial space, and become tissue macrophages. The macrophages take up oxidized LDL, at which point they are called *foam cells*. The macrophages release cytokines, which have two different effects. First, they activate even more macrophages. Second, the cytokines cause smooth muscle proliferation. The proliferated smooth muscle cells migrate to the subendothelial space where they secrete collagen, take up LDL, and may themselves be transformed into foam cells. *(Adapted, with permission, from Hajjar, D.P. and Nicholson, A.C. (1995). Atherosclerosis. Am. Scientist. 83:460.)*

TABLE 7.4 SECONDARY CAUSES OF HYPERTENSION

	Percentage of population
Essential hypertension	91
Renal hypertension	
Renovascular	3
Parenchymal	2
Endocrine hypertension	
Primary aldosteronism	0.3
Cushing's syndrome	0.1
Pheochromocytoma	0.1
Other adrenal forms	0.2
Estrogen treatment ("pill hypertension")	3
Miscellaneous	0.3

Reproduced, with permission, from McPhee, S. et al (eds.). *Pathopathysiology of Disease* (1997). 2nd ed. Stamford, CT, Appleton & Lange, p. 270, as modified from Williams, G.H. and Braunwald, E. (1987). Hypertensive vascular disease. in Braunwald, E. et al (eds.) *Harrison's Principles of Internal Medicine*, 11th ed. New York, McGraw-Hill.

A number of hypotheses have tried to relate essential hypertension to dysfunction of normal mechanisms of salt, water, and blood pressure regulation. However, these remain unproven at present. Regardless of its underlying mechanism of origin, the pathophysiological importance of hypertension is that it is a cause of accelerated atherosclerosis resulting in coronary artery disease, stroke, and renal failure.

The importance of recognizing secondary hypertension is that it becomes possible to treat the underlying disorder and, potentially, cure a problem that would otherwise require life-long therapy (with its own attendant risks).

Furthermore, secondary hypertension is likely to be more resistant to therapy not directed to its underlying cause, than is the case for most patients with essential hypertension.

Coronary artery disease

Regardless of the specific mechanisms by which atherosclerosis of coronary vessels oc-cur, the net result is that the myocardium does not get the blood flow it needs to provide adequate oxygen and nutrients and remove wastes. This condition of oxygen and blood flow insufficiency is known as **ischemia**.

Sometimes inadequacy of coronary blood flow is a gradual process manifest initially upon exertion (e.g., climbing stairs) or redistribution of blood flow (e.g., to the gastrointestinal tract during a meal). The patient then often experiences ischemic pain, termed **angina**. This is a warning that the patient has coronary artery disease, that progression of the underlying disease is likely to result in more and more frequent symptoms with milder and milder exertion as a precipitant, and that there is an increased likelihood of a catastrophic coronary occlusive event. As much as 70% of coronary ischemia may be painless, particularly in patients with diabetes mellitus where neuropathy can impair this warning sign of ischemia.

Other times, the loss of adequacy of blood flow is a sudden occlusive event, again with or without pain. This may be brought on by the propensity of an atherosclerotic plaque to be the nidus for formation of a blood clot formation, a common precipitant of a **myocardial infarction** or heart attack. Another less common mechanism of acute myocardial oxygen insufficiency is **coronary artery spasm**, focal vasoconstriction of a coronary vessel due to release of mediators such as histamine, seratonin, catecholamines and endothelial-derived factors.

Sometimes other factors can exacerbate the situation. For example, someone with an aortic valve that fails to open properly will have to generate very high pressures to maintain a normal cardiac output. Heart muscle, like all muscle, responds to the demand for extra work with **hypertrophy** — increase in the number and size of myocytes and their mass of contractile fibers — until a new steady state is achieved with adequate cardiac output, but at much higher pressures. Not only will the higher pressures result in hypertension that accelerates atherosclerosis, but the hypertrophy of cardiac muscle means that oxygen demand will be higher and therefore that ischemia will occur earlier in the course of progression of atherosclerosis.

Likewise, the patient with poorly controlled hypertension, in addition to accelerating the process of atherogenesis, has an increased afterload. This creates more work for the heart, in order to maintain any given cardiac output. The increased workload also means they are at greater risk of ischemia from any given degree of atherosclerosis. Thus, control of hypertension not only slows the long-term progression of atherosclerosis, it diminishes the short-term risk of myocardial ischemia and its complications (see later). The consequences of ischemia on function of the myocardium depend on the length of time before return of adequate perfusion (see previous discussion of myocardial stunning and hibernation).

When ischemia results in infarction, stunning, or hibernation, the heart loses some of its ability to maintain cardiac output, and more and more blood is left in the heart at the end of systole. In the short run, this increases the pressure in the pulmonary veins. At first, the myocardial response follows Starling's law of the heart: increased myocardial stretch accommodates the extra volume, which moves the heart to a more efficient part of the Starling curve (e.g., as is normally the case in vigorous exercise). However, since the underlying trigger was ischemia due to atherosclerosis, the situation is often unstable and progressing from bad to worse. Soon the heart may be stretched further, to a less efficient part of the Starling curve. But this only worsens the heart's ability to maintain cardiac output, given severe limitations in coronary artery perfusion. The result is also a further increase in pulmonary venous pressure. Eventually the hydrostatic pressure in the pulmonary veins can exceed the oncotic pressure and clearance mechanisms and result in pooling of fluid in the alveolar space, a condition known as pulmonary edema, a manifestation of heart failure. Eventually also, the overstretched myocardium starts to dilate. Myocytes die through apoptosis, and the heart is "remodeled" in a pathological way that results in inability to achieve a good ejection fraction. This syndrome is termed **ischemic cardiomyopathy**, and is another route to heart failure (see Figure 7.21).

Clinical Pearl

○ Lipoprotein (a), called *lipoprotein little a,* is a subspecies of lipoprotein that has been found to vary enormously in different populations and appears to be an independent risk factor for coronary artery disease. It consists of an LDL particle associated with another protein that has homology to a protease that normally inhibits clot formation. One hypothesis is that lipoprotein (a) is particularly atherogenic because it blocks the protease from preventing clot formation in the neighborhood of atherosclerotic plaques. This double negative action (inhibition of an inhibitor of clot formation) may promote clot formation. While promising, the role of lipoprotein (a) measurement in screening the general population for cardiovascular risk factors remains experimental and controversial at present.

Ischemia that triggers angina can also trigger either abnormal cardiac electrical conduction, termed **dysrhythmia**, or abnormal cardiac muscle contraction resulting in **heart failure**.

Dysrhythmia

The normal cardiac conduction system is crucial for the optimal efficiency of cardiac pump

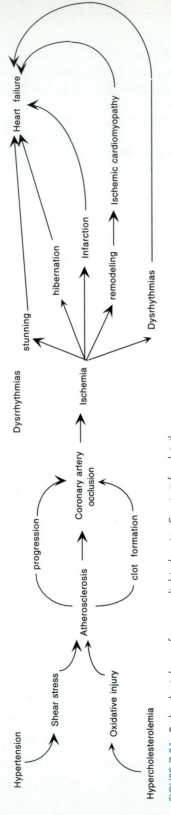

FIGURE 7.21. Pathophysiology of myocardial ischemia. See text for details.

function. A dysrhythmia makes the pump function inefficiently. At the very least, this inefficiency increases the work the heart has to perform and could cause myocardial ischemia. Often, a dysrhythmia results in a fall in cardiac output, sometimes to levels incompatible with life.

Dysrhythmias are of many different types, because of a plethora of mechanisms. They include the following:

- **Tachydysrhythmias** in which the heart beats too fast to fill effectively during diastole.
- **Bradydysrhythmias** in which the heart beats too slowly to maintain cardiac output, including **complete heart block** in which transmission of impulses from atria to ventricles is lost. With complete heart block, the ventricles beat at their own intrinsic rate rather than being entrained by an action potential originating at the SA node. Not only is this beating uncoordinated, inefficient, and generally inadequate to maintain cardiac output, it has the propensity to degenerate to an even less functional rhythm, such as **ventricular fibrillation**, in which the heart muscle contraction is so uncoordinated as to have no cardiac output.

Besides myocardial ischemia, dysrhythmias can be triggered by congenital aberrations of the cardiac conduction system, abnormal stretch, irritation of heart muscle (e.g., by ischemia itself or by drugs, including alcohol), or endocrine or autonomic nervous system disorders.

Heart failure

Heart failure is the inability to maintain cardiac output despite adequate venous preload (the filling pressure in the vena cava just as it enters the heart). Classically, the patient has shortness of breath (**dyspnea**), especially if heart failure develops rapidly, and fatigue, especially if the heart fails more gradually.

Left-sided heart failure results in elevated pulmonary venous pressure as the blood that failed to be pumped backs up into the pulmonary vessels. The elevated pulmonary venous (hydrostatic) pressure, in turn, results in increased interstitial fluid, impaired gas exchange, and hypoxia.

Right-sided heart failure results in elevated systemic venous pressure, often manifest as hepatic engorgement with blood and pedal edema.

In addition to the consequences of backup of blood, heart failure results in a fall in cardiac output. When mild, this may manifest as weakness. When severe, this can result in poor perfusion of tissues, especially the kidneys.

Clinical Pearl

○ Patients with heart and renal disease often walk a fine line between failure of one or the other. Worsening of renal function can sometimes be due to either overtreatment of heart failure (e.g., excessive doses of diuretics) or undertreatment (with insufficient cardiac output to maintain renal perfusion). In these patients careful attention must be paid to other signs of heart failure (S_3; rales, crackling sounds heard on listening to the lungs through a stethoscope), elevated jugular venous pressure, dehydration (skin tenting, low blood pressure, thirst), and the possibility of confounding variables (e.g., Did the patient start taking an over-the-counter nonsteroidal antiinflammatory drug such as ibuprofen which would worsen renal blood flow?). Based on this assessment, a cautious change in medicine regimen (e.g., decreasing diuretics versus increasing afterload-reducing vasodilators) may be necessary to empirically optimize both cardiac and renal function.

Heart failure can occur because of either systolic or diastolic dysfunction. In **systolic dysfunction**, the contractility of the left ventricle is impaired. In **diastolic dysfunction**, the ability of the ventricle to relax so that filling can occur at normal pressures during diastole is compromised. Most patients have a combination of systolic and diastolic dysfunction as the cause of heart failure.

Systolic dysfunction

Three compensatory mechanisms normally prevent systolic dysfunction or work to correct it.

1. Frank-Starling mechanism, with increased stretch to improve contractility
2. Increased heart rate due to release of catecholamines and sympathetic stimulation
3. Hypertrophy of the ventricle

All of these mechanisms will augment cardiac output. However, each is transient and unless the underlying cause of systolic dysfunction is addressed, the ventricle will eventually fail.

Diastolic dysfunction

Diastolic dysfunction involves both passive and active processes. The passive component is **increased stiffness**, **with loss of compliance and decreased elastic recoil** of the left ventricle. This can occur as a result of increased deposition of collagen in normal aging and conditions such as left ventricular hypertrophy and chronic myocardial ischemia. As pressure needed to fill the left ventricle increases, atrial hypertrophy can also passively impair ventricular filling.

The active component of diastolic dysfunction is **impaired rate and degree of left ventricular relaxation**. Left ventricular diastolic relaxation proceeds as calcium is released from binding sites on troponin-C, which allows dissociation of the actin-myosin cross-bridges. Early in diastole, impaired relaxation diminishes the magnitude of the atrial-to-ventricular pressure gradient, hence the ventricle fills more slowly and at higher pressure. Late in diastole, impaired relaxation makes the ventricle more dependent on atrial kick for adequate filling.

Several factors contribute to delayed ventricular relaxation:

- Calcium uptake by the sarcoplasmic reticulum needed for relaxation is energy dependent. Any process, such as ischemia, that decreases ATP levels will impair relaxation.
- Hypertrophy of the left ventricle will impair myocardial contractile protein dissociation.
- Regional mechanical asynchrony may slow global left ventricular relaxation and impair its effectiveness.
- Hypertension, by increasing the work the ventricle has to perform, results in ventricular hypertrophy, which can cause both increased stiffness and decreased relaxation.

Some patients with pure diastolic dysfunction have impaired filling and low cardiac output and fatigue as the predominant findings. Others fill the ventricle adequately, but at higher pressure. In these patients, pure diastolic dysfunction causes as dyspnea and pulmonary edema (as seen in systolic heart failure), because the higher pressure needed to fill the ventricle exceeds the pressure at which fluid leaks out of pulmonary capillaries into the lungs.

Clinical Pearls

Often heart failure is biventricular, with both left and right components, but sometimes it can be predominantly right-sided or left sided.

○ Patients with severe underlying lung disease often display signs of predominantly right-sided heart failure. This is because they require greater than normal right ventricular systolic pressures for normal output, due to the changes in the architecture of their pulmonary vasculature. They often have good left-sided function and little evidence for coronary artery disease, perhaps because the combination of severe lung disease and significant coronary artery disease or left-sided failure is only marginally compatible with life, and as a result, such patients tend to die sooner.

○ Patients who have had a right ventricular myocardial infarction may have impaired right ventricular pump function. As a result they can become exquisitely dependent on preload. Decreases in preload, which would have no effect on a healthy person with good right-sided ventricular contractility and cardiac output, may have a marked effect on cardiac output in the patient with an right ventricular infarct. Of course, if right ventricular output is diminished, so is left ventricular output. Thus it is crucial to provide the patient who presents with an acute right ventricular infarct with adequate intravenous volume to keep his or her central venous pressures very high, because this is the only way they can maintain right-sided cardiac output.

○ The most common cause of right-sided heart failure is left-sided heart failure.

Valvular disease

Inflammation and injury to a heart valve can result in scarring that further impedes either opening or closing of the valve, or both. The result is an increase in the workload of the heart, decrease in the efficiency of its function, or even an absolute inability to maintain cardiac output. Depending on which valve is involved, and whether the major problem is one of valve opening or closure, different signs and symptoms appear:

• If a valve cannot open properly, as occurs in **aortic stenosis**, the resulting obstruction

to flow may prevent the patient from generating an adequate cardiac output. The result may be an episode of heart failure with pulmonary congestion and hypoxia, or of loss of consciousness, termed **syncope**, due to cerebral hypoperfusion.

Aortic stenosis can also cause syncope by other mechanisms. As the left ventricle becomes more and more hypertrophied, increasing the pressure with which it tries to force blood through the stenotic aortic valve, the conduction system can become dysfunctional, resulting in **complete heart block** — failure of an action potential to be transmitted through the AV node to the ventricles, with concomitant loss in cardiac output, and with dizziness or even syncope, as a result of lack of perfusion. Also, the conduction system abnormalities and ischemia observed in aortic stenosis can trigger **ventricular tachycardia**. Because that rhythm is rapid and involves asynchronous activation of the ventricles, it is typically associated with an inadequate cardiac output — especially in a patient with aortic stenosis who has valvular obstruction to blood flow — and syncope. The same myocardial hypertrophy and increased cardiac work, together with some underlying degree of atherosclerosis, can result in myocardial ischemia, which as we have already discussed, can independently result in arrhythmias and poor perfusion.

A key feature of aortic stenosis is that it constrains the intrinsic ability of the heart to match cardiac output to venous return. Thus, it may take little in the way of stress to cause a patient with severe aortic stenosis, who has no symptoms at rest, to develop life-threatening complications.

• In **aortic regurgitation**, also called aortic insufficiency, the aortic valve is unable to close properly and therefore does not form a tight seal between the aorta and the heart. Thus, during diastole, when the ventricle relaxes, some blood flows back into the ventricle from the aorta. In effect, the ventricle gets overfilled (i.e., from both the atria and the aorta). Initially it hypertrophies in an imbalanced way, in response to the uneven increase in wall stress. Later, the ventricle dilate tremendously to accommodate the excessive end-diastolic volume. The degree of symptoms depends on how quickly the aortic regurgitation develops (i.e., whether there is time for these temporizing compensatory mechanisms to develop) and how long the process has been going on (eventually, the heart will fail).

- In **mitral stenosis**, it is the mitral valve that does not open properly. The obstruction to flow into the left ventricle protects it from overload and hypertrophy. Instead, pressures rise in the left atrium, pulmonary veins, and on the right side of the heart (with resulting enlargement and failure of those chambers).

- In **mitral regurgitation**, it is the mitral valve that does not close properly with the onset of systole. The symptoms depend on the rapidity with which disorder develops. Acute mitral regurgitation overloads the left atrium, pulmonary veins, and right side of the heart. Chronic progression of mitral regurgitation presents much like chronic aortic insufficiency, except that the murmur is heard during systole rather than diastole.

Shock

Regardless of the reason, if the heart cannot maintain the necessary cardiac output, the perfusion of many organs becomes inadequate and the patient goes into a state of cardiovascular collapse called **shock**. Shock can occur for a number of underlying reasons, each with its characteristic causes and features (see Table 7.5):

- Inadequate blood volume, as would occur after a severe injury with massive blood loss or in the setting of extreme dehydration

TABLE 7.5   SUBTYPES OF SHOCK AND KEY FEATURES

Hypovolemic shock (decreased blood volume)
   Hemorrhage
   Trauma
   Surgery
   Burns
   Fluid loss associated with vomiting or diarrhea
Distributive shock (marked vasodilation; also called vasogenic or low-resistance shock)
   Fainting (neurogenic shock)
   Anaphylaxis
   Sepsis (also causes hypovolemia due to increased capillary permeability with loss of fluid into tissues)
Cardiogenic shock (inadequate output by a diseased heart)
   Myocardial infarction
   Congestive heart failure
   Arrhythmias
Obstructive shock (obstruction of blood flow)
   Tension pneumothorax
   Pulmonary embolism
   Cardiac tumor
   Cardiac tamponade

Reproduced, with permission, from McPhee, S. et al (eds.). *Pathophysiology of Disease* (1997). 2nd ed. Stamford, CT, Appleton & Lange, pp. 274-275.

such as a patient with 20 L of diarrhea per day due to cholera. This is termed **hypovolemic shock**.

- Inappropriate volume distribution as occurs in overwhelming systemic infection or an anaphylactic reaction (see Chap. 19). Here blood volume is adequate but there has been a loss of vascular tone (e.g., due to the release of cytokines and other mediators) so that the blood volume is no longer adequate for perfusion of tissues. The general term for these conditions is **distributive shock**. Specific subsets include **septic shock** (triggered by severe systemic infection and the cytokines released under those circumstances), **anaphylactic shock** (triggered by the cytokines released in a severe allergic reaction, see Chap. 19), and **neurogenic shock** (due to sudden autonomic activity resulting in vasodilation and pooling of blood in the veins).

- Inappropriate cardiac output as occurs after a massive myocardial infarction with pump failure. This is termed **cardiogenic shock**.
- Inappropriate cardiac output for reasons other than cardiac pump failure, as occurs after a massive pulmonary embolus blocking venous return to the heart, or with severe constrictive pericarditis or critical aortic stenosis. This is termed **obstructive shock**.

Regardless of its cause, if untreated, shock quickly results in multiorgan failure, which rapidly becomes irreversible, leading to death.

Typical findings that characterize the progression from the reversible to the irreversible phases of shock include the following:

- Cerebral hypoperfusion and coma (see Chap. 18).
- Pulmonary vascular congestion, pulmonary edema, and the acute respiratory distress syndrome (see Chap. 8).
- Renal insufficiency progressing to acute tubular necrosis and eventually irreversible acute renal failure (see Chap. 9).

Figure 7.22 summarizes the physiological responses to hypovolemic shock.

Review Questions

25. What are the roles of shear stress and oxidized LDL in the pathogenesis of atherosclerotic plaques?
26. What is complete heart block?
27. What is the difference between systolic and diastolic dysfunction in heart failure?
28. What are some secondary causes of hypertension?
29 Why is it important to identify secondary causes of hypertension?
30. Name four symptoms of aortic stenosis and explain why they develop.

31. Name four categories of shock.
32. What are the features that characterize the progression of shock to the irreversible stage, regardless of its type?

From physiology to medicine: clinical cardiology

We have seen how coronary artery disease is a common process that gives rise to many different disease manifestations of ischemia (e.g., angina, infarction, dysrythmias, heart failure). The immediate physiological issue in a patient with coronary artery disease, is how to optimize myocardial oxygen supply, while minimizing the work that the heart has to do. Current approaches to this problem are as follows:

- Attempt to reverse the underlying atherosclerosis by instituting a very low-fat diet (no more than 10% of total calories as fat, see Ref. 3)
- Treat the patient with drugs to prevent progression of atherosclerosis (e.g., cholesterol-lowering agents) or thrombosis (e.g., aspirin)
- Treat the patient with drugs that decrease the work done by the heart (β-adrenergic blockers or calcium channel blockers)
- Treat the patient with drugs that improve coronary artery blood flow (sublingual nitroglycerine)
- Insert a catheter into an acutely occluded coronary artery and infuse enzymes that dissolve blood clots (**thrombolysis**), after which the patient is treated with anticoagulants for a period to prevent reformation of the clot. To be successful, this therapy must be initiated within a matter of hours after a patient develops the signs and symptoms of coronary artery occlusion (e.g., chest pain and classical ECG findings). Usually this is confirmed by **cardiac catheterization**, which involves squirting some dye into the heart to

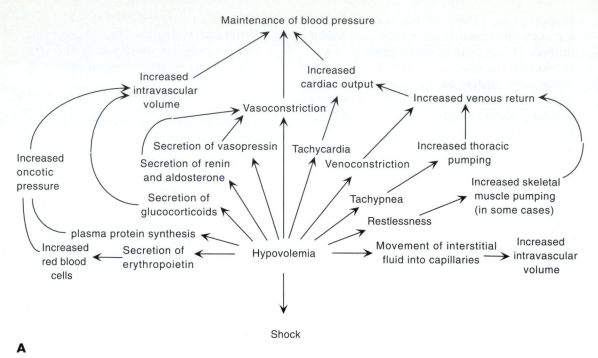

A

FIGURE 7.22. Physiological responses to hypovolemia. Hypovolemia, and the resultant hypoperfusion of tissues, activate a number of compensatory mechanisms (A). Some of these mechanisms in turn have multiple contributing factors. Thus, for example, arteriolar vasoconstriction is itself activated by multiple mechanisms (B), which work over different timescales to correct the perfusion deficit. If the compensatory mechanisms indicated in A are insufficient to maintain blood pressure, the patient will go into shock. (A. Adapted, with permission, from Kusumoto, F. (1997). in McPhee et al. eds. 2nd ed. Stamford, CT, Appleton & Lange, pp. 274-275. B. Adapted, with permission, from Guyton, A.C. and Hall, J.E. Textbook of Medical Physiology, 9th ed. Philadelphia, Saunders, p. 235.)

demonstrate an acute blockage prior to infusing the clot-lysing enzymes. The use of a new class of drugs (inhibitors of glycoprotein IIb/IIIa, the fibrinogen receptor on platelets) is an important new approach to reversal of clot formation in the setting of acute myocardial infarctions. These drugs are designed to block platelet aggregation and thereby prevent an important early step in development of many cases of myocardial infarction.

• Use of a mechanical method to break up a partial or complete atherosclerotic or thrombotic lesion that is causing a fixed obstruction to blood flow. Typically this involves inflating a small balloon at the end of a catheter inserted into the occluded coronary artery, a procedure termed **angioplasty**. Often these procedures are done in conjunction with placement of a **stent**, a piece of tubing that serves to maintain patency of the vessel. However, restenosis remains a significant problem (see Frontiers, in Sec. 6).

• Use of a surgical method to graft a vessel that allows blood to flow around the point of structural obstruction, a procedure termed **coronary artery bypass grafting**. Often sepa-

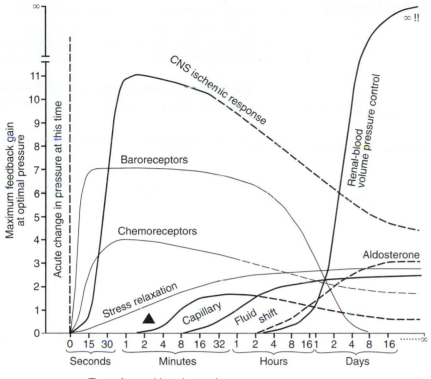

B

FIGURE 7.22 — (continued)

rate grafts are used to bypass obstruction in 2, 3, or even 4 vessels in such a procedure.
- Treat the patient with drugs for complications that are related to ischemia, such as dysrhythmia, heart failure, and cardiomyopathy.
- A patient with heart failure may be treated with digoxin to increase contractility, an afterload reducing agent (arterial vasodilator) and a preload-reducing venous dilator (nitrates) to improve systolic function. Echocardiographic evidence of poor relaxation of ventricular muscle would suggest that diastolic dysfunction contributes substantially to the patient's heart failure) and a different drug regimen may be selected (e.g., a calcum channel blocker).

- In some patients, devices are implanted to deliver a sizable electric shock when a dysrhythmia is sensed. In other patients, **electrical pacemakers** are implanted to deliver an artificial stimulus to replace, back up, or bypass a dysfunctional SA or AV node.
- Nonprocedural and nonpharmacological approaches such as stress reduction through meditation, positive relationships, and exercise.

Depending on the precise "weak link in the chain" in the physiology of any given individual patient, the underlying problem of heart disease can be manifest in different ways, which in turn, modifies the treatment provided.

6. FRONTIERS IN CARDIOVASCULAR RESEARCH

Mouse models for human atherosclerosis

Small animal models of human disease are valuable in that it is possible to carry out in vivo experiments that could not be done ethically on humans, to allow better understanding of disease pathophysiology and preliminary screening of drugs prior to (more expensive) testing in humans. However, the wild-type mouse seems much less susceptible to atherosclerosis than are humans. One approach to developing mouse model systems for atherosclerosis has been to generate "knockout" mice in which sophisticated molecular techniques using homologous recombination generate animals in which both alleles of a particular gene have been deleted.

When apoprotein E deficient mice were created by this means, they were found to have dramatically elevated cholesterol with development of heart disease. Subsequently it was found that crossing these apoprotein E deficient mice with transgenic mice (that is, mice into which an exogenous gene has been introduced into the germline) expressing elevated levels of particular human lipoproteins such as apoprotein A_1 resulted in protection from atherogenicity. Thus, model systems now exist in which antiatherosclerotic physiology can be explored in vivo and used for the rational design of novel therapies that may ultimately be used in humans (see Refs. 4, 5).

Molecular genetics of long Q-T syndromes

The Q-T interval of the ECG can be prolonged in a number of fairly common conditions including hypokalemia, tricyclic antidepressant overdose, and hypothermia. This is a result of prolongation of the action potential and/or delayed ventricular repolarization. These patients are at increased risk for ventricular tachycardia, a life-threatening arrhythmia caused by spontaneous depolarizations as a result of reactivation of sodium or calcium channels.

The long Q-T syndromes are rare genetic disorders in which individuals are at risk for the development of ventricular tachycardia.

Modern molecular techniques were used to identify the gene defect in a subset of patients with long QT syndrome. A 3 amino acid deletion in a specific subtype of sodium channel was identified as the molecular lesion. As a result of this change, there is delayed sodium channel inactivation and altered voltage dependence manifest as increased susceptibility to this arrhythmia (see Ref. 6).

Using this insight, it will now be possible to screen patients and identify those at risk so that they may be monitored more closely or treated prophylactically and followed epidemiologically to determine the best management strategies.

Moreover, model systems can now be constructed (e.g., in transgenic and knockout mice) by which this and other molecular defects that result in arrhythmias can be studied and used to design and test new drugs to prevent the more common conditions in which ventricular tachycardia is seen.

Ironically, since the United States lacks a national health insurance program, such fruits of science could actually be used to harm patients—by allowing insurance companies and HMOs to identify "unprofitable" patients who are more likely to need expensive care in order to deny them coverage or charge them exorbitant premiums. The net result would be that those who most need care would likely not get it.

Ischemia, angiogenesis, and the heart as an organ rather than a pump

Historically, the heart has been viewed as a mechanical pump. Although this concept has been useful and is still of teaching value, it is limited. In our mechanical world, pumps do not sculpt and maintain themselves by a programmed process of development, maturation, and functional renewal. But our bodies do, at least when we are young. The challenge of degenerative disease is to understand why normal repair and renewal stops or goes awry when we get older.

In the science fiction TV series "Babylon 5," the alien spaceships made with Vorlon "organic" technology had the capacity to automatically self-diagnose and repair themselves. This seems to be a much better way of thinking about the organs of the body, such as the heart, rather than in nonliving, mechanical terms as a pump, as we commonly do. If we better understood the fundamental mechanisms by which the heart and its vasculature were formed, perhaps we could intervene far more effectively than we can now to relieve ischemia, repair damage, and improve function.

Mechanism of blood vessel formation

Formation of new blood vessels involves multiple processes. The first step is dissolution of the basement membrane matrix that underlies the endothelium. Then endothelial cells must migrate, reattach, and proliferate. Finally, the endothelial cells must form a tube and lengthen to become a blood vessel. For larger vessels, smooth muscle migration is necessary as well.

A family of growth factors have been described that play various important roles in initial blood vessel development of various tissues of the body, including the heart (see Table 7.3). Based on encouraging animal studies, clinical trials have been initiated to determine whether intracoronary artery injection of various growth factors might improve blood flow and myocardial function in patients whose coronary artery disease is inoperable (e.g., because their disease is too

extensive, involves vessels too small to be bypassed, or because they would be unlikely to survive surgery, given their other medical problems) (see Refs. 7–9).

Mysteries of angiogenesis

A big problem is that we do not understand key processes of heart muscle and blood vessel development, including (just to name a few):

- The role of inflammation. Inflammation accompanies myocardial ischemia. Inflammation is seen in conditions where new blood vessels form. If we understood which inflammatory cells are making or triggering other cells to make which cytokines and how these products interact, we might be able to improve on the normal blood vessel-forming response, which never quite seems to be as good as what was formed originally.
- The way different growth factors interact. Potent endothelial mitogens have been discovered. They appear to interact in complex ways that may account for differences in response to ischemia versus infarction and may involve nongrowth effects of the growth factors.
- The role of necrosis versus apoptosis. Historically, myocardial ischemia has been conceptualized largely in terms of risk for necrosis. But studies suggest that **apoptosis**, nonnecrotic programmed cell death, may be involved particularly where a consequence of heart disease is disordered structure (e.g., hypertrophy or dilatation) and function (decreased cardiac output). How do these changes in structure and function convince cardiac myocytes to shrivel up and die in a programmed fashion (see Refs. 10 and 11)?

Hypercholesterolemia, antioxidants, and the endothelium in heart disease

The current framework for understanding the development of atherosclerosis emphasizes the effects of cytokines in the endothelium of large arterial vessels as a consequence of shear stress and oxidized LDL (see Sec. 5, Atherosclerosis). Once plaques have formed, ischemia can be understood to occur via occlusion and increased risk of clot formation.

However, several lines of evidence suggest that atherogenesis is an even more complex process than might have been imagined. First, studies suggest that, not only does hypercholesterolemia result in more oxidized LDL, but hypercholesterolemia may impair another limb of the defense against reactive oxygen substrates (ROS) by consuming glutathione and promoting formation of peroxinitrite ($ONOO^-$). This reaction generates more damaging ROS such as $ONOO^-$ from nitric oxide, which would otherwise be a vasodilator. The result is to render the vascular endothelium more susceptible to oxidative injury and less able to vasodilate when needed (see Ref. 12).

Other studies suggest that an important dimension of ischemic injury is production of ROS upon reperfusion of ischemic tissues. If this proves to be the case, then the mechanism just outlined would provide an explanation for adding oxidative and vasoconstrictive insult to ischemic injury (see Ref. 13).

Furthermore, studies in LDL receptor-deficient mice suggest that an unexpected consequence of lack of the LDL receptor is a more intense leukocyte-endothelial cell adhesion in response to inflammatory stimuli and cytokines. This mechanism appears to be distinct from the altered expression of adhesion molecules observed in large vessels that has been implicated in the pathogenesis of atherosclerosis (see Ref. 14), suggesting that multiple mechanisms may contribute to atherogenesis.

Finally, the role of endothelins and other products of the vascular endothelium remain shrouded in provocative mystery. Endothelins are peptides secreted by the endothelium that have, at face value, contradictory effects. On the one hand, they cause intense vasoconstriction. On the other hand, they trigger nitric oxide production, which is a vasodilator. As with many other hormones, endothelins may have different effects on one tissue as compared to another, even on the same signaling pathway. Endothelins have also been implicated in affecting the balance of production of ROS and therefore may have an important role in reperfusion injury. Thus, endothelins may do different things in different places (e.g., paracrine versus endocrine) and on different timescales and in the context of different other products (which might antagonize or synergize with one action but not another; see Ref. 16).

Clearly, the interaction of cholesterol metabolism, oxidation-reduction reactions, vasoconstriction and vasodilation, and the hormones regulating these processes are a major uncharted area. We are far from the last — or definitive — word on any of these dimensions to the problem of cardiovascular health and disease.

Estrogen and the heart: some unexpected features

A major controversy in medicine has surrounded postmenopausal estrogen supplementation. On the heart, estrogen has both "good" and "bad" effects. On the one hand, estrogen promotes blood clot formation (in part, through effects on liver protein synthesis, see Chap. 4) and also likely increases the risk of both endometrial and breast cancer. On the other hand, estrogens lower LDL and raise HDL, a change in lipid profile that may protect against the development of atherosclerosis and subsequent heart attacks. Estrogen also has effects on vascular reactivity including effects on endothelin secretion, nitric oxide production, LDL oxidation, and ion channel activity.

Much of the increased cancer risk of estrogens is believed to be eliminated by adding progesterone to estrogen. Until recently, the effect of progesterone supplementation on the cardiovascular risk was unclear.

Data suggest that progesterone does modify the cardiovascular effects of estrogen, but the direction of the effect depends on which of two different progestins is used. These findings raise the possibility that there may exist in nature estrogens and progestins that have subsets of the spectrum of effects associated with one steroid or the other. Thus, a report finds that isoflavones, compounds with a structure similar to estrogen, but which bind weakly to the classical estrogen receptor, may provide cardioprotective effects without effects on breast or uterus (see Refs. 17 and 18).

Other data suggest that there are not only multiple different steroids and steroid-like compounds, but that many steroid hormone effects may be mediated through mechanisms other than that of the classical steroid hormone receptors (see Refs. 19 and 20).

Infections and heart disease

Our thinking about heart disease is dominated by the paradigm that the major risk factors are serum cholesterol (largely influenced by diet), smoking, age, family history, hypertension, and diabetes. Yet these risk factors are absent in nearly 30% of patients with myocardial infarction. What accounts for heart disease in this subset of patients? Whatever that risk factor might be, is it an unrecognized co-factor in patients with the known risk factors?

The role of infectious organisms in human disease has seen movement both in the direction of ascribing an infectious etiology to new diseases (e.g., *Helicobacter pilori* in peptic ulcer) and in showing that some diseases previously thought to be due to infections have a different etiology (e.g., the failure to identify a virus as the cause of prion disorders). The complexity of this question includes the semantic issues of just what does infectious mean and just what is an organism.

With respect to heart disease, two different notions have been raised. First, prior cytomegalovirus infection has been implicated as predisposing to restenosis patients who undergo angioplasty for coronary artery occlusion (see Ref. 21). Second, *Chlamydia* infections have been implicated as a possible trigger of myocardial infarction by enhancing plaque destabilization and disruption (see Ref. 22). The common (and more conventional) theme in both of these ideas is that inflammation is both an important response to infection and contributor to heart disease. Possibly then, the proven value of aspirin in prevention of heart attack is due to more than just its antithrombotic effects.

7. HOW DOES AN UNDERSTANDING OF NORMAL PHYSIOLOGY PROVIDE INSIGHT INTO THE INITIAL CASE PRESENTATION?

Let us revisit N.P., a vigorous 74-year-old retired legal secretary with a syncopal episode.

How did an understanding of the physiology of the heart assist the physician in arguing on behalf of Ms. P.'s best interests in this case?

The physician recognized that several of Ms. P.'s signs and symptoms (syncope, angina, dysrhythmia, and conduction system abnormalities) are all commonly seen as a consequence of aortic stenosis. Furthermore, the murmur got softer because the severity of the obstruction increased over time and, as a result, the flow across the value was decreased (i.e., causing a fall in cardiac output). This was a sign of worsening disease.

The presence of these various symptoms of aortic stenosis should not be taken as an argument against replacing the patient's valve, because they are likely to improve or disappear when the aortic stenosis is corrected. This is especially true since Ms. P. has few medical problems other than those that are, potentially, a consequence of her valvular disease. Contrary to the HMO's argument in this case, correction of the one structural problem (aortic stenosis) might actually make many of the patient's other medical problems get better — and the need to correct the aortic stenosis was getting urgent.

Of course, no medical intervention is without risks. Valve replacement surgery is a major procedure, and the need for postoperative, life-long anticoagulation places the patient at increased risk for future complications. In contrast, without this intervention a patient with severe aortic stenosis is sure to die, most likely within the next year. This is precisely why the health professional must focus on being the advocate of the best interests of the individual patient. To discharge this responsibility competently requires, to the greatest extent possible, that the health professional be free from financial incentives to either treat or not treat. Either could cloud his or her judgment as to what is best for the patient.

SUMMARY AND REVIEW OF KEY CONCEPTS

1. The heart is a 4-chamber pump, connected by valves, which drives the circulation of blood in coordination with the vasculature.
2. Compared to other forms of muscle, cardiac striated muscle has the following:

- Action potentials with a longer period of depolarization, reflecting differences in plasma membrane channels, and a dependence on extracellular calcium to determine force of contraction.

- Automaticity due to spontaneous depolarization of pacemaker cells. This depolarization is caused by back leak of ions to the membrane potential threshold.
- A conduction system composed of specialized cells that entrains the depolarization of heart muscle to provide coordinated contraction of atria and ventricles for efficient pump function.
- More mitochondria, reflecting their need for oxidative phosphorylation, to generate the ATP that allows them to beat regularly for an entire lifetime. This is also why atherosclerosis is commonly first manifested through ischemia in the heart.

3. The ECG allows one to get a surface diagnostic assessment of the heart's conduction system. From this recording one can identify rate and rhythm disturbances, evidence for ischemia or infarction, and metabolic abnormalities.
4. The cardiac cycle can be analyzed in terms of ventricular contraction, termed *systole*, and ventricular relaxation, termed *diastole*. Crucial terms for understanding ventricular function are preload, the filling pressure in diastole, and afterload, the pressure against which the ventricle must work during systole.
5. The Frank-Starling law of the heart reflects the principle that, over the normal range, increased stretch of cardiac muscle fibers better aligns the actin-myosin cross-bridges, thereby increasing the force of contraction. This allows the left side of the heart to accommodate any changes in the amount of blood pumped by the right side. Conversely, an overly stretched heart muscle (e.g., in a patient with dilated cardiomyopathy) may show worsened functional efficiency (decreased cardiac output) with further increased stretch and may benefit from preload and/or afterload reduction with vasodilator drugs.

6. Arteries, capillaries, veins, and lymphatics are the four types of vessels that carry extracellular fluid between the heart and the peripheral tissues. The arteries are muscular, high-compliance vessels that get blood to the tissues. The capillaries are narrow vessels that allow intimate contact exchange of nutrients and wastes between blood and tissues. The veins are conduits back to the heart and capacitance vessels in which excess blood is stored at rest. Lymphatic vessels maintain homeostasis of plasma between tissues and blood vessels.

7. Starling forces provide the basis for fluid dynamics between blood and tissues. The most prominent of these are the hydrostatic force pushing fluid out of blood vessels and the colloid osmotic force holding fluid in the blood vessel. The lymphatics serve to normally maintain the zero sum between these forces without which edema develops.

8. Blood flow is determined by blood pressure, compliance, length, and pressure difference between the ends of a vessel, diameter of the vessel, and viscosity of blood.

9. Cardiac output = heart rate × stroke volume. It is controlled by intrinsic (Frank-Starling), neurogenic, and hormonal mechanisms.

10. Vasomotor tone is important for short-term regulation of blood pressure and operates by a series of neural reflexes that monitor pressure and respond with adjustments of sympathetic innervation to vascular smooth muscle.

11. Atherosclerosis is exacerbated by hypercholesterolemia, hypertension, smoking, and other risk factors. Atherosclerosis results in coronary artery occlusion by plaque or clot and causes ischemia, which can be manifest as angina, myocardial infarction, dysrhythmias, or heart failure.

A CASE OF PHYSIOLOGICAL MEDICINE

J.D. is a 48-year-old sales representative with diabetes mellitus and inadequately treated hypertension who has recently developed shortness of breath on exertion. Two years ago she changed jobs and was denied health insurance at that time, given her preexisting condition of diabetes mellitus. Since she must pay out-of-pocket, her physician visits have been infrequent.

One day, while chasing the bus, she had an acute episode of **dyspnea**. Paramedics were called by a bystander who found her on the ground gasping for air. In the emergency room, her blood pressure was noted to be 180/100 with a heart rate of 110. On her ECG, she had sinus tachycardia with mild ST-T segment abnormalities consistent with ischemia. Acute pulmonary edema was diagnosed on chest x-ray, with a room air O_2 saturation noted to be 84%. She was treated aggressively with diuretics resulting in improvement in her O_2 saturation and dyspnea. However, she felt weak and was unable to walk, and she was admitted to the cardiac care unit to rule out a myocardial infarction and to treat her high blood pressure and congestive heart failure.

Ms. D. was quickly ruled out for myocardial infarction and was transferred to the regular ward. Unfortunately, her lack of insurance caused important aspects of her care to "fall through the cracks." An echocardiogram to assess systolic versus diastolic function was not performed. Ms. D. was placed on the cheapest available medicines for heart failure, which were digoxin and a powerful arteriolar vasodilator. She was discharged with an outpatient clinic appointment.

However, Ms. D. felt far worse on her new medicines than she had previously. She had no energy and felt listless. She woke up too late in the morning to get the three buses she needed to take to get to work on time. Shortly thereafter, she was laid off. Scared and despondent, she saw a physician who spent 12 min with her as a new patient, ordered no testing to evaluate her cardiac function, and simply added an antidepressant.

Two weeks later, feeling more short of breath on exertion than ever, Ms. D. had an argument with her mother, who had berated her for losing her job. That night she took an overdose of antidepressants and was discovered in the morning unresponsive by her roommate, who called the paramedics.

In the emergency room, her uninsured status was noted, and the admitting physician was advised by an administrator to "keep this in mind." Ms. D. was not placed in a bed with a cardiac monitor. This was justified on the grounds that there were no acute changes in her cardiac exam. Unfortunately, a single ECG was done on admission, and serial studies were not performed. They would have demonstrated progressively increased prolongation of the Q-T interval, a known side effect of tricyclic antidepressant overdose.

That night, probably as a complication of her Q-T prolongation, Ms. D. had an episode of ventricular tachycardia. But since she was in an unmonitored bed, neither that dysrhythmia nor its subsequent degeneration into ventricular fibrillation was detected by the hospital staff. Ms. D. was found dead in bed the next morning.

QUESTIONS

1. What physiological explanations might you give for Ms. D.'s initial dyspnea and pulmonary edema?
2. What are the determinants of left ventricular function that might be adjusted to improve cardiac output in such a patient?
3. Explain why Ms. D. might have become subjectively worse with medical therapy for her heart failure.

4. Why does prolongation of the Q-T interval result in an increased risk of ventricular dysrhythmias?
5. What role, if any, might Ms. D.'s preexisting conditions of hypertension and diabetes mellitus have played in the subsequent development of congestive heart failure?

ANSWERS

1. Either systolic or diastolic dysfunction, or both may explain Ms. D.'s initial dyspnea and pulmonary edema.
2. Decreasing ischemia and improving ventricular relaxation would likely have improved her cardiac output; improved ventricular compliance and elasticity are determinants of left ventricular function that would likely improve with these measures.
3. If a significant component of Ms. D.'s heart failure was due to diastolic dysfunction, digoxin, which increases myocardial contractility by increasing intracellular calcium, might actually further delay ventricular relaxation in diastole. A powerful arteriolar vasodilator would result in a reflex tachycardia, further shortening the time of diastole and impairing ventricular filling even more. Fluid retention, another reflex effect of vasodilators can further elevate end-diastolic pressures.
4. Prolongation of the Q-T interval reflects the presence of a longer plateau phase of the ventricular action potential during which reopening of sodium or calcium channels could trigger spontaneous depolarizations, setting in motion the dysrhythmia.
5. Diabetes mellitus increases the risk of atherosclerosis and coronary artery disease. Hypertension results in ventricular hypertrophy and an increased incidence of diastolic dysfunction.

Also (but apparently, not in Ms. D.) hypertensive cardiomyopathy can result in a dilated heart with low cardiac output due to pure systolic dysfunction.

Perhaps if insurance issues had not interfered with her care, Ms. D. would have received proper assessment of her cardiac status (e.g., an echocardiogram to evaluate left ventricular function and an imaging study to assess ischemia). Perhaps if her health care providers had been less rushed and more comfortable thinking physiologically, they would have recognized the error of treating her without regard to her symptoms. Also, they might have placed her in a monitored bed and performed serial ECGs, which would have allowed them to recognize the prolongation of the Q-T interval or, at least, detect the onset of dysrhythmia before her death.

References and suggested readings

REVIEWS

1. Patterson, J.H. and Adams, K.F. (1996). Pathophysiology of heart failure: Changing perceptions. *Pharmacotherapy* 16:29S-36S.
2. Chien, K.R. et al. (1997). Toward molecular strategies for heart disease: Past, present and future. *Jpn. Circ. J.* 61;91-118.
3. Ornish, D. et al. (1998). Intensive lifestyle changes for reversal of coronary heart disease. *JAMA*, Dec 16, 280:2001-2007.

FRONTIERS REFERENCES

4. Plump, A.S. et al. (1992). Severe hypercholesterolemia and atherosclerosis in apolipoprotein E-deficient mice created by homologous recombination in ES cells. *Cell* 71:343-353.
5. Paszty, C. et al. (1994). Apolipoprotein A1 transgene corrects apolipoprotein E deficiency-induced atherosclerosis in mice. *J. Clin. Invest.* 94:899-903.

6. Wang, Q. et al. (1995). SCN5A mutations associated with an inherited cardiac arrhythmia, long QT syndrome. *Cell* 80:805-811.
7. Ware, A. and Simons, M. (1997). Angiogenesis in ischemic heart disease. *Nat. Med.* 3:158-160.
8. Carmeliet, P. et al. (1996). Abnormal blood vessel development and lethality in embryos lacking a single VEGF allele. *Nature* 380:435-439.
9. Isner, J.M. et al. (1996). Clinical evidence of angiogenesis after arterial gene transfer of phVEGF165 in patient with ischemic limb. *Lancet* 348, 370-374.
10. McLellan, W.R. and Schneider, M.D. (1997). Death by design. Programmed cell death in cardiovascular biology and disease. *Circ. Res.* 81:137-144.
11. Teiger, E. et al. (1996). Apoptosis in pressure overload-induced heart hypertrophy in the rat. *J. Clin. Invest.* 97:2891-2897.
12. Ma, X.L. et al. (1997). Hypercholesterolemia impairs a detoxification mechanism against peroxynitrite and renders the vascular tissue more susceptible to oxidative injury. *Circ. Res.* 80:894-901.
13. Maxwell, S.R.J. and Lip, G.Y.H (1997). Reperfusion injury: A review of the pathophysiology, clinical manifestations and therapeutic options. *Int. J. Card.* 58:95-117.
14. Henninger, D.D. et al. (1997). Low-density lipoprotein receptor knockout mice exhibit exaggerated microvascular responses to inflammatory stimuli. *Circ. Res.* 81:274-281.
15. Hocher, B. et al. (1997). The paracrine endothelin system: Pathophysiology and implications in clinical medicine. *Eur. J. Clin. Chem. Clin. Biochem.* 35:175-189.
16. Pernow, J. and Wang, Q-D. (1997). Endothelin in myocardial ischemia and reperfusion. *Cardiovasc. Res.* 33:518-526.
17. Foth, D. and Cline, J.M. (1998). Effects of mammalian and plant estrogens on mammary glands and uteri of macaques. *Am. J. Clin. Nutr.* 68:1413S-1417S.
18. Williams, J.K. and Adams, M.R. (1997). Estrogens, progestins, and coronary artery reactivity. *Nature Med.* 3:273-274.
19. Iafrati, M.D. et al. (1997). Estrogen inhibits the vascular injury response in estrogen receptor

alpha-deficient mice. *Nature Med.* 3:545-548.

20. Gustafsson, J-A. (1997). Estrogen receptor beta — Getting in on the action? *Nature Med.* 3:493-494.

21. Zhou, Y.F. et al. (1996). Association between prior cytomegalovirus infection and the risk of restenosis after coronary atherectomy. *N. Eng. J. Med.* 335:624-630.

22. Sumpter, M.T. and Dunn, M.I. (1997). Is coronary artery disease an infectious disease? *Chest* 112:302-303.

RESPIRATORY PHYSIOLOGY

8

1. INTRODUCTION TO RESPIRATION

Respiration is the set of processes by which:

- Air is brought into the body via the lungs (inhalation), as a result of the action of the diaphragm and other respiratory muscles under control of the central nervous system (CNS).
- Oxygen in the inspired air is carried via the bloodstream to peripheral tissues, where it is used within cells to release energy by metabolically "burning" substrates, a process called *oxidation*. The released energy is stored in chemical form (e.g., through formation of adenosine triphosphate, ATP) and later used to do useful work.
- Carbon dioxide, a waste product generated in peripheral tissues upon oxidation of energy substrates, is carried in the bloodstream back to the lungs and is removed from the body upon exhalation.

The lungs are remarkably efficient at bringing in oxygen-rich air, exchanging gases between blood and air, and releasing from the body CO_2-rich air (see Figure 8.1). The lungs are able to lower the work needed to carry out these critical processes to a level that can be easily sustained by the body, under normal conditions. The major clinical problems involving the lung function are disorders that either *impair gas exchange* or that *increase the work of breathing* needed for adequate gas exchange. In the extreme, either type of disorder is incompatible with life. When less severe, either can result in a new steady state in which the body functions but is less able to get oxygen and eliminate carbon dioxide, with impaired range of activity and quality of life.

Why is understanding respiratory physiology important for medical practice?

The following indicates the importance of respiratory physiology for clinical practice:

- Untreated, respiratory failure is incompatible with life.
- Disorders of the respiratory system, including obstructive and restrictive lung diseases, pulmonary edema, pulmonary embolism,

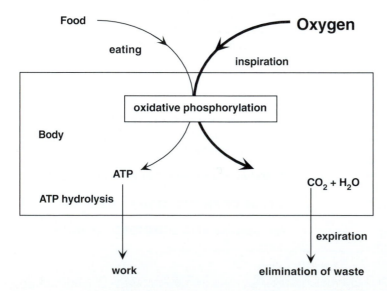

FIGURE 8.1. Role of the lungs. The primary roles of the lungs are to (a) bring in oxygen for oxidative phosphorylation by which the energy stored in food is converted to usable form (e.g., ATP) in order to do work, and (b) eliminate the carbon dioxide generated as a byproduct of this process.

and pneumonia, are major causes of morbidity and mortality throughout the world.

- The incidence of key lung diseases, including asthma, is rising. Furthermore, despite a plethora of powerful new therapeutic drugs, the mortality from asthma is rising.

- Disorders of many other organs (e.g., cardiac, renal, and infectious disease) may have life-threatening manifestations involving the respiratory system that cannot be understood or effectively treated without an understanding of how the lungs work. For example, 1 in 5 people who die in the United States are found at autopsy to have pulmonary emboli (blood clots in the lungs) as a complication of various underlying (usually nonpulmonary) disease. In these cases, the pulmonary emboli typically hastened their deaths.

- Much of chronic lung disease is caused by activities that could be prevented, such as cigarette smoking or environmental pollution. Nevertheless, the manifestation of these diseases varies substantially from patient to patient. Thus, only 10 to 15% of smokers will develop obstructive lung disease. Presumably genetic factors serve to protect the others, but the molecular mechanisms involved remain, fundamentally, unknown.

The needs of the patient for medical attention change with progression of the natural history of lung disease. Early in the course, patient education (e.g., on the effects of smoking and "second hand" smoke, and toward smoking cessation) is paramount and there may be little else for the clinician to do besides reiterate this point (e.g., encourage smoking cessation and offer nicotine replacement medicines). Later, drug therapy for chronic bronchitis and emphysema may be necessary and considerable effort will go into adjusting medical therapy involving principles of pulmonary physiology. Finally, for a patient with end-stage disease despite maximal medical therapy, the focus of medical intervention may be chronic home or nursing care needs. An understanding of respiratory physiology allows the health care provider to readily identify the patient's current status on this continuum of pulmonary disease, meet their current needs, and more effectively anticipate changes in the future.

Case Presentation

G.N. is a 32-year-old man with a long history of mild asthma, who has recently been discharged from the hospital after his first severe asthma exacerbation, which was associated with an episode of bronchitis. On questioning, you learn that he is an intermittent smoker (up to half a pack per day), has a stressful and unpredictable part-time job as a bicycle messenger, and is sometimes homeless, renting cheap rooms in various rundown apartment buildings whenever he can. He noted that he had been feeling progressively more short of breath over the two weeks prior to hospitalization, despite use of inhaled bronchodilators. He states that when he feels well he does not use any anti-asthma medications and is more likely to smoke.

His recent hospitalization scared him much more than prior asthma attacks. He continued to get worse after arriving at the hospital, and it took much longer for him to get better than it did after his previous asthma attacks.

Apparently, he came close to being intubated (having a tube inserted into his trachea to allow mechanical ventilation to treat respiratory failure) shortly after arriving at the emergency room. He relates overhearing the physicians discussing something about "his P_{CO_2} rising from 32 to 45, while his P_{O_2} fell from the high to the low 60s on room air." He wonders why they were more concerned about him than they were about the elderly gentleman in the next bed in the emergency room, whose P_{CO_2} was "only 55"?

He also wonders why he was so sick this time. Apparently, it took 5 days of care in the hospital before he started to get well, and an additional three days before he was well enough for discharge. He feels much better and is quite motivated to prevent another exacerbation if at all possible and now wants to know what he can do to take better care of his lungs.

You take a careful history and physical examination and review the results of spirometry, which reveals an forced expiratory volume in 1 s (FEV_1)/functional vital capacity (FVC) of 0.4 on a recent clinic visit (this is a quantifiable measure of airflow obstruction, as will be discussed later). In the ER, his initial FEV_1/FVC was 0.2. You conclude that there are several possible improvements in management of his disease and have a frank discussion with him.

Review Questions

1. What is respiration?
2. Give four different reasons why understanding respiratory physiology is important.
3. Even though smoking is clearly the major cause of lung disease, why is it that many smokers do not develop lung disease over the course of a full lifetime?

2. COMPONENTS OF THE RESPIRATORY SYSTEM

The respiratory system includes the following:

1. Respiratory muscles
2. The lungs, including both airspaces and the pulmonary vasculature that make efficient gas exchange possible
3. CNS centers, which control respiration,

making adjustments in response to monitored conditions in the body

The respiratory muscles

The respiratory muscles include the diaphragm, the external and internal intercostal muscles, the muscles of the abdominal wall, and the neck muscles (e.g., scalene and sternocleidomastoid, see Figure 8.2).

Normal quiet breathing largely involves contraction of the diaphragm, which lengthens the chest cavity, creating a slight negative pressure in the pleural space, with respect to atmospheric pressure. This negative pressure allows passive expansion of the lungs with air. Relaxation of the diaphragm shortens the chest cavity, which, together with elastic recoil, compresses the lungs, forcing air out.

With forced, rapid (heavy) breathing, the rate of expiration must be increased, so additional muscle groups must be involved. In particular, the abdominal muscles contract to push the abdominal contents up against the diaphragm, thereby providing the additional force needed for rapid expiration.

Another way to expand and contract the lungs is by elevating and lowering the rib cage using the neck and intercostal muscles. Contraction of some muscle groups expands the chest cavity for maximum inspiration; contraction of other muscle groups lowers the rib cage for expiration.

In some lung diseases, the efficiency of the respiratory muscles is decreased, thereby increasing the work of breathing.

Clinical Pearl

○ A health care provider often must make a snap judgment as to the severity of a patient's difficulty breathing. Misjudgment in this situation can be a lethal error and can occur in the emergency room, in the clinic, or at night on a hospital ward.

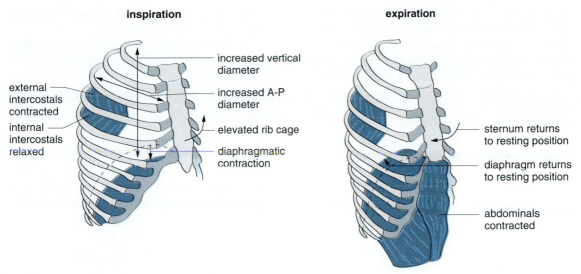

inspiration

increased vertical diameter

external intercostals contracted

increased A-P diameter

internal intercostals relaxed

elevated rib cage

diaphragmatic contraction

expiration

sternum returns to resting position

diaphragm returns to resting position

abdominals contracted

FIGURE 8.2. Inspiration and expiration. Expansion and contraction of the thoracic cage during expiration and inspiration illustrating diaphragmatic contraction, elevation of the rib cage, and function of the intercostal muscles. *(From Guyton, A.C. and Hall, J.E. (1997). Human Physiology and Mechanisms of Disease, 6th ed. Philadelphia, PA, WB Saunders, p. 312.)*

It is easy to be fooled by a patient who is not breathing very fast and is not complaining, simply because of exhaustion. Your first impression might be that the patient is in satisfactory condition — when he or she may in fact be on the way to respiratory failure, imminently requiring mechanical ventilation to prevent death. To determine whether this is the case, you need to assess the arterial blood gases (see Arterial Blood Gases and the A-a Gradient, Sec. 4, and Chap. 10). But what are your criteria for performing this test, which is invasive and painful?

○ One quick means of assessment on physical exam is to look for contraction of neck muscles and nasal flaring occurring in synchrony with breathing at rest. If present, this suggests that the patient's breathing is labored, regardless of the actual respiratory rate. Under these circumstances, failure to elevate the respiratory rate is an ominous sign that the patient may be tiring out with respiratory failure imminent. Such a patient needs to be urgently evaluated further. Another rapid, noninvasive means of assessment is with pulse oximetry, which will be discussed below (see Pulse Oximetry, Sec. 4).

The lungs

The airways of the lungs lead to a honeycomb of airspaces and capillaries separated by the interstitial space (also known as the interstitium). The interstitium is bounded by the capillary endothelium on one side and the airspace epithelium on the other. It normally contains extracellular matrix, mesenchymal cells, and a few immune cells including lymphocytes and mast cells.

The lungs are encased in a double layer of connective tissue termed the **pleura**, with one layer on the lungs and the other layer on the inner wall of the thoracic cavity. Like the pericardium of the heart, the layers of the pleura are normally separated by a small amount of lubricating fluid, which facilitates movement of the lung in the chest cavity with each cycle of inspiration and expiration. Under a variety of pathological circumstances, the volume of this fluid can increase greatly, forming a pleural effusion (see later).

Clinical Pearls

○ Very large pleural effusions can compromise the ability of the lung to expand and thereby interfere with gas exchange, but even a very small pleural effusion is clinically noteworthy. The presence of a pleural effusion on a chest x-ray is an indicator that some aspect of lung homeostasis has been disturbed.

○ Thoracentesis is a procedure in which a needle is passed between the ribs in the back allowing safe removal of a sample of the effusion. Done carefully, the risk of puncturing the lung and causing a pneumothorax (airleak into the chest cavity) is small and more than offset by the benefit of the procedure in selected patients. Such sampling often provides valuable information as to the underlying cause of the effusion and the nature of the disorder in homeostasis. Always remember to do an x-ray with the patient lying on his or her side (called a *decubitus film*) prior to performing thoracentesis, to be sure that the fluid that makes up the pleural effusion is free-flowing. Sometimes, especially with infectious or inflammatory causes of pleural effusion, the fluid can be thick, viscous, trapped, or otherwise not free-flowing. In those circumstances, it may be necessary to carry out the procedure using an imaging system (e.g., ultrasound or computed tomography, CT, scan) to guide placement of the needle.

In particular, thoracentesis must be performed on any patient with a new pleural effusion and fever, because it is important to determine whether the effusion represents a site of infection requiring drainage. The white blood cell count, protein concentration, and culture results are the most important parameters of the effusion, for which determination samples are usually sent. Failure to drain an infected pleural effusion can result in formation of an empyema (a kind of abcess). Not only can this be life-threatening, but even if it resolves on its own, the patient may be left with permanent scarring that causes severe pain and greatly increases the work of breathing (see The Work of Breathing, Sec. 5).

○ After a thoracentesis, it is necessary to get another chest x-ray to rule out pneumothorax as a complication of the procedure (see Pneumothorax, Sec. 9). Sometimes a tension pneumothorax can develop when the pressure of extravasated air acts like a straightjacket to prevent expansion and, therefore, function of the lung. The patient will be acutely short of breath (**dyspneic**), with **hypoxia** (low arterial blood pO_2), **hypercapnea** (high arterial blood pCO_2), and absent breath sounds on the affected side. Emergency placement of a chest tube (or even a simple intravenous catheter) into the affected pleural space, opened under water (so more air does not go into the thorax upon inspiration), results in release of the trapped air, allowing lung expansion.

Airspaces: airways to alveoli

Within the lungs there is a "tree" of branching airways, starting with the trachea and major bronchi and proceeding to passageways that are progressively smaller in diameter (see Figure 8.3A). There are about 27 "generations" of branches from largest to smallest airways. The first 20 or so are conducting airways, which just serve to transport air and do not actually participate in gas exchange. The last 7 comprise terminal respiratory units composed of terminal bronchioles and alveolar ducts, where a gas-blood interface and, hence, gas exchange occur.

The entire airway down to the terminal bronchioles is lined on the lumenal side by a ciliated pseudostratified columnar epithelium (see Figure 8.3B). In the large airways, the epithelial cell walls contain secretory glands and are supported by cartilaginous rings. The walls of medium-sized bronchi contain circumferential smooth muscle that allow their diameter to be regulated (see Sec. 5). Smaller bronchioles and beyond, however, lack such a smooth muscle layer. The terminal bronchioles end in small capillary-lined sacs termed *alveoli*, which are the actual site of gas exchange. The walls of the alveoli consist of an epithelium that separates the airspace from the capillary endothelium. These two cell layers define three compartments: the airspace, the interstitium, and the capillary lumen. The epithelial layer demarcating the airspace is "tighter" than the endothelium that makes up the capillary wall. Thus, fluid leaking from the capillary lumen normally goes into the interstitial space and into the lymphatic drainage rather than into the airspace.

The set of airways and alveoli that make up the lungs are divided into lobes, with each lobe consisting of several segments. At end-expiration, most of the volume of the lungs is air and half of the mass of the lungs is blood within the capillaries.

An important function of the non-gas-exchange portion of the respiratory tree is the filtering out of particles in the air that would otherwise clog and destroy the gas exchange surface of the lungs. Hairs in the nose and cilia and mucus in the upper airways trap large and small particles and sweep them out of the airway.

Pulmonary circulation

A set of branching pulmonary arterioles, progressively smaller in diameter, accompanies the branching bronchial airway tree (Figure 8.3D). When the bronchioles give rise to alveoli, the pulmonary arterioles give rise to capillaries. The capillaries are about 10 μM in diameter, just wide enough for individual red blood cells to squeeze through.

A given pulmonary capillary traverses many alveoli, adding to the efficiency of gas exchange and ensuring that diffusion is complete in only a small fraction of the time that blood is in the lung. This distribution of airspaces and blood vessels is the basis for the effectiveness of gas exchange in the lung. It allows carbon dioxide and oxygen to equilibrate between alveolar air and capillary blood.

The course of the pulmonary veins is different. The flow of many capillaries collects into the pulmonary veins, which run in the interlobar connective tissue of the lung and return oxygenated blood to the left side of the heart.

The pulmonary arteries and veins larger than 50 μM in diameter have a smooth muscle lining and are richly innervated, largely by the sympathetic nervous system. They actively alter their diameter thereby regulating resistance to flow (see Sec. 5).

The structure of the lungs as a delicate air-blood interface is indicated by the fact that the 250 g of alveolar mass that make up the lungs provides a surface area for gas exchange of 75 m^2.

A small bronchial circulation feeds the airways, vessels, connective tissue, and pleura of the lung, and is distinct from the pulmonary arteries and veins. The existence of this small, independent component of lung circulation accounts for much of the observed dis-

A

FIGURE 8.3. Structure of the lungs. A. Conducting airways. The subdivisions of conducting airways and terminal respiratory units. Successive branching produces increasing generations of airways, beginning with the trachea. Note that gas-exchanging segments of the lung occur only after extensive branching with concomitant decrease in airway caliber and increase in total cross-sectional area. B. Bronchial wall anatomy. Structure of a normal bronchial wall. In chronic bronchitis, the thickness of the mucous glands increases and can be expressed as the ratio of (b-c/(a-d), also known as the Reid index. C. The structure of expanded lung. A well-expanded section of lung tissue as it would look under low magnification. The larger central openings are the final branches of the gas exchange airways, also known as alveolar ducts (AD). Surrounding the ducts are the anatomical alveoli (A). There is a great deal of gas exchange and very little tissue. The main function of the anatomical alveoli is to greatly increase the gas exchange surface area. D. Anatomy of the airspaces. Note the close relation between the pulmonary arteries (perfusion) and airways (ventilation). (A. Adapted, with permission, from Weibel, E.R. (1963). Morphometry of the Lung. Springer, as adapted in Prendergast, T.J. and Ruoss, S.J. (1997). Pulmonary disease, in McPhee, S., et al. eds. Pathophysiology of Disease, 2nd ed. Stamford, CT, Appleton & Lange, p. 184. B. Adapted, with permission, from Thurbeck, W.M. (1976). Chronic airflow obstruction in lung disease, in Major Problems in Pathology. Bennington, J.L., ed. Philadelphia, Saunders.)

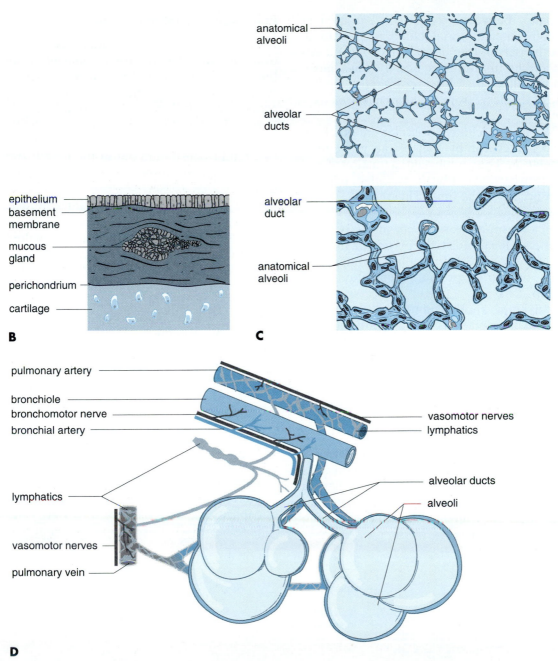

B

C

D

FIGURE 8.3 — (continued)

crepancy between oxygen concentration in alveoli versus arterial blood in a normal, healthy person (see discussion of A-a Gradient and its Implications, Sec. 4). Thus, most, but not all, of the blood returning to the left side of the heart from the lungs has been oxygenated.

Much of the body's vascular endothelium is accounted for by that of the pulmonary circulation. Thus, a substantial fraction of metabolism carried out by the vascular endothelium occurs in the lung. Thus:

- Angiotensin-converting enzyme (ACE), a protease localized to the plasma membrane of vascular endothelium, plays an important role in blood pressure regulation (see Chap. 10).
- Bradykinin, another important peptide involved in regulation of fluid distribution between intravascular and intersitial space, is also inactivated by ACE.
- Prostaglandins are inactivated by other lung enzymes.
- Seratonin and norepinephrine are taken up by the lung.

The pulmonary circulation also serves to filter out any particles, including blood clots that might have formed, before they have a chance to enter the systemic arterial circulation where they might clog end organs such as the brain, causing strokes.

Pulmonary lymphatic vessels

A set of lymphatic vessels is found in association with the conduits for air and blood in the lung. As with other parts of the vascular system (see Chap. 7), the distribution of fluid across the capillary endothelium (i.e., between blood and intersititial fluid) is determined by the balance of hydrostatic forces that tend to push fluid out of the vessel, and colloid osmotic forces that tend to hold fluid in.

Due to the slight negative intrathoracic pressure maintained during inspiration by contraction of the diaphragm, interstitial fluid is normally swept into the lymphatic vessels as rapidly as it is produced. The combination of the tightness of the alveolar epithelium (compared to that of the capillary endothelium) and the forces sweeping it into the lymphatic vessels keeps interstitial fluid out of the alveoli where it would otherwise interfere with gas exchange (Figure 8.4).

Clinical Pearl

○ Under pathological conditions (e.g., disruption of the endothelial barrier), the volume of interstitial fluid in the lungs can increase greatly and eventually exceed the capacity of the lymphatic vessels. Depending on whether the excessive intersti-

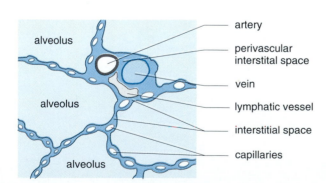

alveolus

alveolus

alveolus

artery

perivascular interstital space

vein

lymphatic vessel

interstitial space

capillaries

FIGURE 8.4. Structure of the alveolar wall.

tial fluid formation is localized or generalized and whether it is associated with a breakdown in the epithelial lining of the alveoli (see Sec. 8), the patient can develop either a pleural effusion (see earlier) or pulmonary edema with gas exchange abnormalities (see Pulmonary Edema and Acute Respiratory Distress Syndrome, Sec. 8).

Pulmonary nervous system

The lungs contain an extensive nervous system that is crucial to regulation of their function. The principal afferent fibers are branches of the vagus nerve that transmit impulses from the following:

- Stretch receptors, which initiate reflex smooth muscle dilation and stimulate an increase in heart rate in response to inhalation
- Irritant receptors, which initiate reflex cough, bronchoconstriction, and mucous production in response to noxious stimuli
- C fibers responding to mechanical and chemical stimuli as part of reflexes affecting the pattern of breathing and slowing heart rate in response to inhalation

The principal efferent fibers are as follows:

- Parasympathetic fibers with cholinergic vagal fibers involved in bronchoconstriction; pulmonary vasodilation, and mucus secretion
- Sympathetic fibers whose stimulation results in bronchiolar smooth muscle relaxation, pulmonary vasodilation, and inhibition of secretory gland activity
- Nonadrenergic, noncholinergic fibers, probably releasing nitric oxide, ATP, and various peptide neurotransmitters that mediate inhibitory activities that balance the cholinergic pathways

Clinical Pearl

○ Dyspnea is a complex sensation that arises from many different causes. For example, patients with chronic lung disease often develop disabling dyspnea that makes their life miserable, leaving them uncomfortable even at rest and unable to sleep. This sets up a vicious cycle of increased fatigue, which worsens their subjective sense of shortness of breath. Sometimes the CNS suppressive effect of codeine and other narcotics can be used to make such individuals more comfortable, with decreased sense of dyspnea, allowing them to sleep without substantially worsening gas exchange.

Medullary respiratory centers

Bilateral nuclei in the medulla and pons provide CNS control over respiration (see Figure 8.5A):

- The dorsal respiratory group in the dorsal medulla can trigger inspiration
- The ventral respiratory group in the ventrolateral medulla contains some neurons that trigger inspiration and others that trigger expiration
- The pneumotaxic center in the dorsal superior pons controls the rate and pattern of breathing

Firing of action potentials from the neurons that control inspiration starts gradually, then increases over about 2 s, then abruptly stops for up to 3 s before starting again. This allows for a steady increase in the volume of the lungs, with time for expiration, rather than bursts of intermittent inspiratory gasps.

Firing of neurons from the pneumotaxic center is responsible for the cessation of action potentials from the other nuclei that trig-

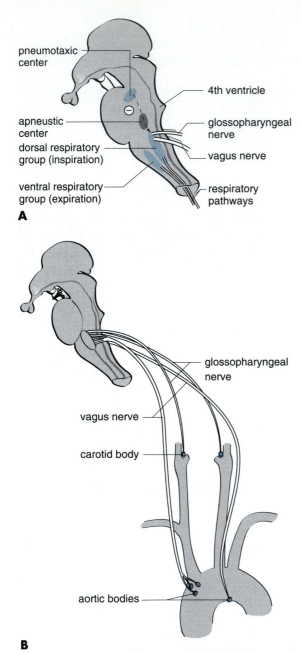

pneumotaxic center

apneustic center

dorsal respiratory group (inspiration)

ventral respiratory group (expiration)

A

4th ventricle

glossopharyngeal nerve

vagus nerve

respiratory pathways

glossopharyngeal nerve

vagus nerve

carotid body

aortic bodies

B

FIGURE 8.5. *A*. Organization of the respiratory center in the brainstem. *B*. Respiratory control by the aortic and carotid bodies. *(From Guyton, A.C. and Hall, J.E. (1997). Human Physiology and Mechanisms of Disease, 6th ed. Philadelphia, PA, WB Saunders, p. 338, 340.)*

ger inspiration. This allows inspiration to last as little as 0.5 s or as long as 5 s.

3. GAS TRANSPORT

Fundamentals of gas transport

Individual molecules are continually in motion, except at a temperature of absolute zero. In either liquid or gaseous form, molecules move from where they have higher concentration (and energy) to where they have a lower concentration (and energy). This is the basis for diffusion. It means, among other things, that dissolved molecules in a liquid are constantly escaping into air, and molecules that make up air are constantly entering liquid at any air-liquid interface. At equilibrium, this movement between liquid and gas phases defines the **vapor pressure** for any given molecule.

One way to measure the amount of various gases is by comparing the pressure they exert on other substances, which is proportional to their concentrations and temperature, and is due to the intrinsic motion of the individual gas molecules. Because the concentrations of gases in air changes with distance from the earth's surface, it is also important to specify the distance from sea level when using pressures to measure gas concentrations.

Air is a mixture of gases (approximately 79% nitrogen, 21% oxygen, with trace amounts of the others). The total pressure of all the gases in air is able to push a column of mercury (Hg) 760 mm, at sea level at 37°C. The contribution of each individual gas in air to the total vapor pressure is called the **partial pressure** for that gas. The composition of inhaled air is also affected by humidity, that is, the partial pressure of water vapor. For water, at 37°C sea level, vapor pressure is 47 mmHg. Since clinically, we are most concerned with the oxygen concentration in air, the fraction of inspired air composed of O_2 molecules is termed the FiO_2. Thus breathing pure, 100% oxygen (partial pressure of 760 mmHg) would provide an FiO_2 of 1.0.

Normal tidal volume, the amount of air moved in and out with quiet breathing, is about 500 mL. Upon maximal inspiration, about 2000 mL of air is taken in and instantly humidified, so its composition is modfied by the vapor pressure of water, which dilutes the other gases present (see Table 8.1). Once humidified, inspired air equilibrates with the air left in the lungs after maximal expiration (about 2400 mL). Only about 350 mL of the 500 mL of air brought in with quiet breathing reaches the alveoli where gas exchange can take place. Thus, at rest, it takes many breaths to replace the "old" air in the lungs with "new" air. Gas in the lungs is replaced gradually over time rather than suddenly, with diffusion playing a key role in eliminating carbon dioxide and bringing in oxygen. Thus we can think of alveolar gas as being in transition from room air to the gases in our bloodstream.

The gases that make up air in the alveoli diffuse into the bloodstream and quickly reach equilibrium, at which point the blood can be said to be saturated. This means that the blood has all of each individual gas that it can hold at a given vapor pressure. Of course, if you were under greater than atmospheric pressure, more of each gas would go into solution. Each gas has its intrinsic solubility in blood based on its physical properties, just as different solids have different intrinsic solubilities in water. The **solubility constant** for a particular gas is a mathematical factor that allows the amount of gas dissolved in a liquid to be determined from its concentration in air. Thus, by the time blood leaves the lung, it contains dissolved gases in proportion to their partial pressures in alveolar air.

In addition, the amount of a gas present in a fluid (e.g., such as blood) is affected by the presence of high affinity binding proteins (as is true for oxygen, see Transport of Oxygen next). **The association constant** (see Chap. 2) is a mathematical factor that allows the amount of a substance (e.g., such as a gas) bound to be determined from the concentrations of binding protein and bound and free gas. The bound fraction serves as an extra reservoir of that particular gas, above and beyond what would dissolve in the liquid based on the solubility constant alone. The size of this extra reservoir is determined by the concentration of the binding sites, their affinity for the gas, and its partial pressure, and is in equilibrium with the fraction of gas in solution.

When blood arrives in the lung, gases present at higher concentration in blood (e.g., CO_2), diffuse into alveolar air, while at the same time, gases present at higher concentration in alveolar air diffuse into the

TABLE 8.1 PARTIAL PRESSURES (mmHg) OF RESPIRATORY GASES AT ENTRANCE TO, AND EXIT FROM, THE LUNGS

	Atmospheric air		Humidified air		Alveolar air		Expired air	
N_2	597.0	(78.62%)	563.4	(74.09%)	569.0	(74.9%)	566.0	(74.5%)
O_2	159.0	(20.84%)	149.3	(19.67%)	104.0	(13.6%)	120.0	(15.7%)
CO_2	0.3	(0.04%)	0.3	(0.04%)	40.0	(5.3%)	27.0	(3.6%)
H_2O	3.7	(0.50%)	47.0	(6.20%)	47.0	(6.2%)	47.0	(6.2%)
TOTAL	760.0	(100.00%)	760.0	(100.00%)	760.0	(100.0%)	760.0	(100.0%)

Reproduced, with permission, from Guyton, A.C. and Hall, J.E. (1997). *Human Physiology and Mechanisms of Disease*, 6th ed. Philadelphia, Saunders, p. 325.

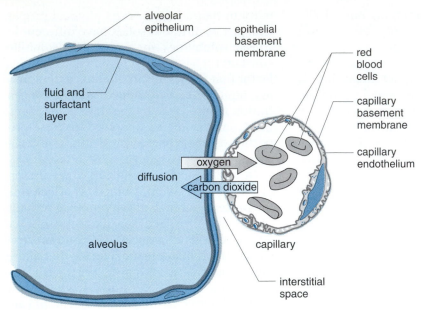

FIGURE 8.6. Gas transport across the respiratory epithelium. *(Adapted from Guyton, A.C. and Hall, J.E. (1997). Human Physiology and Mechanisms of Disease, 6th ed. Philadelphia, PA, WB Saunders, p. 329.)*

bloodstream. Meanwhile, with each breath, gas in the alveoli is gradually exchanged with outside air (Figure 8.6 and Table 8.1).

Biochemistry of gas transport

Transport of oxygen

Oxygen is not very soluble in water. So, to carry oxygen, we have evolved hemoglobin, an iron-containing protein that is present in enormous concentrations in red blood cells. Blood normally contains about 15 g of hemoglobin per 100 mL. This allows oxygen-carrying capacity to increase from the 3 mL O_2 per liter allowed by its solubility in plasma to 200 mL per liter. Since oxygen consumption ranges from 250 to 1500 mL O_2 per min, and cardiac output ranges from 5 to 15 L/min, the extra oxygen-binding capacity of hemoglobin allows the heart and the lungs to com-fortably provide for the oxygen needs of the body.

A given molecule of hemoglobin binds up to 4 mol of oxygen tightly, cooperatively (see Chap. 2), and most importantly, reversibly. That is, oxygen-hemoglobin binding and dissociation is affected by a number of parameters including temperature, pH, the metabolite 2,3 diphosphoglycerate, and the occupancy state of the other oxygen-binding sites (see Figure 8.7). Normally, hemoglobin is almost completely saturated (96%) when exposed to room air ($Fio_2 = 21\%$). This means that there is little to be gained by increasing the ventilatory rate without also increasing cardiac output, since the hemoglobin in blood is already maximally saturated by oxygen. Instead, oxygen concentration (in blood) is generally much more dependent on hemoglobin concentration in red blood cells, red blood cell content of blood (i.e., hematocrit), and adequacy of perfusion of the lungs,

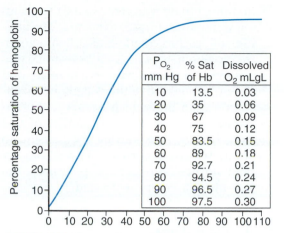

P_{O_2} mm Hg	% Sat of Hb	Dissolved O_2 mLgL
10	13.5	0.03
20	35	0.06
30	67	0.09
40	75	0.12
50	83.5	0.15
60	89	0.18
70	92.7	0.21
80	94.5	0.24
90	96.5	0.27
100	97.5	0.30

FIGURE 8.7. Oxygen-hemoglobin dissociation curve. *(Adapted, with permission, from Ganong, W.F. (1997). Review of Medical Physiology, 18th ed. Stamford, CT, Appleton & Lange.)*

than it is on ventilation rate by itself. Likewise, anemia, acidemia, and other parameters that affect oxygen-hemoglobin binding and dissociation have a major influence on the adequacy of blood O_2 concentration and transport.

In the lung, oxygen diffuses across the epithelial lining of the alveolus, across the interstitial space, across the endothelial wall of the capillary, and across the red blood cell membrane, where it is taken up by unoccupied hemoglobin to be carried to the peripheral tissues of the body. In the periphery, where oxygen tension is low, some of that oxygen is released from hemoglobin. The released oxygen diffuses across the red blood cell membrane, across the capillary endothelium, across the interstitial space, across the basement membrane, and across cell membranes to function in oxidative phosphorylation and generation of ATP in mitochondria.

At rest, only about 25% of the oxygen carried in blood is released to tissues. This allows maintenance of a large gradient of oxygen concentration from blood to cells, which

provides the driving force for diffusion. It also provides a reservoir of oxygen to be called upon when needed. For example, with vigorous exercise, oxygen requirements go up as much as sixfold, while cardiac output may increase only threefold. The balance of oxygen needs can be achieved by simply extracting more oxygen from hemoglobin.

The oxygen content of blood at 37°C and pH 7.4 can be determined by the equation:

$$O_2 \text{ content} = (1.34 \times \text{Hb concentration} \times \%\text{Hb saturation}) + (0.031 \times P_{O_2})$$

where 1.34 mL O_2 is carried per gram of fully saturated hemoglobin; the amount of O_2 dissolved in plasma is proportional to P_{O_2} = 0.031 mL/L of blood per mmHg P_{O_2}. Thus the left hand parenthesis (the hemoglobin bound oxygen) is about 70 times greater than the right hand parenthesis (dissolved O_2).

Clinical Pearl

○ Since hemoglobin in oxygenated blood returning from areas of the lung where gas exchange has occurred is normally largely saturated, hyperventilation of room air will not add much oxygen to the bloodstream. In order to augment oxygen-carrying capacity in, for example, a patient with hypoxia due to a mismatch between ventilation and perfusion (see Sec. 8), the patient must breathe air with a higher percentage of oxygen than that which occurs in room air.

Transport of carbon dioxide

Carbon dioxide (CO_2) is a product of oxidative metabolism of energy substrates (e.g., sugars and fats). CO_2 is extremely soluble in water, and, hence, after diffusing across the cell membrane, interstitium, and endothelium, can be carried back to the lungs simply dissolved in the plasma phase of blood, without needing to be bound to specific carrier protein in red blood cells, as is necessary for oxygen, for adequate alveolar-plasma gas exchange. Once in the lung capillaries, CO_2 dissolved in plasma diffuses down its concentration gradient across the endothelium, interstitium, and epithelium and enters the air spaces of the alveoli, from which it can be removed by exhalation.

The fundamental difference in the way CO_2 and most O_2 are transported in blood, that is, in solution versus bound to hemoglobin, has profound implications. In addition to the greater solubility of CO_2 than O_2 in blood, CO_2 diffuses from airspace to blood 20 times faster than does O_2. Therefore, unlike a fall in blood P_{O_2}, a rise in blood P_{CO_2} can be compensated effectively by an increased ventilatory rate (see preceding Clinical Pearl). Thus, hyperventilation increases the blood-to-air diffusion gradient (difference in P_{CO_2} in blood versus alveolar air), which increases the amount of CO_2 unloaded in the lung.

Clinical Pearl

○ Carbon monoxide (CO) is a gas produced by incomplete combustion of gasoline, or wood, and in the malfunction of home appliances. It has a 200-fold higher affinity for hemoglobin than does oxygen. Hence it will displace oxygen and sequester hemoglobin from participation in oxygen transport, thereby starving tissues for oxygen even when oxygen concentration in the air and lung function are normal. Typically mild symptoms (headache, dyspnea, confusion) begin at about 10 to 20% saturation. Above 60% saturation is often lethal (with symptoms of cerebral and pulmonary edema, coma, hypotension). The first thing to do is to remove a CO poisoning victim from further exposure. The half-life of carboxymethylated hemoglobin (hemoglobin to which carbon monoxide is bound) in room air is 4 to 6 h. Inhalation of pure oxygen (five times higher concentration than that which occurs in air) increases the rate of displacement of CO from hemoglobin, cutting the half-life to about 1 h. In hyperbaric oxygen (higher than normal atmospheric pressure), the half-life can be cut to 15 min.

Review Questions

4. What is the gas composition of air?
5. What is the vapor pressure of water at 37°C at sea level?
6. Explain what vapor pressure and partial pressure mean.
7. Compare and contrast the mechanism for transport of O_2 and CO_2 in the bloodstream.
8. What are the parameters that influence the oxygen-hemoglobin dissociation curve?

4. VENTILATION AND PERFUSION

Ventilation is the process of bringing air in and out of the lungs. Perfusion is the process of permeating the lungs with blood, via the pulmonary capillary bed in order to allow gas exchange between the alveolar air and capillary blood. To achieve the goal for which the lungs exist, two conditions have to be met. First, ventilation has to be efficient enough to allow gas exchange at a level of work that a person can tolerate. Second, perfusion has to be sufficiently well matched to ventilation to allow adequate gas exchange between alveolar air and capillary blood, for any given level of work of breathing.

Much of clinically relevant lung physiology

involves the solution of two fundamental problems that relate back to ventilation and perfusion: How to minimize the work of breathing and how to optimize gas exchange.

Lung volumes and ventilation

Discussion of clinically relevant pulmonary physiology requires that we define some terms with respect to the capacity of the lung to inhale, hold, and exhale air (see Figure 8.8).

All the air that the lungs could theoretically hold is termed the *total lung capacity* (TLC). It is about 6 L in a 70 kg adult. Of this, the amount of air inhaled and exhaled

with each resting breath, about 350 to 400 mL, is termed the *tidal volume* (TV). Functional residual capacity (FRC) is the amount of air left in the lungs after a resting breath, about 4800 mL. Residual volume (RV) is the amount of air remaining in the lungs at the end of a maximal exhalation, about 2400 mL. Vital capacity (VC) is the total amount of air that can be exhaled after a maximal inhalation, normally about 3700 mL. Thus:

$$VC + RV = TLC$$

The forced vital capacity (FVC) is a maneuver that begins with an inhalation from functional residual capacity (FRC, the amount of

FIGURE 8.8. Lung volumes and capacities. The volume of gas in the lungs is divided into volumes and capacities as shown in the bars to the left of the figure. See text for definition of terms. To the right is the change in volume of gas in the lungs during breathing in real time, as measured by spirometry. The first tidal breath shown takes 5 s, indicating a respiratory rate of 12 breaths per minute. FEV_1 (see text) can be measured from the data shown. The spirogram in the figure shows the change in various lung volumes and capacities over time. The forced vital capacity (FVC) maneuver begins with an inhalation from FRC to TLC (lasting about 1 s), followed by a forceful exhalation from TLC to RV (lasting about 5 s). The amount of gas exhaled during the first second of this maneuver is the forced expiratory volume in 1 s (FEV_1). TLC, total lung capacity; VC, vital capacity; RV, residual volume; IC, inspiratory capacity; FRC, functional residual capacity; IRV, inspiratory reserve volume; Vt, tidal volume; ERV, expiratory reserve volume; RV, residual volume. (Adapted, with permission, from Prendergast, T.J. and Ruoss, S.J. (1997), in McPhee, S. et al. eds. Pathophysiology of Disease, 2nd ed. Stamford, CT, Appleton & Lange, p. 183.)

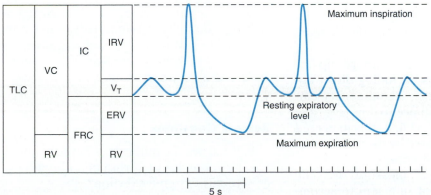

residual air in the lungs after a resting tidal breath) to TLC (taking about 10 s), followed by a forceful exhalation from TLC to RV (taking about 5 s). The amount of air exhaled during the first second of that exhalation is called the FEV_1 (forced expiratory volume in 1 s). A normal individual can expel 70 to 80% of the FVC in the first second. The ratio of FEV_1 to FVC (termed the FEV_1 %) is diminished in patients with obstructive lung disease.

Some of these measurements can be performed with a spirometer, which simply measures amount of air exhaled (e.g., FEV_1 and FVC). Other measurements require equilibration of a tracer gas with air that is not readily expelled (e.g., RV), and thus cannot be quickly assessed at the bedside, requiring instead that the patient be sent to the laboratory for formal pulmonary function studies.

Perfusion pressure

The right ventricle pumps venous blood to the lung at relatively low pressures (mean pressure of 15 mmHg) compared to the left ventricle (mean of 90 mmHg). Since the output of the right side of the heart must match that of the left side, the pulmonary vessels must provide much less resistance to flow than the systemic circulation. This is why the delicate architecture of the lung is so important for proper lung function. There are numerous capillaries that can expand to accommodate right ventricular output, if there is an increased resistance to blood flow in some regions of the lung.

Lung perfusion pressure can go up for many different reasons, including direct obstruction of vessels (e.g., in pulmonary emboli) or increased resistance to flow (e.g., due to interstitial fibrosis). At first, this increased pressure is accommodated by the recruitment and distension of small vessels.

When these "failsafe" measures are fully utilized and are still not sufficient to accom-

modate pulmonary blood flow, pulmonary artery pressure and, hence, right ventricular pressure must go up. This condition is termed **pulmonary hypertension**. Eventually, it can result in pulmonary edema in the subset of patients who develop pulmonary hypertension due to failure of the left side of the heart or cardiogenic shock (with backup of blood resulting in rising pulmonary artery pressure and increased hydrostatic pressure in the capillaries driving fluid into the lung interstitium).

Clinical Pearl

○ While failure of the left side of the heart can result in pulmonary hypertension and pulmonary edema, not all cases of pulmonary hypertension result in pulmonary edema. For example, in primary pulmonary hypertension and pulmonary hypertension due to interstitial lung fibrosis, pulmonary edema is not typically seen. In effect, in these conditions, blood is backing up behind the lungs, elevating pressures in the right side of the heart and often leading to failure of the right side of the heart instead. With interstitial fibrosis, a higher hydrostatic pressure is needed to force fluid out of the vasculature, which is in effect being "reinforced" by the fibrosis. Of course, while protecting against pulmonary edema, interstitial fibrosis diminishes pulmonary blood flow, worsens gas exchange, and increases the work of breathing (see Sec. 5), and therefore is a very bad thing.

Review Questions

9. What are the differences in the respiratory muscles used with quiet breathing versus extreme exertion?

10. Define alveoli.
11. What are the forces that normally keep interstitial fluid from accumulating in the lungs?
12. What is the approximate pressure generated by the right atrium?
13. What is the long-term consequence of increased resistance to right ventricle output?
14. What are the components of the pulmonary nervous system?
15. Where is the respiratory control center located? How does it work?

Arterial blood gases and the A-a gradient

Arterial blood gas determination

Because diffusion is so rapid and complete, concentrations of CO_2 and O_2 in the alveoli are normally reflected in arterial blood P_{CO_2} and P_{O_2} concentrations. Hence one can get a reasonable assessment of adequacy of ventilation and perfusion by obtaining a sample of arterial blood (e.g., by puncture of the radial artery) and determining the P_{O_2} and P_{CO_2} directly.

While arterial blood sampling readily reveals major ventilation and perfusion disturbances, more subtle lesions require calculation of the alveolar to arterial oxygen concentration gradient (A-a gradient).

A-a gradient and its implications

The A-a gradient is a particularly valuable physiological calculation in the case of a patient who has hypoxia (low arterial P_{O_2}) of unclear etiology (see Figure 8.12 later). Hypoxia due to hypoventilation will show high blood P_{CO_2} (hypercapnia), while hypoxia due to inspiration of air lacking O_2 (e.g., at high altitude) will show a low P_{CO_2}, on arterial blood gas determination. However, the dif-

ference between alveolar and arterial blood P_{O_2} will be normal in both of these cases. In contrast, a patient who is hypoxic due to ventilation-to-perfusion mismatch (see later) or due to shunting of venous blood bypassing the lungs, will have an elevated A-a O_2 gradient. Thus, measurement of the A-a gradient in a hypoxic patient will help identify the cause of the hypoxia.

The A-a gradient is elevated in all patients with hypercapnia due to intrinsic pulmonary disease. But a normal A-a gradient in a patient with hypercapnia essentially excludes intrinsic pulmonary disease. Instead, it suggests that the cause of the elevated P_{CO_2} is due to hypoventilation. This perhaps most commonly occurs in patients who have had an overdose of narcotic drugs (e.g., heroin), but may also be due to disease of the chest wall or respiratory muscles, or involve CNS control of respiration, as for example, in response to primary metabolic alkalosis (see Chap. 10).

Calculation of the A-a gradient is most easily done by the alveolar gas equation:

$$P_{AO_2} = F_{IO_2} \times (P_B - P_{H_2O}) - P_{aCO_2}/R$$

where R is the respiratory quotient (ratio of CO_2 production to O_2 consumption) of 0.8, PB is atmospheric pressure of 760 mmHg at sea level, P_{H_2O} is the partial pressure of water in humidified air entering the alveolus, approximately 45 mmHg. P_{AO_2} is the partial pressure of oxygen in alveolar gas. P_{aCO_2} is the partial pressure of CO_2 in arterial blood. Thus, in a patient breathing room air:

$$P_{AO_2} = 150 - 1.25 \times P_{aCO_2}$$

Pulse oximetry

A major advance in ventilation and perfusion monitoring has been the development of technology that allows noninvasive assessment of blood oxygen saturation, based on the difference in wavelength of light reflected from unsaturated versus saturated hemoglobin. Instead of a painful, intermittent and invasive arterial puncture, a simple painless, external finger-clip monitor is worn by the patient. This can be used either continually (e.g., upon hospitalization of a patient needing close monitoring of ventilation or perfusion status), or used intermittently (e.g., for rapid assessment of a clinic patient with known underlying lung disease or symptoms of dyspnea).

Clinical Pearls

Despite its clinical utility, pulse oximetry has several pitfalls that illustrate the importance of approaching clinical findings physiologically:

○ The first 30 point fall in alveolar O_2 partial pressure from normal to a PO_2 of 60 is not very significant to tissues, since the hemoglobin in blood is still about 90% saturated with oxygen at a PO_2 of 60 mmHg. However, at that point the linear part of the hemoglobin-oxygen saturation curve has been reached and any further fall in PO_2 would result in a steep fall in oxygen carrying capacity (see Figure 8.7). Another 30 point drop would be lethal, for instance.

○ In extreme peripheral vasoconstriction (e.g., in shock; see Chap. 7), cutaneous perfusion may be insufficient to allow oxygen saturation to be accurately assessed by a pulse oximeter attached to the patient's finger.

○ Most pulse oximeters are designed to distinguish saturated from unsaturated hemoglobin and do not distinguish *what* hemoglobin is saturated with. Thus a patient with lethal CO poisoning may have an entirely normal value registered by pulse oximetry.

○ O_2 saturation does not reveal the adequacy of CO_2 elimination, which is a linear and hence much more accurate indicator of adequacy of ventilation. An acceptable O_2 saturation may mask an insidious rise in PCO_2 that may be the early warning sign of impending respiratory failure (e.g., due to respiratory muscle fatigue).

Matching ventilation to perfusion

Matching of ventilation ($\dot{V}$) to perfusion ($\dot{Q}$), often referred to by pulmonary physiologists as the $\dot{V}/\dot{Q}$ ratio, is crucial for lung function. It would be futile to provide air to nonperfused segments of lung, because no gas exchange can occur there. Thus, lung that is ventilated but not perfused has a $\dot{V}/\dot{Q}$ ratio of infinity, contributes to dead space, and is a waste of alveoli (see Figure 8.9).

Conversely, pulmonary artery blood flow to lung that is not ventilated has a $\dot{V}/\dot{Q}$ ratio of zero. It is the equivalent of shunting venous blood directly from the right to the left side of the heart and bypassing the lungs, a waste of cardiac output (see Figure 8.9). Of course, in most disease states the lung doesn't go instantly from normal to fully nonperfused or nonventilated. Usually, progression of an underlying disease results in gradual worsening of either ventilation or perfusion, or both (see Figure 8.10).

Blood flow in the lung is never perfectly uniform. First, there is an effect of gravity on pleural pressure that is more negative at the top of the lung than at the bottom (in a standing person). Thus even a completely healthy lung is relatively more expanded at the top than at the bottom. Second, the blood pressure in the pulmonary artery does not perfuse the apex of the lung as well as it does the base. As a consequence of these factors, there is a linear increase in blood flow from top to bottom of the lung.

The third, and in many ways most impor-

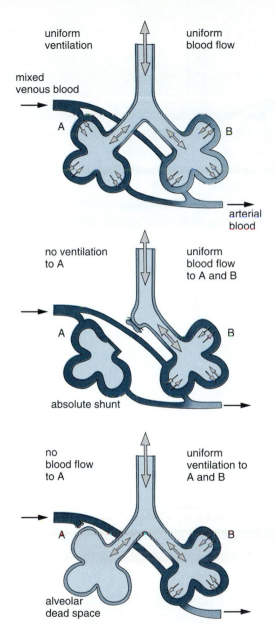

uniform ventilation

uniform blood flow

mixed venous blood

A

B

arterial blood

no ventilation to A

uniform blood flow to A and B

A

B

absolute shunt

no blood flow to A

uniform ventilation to A and B

A

B

alveolar dead space

FIGURE 8.9. Ventilation and perfusion. Three models of the relation of ventilation to perfusion. In this diagram, the circles represent respiratory units, with tubes depicting the conducting airways. The shaded channels represent the pulmonary blood flow, which enters the capillary bed as mixed venous blood (dark) and leaves it as arterialized blood (light). Large arrows show distribution of inspired gas; small arrows show diffusion of O_2 and CO_2. In the idealized case, the P_{O_2} and P_{CO_2} leaving both units are identical.

tant, determinant of pulmonary blood flow is hypoxic pulmonary artery smooth muscle vasoconstriction. In other capillary beds of the body, arterioles vasodilate in response to tissue hypoxia, thereby improving perfusion. In the lung, the smooth muscle of the arterioles is more sensitive to alveolar P_{O_2} than to arterial P_{O_2}, and responds to a fall in alveolar P_{O_2} by vasoconstriction. This allows blood to be shunted away from poorly ventilated regions of the lung, optimizing the match between ventilation and perfusion. Because of the large capacity of the pulmonary circulation and the existence of small vessels that can expand when necessary, hypoxic vasoconstriction usually results in redistribution of blood flow without an increased pulmonary artery perfusion pressure (pulmonary hypertension).

Resting ventilation is about 6 L/min, but only about two-thirds of this is alveolar ventilation. The remaining one-third of ventilation is accounted for by air in large airways that do not participate in gas exchange, the so-called anatomical dead space. Thus, the effective ventilation at rest is about 4 L/min. Resting pulmonary artery blood flow is about 5 L/min. Thus, at rest, the ratio of ventilation to perfusion ($\dot{V}/\dot{Q}$) is 0.8.

Review Questions

16. What is the relation between vital capacity, residual volume, and total lung capacity?
17. Define FEV_1 and describe its clinical significance.
18. Why are the lungs a low-pressure perfusion circuit?
19. What can be learned from arterial blood gas determination?
20. What is the implication of an increase in the A-a gradient?
21. How does pulse oximetry work?
22. What parameters make blood flow through the lungs nonuniform?

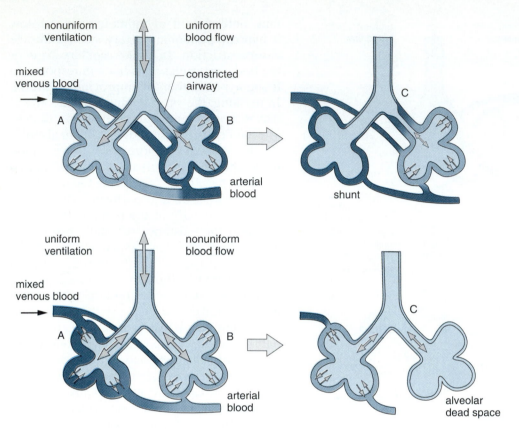

FIGURE 8.10. Ventilation-perfusion mismatching commonly occurs between the extremes indicated in Figure 8.9. Here areas of low $\dot{V}/\dot{Q}$ ratio (Above, A/B) are indicated as being equivalent to lung units in which a certain fraction of cardiac output represents shunted blood (above, C). Areas of high $\dot{V}/\dot{Q}$ ratio (below, A and B) are indicated as being equivalent to lung units in which a certain fraction of alveoli represent dead space (below, C). *(Adapted, with permission, from Comroe, J. (1974). Physiology of Respiration, 2nd ed. Chicago, Year Book.)*

23. Why does hypoxic pulmonary vasoconstriction usually *not* result in elevation of right ventricular and pulmonary arterial pressures?

24. What is the normal resting $\dot{V}/\dot{Q}$ ratio?

25. What are the implications for ventilation and perfusion of an increase in alveolar dead space? Of shunting of blood from the right to the left side of the heart?

5. THE WORK OF BREATHING

Determinants of efficient lung function

As discussed above, a key determinant of efficient lung function is the balance between ventilation of alveoli and perfusion of capillaries that line these airspaces. Neither ventilation to alveoli that are not well perfused nor perfusion of alveoli that are not well ventilated supports effective gas exchange. Thus, when ventilation does not match perfusion, the efficiency of gas exchange falls and the work needed to breathe adequately increases.

Clinical Pearl

○ A significant cause of respiratory failure is respiratory muscle fatigue. Despite otherwise adequate gas exchange at the capillary and tissue level, the inability of the diaphragm and respiratory muscles to carry out the work of breathing results in progressive "slowing of the bellows," fall in oxygenation, and/or rise in carbon dioxide concentration in the blood.

Components of the work of breathing

Because the lung has a delicate structure without rigid walls (except for the largest airways), there is a tendency for small airways and alveoli to collapse and not remain open, especially upon loss of volume with exhalation. Such airway and alveolar collapse would impede air flow and tremendously increase the work of breathing which would have to reopen these structures to get air in.

The work of breathing has two components:

1. Elastic forces and compliance
2. Airway resistance to airflow

Elastic forces and compliance

Compliance of the respiratory system is the ability of the lung and chest wall to change in volume in response to a change in pressure. If compliance is low, more effort must be expended to take in and move out sufficient air for oxygenation of blood, all else being equal.

Elastic recoil is the ability of a structure to return to its baseline shape rather than collapse when it loses volume (upon exhalation). In the case of the lung, elastic recoil is a function of both tissue elasticity and surface tension. If elastic recoil is too low, the airspaces and airways will collapse upon exhalation and the work expended to expand the lung upon inhalation will be much greater.

The normal lung is both highly compliant and has tremendous elastic recoil for the following reasons:

- **Connective tissue**, a multidirectional array of collagen and elastin fibers and connective tissue tend to hold the airways and alveoli open, despite rapid changes in volume of air contained.
- **Surfactant**, a complex secretion of phospholipids and specific proteins produced by type II alveolar cells.

Mechanism of action of surfactant

The molecules of water at the surface of an air-water interface are more strongly attracted to each other than they are to air. This is termed *surface tension* and is what, for example, holds a raindrop together. The same surface tension that tends to make water contract into a droplet would also tend to collapse alveoli during exhalation. For the lungs to work properly, elastic recoil and compliance have to be optimized and balanced. One way to do this is through the use of a surfactant. This phospholipid-protein complex is amphipathic, meaning it has both hydrophobic and hydrophilic surfaces, which allows it to form a thin layer at the air-water interface in which the hydrophobic side faces the air and the hydrophilic surface faces the water, thereby lowering surface tension and preventing alveolar collapse during normal exhalation.

Surfactant serves to achieve the following:

1. Stabilize open alveoli. It does this by lubricating the alveolar surface which allows

surface forces to vary with alveolar surface area. This prevents surface tension-driven collapse of airspaces, termed **atelectasis**, which would otherwise occur with a decrease in alveolar volume upon exhalation.

2. Keep alveoli dry. Surface tension reduces hydrostatic pressure in the alveoli and pericapillary interstitium, increasing the driving force for fluid to move into the alveoli. Surfactant limits this reduction in hydrostatic pressure by reducing surface tension. Without this effect, more interstitial fluid would accumulate in the alveoli, impeding gas exchange and requiring more work of breathing to achieve the same amount of gas exhange.

Clinical Pearl

○ Visible abnormalities of the thoracic cage such as kyphoscoliosis and ankylosing spondylitis can alter lung volumes and compliance and increase the work of breathing, resulting in dyspnea. Part of the assessment of a patient with dyspnea should be to look for such potential predispositions. Likewise, such findings in a healthy patient suggest specific areas for close attention. Thus, aggressive clearing of secretions and expansion of the lung (e.g., through use of a device called an incentive spirometer that encourages the patient to inhale forcefully) will help to prevent atelectasis and related complications in patients who are post-surgery, or recovering from bronchitis or pneumonia.

Airway resistance to airflow

In addition to elastic forces and compliance previously discussed, the work of breathing must overcome airway resistance to airflow. The determinants of flow resistance depend on whether the flow is laminar or turbulent. Laminar flow through a vessel is smooth flow where the molecules in the center move fastest, and those approaching the wall are moving progressively slower with an infinitely thin layer at the vessel wall not moving at all. Turbulent flow is the opposite of laminar flow and occurs beyond a critical velocity, resulting in a noise that can be heard (e.g., with a stethoscope). Laminar flow follows Poiseuille's law (resistance is proportional to length of the airway, viscosity of the gas, and the inverse of the fourth power of the radius). Turbulent flow, however, is proportionate to the square of the flow rate and gas density rather than viscosity. These relations apply both to blood in the vasculature and to gas in the airways.

Most of the resistance to airflow that occurs with normal breathing arises from the medium-sized bronchi rather than from the small airways. Most of the airflow in the airway, at least down to the smallest airways, is turbulent rather than laminar. In small bronchioles airflow becomes laminar. However, in the terminal bronchioles and alveoli there is no bulk flow of air. Instead, air movement occurs by diffusion. The large number of small branches at the level of the bronchioles means that the total cross-sectional area in the respiratory tree increases dramatically, even as the diameter of the airways is decreasing. As a result, the medium-sized bronchi are the "bottleneck" at which airway resistance can change dramatically. Such changes can occur through several mechanisms including:

1. Constriction of the smooth muscle that surrounds medium-sized bronchi (e.g., during an exacerbation of asthma)
2. Hypertrophy of the mucosa and its glands that accompanies mucus oversecretion in response to irritation (e.g., chronic bronchitis due to smoking)

3. Infiltration of the mucosa with immune cells and edema that accompanies inflammatory disorders such as sarcoidosis

When the caliber of medium-sized bronchi decreases for any of these reasons, obstruction to airflow can occur and the work of breathing is increased.

Furthermore, radial traction of the lung interstitium holds the airways maximally open as lung volumes increase. Thus patients with airway obstruction tend to breathe at large lung volumes in an effort to maximize elastic lung recoil and overcome airway resistance.

Forced expiration tends to offset the normal negative intrapleural pressure and thereby exacerbate the tendency of bronchioles to collapse. The phase of exhalation at which this occurs is termed the **equal pressure point** (Figure 8.11). Airway obstruction can occur when this point is reached during exhalation, even with airways of normal caliber; for example, in the patient with emphysema whose lungs have lost elastic recoil. In these patients, the lungs will be overly inflated because that will maximize whatever is left of their elastic recoil. Furthermore, the equal pressure point will be generated at much higher lung volumes than would normally occur. For this reason obstruction to flow is almost always worse during exhalation than during inhalation. This same effect also explains why end-expiratory wheezing (as an indicator of airflow obstruction) is the last component of bronchospasm to resolve (e.g., in a patient recovering from an acute asthma attack).

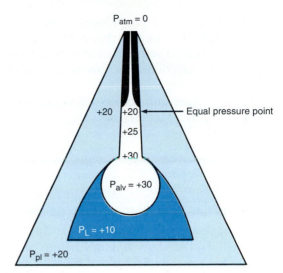

FIGURE 8.11. Concept of the equal pressure point. For air to flow through a tube, there must be a pressure difference between the two ends. In the case of forced expiration with an open glottis, this driving pressure is the difference between alveolar pressure (the sum of pleural pressure and lung elastic recoil pressure) and atmospheric pressure (assumed to be 0). Frictional resistance causes a fall in this driving pressure along the length of the conducting airways. At some point, the driving pressure may equal the surrounding peribronchial pressure. In this event, the net transmural pressure is 0. This defines the equal pressure point. Downstream (toward the mouth) from the equal pressure point, pressure outside the airway is greater than the driving pressure inside the airway. This net negative pressure tends to collapse the airway, resulting in dynamic compression. The more forcefully one expires, the more the pressure surrounding collapsible airways increases. Under these circumstances, flow becomes effort-independent. Ppl, pleural pressure; PL, lung elastic recoil pressure; Palv, alveolar pressure; Patm, atmospheric pressure. (Adapted, with permission, from Prendergast, T.J. and Ruoss, S.J. (1997). Pulmonary disease, in McPhee, S. et al. eds. Pathophysiology of Disease, 2nd ed. Stamford, CT, Appleton & Lange, p. 191.)

Implications of the work of breathing

At rest, the work of breathing is responsible for only about 2% of basal oxygen consumption. In a normal person, total ventilation has to increase tremendously, from resting levels of 6 to 8 L/min to about 70 to 100 L/min, before oxygen utilization for the work of breathing goes up significantly. However, the energy requirements for breathing are dramatically increased for patients with lung disease, both at rest and with exercise. Thus, in patients with severe lung disease, the value of the additional oxygen brought into the body by increased ventilation may be rapidly offset by the additional cost in energy for the work of breathing.

Normally rate and volume of breaths are titrated to achieve the desired minute ventilation with the least work of breathing. In the normal human at rest, this is achieved at a rate of 12 to 15 breaths per minute with a tidal volume of about 500 mL.

The respiratory system is also highly adaptable in response to demand, with a capacity for regulation of ventilation and perfusion. At rest, the lungs take in 4 L/min of air and are perfused by 5 L/min of blood. Upon vigorous exercise, airflow may increase to as much as 100 L/min and pulmonary blood flow to 25 L/min. Normally this range of function is achieved with no more than a 5% variation in arterial carbon dioxide concentration.

Clinical Pearls

○ The contributions of flow resistance to the work of breathing can be minimized by slow, large, tidal volume breaths. Amelioration with this maneuver is an indication that a dyspneic patient has some form of obstructive lung disease.
○ Conversely, rapid, shallow breaths minimizes elastic recoil and would be expected in a patient with severe restrictive lung disease, such as pulmonary fibrosis.

Review Questions

26. What forces must compliance be balanced with for the lungs to function?
27. For efficient gas exchange, with what must ventilation be well matched?
28. What is surfactant and what are its two roles in normal lung function?
29. Describe Poiseuille's law and indicate when it applies in airway airflow?
30. What are the determinants of airflow under conditions where flow is turbulent?
31. Why are the medium-sized bronchioles rather than the small airways the site of maximum resistance to airflow in the lung?
32. What are three mechanisms by which airway resistance to airflow can be increased or decreased?
33. What is the clinical significance of the equal pressure point?
34. How much of an effect on arterial P_{CO_2} is normally seen with maximum exertion, in which ventilation may go up twenty-five-fold and perfusion five-fold?

6. REGULATION OF RESPIRATION

Regulation of the respiratory system normally maintains P_{O_2} and P_{CO_2} within a very narrow range. To achieve this tight regulation, an array of peripheral receptors report to a CNS respiratory center whose output adjusts initiation, duration, and rate of breathing (see Figure 8.12).

Normally, respiration is under both unconscious and voluntary control. You breathe at an internal respiratory rhythm even when you are not thinking about breathing and that rate will automatically change (e.g., in response to activity). In contrast, you can superimpose voluntary controls on the involuntary mechanisms in order to slow, stop, or increase minute ventilation (e.g., for activities such as talking, singing, eating, swimming, and defecation).

The underlying respiratory rhythm is established by respiratory centers in the medulla and brainstem, modified by input from peripheral sensors (Figure 8.5A and Table 8.2).

The lungs inflate passively and deflate actively in response to changes in pleural pres-

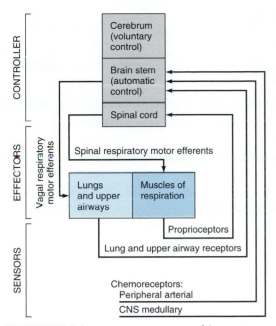

FIGURE 8.12. Schematic representation of the respiratory control system. The interrelations among the central nervous system controller, effectors, and sensors are shown, and the connections among these components. (Adapted, with permission, from Berger, A.J. et al. (1997) Regulation of respiration (3 parts). N. Engl. J. Med. 297:92, 138, 194.)

of arterial oxygenation and increase firing in response to a fall in PaO_2 (hypoxia), especially below 60 mmHg. Either an increase in Pa_{CO_2} (hypercapnia) or a fall in arterial pH (acidemia) will potentiate this response.

- Central chemoreceptors widely distributed throughout the brainstem trigger a response to hypercapnia, probably due to the effect of the CO_2 to decrease cerebrospinal fluid pH.
- Pulmonary stretch receptors in airway smooth muscle and mucosa whose afferents are carried in the vagus nerve respond to lung distention. When lung volume increases, the spontaneous rate of respiration decreases, a phenomenon known as the **Hering-Breuer reflex**.
- Peripheral proprioceptors in joints, muscles, and tendons cause an increase in respiration, which may be important for the automatic response to exercise.
- Spindle receptors in the diaphragm may play a role in monitoring the work of breathing and conveying a sense of dyspnea when the effort is disproportionate to the ventilation achieved.

sures. These changes occur as a result of rhythmic contraction and relaxation of striated muscle in the diaphragm, intercostal muscles, and abdominal wall, in response to neural input from the respiratory center.

Receptors

As mentioned above, control over respiration is mediated by sensory input from a number of different classes of receptors (see Figure 8.5B). The frequency, depth, and timing of spontaneous breathing are modified through this input. These receptors include:

- Chemoreceptors in the peripheral vasculature and in the brainstem. The most important peripheral chemoreceptors are those of the carotid bodies. These function as sensors

Clinical Pearls

○ In humans the hypoxic respiratory drive is entirely due to the carotid bodies located at the bifurcation of the internal and external carotid arteries. Thus, a complication of carotid endarterectomy (a procedure to unclog atherosclerotic carotid arteries to decrease the risk of stroke) is damage or destruction of the carotid bodies and loss of hypoxic respiratory drive. These patients become dependent on hypercapneic respiratory drive, which can itself be lost, perhaps due to desensitization, in chronic lung disease.

○ Similarly, some patients with end-stage chronic obstructive pulmonary disease are dependent on a low PO_2 to drive respira-

TABLE 8.2   CHARACTERISTICS OF VAGAL SENSORY REFLEXES

Receptor	Location	Stimulus	Response
Pulmonary stretch, slowly adapting	Associated with smooth muscle of intrapulmonary airways	Lung inflation Increased transpulmonary pressure	Hering-Breuer inflation reflex Bronchodilation Increased heart rate Decreased peripheral vascular resistance
Irritant, rapidly adapting	Epithelium of (mainly) extrapulmonary airways	Irritants Mechanical stimulation Anaphylaxis Lung inflation or deflation Hyperpnea Pulmonary congestion	Bronchoconstriction Hyperpnea Expiratory constriction of larynx Cough Mucous secretion
Ulcers Pulmonary type (J)	Alveolar wall	Increased interstitial volume (congestion)	Rapid, shallow breathing Laryngeal and tracheobronchial constriction
Bronchial	Airway and blood vessels	Chemical injury Microembolism	Bradycardia Spinal reflex inhibition Mucous secretion

Reproduced, with permission, from Prendergast, T.J. and Ruoss, S.J. (1997). Pulmonary disease, in McPhee, S. et al. eds. *Pathophysiology of Disease*, 2nd ed. Stamford, CT, Appleton & Lange, p. 187.

tion, probably because their relatively high ambient P_{CO_2} has desensitized their hypercapneic drive. Should they develop an exacerbation of their lung disease (e.g., due to a respiratory infection) and become short of breath, the physician might be tempted to place them on high concentrations of inspired O_2, in an effort to make them more comfortable. Paradoxically, giving these patients high concentrations of inspired O_2 could result in cessation of respiratory drive, somnolence, coma, respiratory failure, and death. The correct approach is to give them *low* concentrations of supplemental O_2 to improve their hypoxia without relieving it entirely.

Integrated responses

Normally, central chemoreceptors monitoring hydrogen ion concentration determine the unconscious drive to breathe. Pa_{O_2} is not an important determinant of normal respiratory drive because Pa_{CO_2}-mediated respiration never allows the Pa_{O_2} to get low enough to trigger a response. Ventilation increases 2 to 3 L/min for every 1 mmHg rise in Pa_{CO_2}. This response falls with age, sleep, aerobic conditioning, and with increased work of breathing. Pa_{O_2} has to fall to 50–60 mmHg before the hypoxic stimulus to breathe normally kicks in.

Chronic hypercapnia

While P_{CO_2} is a powerful acute stimulus to breathing, a chronically elevated P_{CO_2} can result in normalization of brain pH due to compensatory alteration in blood bicarbonate concentration as a result of renal compensation (see Chap. 10). The central chemoreceptors are then less sensitive to further changes in arterial Pa_{CO_2}. Such patients may be highly dependent on O_2-sensitive stimulation of respiration from the carotid bodies (see previous Clinical Pearl).

Chronic hypoxia

Individuals who reside at high altitudes (where the oxygen tension in the air is reduced) or who have sleep apnea syndrome (that is, they stop breathing for prolonged periods during sleep) may have a diminished hypoxic drive to breathe. When these people develop lung disease and chronic hypercapnia, they may have even less drive to breathe. Pulmonary hypertension is a common consequence of this syndrome, due to the chronic effects of the pulmonary vasoconstriction triggered by the chronic hypoxia.

Exercise

Exercise can increase minute ventilation enormously, up to twenty-five-fold. In a normal individual, there is relatively little effect on P_{O_2} and only a small fall in P_{CO_2}. The basis for the increased ventilation in response to exercise remains a mystery. It may be that elevated metabolic rate, which increases CO_2 production at the tissue level, somehow stimulates increased ventilatory rate. However, arterial pH, P_{O_2}, and P_{CO_2} remain exactly the same.

Another hypothesis is that body movements excite joint and muscle proprioceptors that stimulate the respiratory center. Finally, it has been suggested that, just as brain centers stimulate the vasomotor center to increase arterial pressure during exercise, so also the brain may send impulses to the respiratory center to increase ventilation.

Review Questions

35. What are some conscious versus involuntary aspects of breathing?
36. Describe the categories of receptors involved in regulation of respiration.

37. Discuss the role of peripheral and central chemoreceptors in regulation of ventilation.

7. LUNG DEFENSES

The intimate nature of the air-blood interface in the lung makes this a potentially high-risk site for invasion of the body by airborne pathogens. Thus a complex set of defenses have evolved. Some of these defenses are physical (e.g., the mechanical roles of mucus and the ciliated respiratory epithelium). Other defenses are biochemical (e.g., secretion of protease inhibitors and peroxidases). Still other defenses are immunological (e.g., the role of macrophages and neutrophils). Table 8.3 summarizes these defenses, some of which are discussed in greater detail elsewhere (see Chap. 19).

Clinical Pearl

○ The high-risk nature of the lung as a site for invasion by pathogens is seen in patients whose immune system has been compromised by AIDS. Many of the AIDS-defining diagnoses involve the lung (e.g., *Pneumocystis carinii* pneumonia). Likewise, AIDS patients are at greater risk for bacterial infections of the lung, including tuberculosis.

Review Questions

38. Summarize the major categories of lung defenses against invasion by pathogens.
39. Give an example of metabolism in the lung necessary to activate a product and one involved in inactivation of a biologically active product.

TABLE 8.3   LUNG DEFENSES

I. Nonspecific defenses
1. Clearance
  a. Cough
  b. Mucociliary escalator
2. Secretions
  a. Tracheobronchial (mucus)
  b. Alveolar (surfactant)
  c. Cellular components (lysozyme, complement, surfactant proteins, defensins)
3. Cellular defenses
  a. Nonphagocytic
    Conducting airway epithelium
    Terminal respiratory epithelium
  b. Phagocytic
    Blood phagocytes (monocytes)
    Tissue phagocytes (alveolar macrophages)
4. Biochemical defenses
  a. Proteinase inhibitors (α_1-protease inhibitor, secretory leukoprotease inhibitor)
  b. Antioxidants (e.g., transferrin, lactoferrin, glutathione, albumin)
II. Specific immunologic defenses
1. Antibody-mediated (B lymphocyte-dependent immunologic responses)
  a. Secretory immunoglobulin (IgA)
  b. Serum immunoglobulins
2. Antigen presentation to lymphocytes
  a. Macrophages and monocytes
  b. Dendritic cells
  c. Epithelial cells
3. Cell-mediated (T lymphocyte-dependent) immunologic responses
  a. Cytokine-mediated
  b. Direct cellular cytotoxicity
4. Nonlymphocyte cellular immune responses
  a. Mast cell dependent
  b. Eosinophil-dependent

Adapted, with permission, from Prendergast, T.J. and Ruoss, S.J. (1997). Pulmonary disease, in McPhee, S. et al. eds. *Pathophysiology of Disease*, 2nd ed. Stamford, CT, Appleton & Lange, p. 188.

8. PATHOPHYSIOLOGY OF RESPIRATORY SYSTEM DISORDERS

Most disorders of the respiratory system involve one or both of the following problems:

1. Impaired ability of the lungs to carry out gas exchange or to match ventilation with perfusion

2. Increased work of breathing due to changes in elasticity or resistance to airflow

As a result of one or both of these functional problems, patients with an extremely wide variety of disorders typically develop symptoms of dyspnea, and arterial blood gas evaluation reveals hypoxia and/or hypercapnea (see Figure 8.13).

As with other organ systems, many different specific causes can present as dysfunction of a particular physiological feature of the respiratory system.

In addition to the functional disorders previously discussed, the lung is a high risk site for development of cancer, perhaps due to the high degree of oxidative stress occurring at this air-aqueous interface (see Chap. 19).

Clinical Pearls

Many respiratory diseases have genetic predispositions and environmental triggers and exacerbators that should be identified by taking a careful history.

○ Cystic fibrosis, α_1 antitrypsin deficiency, and some cases of asthma are examples of diseases affecting the lung that are due to specific gene defects.
○ Stimuli that are known to trigger/exacerbate asthma fall into the following seven categories: allergens (dust mite and cockroach feces, pet dander, pollen), pharmacologic agents (asprin, food coloring, sulfiting chemicals such as sodium bisulfite, β-adrenergic blockers), air pollution (ozone, sulfur dioxide), occupational exposures (wood dust), infections, exercise, and emotional stress.

Asthma and chronic obstructive pulmonary disease

Asthma and **chronic obstructive pulmonary disease** (COPD) are obstructive disorders of

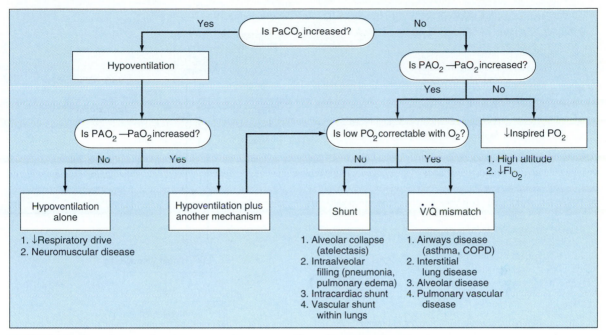

FIGURE 8.13. Flow diagram for diagnosis in hypoxemia. Flow diagram outlining the diagnostic approach to the patient with hypoxemia (PaO$_2$ < 80 mmHg). PAO$_2$-PaO$_2$ is usually < 15 mmHg for subjects < 30 years old and increases by about 3 mmHg per decade after age 30. *(Adapted, with permission, from Fauci, A. et al. eds. (1997). Harrison's Principles of Internal Medicine, 14th ed. New York, McGraw-Hill, p. 1416.)*

the lung. They have in common a decrease in FEV$_1$/FVC, indicating increased resistance to airflow, usually worse on expiration than with inspiration. However, this common clinical picture can be the consequence of a variety of different pathophysiological mechanisms (see Table 8.4).

Patients with asthma have episodes of bronchial smooth muscle hyperreactivity as the cause of obstruction to airflow. Some studies suggest that the pathophysiology of asthma involves a more chronic process of airway inflammation, with leukocyte infiltration of airway epithelium and hypertrophy of mucus-secreting glands and muscle, distinct from the acute finding of smooth muscle hyperreactivity during exacerbations.

In contrast to pure asthma, COPD includes a spectrum of disorders in which the acute

basis for obstruction is not primarily bronchial smooth muscle constriction, although it can be a contributing factor in some cases. In COPD, obstruction occurs primarily for other reasons. At one extreme of the spectrum is **chronic bronchitis**. Here, airflow obstruction is primarily due to mucus overproduction. At the other extreme is **emphysema**, in which alveolar destruction and loss of lung elasticity causes airways to collapse during expiration, trapping air in the lungs that normally would be exhaled (see Figures 8.14 and 8.15). This results in hyperinflation, less driving force to overcome the increased resistance posed by collapsed airways, less capacity for inspiration, and, in sum, poor gas exchange, hypoxia and hypercarbia, and pulmonary hypertension.

In practice, there is considerable overlap in

TABLE 8.4 INFLAMMATORY EVENTS (A) AND PROVOCATIVE FACTORS (B) IN ASTHMA

A. Asthma cellular inflammatory events
 I. Epithelial cell activation or injury
    Cytokine (IL-8) release with neutrophil chemotaxis or activation
    Antigen presentation to lymphocytes
    Secretory epithelial cell hyperplasia and hypersecretion
    Epithelial death; increased magnitude of airway sensory neural reflexes
 II. Lymphocyte activation
    Antigen exposure with lymphocyte proliferation
    Increased cytokine expression: activation of additional effector cells (mast cells, eosinophils, macrophages)
    Activation of B cells; increased IgE synthesis
    Augmented lymphocyte activation by local cytokines
 III. Mast cell and eosinophil activation
    Eosinophil release of cytotoxic and acute proinflammatory mediators
    IgE-mediated mast cell activation, with acute mediator release (e.g., histamine, leukotrienes, platelet-activating factor)
    New expression of multiple cytokines by mast cells, with multiple effector cell activation, as with lymphocytes

B. Asthma: Provocative factors
 I. Physiological and pharmacological mediators of normal smooth muscle contraction
    Histamine
    Methacholine
    Adenosine triphosphate (ATP)
 II. Physicochemical agents
    Exercise: hyperventilation with cold, dry air
    Air pollutants
       Sulfur dioxide
       Nitrogen dioxide
    Viral respiratory infections (e.g., influenza A)
    Ingestants
       Propranolol
       Aspirin; NSAIDs
 III. Allergens
    Low-molecular-weight chemicals, e.g., penicillin, isocyanates, anhydrides, chromate
    Complex organic molecules, e.g., animal danders, dust mites, enzymes, wood dusts

Reproduced, with permission, from Prendergast, T.J. and Ruoss, S.J. (1997). Pulmonary disease, in McPhee, S. et al. eds. *Pathophysiology of Disease*, 2nd ed. Stamford, CT, Appleton & Lange, p. 200.

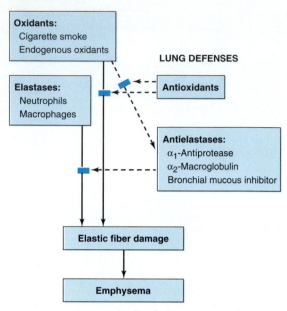

FIGURE 8.14. Proposed role of elastase in emphysema. According to the elastase-antielastase hypothesis of emphysema, the lung is protected from elastolytic damage by α_1-protease inhibitor and α_2 macroglobulin. Bronchial mucus inhibitor protects the airways. Elastase is derived primarily from neutrophils, but macrophages secrete an elastase-like metalloprotease and may ingest and later release neutrophil elastase. Oxidants derived from neutrophils and macrophages or from cigarette smoke may inactivate α_1 protease inhibitor and may interfere with lung matrix repair. Endogenous antioxidants such as superoxide dismutase, glutathione, and catalase protect the lung against oxidant injury. Activation is represented here by solid lines, inhibition by dashed lines. Solid bars represent antagonistic relations. *(Reproduced, with permission, from Prendergast, T.J. and Ruoss, S.J. (1997). Pulmonary disease, in McPhee, S. et al. eds.* Pathophysiology of Disease, *2nd ed. Stamford, CT, Appleton & Lange, p. 204, as modified from Snider, G.L. (1986). Experimental studies on emphysema and chronic bronchial injury. Eur. J. Respir. Dis. 146(suppl):17.)*

presentation of individual patients, although subsets with different predominating features are seen (Table 8.4). Many patients with emphysema, for example, have some degree of bronchial smooth muscle hyperreactivity and

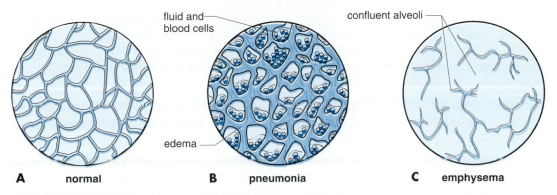

FIGURE 8.15. Pulmonary changes in emphysema and pneumonia. Structure of the normal lung (A), affected lung in lobar pneumonia (B), and affected lung in emphysema (C). Note destruction of architecture of alveoli in C. This greatly decreases the diffusing capacity and increases the compliance of the lung. (Adapted, with permission, from Guyton, A.C. and Hall, J.E. (1997). Human Physiology and Mechanisms of Disease, 6th ed. Philadelphia, Saunders, p. 342.)

some degree of mucus overproduction as contributors to their airflow obstruction. Likewise, worsening of chronic bronchitis is seen in many patients as a precipitant and exacerbant of an attack of asthma.

Clinical Pearl

○ Patients with decompensated left-sided heart failure can have bronchial edema as a result of elevated hydrostatic pressure due to blood backing up behind the left side of the heart. In patients with an underlying predisposition to the development of heart failure, this bronchial edema can result in reflex bronchoconstriction, airway narrowing, and obstructive symptoms including wheezing. This is termed *cardiac asthma*. Unlike conventional asthma, however, treatment must include intervention to improve cardiac function or eliminate excess intravascular volume, either of which will relieve the underlying precipitant of the airflow obstruction. Otherwise, the patient is likely to progress to full-blown pulmonary edema as more and

more fluid extravasates into the alveolar space, impairing gas exchange, resulting in worsening hypoxia and hypercapnea, and even death.

Restrictive lung disease

A number of different disease processes have the effect of increasing elastic recoil, decreasing compliance, and, therefore, decreasing residual lung volumes (see Table 8.5). Dis-

TABLE 8.5 CELLULAR EVENTS IN LUNG INJURY AND FIBROSIS

1. Tissue injury
2. Vascular endothelium activation and permeability changes, with thrombosis and thrombolysis
3. Epithelial injury and activation
4. Leukocyte influx, activation, and proliferation
5. Further tissue injury, remodeling, and fibrosis:
   Perpetuation of tissue inflammation
   Incomplete or delayed resolution of interstitial thrombosis
   Fibroblast proliferation and matrix molecule production or deposition
   Epithelial proliferation and repopulation

Reproduced, with permission, from Prendergast, T.J. and Ruoss, S.J. (1997). Pulmonary disease, in McPhee, S. et al. eds. *Pathophysiology of Disease*, 2nd ed. Stamford, CT, Appleton & Lange, p. 207.

orders with these features can be physiologically characterized as **restrictive lung disease**. Typically, the processes that cause restrictive changes involve an inflammatory response that usually seems to be initiated in the alveoli. Often the term **interstitial lung disease** is used to describe these entities. However, inflammation in these disorders is not limited to the interstitium, but rather progresses beyond the interstitium to involve the airway mucosa and the alveoli as well.

The initiating event in interstitial lung disease is often typically injury to either the capillary endothelium or the alveolar epithelium. Either can respond to injury by changing the adhesion molecules displayed and by secreting cytokines. These changes in turn recruit immune cells, including neutrophils and lymphocytes, to the site of inflammation. Cytokines also change the pattern of gene expression such that the normal quiescent type II epithelial cells of the airspace (which normally make surfactant) are lost and replaced by proliferating type I cells (which do not make surfactant). Thus, intraalveolar surface tension goes up.

Similarly, fibroblasts, a type of mesenchymal cell, respond to the initial release of cytokines by proliferating in the interstitium. They also magnify the inflammatory response through release of cytokines of their own. Finally, they compound the restrictive changes brought about as a result of loss of surfactant secretion, by secreting extracellular matrix molecules including collagen, which are involved in tissue fibrosis. This appears to set up a vicious cycle of lymphocyte and mast cell infiltration, more cytokines, more fibroblast proliferation and more fibrosis, although it often proceeds in a patchy, uneven way, with areas of severely affected lung adjacent to regions with only minor changes.

Unchecked, the fibrosis results in obliteration of airspaces and vasculature, with scar formation. The net effect is stiff lungs, with too much recoil, too much surface tension, small residual volumes and not enough compliance for normal function. Ventilation to perfusion mismatch is also increased.

Pulmonary edema and acute respiratory distress syndrome

Pulmonary edema is the accumulation of interstitial fluid in the alveoli (see Figure 8.16). There are two broad classifications of pulmonary edema. The first is when it occurs because of a pure increase in pulmonary pressures (e.g., due to left-sided heart failure), termed **cardiogenic pulmonary edema**. In the lung, as elsewhere in the body, this form of interstitial fluid accumulation occurs only when the capacity of the lymphatic vessels is exceeded. Thus cardiogenic pulmonary edema can occur in three stages. Early, there is elevation of pulmonary capillary pressures, followed by formation of edema fluid, which is limited to the interstitium and therefore has a small effect on gas exchange and no effect on oxygenation. Later, the fluid starts to leak into alveoli. Once a threshold of edema fluid accumulation in an alveolus has been exceeded, the alveolus becomes completely flooded, perhaps due to impaired surfactant production. Under these conditions oxygenation of the fraction of cardiac output flowing past such alveoli is lost. Importantly, both the endothelial and epithelial layers of the lung are intact in cardiogenic pulmonary edema. The only thing wrong is the ability of the heart to pump with enough force to control hydrostatic pressure. Thus, the edema fluid has a relatively low protein content (<70% of that of plasma) and is termed a **transudate**.

Pulmonary edema can also occur because of changes in the structure of the lung that impair the normal barrier role of the alveolar epithelium to fluid. This second category of pulmonary edema is termed **noncardiogenic**

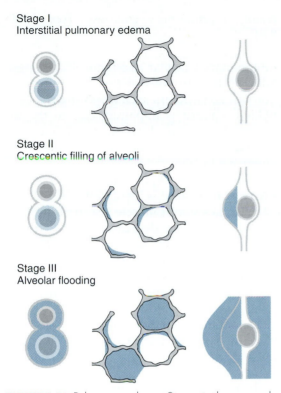

Stage I
Interstitial pulmonary edema

Stage II
Crescentic filling of alveoli

Stage III
Alveolar flooding

FIGURE 8.16. Pulmonary edema. Stages in the accumulation of pulmonary edema fluid. The three columns represent three anatomic views of the progressive accumulation of pulmonary edema fluid. From left to right, the columns represent a cross-section of the bronchovascular bundle showing the loose connective tissue surrounding the pulmonary artery and bronchial wall, a cross-section of alveoli fixed in inflation, and the pulmonary capillary in cross-section. The first stage is eccentric accumulation of fluid in the pericapillary interstitial space. The limitation of edema fluid to one side of the pulmonary capillary maintains gas transfer better than symmetric accumulation. When formation of edema fluid exceeds lymphatic removal, it distends the periobronchovascular interstitium. At this stage, there is no alveolar flooding, but there is some crescentic filling of alveoli. The third stage is alveolar flooding. Note that each individual alveolus is either totally flooded or has minimal crescentic filling. This pattern probably occurs because alveolar edema interferes with surfactant and, above some threshold, there is an increase in surface forces that greatly increases the transmural pressure and causes flooding. (Modified, with permission, from Prendergast, T.J. and Ruoss, S.J. (1997). Pulmonary disease, in

pulmonary edema and is the basis for acute respiratory distress syndrome (ARDS). Common causes of ARDS include toxic inhalations and cytokine release in sepsis or bacterial toxins, which can result in injury to the alveolar epithelium. Here the protein concentration is generally the same as that of plasma and hence the edema fluid is termed an **exudate**.

Once the alveolus is flooded with high protein fluid in ARDS, surfactant is inactivated. The result is increased surface tension, fall in pulmonary compliance, alveolar collapse, and atelectasis. This in turn increases the work of breathing and sets in motion a vicious cycle of increased fluid movement into the collapsed lung and increased susceptibility to infection.

Depending on the time course of its formation and the intactness of the alveolar epithelial barrier, extravasated interstitial fluid can either flow into the alveoli or pool between the pleura (forming a pleural effusion), or both. Carrying around a liter of pleural effusion fluid is like carrying around a liter of culture medium: The risk of infection is greatly increased and what was an isolated problem can quickly become more complicated.

Pulmonary embolism

Pulmonary embolism results in occlusion of pulmonary arterial vessels. Most commonly, a pulmonary embolism results from blood clots that form in the deep veins of the lower extremities above the knees (see Table 8.6), break off, and flow back to the right heart.

FIGURE 8.16 — (continued) McPhee, S. et al. eds. Pathophysiology of Disease, 2nd ed. Stamford, CT, Appleton & Lange, p. 211, as modified in Nunn, J.F. (1993), in Nunn's Applied Respiratory Physiology, 4th ed., Stoneham, MA, Butterworth-Heinemann.)

TABLE 8.6   CAUSES OF PULMONARY EMBOLI

Increased pulmonary capillary transmural pressure
  Increased left atrial pressure
    Left ventricular failure, acute or chronic
    Mitral valve stenosis
  Pulmonary venous hypertension
    Pulmonary venoocclusive disease
  Increased capillary blood volume
    Iatrogenic volume expansion
    Chronic renal failure
  Reduction of interstitial pressure
    Rapid reexpansion of collapsed lung
  Decreased plasma colloid osmotic pressure
    Hypoalbuminemia: nephrotic syndrome, hepatic failure

Increased pulmonary capillary endothelial permeability
  Circulating toxins: bacteremia, acute pancreatitis
  Infectious pneumonia
  Disseminated intravascular coagulation
  Nonthoracic trauma accompanied by hypotension ("shock
    lung")
  High-altitude pulmonary edema
  Following cardiopulmonary bypass

Increased alveolar epithelial permeability
  Inhaled toxins: oxygen, phosgene, chlorine, smoke
  Aspiration of acidic gastric contents
  Drowning and near-drowning
  Depletion of surfactant through high tidal volume positive-
    pressure mechanical ventilation

Reduced lymphatic clearance
  Lymphangitic spread of carcinoma
  Following lung transplant

Mechanism uncertain
  Neurogenic pulmonary edema
  Narcotic overdose
  Multiple transfusions

Adapted, with permission, from Prendergast, T.J. and Ruoss, S.J. (1997). Pulmonary disease, in McPhee, S. et al. eds. *Pathophysiology of Disease*, 2nd ed. Stamford, CT, Appleton & Lange, p. 209.

From there, they are pumped into the pulmonary artery and proceed down the pulmonary arterial tree until the diameter of the vessel is too small for them to pass. The clinical risk factors for pulmonary embolism are venous stasis, injury to blood vessel walls, and increased coagulability (see Table 8.7). As a result of pulmonary embolism (see Table 8.8):

- Pulmonary vascular resistance is increased, due both to the obstruction and to release of vasoconstrictors such as seratonin.
- Gas exchange is impaired, due to the increased alveolar dead space as a consequence of the obstruction, resulting in an increase in P_{CO_2}.
- Reflex alveolar hyperventilation occurs.
- Airway resistance is increased due to reflex bronchial smooth muscle constriction.
- Lung compliance decreases due to edema, hemorrhage, and loss of surfactant. This results in release of mediators and development of atelectasis (areas of lung collapse) as a result of which oxygenation falls.

Sometimes patients have multiple episodes of small pulmonary emboli. In these

TABLE 8.7   RISK FACTORS FOR VENOUS THROMBOSIS

Increased venous stasis
  Bed rest
  Immobilization, especially following orthopedic surgery
  Low cardiac output states
  Pregnancy
  Obesity
  Hyperviscosity
  Local vascular damage, especially prior thrombosis with incompetent valves
  Increasing age

Increased coagulability
  Tissue injury: surgery, trauma, myocardial infarction
  Malignancy
  Presence of a lupus anticoagulant
  Nephrotic syndrome
  Oral contraceptive use, especially estrogen administration
  Genetic coagulation disorders: Factor V Leiden; deficiency of antithrombin III; deficiency of protein C or its cofactor, protein S; deficiency of plasminogen; dysfunctional fibrinogen

Reproduced, with permission, from Prendergast, T.J. and Ruoss, S.J. (1997). Pulmonary disease, in McPhee, S. et al. eds. *Pathophysiology of Disease*, 2nd ed. Stamford, CT, Appleton & Lange, p. 213.

TABLE 8.8   PATHOPHYSIOLOGY OF PULMONARY EMBOLISM

Altered physiology	Effect of thromboembolism	Mechanism
Altered hemodynamics	Increased pulmonary vascular resistance	Vascular obstruction; vasoconstriction by serotonin, thromboxane A_2
Impaired gas exchange	Increase in alveolar dead space	Vascular obstruction; increased perfusion of lung units with high $\dot{V}/\dot{Q}$ ratios
	Hypoxemia	Increased perfusion of lung units with low $\dot{V}/\dot{Q}$ ratios; right-to-left shunting; fall in cardiac output with fall in mixed venous P_{O_2}
Ventilatory control	Hyperventilation	Reflex stimulation of irritant receptors
Work of breathing	Increased airway resistance Decreased pulmonary compliance	Reflex bronchoconstriction; loss of surfactant with lung edema and hemorrhage

Reproduced, with permission, from Prendergast, T.J. and Ruoss, S.J. (1997). Pulmonary disease, in McPhee, S. et al. eds. *Pathophysiology of Disease*, 2nd ed. Stamford, CT, Appleton & Lange, p. 215, as modified from Elliott, C.G. (1992). Pulmonary physiology during pulmonary embolism. *Chest* 101(4 suppl.):1635.)

cases, there may be little effect on either ventilation or perfusion initially. Tachycardia may be the only manifestation. However, eventually enough lung is involved to cause ventilatory disturbances. In the long run these patients may develop pulmonary hypertension as more and more small vessels are occluded and obliterated.

Sometimes patients have a single large embolus that occludes a major pulmonary artery. This form of pulmonary embolism is associated with major perfusion defects and can also cause right-sided heart failure and even cardiogenic shock due to the sudden drop in cardiac output. This is caused by the combination of right-sided heart failure and bulging of the engorged right side of the heart, which obstructs filling of the left ventricle.

Pulmonary embolism is a common complication of a large number of disorders. Between 25 and 50% of hospitalized patients who die are found at autopsy to have pulmonary emboli.

Consideration of the natural history of pulmonary emboli can help us understand the physiology of ventilation perfusion matching. Early in the course of pulmonary embolism,

occlusion of vessels results in areas of high ventilation and poor perfusion, that is, increased dead space. This impairs elimination of CO_2. However, hyperventilation usually prevents or rapidly corrects this abnormality.

After a few hours however, poor perfusion impairs surfactant production and those regions of lung collapse, resulting in atelectasis. At that point, neither ventilation nor perfusion is possible and any residual areas that were still being perfused previously are lost. If the loss of airspaces is now great enough, hypoxia results. Due to the differences in gas exchange properties of CO_2 and O_2, hyperventilation will not be able to correct this, and the patient may need supplemental oxygen if the hypoxia is sufficiently severe.

Clinical Pearls

○ The symptoms of pulmonary embolism can be extremely broad, encompassing symptoms from wheezing to hemoptysis (coughing up blood), to chest pain upon inspiration (called pleuritic chest pain), and signs including infiltrates on chest x-ray (due to pulmonary infarction) and right side of the heart strain on electrocardiogram. Thus, for example, what appears to be a pulmonary embolism often turns out to be pneumonia or a heart attack, and vice versa.

○ Until recently the diagnostic approach upon suspicion of pulmonary embolism was to search for a source of emboli (e.g., a deep venous clot, identifiable by ultrasound) and perform a ventilation versus perfusion scan, looking for areas of subsegmental mismatch. (Unfortunately, these areas are often not very helpful, especially in someone with underlying lung disease who already has large defects in both ventilation and perfusion.) The next step would be to obtain a pulmonary arteriogram. (This was the gold standard diagnostic test, with high sensitivity and specificity, but which is also invasive, expensive, and associated with a high risk of complications from the procedure itself. Hence, this procedure was not usually ordered unless you had both a high clinical suspicion and the other studies were negative.)

For these reasons, knowing when to have a strong enough clinical suspicion to initiate a diagnostic workup for pulmonary embolism used to be a major challenge in clinical judgment. Today, an imaging modality termed **spiral computed tomography** allows rapid, noninvasive diagnosis of pulmonary emboli with high sensitivity and specificity.

Pneumonia

Formally, a pneumonia is any process involving inflammation of the parenchyma of the lung (see Figure 8.14). Most commonly in clinical practice, however, pneumonia refers to infectious diseases of the lung parenchyma. During the course of most lung parenchymal infections (e.g., in contrast to bronchitis, which involves the airway but not the lung parenchyma), alveolar epithelial tightness is disrupted with extravasation of fluid and infected debris into the alveolar space. There is typically poor ventilation of involved regions of lung, resulting in hypoxia. Similar findings with or without infection are seen in patients with localized airway collapse termed *atelectasis*. This entity increases the risk of infection and can result in a pneumonia. As with ARDS, most cases of pneumonia are completely reversible, if the patient survives. Sometimes, however, the patient may be left with residual deficits in lung function. What determines the line between acute disease that can be completely reversed with treatment and the development of chronic complications is at present unknown.

Pneumothorax

Pneumothorax is air in the chest cavity. Typically it occurs due to a hole in the lung through the pleura that connects air spaces with the intrathoracic space. As with fluid, leak of a small amount of air is harmless and is readily resorbed by the body. Provided the leak is small and the body's repair mechanisms are intact, such pneumothoraces are of no consequence. However, if the leak is large or repair mechanisms are "off line," ventilation of the entire lung can be lost as air in the thorax prevents expansion of the lung upon inspiration (see Figure 8.17).

Respiratory failure and mechanical ventilation

Respiratory failure occurs when the lungs are unable to provide adequate O_2 or remove sufficient CO_2. In these circumstances, death can be prevented only by putting a tube in the trachea that establishes an airtight seal with the lungs (endotrachial intubation) and connecting that tube to a machine that deliv-

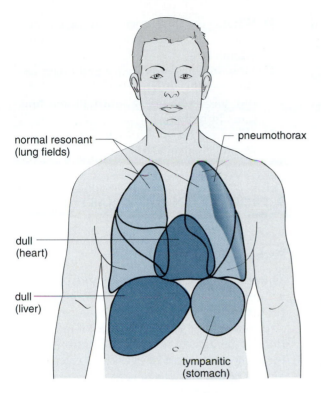

normal resonant
(lung fields)

pneumothorax

dull
(heart)

dull
(liver)

tympanitic
(stomach)

FIGURE 8.17. Pneumothorax. Diagram of normal lung volume (left side of figure) and diminished lung volume with displacement of lung by free air in pneumothorax. *(Adapted, with permission, from Berne, R.M. and Levy, M.N. (1998). Physiology, 4th ed. St. Louis, Mosby, p. 198.)*

ers to the patient's lungs air of defined composition (Fio_2), amount (tidal volume), and frequency (respiratory rate). This intervention is termed **mechanical ventilation**. It almost always requires that the patient be sedated and sometimes even paralyzed, as both the endotracheal tube and the sensation of air being forced into the lungs can be quite unpleasant. Once the patient's breathing is on "autopilot," thanks to this highly technical supportive measure, efforts are focused on identifying and reversing the underlying disorder (e.g., pneumonia, exacerbation of obstructive lung disease).

Clinical Pearls

○ Regardless of the specific disease, patients with sudden, severe respiratory decompensation may require intubation and me

chanical ventilation. The following are some reasons for this intervention:

- Hypoxemia despite high Fio_2 (>60%). Typically this is due to severe pneumonia, pulmonary edema including ARDS, or pulmonary hemorrhage, where treatment of the underlying condition will eventually improve gas exchange and oxygenation.
- Acute hypercarbia (e.g., due to respiratory muscle fatigue in patients with underlying lung disease)
- The need for controlled hyperventilation (e.g., to reduce cerebral blood flow in patients with increased intracranial pressure)
- The need to protect the airway from aspiration in a patient with loss of consciousness (e.g., in suspected drug overdose). This is an indication for intubation, but

not necessarily mechanical ventilation, if they remain strong and able to breathe on their own.

○ Sometimes patients with underlying lung disease who have been intubated during an acute episode of respiratory failure are difficult to extubate. This often leads to discussion of why they are not able to breathe on their own:

- Is it because the underlying process has not resolved sufficiently, that is, one should wait longer before trying to extubate them?
- Is it that they are too weak to breathe on their own and need a period of intensive, intravenous nutritional support to gain back their strength?
- Is it that their underlying lung disease has progressed as a result of the acute disorder (e.g., loss of additional alveoli) to the point that their baseline is now ventilator-dependent?

○ When patients are approaching the end of a long life as a result of a fundamentally irreversible lung disease such as severe emphysema, they may decide that the discomfort of breathing with the help of mechanical ventilation constitutes an unacceptable diminution of their quality of life. In these circumstances, more and more patients opt to not be intubated in the future or to have the tube removed if they have become ventilator-dependent. The physician will often provide opiates to keep the patient comfortable as he or she proceeds to go into respiratory failure and die.

Review Questions

40. What are the common pathophysiological findings in COPD?

41. What is the difference between cardiogenic and noncardiogenic pulmonary edema?
42. How might a pulmonary embolism result initially in hyperventilation, without gas exchange abnormalities, and later in hypoxia?
43. What are the physiological indications for mechanical ventilation of a patient?

9. FRONTIERS IN PULMONARY RESEARCH

Pathophysiology of asthma

The study of the pathophysiological basis for asthma has largely changed from a focus on bronchial smooth muscle hyperreactivity to a recognition of the importance of inflammation in the airway mucosa. Attention is now focusing on the role of cytokines released by airway epithelial cells in response to environmental irritants (see Ref. 3). The epithelial cell-derived cytokines appear to initiate a vicious cycle of inflammation resulting in airway infiltration of mast cells, eosinophils, and lymphocytes. Exploring the details of these relations is an important challenge for the coming period.

An important role for the cytokines IL-13 and IL-4, working via the IL-4 α receptor (IL-4R), has been suggested by studies using a mouse model for experimental asthma (see Refs. 4, 5). While the pathophysiology in mice may be substantially different from that in humans, it is more than intriguing that genetic linkage studies have implicated the region of the human genome in which both of these cytokines and the IL-4R α chain are encoded, in familial susceptibility to asthma (see Refs. 6, 7).

Another dimension of asthma is the role of specific allergens in the environment as triggers of inflammation and bronchial smooth muscle hyperreactivity. But how do they work? A cell culture system was developed to analyze tight junction permeability in response to a protease present in dust mite feces, a known asthmatic allergen (see Ref. 8). What was found was that the dust mite fecal protease specifically cleaved transmembrane proteins that comprise the tight junction, allowing the allergen to cross the epithelial barrier by moving between epithelial cells and thereby be more likely to be seen by the immune system. But how applicable is this elegant study of epithelial tight junction integrity to the in vivo pathophysiology of human asthma? Only further studies will tell. However, this work suggests some intriguing hypotheses with novel therapeutic potential.

Asthmatic bronchial hyperresponsiveness: Back to smooth muscle dysfunction?

The studies that have given rise to the explosion of information on inflammation in the airway were motivated, in part, by frustration at the earlier lack of evidence for an abnormality in bronchial smooth muscle function itself. In the past, bronchial smooth muscle was studied in terms of isometric shortening, which reflects the number of actin-myosin cross bridges (see Chap. 2). Now, even as the plot thickens on the airway inflammation story (see earlier), data suggest that there is, indeed, a molecular defect in airway smooth muscle of patients with asthma. These data implicate *elevated velocity of shortening* rather than increased isometric force generation. In other words, it may have been the *rate* of cycling of cross-bridges rather than their number that is the molecular basis for bronchial smooth muscle hyperresponsiveness. A hypothesis for the difference in smooth muscle dynamics during breathing in normal versus asthmatic individuals that is based on the differences in velocity of contraction (rate of cross-bridge cycling) has been proposed (see Ref. 9). This, in turn, raises the potential for development of new therapeutic modalities in an unexpected area:

changing the velocity of asthmatic bronchial smooth muscle contraction. It is important to remember that diseases with complex pathophysiology likely involve multiple dimensions, pathways, and components. Thus, progress in new directions (e.g., the role of inflammation, see Ref. 10) does not preclude new insights in traditional areas (e.g., bronchial smooth muscle contraction, see Ref. 9).

Growth factors and restrictive lung disease

Restrictive lung disease is typically associated with increased elastic recoil and decreased compliance as a result of pulmonary fibrosis. The pathophysiological mechanism for the pulmonary fibrosis observed in asbestos-induced restrictive lung disease appears to involve recruitment of inflammatory cells including alveolar macrophages and then polymorphonuclear leukocytes (see Ref. 11). These cells produce large amounts of reactive oxygen compounds (also called reactive oxygen species, ROS). These products cause subcellular damage (e.g., they react with proteins, membranes, or DNA). In response to repeated cycles of this sort of damage, the cells of the lung secrete various growth factors that trigger collagen production and progression of fibrosis. Several recent studies highlight diverse aspects of this process. A form of **platelet-derived growth factor** (PDGF) has been strongly implicated as a key contributor to lung fibrosis (see Ref. 12). In another study, apoptosis in the alveoli, as a result of expression of **Fas** and **Fas Ligand**, a cell death-promoting receptor and ligand, also appears to be involved in lung fibrosis (see Ref. 13).

Finally, integrins, the "sticky" molecules on the epithelial cell surface which mediate a range of adhesive interactions between epithelial cells, immune cells, and others, have been implicated in regulation of a key growth factor (TGFβ) involved in pulmonary fibrosis (see Ref. 14). Mice lacking a specific integrin were found to be protected from subsequent development of pulmonary fibrosis, despite having an exaggerated immune response. It appears that a fragment cleaved from the TGF β gene product is a ligand for this integrin. Cells expressing this integrin are able to alter TGFβ activation in a way that somehow potentiates fibrosis.

Endothelin-1 (ET-1) is a fascinating peptide with vasoconstrictive, bronchoconstrictive, and mitogenic properties. Among its many actions is the stimulation of collagen synthesis. Its activation requires proteolytic cleavage by a converting enzyme. It is known to be regulated by proinflammatory cytokines such as IL-8 and TNF α. Studies have localized both ET-1 and its converting enzyme to various cells in the airway and lung during idiopathic pulmonary fibrosis. This has led to the suggestion that ET and its converting enzyme may be involved in the inflammatory cytokine imbalance that contributes to fibrosing lung diseases (see Ref. 15).

The best offense is a good defense

It has been estimated that we expose ourselves to 10^3 to 10^7 pathogenic microbes per cubic meter of air breathed, depending on the environment. Thus, even when we are healthy, the airway must represent quite a war zone. A variety of lines of defense provide constant protection of the airway, and even more lines of defense are activated should infection occur (see Chap. 19). Despite the complexity of currently recognized host defenses, more defenses are being discovered all the time. Two dimensions in "preventive" host defense have recently been appreciated.

One discovery is that a major constituent of normal mammalian airway secretions is a peroxidase made by airway epithelial cells (see Ref. 16). This peroxidase converts hydrogen peroxide, also generated by the air-

way, into hypothiocyanous acid, a toxic compound that kills would-be pathogens. Should pathogens gain a foothold in the airway (in the form of a bronchitis or a pneumonia), neutrophils that represent the first wave of the inflammatory response release a different peroxidase, called myeloperoxidase, which converts hydrogen peroxide into the even more toxic compound, hypochlorous acid (literally the same as Clorox bleach).

Defensins

Another newly appreciated line of defense is the existence of small (30 to 40 amino acid residue) peptides known as **defensins**, which are released both from healthy airway epithelia and from neutrophils during the inflammatory response to infection. The antibacterial action of defensins appears to be mediated by poking a hole in the bacterial plasma membrane (see Ref. 17).

Several observations suggest a complex and, as yet poorly understood, physiology for the defensins. First, they have more than just an antibacterial role: they appear to be a form of early warning system. Work demonstrates that dramatically increased levels of interleukin-8 (IL-8) are released by airway epithelial cells in response to neutrophil defensin (see Ref. 18). IL-8 is an important cytokine involved in recruiting more neutrophils to the airways. Hence, defensins may provide a mechanism by which inflammation begets more inflammation.

Second, it appears that the defensins are designed to work at low salt concentrations. Patients with cystic fibrosis who have impaired Cl$^-$ secretion are unable to maintain the low salt environment needed by airway defensins. As a result, the defensins are inactivated and the airways of cystic fibrosis patients are more easily infected and damaged by pathogens (see Ref. 19).

Third, it appears that defensins and antiproteases neutralize each other (even though defensins are not proteases, (see Ref. 20). This suggests that antiproteases themselves may have a more complex role in host defense than has been previously realized. In this context, the observation that ROS inactivate antiproteases has profound implications. For example, cigarette smoke is loaded with ROS, perhaps 10^{18} molecules per puff (see Ref. 21). Thus, smoking not only potentiates the damage caused by elastase and other proteases released by neutrophils into the airway to clear away debris, it also likely wreaks havoc with the delicate system of checks and balances that make up lines of defense throughout the body in ways that are not currently understood.

10. HOW DOES UNDERSTANDING NORMAL PHYSIOLOGY PROVIDE INSIGHT INTO THE INITIAL CASE PRESENTATION?

Let us look back on G.N., a 32-year-old man with a long history of mild asthma recently discharged from the hospital after his first severe asthma exacerbation, associated with an episode of bronchitis.

As is commonly observed, an asthma exacerbation is triggered by an episode of bronchitis. Often, bronchitis caused initially by a virus is complicated by a subsequent bacterial infection. In addition to bronchodilator medicines, Mr. N. may need steroids (glucocorticoids, see Chap. 13) to calm the underlying inflammatory process that was set in motion by the infection.

Many of these infections are purely viral processes against which conventional antibiotics are no use. Nevertheless antibiotics are often prescribed because it is not easy to distinguish the (probably small) percentage of cases in which subsequent bacterial infection may play a role in perpetuating the asthma exacerbation. Often, clinicians use change in color of sputum (e.g., from white to dark green) as an indicator of bacterial superinfection, for which antibiotics are prescribed.

In response to his question about why the hospital staff were more concerned about him than with the elderly man in the next bed with a higher P_{CO_2}, you can explain how a sudden rise in CO_2 in someone with asthma is of greater immediate concern than a patient with a chronic stable high CO_2 due to emphysema. Mr. N.'s rise in P_{CO_2} was a direct sign of impending respiratory failure, while that of the elderly gentleman with chronic obstructive lung disease and/or emphysema reflects long-term destruction of airways that is probably stable for now.

You can also explain to Mr. N. that he was so sick during this hospitalization because he had an infection in his lungs. You might also point out that the inflammation took about 2 weeks to set in this time. Often, it tends to take an equal length of time for such an inflammatory process to resolve.

Smoking clearly is a terrible thing for Mr. N. (and everyone else). Not only does it maintain the state of airway inflammation responsible for his asthma exacerbations, it independently worsens his lung function by promoting the destruction of alveoli. Stopping smoking completely would be an important step for him to take now, in response to his heightened sense of concern about his health care.

Other factors probably contributing to his worsening lung disease may include the stress of his work, the poor quality of his housing (dust mite feces is a major source of allergens triggering asthma exacerbations), and the intermittent use of his medicines. You should stress the importance of stopping smoking completely, having the apartment properly cleaned, and using inhaled steroids and bronchodilators regularly, not just when he feels ill. Finally, you urge him to come and see you early in the course of an exacerbation and not wait so long before coming in for medical attention.

The spirometry provides you with a "baseline" assessment of his lung function with which to compare objective measurements in the future as an indicator of his condition.

SUMMARY AND REVIEW OF KEY CONCEPTS

1. Respiration involves inhaling O_2-rich air into the lungs, exchanging gases, in particular CO_2 and O_2, between air and blood in the alveoli, and exhaling CO_2-rich air out of the lungs.

2. The components of the respiratory system include the respiratory muscles (diaphragm, abdominals, neck muscles), the lungs from upper airway to alveoli, the pulmonary arteries, capillaries, veins and lymphatics, and the CNS centers involved in control of respiration.

3. Gas transport between alveolar air and pulmonary capillary blood occurs by diffusion. O_2 is transported in blood by binding to hemoglobin, which increases its concentration in blood 70-fold, compared to its intrinsic solubility. CO_2, in comparison, is exceedingly soluble in blood and therefore needs no carrier. This difference explains why CO_2 concentration in blood is directly proportional to minute ventilation, while O_2 is not.

4. The important lung volumes include TLC, TV, RV, and FEV_1. Their measurement allows objective assessment of the degree of obstructive versus restrictive lung disease and the extent to which a patient's acute presentation represents a change from the previous baseline.

5. Arterial blood gases and pulse oximetry provide a monitor for the adequacy of perfusion. The latter has the advantage of being noninvasive, but there are conditions under which it is either misleading or does not tell the whole story in terms of assessing the patient's respiratory status.

6. Normal lung function requires matching of ventilation to perfusion. Ventilation without perfusion increases dead space. Perfusion without ventilation is equivalent to a shunt that wastes a certain fraction of cardiac output.

7. A number of intrinsic mechanisms work to match ventilation to perfusion to the greatest extent possible, such as hypoxic pulmonary vasoconstriction.

8. The work of breathing is determined by the proper balance between elasticity and compliance (both of which are crucial for proper lung function), the degree of airway resistance to airflow, and the effectiveness of gas exchange (which requires that fluid not accumulate in the alveolus and that there be a good match between ventilation and perfusion).

9. Excessive elasticity is seen in restrictive lung disease, while excessive compliance occurs in certain obstructive lung diseases (e.g., emphysema). Other obstructive diseases are due to obstruction to airflow, as, for example, occurs with excessive bronchial smooth muscle constriction in asthma or excessive mucus production and bronchial edema in chronic bronchitis.

10. Perfusion is lost in pulmonary embolism, while ventilation is lost with atelectasis or pneumonia with subsequent redirection of blood flow (e.g., due to hypoxic pulmonary vasoconstriction).

11. A wide array of mechanical and neural regulatory mechanisms give the normal lungs tremendous functional reserve.

12. Various constitutive and inducible defenses protect against disease.

A CASE OF PHYSIOLOGICAL MEDICINE

J.C. was a 44-year-old stockbroker who was admitted to the hospital short of breath and coughing up blood. He was well until the afternoon of the day of admission when, after a transatlantic plane flight, he developed acute left-sided pleuritic chest pain and dyspnea while playing tennis. He then started coughing up blood and was taken to the emergency room for evaluation.

On questioning, he recalled a sore feeling in his left thigh toward the end of the flight. He was noted in the emergency room to have a resting tachycardia (HR = 110), a respiratory rate of 26, with a mild sense of air hunger. Arterial blood gases were pH 7.49, P_{CO_2} 30 mmHg, and P_{O_2} 75 mmHg. An ultrasound study showed a deep venous thrombophlebitis, and spiral CT was positive for multiple pulmonary emboli.

Mr. C. was treated with intravenous heparin, an immediate anticoagulant, and placed on Coumadin, an inhibitor of vitamin K action that inactivates vitamin K-dependent clotting factors, leaving him anticoagulated. His anticoagulation status proved difficult to stabilize, with wild swings from subtherapeutic to an excessively anticoagulated state, and made him unable to be discharged from the hospital for several additional days, resulting in additional complications after discharge. During one of the excessively anticoagulated episodes, the patient was readmitted to the hospital with bleeding complications including pulmonary hemorrhage. During one of the inadequately anticoagulated periods he had a recurrence of pulmonary emboli. Reheparinized, he developed thrombocytopenia (a low platelet count), a known complication of heparinization, which resulted in another episode of pulmonary hemorrhage.

Six months later, Mr. C. again had shortness of breath and hypoxia. This time he was also noted to have no change in his A-a gradient and to have developed a high fever and shaking chills. The diagnosis of pneumonia was established with a sputum smear revealing pneumococcus (a common cause of lobar pneumonia). He was treated and then released.

Two years after the initial episode on the tennis court, Mr. C. has recovered, after a fashion. However, he is no longer able to work, having become disabled by his lung disease. He is dyspneic at rest, having lost a substantial amount of lung capacity between his pulmonary hemorrhages and recurrent pulmonary emboli. His baseline arterial blood gas is now pH 7.39, P_{CO_2} 49, and P_{O_2} 60.

His anticipated home care needs over the next two decades will quickly empty the "medical savings account" he opened 2 years ago. Indeed, he will likely have to spend his assets, including the funds he had set aside to send his children to college, down to the poverty level. Too late, he realizes that the public sector safety net he voted to dismantle is not just for "lazy drug-abusing losers" but also for people like himself.

QUESTIONS

1. What are some notable features of Mr. C.'s initial arterial blood gas determination?
2. Explain the physiological mechanisms behind Mr. C.'s hyperventilation and air hunger.
3. What might have caused Mr. C.'s pulmonary hypertension?
4. Why would the A-a gradient not change with pneumonia unlike the observation with his original pulmonary embolism?
5. Account for the differences between the initial and final arterial blood gas determinations presented, based on your understanding of pulmonary physiology.

ANSWERS

1. Hypoxia with an increased A-a gradient is one notable feature of Mr. C.'s initial arterial blood gas determination.

2. Pulmonary artery obstruction causes a fall in the blood flow from the right to left side of the heart. This decreases left side of the heart filling, which results in reflex tachycardia, in an attempt to augment cardiac output. Hypoxia caused by ventilation perfusion mismatch results in a fall in P_{O_2}. This lowered P_{O_2} stimulates hyperventilation to raise the P_{O_2} to the observed level, with concomitant fall in P_{CO_2}.

3. Recurrent pulmonary emboli cause obstruction and obliteration of small pulmonary arteries. This, in turn, results in elevated pulmonary perfusion pressures, leak of fluid into the lungs, and a chronic sense of shortness of breath.

4. Both ventilation and perfusion are lost with lobar consolidation as occurs in pneumonia. So there is no gradient of oxygen tension between the artery and the alveoli.

5. Mr. C.'s pulmonary fibrosis has caused a chronic ventilation-to-perfusion mismatch, where much of the air that enters the lungs does not reach alveoli in contact with functioning capillaries. This greatly increases the work of breathing in order to oxygenate the blood and eliminate carbon dioxide. Mr. C. is no longer able to keep up with the work required to bring about optimal gas exchange. His body has adjusted, with difficulty, to what he can do.

References and suggested readings

GENERAL REFERENCES

1. McPhee, S., Lingappa, V.R., Ganong, W.F., and Lange, J. eds. (1997). *Pathophysiology of Disease*, 2nd ed. Stamford, CT, Appleton & Lange.
2. Fauci, A., Braunwald, E., Isselbacher, K. et al. eds. (1997). *Harrison's Principles of Internal Medicine*, 14th ed. McGraw Hill, New York.

FRONTIERS REFERENCES

3. Davies, R.J. et al. (1997). New insights into the understanding of asthma. *Chest* 111:2S-10S.
4. Fan, T.M. et al. (1997). Airway responsiveness in two inbred strains of mouse disparate in IgE and IL-4 production. *Am. J. Respir. Cell Mol. Biol.* 17:156-163.
5. Grunig, G. et al. (1998). Requirement for IL-13 independently of IL-4 in experimental asthma. *Science* 282:2261-2263.
6. Postma, D.S. et al. (1995). Genetic susceptibility to asthma–bronchial hyperresponsiveness coinherited with a major gene for atopy. *N. Engl. J. Med.* 333, 894-900.
7. Mitsuyasu, H. et al. (1998). Ile50Val variant of IL4R alpha upregulates IgE synthesis and associates with atropic asthma. *Nature Genet.* 19:119-120.
8. Wan, H. et al. (1999). Der p1 facilitates transepithelial allergen delivery by disruption of right junctions. *J. Clin. Invest.* 104:123-133.
9. Solway, J., and Fredberg, J.J. (1997). Perhaps airway smooth muscle dysfunction contributes to asthmatic bronchial hyperresponsiveness after all. *Am. J. Resp. Cell. Mol. Biol.* 17:144-146.
10. Ohkawara, Y. et al. (1997). Cytokine and eosinophil responses in the lung, peripheral blood and bone marrow compartments in a murine model of allergen-induced airways inflammation. *Am. J. Respir. Cell Mol. Biol.* 16, 510-520.
11. Kamp, D.W., and Weitzman, WA. (1997). Asbestosis: Clinical spectrum and pathogenic mechanisms. *Proc. Soc. Exp. Biol. Med.* 214:12-26.
12. Lasky, A. et al. (1995). Chrysotile asbestos stimulates PDGF-AA production by rat lung fibroblasts in vitro: Evidence for an autocrine loop. *Am. J. Respir. Cell Mol. Biol.* 12: 162-170.
13. Kuwano, K. et al. (1999). Essential roles of the Fas-Fas ligand pathway in the development of pulmonary fibrosis. *J. Clin. Invest.* 104:13-19.
14. Munger, J.S. et al. (1999). The integrin $\alpha v \beta 6$ binds and activates latent TGFbeta 1: A mechanism for regulating pulmonary inflammation and fibrosis. *Cell* 96:319-328.

15. Saleh, D. et al. (1997). Elevated expression of endothelin-1 and endothelin-converting enzyme-1 in idiopathic pulmonary fibrosis: Possible involvement of proinflammatory cytokines. *Am. J. Respir. Cell Mol. Biol.* 16:187-193.

16. Salathe, M. et al. (1997). Isolation and characterization of a peroxidase from the airway. *Am. J. Respir. Cell Mol. Biol.* 17:97-105.

17. McCray, P.B., and Bentley, L. (1997). Human airway epithelia express a beta-defensin. *Am. J. Respir. Cell Mol. Biol.* 16:343-349.

18. Van Wetering, S. et al. (1997). Effect of defensins on interleukin-8 synthesis in airway epithelial cells. *Am. J. Physiol.* 272:L888-L896.

19. Goldman, M.J. et al. (1997). Human beta-defensin-1 is a salt-sensitive antibiotic in lung that is inactivated in cystic fibrosis. *Cell* 88:553-560.

20. Panyutich, A.V. et al. (1995). Human neutrophil defensin and serpins form complexes and inactivate each other. *Am. J. Respir. Cell Mol. Biol.* 12:351-357.

21. Repine, J. E. et al. (1997). Oxidative stress in chronic obstructive pulmonary disease. *Am. J. Resp. Crit. Care Med.* 156:341-357.

RENAL PHYSIOLOGY

9

1. INTRODUCTION TO THE KIDNEYS

The following list shows several crucial roles that the kidneys serve.

• Filter the blood and remove from the blood wastes, in particular, nitrogen-containing compounds such as urea. The **filtrate** is the fluid initially separated from the blood in the kidney. It consists of water with various dissolved substances. Ultimately, part of the filtrate is excreted from the body in the form of **urine**. Complete loss of this function is incompatible with life, unless replaced, for example, by the mechanical process termed **dialysis**.

• Transport specific ions and other substances, including water, from blood to filtrate and from the filtrate back to the bloodstream, as needed to maintain homeostasis. The vigorous but selective activity of renal transporters normally allows reabsorption of all of the glucose and amino acids present in the renal filtrate so that the urine normally contains none of these substances. Also as a result of renal transport activity, urine can be either extremely concentrated or extremely dilute, depending on whether the person is dehydrated (e.g., due to sweating, vomiting, or diarrhea) or has recently drunk a lot of water. Disorders in renal transport function can cause abnormal blood pressure, puffiness of the face, swelling of the extremities, termed **edema**, and fluid and electrolyte imbalances (see Chap. 10).

• Monitor and respond to changes in blood pressure. Some of the most common and effective medications for treatment of high blood pressure work by affecting renal mechanisms. Clinical epidemiological studies suggest that some of these drugs may slow the progression of renal disease, for example, in patients with diabetes mellitus.

• Produce a hormone called *erythropoetin*, which is the key regulator of red blood cell production by the bone marrow. A host of other local mediators are also made in the kidney and participate in a bewilderingly complex array of signaling events whose complexity is only just starting to be appreciated (see Ref. 1).

• Contribute to intermediary metabolism as a major site of amino acid and carbohydrate synthesis and degradation, and detoxification and excretion of many drugs. Failure to adjust the dose of a drug metabolized by the kidney when treating a patient with renal failure may result in needless drug toxicity and side effects.

Why is understanding renal physiology important for medical practice?

• When the kidneys are not functioning normally, the concentration of various substances in blood can change. These changes in the composition of blood directly affect every organ system in the body. Thus, onset of kidney failure is often the beginning of the end for seriously ill patients. Preventing, recognizing (as early as possible), and treating renal failure is often crucial if such patients are to survive.

• Sometimes renal disease develops slowly and insidiously. It is easy to overlook the suggestive findings until the kidneys are too far gone to be saved. At some point in the progression of such renal diseases, changes that were initially adaptive actually hasten further renal disease in the long term. If recognized early enough, treatment can often be started that will slow future renal decline.

• Once substantial, irreversible impairment of kidney function has occurred, the patient is much more fragile and is at high risk for complications of other diseases (such as heart disease and stroke) and illness caused by treatment for other medical conditions. Thus, the elderly patient who has gradually lost renal function over the decades may be harmed by even small doses of over-the-counter medicines (e.g., nonsteroidal anti-inflammatory drugs, called NSAIDs, such as ibuprofen). Physicians must understand these nuances to avoid doing great harm to their patients.

• Sometimes renal disease can proceed very rapidly and the time available to recognize and treat the disorder is extremely short. The physician who understands the kidney, what it does, how it does it, and what happens when it is not working correctly is in a far better position to effectively care for his or her patients.

• Technological innovations have made it possible to replace many functions of the kidney either by various forms of dialysis or by a kidney transplant, albeit nowhere near perfectly. Patients on dialysis can now receive erythropoetin injections to maintain normal red blood cell production, thereby preventing much of the weakness and fatigue that used to accompany renal failure. As a result, patients who used to die of renal failure are often alive and leading near normal lives for decades. Regardless of your area of practice, you will see patients with acute and chronic renal disease. Furthermore, you will have to consider the kidney-related effects of whatever you do (or do not) prescribe on both the healthy kidneys of patients with other disorders, and on the other organs of patients with renal disease.

Case Presentation

F.L. is a 24-year-old woman who has come for medical attention with dyspnea and loss of appetite. She is currently between jobs. Her medical history is notable for frequent urinary tract infections as a child, which were treated occasionally with antibiotics, but never worked up. There is no family history of renal disease. Recently, she slipped and fell getting off a bus and self-treated her injury with bed rest and ibuprofen at home for 2 weeks. All of her symptoms developed afterwards. On exam, blood pressure is noted to be 180/120 and she has evidence of congestive heart failure with an S_3 heard on auscultation of the heart, crackles at the lung bases, and substantial pedal edema in her feet. Arterial blood gases show a pH of 7.25, and blood studies demonstrate renal failure with a creatinine of 9 and potassium of 6.5. Ultrasound shows small shrunken kidneys without renal obstruction, consistent with chronic renal failure. Creatinine clearance is calculated at 15, suggesting that Ms. L. has lost nearly 90% of her renal function. You explain the findings to her and admit her to the hospital for acute dialysis. Ms. L. wants to know what brought on her kidney failure. She finds it incomprehensible that an over-the-counter medicine such as ibuprofen could have contributed to her current condition. She wants you to explain how kidney disease results in difficulty breathing and her loss of appetite. She wonders about the meaning of the abnormal blood tests. She is frightened about what the future holds for her health and her ability to obtain health care with an all encompassing preexisting condition such as renal failure.

Review Questions

1. What are the five major roles of the kidney?
2. Give five reasons why understanding renal physiology is important for medical practice.

2. ANATOMY OF THE KIDNEYS

The kidneys are a pair of encapsulated organs located in the lower back, behind the peritoneal space, surrounded by a protective fat pad (see Figure 9.1A). A renal artery enters and a renal vein exits from each kidney at the hilum connecting the organs to the abdominal aorta and the inferior vena cava, respectively. Also leaving each kidney through the hilum are nerves, lymphatic vessels and a ureter that connects to the urinary bladder in the lower anterior pelvis (see Figure 9.1B).

Within the kidney, an outer region, termed the **cortex** can be distinguished from the inner region, termed the **medulla**. The medulla consists of tissue that forms the **renal pyramids** and terminates in the **renal papillae**. These come together in the renal pelvis and form the ureter (Figure 9.1C).

The functional unit of the kidney is a microscopic tubular structure termed the **nephron** (see Figure 9.2). Each kidney has about a million nephrons. Blood enters the kidney via the renal artery and leaves via the renal vein. After entry into the kidney, the renal artery quickly forms smaller and smaller branches until reaching the level of the individual nephron. Each nephron receives arterial blood via an **afferent arteriole**, with venous blood leaving via a small branch of the renal vein. Between the afferent arteriole and the renal vein are an **efferent arteriole**, as well as two sets of capillary beds. The first capillary bed, termed the **glomerulus**, is interposed between the afferent and efferent arterioles and is the actual point at which blood is filtered in the kidney. The filtrate collects in **Bowman's space**, surrounding the glomerulus (Figure 9.3A). Bowman's space is contiguous with the renal tubule. As the filtrate flows down the **renal tubule**, various substances including salts and water are absorbed or secreted before it finally leaves the kidney as urine. A second capillary bed is termed the **peritubular capillaries** or the **vasa recta** and occurs between the efferent arteriole and the renal veins (see Figure 9.2). The vasa recta encircles the part of the renal tubule termed the **loop of Henle** and plays a crucial role

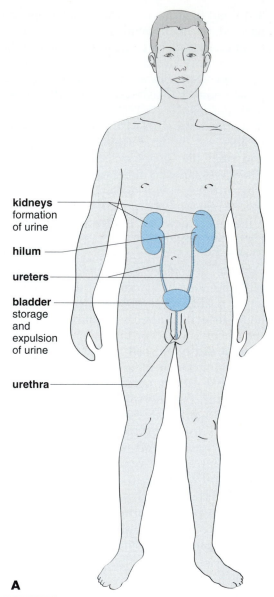

kidneys formation of urine

hilum

ureters

bladder storage and expulsion of urine

urethra

A

FIGURE 9.1. *A.* Schematic diagram indicating the location of the kidney in the body. *B.* Location of the kidneys upon dissection of the retroperitoneum. *C.* Gross anatomy of the kidney.

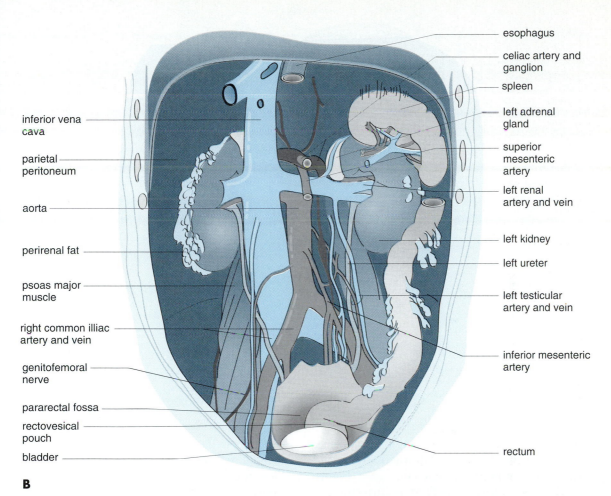

esophagus

celiac artery and ganglion

spleen

left adrenal gland

superior mesenteric artery

left renal artery and vein

left kidney

left ureter

left testicular artery and vein

inferior mesenteric artery

rectum

inferior vena cava

parietal peritoneum

aorta

perirenal fat

psoas major muscle

right common illiac artery and vein

genitofemoral nerve

pararectal fossa

rectovesical pouch

bladder

B

FIGURE 9.1 — (continued)

in regulation of the ability of the kidney to generate a concentrated urine, as will be discussed in Sec. 4. Flow from the vasa recta joins the **renal veins**, and blood exits the kidney via a single large renal vein.

Review Questions

3. Describe the internal organization of the kidney.
4. What is the structural unit of renal function?

5. How many capillary beds does the nephron have? Where are they located?

3. HISTOLOGY AND CELL BIOLOGY OF THE NEPHRON

The tuft of capillaries comprising the **glomerulus** is generally located in the renal cortex. The capillaries of the glomerulus are composed of endothelial cells and are covered

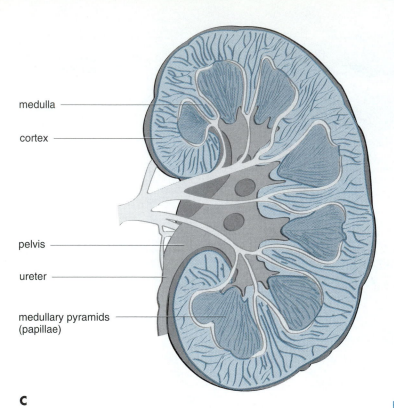

medulla

cortex

pelvis

ureter

medullary pyramids
(papillae)

C

FIGURE 9.1 — (*continued*)

by epithelial cells. A basement membrane separates the capillary endothelial cells and the glomerular epithelial cells (see Figure 9.3B). The epithelial cells that surround the glomerulus form a continuous layer with those of Bowman's capsule, defining Bowman's space and the entryway into the renal tubule. The space between capillaries in the glomerulus is called the **mesangium**. Besides a matrix of collagen and related proteins, the mesangium contains cells that are related to vascular smooth muscle, termed (big surprise) *mesangial cells*, which play a key role in regulation of glomerular function (see Frontiers, in Sec. 9).

The endothelial cells that make up the glomerular capillaries are fenestrated (as were the capillaries in the liver), so they provide no barrier to free-flow of plasma proteins.

Most of the barrier to flow of plasma proteins into the glomerular filtrate is due to the basement membrane whose negative charge is a greater barrier for anionic proteins than cationic proteins. Thus, even though albumin is small enough in diameter to be filtered, under normal conditions, its negative charge effectively sequesters it in the capillary lumen. Finally, the epithelial cells covering the glomerular capillaries have some distinctive features including so-called foot processes or **podocytes**, separated by slit-pores, which may also serve a barrier function.

The renal tubule to which the glomerulus is connected straddles the cortex and medulla (see Figure 9.3A). Each renal tubule consists of several structurally and functionally distinctive parts (see Figure 9.2): a **proximal tubule**, the **loop of Henle** (which in some cases

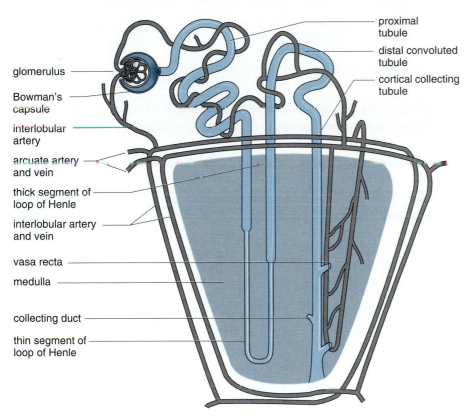

glomerulus

Bowman's
capsule

interlobular
artery

arcuate artery
and vein

thick segment of
loop of Henle

interlobular artery
and vein

vasa recta

medulla

collecting duct

thin segment of
loop of Henle

proximal
tubule

distal convoluted
tubule

cortical collecting
tubule

FIGURE 9.2. Gross anatomy of the nephron. (Adapted, with permission, from Chandrasoma, P. and Taylor, C.E. (1994). Concise Pathology, 2nd ed. Norwalk, CT, Appleton & Lange.)

plunges deep into the renal medulla before coming back up to the cortex), and a distal tubule. The **distal tubule** consists of a **distal convoluted tubule**, which returns to pass close to the glomerulus, (Figure 9.4) and a **cortical collecting tubule**. Finally, the distal renal tubule joins a **medullary collecting duct** to which other nephrons also are connected, which then leads to the ureter. The renal tubules of different nephrons have loops of Henle of different lengths, which reach different depths within the medulla. Each of these variations confers differences in nephron function.

Each functional region of the renal tubule has its own distinctive histologic features (see Figure 9.4). The proximal tubule from which approximately 65% of the electrolytes and water are reclaimed is rich in microvilli and mitochondria, reflecting its need for absorptive surface area and adenosine triphosphate (ATP) to drive active transport. The expansion of apical plasma membrane surface due to microvilli approaches twentyfold. The loop of Henle, where concentration of urine can be achieved, has a so-called **thin segment**, which is highly permeable to water but whose cells lack microvilli and are poor in mitochondria, and a **thick segment**, which is quite active in solute transport but is highly imperme-

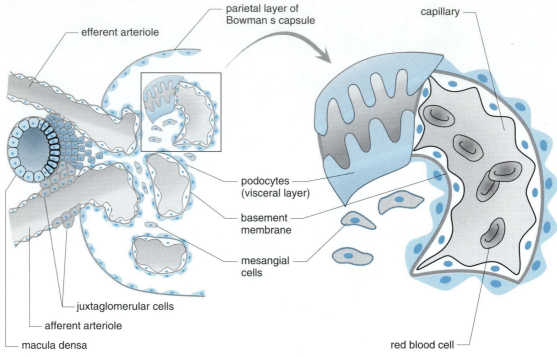

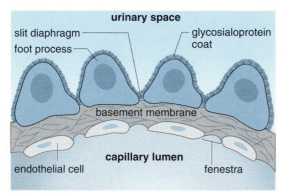

FIGURE 9.3. *A.* Structure of the glomerulus and relation to the renal tubule. *B.* High resolution view of the glomerular membrane. *(B. Adapted, with permission, from Denker, B.M. and Brenner, B.M. Cardinal Manifestations of Renal Disease, in Fauci, A. et al. eds. Harrison's Textbook of Internal Medicine, 14th ed. New York, McGraw-Hill, p. 260.)*

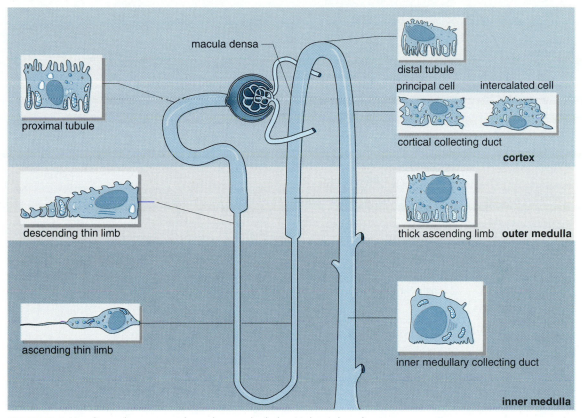

FIGURE 9.4. Histological variation along the renal tubule. *(Adapted, with permission, from Berne, R.M. and Levy, M.N. (1998). Physiology, 4th ed. St. Louis, Mosby, p. 680.)*

able to water. The distal tubule and collecting duct are extensions of the renal tubule beyond the loop of Henle, where additional electrolyte and water adjustments can be made in response to hormonal control, as needed to maintain homeostasis. The late distal tubule consists of two different cell types, the **principal cells** and the **intercalated cells**, each with unique transport properties (see below).

Renal tubular transport requires that transporters be distributed asymmetrically, not only along the length of the renal tubule, but also on the surface of any given renal tubular epithelial cell (see Figure 9.5). For example, Na^+/K^+ ATPase is localized to the basolateral surface of the renal tubular cells and pumps sodium into the interstitium and potassium into the renal tubular cell. The stoichiometry of this pump is 3 sodiums for every 2 potassium ions. The resulting low intracellular sodium creates a gradient favoring passive diffusion of sodium from tubular lumen into tubular cell. Furthermore, the -70 meq intracellular **potential difference** across the plasma membrane that results from this charge distribution favors movement of cations of tubular fluid into the cell, of which

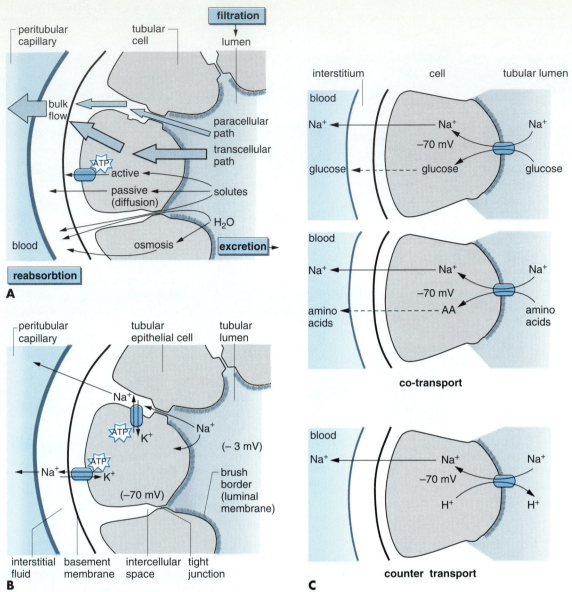

FIGURE 9.5. Active and passive tubular resorptive mechanisms. *A.* Reabsorption of filtered water and solutes from the tubular lumen across the tubular epithelial cells, through the renal interstitium, and back into the blood. Solutes are transported through the cells (transcellular route) by passive diffusion or active transport or between the cells (paracellular route) by diffusion. Water is transported through the cells and between the tubular cell by osmosis. Transport of water and solutes from the interstitial fluid into the peritubular capillary occurs by ultrafiltration (bulk flow). ATP, adenosine triphosphate. *B.* Basic mechanism for active transport of sodium through the tubular epithelial cell. The sodium-potassium pump transports sodium from the interior of the cell across the basolateral membrane, creating a low intracellular sodium concentration and a negative intracellular electrical potential. The low intracellular sodium concentration and the negative electrical potential cause sodium ions to diffuse from the tubular lumen into the cell through the brush border. *C.* Mechanisms of secondary active transport. The upper two cells show the cotransport of glucose or amino acids along with sodium ions through the brush border of the tubular epithelial cells, followed by facilitated diffusion through the basolateral membranes. The third cell shows the countertransport of hydrogen ions from the interior of the cell across the brush border member and into the tubular lumen. Movement of sodium

sodium is predominant. If, instead of being found only on the basolateral surface, the Na^+/K^+ ATPase were uniformly distributed around the tubular cell, or were localized predominantly on the apical surface, the energy released by its hydrolysis of ATP could not be harnessed into net movement of sodium from tubular lumen to blood. Likewise, sodium-binding proteins localized exclusively to the lumenal surface of certain renal tubular epithelial cells allow facilitated diffusion down the concentration gradient generated by Na^+/K^+ ATPase.

The glomeruli, proximal tubules, distal tubules, and early collecting ducts are located in the renal cortex. The individual loops of Henle of various nephrons descend to different degrees into the medulla and then come back up to the cortex in order to allow the **macula densa** of the distal tubule to be located adjacent to the point where the afferent and efferent arterioles enter the glomerulus. Specialized juxtaglomerular cells secrete renin in response to a fall in perfusion pressure (see Chap. 10). These adjacent structures form an important regulatory unit termed the **juxtaglomerular apparatus** (see Figure 9.3).

Review Questions

6. What are the components of a nephron?
7. What is the significance of fenestrations in the glomerular capillary endothelium?
8. What parts of the nephron are located in the renal cortex?

4. PHYSIOLOGY OF THE NEPHRON

Renal blood flow

Approximately 25% of cardiac output goes to the kidneys, which make up only about 1% of the mass of the body. This is far in excess of what is needed for nutrient supply and waste removal and is a higher fraction of cardiac output per unit mass than occurs for the heart, brain, or other tissues. The high throughput of blood reflected by those numbers is necessary to generate the large **hydrostatic pressure** that drives formation of the **glomerular ultrafiltrate** and allows the kidney to carry out extremely fine-tuned regulation of blood electrolytes, water, and volume. Thus, most of the renal blood flow is to the cortex, where the glomeruli are located, and only about 1 to 2% of total renal blood flow goes to the vasa recta.

Filtration in the glomerulus

The blood flowing into the afferent arteriole of an individual nephron is filtered through the **glomerular capillary endothelial cells**, through the underlying **basement membrane**, and through the **epithelial cell** layer. The endothelial cells, being fenestrated, only retain the cells in blood and are not an impediment to protein movement. The basement membrane is a barrier to movement of large proteins (greater than 100,000 Daltons in molecular weight), but would allow the many smaller proteins to be filtered. However, the glomerular epithelial cell layer has negatively charged **filtration slits** that impede movement

FIGURE 9.5 — (continued) ions into the cell, down an electrochemical gradient established by the sodium-potassium pump on the basolateral membrane, provides the energy for transport of the hydrogen ions from inside the cell into the tubular lumen. (Adapted, with permission, from Guyton, A.C. and Hall, J.E. (1997). Human Physiology and Mechanisms of Disease, 6th ed. Philadelphia, Saunders, pp. 224-225.)

of negatively charged molecules such as albumin, the major protein in blood plasma, which would otherwise be small enough to be filtered. Thus, a largely protein-free ultrafiltrate of plasma is normally generated by glomerular filtration. The space in which this fluid ends up is contiguous with the renal tubular lumen. Fairly subtle disorders can alter the size selectivity of the epithelial cells, sometimes resulting in massive proteinuria, which may itself contribute to further progression of renal disease (see Frontiers, in Sec. 9).

Overall, renal blood flow is determined by the pressure gradient between the renal arterial and venous systems:

Renal Blood Flow =

$$\frac{\text{Renal Artery Pressure} - \text{Renal Venous Pressure}}{\text{Total Renal Vascular Resistance}}$$

Review Questions

9. What percentage of cardiac output goes to the kidneys?
10. What percentage of renal blood flow goes to the medulla?
11. What are the determinants of renal blood flow?
12. Describe the two capillary networks in the kidney and the percentage of normal renal blood flow they normally handle.

Glomerular filtration rate

About 20% of the volume of blood plasma flowing through the glomerulus ends up as ultrafiltrate in Bowman's space. Most of that volume is eventually reclaimed, with about 0.5% of the total, about 1 L out of 200, ending up as urine, enriched in wastes and excess electrolytes that are excreted to balance out electrolytes absorbed from the gastrointestinal (GI) tract.

Glomerular filtration rate (GFR) is determined by the net balance of several forces. The relative filterability of substances is a function of both their size and charge. Below a certain size, substances are freely filtered regardless of charge. Above a certain size substances are retained regardless of charge. In the gray zone, roughly the size of an albumin molecule, the charge on the protein determines the extent to which it is filtered. Thus, although albumin is small enough to be filtered, because it has a strong negative charge, 99.5% of it is retained in the capillary lumen. Relative filterability is termed the **capillary filtration coefficient** (K_f). Sometimes small substances that might be expected to be freely filtered are not, simply because they are tightly bound to larger proteins that are not freely filtered.

Another determinant of GFR is **net filtration pressure**, which is the difference between the **hydrostatic pressure** and the **oncotic pressure**. Hydrostatic pressure is the pressure of blood against the capillary wall, which tends to push fluid out of the capillary. Oncotic pressure, also called *colloid osmotic pressure*, is the osmotic pressure from proteins too big to easily leave the capillary lumen which therefore serves to hold fluid in the capillary lumen. These two pressures tend to offset one another, and the distribution of fluid throughout the body represents the balance of these forces in various locations. In the kidney, normally, the filtrate has almost no protein. Thus,

$$\text{GFR} = K_f \times \text{Net Filtration Pressure}$$

In the normal adult human, GFR is about 125 mL/min or 180 L/day.

The major physiological means of regulating GFR is by altering glomerular capillary hydrostatic pressure (normally about 60 mmHg), and glomerular capillary oncotic pressure (normally about 32 mmHg). This is carried out by intrinsic autoregulation and by neurohumoral mechanisms to be discussed below (see Autoregulation of Renal Function and Neural Control of Renal Function, in Sec. 5).

There are three determinants of glomerular capillary hydrostatic pressure:

- Arterial pressure
- Afferent arteriolar resistance
- Efferent arteriolar resistance

Increasing arterial pressure raises GFR, but autoregulatory mechanisms usually limit the variation allowed. Decreasing afferent arteriolar resistance always increases glomerular hydrostatic pressure and increases GFR. However, the effect of changes in efferent arteriolar resistance is more complex. Small increases in efferent arteriolar resistance increase glomerular hydrostatic pressure and thereby increase GFR. Larger increases, however, decrease renal blood flow. When renal blood flow decreases, the fraction of total blood volume filtered increases and glomerular capillary colloid osmotic pressure increases. If the increase in colloid osmotic pressure more than offsets the increased hydrostatic pressure, GFR actually decreases as efferent arteriolar resistance goes up. Such a fall in GFR occurs when the increase in efferent arteriolar resistance is greater than about threefold normal.

Clinical Pearls

○ Elevation of blood urea nitrogen (BUN) and creatinine concentration are often used as laboratory evidence for renal failure. This conclusion is, however, somewhat indirect. Clinicians, therefore, must be attentive to other causes of elevation of BUN (GI bleeding, dehydration, or glucocorticoid or tetracycline therapy) or creatinine (eating a lot of cooked meat). In addition, clinicians must be aware of reasons why creatinine may fail to be substantially elevated despite progression of renal disease (muscle wasting with aging, chronic disease, malnutrition, or chronic glucocorticoid therapy).

○ Failure to perfuse the kidneys with blood accounts for 40 to 80% of cases of acute renal failure. The most common causes are as follows:

- Decreased blood volume (due to volume loss from GI bleeding, burns, diarrhea, excessive diuretic therapy)
- Movement of fluid from intravascular space to tissues (e.g., in pancreatitis, peritonitis, or rhabdomyolysis)
- Decreased blood circulation due to heart failure or peripheral vasodilation as in sepsis
- Volume sequestration in tissues
- A decrease in K_f observed in either diabetes mellitus or hypertension, probably due to altered glomerular basement membrane structure

○ Patients with underlying chronic renal failure are at increased risk for developing acute renal failure. Most likely this is because they have already activated their homeostatic mechanisms to protect renal perfusion and GFR (e.g., prostaglandin-mediated afferent arteriolar vasodilation and angiotensin-II-mediated efferent arteriolar constriction). Thus such patients are particularly sensitive to any new acute insult that further lowers renal perfusion, including any cause of intravascular volume depletion or fluid redistribution. These patients are also at greatest risk for worsening of renal failure upon treatment with either ACE inhibitors (which lower angiotensin II) or NSAIDs such as aspirin or ibuprofen, because those mechanisms have already been activated to maintain homeostasis.

Review Questions

13. What is the fraction of glomerular blood flow that becomes glomerular filtrate normally?
14. How is GFR defined?
15. What are the components of net filtration pressure?
16. How do changes in arterial pressure and afferent and efferent arteriolar resistance each affect GFR?

Renal tubular function

The ultrafiltrate in Bowman's space flows down the lumen of the renal tubule and is modified by active transport processes of **tubular absorption** and **tubular secretion**. Some substances are selectively and actively absorbed from the fluid in the tubular lumen, while other substances return to the bloodstream passively. As a result, relative concentrations of various substances in blood are changed. Some substances are selectively secreted *into* the tubular fluid along the course of the renal tubule, thereby serving to *increase* the concentration gradient for that substance between blood and tubular fluid.

$$\text{Amount Excreted} = \\ \text{Amount Filtered} \\ - (\text{Tubular Absorption} \\ + \text{Tubular Secretion})$$

In the jargon of renal physiology, transport from tubular lumen into the renal interstitium and/or bloodstream is termed **absorption**, while transport from the bloodstream into the tubular lumen is termed **secretion**. For most substances (except potassium and hydrogen ions), tubular absorption is far more important than secretion. Like glomerular filtration, tubular absorption is quantitatively very large (see Table 9.1).

However, whereas glomerular filtration is highly nonselective, tubular absorption is highly selective. Thus, some substances, such as glucose and amino acids, are abundant in the bloodstream and freely filtered, but are normally completely absent from the urine because they are completely reabsorbed.

TABLE 9.1   TUBULAR ABSORPTION

| Substance | Per 24 h | | | | Percentage reabsorbed | Location* |
	Filtered	Reabsorbed	Secreted	Excreted		
Na+ (meq)	26,000	25,850		150	99.4	P, L, D, C
K+ (meq)	600	560[†]	50[†]	90	93.3	P, L, D, C
Cl− (meq)	18,000	17,850		150	99.2	P, L, D, C
HCO₃− (meq)	4,900	4,900		0	100	P, D
Urea (mmol)	870	460[‡]		410	53	P, L, D, C
Creatinine (mmol)	12	1[§]	1[§]	12		
Uric acid (mmol)	50	49	4	5	98	P
Glucose (mmol)	800	800		0	100	P
Total solute (mosmol)	54,000	53,400	100	700	98.9	P, L, D, C
Water (mL)	180,000	179,000		1000	99.4	P, L, D, C

*P, proximal tubules; L, loops of Henle; D, distal tubules; C, collecting ducts.
[†]K+ is both reabsorbed and secreted.
[‡]Urea moves into as well as out of some portions of the nephron.
[§]Variable secretion and probable reabsorption of creatinine in humans.
Reproduced, with permission, from Ganong, F.W. (1997). *Review of Medical Physiology*, 18th ed. Stamford, CT, Appleton & Lange, p. 663.

Others, such as urea, are freely filtered but poorly reabsorbed. The differential and selective absorption of some solutes but not others is a crucial feature of normal renal function.

Transport in the renal tubule is fundamentally no different from what goes on in the GI tract or anywhere else in the body, as every cell has to maintain constancy of its own internal environment within acceptable limits. What is special about the kidney is that the massive amount of transport activity is normally organized in an exquisitely concerted fashion to achieve the enormous task of steady state filtration of total blood volume without marked swings in concentration of water or electrolytes.

Substances can be absorbed either actively or passively (see Chap. 2). Water and some solutes are absorbed passively down their concentration gradients via channels in the plasma membrane. Other substances must be moved actively against a concentration gradient. Active transport can either be primary or secondary. Primary active transport involves the direct expenditure of metabolic energy (usually ATP hydrolysis) for the transport of a specific substance into or out of the renal tubular epithelial cell (see Figure 9.5C).

Secondary active transport is active transport in which uptake of one substance is coupled to uptake of another. Thus, for example, the uptake of glucose and other substances against their concentration gradients does not utilize ATP hydrolysis directly. Rather, the large −70 meq electrochemical gradient, generated through the ATP-consuming action of Na^+/K^+ ATPase, is used to couple movement of sodium down its concentration gradient with movement of glucose *against* its concentration gradient. Similar mechanisms are used for transport of amino acids and hydrogen ions (see Figure 9.5B).

The actual route of transport from the tubular lumen to the bloodstream involves traversing the tubular cell, the renal interstitium, and the capillary endothelial cell. For most substances, both a **transcellular pathway** (across) and a **paracellular pathway** (between) the renal tubular epithelial cells may exist (see Figure 9.5A).

Once in the interstitium, the transport into the capillary lumen is governed by the balance of colloid osmotic (oncotic) forces pulling water and solutes into the capillary lumen and hydrostatic forces pushing them out of the capillary lumen. This is fundamentally no different from the equilibrium between intravascular and interstitial fluid achieved in any peripheral capillary bed, although it has some peculiar features that are of great functional significance for the kidney (see Sec. 5).

The absorption activity changes dramatically over the course of the renal tubule, both in terms of what and how much is absorbed. When active transport moves solutes out of the renal tubular lumen into the interstitium, an osmotic gradient for water movement is created. However, water can move down this gradient only if the membrane of that particular region of the renal tubule is permeable to water. In the proximal tubule, the renal tubular plasma membrane is permeable; however, in the ascending part of the loop of Henle it is *impermeable*. Finally, in the collecting tubule and collecting ducts membrane permeability is hormonally regulated (by antidiuretic hormone, ADH, see Hormonal Control of Renal Function, in Sec. 5).

Absorption of substances

Sodium

Approximately 96 to 99% of all the sodium in the renal filtrate is absorbed. Because almost all cells have Na^+/K^+ ATPase to maintain a low intracellular sodium, renal absorption of sodium is a key regulator of extracellular fluid volume (see Chap. 10).

Sodium is actively transported in all parts

of the renal tubule except the thin segment
of the loop of Henle. Most of the sodium is
absorbed together with chloride, but some is
exchanged for H^+ or K^+. Other transporters
that move sodium include the epithelial sodium channel and thiazide-sensitive sodium
channels. Factors affecting sodium absorption are discussed later.

Chloride

Chloride is highly absorbed along the renal
tubule due to the additive effects of three
mechanisms:

- Uptake of sodium creates an electrical potential gradient that favors passive chloride
absorption by both the transcellular and
paracellular routes.
- As water is absorbed from the tubule by
osmosis, a large gradient of chloride is generated, favoring its passive movement.
- Secondary active transport mechanisms, including a sodium cotransporter, can transport chloride.

Water

Of the 180 L of renal filtrate that a person
normally generates per day, on average, only
about 1 L ends up as urine. Most of the water
in the initial renal filtrate is absorbed passively due to the osmotic effects of absorbed
electrolytes. However, the kidney has a profound ability to regulate water balance *independently* of electrolytes. Concentrated
urine can be excreted due to water retention
when the patient is dehydrated, and dilute
urine can be excreted due to water excretion,
e.g., when the nondehydrated patient has
taken in a water load. Thus the daily load of
dissolved substances (e.g., urea or ions) that
are excreted in the urine could be delivered
in a volume as small as 500 mL or as large
as 20 L.

The **aquaporins** are a set of proteins that
form channels that transport water from renal

tubular lumen to the bloodstream. At least
six members of the gene family that encode
the aquaporins have been identified, each
with a distinctive distribution and function.
Aquaporin-1 is found in the proximal tubule,
while **aquaporin-2** mediates the response to
ADH (see Chap. 10). **Aquaporin-3** is located
on the basolateral side of the renal tubular
collecting duct epithelial cell and mediates
transport of urea and other substances as well
as water.

Urea

Urea is far less permeable to the renal tubular
membrane than are either water or chloride.
Hence only about one-half of the urea
present in the tubule is passively absorbed
along with water, allowing for the excretion
of a substantial amount of urea even when
water and other electrolytes are much more
completely reclaimed from the tubular
lumen.

Clinical Pearls

○ Most substances absorbed from the tubular lumen have a maximum rate of uptake
defined by saturation of available transporters. If the tubular lumenal concentration exceeds a maximum level, the substance will be lost in the urine. A good
example of this is seen with glucose. The
normal blood glucose concentration of 60
to 140 mg/dL is comfortably within the
capacity of the sodium/glucose co-trans-
port system. However, patients with uncontrolled diabetes mellitus (especially
with new onset disease) will have glucosuria (glucose in the urine) as an early symptom due to transporter saturation.
○ Actually, glucose starts to appear in the
urine before total renal transporter saturation for the kidney as a whole is reached.

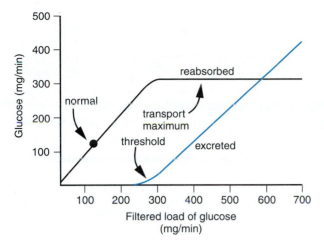

FIGURE 9.6. Renal tubular glucose transport and saturation threshold. Relation between the filtered load of glucose, the rate of glucose reabsorption by the renal tubules, and the rate of glucose excretion in the urine. The transport maximum is the maximum rate at which glucose can be reabsorbed from the tubules. The threshold for glucose refers to the filtered load of glucose at which glucose first begins to appear in the urine. (*Adapted, with permission, from Guyton, A.C. and Hall, J.E. (1997).* Human Physiology and Mechanisms of Disease, *6th ed. Philadelphia, Saunders, p. 226.*)

This is because the kidney is made up of 1 million separate functioning units (nephrons), and not all nephrons have the same maximum capacity for glucose absorption. Thus, those with the least transporter capacity will be saturated first, resulting in glucosuria (see Figure 9.6).

Secretion of substances into renal tubular fluid

A number of substances including various sulfates, steroids, sugars, and amino acid metabolites are secreted into tubular fluid, in contrast to the absorption back into the

bloodstream observed for many of the other products discussed. The physiological significance of secretion of these substances into tubular fluid is not clear. Indeed, we really do not understand well the role of many of those substances in the body, in the first place.

The nonmetabolized carbohydrate inulin is an example of a substance that is not affected by either absorption or secretion. In contrast, glucose, as already mentioned, is normally quantitatively reabsorbed. Para-aminohippuric acid is an organic acid that is used experimentally as an example of a substance that, in addition to being filtered, is also secreted into tubular fluid. Measurement of relative clearance rates compared to inulin indicates whether a substance is partly secreted or absorbed (see Table 9.2).

TABLE 9.2 CLEARANCE RATES OF VARIOUS SUBSTANCES

Substance	Clearance rate (mL/min)
Glucose	0
Sodium	0.9
Chloride	1.3
Potassium	12.0
Phosphate	25.0
Inulin	125
Creatinine	140

Reproduced, with permission, from Guyton, A.C. and Hall, J.E. (1997). *Human Physiology and Mechanisms of Disease,* 6th ed. Philadelphia, Saunders, p. 234.

Review Questions

17. Define renal tubular absorption and secretion.
18. Which is more selective: glomerular filtration or tubular absorption?
19. Contrast electrolyte transport in the GI tract with the nephron.
20. What are three mechanisms of chloride uptake in the renal tubule?

Functions along the length of the nephron

Proximal tubule

Nearly 65% of the sodium and water in the glomerular filtrate are reabsorbed in the proximal tubule. A number of distinctive specializations are seen in the proximal renal tubular cell (see Figure 9.4), including the following:

- High concentrations of mitochondria
- Extensive apical plasma membrane microvilli that serve to expand the surface area
- High concentrations of sodium cotransporters on the apical plasma membrane
- Countertransport mechanisms that absorb sodium while secreting substances including hydrogen ions into the tubular lumen

Loop of Henle

From the proximal tubule, the filtrate enters the loop of Henle (see Figure 9.2), which consists of three functional parts, the descending thin segment, the ascending thin segment, and the thick ascending segment.

The thin segment has very little transport activity, but is made up of epithelial cells that are permeable to water, and about 20% of the water in the filtrate is absorbed there. Once the filtrate arrives in the thick ascending limb of the loop of Henle, it is subjected to vigorous solute transport activity. However the cells that make up this region of the renal tubule are highly impermeable to water, resulting in a very dilute tubular fluid that flows into the distal tubule and is seen by the macula densa. Generation of dilute urine in the thick segment of the loop of Henle is crucial for the ability of the kidney to produce a dilute versus concentrated urine, as will be discussed in Mechanism of Dilute and Concentrated Urine Formation, Sec. 6.

Early distal tubule

By sensing the composition of tubular fluid entering the distal tubule, the macula densa and juxtaglomerular apparatus are able to regulate GFR and renal blood flow within that one nephron (see Sec. 5).

Just beyond the macula densa is the **diluting segment** of the distal tubule, so named because, like the ascending thick segment of the loop of Henle, it has active sodium, chloride and potassium transport activity, but is highly impermeable to water. Thus, tubular fluid entering the second half of the distal tubule is further depleted of electrolytes and therefore is even more dilute.

Late distal tubule

The second half of the distal tubule, includes the cortical collecting tubule and the medullary collecting duct, which are functionally quite similar (see Figure 9.4). They are composed of **principal cells**, which absorb sodium in exchange for potassium, and **intercalated cells**, which absorb potassium and bicarbonate in exchange for hydrogen ions (see Figure 9.7). The activity of these transporters is dependent on the hormone **aldosterone**.

Water channels can be inserted into the plasma membranes of these cells under the influence of the hormone ADH (antidiuretic hormone). Serum potassium concentration and acid-base status also influence the relative activity of the two different cell types.

The collecting duct goes from the cortex of the kidney to the medulla. The part of the renal tubule known as the **medullary collecting duct** is under the influence of ADH, like its cortical counterpart. Although only about 10% of the original volume of glomerular filtrate can be absorbed here, it is a crucial fraction for maintaining fluid and electrolyte homeostasis. Beyond this final segment of the renal tubule, the fluid passes into the ureter as urine and can no longer be reclaimed.

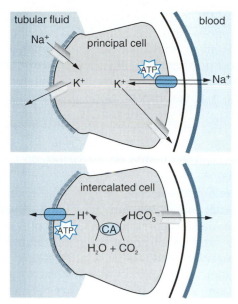

FIGURE 9.7. Transport in the principal and intercalated cells of the distal renal tubule. *(Adapted, with permission, from Berne, R.M. and Levy, M.N. (1998). Physiology, 4th ed. St. Louis, Mosby, p. 710.)*

Also like the cortical collecting tubule, the medullary collecting duct is capable of secreting hydrogen ions against a steep concentration gradient. Hence both of these regions are crucial to the kidney's role in acid-base balance (see Acid-Base Balance, in Sec. 7, and Chap. 10).

Unlike the early distal tubule and the cortical collecting tubule, the medullary collecting duct is somewhat permeable to urea, contributing to the osmolarity of the interstitium and therefore to the kidney's ability to generate a concentrated urine (see Mechanism of Dilute and Concentrated Urine Formation, in Sec. 6).

Clinical Pearls

The renal tubular acidoses (RTAs) are congenital or acquired disorders of acidification out of proportion to the degree of decrease in GFR, involving the renal tubule. Patients present with hyperchloremic metabolic acidosis because the disorder interferes with the ability to excrete an acid load, therefore consuming the body's bicarbonate buffer, with electroneutrality maintained by increased blood chloride concentration.

○ So-called type I or distal tubular RTA involves an inability of the distal nephron to lower tubular pH below about 5.5, either because the tubule is leaky to hydrogen ions or because transport of hydrogen ions into the tubular lumen was impaired. Urinary concentration and potassium excretion also are impaired. Although the metabolic acidosis is generally mild, type I RTA also promotes calcium loss in the urine and, therefore, secondary hyperparathyroidism. Furthermore, in the setting of other illnesses, the acidosis and hypokalemia resulting from loss of these homeostatic mechanisms can be life-threatening. Small daily doses of oral bicarbonate are usually adequate therapy for the acidosis.

○ Type II or proximal RTA involves a defect in bicarbonate absorption from the proximal tubule, often as part of a more general defect in proximal tubular function. Since normally, most bicarbonate is absorbed in the proximal tubule, the volume of bicarbonate delivered to the distal tubule in this disorder overwhelms its absorptive capacity. Eventually, plasma bicarbonate levels fall to a level that is within the capacity of the defective proximal tubule, and a new steady state is reached where normal daily acid excretion is possible, but at a lower serum bicarbonate level. Large doses of bicarbonate need to be given to correct the disorder, because above the altered renal threshold, bicarbonate is lost in the urine.

○ Type IV RTA, often seen in patients with diabetes mellitus, is characterized by loss of distal tubular hydrogen and potassium secretion, resulting in hyperkalemia. Hypoaldosteronism is one common etiology of type IV RTA, often due to inadequate renin production due to progression of underlying renal disease (see Chap. 10).

Review Questions

21. What are the regions of the renal tubule? What are some of their distinguishing characteristics? What percent of glomerular filtrate is absorbed in each?
22. What is a functional similarity between the thick ascending limb of the loop of Henle and the diluting segment of the distal tubule, just beyond the macula densa?
23. How are the cortical collecting tubule and medullary collecting duct similar in properties?

5. REGULATION OF RENAL FUNCTION

Since the kidneys are central to so many different dimensions of systemic homeostasis including fluids, electrolytes, acid-base balance, and blood pressure, it should not be surprising that renal function is heavily regulated. Some aspects of regulation are built into the physical structure of the kidney and its functional units, the nephrons (see below). Other aspects of regulation are mediated by nerves, hormones, and locally acting factors whose precise integration into the overall scheme of renal homeostasis has yet to be well understood.

Autoregulation of renal function

Normally, GFR is 180 L/day, of which 178.5 L is reabsorbed with a daily urine volume of 1.5 L. If renal function is dependent on GFR and GFR is dependent on the renal arterial-to-venous pressure gradient, what prevents GFR from varying wildly with changes in blood pressure? To illustrate the magnitude of the problem, consider an unregulated system: A trivial rise in blood pressure from a mean of 100 to 110 mmHg would cause a 10% rise in GFR from 180 to 198 L/day. If tubular absorption were constant at 178.5 L, urine volume would rise to nearly 20 L.

All else being equal, this does not happen for two reasons:

First, much, but not all, of the effect of systemic blood pressure on GFR is prevented by a form of autoregulation termed **tubuloglomerular feedback** that adjusts arteriolar resistance to maintain a near-constant GFR as long as mean blood pressures are in the range of 75 to 160 mmHg.

Second, because even when there is a change in GFR, other mechanisms exist to alter tubular absorption as needed to match the change in GFR in direction and magnitude, and thereby maintain fluid and electrolyte homeostasis (see below).

Tubuloglomerular feedback in autoregulation of glomerular filtration rate

Changes in systemic arterial pressure are reflected in corresponding changes in afferent renal arteriole perfusion pressure at the level of individual nephrons. Consider a fall in systemic blood pressure. This results in a decrease in renal afferent arteriole perfusion pressure, which lowers glomerular capillary hydrostatic pressure — a key determinant of filtration fraction — and therefore decreases GFR.

As GFR decreases, the amount of sodium and water delivered to the renal tubule also decreases. This is because, all else being equal, the transporters are working as hard as they can and when the volume they have to work on decreases, there will be less salt left by the time what is left of the filtrate gets to the macula densa. When the macula densa senses a decreased concentration of sodium, it triggers two changes:

- Dilation of the afferent arteriole, which decreases its resistance and increases glomerular capillary hydrostatic pressure, filtration fraction, and GFR.
- Renin release from the juxtaglomerular cells. Through a pathway described elsewhere (see Chap. 10), renin results in an increase in angiotensin II, a powerful constrictor of the efferent arteriole, thereby further increasing glomerular capillary hydrostatic pressure, filtration fraction, and GFR.

Thus these two homeostatic changes work to offset the decrease in GFR that occurred in response to the fall in systemic arterial pressure. Precisely the opposite changes are triggered by a rise in systemic arterial pressure.

Glomerular-tubular balance

The autoregulatory mechanisms involving the macula densa and juxtaglomerular apparatus are involved in the homeostatic maintenance of GFR. But sometimes there is a change in GFR, for example, because the change in systemic blood pressure is very marked, or because the autoregulatory mechanisms of tubuloglomerular feedback are not instantaneous and it takes some time to achieve their full effect. In those circumstances, another set of regulatory mechanisms comes into play to alter tubular absorption in the direction and magnitude to offset the effect of the change in GFR.

In part, glomerular-tubular balance is simply a consequence of physical forces. The very increase in afferent arteriolar perfusion pressure that increased filtration fraction and GFR will increase the colloid osmotic pressure pulling fluid back into the capillaries of the vasa recta.

In part, neural and hormonal mechanisms also play a role in glomerular-tubular balance. Table 9.3 indicates the hormones, sites, and actions that respond to an increase or a decrease in blood pressure by altering tubular absorption.

Despite these multiple regulatory mechanisms to prevent changes in GFR and when GFR does change, to match the tubular absorption to GFR, small effects of arterial blood pressure on urine output are observed, a phenomenon termed **pressure natriuresis**. In part, this is because increased blood pressure slightly increases the hydrostatic pressure in the vasa recta that partly offsets the tendency of colloid osmotic forces to promote

TABLE 9.3 HORMONES, SITES, AND ACTIONS THAT RESPOND TO AN INCREASE OR A DECREASE IN BLOOD PRESSURE BY ALTERING TUBULAR RESORPTION

Hormone	Site of action	Effects
Aldosterone	Distal tubule/collecting duct	↑ NaCl, H_2O reabsorption, ↑ K^+ secretion
Angiotensin II	Proximal tubule	↑ NaCl, H_2O reabsorption, ↑ H^+ secretion
Antidiuretic hormone	Distal tubule/collecting duct	↑ H_2O reabsorption
Atrial natriuretic peptide	Distal tubule/collecting duct	↓ NaCl reabsorption
Parathyroid hormone	Proximal tubules, thick ascending loop of Henle/distal tubules	↓ PO_4^- reabsorption, ↑ Ca^{++} reabsorption

Reproduced, with permission, from Guyton, A.C. and Hall, J.E. (1997). *Human Physiology and Mechanisms of Disease*, 6th ed. Philadelphia, Saunders, p. 232.

an increase in tubular absorption. Another part of this phenomenon is that production of angiotensin II, a key hormone in autoregulation of GFR, falls in response to an increase in blood pressure, resulting in a loss of its sodium-retaining effects. Thus the system is set up to maintain GFR, with both a fallback position and a safety valve. The fallback position is to alter tubular absorption when GFR changes. The safety valve is to alter fluid and electrolyte handling in response to changes in blood pressure. Since one way to correct a potentially dangerous rise or fall in blood pressure is to decrease or increase intravascular volume, such changes in sodium absorption are entirely appropriate from the point of view of maintaining homeostasis (see Figure 9.8).

Diuretics are drugs that have as one of their effects the inhibition of one or another transport mechanism in the renal tubule. As a result, diuretics promote salt (and with it water) loss in the urine. Clinically, they are valuable in the treatment of various fluid and electrolyte disorders (see Chap. 10). Table 9.4 and Figure 9.9 summarize the major classes of diuretics and their mechanisms of action, including agents that are not used clinically but that illustrate a physiological point.

TABLE 9.4 DIURETICS AND THEIR PRINCIPAL MECHANISMS OF ACTION ON RENAL TUBULAR TRANSPORT

Agent	Mechanism of action
Water	Inhibits vasopressin secretion
Ethanol	Inhibits vasopressin secretion
Antagonists of V_2 vasopressin receptors	Inhibit action of vasopressin on collecting duct
Large quantities of osmotically active substances such as mannitol and glucose	Produce osmotic diuresis
Xanthines such as caffeine and theophyline	Decrease tubular reabsorption of Na^+ and increase GFR
Acidifying salts such as $CaCl_2$ and NH_4Cl	Supply acid load; H^+ is buffered, but an anion is excreted with Na^+ when the ability of the kidneys to replace Na^+ with H^+ is exceeded
Carbonic anhydrase inhibitors such as acetazolamide (Diamox)	Decrease H^+ secretion, with resultant increase in Na^+ and K^+ excretion
Metolazone (Zaroxolyn), thiazides such as chlorothiazide (Diuril)	Inhibit Na^+ and K^+ reabsorption in the proximal tubule (minor effect) and in the early portion of the distal tubule (major effect)
Loop diuretics such as furosemide (Lasix), ethacrynic acid (Edecrin), and bumetanide	Inhibit Na^+-K^+-$2Cl^-$ cotransport in the medullary thick ascending limb of the loop of Henle
K^+-retaining natriuretics such as spironolactone (Aldactone), triamterene (Dyrenium), and amiloride (Colectril)	Inhibit Na^+-K^+ "exchange" in the collecting ducts by inhibiting the action of aldosterone (spironolactone) or by inhibiting Na^+ reabsorption (triamterene, amiloride)

Modified and reproduced, with permission, from Ganong, F.W. (1997) *Review of Medical Physiology*, 18th ed. Stamford, CT, Appleton & Lange, p. 677.

FIGURE 9.8. Glomerular tubular balance and tubuloglomerular feedback. *(Reproduced, with permission, from Ganong, F.W. (1997).* Review of Medical Physiology, *18th ed. Stamford, CT, Appleton & Lange, p. 666.)*

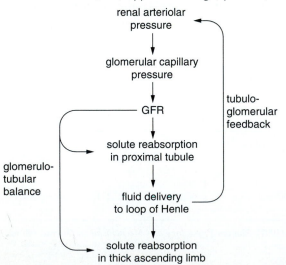

Clinical Pearl

○ Some of the most powerful diuretics are those that block active transport of Cl⁻, and with it water, in the ascending loop of Henle. Hence they are termed *loop diuretics*, the most common being the drug furosemide. However, in patients, for example, with heart failure and peripheral edema who have a falling GFR, these agents work less and less well. This is because, as GFR falls, a larger and larger fraction of total solute is reabsorbed in the proximal tubule, with less and less filtrate delivered to the furosemide-sensitive ascending limb of the loop of Henle. Also, compensatory responses in the distal tubule partly offset the effect of furosemide on the loop of Henle. Thiazide-type diuretics are, by themselves, mild diuretics in a patient with normal renal function. This is because their (minor) action at the proximal tubule simply shifts solute absorption preferentially to the loop of Henle, and their (major) action on the distal tubule involves a very small percentage of total filtrate. However, in patients with a low GFR on a loop diuretic, the fraction of solute reabsorbed distally is much larger. Because the combination of thiazide and loop diuretics blocks both proximal and distal tubular and loop sites of solute reabsorption, together a thiazide and loop diuretic result in a far greater diuretic effect than either agent alone, especially in patients with low GFR.

Review Questions

24. Describe the homeostatic mechanisms that prevent a fall in GFR when systemic blood pressure falls.
25. Describe the homeostatic mechanisms to match a rise in GFR due to a rise in systemic blood pressure, with increased tubular absorption.

26. What is pressure natriuresis, and what is its relation to autoregulation and glomerulotubular feedback?

Neural control of renal function

The renal blood vessels are heavily innervated by the sympathetic nervous system. Essentially all aspects of regulation of renal function discussed could, in principle, be controlled by the action of renal nerves. Thus activation of sympathetic innervation to the kidney will achieve the following:

- Vasoconstrict the afferent and efferent arterioles and thereby reduce GFR.
- Increase sodium reabsorption in the proximal tubule and thick ascending limb of the loop of Henle.
- Increase renin secretion and therefore angiotensin II formation, which will further increase absorption of tubular sodium.

However, a normal person at rest has little sympathetic tone to the kidneys. Thus this mechanism is probably only involved in the defense against severe and sudden hypovolemia (e.g., from hemorrhage).

Hormonal control of renal function

A variety of hormones and locally released regulatory substances can substantially affect renal blood flow, GFR, and, therefore, tubular absorption (see Table 9.5). These are discussed in more detail in Chapter 10.

Clinical Pearl

○ NSAIDs are particularly dangerous in patients who are elderly or who have some degree of underlying renal impairment, because these patients may be particularly dependent on prostaglandins to offset otherwise excessive sympathetic vasocon-

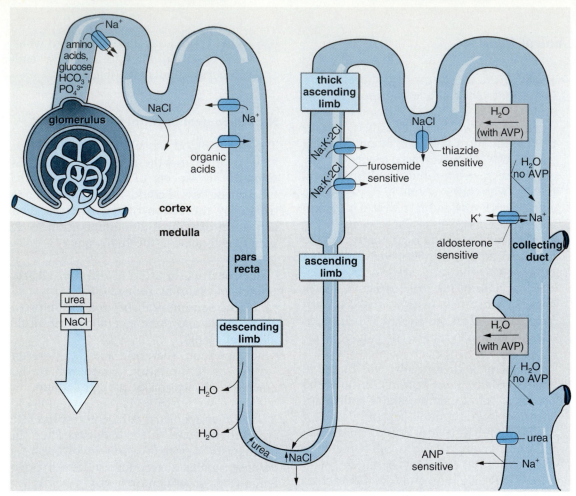

FIGURE 9.9. Major sites of action of diuretics along the course of the nephron. Fluid reabsorption across the proximal tubule is isosmotic and accounts for reabsorption of approximately two-thirds of the filtered sodium and water. The major portions of the filtered bicarbonate, amino acids, glucose, and phosphate are reabsorbed in the early proximal convoluted tubule. Reabsorption of glucose and amino acids is coupled to sodium transport and generates a negative potential difference within the tubular lumen. At the same time, bicarbonate is reabsorbed by a nonelectrogenic mechanism, via H^+ secretion. The active transport of these solutes results in transepithelial concentration and effective osmotic pressure gradients promoting water flow across the proximal tubule, into the peritubular capillaries. The rise in tubular fluid Cl^- concentration is a necessary reciprocal consequence of the decreased lumenal bicarbonate concentration. The resultant high concentration of Cl^- becomes an important force for the outward passive transport of Cl^- down its concentration gradient, resulting in a lumen-positive potential difference in the late proximal convoluted tubule. The pars recta of the proximal tubule is capable of active electrogenic transport of sodium independent of organic solute transport. Under normal conditions, approximately one-third of the glomerular filtrate enters the descending limb of the loop of Henle. Because the thin descending limb is incapable of active outward sodium chloride transport and is characterized by low permeability to sodium but high water permeability, water is abstracted passively as the fluid approaches the bend of Henle's loop. Hypertonic fluid with a greater sodium chloride concentration but lower urea concentration than the surrounding medullary interstitium thus enters the thin ascending limb of Henle, which is largely impermeable to water and urea but is highly permeable to sodium chloride. This permits passive outward diffusion of sodium chloride. Active Na : K : 2Cl transport across the water-impermeable

TABLE 9.5   HORMONES AND LOCAL MEDIATORS THAT REGULATE GFR

Hormone or autacoid	Effect on GFR
Norepinephrine	↓
Epinephrine	↓
Endothelin	↓
Angiotensin II	↔ (prevents ↓)
Endothelium-derived nitric oxide	↑
Prostaglandins	↑

Reproduced, with permission, from Guyton, A.C. and Hall, J.E. (1997). *Human Physiology and Mechanisms of Disease*, 6th ed. Philadelphia, Saunders, p. 220.

striction. Without the prostaglandin effects, renal blood flow in these patients may diminish to the point where acute tubular necrosis occurs, setting in motion further irreversible deterioration in their renal function.

Review Questions

27. What are three effects of the sympathetic nervous system on the kidney?
28. How important is the sympathetic nervous system for normal kidney function at rest?
29. Name five hormones that affect the kidney and summarize their actions.
30. What is the special role of angiotensin II in regulation of renal function in response to a drop in systemic blood pressure?
31. What is a possible role of prostaglandins in the setting of increased sympathetic activity to the kidneys?

6. MECHANISM OF DILUTE AND CONCENTRATED URINE FORMATION

Sometimes we drink more water than we need, and have to excrete a water load to maintain homeostasis. Other times, water is hard to get, and we must conserve water while we seek it. One way to conserve water is to generate a very concentrated urine. Human urine can be as dilute as 50 mosmol/L or as concentrated as 1400 mosmol/L, depending on the needs of homeostasis. Remarkably, these extremes of concentration can be achieved while independently maintaining sodium and potassium balance. The monitoring and coordination of the various responses to these diverse needs is the domain of the hypothalamus (see Chap. 11). In response to

FIGURE 9.9 — (*continued*) thick ascending limb of the loop of Henle allows for separation of solute and water. In consequence, tubular fluid becomes dilute and the medullary interstitium hypertonic. Irrespective of the final molarity of the urine, the fluid that enters the distal convoluted tubule is always hyposmotic. This segment exhibits active sodium reabsorption. All but the terminal portion of the distal convoluted tubule is water-impermeable, even in the presence of vasopressin (see Chap. 10). Aldosterone exerts its effect in this segment by enhancing sodium reabsorption, which is variably coupled to K+ and H+ secretion. The cortical and papillary portions of the collecting duct are sites where vasopressin exerts its principal effect. The permeability of these segments to water in the absence of vasopressin is very low but can be greatly enhanced in its presence. These segments are also characterized by active sodium resorption, which appears to depend on the presence of mineralocorticoid. In the absence of vasopressin, the collecting tubule is water-impermeable so that hypotonic tubular fluid flows through into the urine. In the presence of vasopressin, water is avidly resorbed here, resulting in hypertonic final urine. Major sites of action of furosemide, thiazide diuretics, aldosterone, and atrial natriuretic peptide (ANP) are shown. (*Adapted, with permission, from Brenner, B.M. and Mckenzie, H.S. (1998),* Disturbance of Renal Function, *in Fauci, A. et al. (eds.)* Harrison's Textbook of Internal Medicine, *14th ed. New York, McGraw-Hill, p. 1501.*)

a) water diuresis

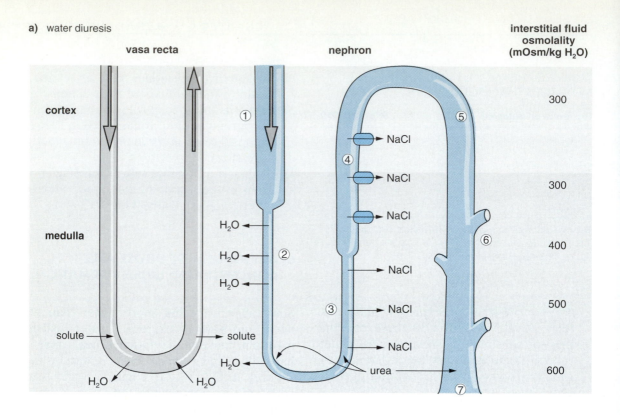

b) antidiuresis

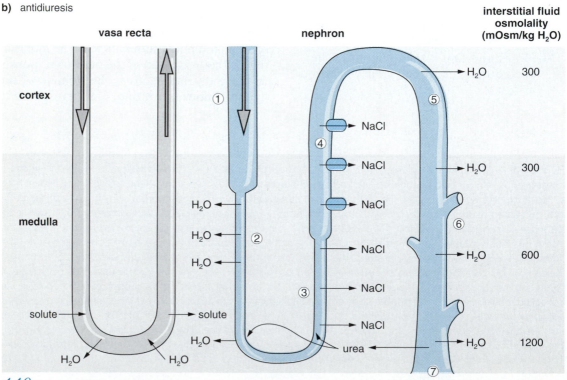

signals from the hypothalamus, the kidney generates either a dilute or concentrated urine. The following explains how this is achieved.

The osmolarity of glomerular ultrafiltrate is about 300 mosmol/L, the osmolarity of blood plasma. Since both solutes and water are proportionately absorbed in the proximal tubule, the osmolarity does not substantially change. However, in the thin segments of the loop of Henle, water absorption by osmosis makes the filtrate more concentrated, about 600 mosmol/L, due to the hypertonicity of the interstitium. Thus, the first requirement of a concentrated urine is an intact hypertonic medullary interstitium.

The **countercurrent multiplier** is a term used to describe the mechanism by which a hypertonic medullary interstitium is achieved and maintained in the kidney. The vasa recta play a crucial role in this process (see Figure 9.10). The basic idea here is that since sodium but not water is absorbed in certain parts of the renal tubule (e.g., the ascending thick segment of the loop of Henle) and since there is a constant flow of tubular fluid delivering more sodium to this region of the tubule, a diffusional gradient is formed in both the tubule and the interstitium whose maximum interstitial and tubular osmolarity is achieved at the tip of the loop of Henle, at steady state (see Figure 9.10).

Other contributors to the high medullary interstitial osmolarity include the following:

• Active transport of ions from collecting duct to medullary interstitium

• Passive diffusion of urea from the inner medullary collecting ducts into the medullary interstitium.

Subsequently, in the ascending thick segment of the loop of Henle, solute absorption occurs without movement of water, making the tubular fluid more dilute, down to about 100 mosmol/L. Regulation of the final osmolality of urine is largely dependent upon even later events in the distal tubule, collecting tubule, and collecting ducts, which are sensitive to ADH. When ADH is absent, the cells of the distal tubule, collecting tubule, and collecting ducts are highly impermeable to water, just as the cells that make up the ascending limb of the loop of Henle. Continued solute absorption leads to a very dilute urine. When ADH is present, water channels are inserted into the apical plasma membrane allowing uptake of water from the tubular fluid. Depending on how concentrated a urine is desired, more and more water channels can be inserted, in response to more and more ADH in the bloodstream. In the extreme, a very concentrated urine can be generated by reabsorbing the maximum amount of water from tubular fluid. Thus, the second requirement for a concentrated urine is the presence of ADH (and the ability to respond to it).

A crucial feature of the countercurrent mechanism is that the most ADH-sensitive locations for water uptake are in the parts of the tubule that are in the cortex. Thus, in response to ADH, water rapidly moves from the tubular lumen through the tubular cell

FIGURE 9.10. Countercurrent multiplier and function of the vasa recta. a. Mechanism for the excretion of dilute urine (water diuresis). Vasopressin is absent and the collecting duct is essentially impermeable to water. Note that the osmolality of the medullary interstitium is reduced during water diuresis. b. Mechanism for the excretion of a concentrated urine (antidiuresis). Plasma ADH levels are maximal, and the collecting duct is highly permeable to water. Under this condition, the medullary interstitial gradient is maximal. *(Adapted, with permission, from Berne, R.M. and Levy, M.N. (1998). Physiology, 4th ed. St. Louis, Mosby, p. 725.)*

into the interstitium and then enters the bloodstream from which it leaves the kidney without disturbing or "washing out" the hypertonicity of the medullary interstitium. Remember, as mentioned previously, blood flow to the medulla is only about 1 to 2% of renal blood flow, further preserving the medullary interstitial concentration gradient.

Finally, the vasa recta capillary system plays a crucial role in maintaining the hypertonic osmolar gradient of the renal medulla. Because these capillaries follow the course of the loops of Henle, the medullary salt and urea osmolar gradient in the medullary interstitium is not dissipated as rapidly as would occur if the capillaries flowed "straight" to the renal veins (see Figure 9.10).

The effects of the various transport activities of the renal tubule are summarized in Figure 9.11.

Clinical Pearl

○ Despite the homeostatic mechanisms described to preserve the hypertonicity of the renal medullary interstitium, it is possible to generate renal disease by dissipation of the hypertonicity. An example of this phenomenon occurs in patients who have a prolonged period of massive diuresis (e.g., diabetes insipidus due to a central nervous system lesion).

These patients initially have one etiology for defective urinary concentration (lack of ADH to trigger insertion of channels for water absorption into the apical distal tubular and collecting duct membrane). Later they develop another lesion as a complication of dissipation of medullary interstitial hypertonicity (termed **medullary washout**). Thus, once washout has occurred, they will continue to have dilute urine even if provided ADH, until hypertonicity of the renal medullary interstitium is reestablished over the next day or so.

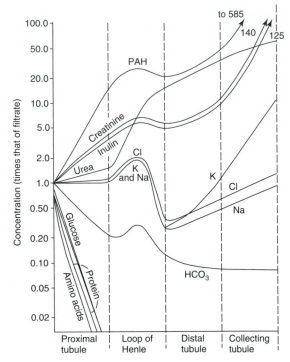

FIGURE 9.11. Summary of concentrations in the renal filtrate along the course of the renal tubule. Changes in average concentrations of different substances at different points in the tubular system relative to the concentrations of each substance in the glomerular filtrate. A value of 1.0 indicates that the concentration of the substance in the tubular fluid is the same as the concentration of that substance in the glomerular filtrate. Values below 1.0 indicate that the substance is reabsorbed more avidly than water; values above 1.0 indicate that the substance is reabsorbed to a lesser extent than water. (Adapted, with permission, from Guyton, A.C. and Hall, J.E. (1997). Human Physiology and Mechanisms of Disease, 6th ed. Philadelphia, Saunders, p. 229.)

Review Questions

32. What are the two requirements to achieve a concentrated urine?
33. How does the countercurrent multiplier mechanism work?
34. Where is the maximal solute concentration in the kidney?

7. OTHER RENAL FUNCTIONS

Erythropoetin secretion

Another function of the kidney is to secrete erythropoietin, the trophic hormone involved in red blood cell production and maturation in the bone marrow. In anemia, oxygen-carrying capacity of the blood is reduced. Since the renal tubule operates under low oxygen tension, particularly in the medulla, it is a good location for a sensor of oxygen-carrying capacity and hence the need for additional red blood cells. Erythropoietin travels via the bloodstream to the bone marrow where it stimulates erythropoiesis (synthesis of red blood cells), raising the hematocrit and therefore the oxygen-carrying capacity of the blood. This response relieves the hypoxia/anemia that triggers erythropoietin release in the first place, constituting a simple endocrine negative feedback loop (see Chap. 3).

Clinical Pearls

○ Anemia due to lack of erythropoietin production is a typical finding in patients with severe chronic renal failure, with a hematocrit in the low 20 range. The anemia of renal failure causes the hematocrit to fall into the low 20's but not lower because at that point other triggers of hematopoesis besides erythropoetin are maximally actuated. Erythropoietin treatment of anemia in patients with renal failure leads to numerous benefits including the following:

  • Improved muscle function
  • Enhanced immune response to hepatitis vaccine
  • Decreased left ventricular hypertrophy
  • Improved brain electrophysiology

  It is not clear to what extent these improvements reflect poorly understood consequences of erythropoietin action versus amelioration of poorly understood complications of anemia.

○ Patients treated with erythropoietin often display worsened hypertension. Although this is partly due to increased intravascular volume, it may also be a consequence of erythropoietin stimulation of secretion of endothelin, a powerful vasoconstrictor.

Gluconeogenesis

The kidney is a secondary site, after the liver, of various intermediary metabolic pathways, including gluconeogenesis, urea synthesis, and transamination of amino acids, in particular glutamine. This allows flux of intermediary metabolites between the pathways of carbohydrate and protein metabolism.

Calcium homeostasis

The kidney plays a number of important roles in calcium and phosphate homeostasis, which are discussed in more detail in Chapter 14. To briefly summarize, the kidney is the site of the following actions:

• Activation or inactivation of vitamin D, depending on whether the regulated enzymes 1, 25 hydroxylase (which generates an active vitamin D metabolite) or 24, 25 hydroxylase (which generates an inactive vitamin D metabolite) are active.
• Action of parathyroid hormone (PTH), resulting in calcium retention and phosphate wasting in the urine.

Clinical Pearl

○ Renal failure results in difficulty in phosphate excretion and, perhaps, insensitivity to PTH action. As a result of these and other effects, renal failure is characterized by increased PTH secretion and calcium loss from bone. This so-called secondary hyperparathyroidism results in substantial bone loss and severe secondary complications of renal failure if not adequately treated. Treatment involves restriction of dietary phosphate and supplementation of dietary calcium.

Acid-base balance

Acid-base balance is the domain of more than just the kidneys. Without proper heart, lung, and liver function, acidosis or alkalosis may develop, even with normal kidneys. Nevertheless, the kidneys normally play a crucial role in long-term acid-base homeostasis, discussed in more detail in Chapter 10.

Review Questions

35. What is the role of the kidney in secondary hyperparathyroidism, and how can this condition be treated?
36. Where does erythropoetin have its major actions?
37. What are four consequences of treating the anemia of chronic renal failure with erythropoetin?

8. PATHOPHYSIOLOGY OF RENAL DISORDERS

How normal kidney structure and function can be altered in disease

Renal disease can be categorized either by the site of the lesion (e.g., vascular, glomerular, or tubular disease) or by the nature of the factors that have led to kidney disease (e.g., immunological, metabolic, infiltrative, infectious, hemodynamic, or toxic/drug effects). Some regions of the kidney are particularly susceptible to certain kinds of injury:

- The renal medulla is a low-oxygen-tension environment. This makes it more susceptible to ischemic injury.

- Because of its role as the initial filter of blood entering the kidney, the glomerulus is a particularly prominent site of injury related to excessive or inappropriate immune complex formation and clearance, and complement fixation.
- Hemodynamic factors regulating blood flow have a profound effect on the kidney because GFR, a primary determinant of renal function, depends on blood flow and because of the susceptibility of the kidney to hypoxic injury.

It is important to recognize that renal disease lies on a continuum from mild abnormalities to necrosis of renal tubules. Ischemic, toxic, infectious, and other forms of injury often start as a mild abnormality which, if uncorrected, can proceed to severe disease. Thus, your patient's status along the expected natural history of the disorder is an extremely important consideration that will guide your therapy and better allow you to anticipate complications.

One useful organizing scheme that combines a consideration of both the site and cause of renal disease in approaching patients with newly discovered renal failure is first to categorize the cause of renal failure as prerenal, intrarenal, or postrenal, and then to subdivide these categories as to specific etiology and location (see Table 9.6).

Prerenal causes are those resulting from inadequate blood flow to the kidney, whether due to intravascular volume depletion, a structural lesion of the renal arteries, drug effects on renal blood flow, or hypotension from any cause resulting in renal hypoperfusion. More than two-thirds of all cases of acute renal failure are due to prerenal causes.

Under conditions where renal perfusion is inadequate, that is, due to prerenal causes of renal dysfunction, the kidney will be maximally stimulated to retain sodium (e.g., relative to creatinine). However, once acute tubular necrosis has occurred, nothing (including sodium) will be absorbed. Thus, the

TABLE 9.6   CATEGORIES OF RENAL DISEASE

Prerenal disease
- A. True volume depletion due to gastrointestinal, renal, or third-space losses
- B. Congestive heart failure
- C. Hepatorenal syndrome in advanced hepatic cirrhosis
- D. Bilateral renal artery stenosis, particularly after the administration of an angiotensin converting enzyme inhibitor
- E. Use of a nonsteroidal antiinflammatory drug in certain clinical settings
- F. Shock due to fluid loss, sepsis, or cardiac failure — frequently progresses to acute tubular necrosis

Intrarenal disease
Glomerular disease
- A. Acute glomerulonephritis, including postinfectious glomerulonephritis and lupus nephritis
- B. Crescentic or rapidly progressive glomerulonephritis

Vascular disease
- A. Vasculitis, usually associated with systemic symptoms
- B. Atheroemboli to the kidney, most often following surgical or radiologic manipulation of a markedly atheromatous aorta

Tubulointerstitial disease
- A. Acute tubular necrosis
  1. Postischemic — following any cause of severe renal ischemia
  2. Toxic — aminoglycoside antibiotics, radiocontrast agents (primarily in those with diabetes with renal insufficiency), the chemo-
     therapeutic agent cisplatin, or the excretion of heme pigments with hemolysis or rhabdomyolysis
- B. Acute, usually drug-induced interstitial nephritis
- C. Intratubular obstruction, due to immunoglobulin light chains in multiple myeloma, calcium in hypercalcemia, the antiviral drug
     acyclovir, or uric acid crystals following excess tissue breakdown and release of purines after chemotherapy or radiation therapy of
     a hematologic malignancy

Postrenal disease
Urinary tract obstruction
- A. Prostatic disease in older men
- B. Pelvic or retroperitoneal malignancy
- C. Unilateral ureteral obstruction (e.g., by a kidney stone)

Modified and reproduced, with permission, from Rose, B.D. and Rennke, H.G. (1994). *Renal Pathophysiology*. Baltimore, Williams & Wilkins, p. 238.

fractional excretion of sodium (FENa) is a useful index by which to distinguish the early stage of prerenal azotemia from the later stage of acute tubular necrosis (see Table 9.7).

Postrenal causes are those related to urinary tract obstruction, either due to kidney stones, structural lesions of the urinary tract (tumors, prostatic hypertrophy, strictures, etc.), or functional abnormalities (e.g., spasm, drug effects). Only about 5% of cases of acute renal failure have a postrenal cause. However, their importance comes from the fact that these are some of the most readily reversible causes of renal failure if detected early enough. The actual mechanism of renal failure in obstruction is probably due to elevation of pressure in Bowman's space, thereby dropping GFR.

Intrarenal causes are those disorders that cause direct damage to the nephron rather than resulting in damage to nephrons as a consequence of inadequate perfusion or obstruction (see Table 9.7). As mentioned earlier, intrarenal causes include specific disorders of the kidney as well as systemic diseases with prominent manifestations in the kidney. Some of these disorders manifest as glomerular injury and others involve primarily the tubules. Within each category, disorders can be further categorized by either specific cause or by manifestations.

TABLE 9.7 FRACTIONAL EXCRETION OF SODIUM IN PRERENAL STATES VERSUS ACUTE TUBULAR NECROSIS

Diagnostic index	Typical findings	
	Prerenal azotemia	Intrinsic renal azotemia
Fractional excretion of sodium (%)* $$\frac{U_{Na} \times P_{Cr}}{P_{Na} \times U_{Cr}} \times 100$$	<1	>1
Urine sodium concentration (mmol/L)	<10	>20
Urine creatinine to plasma creatinine ratio	>40	>20
Urine urea nitrogen to plasma urea nitrogen ratio	>8	<3
Urine specific gravity	>1.018	<1.015
Urine osmolality (mosmol/kg H$_2$O)	>500	<300
Plasma BUN : creatinine ratio	>20	<10–15
Renal failure index* $$\frac{U_{Na}}{U_{Cr}/P_{Cr}}$$	<1	>1
Urine sediment	Hyaline casts	Muddy brown granular casts

*Most sensitive indices

Note: U_{Na}, urine sodium concentration; P_{Cr}, plasma creatinine concentration; P_{Na}, plasma sodium concentration; U_{Cr}, urine creatinine concentration; BUN, blood urea nitrogen.

Reproduced, with permission, from Brady, H.R. and Brenner, B.M., (1998). Acute Renal Failure, in Fauci, A. et al. eds. *Harrison's Textbook of Internal Medicine*, 14th ed. New York, McGraw-Hill, p. 1510.

Manifestations of altered kidney function

The major manifestations of altered kidney function are as follows:

- Electrolyte and acid-base disturbances (discussed in Chap. 10).
- Signs and symptoms of *uremia*, a term used to describe the complex of findings due to accumulation of toxic wastes (such as urea) that would normally be eliminated by the kidney (see Table 9.8).
- Intravascular volume expansion resulting in congestive heart failure and eventually pul-

monary edema, due to the inability to excrete sodium and water (e.g., absorbed from the GI tract or infused intravenously).
- Anemia with a hematocrit in the mid-20s, which is typically seen with renal failure due to lack of erythropoietin production, unless the patient is treated with exogenous erythropoietin injections.

Review Questions

38. What characteristics of various parts of the nephron make it particularly susceptible to certain types of injury?

TABLE 9.8 SIGNS AND SYMPTOMS OF UREMIA

Clinical abnormalities in uremia*

Fluid and electrolyte disturbances
  Volume expansion and contraction (I)
  Hypernatremia and hyponatremia (I)
  Hyperkalemia and hypokalemia (I)
  Metabolic acidosis (I)
  Hyperphosphatemia (I)
  Hypocalcemia (I)

Endocrine-metabolic disturbances
  Secondary hyperparathyroidism (I or P)
  Aluminum-induced osteomalacia (D)
  Vitamin D–deficient osteomalacia (I)
  Carbohydrate intolerance (I)
  Hyperuricemia (I or P)
  Hypertriglyceridemia (P)
  Increased Lp(a) level (P)
  Decreased high-density lipoprotein
    level (P)
  Protein-calorie malnutrition (I or P)
  Impaired growth and development (P)
  Infertility and sexual dysfunction (P)
  Amenorrhea (P)
  Hypothermia (I)
  Dialysis-induced β_2-microglobulin amy-
    loidosis

Neuromuscular disturbances
  Fatigue (I)[†]
  Sleep disorders (P)
  Headache (I or P)
  Impaired mentation (I)[†]
  Lethargy (I)[†]
  Asterixis (I)
  Muscular irritability (I)
  Peripheral neuropathy (I or P)
  Restless legs syndrome (I or P)
  Paralysis (I or P)
  Myoclonus (I)
  Seizures (I or P)
  Coma (I)
  Muscle cramps (D)
  Dialysis disequilibrium syndrome (D)
  Dialysis dementia (D)
  Myopathy (P or D)
Cardiovascular and pulmonary distur-
    bances
  Arterial hypertension (I or P)
  Congestive heart failure or pulmonary
    edema (I)
  Pericarditis (I)
  Cardiomyopathy (I or P)
  Uremic lung (I)
  Accelerated atherosclerosis (P or D)
  Hypotension and arrhythmias (D)

Dermatologic disturbances
  Pallor (I)[†]
  Hyperpigmentation (I, P, or D)
  Pruritus (P)
  Ecchymoses (I)
  Uremic frost (I)
Gastrointestinal disturbances
  Anorexia (I)
  Nausea and vomiting (I)
  Uremic fetor (I)
  Gastroenteritis (I)
  Peptic ulcer (I or P)
  Gastrointestinal bleeding (I, P, or D)
  Hepatitis (D)
  Idiopathic ascites (D)
  Peritonitis (D)
Hematologic and immunologic distur-
    bances
  Normocytic, normochromic anemia (I)[†]
  Microcytic (aluminum-induced) anemia
    (D)
  Lymphocytopenia (P)
  Bleeding diathesis (I or D)[†]
  Increased susceptibility to (I or P)
  Splenomegaly and hypersplenism (P)
  Leukopenia (D)
  Hypocomplementemia (D)

*Virtually all abnormalities in this table are completely reversed in time by successful renal transplantation. The response of these abnormalities to hemodialysis or peritoneal dialysis therapy is more variable. (I) denotes an abnormality that usually improves with an optimal program of dialysis and related therapy; (P) denotes one that tends to persist or even progress, despite an optimal program; (D) denotes one that develops only after initiation of dialysis therapy.
†Improves with dialysis and erythropoietin therapy.
Reproduced, with permission, from Lazarus, J.M. and Brenner, B.M. (1998), Chronic Renal Failure, in Fauci, A. et al. eds. *Harrison's Textbook of Internal Medicine*, 14th ed. New York, McGraw-Hill, p. 1516.

39. Define prerenal, intrarenal, and postrenal causes of renal failure.
40. What are the major clinical manifestations of inadequate renal function?

9. FRONTIERS IN KIDNEY RESEARCH

The expansion of knowledge in cell and molecular biology of the last two decades has substantially affected kidney research. Thus, there has been a major shift in the focus of research from studies of the physiology of individual nephrons and characterization of pathological processes in descriptive terms, to the study of subcellular signaling, including the study of mechanisms of action of hormones, chemokines, and local factors and their receptors in different renal cell types. New directions have been opened up by application of new technologies in which specific genes affecting intrarenal signaling are eliminated (**knockout mice**) or in which specific gene mutations are introduced (**transgenic mice**).

Protein filtration, proximal tubule cells, and progression of renal failure

A fundamental renal function is to filter blood at the glomerulus, allowing small substances to enter the renal tubule while large substances such as proteins are retained in the bloodstream. What if this filter is damaged? Naively, one might expect loss of filtration function to be the only consequence. But if we think about it, biologically active growth factors, cytokines, and other products would inappropriately see the renal tubular cell apical plasma membrane. Since a recurring theme in evolution and biology is to make use of such situations, might inappropriate cross-talk via receptor-mediated actions of filtered proteins be a problem? Work suggests that toxic effects of filtered proteins as biologically active molecules may be a cause of progression of renal injury (see Refs. 6 and 7).

Mesangial cells and the regulation of glomerular filtration rate

Using a rat model for glomerulonephritis, investigators have discovered a new function of the juxtaglomerular apparatus to serve as a reservoir for production of mesangial cells. When mesangial cells are damaged or destroyed, it appears that mesangial cells in the juxtaglomerular apparatus (distinct from renin-secreting cells) are relatively protected (e.g., from antibody-mediated attack) and respond by proliferating and migrating out to repopulate the mesangial cell-depleted glomerulus. Perhaps an overexuberant response accounts for renal disease involving excessive mesangial cell function (see Ref. 8).

What is the role of the mesangial cell? A growing body of evidence suggests that, among other things, mesangial cells regulate GFR by controlling the filterable surface area of the glomerular capillary. Normally the contractile tone of the mesangial cell is set by the balance of factors promoting contraction versus relaxation of smooth muscle (to which mesangial cells are related). Evidence suggests that a variety of intraglomerular sources of nitric oxide (e.g., from macrophages and endothelial cells), in response to inflammatory cytokines, mechanical stress, and other mediators (e.g., acetylcholine or bradykinin), affects the contractile state and therefore the physiological function of the mesangial cells (see Ref. 9).

Angiotensin receptors: A balance of forces in the kidney

A key theme in biology that is readily apparent in the kidney is that the normal resting condition represents a balance of forces that are intended to buffer changes and maintain homeostasis. A remarkable new dimension to this theme appears to be emerging from data on the role of the two different isoforms of the angiotensin II receptor. One form, termed *type 1*, is the trigger of vasoconstriction in response to angiotensin II, the conventional role. As with many hormones, activation of this receptor also has growth-promoting effects on the tissues that express it. There is also a second form of the angiotensin II receptor, termed the *type 2 receptor*, whose function has been unknown. Now studies suggest that activation of the type 2 receptor blocks at least the growth-promoting effects of the type 1 receptor. Data in transgenic mice have extended this observation to the vascular effects believed to be the most important consequences of activation of the angiotensin II receptor type 1 (see Refs. 10 to 12). Thus, type 2 angiotensin II receptors appear to be broad antagonists of the function of type 1 receptors.

Endothelin, the endothelial cell, and glomerulosclerosis

Another recurring theme in modern molecular medicine is the notion that local synthesis of various mediators can have local, organ-specific effects through activation of cascades of gene expression that would not be detected by measuring systemic levels of hormones and mediators. Precisely this phenomenon is believed to be the basis for at least some forms of progressive glomerulosclerosis. This form of chronic renal disease occurs as a consequence of various disorders including diabetes mellitus. It results, at least in part, from accumulation of extracellular matrix proteins, as well as changes in gene expression by mesangial cells, endothelial cells, and other components of the nephron. Studies suggest that an injured endothelium is activated to synthesize angiotensinogen locally, with resulting locally generated angiotensin II. Angiotensin II, besides its vasoconstrictive effects, appears to activate expression of transforming growth factor β (TGFβ) by endothelial cells. TGFβ in turn alters the pattern and quantity of extracellular matrix protein synthesis and other steps in the final common pathway leading to sclerotic destruction of the glomerulus. Within this overall framework, there remains plenty of room for additional contributors and intermediate steps in the pathophysiological process, possibly varying according to trigger, consequences, location of the lesion, or other parameters. For example, endothelin, a powerful local mediator, has been implicated in both vasoconstriction and cytokine activities (see Ref. 13).

Cell adhesion molecules and acute renal failure

Cell adhesion molecules, the biological equivalent of "Velcro," appear to play diverse and interesting roles in the pathogenesis of acute renal failure. Consider first the paradigm of reperfusion injury. It appears that upon reperfusion of ischemic tissue, there is a change in the adhesion molecules expressed by injured endothelium allowing inflammatory cells (such as polymorphonuclear leukocytes [PMNs]) to be recruited to these tissues. The inflammatory cells then release free radicals that cause oxidative injury to tissues. Since a switch in adhesion molecule interactions appears to be a key step in this process, treatments that prevent the characteristic change in adhesion molecule expression might be expected to mitigate the inflammatory injury. Possible therapeutic approaches include injection into the bloodstream of antibodies to block adhesion molecules' function or uptake into cells of antisense oligonucleotides to block adhesion molecule expression. These are sequences of DNA that are complementary to the sequence of a particular gene and which therefore hybridize to messenger RNAs expressed from that gene, thereby preventing their translation (see Ref. 14). This is often an effective way of decreasing expression of the particular gene product in cells, and perhaps can be used to alter the pattern of adhesion molecule displayed by the kidney.

The role of cell adhesion molecules is not limited to the endothelium and recruitment of inflammatory cells, however. An early event in acute tubular necrosis in response to ischemia is depletion of ATP and resultant rearrangement of the cytoskeleton (see Chap. 2). As a result, adhesion molecules that used to be limited to one side of a cell are now redistributed all around the cell. With these changes, not only is the epithelial barrier disrupted with sloughing of living cells (which have actually been cultured from the urine of patients with acute tubular necrosis), but the sloughed cells attach to each other, due to the change in distribution of adhesion molecules. This subsequent reaggregation is why sloughed epithelial cells form "renal casts" seen in acute tubular necrosis. These casts may cause obstruction of the renal tubule and elevated back pressure in individual renal nephrons, causing further damage. Thus, intrinsic and prerenal disease may in fact destroy nephrons by a mechanism that at the molecular level resembles "postrenal" obstruction (see Refs. 15 and 16).

10. HOW DOES AN UNDERSTANDING OF NORMAL PHYSIOLOGY PROVIDE INSIGHT INTO THE INITIAL CASE PRESENTATION?

You explain to Ms. L., the 24-year-old woman with shortness of breath and loss of appetite, that the kidney is a delicate and somewhat fragile structure and that many things can damage it and cause it to stop functioning. Although you do not know for sure at this time why her kidneys do not work, there are several possibilities. Recurrent, persistent, or inadequately treated urinary tract infections, which she may have had as a child, are a frequent cause of renal failure. Renal failure is sometimes caused by genetic problems, such as polycystic kidney disease, which are inherited. This is unlikely to be what happened to her, because she has no family history of renal disease. Sometimes high blood pressure damages the kidney, and her current high blood pressure may be either a cause or a result of the kidney damage. Sometimes the body's immune system attacks the kidney, and you will do tests to look for evidence of this.

Muscle injury results in proteins released from the damaged muscle precipitating in and clogging the renal tubules. The reason that the combination of ibuprofen and muscle injury brought on her current symptoms is that a small acute injury is often enough to dramatically worsen slowly progressing chronic renal failure. Probably this is because her body's ability to function normally in spite of limited kidney function (through utilization of homeostatic mechanisms) had been stretched to the limit and could not further adapt to additional acute injury. The current symptoms developed because her remaining level of renal function is simply below that to which her body can adapt. The public has no idea how dangerous certain over-the-counter medicines can be especially to particular subsets of individuals whose homeostatic defenses are impaired, as in her case.

Because her kidneys can no longer filter and remove excess fluid from her body, she has become volume overloaded. The excess fluid is backing up into her legs, causing swelling, and into her lungs, causing difficulty breathing. This is a form of congestive heart failure in which the problem is not with the heart but rather the kidneys and volume regulation. Physical signs of this process are an S_3 heart sound, crackles in the lungs, edema, acidosis, and hypoxia. Loss of appetite reflects, at least in part, the fact that toxins and wastes that would normally be filtered out of the bloodstream by the kidney are accumulating in her body (uremia) and interfere with appetite regulation.

Volume overload, acidosis, and elevated potassium are three important parameters used to determine when a patient with deteriorating renal function needs to go on dialysis. You explain to Ms. L. that she has signs of needing dialysis soon and she will probably feel much better when she is dialyzed. It remains to be seen whether or not her kidneys will regain sufficient function to avoid the need for chronic dialysis in the near future. She will need a low-protein diet that minimizes workload and toxin exposure to the kidney. Her diet will also need to be low in phosphorous and high in calcium and vitamin D to compensate for changes in kidney function. She will need thorough education about what is involved in chronic dialysis and how that compares to the option of a kidney transplant. Living with chronic renal failure will involve major adaptations in her life for which she will need much support.

SUMMARY AND REVIEW
OF KEY CONCEPTS

1. The primary role of the kidneys is to filter the blood, removing wastes and adjusting the concentration of electrolytes and water to maintain homeostasis. Secondary roles include stimulation of red blood cell production and adjustment of blood pressure. Signs and symptoms of kidney failure include dyspnea and fatigue, loss of appetite, altered mental status, anemia, and accelerated atherosclerosis.

2. The functional unit of the kidney is the nephron, a microscopic tubular structure that consists of many regulated parts. The glomerulus is a tuft of capillaries at which an initial ultrafiltrate of blood, normally free of cells and most proteins, is achieved. The renal tubule is a multicomponent structure through which the ultrafiltrate flows, with various transporters in various regions altering the composition of the tubular fluid by taking up electrolytes with or without water. Most of the volume is reclaimed in the proximal renal tubule, but most of the regulation of salt and water balance occurs at the distal renal tubule where aldosterone-sensitive sodium, potassium, and hydrogen ion transporters and antidiuretic hormone-sensitive water channels occur.

3. The GFR is a key determinant of renal function, because, if the blood is not filtered in the first place, there is little the kidney can do about it later.

4. A countercurrent multiplier mechanism allows the renal medulla to maintain a hypertonic interstitium that is important for concentration of urine.

5. A special structure, the juxtaglomerular apparatus, monitors and regulates renal blood flow and glomerular capillary perfusion pressure, as well as distal tubular fluid composition. Intrarenal regulatory mechanisms involve hormones such as the renin-angiotensin-aldosterone system; local mediators such as prostaglandins, endothelins, and nitric oxide; and neural input from the sympathetic nervous system.

6. Acute renal disease can be categorized as prerenal (involving events outside of the kidney that result in hypoperfusion), intrarenal (mechanisms involving direct damage to the kidney itself), and postrenal (consequences of obstruction with damaging consequences of elevated back-pressure on nephron function). Chronic renal disease renders the kidney particularly sensitive to acute insults because homeostatic mechanisms are stretched to the limit.

A CASE OF PHYSIOLOGICAL MEDICINE

E.B. is a 52-year-old car mechanic with diabetes mellitus and unsuccessfully treated hypertension, who is admitted to the hospital with lower extremity cellulitis, total body edema, and progression of chronic renal failure. He has been treated for diabetes mellitus for the past 12 years. Eight years ago he was placed on twice-daily insulin injections, with fasting blood glucose in the range of 150 to 350 mg/dL (normal, 60 to 140 mg/dL). He has had proteinuria for over 5 years. About one month ago he noted swelling in his feet, for which he was prescribed furosemide and leg elevation, which resulted in some improvement. Blood chemistries at that time noted a white blood cell count of 6×10^3 per milliliter (normal is 4.8 to 10.8×10^3 per milliliter), a hematocrit of 33% (normal is 42 to 52%), blood urea nitrogen (BUN) level of 36 mg per dL (normal is 8 to 25 mg/dL), and a creatinine level of 2.5 mg/dL (normal is 0.8 to 1.3 mg/dL), with a creatinine clearance of 70 mL (normal is 90 to 140 mL).

Physical examination now is notable for fever to 38.5°C and an elevated blood pressure at 180/100. Mr. B. has severe swelling all over his body, an edematous condition termed *anasarca*, with red discoloration of the skin over his left lower extremities, extending all the way to his swollen scrotum. Several small, weeping, purulent lesions were noted on the left leg. Stool was negative for gross or occult blood. Blood analysis now demonstrates a white blood cell count of 16 $\times 10^3$ per milliliter with 85% neutrophils, a hematocrit of 28%, sodium of 129 mg/dL (normal is 135 to 145 mg/dL), potassium of 3.7 mg/dL (normal is 3.5 to 4.5 mg/dL), glucose of 480 mg/dL (normal is 60 to 140 mg/dL), BUN level of 58 mg/dL, and creatinine level of 5.6 mg/dL. Urinalysis revealed 4+ protein and is otherwise normal. Chest x-ray revealed small pleural effusions bilaterally, with an enlarged heart. The electrocardiogram was remarkable only for left ventricular hypertrophy.

Blood and lower extremity wound cultures were taken, and Mr. B. was treated with intravenous antibiotics. His insulin requirements, which a month ago had been 45 U daily, were noted initially in the hospital to be up to 80 U a day. As his cellulitis responded to antibiotic therapy, his insulin requirements also fell to a total of 20 U, substantially less than he required a month ago.

While he was in the hospital he was evaluated with a 24-h urine collection, which revealed 8 g of protein (normal is < 150 mg) per 24 h and a creatinine clearance of 10. Prior to discharge, an arteriovenous fistula was placed in anticipation of the need for hemodialysis in the near future.

QUESTIONS

1. What is the relation between Mr. B.'s underlying diabetes mellitus, his new finding of total body edema, and dramatically worsening renal function?
2. Mr. B.'s hematocrit has dropped 5 points in a month, without an obvious source of blood loss? How do you account for this change?
3. There seems to be a discrepancy between the dramatic fall in creatinine clearance and the less dramatic rise in serum creatinine. Explain this.
4. Mr. B.'s insulin requirements first went up, presumably due to the combination of stress-induced increase in counterregulatory hormone production, as well as the effects of poor blood glucose control on his remaining β cells of the endocrine pancreas (see Chap. 6). Subsequently, Mr. B. was able to achieve a lower blood glucose level on less insulin than he had needed a month ago. How do you explain the discrepancy between insulin needs a month ago versus now?
5. What is the role of poor hypertension control in the progression of Mr. B.'s renal disease? How should he have been treated previously?

ANSWERS

1. Diabetes mellitus damages the kidneys chronically. Besides the progressive renal failure, a hallmark of diabetic renal disease is profound proteinuria, because the selective mechanism that normally prevents filtration of albumin is lost. Loss of albumin in the urine (8 g per 24 h) results in falling oncotic pressure in the vasculature, and, therefore, more fluid in the extravascular extracellular space (seen as edema).
2. This change can be accounted for by the loss of erythropoetin production by his failing kidneys.
3. Creatinine is a useful measure of renal function; however, its level of accumulation in the bloodstream does not correspond to glomerular function as well as does creatinine clearance. This is due to various factors. For example, creatinine is not just filtered at the glomerulus, but also

secreted into the renal tubule. As glomerular filtration rate falls very low, tubular secretion of creatinine becomes proportionately greater and causes the serum creatinine to be less and less representative of the fall in glomerular filtration (i.e., of the degree of renal failure). Furthermore, the amount of creatinine produced is related to muscle mass, thus a small rise in creatinine in a thin elderly patient with poor muscle mass may reflect a substantial loss of renal function, which would be more accurately revealed by the creatinine clearance. Thus, creatinine clearance which corrects for various confounding factors, gives a better assessment of renal function than the isolated measurement of creatinine.

4. Insulin is in part eliminated by the kidneys. Therefore, the discrepancy is a consequence of the fact that progression of renal failure resulted in a longer half-life for his injected insulin than previously.

5. Glomerular hyperfiltration and elevated afferent arteriole perfusion pressures are believed to contribute to the destruction of individual nephrons. The high blood pressure exacerbates the underlying renal damage caused by diabetes mellitus. Mr. B. should have been placed on an angiotensin converting enzyme inhibitor to treat his high blood pressure. These medicines have been shown to slow the progression of diabetic renal disease.

References and suggested readings

GENERAL REFERENCES

1. Navar, L.G. (1998). Integrating multiple paracrine regulators of renal microvascular dynamics. *Am. J. Physiol.* 274:F433-444.
2. Lee, M.D. et al. (1997). The aquaporin family of water channel proteins in clinical medicine. *Medicine* 76:141-156.
3. Fauci, A., Braunwald, E., Isselbacher, K. et al. (eds.) (1997). *Harrison's Principles of Internal Medicine*, 14th ed. McGraw Hill, New York.
4. Rose, B.D. (1994). *Clinical Physiology of Acid-Base and Electrolyte Disorders*, 4th ed. New York, McGraw-Hill.
5. Valtin, H. and Schafer, J.A. (1995). *Renal Function*, 3rd ed. Boston, Little Brown.

FRONTIERS REFERENCES

6. Remuzzi, G. et al. (1997). Understanding the nature of renal disease progression. *Kidney Int.* 51:2-15.
7. Zoja, C. et al. (1995). Proximal tubular cell synthesis and secretion of endothelin-1 on challenge with albumin and other proteins. *Am. J. Kidney Dis.* 26:934-941.
8. Hugo, C. et al. (1997). Extraglomerular origin of the mesangial cell after injury: A new role of the juxtaglomerular apparatus. *J. Clin. Invest.* 100:786-794.
9. Stockand, J.D. and Sansom, S.C. (1997). Regulation of filtration rate by glomerular mesangial cells in health and diabetic renal disease. *Am J. Kidney Dis.* 29:971-981.
10. Yoshida, H. et al. (1995). Role of the deletion polymorphism of the angiotensin converting enzyme gene in the progression and therapeutic responsiveness of IgA nephropathy. *J. Clin. Invest.* 96:2162-2169.
11. Nakajima, M. et al. (1995). The angiotensin II type 2 (AT2) receptor antagonizes the growth effects of the AT1 receptor: Gain-of-function study using gene transfer. *Proc. Natl. Acad. Sci. USA* 92:10663-10667.
12. Ichiki, T. et al. (1995). Effects on blood pressure and exploratory behaviour of mice lacking angiotensin II type-2 receptor. *Nature* 377:748-750.
13. Rabelink, T.J. et al. (1996). Endothelin in renal pathophysiology: from experimental to therapeutic application. *Kidney Int.* 50:1827-1833.
14. Lee, L.K. et al. (1995). Endothelial cell injury initiates glomerular sclerosis in the rat remnant kidney. *J. Clin. Invest.* 96:953-964.
15. Rabb, H. et al. (1997). Leukocytes, cell adhesion molecules and ischemic acute renal failure. *Kidney Int.* 51:1463-1468.
16. Goligorsky, M.S. et al. (1993). Integrin receptors in renal tubule epithelium: new insights into the pathophysiology of acute renal failure. *Am. J. Physiol.* 264:F1.

FLUID, ELECTROLYTE, ACID–BASE, AND BLOOD PRESSURE REGULATION

10

1. INTRODUCTION TO FLUID, ELECTROLYTE, ACID–BASE, AND BLOOD PRESSURE REGULATION

The concentration of particular ions in body fluids has a major effect on the function of many cellular enzymes, and hence on cells and organ systems. Thus, these ions, also called **electrolytes**, must be closely regulated for survival. Patients whose illnesses result in major deviations of blood ionic concentration are at great risk of further complications and even death as a consequence of these abnormalities.

Regulation of acid–base balance, electrolyte concentration, fluid distribution, and blood pressure falls outside of the realm of any one organ system. Thus:

- The acid–base composition of blood is regulated primarily by the lungs (see Chap. 8) and the kidneys (see Chap. 9). The liver also plays a major role because it normally removes products such as lactic acid (e.g., generated by intense muscle activity) from the bloodstream (see Chap. 3). Likewise, since the gastrointestinal (GI) tract generates large volumes of acid and base, its dysfunction (e.g., in vomiting and diarrhea) has significant effects on acid–base, fluid, and electrolyte homeostasis.
- The concentrations of the electrolytes sodium and potassium in blood are regulated in large measure by the kidney, with help from certain hormones, which will be discussed later in this chapter. But the kidney could not play its crucial role if sodium-potassium ATPase (Na^+/U^+ ATPase) in the plasma membrane of most cells of the body were not expending massive amounts of metabolic energy to keep potassium inside and sodium outside of cells.
- Water homeostasis is partly a passive consequence of the distribution of sodium in the body, partly under the direct control of the antidiuretic hormone (ADH) and partly dependent on our response to thirst. A hypothalamic osmoreceptor plays a crucial role in that response (see Chap. 11).
- Blood pressure results from contributions by many different organs, including the heart, the vasculature, the sympathetic nervous system, the kidneys, and various hormones and their activators, made in the adrenal gland, the liver, and elsewhere.

Role of fluid, electrolyte, and blood pressure physiology in medicine

Disorders of fluid, electrolyte, and acid–base regulation illustrate the importance of circulatory system homeostasis in our lives. Even mild electrolyte and acid–base abnormalities may make patients feel "lousy." Presumably this is because various organ systems do not function as well as they should when there is even a small deviation of these parameters from the normal range. Severe electrolyte or acid–base disorders, on the other hand, can have life-threatening consequences, such as causing cardiac dysrrhythmias (see Chap. 7). Blood pressure is also closely regulated in ways that substantially overlap with the mechanisms by which fluid and electrolytes are controlled. Several mechanisms normally come into play to maintain blood pressure under conditions where it would otherwise fall excessively. Patients whose blood pressure is too low, a condition known as **hypotension**, will feel dizzy and weak, especially upon standing. A more severe fall in blood pressure can result in damage to organ systems — resulting, for example, in renal failure.

In the modern world, high blood pressure, termed **hypertension**, is a far more common problem than hypotension. Indeed, in modern, high-stress societies, it occurs in epidemic proportions, affecting up to half of the adults in suburban America. Even mild hypertension, with which patients feel perfectly fine in the short run, can ultimately have serious consequences if not corrected, as it increases the long-term likelihood of heart attacks, strokes, and kidney disease.

Why is understanding fluid, electrolyte, and blood pressure regulation important for medical practice?

- A number of common health problems, including heart, liver, kidney, and psychiatric disease, are often associated with significant fluid and electrolyte complications. Appreciation of fluid and electrolyte homeostasis can allow the clinician to anticipate and sometimes even prevent them.
- Certain disorders of acid–base and fluid and electrolyte balance are interrelated. Often, one will be difficult to resolve until the other is also recognized and corrected.
- Secondary causes of hypertension can often be cured. Some 5 to 10% of the millions of people with hypertension have a specific identifiable cause for elevated blood pressure (these cases are called *secondary* because there is some other *primary* problem). If the health care provider thinks physiologically about hypertension, these underlying causes can often be identified and corrected, thereby sparing the patient potentially lifelong antihypertensive therapy and its complications, as well as addressing the primary problem, which would eventually have caused the patient other problems as well.
- Powerful pharmacologic tools are available to manipulate blood pressure. However, these can be misused and cause harm to the patient, especially if the clinician does not have a physiological understanding of what, besides a particular number (e.g., for blood pressure), he or she is trying to achieve. Consider the following case.

Case Presentation

G.D. is a 68-year-old retired salesman who has just been admitted to the intensive care unit (ICU) after presenting to the emergency room with pulmonary edema. His systemic (peripheral) vascular resistance is high, and his cardiac output is low. These values are routinely measured in desperately ill patients by inserting a catheter into a large vein and guiding it with the flow of venous blood back to the right side of the heart. A transducer at the end of the catheter allows measurement of these and other important variables of cardiovascular function. Despite his serious medical condition, Mr. D is alert and oriented and has no chest pain or electrocardiographic changes suggesting myocardial ischemia. He is started on afterload reducing agents, vasodilators, and diuretics, all medicines that should help to optimize his cardiac output, but may also run the risk of making him hypotensive (see Chap. 7). With these orders written, the physician decides to go home for the night and signs Mr. D out to the care of the resident in charge of the ICU.

On her way out the door, Mr. D's physician hears an emergency page calling the resident to the ICU. Returning to the ICU out of curiosity (anxiety, really), she finds the resident about to start Mr. D on high-dose dopamine. It seems that it has just been noticed that Mr. D has no detectable blood pressure. The resident's reasoning is that high-dose dopamine is one way to boost the patient's blood pressure, as the effects of this catecholamine are to increase heart rate, contractility, and peripheral vasoconstriction.

Taking 30 s to reassess Mr. D, the physician points out that he is actually still perfusing his brain, heart, kidneys, and extremities adequately (how did she assess these?), and therefore the lack of a blood pressure reading is somewhat inconsistent with his clinical picture.

Instead of high-dose dopamine, she suggests a somewhat more conservative approach: (1) putting further afterload reducing, vasodilator, and diuretic therapy on hold, while (2) monitoring the patient closely in the Trendelenberg position (lying flat with the head of the bed lowered slightly below the feet) and (3) checking the equipment to make sure the blood pressure readings are accurate. Finally, a small amount of normal saline might be given, on the possibility that an excessive degree of diuretic therapy is responsible for the patient's hypotension.

Sure enough, while low (60/40), the patient's blood pressure is detectable manually. Over the next hour, the blood pressure gradually improves with the various instituted measures, and a faulty microprocessor in the high-tech intraarterial blood pressure monitor is identified and replaced. Soon Mr. D's blood pressure has improved to 90/60 sitting up, and the various medicines are restarted at a lower dose without incident.

Suppose the initial physician had not been present to dissuade the covering resident, and the high-dose dopamine infusion had been initiated. To what untoward events might the patient have been unnecessarily subjected? By what mechanisms?

2. THE DETERMINANTS OF ELECTROLYTE AND ACID–BASE BALANCE

Fluid and electrolyte homeostasis

The body consists of the space within cells (*intracellular space*) and the space outside of cells (*extracellular space*). The extracellular space can be further divided into the space within blood vessels (*intravascular space*) and the *extravascular extracellular space* (see Figure 10.1). Electrolytes and water are in a dynamic equilibrium between these different compartments.

The distribution of water between intracellular and extracellular compartments is determined largely by the distribution of *osmotically active particles* across the plasma membrane. Sodium (Na^+), chloride (Cl^-), potassium (K^+), and bicarbonate (HCO_3^-) are the major ions in the body. Because of the high levels of sodium-potassium ATPase (Na^+/K^+-ATPase) in the plasma membrane of all mammalian cells, most of the Na^+ in the body is located outside of cells, while K^+ is largely sequestered inside of cells. In large measure, Cl^- follows the flow of **cations** to maintain **electroneutrality** (equivalence of positive and negative charges). The kidney has various mechanisms by which it is able to retain or eliminate sodium, and with it water (see Chap. 9 and below). Largely because of the action of Na^+/K^+-ATPase and these renal mechanisms, Na^+, the major extracellular cation, is also the major determinant of extracellular volume (see Figure 10.2).

The electrolyte concentrations in the blood represent a steady-state balance of several processes involving water and electrolytes (see Table 10.1):

- Input into the GI tract (i.e., from food and drink).
- Absorption from the GI tract (of ingested and secreted substances).
- Distribution across the plasma membrane of proteins and other charged or osmotically active substances.
- Activity of various transporters, pumps, and channels, some of which maintain highly asymmetric distributions of particular electrolytes across the plasma membrane (e.g., Na^+/K^+-ATPase).
- Intracellular signaling via pathways that use particular electrolytes (e.g., calcium) as a second messenger. Most of the calcium in the cell is tightly bound to proteins, with the physiologically active ionized free calcium

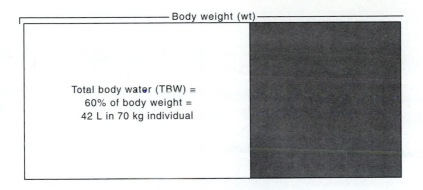

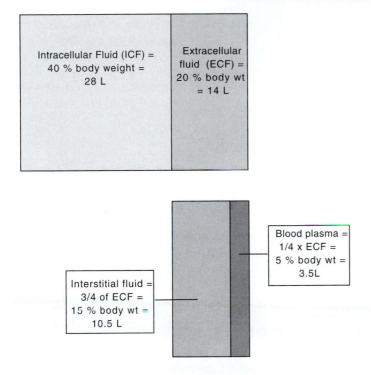

FIGURE 10.1. Fluid compartments of the body. The body weight of a hypothetical 70-kg individual is represented by the entire top rectangle, with total body water (TBW) shown as a white box (left) and total body solids as a dark gray box (right). The middle rectangle resolves TBW into intracellular fluid (ICF, light gray box on left) and extracellular fluid (ECF, darker gray box on the right). The lowest rectangle resolves ECF into interstitial fluid (lighter gray box on left) and intravascular volume (blood plasma, darker gray box on right). For each box representing a different fluid compartment, the percentage of body weight and the approximate volume in liters in a 70-kg individual are indicated. (Adapted with permission, from Ganong WF (1999). Review of Medical Physiology, 19th ed. Stamford, CT, Appleton & Lange, p. 2.)

concentration tightly regulated and subject to transient local fluctuations that effect signal transduction.

• Elimination or reclamation of salts and water by the kidneys.
• Elimination of fluid and electrolytes in stool.
• Loss via evaporation of water and salt from skin (as sweat) and mucous membranes.

The kidneys are able to exert a large degree of control over extracellular volume simply by controlling the level of filtered sodium in the renal tubular fluid. When sodium is reclaimed from the renal tubule, extracellular fluid volume increases, as water follows the osmotically active sodium ions. When sodium, and with it water, stays in the renal

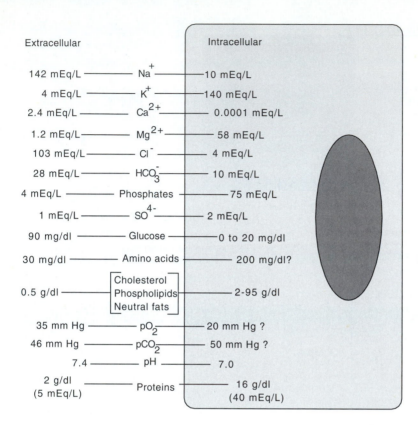

Extracellular		Intracellular
142 mEq/L	Na$^+$	10 mEq/L
4 mEq/L	K$^+$	140 mEq/L
2.4 mEq/L	Ca^{2+}	0.0001 mEq/L
1.2 mEq/L	Mg^{2+}	58 mEq/L
103 mEq/L	Cl$^-$	4 mEq/L
28 mEq/L	HCO$_3^-$	10 mEq/L
4 mEq/L	Phosphates	75 mEq/L
1 mEq/L	SO^{4-}	2 mEq/L
90 mg/dl	Glucose	0 to 20 mg/dl
30 mg/dl	Amino acids	200 mg/dl?
0.5 g/dl	Cholesterol Phospholipids Neutral fats	2-95 g/dl
35 mm Hg	pO$_2$	20 mm Hg ?
46 mm Hg	pCO$_2$	50 mm Hg ?
7.4	pH	7.0
2 g/dl (5 mEq/L)	Proteins	16 g/dl (40 mEq/L)

FIGURE 10.2. Concentrations of various ions and electrolytes in the body. The major differences between intracellular and extracellular fluid compartment concentrations of various ions and solutes is indicated. (Adapted with permission from Guyton AC, Hall JE, Human Physiology and Mechanisms of Disease, 6th ed. Philadelphia, PA, Saunders, p. 35.)

filtrate, it leaves the kidney as urine, and extracellular fluid volume decreases. This simple relationship between sodium excretion and extracellular volume depends on Na$^+$/K$^+$-ATPase, as mentioned earlier.

Clinical Pearls

○ The kidney's ability to reclaim sodium from tubular fluid can be very efficient, but it is not perfect. If a patient drinks really *huge* amounts of water (e.g., 20 L/day for a number of days), as sometimes occurs in patients with certain psychiatric disorders or those with diabetes insipidus (see Chap. 11), he or she can eventually lose enough sodium in maximally dilute urine to cause a fall in serum sodium.

Furthermore, such a large amount of water ingestion, absorption, and excretion may result in sufficiently large urine flow to at least partially wash out the interstitial urea gradient in the renal medulla, which is necessary for renal concentrating mechanisms. Until this urea gradient is reestablished, the patient will have a defect in the ability to concentrate urine (see Chap. 9).

○ A more common cause of low serum sodium (called *hyponatremia*) occurs when other osmotically active substances are elevated in the bloodstream. Consider the example of elevated blood glucose, as occurs in a patient with uncontrolled diabetes mellitus. The high blood glucose will result in water moving out of cells, diluting the sodium and hence making it appear low, when the reality is that the amount of water outside of cells is high.

TABLE 10.1 WATER GAIN AND LOSS

Normal Routes of Water Gain and Loss in Adults at Room Temperature (23°C)

Route	mL/day
Water intake	
Fluid[a]	1200
In food	1000
Metabolically produced from food	300
TOTAL	2500
Water output	
Insensible	700
Sweat	100
Feces	200
Urine	1500
TOTAL	2500

[a]Fluid intake varies widely for both social and cultural reasons.

Effect of Environmental Temperature and Exercise on Water Loss and Intake in Adults (in mL/day)

	Normal temperature	Hot weather
Water loss		
Insensible loss:		
Skin	350	350
Lungs	350	250
Sweat	100	1400
Feces	200	200
Urine	1500	1200
Total loss	2500	3400
Water intake to maintain water balance	2500	3400

In hot weather and during prolonged heavy exercise, water balance maintained only if the individual increases water intake to match increased loss of water in sweat. Decreased water excretion by kidneys alone is insufficient to maintain water balance.

From Stanton BA and Koeppen BM, The Kidney, in Berne MN and Levy, MN, eds. (1998). *Physiology.* 4th ed. St. Louis, MO, Mosby, p. 718.

The resulting expansion of intravascular volume will increase glomerular filtration rate and with it, filtration of glucose into the tubular fluid. Above the average maximum rate at which renal transporters can reclaim glucose from tubular fluid, it will be lost in the urine. This starts to occur at a blood glucose of about 200 mg/dL. The excess glucose that is lost in the urine takes water with it. This loss of water with a filtered osmotically active substance (such as glucose) is termed an **osmotic diuresis**. As the body becomes depleted of water (lost in the urine), the hypothalamus senses hypovolemia and secretes ADH in an attempt to maintain intravascular volume by retaining water, even at the expense of decreased serum osmolality, thus providing another mechanism for hyponatremia in this condition.

Fluid compartments and volume of distribution within the body

While the activity of Na^+/K^+-ATPase is normally responsible for the equilibrium distribution of water between the intracellular and extracellular compartments, it does *not* determine the distribution of extracellular water between intravascular and extravascular compartments.

Instead, the distribution between intravascular and extravascular extracellular fluid is determined by the fact that the proteins in plasma are substantially impeded from leaving most blood vessels. This is in contrast to the unusual situation observed in the liver, where the capillaries (termed sinusoids) have fenestrations and no basement membrane, and hence plasma proteins are freely in contact with hepatocytes (see Chap. 4).

Since plasma proteins are osmotically active, they hold water with them in the intravascular space. This tendency of plasma proteins to hold water in the intravascular space is called **oncotic pressure**. The oncotic pressure resulting from plasma proteins is offset by the force of intravascular fluid against the vessel wall, called **hydrostatic pressure**, which drives water out of the vessel and into the spaces between cells.

The balance between these two forces is different in different parts of the body and under different physiological and pathophysiological states. One of the roles of lymphatic drainage is to return to the intravascular volume the fluid (water, electrolytes, and plasma proteins) that extravasated out of the vessel as a result of the (usually small) net imbalance between oncotic and hydrostatic pressures in tissue capillaries. Edema develops only when the net flow occurring as a result of the difference between oncotic and hydrostatic pressure is greater than the capacity of the lymphatic vessels to return extravasated fluid to the intravascular space. These so-called **Starling forces** are discussed more extensively in Chapter 7.

Clinical Pearls

○ In portal hypertension (see Chap. 4), an increase in hydrostatic pressure, perhaps combined with decreased oncotic pressure due to less albumin being made by a cirrhotic liver, results in extravasation of fluid into the peritoneal space, the phenomenon termed ascites.

○ In the protein-calorie malnutrition disease termed kwashiorkor, inadequate dietary protein impairs the liver's ability to synthesize albumin, the major determinant of plasma oncotic pressure. As a result, starving children develop an imbalance in hydrostatic and oncotic pressures of the portal vein solely as a result of inadequate oncotic pressure. Since the determinant of intravascular volume is the balance of oncotic and hydrostatic pressures, this condition results in ascites formation without portal hypertension and the appearance of bloated bellies on emaciated bodies.

○ Prolonged standing results in the veins of the legs becoming engorged with blood (varicose veins). This increases the hydrostatic pressure and can force enough water out of the vessels and into the extravascular extracellular space to cause swelling of the feet, termed pedal edema. Staying off one's feet and elevating them (e.g., on a pillow in bed at night) is one way to get the excess fluid to flow out of the tissues of the feet so that it can be reabsorbed from the extracellular extravascular space into the circulation. Once it is back in the blood vessels of the circulation, the excess fluid can be eliminated through the kidneys. The kidneys can act either on their own or with the assistance of a diuretic, a drug that impairs the renal tubule's ability to reclaim water or salt (and with it, water), promoting loss of fluid in the urine and thereby contributing eventually to the resolution of edema.

Determinants of acid–base balance

The hydrogen ion (H^+) concentration in a solution is a measure of its *acidity* and is usually expressed in terms of pH, the negative log of the H^+ concentration, which is an inverse relationship. The normal pH of blood is approximately 7.4, which is an H^+ concentration of 40 nM (0.0000004 mole/L).

Conditions in which the blood H^+ concentration exceeds this value are termed **acidosis** and refer to a *lower* than normal pH. Conditions in which the blood H^+ ion concentration falls below this level are termed **alkalosis** and refer to a *higher* than normal pH. Acids can also be categorized by their *strength.* A strong acid (AH) is one that dissociates more completely into H^+ and the corresponding anion A^-. The range of H^+ concentration that is compatible with life ranges from a low of 16 nM to a high of 160 nM, a pH range of 7.8 to 6.8.

Hydrogen ions (H^+) are constantly being generated by metabolic reactions in tissues.

Nevertheless, the normal blood H^+ concentration is approximately a millionfold lower than the concentration of ions such as Na^+. It is extremely important for the proper functioning of the body that hydrogen ions not build up to high concentrations. This is because the H^+ ion is smaller and more reactive than most other electrolytes. If the H^+ ion were present at high concentrations, its high-affinity binding to negative charges on proteins would disrupt protein folding and consequently protein function. Proteins whose folding has been altered sufficiently to make them nonfunctional are said to be **denatured**. This is why many cellular enzymes, and therefore organ systems, will not function well at a substantial deviation from normal pH.

Beyond that general statement as to why deviations from normal pH are harmful, certain sorts of organ system dysfunction are particularly prominent in individuals who develop acidosis or alkalosis (see Table 10.2). Which of these complications occurs first or most prominently in any given individual patient will be a consequence of genetic differences and differences in the extent of underlying disease that make one organ system or another more sensitive to disordered acid–base homeostasis (see Ref. 1).

Buffers

While the lungs and kidneys are remarkably efficient acid–base regulators, they do not work instantaneously, and the body simply can't afford to have H^+ ions floating around by themselves for even the few minutes that it might take for elimination by respiration or renal excretion. Buffers allow the body to tolerate a small excess or deficiency of acid while homeostatic corrective measures are in progress, without significant alteration in cellular or blood pH.

Buffers are substances that can dissociate into an anion and a hydrogen ion, which tends to maintain pH in a particular range (which

TABLE 10.2 ADVERSE CONSEQUENCES OF SEVERE ACID–BASE DISTURBANCES

Major Adverse Consequences of Severe Alkalemia

Cardiovascular
  Arteriolar constriction
  Reduction in coronary blood flow
  Reduction in anginal threshold
  Predisposition to refractory supraventricular and ventricular arrhythmias

Respiratory
  Hypoventilation with attendant hypercapnia and hypoxemia

Metabolic
  Stimulation of anaerobic glycolysis and organic acid production
  Hypokalemia
  Decreased plasma ionized calcium concentration
  Hypomagnesemia and hypophosphatemia

Cerebral
  Reduction in cerebral blood flow
  Tetany, seizures, lethargy, delirium, and stupor

Major Adverse Consequences of Severe Acidemia

Cardiovascular
  Impairment of cardiac contractility
  Arteriolar dilatation, venoconstriction, and centralization of blood volume
  Increased pulmonary vascular resistance
  Reductions in cardiac output, arterial blood pressure, and hepatic and renal blood flow
  Sensitization to reentrant arrhythmias and reduction in threshold of ventricular fibrillation
  Attenuation of cardiovascular responsiveness to catecholamines

Respiratory
  Hyperventilation
  Decreased strength of respiratory muscles and promotion of muscle fatigue
  Dyspnea

Metabolic
  Increased metabolic demands
  Insulin resistance
  Inhibition of anaerobic glycolysis
  Reduction in ATP synthesis
  Hyperkalemia
  Increased protein degradation

Cerebral
  Inhibition of metabolism and cell-volume regulation
  Obtundation and coma

Reproduced, with permission, from Adrogue HJ and Madias NE (1998). Management of Life-Threatening Acid-Base Disorders. *New Eng. J. Med.* 338:26–34 (part 1) and 107–111 (part 2).

varies from buffer to buffer). The particular concentration of H$^+$ ions at which a particular buffer has the greatest buffering capacity is termed its pK. This is simply the pH at which the concentration of dissociated buffer molecules is equal to the concentration of the undissociated buffer molecules. Putting this in mathematical terms, where [A$^-$] represents the concentrations of dissociated buffer and [HA] the concentration of undissociated buffer,

$$HA \leftrightharpoons [H^+] + [A^-] \qquad (1)$$

The pK is the point where half of the buffer has dissociated and half has not, that is, where

$$[A^-]/[HA] = 1 \qquad (2)$$

Buffers maintain homeostasis by preventing changes in H$^+$ concentration that would affect the function of enzymes and hence of cells. Consider a buffer solution at its pK. Addition of an H$^+$ ion to the solution [i.e., to the right-hand side of Eq. (1)] will, by the law of mass action (see Chap. 2), shift the equilibrium slightly in the direction of the undissociated form [left-hand side of Eq. (1)]. But formation of a molecule of undissociated buffer can occur only if a free hydrogen ion is removed from the solution, which would exactly offset the increase in the H$^+$ ion concentration caused by adding an H$^+$ ion to the solution in the first place. Thus, the presence of the buffer will have prevented an increase in the total number of free H$^+$ ions, despite the fact that a free H$^+$ ion was just added to the solution.

Conversely, adding a molecule of an alkali or base uses up a molecule of H$^+$. But again, the law of mass action will result in a molecule of undissociated buffer separating into the anion and the H$^+$ molecule, replacing the molecule of H$^+$ lost upon addition of the base. In order to affect the pH of a buffer solution in a major way, a relatively large amount of acid or base must be added. The buffer is then said to be consumed, and the further the pH is moved away from the pK, the less effective the buffer is at accommodating or generating H$^+$ ions and the greater the change in pH.

The Henderson-Hassellbach equation [Eq. (3)] converts this concept of buffering into a mathematical equation and explains how the pH system for measuring hydrogen ions is actually derived:

$$pH = pK + \log([A^-]/[AH]) \qquad (3)$$

Negatively charged (anionic) proteins within cells can take up excess protons so as to keep the free H$^+$ concentration at or close to its normal value. Since the protein concentration within cells is extremely high, these are the major intracellular buffers.

The major extracellular buffer is normally HCO$_3^-$. Since its concentration is not terribly high (approximately 24 mM), and its pKa is substantially lower than normal blood pH, you might not expect HCO$_3^-$ to be a terribly effective or important body buffer. However, the fact that it is in equilibrium with CO$_2$, which is rapidly eliminated via the lungs, makes HCO$_3^-$ extremely effective and important as an extracellular buffer [see Eq. (4)].

$$CO_2 + H_2O \leftrightharpoons H_2CO_3 \leftrightharpoons H^+ + HCO_3^- \qquad (4)$$
$$\text{(carbonic acid)} \qquad \text{(bicarbonate ion)}$$

The enzyme carbonic anhydrase, which is particularly active in the lung and kidney, serves to catalyze this reaction, thereby facilitating interconversion between gaseous CO$_2$ and soluble HCO$_3^-$, depending on which concentration is higher (i.e., following the law of mass action).

Given the dominant role of P$_{CO_2}$ and HCO$_3^-$ in determining blood pH, it is sometimes useful to note that

$$H^+ = 24 \times P_{CO_2}/[HCO_3^-] \qquad (5)$$

or

$$pH = 6.10 + \log[HCO_3^-]/0.03 P_{CO_2} \quad (6)$$

where 6.10 is the negative log of the pK of Eq. 4 and 0.03 is the percent solubility of P_{CO_2} in plasma.

Should the major intracellular and extracellular buffering capacity of the body be used up, calcium phosphate salts are released from bone, generating phosphate that serves to buffer additional H^+ ions — but at the cost of bone loss.

Defense of blood pH

To safeguard against the potentially damaging effects of H^+ ions, the body has three lines of defense:

- The immediate, essentially instantaneous defenses are the intracellular and extracellular **buffers**.
- A second line of defense operating on a time scale of minutes is the lungs. As was discussed in Chapter 8, the lungs efficiently eliminate carbon dioxide (CO_2) from the body. Since most CO_2 is a dissolved gas in equilibrium with carbonic acid [see Eq. (4)], elimination of CO_2 is a very effective means of ridding the body of acid.

  The body generates about 20 mol of H^+ daily, most of which is eliminated in this manner by the lungs. Carbonic acid is termed a **volatile acid** because of the relationship described in Equation (4), by which acid can be excreted as carbon dioxide and water. The respiratory control centers in the medulla respond to either a fall in pH or a rise in P_{CO_2} [which, from Eq. (4), are in equilibrium] by stimulating ventilation, and eliminating more CO_2, with water eliminated by the kidneys.
- A third line of defense, operating on a time scale of hours to days, is provided by the kidneys. The kidneys have the capacity to absorb bicarbonate throughout the renal tubule (see Figure 10.3A). The magnitude of bicarbonate reabsorption or loss from the kidney is controlled to maintain acid–base homeostasis by several processes.

Besides absorbing or eliminating bicarbonate as a means of regulating the pH of the blood, the kidney can form "new" bicarbonate by eliminating ammonium ions (NH_4^+) formed by breakdown of glutamine to glutamate (see Figure 10.3B). Excretion of (NH_4^+) is another means of eliminating acid. From Equation (4), we see that eliminating acid is the same as retaining bicarbonate ions (HCO_3^-) that would otherwise be lost in the renal tubular fluid.

In addition, the kidneys are the only way of removing from the body nonvolatile so-called **fixed acids**, those ions that cannot be removed by the lungs. The lungs are not able to remove fixed acids because, unlike CO_2, these ions exist largely as liquids under conditions of standard pressure and temperature. Examples of fixed acids include phosphoric acid and sulfuric acid, generated by protein metabolism. Normally, about one-third of the acid eliminated by the kidneys is fixed acid and two-thirds is due to excretion of NH_4^+. The kidneys actually excrete the fixed acids themselves as salts and eliminate the hydrogen ions generated from those fixed acids in the form of various urinary buffers whose pKs are in the range of hydrogen ion concentration achievable in the kidney (pH no lower than about 4). The renal mechanisms involved in using urinary buffers such as HPO_4^{-2} to excrete the hydrogen ions generated from fixed acids are described in Figure 10.3C.

Clinical Pearls

○ The diet is a major determinant of daily acid load. Generally, a diet high in protein and nucleic acids is a greater source of

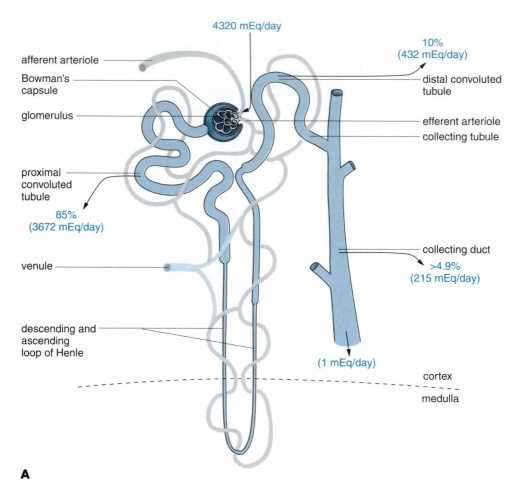

A

FIGURE 10.3. Renal mechanisms of acid–base balance. *A.* Resorption of bicarbonate in the different segments of the renal tubule. The percentages of the total filtered load of bicarbonate reabsorbed and the total number of miliequivalents are shown. Absorption in the proximal tubule is dependent on a Na^+/H^+ transporter. Thus, factors that affect sodium balance will affect bicarbonate absorption. In volume-expanded states where Na reabsorption is diminished, so will be the capacity to resorb HCO_3^-. In volume-contracted states where Na is actively being reclaimed, so will be HCO_3^-.

fixed acid because it is rich in sulfur- and phosphate-containing substances that cannot be eliminated by respiration and therefore require involvement of the kidneys.

Conversely, a fruit- and vegetable-rich diet can be thought of as high in alkali because it contains relatively little sulfur and phosphate. Instead, almost all of the acid generated by a vegetarian diet is carbonic acid. In the blood, this is carried as H_2CO_3. Through the action of carbonic anhydrase, this dissociates into H_2O and CO_2, with the CO_2 being eliminated by the

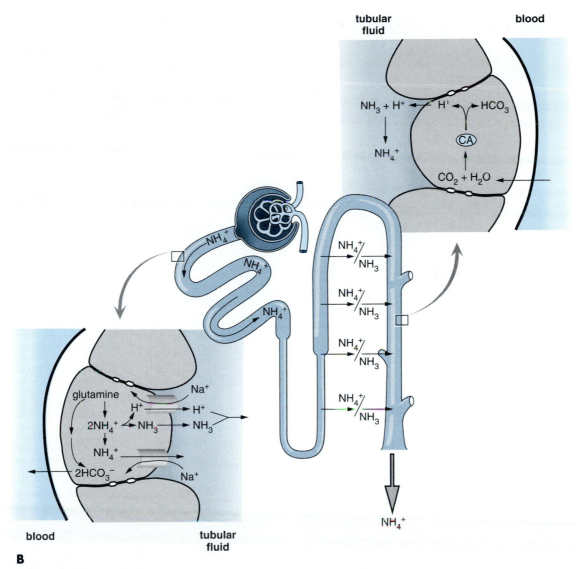

B

FIGURE 10.3 — (*continued*) *B.* Ammonium ion production, transport, and excretion by the kidney. Glutamine is metabolized in the kidney to NH_4^+ and HCO_3^-. The NH_4^+ is secreted into the lumen, and the HCO_3^- enters the bloodstream. The secreted NH_4^+ is reabsorbed in the loop of Henle and accumulates in the medullary interstitium in the form of both NH_3 and NH_4^+. The NH_3 diffuses back into the tubular fluid and reaches the collecting duct, where H^+ secretion forms NH_4^+, which is trapped and eliminated in the urine. For every molecule of NH_4^+ so excreted, a molecule of HCO_3^- is returned to the systemic circulation. NH_4^+ in the urine is thus a marker of proximal tubule glutamine metabolism, which in turn determines new HCO_3^- formation.

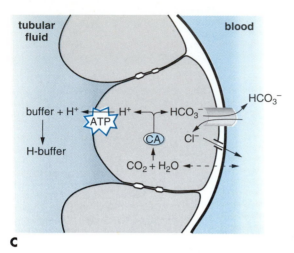

c

FIGURE 10.3 — (continued) C. Excretion of fixed acids by the kidney. Urinary buffers such as HPO_4^{-2}, with a pK in the range of acidity achievable in the kidney, are used to eliminate fixed or titratable acid in the urine. Shown are cells of the proximal renal tubule. CA = carbonic anhydrase; ATP = adenosine triphosphate.

lungs, leaving only water, which can be easily eliminated by the kidneys or other organs [see Eq. (4)].

○ The effectiveness of bicarbonate as a buffer is dependent on (1) carbohydrate and fat metabolism proceeding to completion (i.e., generation of CO_2) and (2) adequacy of ventilation. Under conditions of starvation (ketosis), uncontrolled diabetes mellitus (ketoacidosis), or hypoperfusion (lactic acidosis), incompletely metabolized, nonvolatile intermediates accumulate (ketones and lactate, respectively, instead of carbonic acid). If the metabolic abnormality is resolved (e.g., correction of insulin deficiency in ketoacidosis or hypoperfusion in lactic acidosis), ketones and lactate can be quickly metabolized to bicarbonate, allowing rapid respiratory correction of blood pH by elimination of volatile CO_2. If the metabolic abnormality is not resolved, ketones and lactate act as if

they were fixed acids, and blood pH can drop dangerously.

○ Fixed acids accumulate in renal failure. Without dialysis (mechanical filtration of blood), an individual who has lost all kidney function is unable to survive because accumulation of fixed acids consumes the buffering capacity of the body, resulting in organ failure (e.g., cardiac arrhythmias, etc.) and death.

Generally, an imbalance in acid generation or elimination that is due to inadequacy of either the lungs or the kidneys is compensated by a nearly equal and opposite change in the other organ.

○ For example, diarrhea with loss of bicarbonate-containing fluids will cause a metabolic acidosis, which will automatically trigger development of respiratory alkalosis and hyperventilation to eliminate enough CO_2 gas via the lungs to nearly compensate for the bicarbonate loss in the stool. This respiratory compensation is an integral part of the body's response to the primary disturbance. If the respiratory compensation is not sufficient, renal bicarbonate conservation will also come into place over the next period of hours to come very close to completing the correction.

○ Conversely, vomiting, with loss of stomach hydrochloric acid, results in a metabolic alkalosis, for which hypoventilation and a rising blood CO_2 is corrective.

○ A patient with deteriorating respiratory function (e.g., due to severe air trapping in asthma or chronic obstructive lung disease) will manifest a respiratory acidosis (with a rising blood CO_2). To conserve body buffers, the kidney will respond by eliminating acid, causing a metabolic alkalosis to partially correct for the rising blood CO_2.

Review Questions

1. What are the fluid compartments of the body?
2. What determines the distribution of sodium and water between the intracellular and extracellular spaces?
3. What determines the distribution of sodium and water between the intravascular and extravascular spaces within the extracellular compartment?
4. What is an acid? a base? a buffer?
5. What is the pK of a buffer?
6. What is the effect of a buffer on the pH of a solution in which that buffer is dissolved, upon addition of acid? of base?
7. Why is acid generated by metabolism?
8. What is the difference between volatile and fixed acids?
9. What is normal blood pH?
10. How does the body handle acids generated during the course of metabolism?

3. THE DETERMINANTS OF BLOOD PRESSURE

The term *blood pressure* has two different meanings for physiological medicine. First, there is what we would *like* to measure, namely, the effectiveness with which organs are perfused with oxygenated blood, following which the blood is returned to the heart and lungs, where oxygen is replenished and CO_2 eliminated. Then there is what we are able to easily measure, which is the pressure at which blood courses through the brachial artery, the largest artery in the arm. Usually this measured blood pressure is an accurate reflection of perfusion pressure — but sometimes it is not, as, for example, in the initial case presentation.

Three physical features of the circulatory system that are crucial to both meanings of blood pressure are:

- **Adequate blood volume**, normally about 5 L, to allow various parameters (discussed later in this section) to regulate blood pressure. Adequacy of blood volume is monitored by various baroreceptors on both the venous and arterial sides of the circulation (see Chap. 7). These baroreceptors respond by either sending signals to the brain to alter sympathetic nervous system activity or affecting the release of hormones directly.
- **Adequate cardiac structure and function** (see Chap. 7), allowing the heart to pump sufficient blood to generate blood pressure. This requires appropriate cardiac chamber volume, relaxation for diastolic filling, contraction during systole, and competent cardiac valves, so that a substantial volume of blood is not lost backward during systolic ejection.
- **Adequate compliance of blood vessels**, allowing them to be distended, which transmits pressures generated by the heart down through the entire arterial tree (see Chap. 7).

Assuming that these three physical requirements are met (see Figure 10.4), the actual blood pressure achieved is determined by three physiological parameters over which hormones and nerves have control:

- **Cardiac output** (heart rate × stroke volume)
- **Peripheral resistance** (vascular smooth muscle tone)
- **Sodium and water balance** (as regulated by the kidney)

Because these three variables are interconnected, the body rapidly compensates for a change in one by alteration of the other two, thereby minimizing perturbation of blood

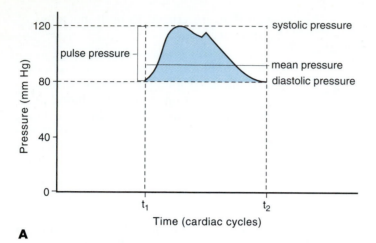

A

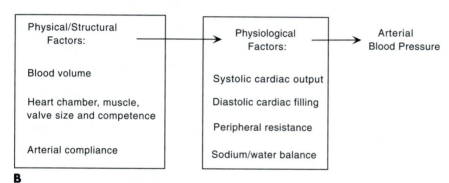

B

FIGURE 10.4. Physical and physiological determinants of blood pressure. *A*. Arterial systolic, distolic, pulse, and mean pressures. The mean arterial pressure represents the area under the arterial pressure curve (shaded) divided by the cardiac cycle duration $(t_2 - t_1)$. *B*. The primary physical/structural prerequisites and physiological parameters that determine arterial pressure. Clinically significant hypotension can generally be categorized as resulting from disorder of one of these parameters. In contrast, the pathophysiology of hypertension is far less well understood. *(A and B. Adapted, with permission, from Berne RM, Levy MN (1998). Physiology, 4th ed. St. Louis, MO, Mosby, p. 420.)*

pressure and tissue perfusion. This homeostatic response involves

1. Sensing the change in effective circulating volume through strategically located volume receptors
2. Responding to offset the change through effectors including hormones and nerves

Thus,

- A change in cardiac output results in reflex changes in both vascular tone and water and sodium excretion.
- A change in vascular tone results in both cardiac and renal compensation.
- A change in renal function results in in-

creased or decreased intravascular volume, with reflex changes in cardiovascular functions (e.g., heart rate and peripheral vasoconstriction).

Several classical hormone systems, and some newly appreciated ones, are involved in the control of the physiological parameters of blood pressure.

- The **catecholamines** contribute to control of blood pressure by directly affecting vascular smooth muscle tone, increasing cardiac output, or both.
- The **renin-angiotensin-aldosterone** system generates products that have direct vasoconstrictive effects on vascular smooth muscle (**angiotensin II**) and that affect renal function (**aldosterone**) to cause changes in fluid and electrolyte balance. Members of this family are believed to function in both endocrine and paracrine modes of action.
- **Antidiuretic hormone** (ADH), also known as **vasopressin**, is both an activator of water channels in the distal renal tubule and, at higher concentration, a powerful direct vasoconstrictor of vascular smooth muscle.
- **Atrial natriuretic peptide** (ANP) affects renal sodium transport and thereby affects intravascular volume.
- The **endothelins** are a set of powerful but poorly understood peptides made in many different places in the body that have paracrine effects on vascular smooth muscle, renal function, and cardiac function. Many of their actions are mediated by **nitric oxide**.
- **Prostaglandins** are a class of lipid-derived local mediators that serve as signaling molecules in a number of organs, including the kidney and various vascular beds. Some prostaglandins are believed to mediate vasoconstriction, while others may mediate vasodilation.
- **Kallikrein** is a protease secreted by the kidney that cleaves the circulating protein precursor **kininogen** to generate the locally va-

sodilating peptide **bradykinin**. Bradykinin, in turn, may work by generating nitric oxide and/or prostaglandins in various cells of the kidney.

- The **sympathetic nervous system** serves to integrate the function of various different components of blood pressure regulation through direct effects on the heart, blood vessels, and kidney.

Clinical Pearls

○ Blood pressure is measured in the brachial artery by inflating a cuff on the upper arm to approximately 250 mmHg (i.e., above the patient's blood pressure). The cuff is then released and the examiner listens for the point at which the turbulent flow of blood rushing into the brachial artery is first heard. This is the **systolic pressure**. As the pressure in the cuff continues to go down, a point is reached where there is no longer a gradient for turbulent flow at any point in the cardiac cycle, and hence no sound is heard. This point is known as the **diastolic pressure**.

○ Even though we do not know the cause of hypertension in most cases, we know that we can affect blood pressure with drugs that modify one or more of the factors indicated previously. Thus, when a patient's blood pressure is too low, it can be raised by drugs that increase cardiac output or vascular tone (e.g., norepinephrine). Conversely, blood pressure can be lowered by drugs affecting the heart (e.g., β-adrenergic blockers such as metoprolol), kidney (e.g., diuretics such as furosemide), or blood vessels (e.g., angiotensin converting enzyme inhibitors like benazepril or α-adrenergic blockers such as prazosin).

○ Besides the risk of catastrophic events such as a heart attack or a stroke, untreated hypertension takes a terrible toll in terms of slowly progressing injury to the brain (lacunar infarcts) and the kidneys (hypertensive nephropathy resulting in chronic renal failure).

Review Questions

11. What are the determinants of blood pressure?
12. How are heart rate and contractility controlled?
13. How does the kidney contribute to maintenance of correct intravascular volume?
14. What are the major hormones controlling blood pressure?

4. THE RENIN-ANGIOTENSIN SYSTEM

Renin is a protease secreted by the **juxtaglomerular cells** of the *renal afferent arteriole*

(see Figure 10.5) in response to several different stimuli (see Table 10.3).

Either a decrease in renal perfusion, as measured by renal baroreceptors, or a decrease in tubular sodium concentration, detected by the macula densa of the distal renal tubule (adjacent to the juxtaglomerular cells), triggers renin release. Renin increases blood pressure by initiating a cascade of proteolysis, ultimately generating the potent vasoconstrictor angiotensin II (see Figure 10.6).

Angiotensin II causes:

- Vascular smooth muscle constriction
- Stimulation of aldosterone secretion
- A direct effect on proximal tubule sodium reabsorption
- Thirst through an action on the hypothalamus centrally

Additional regulators of renin secretion are the catecholamines, both in the circulation and via the renal sympathetic innervation (see Sec. 7).

FIGURE 10.5. Juxtaglomerular apparatus and the anatomy of renin release. Diagram of a glomerulus indicating the afferent and efferent arterioles, the macula densa, and juxtaglomerular apparatus, where the distal tubule comes close to these structures.

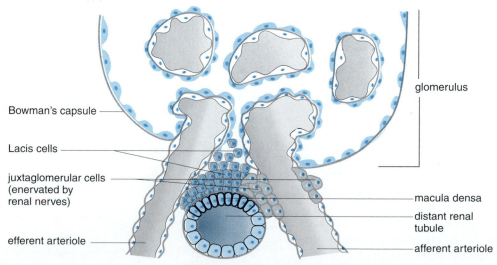

Bowman's capsule

Lacis cells

juxtaglomerular cells (enervated by renal nerves)

efferent arteriole

glomerulus

macula densa

distant renal tubule

afferent arteriole

TABLE 10.3   REGULATORS OF RENIN RELEASE

Factors That Affect Renin Secretion

Stimulatory
  Increased sympathetic activity via renal nerves
  Increased circulating catecholamines
  Prostaglandins

Inhibitory
  Increased Na^+ and Cl^- reabsorption across macula densa
  Increased afferent arteriolar pressure
  Angiotensin II
  Vasopressin

Conditions That Increase Renin Secretion

Sodium depletion
Diuretics
Hypotension
Hemorrhage
Upright posture
Dehydration
Cardiac failure
Cirrhosis
Constriction of renal artery or aorta
Various psychologic stimuli

Reproduced, with permission, from Ganong WF (1997). *Review of Medical Physiology.* 18th ed. Stamford, CT, Appleton & Lange, p. 429.

Generation of angiotensin II

Renin cleaves angiotensinogen (a protein containing over 400 amino acid residues that is synthesized in, and secreted from, the liver) to generate the 10-amino-acid-residue peptide **angiotensin I**.

Angiotensin I is further cleaved by a protease in the vascular endothelium called **converting enzyme** to generate the 8-amino-acid-residue peptide **angiotensin II**, which is a direct vasoconstrictor and a major stimulant of the secretion of **aldosterone**, the major mineralocorticoid involved in sodium reabsorption and thus extracellular fluid expansion (see Figure 10.7). Angiotensin II is also a feedback inhibitor of renin secretion, thereby closing a negative feedback loop of blood pressure regulation.

Inhibitors of converting-enzyme such as captopril are currently some of the most efficacious drugs for control of blood pressure. Part of the efficacy of converting-enzyme inhibitors may be due to the fact that in addition to cleaving angiotensin I to angiotensin II, converting enzyme is also responsible for degradation of bradykinin, an important renal vasodilator. Thus, converting-enzyme inhibitors not only inhibit angiotensin II action, they also *potentiate* bradykinin action.

There are at least two different receptors for angiotensin II, and they differ in anatomic distribution, the second messenger systems by which they function, and homeostatic regulation. One, known as the AT_1 receptor, mediates the conventional vasoconstrictive and growth-promoting effects for which angiotensin is generally known. It appears that the subtype of AT_1 receptors found on arterioles is *downregulated* in the presence of high angiotensin II levels, perhaps as a fail-safe to prevent excessive vasoconstriction. The AT_1 receptor works via a G-protein to activate phospholipase C. Phosphatidyl inositol turnover triggered by AT_1 receptor activation, with the resulting formation of diacyl glycerol and release of arachidonic acid, ultimately generates prostaglandins, which may be the actual mediator of many of angiotensin II's vasoconstrictive effects. AT_1 receptors found in the adrenal cortex are regulated quite differently. These angiotensin II receptors are *upregulated* by high angiotensin II levels, making the adrenal cortex *more* sensitive to the effect of angiotensin II as a stimulus of aldosterone secretion under conditions in which angiotensin II levels are high.

The AT_2 receptor is found in the brain and elsewhere; it seems to be more prevalent in embryonic and neonatal life, but it is also present in the adult. At least some of its actions seem to promote apoptosis. To this extent, it seems to mediate the opposite of the growth-promoting effects of AT_1 receptors. Thus an important frontier of angiotensin II research is exploration of the possibility that

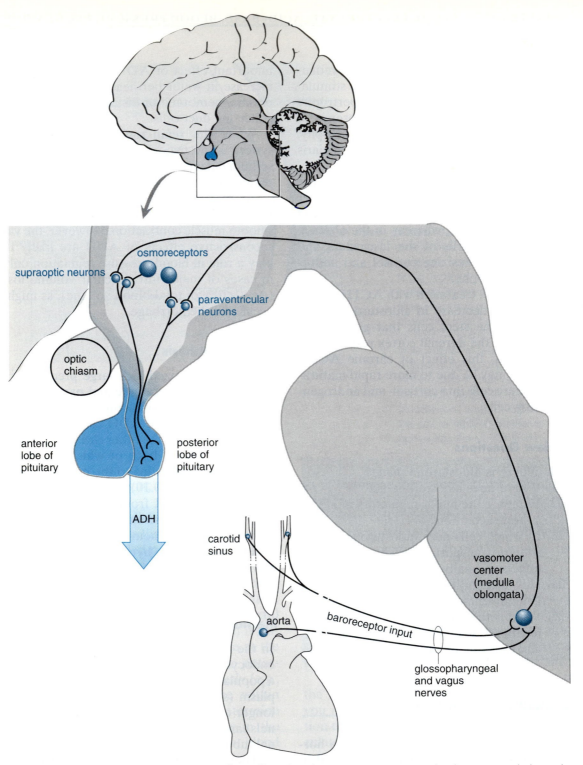

FIGURE 10.9. Regulation of ADH secretion. Afferent fibers from baroreceptors are carried in the vagus and glossopharyngeal nerves to the vasomotor center in the medulla. From there, fibers to the hypothalamus trigger ADH secretion

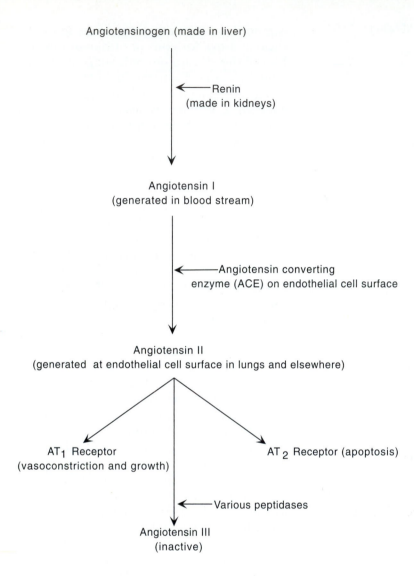

Angiotensinogen (made in liver)

Renin
(made in kidneys)

Angiotensin I
(generated in blood stream)

Angiotensin converting
enzyme (ACE) on endothelial cell surface

Angiotensin II
(generated at endothelial cell surface in lungs and elsewhere)

AT$_1$ Receptor
(vasoconstriction and growth)

AT$_2$ Receptor (apoptosis)

Various peptidases

Angiotensin III
(inactive)

FIGURE 10.6. Proteolytic cascade of the renin-angiotensin system. Angiotensinogen is a 453-amino-acid protein secreted from the liver that is cleaved in the bloodstream by renin secreted from the kidney, to generate angiotensin I, which comprises the amino terminal 10 amino acid residues of angiotensinogen. Two amino acid residues are removed from the carboxy terminus of angiogensin I by angiotensin converting enzyme (ACE), a membrane-bound enzyme of the endothelial cell surface, to generate angiotensin II. Much, but not all, of this conversion is believed to occur at the capillary endothelium in the lungs. Angiotensin II binds to at least two receptor subtypes, called AT$_1$ and AT$_2$, whose currently known actions are indicated. The half-life of angiotensin II in the bloodstream is extremely short, about 1 to 2 min. Angiotensin II is rapidly inactivated by proteases in blood. (*Adapted, with permission, from Ganong WF (1999). Review of Medical Physiology, 19th ed. Stamford, CT, Appleton & Lange, p. 426.*)

different subtypes of receptors are involved in very different actions, perhaps operating on various time scales (see Table 10.4).

Review Questions

15. Where is renin made?
16. What does renin do?
17. What are the major regulators of renin secretion?

18. Where is angiotensinogen made?
19. Where is converting enzyme located, and what *two* actions does it have?

Aldosterone

Aldosterone is the primary mineralocorticoid of the body. It is synthesized in cells of the *zona glomerulosa*, the region of the adrenal

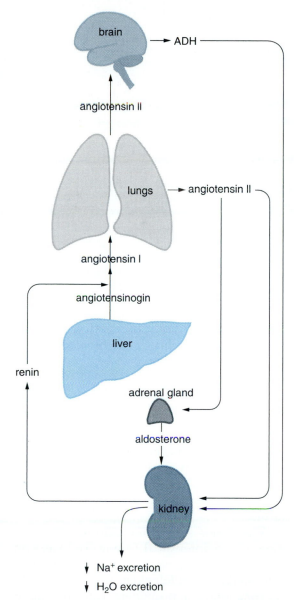

FIGURE 10.7. Schematic representation of the renin-angiotensin-adosterone system. The primary effect of angiotensin II is to stimulate vascular smooth muscle constriction and aldosterone synthesis and secretion from the adrenal cortex. Angiotensin II also has effects on the brain to potentiate the pressor effect of angiotensin II. It also stimulates ADH and ACTH secretion, most likely via the circumventricular organs of the brain that are excluded from the blood-brain barrier. Angiotensin II also works via the hypothalamus to stimulate thirst and has a

TABLE 10.4   ACTIONS OF ANGIOTENSIN II

Tissue Affected	Action
Artery	Stimulates contraction, growth
Adrenal zona glomerulosa	Stimulates secretion of aldosterone
Kidney	Inhibits release of renin
	Increases tubular reabsorption of sodium
	Stimulates vasoconstriction[a]
	Releases prostaglandins
	Affects embryogenesis
Brain	Stimulates thirst and the release of vasopressin
Sympathetic nervous system	Increases central sympathetic outflow
	Facilitates peripheral sympathetic transmission
	Increases adrenal release of epinephrine
Heart	Increases contractility and ventricular hypertrophy

[a]Angiotensin II is a more active vasoconstrictor of efferent glomerular arterioles than of afferent arterioles.
Reproduced, with permission, from Goodfriend TL et al. (1996). Angiotensin receptors and their antagonists. *New Eng. J. Med.* 334:1649–1654.

cortex that lies just under the capsule of the adrenal gland (see Chap. 13).

Aldosterone's action is to bind mineralocorticoid receptors in the cytosol of various epithelial cells to activate transcription of genes whose encoded products are involved in stimulating sodium uptake across their apical surface (see Figure 10.8). The most important site of action of aldosterone is in the distal tubule of the nephron (see Chap. 9). However, aldosterone also has effects at other

FIGURE 10.7 — (continued) direct effect on sodium resorption in the proximal tubule. All of the effects of angiogensin II, both direct and indirect, work to increase blood pressure and intravascular volume. *(Adapted, with permission, from Berne RM, Levy MN (1998). Physiology, 4th ed. St. Louis, MO, Mosby, p. 733.)*

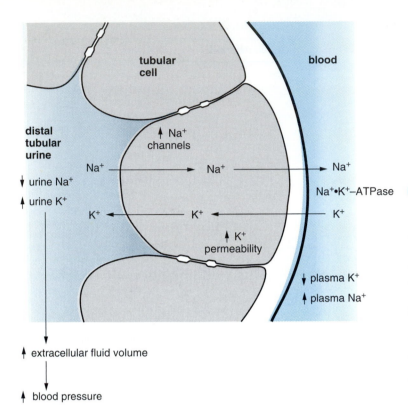

FIGURE 10.8. Mechanism of aldosterone action. Aldosterone, a steroid hormone, works via the mineralocorticoid receptor to affect electrolyte transport in the distal renal tubule. One effect is to increase sodium reabsorption from the distal renal tubular fluid. A second effect is to promote potassium secretion. Na^+/K^+-ATPase activity is also stimulated, so that the extra sodium absorbed from the renal tubular fluid enters the bloodstream, while potassium enters the cell to replace potassium transported into the tubular fluid.

sites, including the gut, salivary, sweat, and mammary glands.

In the case of the distal renal tubule, aldosterone increases sodium influx from the urine into the so-called principal cells. Water follows the sodium leaving the urine, and electroneutrality is maintained by either chloride uptake from, or potassium secretion into, the urine. Na^+/K^+-ATPase on the basolateral surface transfers the sodium, and with it water, into the extracellular space, while at the same time replenishing intracellular potassium. Other forces discussed previously (e.g., hydrostatic versus oncotic pressure within blood vessels, see Chap. 7) will determine whether the sodium and water stay in the interstitial space or move into the blood vessels.

When potassium concentration is below normal, hydrogen ions rather than potassium ions are transferred to the urine in response to aldosterone-mediated uptake of sodium (see Figure 10.8). The basis for this effect is a different cell type of the distal renal tubule whose response to aldosterone (and acidemia) is to secrete hydrogen ions into the urine.

The major stimuli for aldosterone secretion are angiotensin II (a powerful vasoconstrictor, see Sec. 9) and K^+ concentration. This makes great teleologic sense, since aldosterone plays a prominent role in maintenance of both volume and potassium balance.

Since aldosterone is made by a region of the adrenal cortex (the zona glomerulosa), you might have expected aldosterone secretion to be regulated by ACTH, like the fasciculata and reticularis layers of the adrenal cortex. Reality proves more complex.

Acutely, ACTH *will* also stimulate aldosterone secretion. However, ACTH is not trophic for the zona glomerulosa, in the same way that it is for the fasciculata and reticularis. This means that with ACTH stimulation, glomerulosa cells do not hypertrophy and multiply. Conversely, in the absence of ACTH, the glomerulosa cells do not atrophy, as do the cells of the fasciculata and reticularis layers of the adrenal cortex.

Thus, even in the absence of ACTH, the glomerulosa will still respond to the other stimuli (angiotensin II and potassium) and secrete aldosterone, whereas in the absence of ACTH, the cells of the fasciculata and reticularis (synthesizing cortisol and androgens), will atrophy.

Chronically, treatment with ACTH results in a gradual decrease in aldosterone secretion. Since the stem cells that give rise to the layers of the adrenal cortex reside in the glomerulosa, this effect of chronic ACTH treatment may be due to more rapid maturation of these cells into cortisol- and androgen-secreting cells.

Review Questions

20. Where is aldosterone made?
21. Where does aldosterone act?
22. What are the major regulators of aldosterone secretion?
23. In which cells does aldosterone affect sodium transport, and what are these effects normally?
24. How do conditions of acidosis or hypokalemia change aldosterone's effects?
25. What is the difference between the effect of ACTH on aldosterone secretion and that on cortisol secretion?

5. ANTIDIURETIC HORMONE

ADH, also known as vasopressin, is a hormone made in the hypothalamus, stored in the posterior pituitary, and released into the systemic circulation in response to neural or hormonal stimuli (see Figure 10.9). The most important effect of ADH is to stimulate an increase in water permeability of the apical plasma membrane of distal renal tubule and collecting duct cells.

While the renin-angiotensin-aldosterone system is the major hormonal modulator of sodium balance, ADH is the major hormonal regulator of water balance.

As its alternative name, vasopressin, implies, ADH also plays a role in vascular smooth muscle contraction. However, the vasoconstrictive effects of ADH are likely to play a role in blood pressure regulation only in cases of major intravascular volume loss (e.g., >10% of total blood volume), as might occur with hemorrhage.

ADH biosynthesis

ADH is synthesized as a large precursor in neurons of the supraoptic and paraventricular nuclei of the hypothalamus. The large precursor is cleaved into ADH and neurophysin (the name given to the other cleavage product of the precursor), both of which are transported down the axons to the posterior pituitary (see Figure 10.10).

Release of ADH from these nerve terminals into the bloodstream occurs as part of a posterior pituitary neuroendocrine feedback loop in response to hyperosmolality and hypovolemia. A function for neurophysin is not yet known.

Mechanism of ADH action

In the absence of ADH, water channels are endocytosed and stored in the membranes of a population of endocytic vesicles in the cytoplasm (see Figure 10.11). Since they are no longer on the cell surface, these water channels cannot mediate water uptake from the renal tubular fluid.

There are two different receptors for ADH, so-called V_1 and V_2 receptors, which differ in their anatomic distribution and effects. The V_1 receptor appears to mediate the

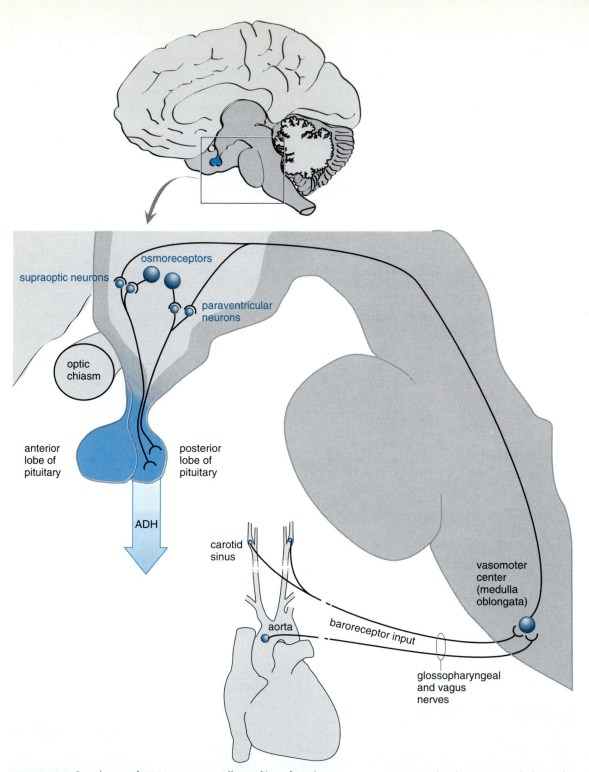

FIGURE 10.9. Regulation of ADH secretion. Afferent fibers from baroreceptors are carried in the vagus and glossopha-ryngeal nerves to the vasomotor center in the medulla. From there, fibers to the hypothalamus trigger ADH secretion

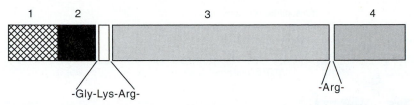

FIGURE 10.10. Biosynthesis of ADH. ADH is made as a larger precursor termed prepropressophysin consisting of a cleaved signal peptide (1), the 9-amino-acid mature vasopressin (ADH, 2), neurophysin II (3), and a glycopeptide (4). Neurophysin II and the glycopeptide are both secreted along with mature ADH, but their physiological roles are unknown. Glycine (Gly) in position 10 is necessary for amidation of the Gly in position 9, a modification found in the mature ADH molecule. ADH is also generated in the gonads and adrenal cortex, but its significance in those locations is unknown. *(Adapted, with permission, from Ganong WF (1999). Review of Medical Physiology, 19th ed. Stamford, CT, Appleton & Lange, p. 230.)*

vasoconstrictive actions of ADH/vasopressin via a signaling pathway involving phosphatidyl inositol turnover. The V_2 receptor stimulates cyclic-AMP production; this mediates the effects on the distal renal tubule, which is where it is found.

Upon ADH release and binding to the V_2 receptor in the basolateral plasma membrane of the cortical and medullary collecting tubules of the distal nephron, the water channel–rich vesicles are triggered via cyclic-AMP-mediated signaling to fuse to the plasma membrane. There, on the cell surface, the water channels are able to mediate transport of water from tubular lumen to tubular cell cytosol (see Figure 10.11).

ADH also has a number of other effects that reinforce its effect on water permeability. One of these is the enhancement of sodium chloride and urea accumulation in the renal medullary interstitium. This augments the generation of medullary hypertonicity and thereby promotes increased renal water reabsorption and urinary concentration.

ADH has several effects on electrolyte transport. Most of these are of unclear clinical significance, but one, stimulation of potassium secretion, is worth mentioning because it appears to simplify matters. You might have expected ADH-stimulated water reabsorption to indirectly *diminish* potassium secretion by diminishing the distal flow of water in the renal tubular lumen. This consequence is offset by a direct effect of ADH to *stimulate* potassium secretion. Thus, you can think of the net effect of ADH as being on water balance alone.

Stimuli for ADH secretion

Change in osmolality is the stimulus to which ADH secretion is most sensitive. A change of as little as 1% in osmolality triggers two homeostatic mechanisms:

FIGURE 10.9 — *(continued)* in response to substantial intravascular volume loss. Box shows how the supraoptic and paraventricular nuclei in the hypothalamus get input from both the vasomotor center and the hypothalamic osmoreceptors, which are integrated to determine the magnitude of ADH response. *(Adapted, with permission, from Berne RM, Levy MN (1998). Physiology, 4th ed. St. Louis, MO, Mosby, p. 720.)*

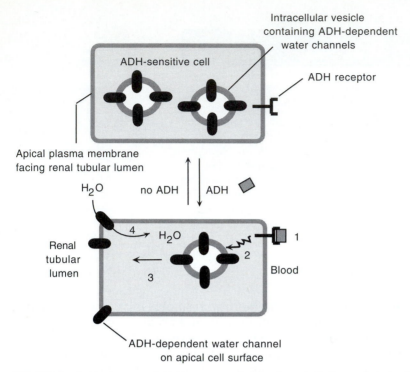

FIGURE 10.11. Mechanism of ADH action on the distal renal tubular epithelial cell. Depicts an ADH-sensitive cell in the distal renal tubule in the absence (top) and presence (bottom) of ADH. Analogous to the response of glucose transporters in muscle or adipose tissue to insulin (see Fig. 6.6), ADH-sensitive cells in the distal renal tubule contain intracellular vesicles bearing water channels. Binding of ADH to its receptor on the basolateral surface (1) triggers signaling to the intracellular vesicles that contain water channels (2) to fuse to the apical plasma membrane (3) and begin water uptake into the cell (4). Not shown in this cartoon is the fact that the occupied ADH receptor is endocytosed and transported to an acidic compartment, where signaling is terminated with recycling of the receptor back to the cell surface. Termination of signaling results in re-internalization of water channels into internal endosomal vesicles, where they will wait for the next cycle of ADH-stimulated vesicular transport.

- Thirst, which provides more free water
- ADH secretion, which allows the kidney to reclaim free water that would otherwise be lost in the urine

The osmotic stimulus to ADH secretion is actually mediated by **tonicity** rather than osmolality. Tonicity refers to the concentration of solutes that are *not* freely permeable across the plasma membranes of most cells, such as sodium, chloride, and glucose. Solutes, such as urea, that contribute to osmolarity but are freely permeable across cell membranes are not a stimulus to ADH secretion.

Thus, ADH is secreted into the bloodstream in response to a change in tonicity. ADH then binds to receptors on the basolateral surface of the epithelial cells of the renal collecting ducts. ADH binding activates these receptors and a signaling cascade that raises cyclic AMP, which in turn triggers fusion of vesicles containing water channels to the apical plasma membrane.

The resulting increase in the magnitude of water transport results in a dramatic increase in the **concentration of the urine**, up to twentyfold over the unstimulated state. This action conserves water that would otherwise be lost in the urine. As a result of this water conservation, there is a *dilution of body fluids.*

From a mechanistic perspective, it is interesting to note that the way ADH works is to increase the amount of water taken up by increasing the number of transporters rather than by increasing the number of water molecules transported by any individual water channel. In enzymologic terms (see Chap. 2), this is an effect on V_{max} rather than K_m.

The other important parameter governing ADH secretion is blood volume. ADH is not terribly sensitive to small changes in blood volume, in contrast to its exquisite sensitivity to tonicity (effective osmolality). However, when there is a major (greater that 5 to 10%) fall in blood volume, left atrial baroreceptors sense the change in filling pressure and signal the hypothalamus via vagal afferents, which trigger a large burst of ADH release. Thus, although the response of ADH secretion to hypovolemia is less sensitive than the response to osmotic stimuli, once activated, it is larger in magnitude and will continue even in the face of hypotonicity, thus overriding the osmolar signals that control ADH secretion.

Another way of thinking about the difference in sensitivity of ADH to osmotic versus volume stimuli is that changes in volume alter the "set point" for ADH response to hypertonicity (see Figure 10.12). Other regulators

FIGURE 10.12. Principles of ADH response. Diagram illustrates the influence of hemodynamic status on the osmoregulation of ADH in humans. The numbers in the center circles refer to the percentage change in volume or pressure; N refers to the normovolemic normotensive individual. Note that the hemodynamic status affects both the slope of the relationship between the plasma ADH and osmolality and the osmotic threshold for ADH release. *(Adapted, with permission, from Robertson GL, Shelton, RL, Athar, S. (1976). Kidney Int 10:25. Reproduced by permission from Kidney International.)*

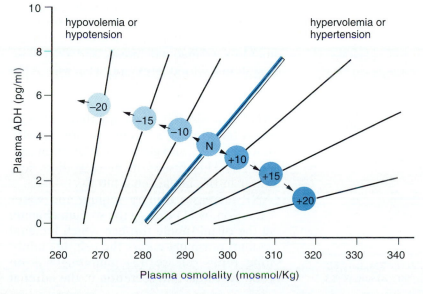

of ADH secretion are indicated in Table 10.5.

Teleologically, the ADH response to tonicity versus volume makes sense because the osmotic control is in operation constantly to optimize the internal environment, whereas the change in sensitivity in response to volume loss provides an emergency response to critical situations when all hell has broken loose — and you'd rather perfuse your tissues with hypotonic blood than with no blood at all.

The ADH system's response to a major volume loss is reinforced by the other regulatory systems. For example, volume loss also triggers the sympathetic nervous system, which:

1. Increases the heart rate to compensate for the loss of stroke volume.
2. Triggers peripheral vasoconstriction.
3. Stimulates renin release via the renal nerves. This renal effect not only generates

TABLE 10.5   REGULATORS OF ADH SECRETION

Stimulation	Inhibition
Extracellular fluid osmolality increase	Extracellular fluid osmolality decrease
Volume decrease	Volume increase
Pressure decrease	Temperature decrease
Cerebrospinal fluid sodium increase	α-Adrenergic agonists
Angiotensin II	γ-Aminobutyric acid (GABA)
Pain	Ethanol
Nausea and vomiting	Cortisol
Stress	Thyroid hormone
Hypoglycemia	Atrial natriuretic peptide
Cytokines	
Temperature increase	
Senescence	
Drugs	
Nicotine	
Opiates	
Barbiturates	
Sulfonylureas	
Antineoplastic agents	

Reproduced, with permission, from Berne RM, Levy MN (1998). *Physiology,* 4th ed. St. Louis, MO, Mosby, p. 903.

another vasoconstrictor in its own right (angiotensin II), it also triggers aldosterone release, which mediates an increase in the osmolality of the extracellular fluid to compensate for the hypoosmolar effects of ADH-mediated water reabsorption.

Review Questions

26. Where is ADH made?
27. What does ADH regulate?
28. What are the major stimuli to ADH secretion?
29. Describe the effects of activation of V_1 versus V_2 receptors for ADH.
30. Where are each of these receptor types located?

6. ATRIAL NATRIURETIC PEPTIDE AND RELATED PRODUCTS

ANP is a peptide made and secreted by the heart that provides a system of "counterregulation" to the actions of the renin-angiotensin-aldosterone system discussed previously. Whereas, in response to renal hypoperfusion, activation of the renin-angiotensin-aldosterone system serves to retain sodium and raise blood pressure, ANP is secreted in response to left atrial stretch and promotes renal sodium loss, termed **natriuresis**, and a decrease in systemic blood pressure. The way ANP does this is as follows:

- ANP is a direct vasodilator that increases renal blood flow, afferent arteriolar perfusion pressure, and glomerular filtration rate (GFR). This results in more sodium and water in the initial renal filtrate.
- ANP increases urinary sodium and water excretion by (1) closing the sodium channel in the distal tubule through which lumenal sodium normally enters the cell, (2) inhibiting renin release, (3) inhibiting aldosterone synthesis and secretion in the adrenal

zona glomerulosa, and (4) interfering with ADH action.

Each of these and other actions contributes to a loss of sodium in the urine, i.e., a natriure-

sis. In addition, a number of other natriuretic peptides have been identified. Figure 10.13 summarizes the effects of ANP.

Urodilatin is an ANP-like product that is made by the distal renal tubule in response

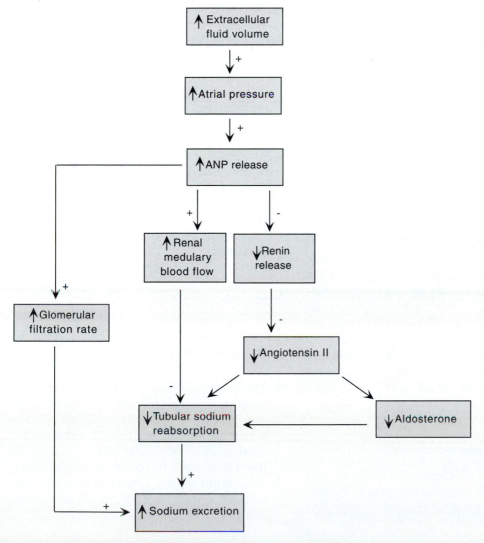

FIGURE 10.13. ANP as a counterregulatory factor in fluid homeostasis. Pathways by which increases in extracellular fluid volume lead to increased sodium excretion and homeostatic correction of volume status. + indicates a stimulatory effect; − indicates an inhibitory effect. Some effects are due to diminution of an otherwise stimulatory effect, in which case + or − is not indicated. *(Adapted, with permission, from Rhodes RA and Tanner GA (1995). Medical Physiology, Boston, Little, Brown, p. 454.)*

to a rise in blood pressure or an increase in effective circulating volume. It is a local mediator whose effects are limited to the kidney.

Clinical Pearl

○ While important aspects of ANP physiology remain poorly understood, it appears that ANP plays an important counterregulatory role in the pathophysiology of congestive heart failure (CHF). CHF is a low cardiac output state in which the backup of blood behind the left heart results in elevated hydrostatic pressure and fluid extravasation into the lungs (see Chap. 7). This fluid and electrolyte disturbance is often exacerbated by the renal response to the low cardiac output state. The kidney retains sodium and triggers peripheral vasoconstriction (see Chap. 9). Sodium retention expands the intravascular compartment, worsening the fluid overload state in the lungs. The vasoconstriction elevates peripheral vascular resistance, further diminishing the perfusion and further impairing cardiac output by increasing the afterload against which the heart must work. Both of these processes will exacerbate left atrial stretch, triggering more release of ANP, which *promotes* renal sodium loss and lowering of peripheral resistance (see the preceding discussion). Thus, ANP potentially can play a self-correcting role in CHF.

Review Questions

31. What are the effects of ANP?
32. The actions of which hormones are antagonized by ANP?

7. CATECHOLAMINES

The catecholamines are important contributors to fluid, electrolyte, and blood pressure regulation in several ways. Released from the adrenal medulla and the sympathetic nerves, respectively, epinephrine and norepinephrine have effects on both the heart and the vasculature. The most important effects of the catecholamines are those of the sympathetic nervous system. The catecholamines of the adrenal medulla seem to be dispensible under normal circumstances.

A variety of different adrenergic receptors exist, with different tissue distributions, different affinities for the various catecholamines, and different effects (see Table 10.6). Thus,

- α-adrenergic receptors mediate vasoconstriction.
- β_1 receptors mediate cardiac inotropic and chronotropic effects and renal activation of the renin-angiotensin-aldosterone system.
- β_2 receptors mediate bronchiolar smooth muscle dilatation and peripheral vasodilation.
- Dopaminergic d_1 receptors mediate renal vasodilatation.
- Dopaminergic d_2 receptors in the brain are associated with nausea and inhibition of prolactin release.

Catecholamines stimulate renal sodium resorbtion by three mechanisms:

1. Direct increase in proximal tubule and loop sodium absorption from the renal filtrate.
2. An increase in arteriolar resistance, which results in altered peritubular capillary hemodynamics and increased return of sodium and water to the intravascular space.
3. Activation of the renin-angiotensin-aldosterone system through β_1-adrenergic receptors.

TABLE 10.6 CATECHOLAMINE RECEPTORS[1]

Organ or Tissue	Adrenergic Receptor	Effect
Heart (myocardium)	β_1	Increased force of contraction (inotropic)
	α_1, β_1	Increased rate of contraction (chronotropic)
	β_1	Increased excitability (predisposes to arrhythmia)
	β_1	Increased AV nodal conduction velocity
Blood vessels (vascular smooth muscle)	α_1, α_2	Vasoconstriction, hypertension
	β_2	Vasodilation
Kidney (juxtaglomerular cells)	β_1	Increased renin release
Gut (intestinal smooth muscle)	α_1	Increased sphincter tone (hyperpolarization); decreased motility (relaxation)
	β_2	Decreased motility (relaxation)
Pancreas (B cells)	α_2	Decreased insulin release Decreased glucagon release
	β_2	Increased insulin release Increased glucagon release
Liver	α_1, β_2	Increased gluconeogenesis Increased glycogenolysis Release of potassium
Adipose tissue	α	Decreased lipolysis
	β_1, β_3	Increased lipolysis
Skin (apocrine glands on hands, axillas, etc.)	α_1	Increased sweating
Lung (bronchial smooth muscle)	β_2	Dilation of bronchi and bronchioles
Uterus (genitourinary smooth muscle)	α_1	Contraction
	β_2	Relaxation
Bladder (genitourinary smooth muscle)	α_1	Contraction
	β_2	Relaxation
Skeletal muscle	β_2	Vasodilation Increased glycogenolysis Increased release of lactic acid
Platelets	α_2	Aggregation
Central nervous system	α	Increased alertness, anxiety, fear
Peripheral nerves	α_2	Decreased norepinephrine release
Most tissues	β	Increased calorigenesis Increased metabolic rate

[1]Reproduced, with permission, from Ganong WF in McPhee S et al., eds. (1997). *Pathophysiology of Disease,* 2nd ed. Stamford, CT, Appleton & Lange, p. 280, as modified from Greenspan FS and Strewler GJ, eds. (1997). *Basic and Clinical Endocrinology,* 5th ed. Stamford, CT, Appleton & Lange.

In states of effective circulatory volume depletion, endogenous norepinephrine is a potent vasoconstrictor, acting via α_1-adrenergic receptors to reduce renal blood flow and thereby preserve perfusion to the coronary and cerebral beds.

When catecholamines are used pharmacologically, consideration of their dose is crucial. At progressively higher doses, catecholamines lose their selectivity as a result of cross-activation of receptors (e.g., α vs. β). Thus, at low doses, at which it activates d_1 receptors but not alpha receptors, dopamine is an effective and selective renal vasodilator that can improve perfusion of the kidneys in a patient in shock. However, at higher doses, dopamine will activate α receptors. The resulting vasoconstriction may maintain the patient's blood pressure, but may lead to renal failure due to hypoperfusion of the kidneys, and necrosis of fingers and toes due to hypoperfusion of the extremities.

Review Questions

33. What are the major classes of effects of the catecholamines?
34. By which receptor types does each occur?
35. Epinephrine and norepinephrine are both catecholamines. What is the basis for the difference in their functions?
36. When do catecholamines lose their receptor subtype specificity?
37. What are some mechanisms by which catecholamine desensitization might occur? *Hint:* review the discussion of desensitization in Chapter 3.

8. PROSTAGLANDINS AND OTHER LOCAL MEDIATORS OF RENAL BLOOD FLOW

Prostaglandins are members of a family of signaling lipids derived from the 20-carbon fatty acid **arachidonic acid** (see Figure 10.14). A distinctive feature of the prostaglandins is that they are local mediators, affecting cells in the immediate vicinity of the synthesizing cell.

A number of hormones that regulate blood pressure, including angiotensin II, may work, at least in part, via generation of prostaglandins. It now appears that not only are there different prostaglandins mediating different effects (e.g., vasodilation vs. vasoconstriction), but prostaglandins carrry out different *types* of functions in different regions of the kidney. Thus, renal medullary prostaglandin production appears to be involved in salt and water excretion in response to volume overload, whereas production of prostaglandins in the renal cortex serves to protect glomerular circulation under conditions of volume depletion.

The mechanisms of action of, and interaction between, the various local mediators, including prostaglandins, bradykinin, the endothelins, dopamine, nitric oxide, and others, is currently poorly understood but the subject of intense investigation (see Ref. 1).

Review Questions

38. What are prostaglandins?
39. Where are prostaglandins made?
40. How do prostaglandins work?

9. HOMEOSTATIC CORRECTION OF ALTERED FLUID AND ELECTROLYTE STATES

The role of the hormonal systems that integrate fluid, electrolyte, and blood pressure control is to maintain homeostasis. Let us consider how the body responds to particular deviations from the normal range of overall volume and specific electrolytes.

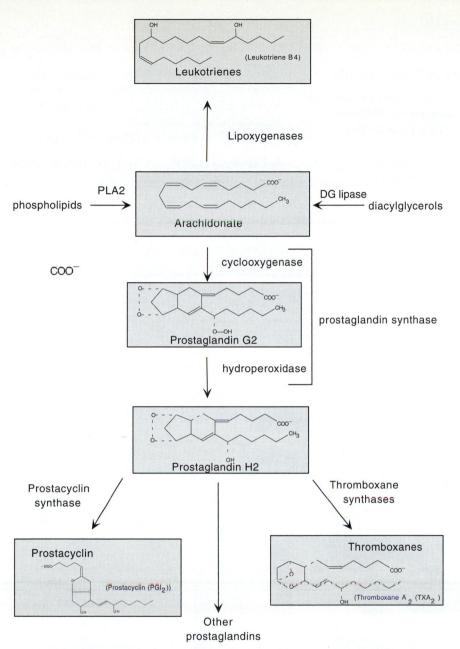

FIGURE 10.14. Relationship of arachidonic acid to other pathways of signaling lipids. Arachidonate is the major precursor of eicosanoid hormones. Prostaglandin synthase is the enzyme that catalyzes the first step in a pathway leading to prostaglandins, prostacyclins, and thromboxanes. Lipoxygenase is the enzyme that catalyzes the initial step in a pathway leading to leukotrienes. Prostaglandin synthase has both a cyclooxygenase and a hydroperoxidase activity, as indicated. PGH2 is a precursor from which other prostaglandins are made. PLAZ = phospholipase Az; DG lipase = diacylglycerol lipase. *(Adapted, with permission, from Stryer L (1995). Biochemistry, 4th ed. New York, Freeman, pp. 624–625.)*

Integrated response to hypervolemia

In response to *too much* intravascular volume, volume sensors signal the kidney to excrete salt and water. This is done by:

1. Stimulation of ANP secretion
2. Inhibition of renin secretion
3. Inhibition of ADH secretion

The rise in ANP secretion in response to left atrial stretch promotes renal salt and water loss by affecting the macula densa and tubuloglomerular feedback.

The fall in renin secretion is due to:

1. Elevated renal arterial perfusion pressure sensed by the juxtaglomerular apparatus

FIGURE 10.15. *A.* Integrated response to hypervolemia. 1. When intravascular volume expands, sympathetic nerve endings to the renal arterioles decrease their firing, resulting in smooth muscle relaxation and dilation of the arterioles. This effect is greater on the afferent than on the efferent arteriole, resulting in increased hydrostatic pressure in the glomerulus and hence increased glomerular filtration rate (GFR). ANP also dilates the afferent and constricts the efferent arteriole, contributing to this effect. With increased GFR, the filtered load of sodium increases, and with it goes water, resulting in an increased volume of urine to correct the hypervolemia. 2. Another effect contributes to correction of hypervolemia. The sympathetic innervation of the kidney also controls renin release. Thus, decreased sympathetic activity results in decreased renin secretion; this results in a decrease

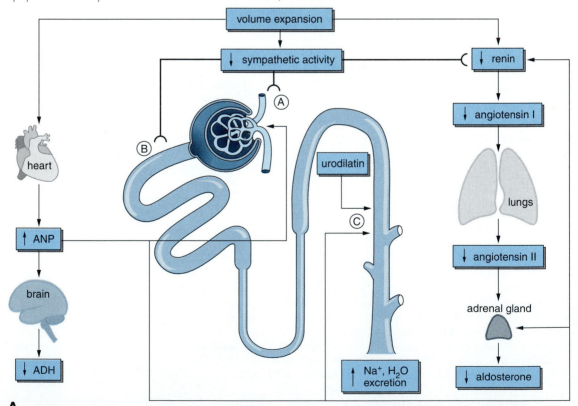

A

2. Decreased stimulation by the renal sympathetic nerves
3. A direct effect of ANP on renin secretion

Lower plasma renin results in decreased generation of angiotensin II and therefore in less aldosterone secretion (see Figure 10.15A).

The fall in renal sympathetic nervous stim-

ulation results in more dilation of the afferent than of the efferent arteriole, which increases the pressure within the glomerulus, and therefore increases GFR and, with it, increases the filtered load of sodium. ANP also contributes to this effect.

The fall in renal sympathetic nervous system activity, along with the fall in angiotensin

FIGURE 10.15 — (continued) in angiotensin II production, which would otherwise stimulate proximal tubular sodium resorption. 3. Through the aforementioned effects, more sodium is delivered to the distal tubule; hence, all else being equal, more sodium, and with it water, will be lost. The decrease in aldosterone resulting from decreased angiotensin II results in a further increase in loss of sodium, until correction of the hypervolemia. B. Integrated response to hypovolemia. Each of the aforementioned mechanisms operates in the opposite direction to decrease GFR, decrease sodium delivery to the renal tubule, and increase sodium and water reabsorption from the renal tubular fluid, thereby correcting the hypovolemia. (Adapted, with permission, from Berne RM, Levy MN (1998). Physiology, 4th ed. St. Louis, MO, Mosby, pp. 736–737.)

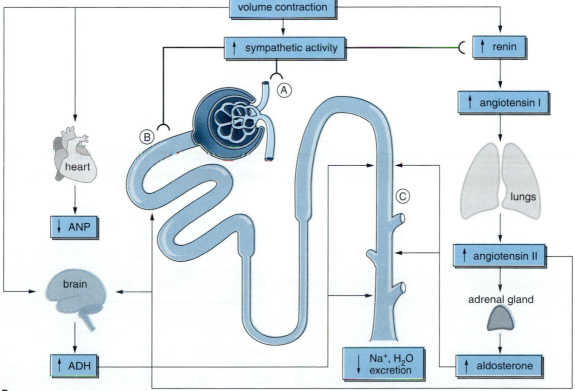

B

II, decreases sodium resorption from the proximal tubule. This, in turn, means that more sodium will be delivered to the distal tubule, which will not resorb the sodium as efficiently, both because more has been delivered and because aldosterone needed for sodium/potassium exchange has decreased. Finally, the fall in ADH levels, both due to increased ANP and due to correction of hyperosmolarity, allows excretion of more water.

Integrated response to hypovolemia

In response to *too little* intravascular volume, volume sensors trigger renal salt and water conservation. This occurs through

1. Increased activity of the renal sympathetic nerves, which affect the macula densa and the juxtaglomerular apparatus and, therefore, tubuloglomerular feedback (see Chap. 9)
2. Increased secretion of renin, and therefore increased levels of angiotensin II and aldosterone
3. Increased ADH secretion by the posterior pituitary in response to both the baroreceptor response to hypovolemia and the high levels of angiotensin II
4. Inhibition of ANP secretion by the atrium and of urodilatin secretion by the distal tubule.

Figure 10.15B summarizes the integrated response to hypovolemia. The effects include a fall in GFR as a result of afferent and efferent arteriole vasoconstriction, in response to the renal sympathetic nervous activity. Since the vasoconstrictive effect is greater on the afferent than on the efferent arteriole, intrarenal hydrostatic pressure, and therefore GFR, falls, reducing the filtered load of Na^+.

Both the increased sympathetic nervous system activity and the rise in angiotensin II brought about by increased renin secretion promote greater proximal tubule sodium resorption. Since GFR has gone down, there is less Na^+ to be absorbed. Therefore, both the relative fraction absorbed and total amount absorbed increase.

The fall in intrarenal hydrostatic pressure probably also favors resorption of fluid into the peritubular capillaries as a result of Starling forces (see Chap. 7).

The rise in angiotensin II causes more aldosterone secretion, which promotes distal tubular and collecting duct sodium reabsorption. Both ANP and urodilatin, which would otherwise have inhibited collecting duct reabsorption, are absent.

Together these effects can succeed in lowering filtered sodium in the urine to almost zero.

The increased ADH secretion causes increased water reabsorption from the distal tubule and collecting duct.

Integrated response to hypernatremia

Elevated intravascular volume (via baroreceptors and sympathetic nervous system activity) or elevated blood sodium (via the macula densa) leads to a decrease in renin secretion. The fall in renin level results in less angiotensin II generation and hence diminished aldosterone secretion and diminished sodium resorption, with consequent increased urinary sodium loss to correct hypernatremia.

Also, elevated blood sodium is an osmotic signal to the hypothalamus to trigger both thirst and ADH release. Thirst results in more water intake and ADH results in more water reabsorption from tubular fluid in the distal nephron. These effects further diminish the blood sodium concentration until both sodium concentration and blood volume/pressure approach the normal range. This homeostatic mechanism breaks down, for example, when ADH is lacking and hence free water cannot be reclaimed from the renal

TABLE 10.7   CAUSES OF HYPERNATREMIA

Water loss
- A. Insensible loss
  1. Increased sweating: fever, exposure to high temperatures, exercise
  2. Burns
  3. Respiratory infections
- B. Renal loss
  1. Central diabetes insipidus
  2. Nephrogenic diabetes insipidus
  3. Osmotic diuresis: glucose, urea, mannitol
- C. Gastrointestinal loss
  1. Osmotic diarrhea: lactulose, malabsorption, some infectious enteritides
- D. Hypothalamic disorders
  1. Primary hypodipsia
  2. Reset osmostat due to volume expansion in primary mineralocorticoid excess
  3. Essential hypernatremia with loss of osmoreceptor function
- E. Water loss into cells
  1. Seizures or severe exercise
  2. Rhabdomyolysis

Sodium retention
- A. Administration of hypertonic $NaCl$ or $NaHCO_3$
- B. Ingestion of sodium

Reproduced, with permission, from Rose BD (1994). *Clinical Physiology of Acid-Base and Electrolyte Disorders,* 4th ed. New York, McGraw-Hill, p. 696.

tubular fluid (see Sec. 10). Causes of hypernatremia are summarized in Table 10.7.

Integrated response to hyponatremia

A fall in blood sodium is detected by the macula densa, leading to an increase in renin secretion and hence more angiotensin II generation. Angiotensin II stimulates aldosterone secretion, which increases sodium resorption from the urine, thereby correcting the hyponatremia. Simultaneously, if hyponatremia is accompanied by a fall in osmolality, this will result in a diminished stimulus for ADH secretion, thereby decreasing the number of water channels in the distal nephron and hence generating a more dilute urine and excreting the excess free water. Condi-

tions that result in hyponatremia, as a result of failure of homeostatic mechanisms, are summarized in Table 10.8.

Integrated response to hyperkalemia

Since most K^+ in the body is inside cells, the elevation of blood K^+ occurring as a result of absorption of a K^+ load from the GI tract gets substantially dampened almost immediately by movement of most of the excess K^+ into cells. Both catecholamines (via the β-adrenergic receptor system) and insulin (via the insulin receptor) will have this effect in part by stimulation of Na^+/K^+-ATPase.

During intense exercise, potassium leaves muscle cells, resulting in a transient increase in blood potassium concentration by as much as 1 to 1.5 meq/L.

TABLE 10.8   CAUSES OF HYPONATREMIA

Disorders in which renal water excretion is impaired
- A. Effective circulating volume depletion
  1. Gastrointestinal losses: vomiting, diarrhea, tube drainage, bleeding, intestinal obstruction
  2. Renal losses: diuretics, hypoaldosteronism, Na^+-wasting nephropathy
  3. Skin losses: ultramarathon runners, burns, cystic fibrosis
  4. Edematous states: heart failure, hepatic cirrhosis, nephrotic syndrome with marked hypoalbuminemia
  5. K^+ depletion
- B. Diuretics
  1. Thiazides in almost all cases
  2. Loop diuretics
- C. Renal failure
- D. Nonhypovolemic states of ADH excess
  1. Syndrome of inappropriate ADH secretion
  2. Cortisol deficiency
  3. Hypothyroidism
- E. Decreased solute intake
- F. Cerebral salt-wasting

Disorders in which renal water excretion is normal
- A. Primary polydipsia
- B. Reset osmostat: effective volume depletion, pregnancy, psychosis, quadriplegia, malnutrition

Reproduced, with permission, from Rose BD (1994). *Clinical Physiology of Acid-Base and Electrolyte Disorders,* 4th ed. New York, McGraw-Hill, p. 654.

Blood K^+ is a major stimulus to aldosterone secretion, which enhances sodium-for-potassium exchange with renal tubular fluid, thereby eliminating K^+ and correcting an elevation in blood K concentration, termed hyperkalemia (see Figure 10.16).

Common syndromes in which homeostatic regulation of potassium may malfunction include renal failure, in which excess fixed acids generated by metabolism enter cells throughout the body (see Table 10.9). Since the chloride ion, with which these acids are largely associated, does not readily enter cells, electroneutrality requires that K^+, the major intracellular cation, leave cells. Thus, hyperkalemia is exacerbated by the metabolic acidosis in renal failure.

This phenomenon appears to be less apparent in the case of organic anion acidoses such as those due to lactic acid (e.g., due to hypoperfusion of tissues) or ketoacids (e.g., in diabetic ketoacidosis). In these cases, the excess organic anions can be taken up to maintain electroneutrality without exit of K^+.

FIGURE 10.16. Overall body potassium balance. Increased plasma insulin, epinephrine, and aldosterone all stimulate potassium movement into cells and decrease plasma potassium (K^+). The amount of K^+ in the body is determined by the difference between dietary intake and output from the kidney and GI tract. Renal potassium excretion is regulated primarily by plasma K^+ and aldosterone. *(Adapted, with permission, from Berne RM, Levy MN (1998). Physiology, 4th ed. St. Louis, MO, Mosby, p. 746.)*

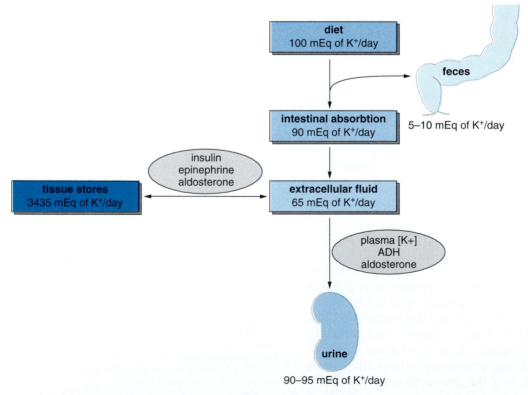

TABLE 10.9   CAUSES OF HYPERKALEMIA

Increased intake[a]

  A. Oral

  B. Intravenous

Movement from cells into extracellular fluid

  A. Pseudohyperkalemia[a]

  B. Metabolic acidosis

  C. Insulin deficiency and hyperosmolality in uncontrolled diabetes mellitus,[a] also acute hyperosmolality due to hypernatremia or the administration of hypertonic mannitol

  D. Tissue catabolism[a]

  E. β-Adrenergic blockade

  F. Severe exercise

  G. Digitalis overdose

  H. Periodic paralysis — hyperkalemic form

  I. Cardiac surgery

  J. Succinylcholine

  K. Arginine

Decreased urinary excretion

  A. Renal failure[a]

  B. Effective circulating volume depletion[a]

  C. Hypoaldosteronism[a]

  D. Type 1 renal tubular acidosis — hyperkalemic form

  E. Selective potassium secretory defect

[a]Most common causes.

Reproduced, with permission, from Rose BD (1994). *Clinical Physiology of Acid-Base and Electrolyte Disorders.* 4th ed. New York, McGraw-Hill, p. 826.

Hyperkalemia is nevertheless often observed in these patients, probably due to intracellular dehydration, accompanied by a movement of K^+ ions out of cells. Also, since it promotes aldosterone secretion, whose action will eliminate the excess potassium, the hyperkalemia that occurs in metabolic acidosis is generally mild, assuming normal kidney function.

The osmotic diuresis associated with many of these syndromes (e.g., due to hyperglycemia in diabetic ketoacidosis) causes a net potassium loss. This is masked as long as acidosis is present, because hydrogen ions displace potassium from the large intracellular reservoir. However, once the acidosis and volume depletion are corrected, potassium rapidly moves back into cells, and the patient can develop profound and dangerous hypokalemia (see Figure 10.17).

Clinical Pearls

○ The large discrepancy between intracellular and extracellular potassium ion concentration means that lysis of even a relatively small number of cells (e.g., red blood cells) can result in a falsely elevated blood potassium. Hence, before reacting to a "panic value" of elevated serum potassium that seems unexpected given the patient's clinical picture, consider hemolysis. This is a common problem when blood is drawn through very small needles or is drawn under strong suction.

○ Distention of the veins below a tourniquet is often promoted by opening and closing of the fist. When excessive, this manuver can mimic the effect of exercise (see above) and raise blood potassium by as much as 1 to 1.5 meq compared to the systemic venous blood potassium concentration.

○ An electrocardiogram (ECG) is a simple way to determine whether an elevated blood potassium level is likely to need immediate therapy or whether a slower approach to correction — or a repeat test to rule out a false value due to hemolysis — is appropriate. The ECG in hyperkalemia is notable for peaking and narrowing of the T wave and shortening of the QT interval as potassium rises above 6 meq/L. At even higher potassium levels, delayed depolarization results in widening of the QRS complex, impaired cardiac conduction, and risk of ventricular dysrrhythmias.

○ The fastest initial therapy for a life-threatening potassium concentration (confirmed by ECG changes) is intravenous infusion of calcium to antagonize the effects of potassium at the myocardial plasma membrane. At the same time, initiation of an insulin and glucose infusion will drive excess po-

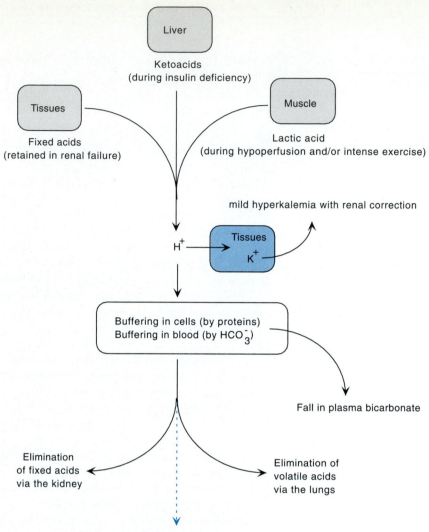

A

FIGURE 10.17. A. Response to acidosis. Acidosis occurs when either production of acids exceeds the body's ability to excrete them or the acid excretory mechanisms are impaired. Shown are three major sources of acid, namely, ketoacids from the liver, fixed acids from tissue metabolism, and lactic acid from muscle. As acid rises, body buffers are consumed, resulting in a fall in plasma bicarbonate (and eventually calcium loss from bone), which mitigates the fall in pH. Nevertheless pH does fall, albeit far more slowly than it would in the absence of the body buffers. As pH falls, H^+ enters cells and K^+, the predominant intracellular cation, leaves to maintain electroneutrality. The extracellular potassium is excreted by the kidneys (assuming normal renal function); hence the blood potassium level will appear normal even though the body may be substantially potassium depleted within cells, an effect that is being masked by the acidosis.

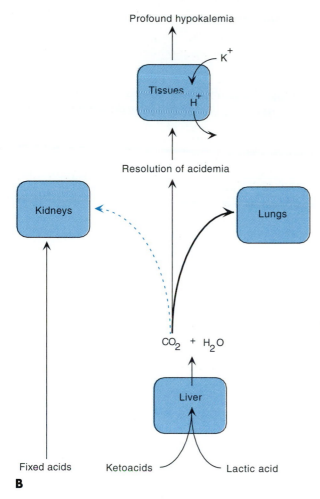

B

FIGURE 10.17 — (*continued*) *B*. Response to correction of acidosis. Hepatic metabolism of ketoacids and lactic acid generates bicarbonate, which is in equilibrium with carbon dioxide and water, the former eliminated via the lungs, the latter via the kidneys, which are also responsible for the elimination of fixed acids. As acidosis is resolved, H+ ions leave cells, and potassium returns. However, since hundreds of milliequivalents of potassium may have been lost in the urine, depending on the time frame over which the acidosis developed, profound hypokalemia can suddenly occur as the pH rapidly is normalized.

tassium into cells, as will respiratory alkalosis caused by hyperventilation (e.g., in the case of a patient on mechanical ventilation). These acute measures should be followed up with a slower but more definitive therapy, such as oral or rectal administration of potassium-binding resins or hemodialysis.

Integrated response to hypokalemia

When serum K^+ is low, the stimulus for aldosterone secretion is diminished, re-sulting in a self-correcting conservation of potassium. If angiotensin II is elevated (e.g., due to secretion of renin in response to volume loss), aldosterone will still be secreted even in the presence of hypokalemia. However, its action will cause loss of hydrogen ions rather than potassium ions. This will allow sodium retention while preventing further potassium loss, but will also generate a metabolic alkalosis. This metabolic alkalosis will be resolved only upon correction of the original volume deficit that resulted in elevated angiotensin II in the first place. Table 10.10 summarizes the con-

TABLE 10.10   CAUSES OF HYPOKALEMIA

Decreased net intake
    A. Low dietary intake or K^+-free intravenous fluids
    B. Clay ingestion

Increased entry into cells, leading to transient hypokalemia
    A. Elevation in extracellular pH
    B. Increased availability of insulin
    C. Elevated β-adrenergic activity:[a] stress, coronary ischemia, delirium tremens, administration of β-adrenergic agonists for asthma or heart failure
    D. Periodic paralysis — hypokalemic form
    E. Treatment of megaloblastic anemias with vitamin B_{12} or folic acid, or of neutropenia with granulocyte-macrophage colony-stimulating factor
    F. Pseudohypokalemia
    G. Hypothermia

Increased gastrointestinal losses[a]

Increased urinary losses
    A. Loop and thiazide-type diuretics[a]
    B. Mineralocorticoid excess
    C. Increased flow to the distal nephron
        1. Salt-wasting nephropathies
        2. Loop and thiazide-type diuretics
    D. Sodium reabsorption with a nonreabsorbable anion
        1. Vomiting or nasogastric suction[a]
        2. Metabolic acidosis
        3. Penicillin derivatives
    E. Amphotericin B
    F. Hypomagnesemia[a]
    G. Polyuria
    H. L-dopa

Increased sweat losses

Dialysis

Potassium depletion without hypokalemia

[a]Most common causes.
Reproduced, with permission, from Rose BD (1994). *Clinical Physiology of Acid-Base and Electrolyte Disorders*. 4th ed. New York, McGraw-Hill, p. 777.

ditions under which hypokalemia often occurs.

Remember that typically, the corrective mechanisms discussed here are activated by minuscule deviations of electrolytes from the normal range. Thus, when a patient has profound abnormalities of serum electrolytes, the nature of those abnormalities often provides an important clue as to the underlying disease process.

Review Questions

41. What is the homeostatic response to hypernatremia?
42. What is the homeostatic response to hypervolemia?
43. What is the homeostatic response to hyponatremia?
44. What is the homeostatic response to hyperkalemia?
45. What is the homeostatic response to hypokalemia?

Integrated response to metabolic acidosis

This is a disorder of acid–base balance in which acidosis is accompanied by a fall in the plasma HCO_3^- concentration. The normal homeostatic response is hyperventilation, as the lungs attempt to compensate for the acidosis by dropping the blood P_{CO_2} concentration. Some of the conditions in which metabolic acidosis is observed are indicated in Table 10.11.

When metabolic acidosis is fully compensated, the pH is close to normal, but both HCO_3^- and P_{CO_2} are low. The tip-off as to which came first, the metabolic acidosis or the respiratory alkalosis, is that compensatory reactions usually do not quite correct completely, so if the underlying problem is metabolic acidosis, the pH will probably be slightly *lower* than 7.4.

Integrated response to metabolic alkalosis

In the metabolic alkaloses, blood pH rises (H^+ ion concentration falls) as a result of a rise in plasma HCO_3^-, which by the law of

TABLE 10.11 CAUSES OF METABOLIC ACIDOSIS WITH AND WITHOUT AN ANION GAP

Causes of Metabolic Acidosis

Inability to excrete the dietary H^+ load
A. Diminished NH_4^+ production
  1. Renal failure[a]
  2. Hypoaldosteronism (type 4 renal tubular acidosis)[a]
B. Diminished H^+ secretion
  1. Type 1 (distal) renal tubular acidosis

Increased H^+ load or HCO_3^- loss
A. Lactic acidosis[a]
B. Ketoacidosis[a]
C. Ingestions
  1. Salicylates
  2. Methanol or formaldehyde
  3. Ethylene glycol
  4. Paraldehyde
  5. Sulfur
  6. Toluene
  7. Ammonium chloride
  8. Hyperalimentation fluids
D. Massive rhabdomyolysis
E. Gastrointestinal HCO_3^- loss
  1. Diarrhea[a]
  2. Pancreatic, biliary, or intestinal fistulas
  3. Ureterosigmoidostomy
  4. Cholestyramine
F. Renal HCO_3^- loss
  1. Type 2 (proximal) renal tubular acidosis

Anion Gap in Major Causes of Metabolic Acidosis

High anion gap[b]
A. Lactic acidosis: lactate, D-lactate
B. Ketoacidosis: β-hydroxybutyrate
C. Renal failure: sulfate, phosphate, urate, hippurate
D. Ingestions
  1. Salicylate: ketones, lactate, salicylate
  2. Methanol or formaldehyde: formate
  3. Ethylene glycol: glycolate, oxalate
  4. Paraldehyde: organic anions
  5. Toluene: hippurate (usually presents with normal anion gap)
  6. Sulfur: SO_4^{2-}
E. Massive rhabdomyolysis

Normal anion gap (hyperchloremic acidosis)
A. Gastrointestinal loss of HCO_3^-
  1. Diarrhea
B. Renal HCO_3^- loss
  1. Type 2 (proximal) renal tubular acidosis
C. Renal dysfunction
  1. Some cases of renal failure
  2. Hypoaldosteronism (type 4 renal tubular acidosis)
  3. Type 1 (distal) renal tubular acidosis
D. Ingestions
  1. Ammonium chloride
  2. Hyperalimentation fluids
E. Some cases of ketoacidosis, particularly during treatment with insulin

[a]Most common causes.
[b]The substances after the colon represent the major retained anions in the high-anion-gap acidoses.
Reproduced, with permission, from Rose BD (1994). *Clinical Physiology of Acid-Base and Electrolyte Disorders*. 4th ed. New York, McGraw-Hill, pp. 545–546.

mass action drives Equation (4) (see Sec. 2) to the left:

$$CO_2 + H_2O \rightleftharpoons H_2CO_3 \rightleftharpoons H^+ \text{ and } HCO_3^- \quad (4)$$

In response, hypoventilation occurs, resulting in a rise in P_{CO_2}, a compensatory respiratory acidosis to bring the pH back close to normal. As discussed previously, individuals in which the metabolic alkalosis was the primary problem will have a slightly elevated blood pH to go with the higher than normal HCO_3^- and P_{CO_2}, as, again, the primary acid–base disturbance is not quite fully offset by the compensatory response. The causes of metabolic alkalosis are summarized in Table 10.12.

Integrated response to respiratory acidosis

Respiratory acidosis occurs when P_{CO_2} increases as a result of hypoventilation. In Equation (4), as P_{CO_2} goes up, the equation is driven to the right, generating more H^+.

This can occur either as a primary disorder (e.g., due to respiratory failure) or as a way of compensating for a metabolic alkalosis. When respiratory acidosis is a primary disorder, the patient's response depends on whether the acidosis develops quickly or slowly, because the renal compensation (retention of HCO_3^-) takes a few days to be fully manifest. Thus, a patient with rapid-onset respiratory failure (e.g., occurring in minutes to hours, as in a patient with a bad asthma attack) can have a dramatic fall in pH because there has not been enough time for renal compensation to occur. In contrast, a patient with chronic respiratory acidosis (for example, a patient with emphysema, see Chap. 8) will have a near normal (but slightly low) pH and a substantial elevation of plasma HCO_3^-, reflecting renal compensation. Table 10.13 summarizes the common causes of respiratory acidosis.

TABLE 10.12

Causes of Metabolic Alkalosis

Loss of hydrogen
- A. Gastrointestinal loss
  1. Removal of gastric secretions — vomiting or nasogastric suction[a]
  2. Antacid therapy, particularly with cation-exchange resin
  3. Chloride-losing diarrhea
- B. Renal loss
  1. Loop or thiazide-type diuretics[a]
  2. Mineralocorticoid excess[a]
  3. Postchronic hypercapnia
  4. Low chloride intake
  5. High-dose carbenicillin or other penicillin derivative
  6. Hypercalcemia, including the milk-alkali syndrome
- C. H$^+$ movement into cells
  1. Hypokalemia[a]
  2. Refeeding (?)

Retention of bicarbonate
- A. Massive blood transfusion
- B. Administration of NaHCO$_3$
- C. Milk-alkali syndrome

Contraction alkalosis
- A. Loop or thiazide-type diuretics
- B. Gastric losses in patients with achlorhydria
- C. Sweat losses in cystic fibrosis

Causes of Impaired HCO$_3^-$ Excretion That Allow Metabolic Alkalosis to Persist

Decreased glomerular filtration rate
- A. Effective circulating volume depletion
- B. Renal failure (usually associated with metabolic acidosis)

Increased tubular reabsorption
- A. Effective circulating volume depletion
- B. Chloride depletion (also decreases bicarbonate secretion)
- C. Hypokalemia
- D. Hyperaldosteronism

[a]Most common causes.
Reproduced, with permission, from Rose BD (1994). *Clinical Physiology of Acid-Base and Electrolyte Disorders.* 4th ed. New York, McGraw-Hill, pp. 516, 518.

TABLE 10.13   CAUSES OF RESPIRATORY ACIDOSIS

Inhibition of the medullary respiratory center
- A. Acute
  1. Drugs: opiates, anesthetics, sedatives
  2. Oxygen in chronic hypercapnia
  3. Cardiac arrest
  4. Central sleep apnea
- B. Chronic
  1. Extreme obesity (Pickwickian syndrome)
  2. Central nervous system lesions (rare)
  3. Metabolic alkalosis (although hypercapnia is an appropriate response to the rise in pH in this setting)

Disorders of the respiratory muscles and chest wall
- A. Acute
  1. Muscle weakness: crisis in myasthenia gravis, periodic paralysis, aminoglycosides, Guillain-Barré syndrome, severe hypokalemia or hypophosphatemia
- B. Chronic
  1. Muscle weakness: spinal cord injury, poliomyelitis, amyotrophic lateral sclerosis, multiple sclerosis, myxedema
  2. Kyphoscoliosis
  3. Extreme obesity

Upper airway obstruction
- A. Acute
  1. Aspiration of foreign body or vomitus
  2. Obstructive sleep apnea
  3. Laryngospasm

Disorders affecting gas exchange across the pulmonary capillary
- A. Acute
  1. Exacerbation of underlying lung disease (including increased CO$_2$ production with high-carbohydrate diet)
  2. Adult respiratory distress syndrome
  3. Acute cardiogenic pulmonary edema
  4. Severe asthma or pneumonia
  5. Pneumothorax or hemothorax
- B. Chronic
  1. Chronic obstructive pulmonary disease: bronchitis, emphysema
  2. Extreme obesity

Mechanical ventilation

Reproduced, with permission, from Rose BD (1994). *Clinical Physiology of Acid-Base and Electrolyte Disorders.* 4th ed. New York, McGraw-Hill, p. 607.

Integrated response to respiratory alkalosis

Respiratory alkalosis occurs as a result of hyperventilation that causes a fall in Pco$_2$ below the normal range. As with a respiratory acidosis (but with pH moving in the opposite direction), respiratory alkalosis can occur either suddenly or gradually. When it is sudden, the fall in Pco$_2$ occurs much faster than the renal compensatory response of HCO$_3^-$ loss in the urine, and thus blood pH may rise dramatically. A chronic respiratory alkalosis,

TABLE 10.14   CAUSES OF RESPIRATORY ALKALOSIS

Hypoxemia
  A. Pulmonary disease: pneumonia, interstitial fibrosis, emboli, edema
  B. Congestive heart failure
  C. Hypotension or severe anemia
  D. High-altitude residence

Pulmonary disease

Direct stimulation of the medullary respiratory center
  A. Psychogenic or voluntary hyperventilation
  B. Hepatic failure/urea cycle defects, hyperammonemia
  C. Gram-negative septicemia
  D. Salicylate intoxication
  E. Postcorrection of metabolic acidosis
  F. Pregnancy and the luteal phase of the menstrual cycle (due to progesterone)
  G. Neurologic disorders: cerebrovascular accidents, pontine tumors

Mechanical ventilation

Reproduced, with permission, from Rose BD (1994). *Clinical Physiology of Acid-Base and Electrolyte Disorders.* 4th ed. New York, McGraw-Hill, p. 632.

occurring over days, will be well compensated by the kidneys, and hence pH will be (nearly) normal, but HCO_3^- will be low. Table 10.14 summarizes the common causes of respiratory alkalosis. Table 10.15 provides some simple "rules of thumb" that allow estimation of the contributions to various mixed acid–base disorders.

Clinical Pearls

○ In a patient with a metabolic acidosis, it is useful to distinguish causes that result in a so-called anion gap, that is, a discrepancy between the sodium plus potassium ion concentrations of the major cation (Na^+) and the major anions (Cl^- and HCO_3^-) in blood. Normally the anion gap should be less than 5 to 11, reflecting the concentration of various other anions in plasma. Patients with anion-gap metabolic acidoses often have values of 15 to 20 or higher.

When the anion gap is elevated, that means that some substance (the unmeasured anion) has accumulated in the bloodstream and is the likely cause of the metabolic acidosis (e.g., lactate as a result of glycolysis in hypoperfused tissues, ketones in diabetic ketoacidosis, fixed acids in renal failure, myoglobin in crushed tissue injuries, or salicylate in aspirin overdose, see Table 10.11). If there is no anion gap, then the metabolic acidosis is most likely caused by bicarbonate loss (e.g., due to diarrhea or renal tubular dysfunction). A simple formula to calculate the anion gap from readily available serum electrolyte values is:

$$\text{Anion gap} = [Na^+] - ([Cl^-] + [HCO_3^-])$$

○ The intravascular volume status and potassium ion concentration are important determinants in patients with metabolic alkalosis. Intravascular volume depletion will activate the renin-angiotensin-aldosterone system, and aldosterone will be a powerful stimulus to sodium retention by exchange of potassium or, in the case of potassium deficiency, hydrogen ion. Thus, the patient with potassium deficiency and intravascular volume depletion (e.g., as a result of vomiting or diarrhea) will continue to lose H^+ ions in the urine in order to retain sodium, making the metabolic alkalosis difficult to correct unless the intravascular volume and potassium ion depletion are addressed (e.g., by providing Na^+- and Cl^--rich intravenous fluids supplemented with K^+).

○ Hypercapnea (elevated P_{CO_2}) could be either a primary respiratory acidosis or a respiratory compensation for a metabolic alkalosis. To distinguish between the two, calculate the alveolar-arterial O_2 gradient (see Chap. 8). This is always increased in a primary respiratory acidosis. If, instead, the A-a gradient is normal, intrinsic lung

TABLE 10.15   COMPENSATION AND CORRECTIONS FOR FIXED ACID–BASE DISORDERS

Characteristics of the Primary Acid–Base Disturbances

Disorder	pH	[H$^+$]	Primary disturbance	Compensatory response
Metabolic acidosis	↓	↑	↓ [HCO$_3^-$]	↓ P$_{CO_2}$
Metabolic alkalosis	↑	↓	↑ [HCO$_3^-$]	↑ P$_{CO_2}$
Respiratory acidosis	↓	↑	↑ P$_{CO_2}$	↑ [HCO$_3^-$]
Respiratory alkalosis	↑	↓	↓ P$_{CO_2}$	↓ [HCO$_3^-$]

Renal and Respiratory Compensations to Primary Acid–Base Disturbances in Humans

Disorder	Primary change	Compensatory response
Metabolic acidosis	↓ [HCO$_3^-$]	1.2 mmHg decrease in P$_{CO_2}$ for every 1 meq/L fall in [HCO$_3^-$]
Metabolic alkalosis	↑ [HCO$_3^-$]	0.7 mmHg elevation in P$_{CO_2}$ for every 1 meq/L rise in [HCO$_3^-$]
Rrespiratory acidosis	↑ P$_{CO_2}$	
Acute		1 meq/L increase in [HCO$_3^-$] for every 10 mmHg rise in P$_{CO_2}$
Chronic		3.5 meq/L elevation in [HCO$_3^-$] for every 10 mmHg rise in P$_{CO_2}$
Respiratory alkalosis	↓ P$_{CO_2}$	
Acute		2 meq/L reduction in [HCO$_3^-$] for every 10 mmHg fall in P$_{CO_2}$
Chronic		4 meq/L decrease in [HCO$_3^-$] for every 10 mmHg reduction in P$_{CO_2}$

Reproduced, with permission, from Rose BD (1994). *Clinical Physiology of Acid-Base and Electrolyte Disorders.* 4th ed. New York, McGraw-Hill, pp. 506, 508.

disease is extremely unlikely. Rather, a normal A-a gradient suggests that either (1) the hypercapnea is compensatory, (2) the primary problem is in the medullary respiratory control centers of the brain, or (3) there is chest wall/inspiratory muscle dysfunction.

○ Because calcium binding to albumin is highly pH-dependent, one of the dramatic manifestations of respiratory alkalosis (e.g., in an anxious, hyperventilating patient) is a fall in ionized free calcium to the point where muscle spasms occur. This, of course, frightens the patient even more, resulting in more anxiety, more hyperventilation, and worsened symptoms. The appropriate maneuver is to calm the patient down and have him or her rebreath in a paper bag to try and bring up the P$_{CO_2}$, which will result in an equally dramatic resolution of the symptoms and a most grateful patient.

Review Questions

46. How do you distinguish a primary metabolic acidosis from compensation for a respiratory alkalosis?

47. What is the importance of time frame in the homeostatic response to acidosis or alkalosis, i.e., whether it develops rapidly or slowly?

48. What is the meaning of an anion gap in a patient with a metabolic acidosis?

49. Why is the alveolar-arterial oxygen gradient useful in evaluating a patient with a respiratory acidosis?

10. COMMON CLINICAL DISORDERS IN ENDOCRINOLOGY OF FLUID, ELECTROLYTE, AND BLOOD PRESSURE CONTROL

The disorder **diabetes insipidus** results from lack of ADH effect due to either central causes (e.g., pituitary stalk transection) or peripheral causes (lack of ADH receptors, etc.). It manifests as an inability to excrete a concentrated urine. The patient may have 20 L or more of dilute urine per day but is otherwise well as long as oral intake matches urine output. In untreated patients, oral intake eventually falls behind, and they present with dehydration and hypernatremia.

The **syndrome of inappropriate ADH secretion** (SIADH) is a common finding in patients with a variety of different brain or lung lesions, including (but not limited to) tumors. It results in water retention and hyponatremia. It does *not* usually result in volume expansion and edema because various mechanisms (e.g., ANP) mediate correction of the volume status, leaving hyponatremia as the sole major manifestation. Indeed, the diagnosis cannot really be made in the presence of edema because, even if ADH secretion is elevated, it may be an *appropriate* response to intravascular volume depletion with a shift in fluid to the extravascular extracellular compartment.

This syndrome can usually be effectively treated by restricting patients' free water intake of (in effect, letting a small degree of dehydration occur to convert the unregulated secretion of ADH from inappropriate to appropriate).

Primary hyperaldosteronism, usually due to an adrenal tumor, results in enhanced potassium and hydrogen ion secretion, resulting in hypokalemia and metabolic alkalosis. Sodium and water retention are often partly mitigated by counterregulatory mechanisms, perhaps including ANP. This entity should always be considered in a patient with hypertension and hypokalemia in whom secondary causes of hypertension have not been previously explored. An imaging study of the abdomen would probably be the next diagnostic procedure, in search of an adrenal tumor.

Primary hypoaldosteronism is often accompanied by **hyperkalemia** and **metabolic acidosis**. Sodium wasting also occurs, but it is not prominent because other antinatriuretic mechanisms such as angiotensin II and reduced renal perfusion pressure are activated by the initial volume depletion. A form of this syndrome termed hyporeninemic hypoaldosteronism is seen commonly in diabetic patients consequent to their renal vascular disease. The resulting renal disorder is also termed a type IV renal tubular acidosis (type IV RTA, see Chap. 9).

Hypertension is the elevation of resting blood pressure above the normal range. The limits for normal blood pressure increase somewhat with age. Physiologically, hypertension can be caused by a variety of cardiovascular, renal, and neuroendocrine derangements. These include sodium or fluid overload and excessive sympathetic neural activity. In most cases, patients with hypertension have **essential hypertension**, which simply means that we have no ready understanding of the abnormalities responsible for development of the disorder. Endocrine causes of hypertension are relatively rare. Nevertheless, most cases of essential hypertension will respond to drugs that work by interfering with the endocrine components of blood pressure control. Thus, drugs that block β-adrenergic receptors (propranolol, metoprolol, nadolol) and drugs that block angiotensin I to angiotensin II conversion (captopril, enalapril) are effective antihypertensive agents. Recently, it has been observed that patients with essential hypertension can be sorted by whether they have "low renin" or "high renin," with certain characteristics associated with each group (see Chap. 14).

Heart failure occurs when the heart is no longer able to respond to changes that would normally trigger an increase in cardiac output. A common cause is the consequences of long-term, poorly controlled hypertension. The initial cardiac response to prolonged high afterload (hypertension) is hypertrophy. Eventually, the heart can no longer make up for the high afterload by a "harder squeeze" and fails to sufficiently empty the ventricle in the course of systole. As a result, the heart starts to dilate to accommodate the residual volume. This sets in motion a vicious cycle in which the heart moves to a less efficient part of the Starling curve, which means it has to do more work to achieve a given cardiac output, which makes it fall further behind, eventually resulting in dilated cardiomyopathy (see Chap. 7). In such a patient, the fall in forward cardiac output results in a fall in renal perfusion, which activates the renin-angiotensin-aldosterone and ADH systems. Activation of the renin-angiotensin-aldosterone system will increase sodium retention (and with it water), while ADH will retain even more water, resulting in hyponatremia.

The stretch of the left atrium by an overfilled heart will also trigger ANP release and natriuresis, but this may not be sufficient to counteract the stronger drive to retain sodium and expand intravascular volume. In any case, the underlying cardiac dysfunction prevents normal homeostatic correction.

Meanwhile, a consequence of decreased cardiac output is that blood pools on the venous side, resulting in increased hydrostatic pressure. Increased hydrostatic pressure imbalances the Starling forces in favor of moving more fluid into the interstitial space (see Chap. 7). Lymphatic vessels will return the excess interstitial fluid to the circulation, but their capacity is limited and can easily be exceeded, resulting in excess interstitial fluid, termed edema.

As a result, despite the fact that they have *effective* circulatory volume depletion, these patients become *total* body sodium and water overloaded, with development of hyponatremia and edema (see Figure 10.18).

Furthermore, if the patient happens, for some reason, to develop an increase in blood pressure, and hence afterload, he or she may develop pulmonary edema as fluid backs up into the lungs as a result of elevated cardiac filling pressures behind a heart that cannot respond by more forceful contraction to increase cardiac output (see Chap. 7).

Clinical Pearl

○ What are some of the mechanisms by which hypertension causes disease? There are several:

- Shear stress (the damaging effects of turbulent flow and high pressure) on the endothelium, which potentiates oxidative injury. Together, these forces cause thickening of basement membranes, making for inefficient nutrient and waste exchange. This, in turn, results in formation of scar tissue and a steady loss of organ function.
- Acceleration of atherosclerotic plaque formation, which impedes perfusion. Plaque material can break off from the vessel walls and occlude the vessel further along as it narrows.
- Catastrophic rupture of a blood vessel whose wall was weakened by plaque formation and scarring (e.g., in the brain, resulting in a stroke).

Review Questions

50. Why might a patient develop diabetes insipidus?
51. What is the significance of edema in a patient with hyponatremia?
52. What findings suggest primary hyperaldosteronism?

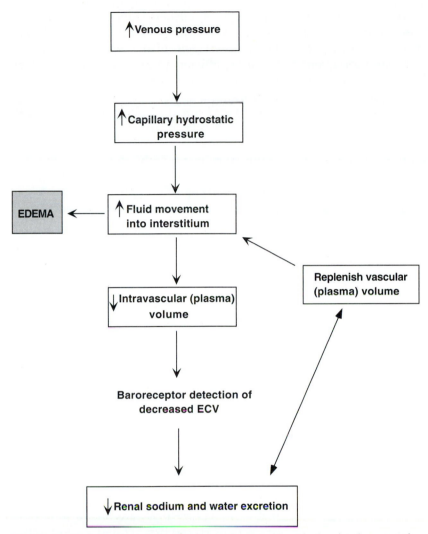

FIGURE 10.18. Pathophysiology of edema. Steps involved in the development of edema as a result of increased venous pressure, as occurs in heart failure, for example. Sodium chloride and water retention by the kidney maintains plasma volume with increase in interstitial fluid. *(Adapted, with permission, from Berne RM, Levy MN (1998). Physiology, 4th ed. St. Louis, MO, Mosby, p. 746.)*

11. FRONTIERS IN FLUID, ELECTROLYTE, ACID–BASE, AND BLOOD PRESSURE PHYSIOLOGY

Traditional thinking about the hormones and organ systems involved in fluid, electrolyte, and blood pressure regulation is changing in ways that will dramatically affect future medical practice:

• Mechanical views of the heart as a pump and blood vessels as plumbing are giving way to a more modern "organic" view in which *both* structure and function can change over time. From the modern perspective, growth control, proliferation, and apoptosis of specific cell types — events that result in "remodeling" of organs — occur as a consequence of signaling cascades (see Ref. 3). These signaling events are sometimes triggered by hormones whose actions were previously thought of only in terms of opening one sort of channels or another to regulate electrolyte concentrations.

- Cell volume is being recognized as a trigger of cell division, suggesting that volume-sensitive pathways may be a therapeutic target in unregulated cellular proliferation (see Ref. 4).
- In sickle cell anemia, a mutation in the oxygen-carrying protein hemoglobin renders the protein highly sensitive to polymerization in response to insults — including dehydration. Blocking electrolyte, and hence fluid, shifts may be a means of preventing some of the most serious complications of this disease.

Some aspects of the changing nature of fluid and electrolyte physiology are highlighted in more detail in the following section.

Type 3 β-adrenergic receptors and cardiovascular disease

Recently, a third type of β-adrenergic receptor has been discovered (see Ref. 5). The interesting thing about this receptor is that its actions seem to be counter to those of β_1 receptors. Furthermore, it appears that it is induced to some extent in chronic heart failure — in effect, serving as nature's own beta-blocker therapy. Of course, as in pharmacologic beta-blocker therapy, there is a fine line between the beneficial effects of beta

blockade in cardiac ischemia (preventing overwork on the part of the ischemic and failing heart; optimizing contractility to give the most efficiency) and the harmful effects (weakness and fatigue; congestive heart failure).

Perhaps some patients (e.g., those with severe congestive heart failure due to β_3 receptors) will benefit from a means of inactivating this third limb of the β-adrenergic system, while others (e.g., those with severe angina) will get selective benefit from β_3 agonists.

Genetic programming of the propensity for adult hypertension in utero

Studies in a line of spontaneously hypertensive rats suggest an intriguing basis for this genetic predisposition to hypertension (see Ref. 6). It appears that excessively low levels of maternal (placental) β-hydroxysteroid dehydrogenase result in failure to completely inactivate maternal cortisol. The resulting excess mineralocorticoid effects of maternal cortisol somehow program the fetus in ways that result in spontaneous hypertension as an adult.

The next step is to identify the genes being activated and the pathways by which they work. Furthermore, studies need to be done to see if, how, and to what human population these animal studies apply.

What is exciting about this work is that it provides a model system that may make it possible to dissect the genetics of at least a subset of hypertension. It also reveals an unexpected connection between fetal biology and adult pathophysiology and another role for the adrenal steroids. As is often the case, pathologic observations (e.g., spontaneous hypertension) highlight the existence of physiological functions that were not previously appreciated.

Nitrosohemoglobin: a built-in blood pressure–lowering buffer system

Nitric oxide (NO) gas has been recently recognized as the likely mediator of the vasodilatory effects of nitrates. However, what has not been realized until very recently is that there is a complex relationship between NO and hemoglobin. It appears that the O_2-loaded hemoglobin molecule is also loaded with NO. Release of the NO in the periphery provides a vasodilatory stimulus that has the effect of promoting tissue oxygenation by increasing blood flow in areas that need to be oxygenated (see Ref. 7).

It has long been appreciated that one drawback of artificial blood products is that they have a propensity to cause hypertension; however, the mechanism has been obscure. Perhaps loading NO onto the hemoglobin in artificial blood might serve to offset the undesired hypertensive side effect.

Genetics of salt-sensitive hypertension

For reasons unknown, some people respond to a salt load by excreting all of the excess salt without an increase in arterial pressure. In others, some of the salt load is retained, and hence intravascular volume expands and blood pressure goes up. If we knew to which subset any given patient belonged, we would know whether that patient's hypertension might respond to dietary salt restriction. But this is not easy to determine directly in large numbers of people in a cost-effective manner, and given the complex polygenic nature of hypertension, it is unlikely to be determinable in the future with a simple screening blood test.

One approach to this problem has been the development of salt-sensitive, spontaneously hypertensive strains of rats, that is, animals whose genes impair their ability to respond optimally to increased sodium intake. Re-

markably, some of these rat strains display a constellation of findings reminiscent of those in salt-sensitive hypertensive humans: They are insulin-resistant, are hyperlipidemic, and have low serum renin levels, and they tend to be relatively refractory to angiotensin converting enzyme inhibitors. Instead, both the rats and these patients respond better to diuretics. Also like the patients, the rats are prone to development of severe progressive hypertensive renal disease, which may be what makes the disorder eventually irreversible, even if they are placed on a low-salt diet.

Study of these animal models and the genes responsible for this phenotype may ultimately allow more effective separation of patients into subsets that respond better to one medicine than to another (see Ref. 8).

12. HOW DOES AN UNDERSTANDING OF NORMAL PHYSIOLOGY PROVIDE INSIGHT INTO THE INITIAL CASE PRESENTATION?

This patient presented to the hospital with pulmonary edema, and his initial findings are consistent with cardiogenic shock (see Chap. 7), in which his heart muscle is too weak (e.g., due to ischemia) to maintain an adequate cardiac output.

The afterload reducing agent, vasodilator, and diuretic were treatments intended to improve his cardiac output without increasing the workload of the heart.

By decreasing afterload, you increase the amount of blood the heart can pump for a given amount of work, because the pressure against which it must work goes down.

By decreasing preload with vasodilators, you allow the heart to be less engorged with blood and therefore work with less wall tension, which would otherwise make it contract less efficiently.

The diuretic promotes sodium and water loss via the kidneys, thereby decreasing intravascular volume and making the workload on the heart easier by both of the previously mentioned mechanisms.

The problem is that if you overdo these treatments, you will lower blood pressure too much and cause inefficient and inadequate cardiac output for a different reason: inadequate filling of the heart. Thus, patients with diminished cardiac reserve walk a fine line between congestive heart failure, hypertension, and pulmonary edema, on the one hand, and hypotension, poor perfusion, and worsened ischemia and renal failure, on the other. The challenge is to treat the former without causing the latter.

The effect of high-dose dopamine on a normal heart would be to increase heart rate, contractility, and cardiac output (effects via β receptors). Its effects on the vasculature would be to cause vasoconstriction (α-receptor effects). But in a patient (like this one!) whose heart was already functioning marginally, perhaps because of ischemia, and whose peripheral resistance was already high because of a low output state, the effects of high-dose dopamine could be disastrous: worsened ischemia, worsened cardiac output, worsened tissue perfusion.

Furthermore, the resident failed to use common sense: a 30-s assessment of brain perfusion (mental status), heart perfusion (whether the patient had chest pain or ECG changes suggestive of ischemia), kidney perfusion (urine output of at least 20 cc/hr from the Foley catheter), and extremity perfusion (warm extremities of normal color with capillary filling in the fingertips) was not consistent with the lack of a detectable blood pressure. As long as the patient is perfusing vital organs well, there is time to identify the real problem and think through the physiology so that the further treatment does not make things worse (as high-dose dopamine might well have done). Perhaps the blood pressure monitor was not functioning properly (in the real world machines often fail us at the worst possible times!). Did the ICU staff measure the blood pressure manually with a blood pressure cuff to confirm the results displayed on the monitor? Perhaps the hypotension was a transient effect of too much vasodilator (some diuretics are known to have a transient, immediate vasodilating effect even before their intended effect on the kidney is manifest)?

The strategy suggested by the first physician, namely, to (1) place the patient in a position that would safeguard blood flow to the brain (Trendelenberg position), (2) stop giving the drugs that might have caused the problem (the vasodilator and diuretic) for now, and resume them at a lower dose later, (3) check for equipment error, and (4) consider giving small amounts of fluid to expand intravascular volume gingerly, was a far more prudent strategy. When in doubt, *look at the patient.*

Clinical Pearls

○ Sometimes a patient may present in clinic with an extremely low blood pressure or heart rate. However, if the patient is feeling fine; gives no history of falling, fainting, or other such events; is having no dysrrhythmia on ECG; has had no symptoms referable to low blood pressure or poor perfusion; does not display *orthostatic changes* (a fall in measured blood pressure with rise in heart rate upon moving from a recumbent to a standing position), then he or she is perfusing adequately and there is no need for any treatment.

○ The converse of this point is that even if blood pressure is normal and large, palpable pulses are good, this does not guarantee that tissue perfusion is good or that nutrient and waste exchange between capillaries and tissues is normal. Even with normal blood pressure and pulses, patients may have bad small-vessel and capillary atherosclerosis or thickened capillary basement membranes that impair tissue perfusion and exchange, respectively. Such small-vessel disease is a common finding in patients with diabetes mellitus — who can also have large-vessel atherosclerosis.

SUMMARY AND REVIEW OF KEY CONCEPTS

1. Acid–base regulation involves instantaneous defense of blood pH by body buffers, including bicarbonate, proteins, and, when necessary, calcium salts released from bone. Volatile acids are subsequently rapidly eliminated (in minutes) by exhaling CO_2. Renal acid excretion occurs more gradually (over hours), involving, in part, elimination of NH_4^+ and regeneration and return of bicarbonate to the bloodstream. The kidney is the only site of elimination of fixed acids, such as phosphoric and sulfuric acids, which are derived largely from protein metabolism.

2. Electrolyte and water distribution across the plasma membrane, and thus intracellular versus extracellular volume, is determined by sodium concentration and the activity of Na^+/K^+-ATPase, with water following the sodium. Hence, renal conservation of sodium and water is a crucial determinant of fluid homeostasis.

3. Intravascular versus extracellular extravascular fluid distribution is determined by the difference between the oncotic pressure and the hydrostatic pressure, with the lymphatic drainage returning to the circulation extracelluler extravascular fluid that was extruded from blood vessels because of an imbalance between these forces.

4. A variety of hormones and their receptors control the actions of the heart, lungs, and kidneys in fluid, electrolyte, acid–base, and blood pressure regulation, including:

   • The renin-angiotensin-aldosterone system (which activates sodium retention by the kidney)
   • The catecholamines (and the sympathetic nervous system, to which they are related)
   • ADH, which triggers distal renal tubular water channel insertion and action in response to osmolar and volume stimuli
   • ANP, which promotes natriuresis by the kidney in response to left atrial stretch

5. In addition to these major hormone systems, there are a host of poorly understood local mediators such as prostaglandins, nitric oxide, and peptides such as endothelins and bradykinin that participate in regulation of renal blood flow and salt and water balance.

6. Appropriate blood volume, vascular compliance, and cardiac efficiency are underlying features necessary for fluid and electrolyte homeostasis. Given adequacy of these features, regulation will be determined by cardiac output (heart rate × stroke volume, stimulated by catecholamines), peripheral resistance (controlled by hormones and sympathetic nervous system tone), and various mechanisms by which the kidneys conserve salt and water.

7. There are a number of classic fluid, electrolyte, and blood pressure dysfunction syndromes that highlight the key features of normal homeostatic mechanism:

   • Metabolic acidosis (either with or without an anion gap), with compensatory respiratory alkalosis
   • Metabolic alkalosis with a compensatory respiratory acidosis
   • Respiratory acidosis, with or without a compensatory metabolic alkalosis, de-

pending on the rapidity of onset (meta-bolic compensation takes a few days)
- Respiratory alkalosis, with or without a compensatory metabolic acidosis, de-pending on the rapidity of onset (meta-bolic compensation takes a few days)

In all cases, the primary disorder can be distinguished because compensation is never complete, leaving a slight shift in blood pH in the direction of the primary abnormality.

- Diabetes insipidus, due to lack of ADH, with large volumes of dilute urine and a risk of hypernatremia and dehydration should the patient fail to maintain wa-ter intake
- Syndrome of inappropriate ADH secre-tion, characterized by hyponatremia, usu-ally without edema, and responsive to free water restriction

A CASE OF PHYSIOLOGICAL MEDICINE

Acid–Base Balance

J.M. is a 32-year-old part-time history student with cystic fibrosis (CF). After a recent exac-erbation of his CF, the patient is now sub-stantially more short of breath than pre-viously. As a result of this debilitating lung disease, he has an arterial blood gas reading of pH = 7.4, P_{CO_2} = 71, P_{O_2} = 61, and HCO_3 = 44 (normal: pH = 7.4, P_{CO_2} = 40, P_{O_2} = 90, HCO_3 = 24).

One concern is that perhaps the high P_{CO_2} has resulted in his brain becoming acclimated to this condition, and since he has metaboli-cally compensated fully, his respiratory drive is being impaired at the same time that he is hypoxic.

As a manuever to increase his respiratory drive, the physicians treat the patient with acetazolamide, a carbonic anhydrase inhibi-tor that will effectively shift the equilibrium in favor of loss of bicarbonate in the urine. As a result, the patient will have a change in his acid–base status that will maximize his respiratory drive. They reason that the more CO_2 he is able to eliminate via his lungs, the more oxygen he will be able to carry, thereby improving his oxygenation and relieving his dyspnea.

Sure enough, 3 days after initiating the acetazolamide therapy, the patient's blood gas reading was found to be pH = 7.28, P_{CO_2} = 61, P_{O_2} = 73, HCO_3 = 29, and the patient was more comfortable, with less dyspnea.

Unfortunately, a day later Mr. M. devel-oped an excruciating headache, a known complication of acetazolamide therapy.

QUESTIONS

1. Characterize the nature of his acid–base disorder at the beginning of the case.
2. How did the acetazolamide therapy change the nature of his acid–base disorder?

ANSWERS

1. Mr. M. has a chronic respiratory acidosis due to carbon dioxide retention, and a compensating metabolic alkalosis with re-tention of bicarbonate.
2. His ability to compensate with a metabolic alkalosis was blocked. The resulting un-compensated respiratory acidosis served as a further stimulus to his respiratory centers to optimize his ventilation.

Fluid, electrolyte, and blood pressure regulation

The patient is an 83-year-old woman who has been caring for herself without help and living alone at home. Two nights ago, she slipped and fell while getting out of the bathtub, hitting her head and losing consciousness briefly. She lay there for nearly 24 h, unable to get up, until she was found by a neighbor, who called paramedics.

On arrival in the emergency room, her blood pressure is 60/40, with a heart rate of 120. Physical exam and x-ray studies reveal a hip fracture and substantial blood loss. ECG and chest x-ray are normal. Electrolytes are notable for a sodium of 155 meq/L (normal is 134 to 144 meq/L) and a potassium of 3.5 meq/L (normal is 3.5 to 4.6 meq/L). Blood urea nitrogen (BUN) is 90 mg/dL (normal is 5 to 15 mg/dL), and creatinine is 2.5 (normal is 0.6 to 1.4), with strongly heme positive urine with no red or white blood cells seen. Apparently, 2 years ago the patient had routine laboratory studies, including all of the above, that were normal.

QUESTIONS

1. Why is the patient hypotensive?
2.a. What endocrine mechanisms normally contribute to regulation of blood pressure and volume homeostasis?
   b. Which of these do you think are likely to have been activated in this patient?
3.a. If separate receptors exist that mediate the antidiuretic and vasoconstrictive effects of vasopressin/antidiuretic hormone, how is it that normally (i.e., in the absence of profound volume depletion), only the osmolar effects are seen?
   b. How come her serum sodium is not *below* normal if she is holding on to free water due to ADH?
   c. Suppose she had had access to free water while on the floor at home. Would her blood pressure be likely to be higher? How else might her blood sodium and potassium values have been different?

4. Can you explain the elevation in BUN and Cr and the "heme positive" urine that had no red blood cells seen?

ANSWERS

1. Blood loss and dehydration. There is no evidence for infection (septic shock) or myocardial infarction (cardiogenic shock) in this history.
2.a. Renin-angiotensin-aldosterone, catecholamines, ADH/vasopressin
   b. All of them.
3.a. The levels of ADH released in response to osmotic stimuli are normally not sufficiently high to occupy the (lower-affinity) vasoconstrictive receptors.
   b. The patient has presumably been unable to take in free water, but has been losing water through insensible losses. The water reclaimed through ADH action minimizes the extent to which she loses water in the urine but does *not* do anything for the insensible losses (e.g., due to evaporation during breathing, etc.). Thus, she was getting inexorably dehydrated lying there on the floor.
   c. Yes, her pressure might be somewhat higher, but it probably would not be up to normal, because she would need to take in *sodium* to preferentially expand her intravascular volume.

   Presumably, if she were taking in free water and holding on to it thanks to ADH, her serum sodium would be lower.

   Furthermore, an increase in GFR due to improved renal perfusion due to a somewhat higher blood pressure might have resulted in more aldosterone-mediated sodium retention, thereby driving her potassium lower than the value in the case as presented.

   However, if she drank enough, GFR might increase sufficiently to shut off renin secretion, therefore generating no more angiotensin II and removing the stimulus for aldosterone secretion, and her potassium would then tend to stay the same.

4. Because of dehydration and blood loss, her blood pressure may have dropped below the level needed to maintain renal perfusion, resulting in so-called prerenal azotemia (elevation of BUN), followed by acute renal tubular necrosis.

Furthermore, crush injury to muscle (which can occur from just lying on a hard surface in one position for a long time) releases myoglobin, which precipitates in the renal tubules, exacerbating the renal tubular necrosis.

The positive test for heme in the urine is due to (1) cross-reactivity of myoglobin with hemoglobin and (2) perhaps some degree of hemolysis with filtration of released hemoglobin in the urine. Never forget that tests that are in widespread use must balance accuracy vs. ease of use versus cost.

From the data presented, it is impossible to know how bad a case of acute tubular necrosis she has. In the hospital, renal obstruction would be ruled out by an ultrasound examination, she would be gently hydrated, and her renal function would be monitored (by measuring the daily change in her serum creatinine). As long as she was still making adequate urine, intravenous hydration could be more vigorous and sodium bicarbonate could be added to the intravenous fluid to alkalinize her urine. This tends to minimize further myoglobin precipitation, and thereby may prevent her renal function from further deterioration by this mechanism. She might need hemodialysis, at least until renal recovery, which might take some weeks — or might not occur at all.

References and suggested reading

1. Rose BD (1994). *Clinical Physiology of Acid-Base and Electrolyte Disorders,* 4th ed. New York, McGraw-Hill.
2. Adrogue HJ, Madias NE (1998). Management of life-threatening acid-base disorders. *New Engl J Med* 338:26–34 (part 1) and 107–111 (part 2).
3. Navar LG (1998). Integrating multiple paracrine regulators of renal microvascular dynamics. *Am J Physiol* 274:F433–444.
4. McManus ML et al. (1995). Mechanisms of Disease: Regulation of cell volume in health and disease. *New Engl J Med* 333:1260–6.
5. Gauthier C et al. (1996). Functional beta 3-adrenoceptor in the human heart. *J Clin Invest* 98:556–562.
6. Seckl JR et al. (1995). Placental 11 beta hydroxysteroid dehydrogenase and the programming of hypertension. *J Steroid Biochem Molec Biol* 55:447–455.
7. Jia L et al. (1996). S-nitrosohaemoglobin: A dynamic activity of blood involved in vascular control. *Nature* 380:221–225.
8. Cowley AW Jr (1997). Genetic and nongenetic determinants of salt sensitivity and blood pressure. *Am J Clin Nutr* 65(suppl):587S–593S.

PHYSIOLOGY OF THE HYPOTHALAMUS AND PITUITARY

11

1. INTRODUCTION TO THE HYPOTHALAMUS AND PITUITARY GLAND

Growth, reproduction, metabolism, and response to stress are examples of intricate physiological processes that are too complex to control with a single set of instructions. There are just too many contingencies ("if this, do that; if something else, do another thing . . .") for these systems to be controlled by a simple "on-and-off" switch.

With the evolution of vertebrate organisms, this problem was solved, in part, by the introduction of new levels of control between the brain and the body, including the **hypothalamus** and the **pituitary gland**. These structures serve as points where competing signals can be integrated, and thus where decisions as to what to do in the short, medium, and long term can be made and modified.

Inputs from many different regions of the brain are interpreted by the hypothalamus, which then instructs the pituitary gland, which then instructs a particular endocrine end organ, which then directs specific changes in the activity of various target tissues. The goal of this system is to make sure that the final outcome is as close to the present needs of the body as possible, while providing a means of modifying output in response to many different variables. Each of these complex cascades of information flow and feedback is termed a **neuroendocrine axis**.

Role in Overall Physiology

The role of the hypothalamus and pituitary gland is:

- To provide **hormones** that control key physiological processes needed for the survival of complex multicellular organisms, including growth, reproduction, metabolism, and response to stress. Hormones are a good way of getting various organ systems involved in a particular physiological process "on the same page" with respect to short-, medium-, and long-term goals, in response to a change in the environment. For example, a high-stress time might not be the best situation in which to raise offspring. So during those times, in response to environmental or physiological cues or to input from higher centers of the brain, the hypothalamus blocks production of key pituitary hormones, and as a result the chances of becoming pregnant are greatly diminished (see Chap. 16).

- To ensure appropriate response to deviations from internal set points governing parameters such as body temperature, energy stores, and osmolality (ionic concentrations in the blood). The hypothalamus monitors these parameters and triggers various forms of timely corrective action as needed to maintain them within an acceptable range, thereby maintaining homeostasis. This is why, for example, when we sense the environment to be cold, our peripheral blood vessels vasoconstrict (minimizing further body heat loss), we shiver (generating more heat), and we have the urge to seek shelter (to get warm).

- To achieve emotions and behaviors that are appropriate for the current physiological plan–integration of the voluntary with the automatic. For example, when you see a tiger chasing you, it is a good thing that you feel scared and have the urge to run away, and that at the same time your heart is racing to maximize your cardiac output toward that goal. Without this, your survival might be in jeopardy.

- To serve as pacemaker for **circadian rhythms**, including sleep-wake cycles, body temperature cycles, and cyclical changes in the magnitude of secretion of various hormones during the course of the day. The **suprachiasmic nuclei (SCN)** is the region of the hypothalamus that generates circadian rhythms, including those involving the hormone **melatonin** from the pineal gland. Inputs from the SCN and other regions are coordinated in the hypothalamus. Disruption of these rhythms is responsible for jet lag, insomnia, and other disturbances that, while not intrinsically life-threatening, can make us miserable.

- To triage competing demands so that the most important things are done first. Otherwise you might be "paralyzed" by contradictory dictates from different parts of your brain. For example, you are not forced to interrupt whatever you are doing to look for a drink of water every time there is a minuscule drop in your blood osmolarity. Instead, via the hypothalamus, the brain is able to first activate renal water conservation measures. These measures delay the time when dehydration is sufficiently severe to interrupt whatever you are doing with the awareness of thirst and the urge to seek water.

Why Is Understanding the Hypothalamus and Pituitary Important for Medicine?

- The hypothalamus and pituitary gland are key links in the chain of command for the physiology of a number of organ systems. Thus, for example, a patient with inadequate adrenal function (see Chap. 13) could, in principle, have a problem either with the adrenal glands, or with the pituitary gland that controls the adrenal glands, or with the cells of the hypothalamus that control the relevant cells in the pituitary gland. You must always remember that end organ failure (such as of the adrenal gland) could be due entirely to disease higher up the chain of command (e.g., in the pituitary gland or hypothalamus). Furthermore, long-standing failure higher up the chain of command,

or long-standing replacement of the final hormone of an endocrine gland that is part of a neuroendocrine axis, often results in atrophy of one or more levels of that particular neuroendocrine axis. This is seen, for example, with chronic steroid therapy in a patient with bad lung disease or rheumatoid arthritis. Neglect of these features of physiological function of the hypothalamus and pituitary gland is occasionally responsible for the unnecessary death of patients, even in the best of hospitals.

- In clinical practice, the output from the pituitary gland is often used as the quickest and cheapest means to determine the functional state of an end organ (e.g., the thyroid gland). However, failure to understand how communication within each of the hypothalamic–pituitary–end organ neuroendocrine axes works can result in a clinician's being fooled into mistaking one problem (e.g., sick euthyroid syndrome) for another (e.g., thyroid failure), where the appropriate treatment for the two conditions are quite different (see Chap. 12).

- Many of the patient's presenting complaints may relate to hypothalamic functions. Thus, pain, fever, and loss or gain of weight are common "nonspecific" complaints and findings in human disease in which the hypothalamus often plays a key role.

- From a practical clinical perspective, a patient's state of mind tremendously influences how he or she thinks and behaves. A patient's perception of illness and the degree to which the illness disrupts the patient's daily life are probably influenced by output from the hypothalamus. This, in turn, affects not only the complaints brought to the health care provider, but also the effectiveness of therapies that might be prescribed. The hypothalamus is at the center of this web, and the hormones of the pituitary gland constitute some of its major forms of output. Failure to consider its role can foil an otherwise effective therapy.

Case Presentation

RB is a 33-year-old woman survivor of a hit-and-run traffic accident in which she received substantial head injuries, including damage to the hypothalamus and pituitary stalk transection. Postrecovery, she has noted a 50-lb weight gain over 6 months, and she is left with a waxing and waning pattern of somnolence, irritability, and emotional lability that was not present prior to the accident. She has been prescribed anterior and posterior pituitary hormone replacement. Twice she has forgotten to take some or all of her hormone replacement medications. Both times she became comatose, with her serum sodium elevated to over 160 meq/L. A third episode of coma 1 month ago was unexplained. A friend found her in bed at home with profound hypothermia and obtundation. A workup for sepsis was negative, and she was back to her baseline condition one day later.

Ms. B has just received a letter in the mail announcing that the insurance company covering her accident-related care is terminating her indemnity coverage and is reassigning her to a managed care plan. This means that the funds that have paid for her dozen prescription drugs and a visiting nurse to monitor her care three times a week since her last hospitalization are no longer available. She will now be allowed a maximum of four prescriptions a month. Instead of being called on by the visiting nurse, she will be mailed two bus vouchers per month to go to the clinic. Instead of being allowed to see her regular doctor as needed, she is being assigned to a for-profit HMO with a record of being primarily interested in enrolling healthy patients.

She wishes to appeal these changes in her health insurance coverage, and she turns to you for help in explaining to her insurance company representative why she needs each of her hormone replacement medications. She also needs help in making a convincing argument as to why she needs closer medical supervision than the new program allows.

Clinical Pearls

○ Recognizing the role of the hypothalamus in perception can help us care for the patient whose behavior is challenging with greater compassion. Often, a more sympathetic manner on the part of the health care provider can itself be therapeutic for a patient who is frustrated and demoralized, perhaps because previous providers expressed skepticism as to whether the symptoms were "real" or really "that bad." In the not-too-distant future it may actually be possible to alter hypothalamic output in ways that make it easier for patients to lose weight, live with chronic pain, control their emotions, and otherwise improve the quality of their lives. Until then, it helps to be aware of why different people with the same illness might be more or less miserable. Helping the patient to change his or her perception of the symptoms may be the most effective course of action in the meantime.

○ Sometimes health care providers are lulled into underestimating the severity of an illness because the patient is stoic, suffering in relative silence. Sometimes, just the opposite occurs. An extremely histrionic patient who "cries wolf" regularly may be ignored early in an acute, new disease process, costing valuable time and possibly leading to a medical catastrophe that could have been avoided had their symptoms been taken more seriously. Both of these are examples of how the hypothalamus greatly complicates the interaction of patients with their health care providers—and makes it unlikely that perceptive clinicians will be replaced by computers any time soon.

Review Questions

1. What is the role of the hypothalamic-pituitary unit in the overall scheme of body physiology?
2. Why might the same objective amount of pain manifest differently in two individuals?

2. ANATOMY AND HISTOLOGY OF THE HYPOTHALAMUS AND PITUITARY GLAND

Hypothalamus

The hypothalamus is a remarkably small, poorly demarcated area in the floor of the third ventricle that comprises less than 1% of the area of the brain (Figure 11.1). It is contiguous with the pituitary gland, to which it is structurally and functionally connected. The special structural relationship of the hypothalamus to the pituitary can be appreciated by a consideration of their embryologic origins (see Figure 11.2).

The hypothalmus is one of the few areas of the brain that is not sealed off from the body by tight junctions between the endothelial cells of its blood vessels. Thus, whereas most areas of the brain get only small-molecule nutrients such as glucose from the bloodstream, the hypothalamus can monitor and respond to higher-molecular-weight substances, such as hormones and cytokines. This feature allows the hypothalamus to play the role of regulator of various body processes, such as temperature and feeding, that respond to proteins produced elsewhere in the body (see the following).

Viewed anteriorly to posteriorly (see Figure 11.3 and Table 11.1):

- The anterior third of the hypothalamus, containing the so-called anterior hypothalamic and preoptic areas, is involved in integration of fluid-electrolyte, thermoregulatory, and nonendocrine reproductive functions.
- The middle third of the hypothalamus (behind the anterior third) contains nuclei responsible for the endocrine and autonomic regulatory mechanisms and gives rise to the pituitary stalk.
- The posterior third of the hypothalamus, including the mamillary body (whose function is unknown), contains posterior, lateral, and premamillary nuclei involved in thermoregulatory and emergency response integration.

The above functional "map" of the hypothalamus presents the broad brush stroke, but is not to be taken as absolute. For example, thyrotropin-releasing hormone (TRH) is made in neurons of nuclei in different parts of the hypothalamus, probably serving different functions in each case (see below).

Review Questions

3. What is the role of the medial zone of the hypothalamus?
4. Where in the hypothalamus are thermoregulatory and fluid and electrolyte homeostasis integrated?

Clinical Pearls

○ Because the hypothalamus is such a small and poorly demarcated structure, hypothalamic disease (e.g., a tumor) often has a distinctive presentation as a disorder of

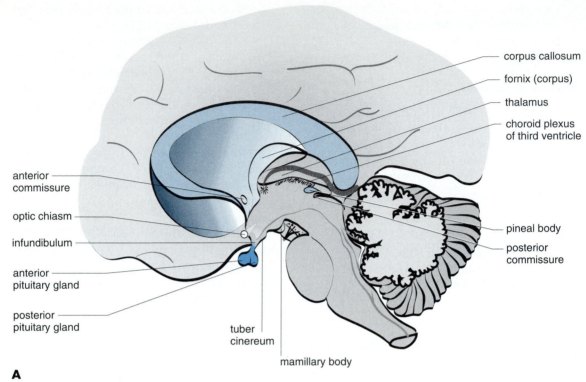

A

FIGURE 11.1. *A.* Sagittal section through the brain, showing the hypothalamus and surrounding structures.

one of the surrounding structures (see Figure 11.4). Thus:

- Headaches can occur as a result of stretch of the dura.
- Upward impingement on the optic chiasm can produce visual field defects, classically including homonymous hemianopsia.
- Forward impingement on the cavernous and sphenoid sinuses can result in blood clots and strokes.
- Sideward impingement can result in cranial nerve palsies.
- Erosion or trauma resulting in a connection between the third ventricle and the pharynx can result in a cerebrospinal fluid (CSF) leak presenting as "postnasal drip."

○ Cells secreting gonadotropin-releasing hormone (GnRH) originate embryologically in the olfactory placode and migrate into the hypothalamus. Thus the defect in the entity known as Kallman syndrome combines loss of smell with infertility.

Anterior Pituitary

The pituitary gland consists of two functionally and embryologically distinct parts (Figures 11.2 and 11.3). The **anterior lobe** contains discrete populations of cells, each

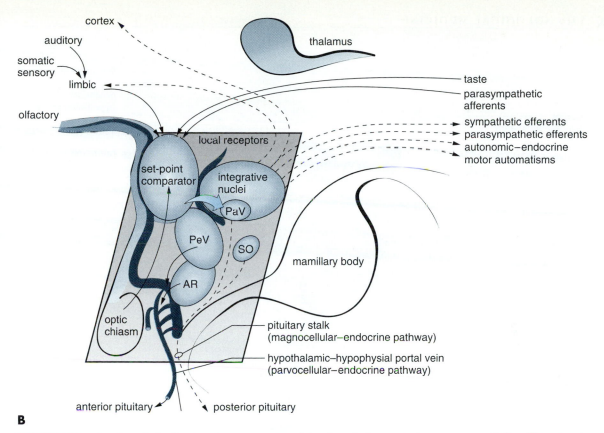

B

FIGURE 11.1 — *(continued)* B. Functional organization of the hypothalamus, indicating some of the afferent and efferent pathways. SO = supraoptic nucleus; AR = arcuate nucleus; PeV = periventricular nucleus; PaV = paraventricular nucleus. *(B adapted, with permission, from Saper CB, in Pearlman AL, Collins RC (eds):* Neurobiology of Disease. *New York, NY, Oxford University Press, 1990.)*

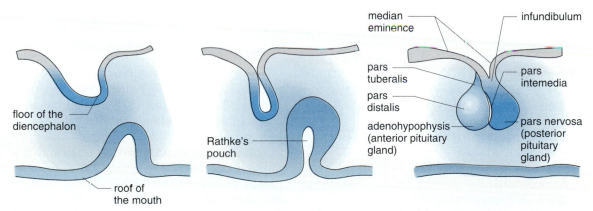

FIGURE 11.2. Embryology of the hypothalamus and pituitary gland. Diagram of the development of the anterior and posterior pituitary gland, indicating how the anterior pituitary is derived from the ectoderm of the roof of the mouth, while the posterior pituitary is an extension of neural ectoderm from the floor of the diencephalon. *(Adapted, with permission, from Junqueira LC, et al.,* Basic Histology, *8th ed. Norwalk, CT: Appleton & Lange, 1995.)*

517

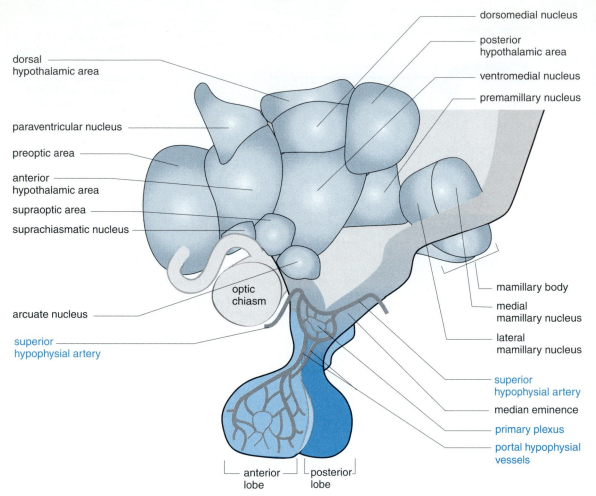

dorsal hypothalamic area

paraventricular nucleus

preoptic area

anterior hypothalamic area

supraoptic area

suprachiasmatic nucleus

arcuate nucleus

superior hypophysial artery

dorsomedial nucleus

posterior hypothalamic area

ventromedial nucleus

premamillary nucleus

optic chiasm

mamillary body

medial mamillary nucleus

lateral mamillary nucleus

superior hypophysial artery

median eminence

primary plexus

portal hypophysial vessels

anterior lobe

posterior lobe

FIGURE 11.3. Another view of the organization of the hypothalamus.

uniquely involved in the synthesis and secretion of a particular polypeptide hormone, including

- Growth hormone (GH), also called somatotropin
- Prolactin
- Adrenocorticotropic hormone (ACTH), also called corticotropin
- Luteinizing hormone (LH) and follicle-stimulating hormone (FSH)
- Thyroid-stimulating hormone (TSH), also called thyrotropin

The anterior pituitary has a rich blood supply, and its cells are bathed by a peculiar venous drainage from the hypothalamus termed the **hypothalamic-pituitary portal system** (see Figure 11.5A). This vascular arrangement is derived from the superior hypophyseal artery and consists of a **primary plexus** of capillaries formed in the median eminence which then flows via portal veins to the anterior pituitary. There, another capillary network termed the **secondary plexus** is formed and drains into the systemic venous circulation.

TABLE 11.1 FUNCTIONS OF HYPOTHALAMIC NUCLEI

Hypothalamic Region	Location and Description	Function
Periventricular zone	Most medial part of the hypothalamus; adjacent to third ventricle	Production of releasing factors for anterior pituitary hormones
Paraventricular and supraoptic nuclei	Medial zone (just lateral to periventricular zone)	Production of oxytocin and vasopressin stored in posterior pituitary
Medial preoptic nucleus, dorsomedial, ventromedial, premamillary, anterior and posterior hypothalamic nuclei	Medial zone	Controlling behavior for homeostasis
Medial forebrain bundle	Lateral zone tracts	Connect cells of the hypothalamic nuclei to both the brain stem and the forebrain
Anterior hypothalamic and preoptic areas	Anterior third of the hypothalamus	Integration of fluid and electrolyte, thermoregulatory, and nonendocrine reproductive functions
Tuberal region	Middle third of hypothalamus just posterior to the anterior area; gives rise to the pituitary stalk	Contain nuclei responsible for the endocrine and autonomic regulatory mechanisms and integration of energy, metabolic, and reproductive responses
Posterior, lateral, and premamillary nuclei	Posterior third of the hypothalamus	Involved in thermoregulatory and emergency response integration

Reproduced, with permission, from Saper, C.B.: Hypothalamus. In: *Neurobiology of Disease.* Pearlman AL, Collins, R.C. (eds). New York, NY: Oxford Univ. Press, 1990.

This organization of blood supply is crucial for the function of the anterior lobe, since it allows tiny amounts of short-lived peptides released from the hypothalamus (into the primary plexus) to rapidly reach the cells of the anterior pituitary (via the secondary plexus) without dilution into the systemic circulation. These hypothalamic peptides control secretion of the anterior pituitary hormones (see Table 11.2).

Generally, a given anterior pituitary cell is specialized for synthesis and secretion of a particular polypeptide hormone. It also usually has receptors for the appropriate hypothalamic releasing factor. Activation of those receptors by hypothalamic hormone binding triggers hormone synthesis and release. Thus, separate populations of cells within the anterior pituitary can be identified as **somatotrophs, lactotrophs, corticotrophs, gonadotrophs,** and **thyrotrophs**. Particular lesions may affect secretion by one subpopulation of cells more than another. The venous drainage from the anterior pituitary flows into the systemic circulation, carrying the anterior pituitary hormones to their specific target organs (see Figure 11.5A).

Clinical Pearl

○ Because hypothalamic hormones are released into the pituitary portal circulation, their concentrations are relatively high when they reach their target cells in the anterior pituitary. This allows them to occupy sufficient receptors to have an effect, despite their relatively low affinity for their receptors. Conversely, the dilution into systemic circulation lowers the concentration, so that they do *not* have effects on the periphery even if their receptors are present, because their concentrations are now too low to occupy sufficient numbers of receptors, given their low affinity. Thus, the body may be able to use peripheral receptors for various hypothalamic peptides to serve other functions. This would be triggered by local paracrine production of the same peptides without the two systems getting in each other's way. This may account for why corticotropin-releasing hormone (CRH), a hypothalamic peptide that releases ACTH from the anterior pituitary, is also found as a product synthesized locally in the endometrium of the uterus (see Chap. 16), or why somatostatin, a hypothalamic peptide that inhibits growth hormone secretion, is also found in the brain, the GI tract, and elsewhere (see Chaps. 5 and 6). However, it also means that pharmacologic use of these products, typically at far higher concentrations in the peripheral bloodstream than would occur physiologically, runs the risk of unintended consequences. Some of these side effects may occur on a very different time scale from the intended consequence of treatment with the hormone.

Posterior Pituitary

The **posterior pituitary** is composed of neurons whose cell bodies lie in the paraventricular and supraoptic nuclei of the hypothalamus. Thus the posterior pituitary is, literally, a part of the brain. These peptides, **oxytocin** and **vasopressin** [also called antidiuretic hormone (ADH)], are synthesized as larger precursors. The precursor proteins are cleaved to generate the hormone, which is packaged into granules and transported down the axons from the hypothalamus to terminals in the posterior pituitary. These terminals abut along a capillary bed that feeds directly into

headaches

a) stretching of dura by tumor

b) hydrocephalus (rare)

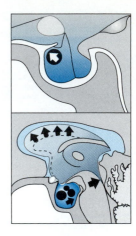

visual field defects

c) nasal retinal fibers compressed by tumor

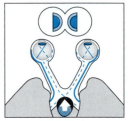

cranial nerve palsies and temporal lobe epilepsy

d) lateral extension of tumor

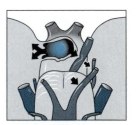

cerebrospinal fluid rhinorrhea

e) downward extension of tumor

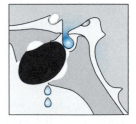

A

FIGURE 11.4. A. Various symptoms of a pituitary tumor. Arrows indicate location of the tumor and direction of its local invasion of surrounding tissues. Visual field defects shown in third panel from top are plotted with the Goldmann perimeter.

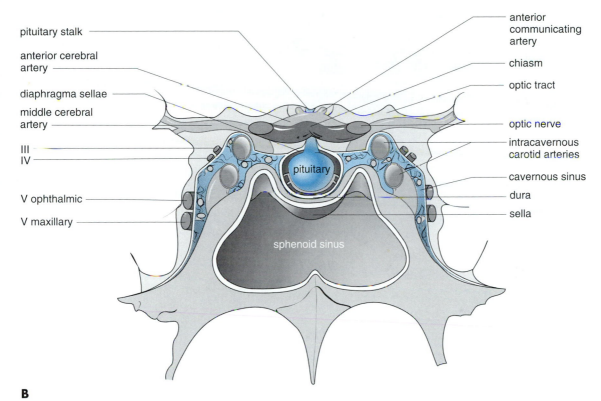

B

FIGURE 11.4 — (continued) B. Structures around the hypothalamus and pituitary gland. Indicated are the relationship between the pituitary gland and the cranial nerves and cavernous sinus as seen in coronal section through the pituitary. (A. Adapted, with permission, from Wass JAH, Hypopituitarism, in Clinical Endocrinology: An Illustrated Text, Gower, 1987. B. Adapted, with permission, from Taren JA, in Schneider et al. (eds), Correlative Neurosurgery, 3d ed. Springfield, IL, Charles C Thomas, 1982.)

the systemic circulation, unlike the portal system that serves the anterior pituitary circuit. Upon neural stimulation of the hypothalamus, these peptides are released into the bloodstream (see Figure 11.5B).

Anterior and posterior pituitary hormone secretion is regulated by various stimuli from both the brain and the environment, but in somewhat different ways.

The mechanism of regulation from the brain is usually by altering the inputs to the hypothalamus. This alters the rate or amount of hypothalamic hormone secreted which in turn have their effects on hormones from the anterior lobe. For posterior pituitary hormones, which are made in hypothalamic neurons, brain inputs affect secretion directly.

Regulation from the environment in the case of anterior pituitary hormones includes feedback inhibition by the end organ hormone. In the case of posterior pituitary hormones, often the autonomic nervous system transmits signals back to the brain that alter the inputs to the hypothalamus.

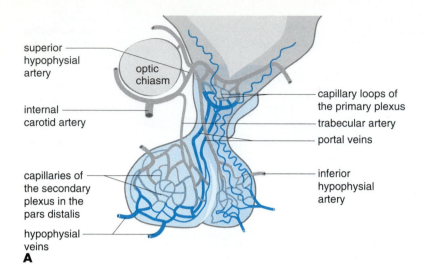

superior hypophysial artery

optic chiasm

internal carotid artery

capillaries of the secondary plexus in the pars distalis

hypophysial veins

A

capillary loops of the primary plexus

trabecular artery

portal veins

inferior hypophysial artery

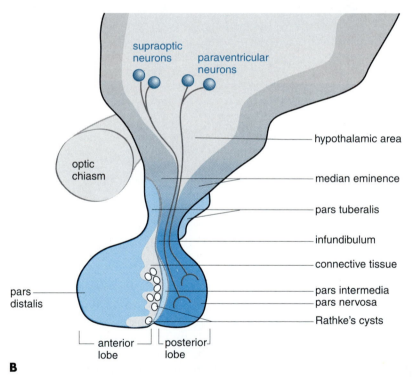

supraoptic neurons

paraventricular neurons

optic chiasm

pars distalis

anterior lobe

posterior lobe

B

hypothalamic area

median eminence

pars tuberalis

infundibulum

connective tissue

pars intermedia
pars nervosa

Rathke's cysts

FIGURE 11.5. *A.* Anatomy of and blood supply to the pituitary gland. Blood flow from the arterial system enters the primary venous plexus in the hypothalamus and drains into the portal vein, which then breaks up into the secondary plexus of the pituitary portal system in the anterior lobe, which drains into the hypophysial veins and returns to the systemic venous circulation. *B.* The component parts of the pituitary gland and their relationship to the hypothalamus. Note that neurons of the paraventricular and supraoptic nuclei of the hypothalamus extend into the posterior pituitary. *(Adapted, with permission, from the Ciba Collection of Medical Illustrations by Frank H. Netter, M.D.)*

TABLE 11.2   STRUCTURE OF HYPOTHALAMIC RELEASING FACTORS IN HUMANS

TRH	(pyro)Glu-His-Pro-NH$_2$
GnRH	(pyro)Glu-His-Trp-Ser-Tyr-Gly-Leu-Arg-Pro-Gly-NH$_2$
Somatostatin	Ala-Gly-Cys-Lys-Asn-Phe-Phe-Trp-Lys-Thr-Phe-Thr-Ser-Cys
CRH	Ser-Glu-Glu-Pro-Pro-Ile-Ser-Leu-Asp-Leu-Thr-Phe-His-Leu-Leu-Arg-Glu-Val-Leu-Glu-Met-Ala-Arg-Ala-Glu-Gln-Leu-Ala-Gln-Gln-Ala-His-Ser-Asn-Arg-Lys-Leu-Met-Glu-Ile-Ile-NH$_2$
GHRH	Tyr-Ala-Asp-Ala-Ile-Phe-Thr Asn-Ser-Tyr-Arg-Lys-Val-Leu-Gly-Gln-Leu-Ser-Ala-Arg-Lys-Leu-Leu-Gln-Asp-Ile-Met-Ser-Arg-Gln-Gln-Gly-Glu-Ser-Asn-Gln-Glu-Arg-Gly-Ala-Arg-Ala-Arg-Leu-NH$_2$
PIF	Dopamine

For the Somatostatin row, a disulfide bridge (S—S) connects the two Cys residues.

Preprosomatostatin is processed to a 14-amino-acid peptide and also to a 28-amino-acid residue polypeptide.
Reproduced with permission from Ganong WF, *Review of Medical Physiology*, 19th ed. Stamford, CT: Appleton & Lange, 1998.

Like all hormones, those of the anterior and posterior pituitary carry out their actions by binding to specific receptor proteins on the surface of hormone-responsive cells. This binding is transduced in diverse ways (discussed in Chap. 3) to generate tissue-specific effects.

Review Questions

5. What are the major hormones secreted by the anterior pituitary gland?
6. Where do the neurons whose axons comprise the substance of the posterior pituitary originate?

3. FUNCTIONAL ORGANIZATION OF THE HYPOTHALAMUS AND PITUITARY

The characteristic functional programs of the hypothalamus involve integrative functions that interface the central and peripheral nervous systems and neuroendocrine feedback loops that control the secretion of pituitary hormones.

Integrative Functions

The neurons of the hypothalamus have a bewildering array of connections to other parts of the brain. These include connections that (i) inform the brain of the status of certain homeostatic parameters, (ii) interface with the brain to determine the appropriate response, and (iii) inform the body exactly what has been decided and what it is to do. Thus the hypothalamus integrates the voluntary and involuntary actions, so that:

• In survival-threatening situations, we get scared, develop a fast heart rate, and have the impulse to run away.
• In a low-temperature environment, we feel cold, start shivering, and have an impulse to look for appropriate shelter.
• When we get dehydrated, we develop a dry mouth, feel thirsty, and look for something to drink.

Neuroendocrine Feedback Loops

The hypothalamus has a characteristic molecular mechanism by which it maintains the hierarchy of command and control from brain to hypothalamus to pituitary to endocrine gland to end organ or target tissue and back again. These **neuroendocrine feedback loops** allow the brain (via neurotransmitters) to interface with the body (via hormones) in a way that is optimized for both flexibility and speed. Neuroendocrine feedback loops occur in two general forms (see Figure 11.6).

Neuroendocrine feedback loops involving the anterior pituitary

These neuroendocrine feedback loops comprise a cascade of hormones that trigger other hormones, which trigger still other hormones. As previously discussed, hypothalamic releasing factors travel via the pituitary portal blood flow to the nearby anterior pituitary. There, the releasing factors trigger the specific anterior pituitary cells that have receptors for a particular releasing factor to secrete other, longer-lived hormones, which travel into the systemic circulation.

Once in the peripheral circulation, the anterior pituitary hormones bind to and activate receptors on specific peripheral end organ endocrine glands (e.g., the thyroid, the adrenal, the gonads, and the liver) to secrete yet other hormones. These hormones, in turn, activate receptors on various *target tissues* that maintain various differentiated functions. In addition to their effects on target tissues, the hormones secreted into the bloodstream by the peripheral endocrine glands feed back to the hypothalamus and pituitary gland and turn off the stimuli that initiated the cascade of secretion.

In addition to the "long" feedback loops by which the final hormone in a cascade shuts off secretion of the hormones of the earlier steps in the axis, there is evidence for "short" feedback loops in which hypothalamic or pituitary hormones feed back to inhibit the stimulus for their own secretion (see Figure 11.6).

The crucial role of the hypothalamus lies in its interface with the rest of the brain. Thus, neurotransmitters released at the hypothalamus from neurons arising in various parts of the brain can greatly influence the sensitivity and magnitude of the responses that constitute these hormonal feedback loops. Conversely, changes in the body, reflected in the neuroendocrine feedback loop, can be communicated back to the brain by the hypothalamus. In these ways, the body responds to the brain, and vice versa.

Four different anterior pituitary neuroendocrine feedback loops are well described. They are involved in the control of

1. Development and metabolism: TRH, thyrotropin (TSH), and thyroid hormone (see Chap. 12).
2. The response to stress: CRH, ACTH, and cortisol (see Chap. 13).
3. Growth: Growth hormone–releasing hormone (GHRH), GH, insulin-like growth factor (IGF-1), and somatostatin.
4. Reproduction: GnRH, LH, FSH, and estradiol/testosterone (see Chaps. 15 and 16).

Neuroendocrine feedback loops involving the posterior pituitary

There are two additional neuroendocrine feedback loops that do not involve hypothalamic releasing factors acting via the pituitary portal blood flow. In these two cases, the hormone is released directly into the systemic circulation from the posterior pituitary, as discussed above.

One involves the peptide hormone **vasopressin** (also known as ADH). A region of the hypothalamus senses a rise in blood osmolality (e.g., due to dehydration) and triggers release of ADH, which retains water from the renal tubule (see Chap. 9), thereby correcting the rise in osmolality and shutting off further ADH secretion. At the same time, the hypothalamus sends a signal to other

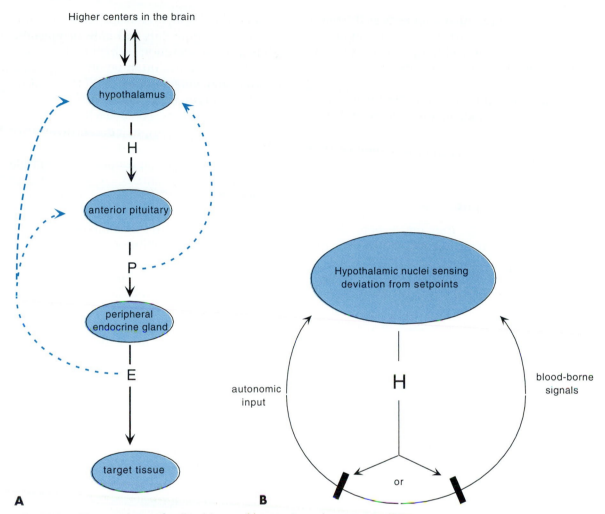

FIGURE 11.6. Neuroendocrine feedback loops of the anterior and posterior pituitary.
A. Anterior pituitary feedback loops involve secretion from the hypothalamus into
the pituitary portal blood flow to the anterior pituitary, triggering release of products
into the systemic circulation; when these products reach the peripheral endocrine
glands, they trigger secretion of hormones that affect peripheral target tissues as
well as feed back onto the hypothalamus and pituitary to inhibit further secretion.
B. Posterior pituitary feedback loops sense either deviations from set points by
specific nuclei in the hypothalamus (e.g., as in the case of osmoregulation; see
Chap. 10) or stimulation from afferent neural pathways arising in peripheral tissues
(e.g., in the case of volume depletion or nipple stimulation in the suckling reflex;
see Chap. 17). These receptors in turn trigger secretion of hormones from neurons
in specific hypothalamic nuclei whose terminals comprise the posterior pituitary
gland. These products flow directly into the systemic circulation, where they bind
to receptors that relieve the initial stimulus for hormone secretion.

parts of the brain that manifests as the sensation of thirst and triggers water-seeking behavior. This feedback loop is most sensitive to osmolality, but also responds to large changes in volume (see Chap. 10).

The other posterior pituitary neuroendocrine feedback loop involves the peptide hormone **oxytocin** and controls specialized muscles involved in childbirth and milk ejection during breast feeding (see Chap. 17).

Review Questions

7. What are the four major neuroendocrine feedback loops of the anterior pituitary?
8. What are the two major neuroendocrine feedback loops of the posterior pituitary?
9. Contrast the neuroendocrine feedback loops of the anterior and posterior pituitary.

4. BIOSYNTHESIS AND PROCESSING OF HYPOTHALAMIC RELEASING FACTORS AND PITUITARY HORMONES

Most of the hypothalamic and pituitary hormones are polypeptides exported out of specific cells through the secretory pathway. Thus, they share with the secretory proteins of all other tissues universal features, including synthesis on membrane-bound ribosomes of the endoplasmic reticulum (ER), translocation across that membrane into the ER lumen, and trafficking by vesicle fission and fusion through the compartments of the secretory pathway. Ultimately, they are packaged in secretory vesicles that can condense into granules and are released outside of the cell upon fusion of the granule to the plasma membrane, upon specific stimuli for secretion (see Chap. 3).

Secretion of hypothalamic and pituitary hormones is generally **pulsatile** or **episodic**. Thus, proper secretion of hypothalamic and pituitary hormones often involves a particular *rate* and *magnitude* of secretory pulses, and is different at different times or under different conditions. Too much hormone may result in downregulation or desensitization of receptors on a target cell. Too little hormone may not trigger the appropriate magnitude of response (see Chap. 3).

The one well-characterized non-peptide released from the hypothalamus to affect the anterior pituitary is **dopamine**, which serves as a tonic inhibitor of prolactin secretion.

All of the pituitary hormones are proteins or peptides derived from larger proteins:

• GH and prolactin are nonglycosylated single-subunit proteins whose only posttranslational processing is the removal of the signal sequence for translocation into the ER lumen.
• LH, FSH, and TSH each consist of two glycosylated subunits. The alpha subunit is identical among all three of these hormones. Biologic specificity (recognition of one receptor rather than another) in this family is conferred by the beta subunit, which is different in each case.
• Several pituitary hormones are generated by cleavage of a single large precursor called proopiomelanocortin (POMC, see Figure 11.7). ACTH, melanocyte-stimulating hormone (MSH), and endorphin are examples of biologically active peptides generated from this single precursor.

Histologically, the subtypes of endocrine cells involved in secretion of different hormones stain differently with PAS/orange G stain. Prolactin and growth hormone secreting cells, termed acidophils, stain green. LH, FSH, TSH, and ACTH secreting cells, termed basophils, stain pink, while other cells with

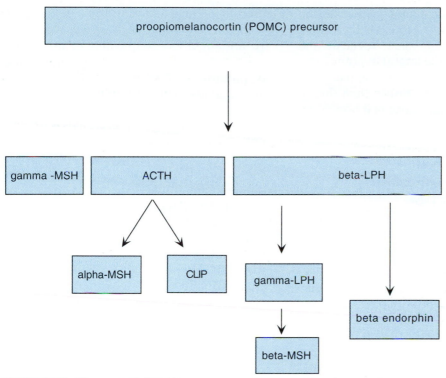

FIGURE 11.7. Cleavage of POMC into various active peptides. A single large precursor protein, proopiomelanocortin, synthesized in specific cells of the anterior pituitary, is processed into a variety of active peptides, which are secreted. These cleavage events may themselves be regulated, to some extent, in a cell-specific manner. MSH = melanocyte stimulating hormone; LPH = lipotropin; CLIP = fragment of ACTH. *(From Speroff L, et al., Clinical Gynecologic Endocrinology and Infertility, 5th ed. Baltimore, MD: Williams & Wilkins, 1994.)*

little visible cytoplasm are termed chromophobes. The biologic functions of many of these hormones will be discussed in subsequent chapters. Alternative pathways of precursor cleavage may generate additional hormones whose functions we as yet know nothing about.

Review Questions

10. What is the biosynthetic relationship of ACTH to β-endorphin?
11. What is a similarity in biosynthesis and structure of LH, FSH, and TSH?

5. ROLE OF THE HYPOTHALAMUS AND PITUITARY IN CENTRAL CONTROL OVER ENDOCRINE GLANDS

In addition to their role in control of neuroendocrine feedback loops of the anterior and posterior pituitary and in thermoregulation, the ventromedial nuclei and lateral hypothalamic area play an important role in satiety and hunger, respectively. Thus, destruction of the ventromedial nuclei results in hyperphagia and weight gain. Similar effects are seen upon excess stimulation of the lateral hypothalamic area. Conversely, destruction of the lateral hypothalamus can result in aphagia (a lack of desire to eat). This effect can be severe enough to cause cachexia and death. The effects of the lateral hypothalamic lesions are believed likely to be on pathways passing through the area rather than due to destruction of neurons whose cell bodies actually reside there.

6. CLINICAL ASSESSMENT OF HYPOTHALAMIC AND PITUITARY FUNCTION

Knowledge of the neuroendocrine feedback loops is important not only for an understanding of how these systems work, but also in order to clinically assess and treat specific disorders. As a general rule, a partial or complete lesion at any given step of a neuroendocrine feedback loop (with the brain defined as the top step and the end organ/target tissue as the bottom step) results in a correspondingly partial or complete loss in secretion of hormones at all lower steps. At the same time, it results in elevation of the level of hormones at all higher steps (see Figure 11.6). This makes teleologic sense, since the lower steps are no longer being stimulated and the higher steps are therefore no longer getting feedback, and so they are frantically trying to trigger secretion of the missing hormone. Similarly, an excess of hormone secreted at a given step of the axis will result in suppression at all higher steps in the axis and an excess of hormone secreted at all lower steps of the feedback loop, for exactly the opposite reasons.

However, simple measurement of peripheral blood levels of hormones can be misleading for the assessment of neuroendocrine feedback loops, because:

- Hypothalamic hormones are extremely short-lived and may not be detectable in the peripheral circulation, even if they were present at high concentration in the pituitary portal circulation.
- A random blood sample may be taken during a "peak" or "valley" in the time course of pulsatile or episodic secretion, giving a misleadingly high or low blood value for the hormone. Thus, a more reliable approach in assessing a neuroendocrine axis is to carry out a **provocative test**: Administration of a stimulus to hormone secretion will result in a measurable burst of its release into the bloodstream—unless there has been a lesion of that gland.
- Some cells (e.g., gonadotrophs) are very sensitive to the particular pulsatile pattern of stimulation they receive (e.g., by GnRH from the hypothalamus). Thus, too much stimulation results in downregulation of the GnRH receptors and shutdown of gonadotrophin secretion. Note that this is the same final outcome as would occur with no GnRH secretion except that GnRH receptors on gonadotropes would likely be upregulated in that case.
- Many hypothalamic and pituitary hormones are trophic for their target tissues, meaning that in addition to stimulating hormone secretion, they are required to maintain the health of their targets. Thus, lack of a hypothalamic or pituitary hormone not only results in an immediate deficit in secretion, it reduces the "secretory reserve" that could be called upon in special circumstances as the cells undergo atrophy. Conversely, excessive stimulation will often (at least initially) result in hypertrophy of the target gland, as well as excessive secretion of the target gland's hormone.

Clinical Pearls

○ During pregnancy, the lactotrophs increase from comprising 15% of the weight of the anterior pituitary gland to about 70% exogenous in anticipation of the need for prolactin to support postpartum milk synthesis. So, before concluding that a patient (presenting, for example with headaches, and noted on head CT scan to have an enlarged pituitary) has a brain tumor . . . check to make sure she is not just pregnant!

○ Patients who require prolonged treatment with glucocorticoids (e.g., patients with severe reactive airway disease or autoimmune disorders) develop adrenal atrophy because the CRH-ACTH-cortisol neuroendocrine axis has been shut down. The exogenous glucocorticoids inhibit the hypothalamus and pituitary, preventing release of ACTH, which, in addition to being needed for endogenous adrenal corticosteroid production, is crucial for maintenance of the adrenal cortex. The process of weaning these patients off glucocorticoids can be difficult, slow, and subject to frequent setbacks—every time they are under stress (e.g., infection or trauma), they need to take additional "stress dose" glucocorticoids to make up for what their atrophied adrenals are unable to provide. But that further delays the progress of their adrenal recovery.

Review Questions

12. What regions of the hypothalamus control satiety and hunger?
13. What are four potential pitfalls in assessment of neuroendocrine feedback loops?

7. NORMAL THERMOGENESIS AND THE ENDOCRINOLOGY OF FEVER

Normal Thermogenesis

Homeotherms are those organisms, including mammals such as ourselves, that, unlike reptiles, amphibians, and fish, regulate their core body temperature. Metabolism always generates heat because no process of either work or moving energy from one chemical form to another occurs with 100% efficiency. A substantial amount of energy (about 20–40% generally) gets dissipated as heat. Homeotherms have taken advantage of this "fact of life" and put it to good use by evolving enzymes and other mechanisms whose sophistication *requires* that the temperature be kept in a narrow range most of the time. Thus the "waste" heat of metabolism contributes to making our more complex metabolism possible (see Figure 11.8).

The anterior hypothalamus contains the **thermostat** that sets the core body temperature to be maintained. The heat generated by metabolism is dissipated by vasodilation and sweating when heat generation is in excess of what is needed to maintain core body temperature. Vasoconstriction is used to conserve heat when the environment is somewhat colder than the body. Sometimes, however, the heat needed to maintain a constant body temperature exceeds that which is a "free" byproduct of metabolism. In these cases, other mechanisms are used to augment heat generation:

• In situations where the environment is much colder than the body, shivering increases muscle contraction and with it heat generation.
• Another mechanism is through the action of so-called **uncoupling proteins**. Recall that most usable chemical energy in most eukaryotic cells is generated by "burning" food fuels in mitochondria. That process involves controlled release of stored chemcial energy (e.g., from glucose) and reharnessing a substantial part of the released energy in a different chemical form (e.g., as ATP, see Chaps. 1 and 2). As an intermediate between the two forms of chemical energy (starting foodstuffs versus ATP generated),

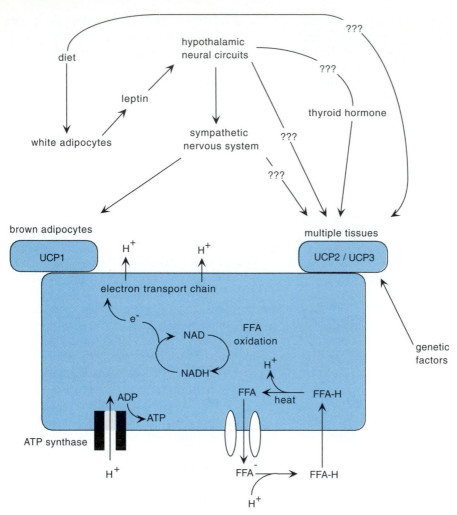

FIGURE 11.8. Pathways of normal thermogenesis. This indicates how uncoupling proteins can serve as a final common pathway for responding to various signals, including leptin levels, the sympathetic nervous system, and thyroid hormone, resulting in an integrated response to the energy, heat, and oxygen status of the cell. (Adapted, with permission, from Fleury et al. (1997). Uncoupling protein-2: a novel gene linked to obesity and hyperinsulinemia. Nat. Genet. 15:269–272.)

the energy is stored as potential energy in a hydrogen ion gradient formed across the inner mitochondrial membrane. Uncoupling proteins dissipate the potential energy in the hydrogen ion gradient as heat, before it can be recaptured in chemical form by making ATP through the process of oxidative phosphorylation. The best-studied example of uncoupling protein action occurs in brown fat in rodents and neonates. Recently, additional members of this family of proteins have been identified (see Sec. 10).

• A third mechanism of heat generation is through **futile cycles**. These are offsetting metabolic pathways that produce and consume energy while moving substrates in opposite directions, such that the sole net consequence of their action is the generation of heat. An example is running a molecule of glucose through glucolysis and then right away turning around and running the end products back through gluconeogenesis. You end up with what you started with (one molecule of glucose), but a substantial amount of energy is dissipated as heat—"paid for" by the utilization of other molecules of ATP within the cell to carry out those enzymatic pathways.

These mechanisms of normal thermogenesis involving general metabolism, uncoupling proteins, and futile cycles are affected by thyroid hormone (see Chap. 12), which integrates all of these pathways at any given set point of the hypothalamic thermostat.

Fever

In contrast to normal thermogenesis, **fever** is a condition in which the thermostat within the hypothalamus is reset to a higher level. All the same mechanisms of heat generation and conservation still apply, but this time they are defending a higher core body temperature. The most common trigger of fever is infection, but fever can also be seen as a host's reaction to certain drugs, hemorrhage, **thrombophlebitis** (blood clots), cancer, trauma, and a variety of immunologic disorders (see Chap. 19).

Fever is a complex, integrated physiological response that is part of the so-called **acute-phase reaction** to immune challenge (see Ref. 1). It involves autonomic, neuroendocrine, and behavioral changes in conjunction with a resetting of the hypothalamic thermostat that regulates body temperature. The goal of these changes can be thought of as creating an internal environment that is inhospitable to an invader. For example, anorexia (loss of appetite) minimizes blood glucose that an invader could have used just as easily as could the host and stimulates lipolysis and proteolysis-based metabolism. Likewise, slightly elevated temperature is believed to improve the efficiency of killing invading bacteria by macrophages and to impair microbial replication.

Fever is initiated by the release of *endogenous pyrogens*. Some of these endogenous pyrogens are actually **cytokines**, such as interleukin-1 and interleukin-6, tumor necrosis factor, and interferons α and β. However, not all cytokines are endogenous pyrogens. Interleukin-1 β is an example of an endogenous pyrogen released by macrophages that are activated by invading infectious organisms such as bacterial pathogens.

Prostaglandins are released by endothelial cells and/or neurons, in response to endogenous pyrogens. The prostaglandins enter the neurons of the anterior hypothalamus and trigger a change in the set point of the thermostat so that all of the normal thermoregulatory processes (e.g., vasoconstriction, vasodilation, shivering, etc.) occur in order to maintain a higher temperature. It appears that prostaglandins are not involved in maintaining the normal temperature, since drugs that block their production do not cause hypothermia.

Endogenous Pyrogens and the Blood-Brain Barrier

The blood-brain barrier is due to the presence of tight junctions between endothelial cells of the capillaries in the brain. As a result of these tight junctions, substances are prevented from leaking out of capillaries and into contact with the neurons of the brain.

There are two different mechanisms, one direct, the other indirect, by which elevation of blood levels of cytokines can result in cytokine elevation in the brain, despite the existence of the blood-brain barrier.

• The direct mechanism involves groups of cells that line the brain's ventricles, whose capillaries lack tight junctions and which therefore have no blood-brain barrier. Termed the **circumventricular organs**, they are able to serve as a window by which the generation of endogenous pyrogens in the systemic bloodstream can be monitored by selected groups of cells in the brain.

Many of these neurons use the very peptides and proteins that they respond to as neurotransmitters to trigger the hypothalamus to coordinate a response. There is, however, a brain-CSF barrier that prevents cytokines that reach neurons of the hypothalamus in this way from leaking into the CSF, from which they might indiscriminately travel throughout the rest of the brain.

• The indirect mechanism involves cytokines in the blood activating the endothelial cells that make up the capillary wall. The activated endothelial cells, which are simultaneously in contact with the bloodstream on one side and the brain on the other, then secrete cytokines into the brain directly (see Figure 11.9). Thus, cytokines do not always need to travel from the bloodstream to get to the brain.

• The extent to which fever is controlled by direct versus indirect mechanisms of

FIGURE 11.9. Blood-brain-CSF barrier. Schematic diagram of the blood-brain barrier, which separates neurons from substances unable to traverse endothelial cells because of their tight junctions in most of the brain. An exception to this rule is the so-called circumventricular organs, including the hypothalamus, where the capillary endothelium lacks tight junctions. Also indicated is the capacity of brain endothelium to secrete cytokines, prostaglandins, and other products directly into the substance of the brain, bypassing the need for these products to negotiate the blood-brain barrier.

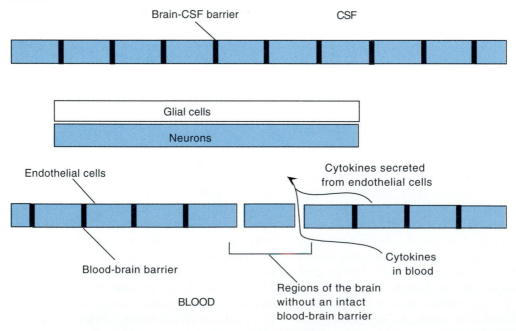

cytokine and prostaglandin communication has not been established. Regardless, the neurons of the hypothalamus respond to cytokines and prostaglandins by triggering activation of a plethora of autonomic, endocrine, and behavior control pathways.

• The autonomic changes result in selective vasoconstriction and redistribution of blood flow away from the skin. As a result, metabolically generated heat is not diffused, and the temperature of the body rises.

• Pathways to the thermoregulatory preoptic area of the hypothalamus reset the thermostat, so that a higher temperature is seen as "normal."

• The paraventricular nucleus of the hypothalamus releases CRH to *stimulate adrenal glucocorticoid secretion* (an appropriate response to stress) and alter vasopressin release.

• Behavior changes include *shivering*, which increases heat generation, *chills*, which induce a search for warmth, *anorexia, malaise,* and *somnolence*, which induce rest and diminish nonessential activity.

There is a growing opinion that perhaps clinicians should not be so quick to treat fever and that fever below 40°C may actually assist recovery from infection, for the reasons mentioned.

It is important to distinguish fever from hyperthermia. In physiologic fever, an adaptive response has purposely reset the thermostat to a higher, but still safe, level. Temperature is elevated 1 to 4°C in a response that probably helps the organism overcome infection or other cause of fever. In hyperthermia, the ability of the thermostat to regulate body temperature has been overwhelmed (e.g., in heatstroke). Body temperature can rise beyond 41°C, potentially causing brain damage or life-threatening cardiac arrhythmias. Figure 11.10 summarizes the mechanism controlling fever.

Review Questions

14. What are endogenous pyrogens?
15. What is their mechanism of action?
16. What are some direct and indirect mechanisms by which the hypothalamus can receive a message from the systemic circulation triggering the febrile response?
17. What are four ways in which the hypothalamus can respond to endogenous pyrogens?

Clinical Pearls

○ How do antipyretics (fever-reducing medicines) work?

• Acetaminophen itself actually has no activity against cyclooxygenase, the enzyme that generates prostaglandins. However, brain cytochrome P450 is able to oxidize acetaminophen into a product that is inhibitory of brain cyclooxygenase, thereby diminishing prostaglandin production and lowering fever.

• Nonsteroidal anti-inflammatory drugs (NSAIDs), such as aspirin and ibuprofen, also block cyclooxygenase. However, they act on all cyclooxygenase and do not require oxidation to become active. Hence, they are effective in a wider range of inflammatory conditions. The inhibition of cyclooxygenase by NSAIDS such as ibuprofen is reversible; that by aspirin is irreversible.

• Glucocorticoids such as prednisone are more profound anti-inflammatory agents than the NSAIDs. First, they induce expression of proteins termed lipocortins or annexins that block activation of phospholipase A_2, thereby preventing formation of arachidonic acid, the precursor of not just the prostaglandins and throm-

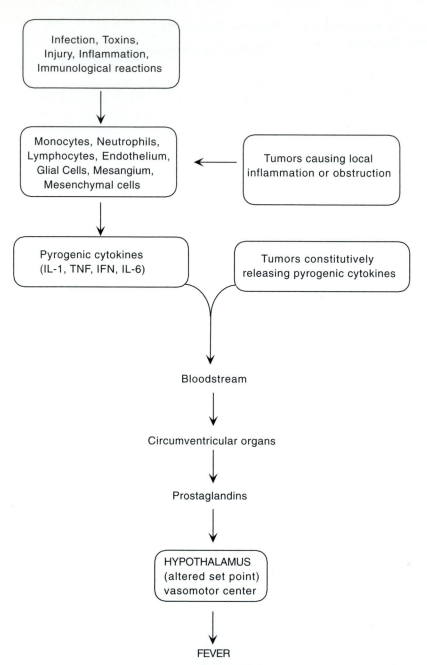

FIGURE 11.10. Pathogenesis of fever. *(Adapted, with permission, from Dinarelo CA, Bunn PA. (1997). Fever. Semin. Oncol. 24:288–298.)*

boxanes, but the leukotrienes as well. Second, the glucocorticoids block transcription of various pyrogenic cytokines.
- Some drugs, such as phenothiazines, interfere with vasoconstriction and hence can block fever, as can drugs that block muscle contraction. They are not true antipyretics because they will lower even normal core temperature. They do not actually affect the set point of the hypothalamic thermostat, but rather interfere with its function.

8. CONTROL OF SATIETY AND PATHOPHYSIOLOGY OF OBESITY

Normal Control of Body Weight

Normally, body weight is quite well maintained, both in the short term and over longer periods of time. Various physiological control mechanisms, integrated by the hypothalamus, work to maintain body weight over the short and long term (see Figure 11.11 and Ref. 2).

Short-term maintenance of body weight

The key parameters of short-term regulation of body weight are

- Amount and composition of ingested food
- Satiety (a complex response to food intake that has mechanical, neural, and humoral components)
- Nutrient absorption and assimilation

Given an unlimited supply of food, most of us stop eating when we develop a sense of satiety. This occurs because

1. Gastric distention triggers an autonomic reflex to the hypothalamus.
2. Hormones secreted in response to food ingestion and absorption can have direct and indirect effects on the hypothalamus. For example, the hormone cholecystokinin (CCK) affects the hypothalamus directly as a satiety factor, quite separate from its effects (discussed in Chap. 5) on pancreatic enzyme secretion and gallbladder motility.
3. Various substrates, including glucose, free fatty acids, and amino acids, are sensed directly at the hypothalamus and may serve as satiety factors. It is likely that these direct effects are reinforced by indirect effects on hormones and neural pathways mediating satiety.

The effects of hormones that affect substrates can be complex. For example, insulin can both serve as a satiety factor and provoke hunger, depending on whether it is secreted physiologically, in a way that lowers blood glucose into the normal range, or pharmacologically, in a way that may cause hypoglycemia, thereby triggering an compensatory hunger response via the hypothalamus.

Long-term maintenance of body weight

In contrast to short-term maintenance, long-term regulation of body weight is largely influenced by substrate storage (degree of fatness) and energy expenditure (physical activity and metabolic rate). The fat cell, or **adipocyte**, long viewed as a simple repository for excess calories in the form of triglyceride, has been found to participate actively in the feedback loop of satiety in a way that directly involves the hypothalamus and integrates short- and long-term control.

In response to a particular level of triglyceride storage, the adipocyte secretes a hormone called **leptin**, which binds to receptors in the arcuate nucleus of the hypothalamus, thereby lowering levels of neuropeptide Y (NPY) and triggering the sense of satiety. The level of *sympathetic tone* and the activ-

Afferent signals decreasing appetite or increasing energy expenditure

Afferent signals increasing appetite or decreasing energy expenditure

GI tract
Glucagon, cholecystokinin, glucose, glucagon-like peptides, bombesin peptides

GI tract
Opiods, neurotensin, somatostatin, growth hormone-releasing hormone

Endocrine System
Epinephrine (beta-adrenergic effect), estrogens

Endocrine System
Epinephrine (alpha-adrenergic activity), androgens, glucocorticoids, insulin, progesterone

Adipose Tissue
Leptin

H

Peripheral Nervous System
Norepinephrine (beta adrenergic effect)

Peripheral Nervous System
Norepinephrine (alpha adrenergic activity)

Central Nervous System
Dopamine, gamma-aminobutyric acid seratonin, cholecystokinin, CRH

Central Nervous System
Galanin, opiods, somatostatin, growth hormone-releasing hormone

Norepinephrine, seratonin, NPY, MCH, GLP, CRH

Efferents

Integrated Change in Energy Intake and Expenditure

A

FIGURE 11.11. A. Molecules from various tissues that affect energy intake and expenditure through the hypothalamus. Many afferent signals, reflecting the nutritional state and other parameters of the host, affect the levels of various neurotransmitters in the hypothalmus, whose output titrates energy intake and expenditure by the host. *(Adapted, with permission, from Rosenbaum M et al. (1997). Obesity. N. Engl. J. Med. 337:396–407.)*

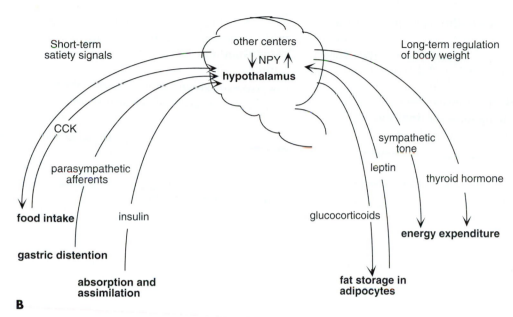

B

FIGURE 11.11 — (*continued*) B. Parameters controlling normal body weight, indicating short-term (left) and long-term (right) components. (*Adapted, with permission, from McPhee SJ et al., eds. (1999). Pathophysiology of Disease, 3rd ed. New York, McGraw-Hill.*)

ity of pathways that affect glucocorticoid, thyroid hormone, and catecholamine secretion are altered in response to changes in NPY in the hypothalamus. These hormones are crucial for weight regulation, in part, because they have effects on the extent to which calories are "burned" without harnessing work, which is one way of responding to an imbalance between food input and energy output. Thus, at least in animal models, adrenalectomy (which eliminates glucocorticoids and diminishes catecholamines) reverses many forms of weight gain, including that which results from hypothalamic lesions.

Insulin can also contribute to long-term hormonal regulation of satiety through effects that are distinct from, and counterregulatory to, its short-term ability to stimulate hunger pharmacologically (see the previous section). It does this by a direct effect on the brain, which it can enter via the circum-

ventricular organs, where it affects leptin-mediated signaling.

Under normal circumstances, the hypothalamus presumably integrates all of these short- and long-term reflexes to achieve homeostasis. The precise mechanisms within the brain are complex and currently not well understood. In addition to the interaction of many different hormones and neurotransmitters, there are many different forms of receptors for these hormones and neurotransmitters. The process of sorting out which receptors mediate which effects via which ligands is currently in progress. NPY seems to play a crucial role in promotion of feeding behavior. Thus, the net effect of the autonomic and hormonal input to the hypothalamus in response to food intake appears to be to decrease the levels of NPY and thereby promote satiety.

The interaction of NPY with the leptin

signaling system is different in response to starvation and weight loss from that in response to excessive food intake and weight gain (see Figure 11.12). A particular subtype of receptor for the peptide melanocortin is involved in the response to increase in weight, with different ligands serving poorly understood stimulatory and inhibitory functions (see Sec. 10.).

Disorders of body weight regulation can occur through alteration of several variables, including

1. The amount and type of food ingested
2. The central control of satiety
3. Hormonal control of assimilation and/or storage
4. Physical activity or metabolic rate

Obesity: Definition and Relationship to Disease

Obesity can be defined as excess body weight sufficient to increase overall morbidity and mortality. When individuals are compared with respect to height and weight in a way that some believe measures "fatness" [body mass index (BMI) = weight/height^2, with normal being 22 to 24 kg/m^2], it is observed that nearly 20% of the population suffers some increased morbidity or mortality attributable to obesity. Moreover, the incidence of morbidity and mortality increases dramatically with increasing obesity, such that individuals with a BMI of 150% of normal have double the risk, while those that are 200% of normal BMI have 10 times the risk (see Refs. 4 and 5).

Pathophysiology of obesity

The pathophysiology of obesity is both extraordinarily complex and poorly understood. Much of the recognition of obesity in the pathophysiology of disease comes from epidemiologic studies that identify obesity as a risk factor for increased morbidity and mortality from various diseases, but do not provide insight into the mechanism by which this happens. Figure 11.13 summarizes some of the ways in which obesity is thought to contribute to a variety of disease states.

There appear to be multiple mechanisms by which obesity can develop. Thus obesity may be either a cause or a consequence of disease, depending on the disorder. For example, non-insulin-dependent diabetes mellitus is sometimes first manifest clinically upon sudden weight gain and can be difficult to control without weight loss, reflecting the insulin-resistant character of the obese state. Moreover, if the weight can be lost, the diabetes may once again become latent, controlled by diet and exercise alone. In such cases, obesity seems clearly to be an etiologic factor in the development of diabetes mellitus. Yet insulin injections, which may be necessary to control the symptoms of diabetes in such a patient, will further exacerbate the weight gain that precipitated the disorder in the first place by causing the deposition of fuel substrates as fat. Such "chicken-or-egg" relationships make the pathophysiology of obesity difficult to dissect. Nevertheless, important progress has been made in recent years toward developing a coherent framework in which to view obesity as both cause and consequence of disease. Some of these observations are noted here.

• The hypothalamus has distinct satiety and feeding centers because lesions in the ventromedial hypothalamus result in hunger and obesity, whereas lesions in the lateral hypothalamus result in loss of appetite and profound weight loss. A family of peptide neurotransmitters called the **orexins** and another family including **melanin-concentrating hormone** appear to be made in the lateral hypothalamus. When injected into the brain of laboratory animals, these peptides stimulate appetite. Clearly a complex regu-

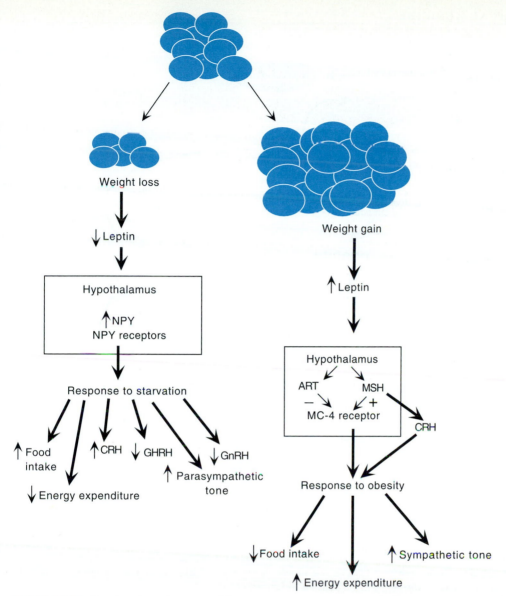

FIGURE 11.12. Postulated mechanisms of homeostatic response to weight loss (starvation) and weight gain (excessive feeding). Loss of body fat (e.g., in starvation, left-hand panel) leads to a decrease in blood leptin concentration, which is integrated in the hypothalamus with other signals and results in many different adaptive responses, including increased food-seeking behavior, decreased energy expenditure, increased CRH (starvation is a stress), decreased GnRH (starvation is not a good time to get involved in reproductive functions), and increased parasympathetic tone. In the presence of weight gain due to increased body fat, leptin levels in the blood increase, and there is competition between MSH (a positive regulator) and ART (a negative regulator) for MC-4 receptor occupancy. Activation of this receptor (e.g., by MSH) triggers a programmed response to obesity, including decrease in food intake, increase in energy expenditure, and increase in sympathetic tone. Directly and indirectly, uncoupling protein levels in the mitochondria also increase. (Adapted, with permission, from Friedman JM, Halaas JL (1998). Leptin and the regulation of body weight in mammals. Nature 395:763–770.)

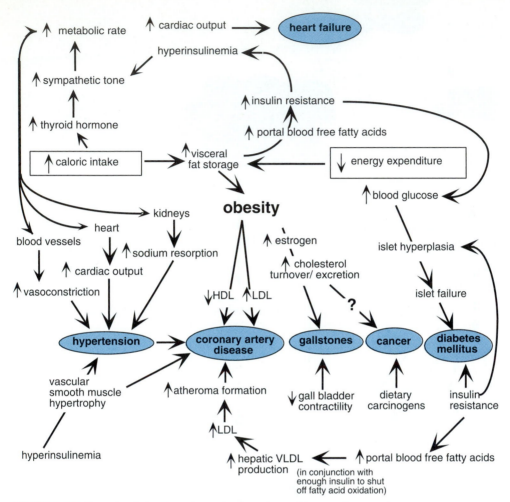

FIGURE 11.13. The role of obesity in the pathophysiology of human disease. Some ways by which obesity may contribute to disease are shown. Short arrows refer to a change in the indicated parameter, and long arrows indicate a consequence of that change. In some cases, evidence is epidemiologic in nature; in other cases, it is experimental. *(Adapted, with permission, from Bray GA (1992). Pathophysiology of obesity. Am J Clin Nutr 55:4885.)*

lation is involved, since neurons containing the appetite-suppressing **alpha-melanocyte stimulating hormone** (MSH) also project to the lateral hypothalamus. MSH activates the MC4 receptor, an effect that is blocked by a natural antagonist of MSH called **agouti-related protein** (ART) (see Table 11.3). In mice, deletion of the agouti gene results in an obesity syndrome.

• The number of fat cells in the body is probably established during infancy. One hypothesis is that obesity appearing during adulthood results from enlargement of individual fat cells (hypertrophy) rather than an in-

TABLE 11.3 HYPOTHALAMIC PEPTIDES
REGULATING FOOD INTAKE

Increase Food Intake	Decrease Food Intake
NPY	CART
MCH	CCK
Galanin	CRH
Orexin a and b	α-MSH
Peptide YY	Insulin
Noradrenaline	GLP-1
(α2 receptor)	Bombesin
	Urocortin
	Serotonin

Many other peptides are likely to be discovered, and the precise pathways of stimulation inhibition and feedback are
likely to be elucidated, in the years to come. NPY = neuropeptide Y; MCH = melanocortin; ART = agouti-related protein; CCK = cholecystokinin; CRH = corticotropin releasing
hormone; α-MSH = α-melanocyte stimulating hormone;
GLP-1 = glucagon-like peptide-1.
Reproduced, with permission, from Friedman JM, Halaas JL
(1998). *Nature* 395:763–770.

creased number of fat cells (hyperplasia).
Obesity due to fat cell hypertrophy appears
to be much more easily controlled than obesity due to fat cell hyperplasia. Perhaps feedback signals in response to the degree of
fat cell hypertrophy are important to the
hypothalamic "lipostat."

- It is now recognized that *where* fat is deposited is a more important determinant of
health risk than *how much* is deposited.
Thus, so-called visceral or central obesity
(omental fat in the distribution of blood flow
draining into the portal vein) seems far
more important as a risk factor for obesity-
related morbidity and mortality than so-
called subcutaneous, gynoid (lower body),
or peripheral fat. It appears that visceral
fat (which gives middle-aged men their pot-
bellies) is more sensitive to catecholamines
and less sensitive to insulin, making it a
marker of insulin resistance. Consistent with
these findings is the observation that obese
individuals who engage in vigorous physical
activity and whose obesity is largely due

to high caloric intake (e.g., sumo wrestlers)
have subcutaneous rather than visceral fat
and do not demonstrate substantial increased insulin resistance. In contrast, the
obesity associated with a sedentary lifestyle,
which carries a much higher risk and is associated with a greater degree of insulin resistance in patients both with and without a
diagnosis of diabetes mellitus, is believed to
be largely visceral obesity.

- It has been demonstrated that the genetically obese *ob/ob* strain of rats has a defective leptin gene. The resulting loss of a normal hormonal cue to long-term satiety
seems to be a critical feature of this particular model of excessive weight gain. When
these animals are treated with leptin, they
lose weight—and gain fertility. In contrast,
genetically obese *db/db* mice, which have a
defective leptin receptor, do not benefit
from leptin treatment.

- In the vast majority of obese humans, excessive rather than deficient leptin levels are
observed. Thus, it appears that the most
common form of human obesity involves
leptin resistance in the face of high endogenous leptin levels, rather than defective leptin secretion as observed in the *ob/ob* rat.
Whether apparent leptin resistance represents downregulation or desensitization of
receptors, defects in leptin receptor–
mediated signal transduction or some other
mechanism remains to be determined (see
Chap. 3). As with insulin resistance, there
may be a wide range and mix of mechanisms
involved, differing from individual to individual, due to genetic and environmental
factors.

- Psychological factors also make an important contribution to the development of
obesity in humans. For example, obese individuals appear to regulate their desire
for food by greater reliance on external
cues (e.g., time of day, appeal of the food)
than on endogenous signals (e.g., feeling
hungry).

Clinical Pearls

○ Clinicians, researchers, and patients often inappropriately "medicalize" obesity. In fact, there is little evidence that mild obesity—up to 30% over normal BMI—is harmful. Recent clinical epidemiologic studies suggest that excessive dieting, restriction of fat intake, and weight loss can be distinctly harmful (see Ref. 6). Thus, while regulating weight is an important part of disease prevention, it is important to recognize that how weight gain is controlled is even more important. When weight regulation results from good dietary and exercise habits, the result will be beneficial. However, pharmacologic approaches to mild or moderate obesity may do more harm than good (see Ref. 7). Our society has accepted fashion-driven ideals of thinness that bear no relationship to health. The lack of attainment of these ideals can do great harm to the self-image of patients, and consequently negatively affect their health. Health care providers have a responsibility not to promote fashion standards, but rather to help patients achieve a more physiological approach to diet, exercise, and weight maintenance.

○ Part of the problem in weight control is that the hypothalamus seems to get "on the wrong page" and works against the wishes of the individual because it "thinks" it is trying to prevent further loss of body weight as it is supposed to do in times of real starvation.

○ At least in animal models, adrenalectomy (which eliminates glucocorticoids) reverses many forms of weight gain including that which results from hypothalamic lesions. Of course, this would be an inappropriately draconian way to deal with most human obesity, but it suggests that there are mechanisms involving hypothal-

amic output to peripheral endocrine glands that may one day be beneficially manipulated by pharmacological or other means.

○ It is commonly observed that patients with type II diabetes mellitus who are placed on insulin gain weight, which only worsens their insulin resistance. This is because most obese humans are leptin resistant. In effect, they are more sensitive to the fuel storage effects of insulin than they are to its ability to promote satiety. Thus, a successful program of exercise and weight loss may be more effective than insulin injections to improve diabetes control in these patients.

Review Questions

18. What are the short- and long-term factors involved in normal control of body weight?
19. Define obesity.
20. What diseases are associated with obesity?
21. Outline several pathophysiological mechanisms by which obesity contributes to disease.
22. Why do some observers think that the medical profession is overdoing its advocacy of weight reduction?

9. EFFECTS OF HYPOTHALAMIC/PITUITARY DISEASE ON HOMEOSTASIS

Because the hypothalamic nuclei are present in pairs and are surrounded and fed by the vessels of the circle of Willis (see Figure 11.4), isolated hypothalamic disease due to trauma or vascular insufficiency is exceedingly rare. However, the stalk that connects the hypothalamus to the pituitary is quite susceptible to traumatic transection (e.g., during surgery or in a car accident), with acute loss of communication between hypothalamus and pituitary. Since pituitary portal blood flow is interrupted, stimulation by hypothalamic releasing hormones is lost, and hence the neuroendocrine axes are terminated. Of the pituitary hormones, only the secretion of prolactin continues—in fact, it increases. This is because prolactin's control from the hypothalamus is largely through tonic *inhibition* of prolactin secretion by dopamine. Thus its blood levels are dramatically and diagnostically elevated in stalk transection.

Similarly, transection of axons to the posterior pituitary results in loss of fluid and electrolyte homeostasis, with development of diabetes insipidus, characterized by an inability to concentrate urine. These findings are often observed after brain surgery. The symptoms often resolve, either rapidly, as edema resolves, or more gradually, with regeneration of adequate neural and vascular connections over time. In some cases, however, restoration of water homeostasis never adequately occurs, and hormone replacement is necessary to maintain homeostasis (see introductory case).

Children with the diencephalic syndrome typically have a brain tumor in the anterior hypothalamus, resulting in weight loss and emaciation in spite of normal food intake. They maintain an alert and cheerful disposition in spite of their progression to death. Paradoxically, very similar lesions in adults seem to cause a different syndrome of obesity, somnolence, and spontaneous rage.

Finally, hypothalamic lesions may cause disorders of consciousness. However, it is difficult to distinguish loss of specific hypothalamic functions residing in specific nuclei from the effects of a general interruption of communication between the brain and body, either due to lesions in tracts passing through a given area or due to pressure effects, etc.

Review Questions

23. What is a common complication involving the hypothalamic-pituitary unit that can occur either transiently (as an indirect result of edema postoperatively) or permanently (as a result of direct trauma)?

24. In what ways would transection of the hypothalamic stalk be functionally similar to or different from complete destruction of the pituitary gland?

10. FRONTIERS IN NEUROENDOCRINOLOGY

Molecular Biology of Gene Expression in the Pituitary Gland

The pituitary gland provides a model system in which to study organogenesis. It appears that a specific transcription factor termed Pit-1 serves as a developmental regulator by which several of the specific cell types in the anterior pituitary are determined. Pit-1 also controls proliferation of these cell types and transcription of the hormones they make. This appears to be a general strategy by which cell differentiation and organ development are regulated (see Ref. 8).

Psychoneuroendocrinology: Oxytocin and Behavior

Many peptide hormones that have defined effects on peripheral tissues are also found in the brain, where they may be used as neurotransmitters by specific subsets of neurons. In most of these cases, the role in the brain is unknown. What little is known suggests intriguing possibilities. Consider oxytocin, for example. Neurons of the hypothalamus that synthesize the peptide oxytocin not only store it in the posterior pituitary for release into the systemic circulation, but also project it to various parts of the brain where neurons displaying oxytocin receptors can be found. These include areas within the limbic system (including the amygdala and hippocampus), autonomic centers of the midbrain (including the locus caeruleus), the brainstem, and the spinal cord. Some neurons release oxytocin directly into the cerebrospinal fluid.

Studies in rats have started to indicate some of the roles these central oxytocin receptors may play that are quite different from the role of oxytocin in peripheral tissues (e.g., affecting function of the uterus and mammary gland; see Chap. 17). It appears that oxytocin in the brain has a complex effect on memory. At low concentrations, oxytocin may improve memory, while at high concentrations, it worsens it. Oxytocin administered in the brain also affects a range of behavior. It stimulates stereotyped self-grooming and initiates maternal behavior (but only when the animals are in a novel environment). Some data have been interpreted to suggest a role for oxytocin in development of pair bonding and the formation of monogamous relationships.

Human obsessive-compulsive disorder is a chronic disabling psychiatric condition in which the patient repeatedly experiences the sudden intrusion into consciousness of unwanted thoughts or images and has repeated urges to perform seemingly senseless acts. A recent study found elevated levels of oxytocin, but not of vasopressin, in cerebrospinal fluid in such patients. The precise role of oxytocin in these psychiatric disorders remains to be determined (see Ref. 9).

Peripheral versus Central Actions of Leptin

We think of the primary actions of leptin as being in the hypothalamus, where it affects pathways that control feeding behavior, satiety, and thermogenesis. However, in addition, leptin has powerful effects on adipose tissue, where it promotes lipolysis and glucose utilization (see Ref. 10). Likewise, leptin has been shown to be a powerful inhibitor of insulin secretion, providing another feedback loop for control of carbohydrate utilization (see Ref. 11). Indeed, recent studies suggest that cytokines play a role in leptin release (see Ref. 12). These and other findings raise the possibility that leptin is controlled by a network of factors, including autocrine and paracrine interactions, which serve to integrate central and peripheral, behavioral and metabolic aspects of fuel homeostasis in ways far more complex than we can currently fathom. Furthermore, leptin's action appears to include effects on adipocyte differentiation, at least at pharmacologic doses, such that leptin treatment causes fat cells not only to lose their fat content, but also to lose their ability to make fat (see Ref. 13).

Energy Metabolism, Oxidative Stress, and the Immune System

The presence of oxygen in the atmosphere was both a boon and a bane to life on earth. By allowing much more complete release of chemical energy from foods through the mechanism of oxidative phosphorylation, oxygen made possible the higher level of energy economy necessary to sustain multicellular organisms and made possible the evolution of a variety of energy-intensive activities, including running, thinking, pumping blood, and filtering urine. Can you imagine our existence without any one of these functions? On the other hand, oxygen is a highly toxic, reactive molecule that can damage proteins, lipids, nucleic acids, and other structures that are the basis for life itself. Indeed, evolution has harnessed even this negative aspect of oxygen through the biology of neutrophils, those suicidally ferocious warriors of the immune system that engulf invading organisms and then destroy them by generating reactive oxygen species (see Chap. 19). Thus it is clear that a fine, highly regulated balance must be maintained between the good and the bad sides of oxygen with respect to energy generation, thermogenesis, immune function, and oxidative injury (a key step implicated in cancer, heart disease, and neurodegenerative diseases such as Alzheimer's disease; see Chap. 20).

In this light, several recent observations are particularly intriguing. First, it appears that there are not one, not two, but three different uncoupling protein genes in the mitochondria of various human tissues (see Refs. 14, 15). One role for uncoupling proteins is in nonshivering thermogenesis, the mechanism by which we maintain our bodies at the optimum temperature at which our enzymes work best. Another role for uncoupling proteins may be to dissipate excess energy as heat to prevent excessive weight gain. Consistent with this role, leptin appears to increase mRNA for two of the uncoupling proteins. A third role for uncoupling proteins may be to prevent oxygen toxicity. Teleologically speaking, when the cell is replete with ATP, it would rather not allow oxygen to hang around waiting for ATP depletion, when it will once again be needed to drive oxidative phosphorylation. This is because in the meantime, the oxygen can only do bad things to the cell, reacting with and damaging precious, expensive macromolecules. Thus, another role for uncoupling proteins may be to use up the oxygen in futile cycles of heat generation and dissipation in order to maintain oxygen levels, and hence reactive oxygen radical species, within strict limits that other lines of defense against oxidative damage can handle (see Chap. 19).

Another intriguing, but still mysterious, connection between energy metabolism and the immune system comes from experiments in mice. A recently identified gene termed *magohany*, which suppresses the effect of deletion of the *agouti* gene, has been found to be a transmembrane homologue of the protein **attractin**, made by activated T cells and involved in immune cell interaction (see Refs. 16, 17). Are these molecular examples of overlap between the programs of energy me-

tabolism, thermogenesis, and immune function simply a coincidence? Or are there feedback loops, conceptual connections, and evolutionary rationales that we currently do not understand? Clearly, one of the great challenges for the future is to synthesize the tremendous explosion of knowledge about isolated systems to generate insight into how they interact in ways that have implications for human health and disease.

Neuronal–Glial Cell Interactions in Hypothalamic Function

Glial cells are often thought of as simply providing structural and metabolic support for neurons, which do the real work of the central nervous system. Recent studies on neuronal–glial cell interactions in the hypothalamus suggest the importance of glial cell activation in controlling the function of neurons. It appears that a substantial degree of plasticity—function-dependent structural changes—occurs in the hypothalamus, mediated by glial cell signaling. While the precise role of glial cells in hypothalamic function remains unknown, major insights into how the hypothalamus works may eventually emerge from this new area of research (see Ref. 18).

11. HOW DOES AN UNDERSTANDING OF NORMAL PHYSIOLOGY PROVIDE INSIGHT INTO THE INITIAL CASE PRESENTATION?

Let us once again consider the predicament of RB, the 33-year-old woman survivor of a hit-and-run traffic accident in which she received substantial head injuries, including damage to the hypothalamus and pituitary stalk transection.

Ms. B has a serious and chronic condition. Hormone replacement to maintain ADH, adrenal, thyroid, and estrogen action is mandatory if hypernatremia, shock, hypothyroidism, and osteoporosis, respectively, are to be avoided. Failure to provide Ms. B with adequate support services is tantamount to a death sentence. It will result in repeated life-threatening episodes like those that have already occurred, on an unpredictable basis. These are most likely due to the hypothalamic injuries and are beyond her control.

Many clinicians regularly need to appeal denials of care from their patients' insurance companies. A good understanding of physiology can help you argue the patient's case more cogently than you could if you based your argument on treatment algorithms or compassion alone.

SUMMARY AND REVIEW OF KEY CONCEPTS

1. The hypothalamus provides hormones that control the pituitary and, through it, various processes including growth, reproduction, metabolism, and responses to stress.

2. The hypothalamus monitors and triggers appropriate responses to deviations from baseline of body temperature, osmolality, and energy stores and serves as the pacemaker for circadian rhythms such as fluctuations in hormone secretion and sleep-wake cycles.

3. The hypothalamus integrates emotions and behaviors with appropriate automatic physiological responses and serves as a clearinghouse for competing demands that would otherwise affect processes it controls.

4. The hypothalamus is a poorly demarcated region in the floor of the third ventricle of the brain that consist of nuclei. Most medially, the periventricular and medial paraventricular nuclei secrete factors that control the anterior pituitary. The adja-

cent medial zone gives rise to most of the neurons of the posterior pituitary. The lateral zone has neurons whose axons connect the hypothalamus to both the brainstem and the forebrain. Viewed anterior to posterior, the anterior one-third of the hypothalamus controls fluid, electrolyte, and thermoregulatory functions. The middle third controls endocrine and autonomic regulatory functions. The posterior third of the hypothalamus is involved in thermoregulatory and emergency response integration. In general, these functional correlations to specific hypothalamic nuclei should be taken as an approximation, because the demarcations are not precise or absolute.

5. Hypothalamic hormones are TRH, CRH, somatostatin, dopamine, LHRH, GHRH (controls anterior pituitary), oxytocin, vasopressin (posterior pituitary).

6. The anterior pituitary hormones are growth hormone, prolactin, ACTH, LH, FSH, and TSH.

7. The pituitary portal system is important in that it allows relatively high concentrations of hypothalamic releasing factors to be seen in a localized blood flow (of the anterior pituitary).

8. Organization of anterior and posterior pituitary neuroendocrine feedback loops and inhibitory vs. stimulatory control: Anterior pituitary feedback loops are cascades of hormones. Those of the posterior pituitary interface with the autonomic nervous system.

9. Biosynthesis, processing, and regulated secretion of anterior pituitary hormones: These hormones are often made as precursors, modified by proteolysis or glycosylation, and secreted in a pulsatile fashion in response to specific stimuli (e.g., hypothalamic releasing factors).

10. Implications of half-life, pulsatility, and trophic actions of various hypothalamic and pituitary hormones: These define the

physiological role of a hormone and are the basis for many diseases in which one aspect or another is dysregulated.

11. Normal thermogenesis involves heat production as a by-product of normal metabolism, futile cycles, and uncoupled energy generation. Heat is dissipated or conserved by sympathetic nerve-mediated peripheral vasoconstriction/vasodilation.

12. Fever involves a resetting of the physiological thermostat to a higher level through the effects of prostaglandins released in response to pyrogenic cytokines that cross or signal across the blood-brain barrier. Fever is distinct from hyperthermia.

13. Normal body weight is regulated by separate but integrated mechanisms in the short and long terms. Parameters of short-term control include amount and composition, satiety, nutrient absorption, and assimilation. Satiety is triggered by gastric distention, hormones (especially CCK), and autonomic/higher input to the hypothalamus that decreases levels of NPY. Long-term control involves leptin produced by adipose tissue and feeding back on the arcuate nucleus to lower NPY levels and increase sympathetic tone.

14. Extreme obesity is associated with substantial increased risk of various diseases.

A CASE OF PHYSIOLOGICAL MEDICINE INVOLVING THE HYPOTHALAMUS AND PITUITARY GLAND

EF is a 43-year-old scout leader who was quite healthy until 2 years ago, when he developed loss of libido, lethargy, and severe headaches. Three months later he developed visual changes, for which he sought medical attention. A CT scan demonstrated pituitary enlargement, most likely due to a tumor.

Blood testing at that time showed an elevated prolactin level, but no other abnormalities of pituitary function. Because Mr. F's clinician was attentive to details (and understood the physiology), she followed up the random blood hormone levels with provocative testing of his adrenal axis. The results were abnormal, suggesting that the prolactin-secreting tumor was compressing the rest of the pituitary gland.

Mr. F was tried on a dopamine agonist to control his hyperprolactinemia, with some benefit in symptoms. However, 6 months later, his pituitary mass was noted to be enlarging, and so authorization for surgery was requested from his HMO.

While waiting for a response, Mr. F decided to take a long-planned vacation to Switzerland. There, while rock climbing, he fell, resulting in a fractured pelvis. He was taken to the operating room of the local Swiss hospital, but did not inform his new Swiss clinicians about his pituitary condition. During the surgery, Mr. F was noted to have a difficult-to-maintain blood pressure. Postoperatively he had a stormy course in the intensive care unit. At this point, a thoughtful resident ordered additional provocative testing and found that Mr. F was profoundly adrenally insufficient.

Appropriate replacement was initiated, with stabilization of his hospital course. Three months later, Mr. F underwent a successful pituitary resection.

QUESTIONS

1. The patient's clinical course displayed a progression from headaches to visual field defects to generalized pituitary hormone insufficiency. Is this the course you would expect from a pituitary tumor? Why or why not?

2. Why was the defect in the adrenal axis only picked up by provocative testing and not by simply measuring blood levels of ACTH?

3. What is the rationale for treatment with a dopamine agonist?

4. The patient apparently developed adrenal insufficiency in the window of time between his initial diagnosis and his emergency surgery in Switzerland.

   a. What other conditions would you want to test for, based on your knowledge of what the pituitary makes?

   b. What pituitary products might also be abnormal but are likely to be irrelevant to management of the patient's current clinical condition?

ANSWERS

1. This is a classic presentation for an expanding pituitary mass. Initially, the mass causes increased intracranial pressure resulting in headaches. Later, the close relationship between the optic chiasm and the pituitary gland results in visual field defects, typically bitemporal hemianopsia, as crossing fibers are impinged by the upward expanding mass. Eventually, the other cells of the pituitary gland are squeezed against the surrounding capsule and destroyed as the mass continues to expand.

2. ACTH and cortisol secretion are episodic and have a short half life so random blood levels can be misleading. Provocative testing is a way of seeing if the axis can respond to a stress as it is supposed to, and is a far more sensitive "real life" way of picking up defects relatively early in the course of the disease.

3. Prolactin is normally under negative control by dopamine, meaning that dopamine blocks its secretion. Sometimes, a tumor that secretes prolactin has not completely lost its capacity to respond to physiological controls but may not be as sensitive to them as normal. Hence treatment with a drug that augments dopamine effects *may* result in inhibition of prolactin secretion from the tumor.

4a. The other major anterior pituitary hormones are LH and FSH involved in reproductive function, TSH involved in metabolism, and growth hormone. The possibility of hypothyroidism could be assessed either with a TSH level or a free T4 level. Given the long half life in blood and the large reservoir in the gland, there is no point in provocative testing of thyroid function. If the patient were trying to father a child or had complaints regarding libido, a low LH level or more importantly a low testosterone level might reveal utility of LH and FSH (for fertility) or testosterone (for libido but not fertility, see Chapter 15).

4b. Growth hormone deficiency is treated only in children capable of linear growth. Once the epiphyses have closed, the utility of growth hormone therapy is unclear. The posterior pituitary is less likely to be involved, given its embryological distinctness. However if it were involved, this would be indicated by hypernatremia and large urine volumes, signs of ADH deficiency (see Chapter 10). There is no known clinical significance of lack of oxytocin secretion in a male.

References and suggested readings

GENERAL REFERENCES

1. Dinarelo CA, Bunn PA (1997). Fever. *Semin Oncol* 24:288–298.

2. Friedman JM, Halaas JL (1998). Leptin and the regulation of body weight in mammals. *Nature* 395:763–770.

3. Wurtman RJ (1996). What is leptin for and does it act on the brain? *Nat Med* 2:492–493.

4. Rosenbaum M, et al (1997). Obesity. *N Engl J Med* 337:396–407.

5. Pi-Sunyer FX (1993). Medical hazards of obesity. *Ann Intern Med* 119:665.

6. Angell M, Kassirer J (1998). Losing weight—an ill-fated new year's resolution. *N Engl J Med* 338:52–54.

7. Conolly HM, et al (1997). Valvular heart disease associated with fenfluramine-phentera-mine. *N Engl J Med* 337:581–588.

FRONTIERS REFERENCES

8. Andersen B, Rosenfeld MG (1994). Pit-1 determines cell types during development of the anterior pituitary gland. *J Biol Chem* 269, 29335–29338.

9. Leckman JF, et al. (1994). The role of central oxytocin in obsessive compuslive disorder and related normal behavior. *Psychoneuroendocri-nol* 19:723–749.

10. Siegrist-Kaiser CA, et al. (1997). Direct effects of leptin on brown and white adipose tissue. *J Clin Invest* 100:2858–2864.

11. Kulkarni RN, et al. (1997). Leptin rapidly suppresses insulin release from insulinoma cells, rat and human islets, and in vivo, in mice. *J Clin Invest* 100:2729–2736.

12. Kirchgessner RG, et al. (1997). Tumor necrosis factor alpha contributes to obesity-related hyperleptinemia by regulating leptin release from adipocytes. *J Clin Invest* 100:2777–2782.

13. Zhou Y-T, et al. (1999). Reversing adipocyte differentiation: Implications for treatment of obesity. *Proc Natl Acad Sci USA* 96:2391–2396.

14. Fleury C, et al. (1997). Uncoupling protein-2: A novel gene linked to obesity and hyperinsuli-nemia. *Nat Genet* 15:269–272.

15. Boss O, et al. (1998). The uncoupling proteins, a review. *Eur J Endocrinol* 139: 1–9.

16. Gunn TM, et al. (1999). The mouse mahogany locus encodes a transmembrane form of human attractin. *Nature* 398:152–155.

17. Nagle DL, et al. (1999). The mahogany protein is a receptor involved in suppression of obesity. *Nature* 398:148–152.

18. Theodosis DT, MacVicar B (1996). Neurone-glia interactions in the hypothalamus and pituitary. *Trends in Neurosciences* 19:363–366.

PHYSIOLOGY OF THE THYROID GLAND

12

1. INTRODUCTION TO THE THYROID GLAND

The significance of the thyroid gland and its hormones

The thyroid gland synthesizes and secretes thyroid hormone in response to appropriate stimulation. Thyroid hormone has three distinct roles:

1. Thyroid hormone is a crucial determinant of normal growth and development, affecting virtually every tissue of the body.
2. Thyroid hormone is a regulator of overall cellular energy expenditure and substrate utilization.
3. Thyroid hormone serves to optimize the sensitivity of particular tissues to various other hormones and other influences. Thus, lack or excess of thyroid hormone can have dramatic effects on the brain, the bones, and the cardiovascular system, to name just a few.

Understanding of thyroid hormone action is complicated by several features:

- First, there is no one target tissue from which a full appreciation of thyroid hormone's actions and importance can be gleaned — thyroid hormone affects lots of different organ systems in important and diverse ways.
- Second, as indicated previously, much of what thyroid hormone does is **permissive**, serving to facilitate the actions of other hormones and pathways. Thus it is easy to forget the role of thyroid hormone in making other hormones "work just right."
- Third, patients with the same thyroid disorder can present with very different manifestations. Presumably this reflects the combinatorial possibilities for effects of thyroid hormone excess or deficiency on a host of other organ and endocrine systems that vary from one person to the next due to genetic and/or environmental differences.

Why is understanding thyroid physiology clinically important?

A practical appreciation of thyroid physiology is important for clinicians because disorders of the thyroid gland are both common and treatable, and can be devastating to the patient if they are not appreciated early in the course of disease.

Also, thyroid disorders can be quite subtle and insidious in their onset and even in their full-blown presentation. The image of a hyperthyroid patient "bouncing off the walls" describes only one subset of patients. Patients with "apathetic thyrotoxicosis" seem at first glance to have a very different presentation — although on closer inspection, their symptoms make perfect physiological sense (see Clinical Pearl in Sec. 4).

Likewise, hypothyroidism can be very slow to develop — over many months or even years — making it difficult for family members to pinpoint the onset of behavioral changes. Although typically hypothyroidism presents with somnolence and slowing of affect and metabolism, sometimes the patient can act quite crazed — the syndrome of "myxedema madness" (see Sec. 4).

All of this also means that the clinician can easily be fooled and miss thyroid disease, unless he or she appreciates its physiological basis and specifically considers the possibility.

Case Presentation

L.F. is a 52-year-old seamstress who has undergone extensive evaluation for atrial fibrillation refractory to medical management. Evaluation of her condition has included a cardiac catheterization, which revealed no significant coronary artery disease and no evidence of pulmonary emboli. She was admitted to the hospital by her cardiologist for invasive cardiac electrophysiologic studies and ablation of the tracts responsible for the dysrhythmia. However, an astute resident noted the presence of a mild tremor on physical exam and a history of heat intolerance whose onset was a few months prior to development of cardiac symptoms. The resident also found a significant drop in Ms. F.'s recent serum cholesterol compared to 3 years ago, and a lack of thyroid function tests in her previous medical workup. The invasive testing was delayed in order to carry out thyroid function testing, and after the results became known, the plans for further evaluation of her heart were canceled.

Health care providers are committed to "first, do no harm." Yet with the development of more and more sophisticated, invasive things that can be done to patients (most of which carry a significant risk of complications), the risk that the health care provider will, in fact, harm patients by doing things for them has increased. An important line of defense against such iatrogenesis (complications inadvertently caused by the health care provider through diagnostic studies or therapeutic interventions) is to make sure that explanations for what is going on with the patient that may *not* require invasive studies or high-risk treatment have been adequately considered. That means the health care provider must understand normal physiology and how it is changed in the setting of disease. The thyroid provides some classic examples, as in this case.

Review Questions

1. What are the three roles of thyroid hormone?
2. Give three reasons why clinicians need to have a good understanding of thyroid physiology.

2. ANATOMY AND HISTOLOGY OF THE THYROID GLAND

The thyroid gland is located in the anterior part of the neck, adjacent to, and just below, the thyroid cartilage (see Figure 12.1). Embryologically, it is derived from an outpouching of the floor of the pharynx that grows downward, in front of the trachea, bifurcating to form the two lobes of the thyroid gland. In a normal adult, the thyroid gland weighs about 20 g. The thyroid gland has a rich blood supply, about 5 mL/g/min, arising from the superior and inferior thyroid arteries and exiting via the thyroid veins.

At the cellular level, thyroid tissue is organized into groups of cells called **follicles**. The cells of each follicle form a round shell surrounding a lumen filled with secreted material called **colloid**. This colloid mainly consists of modified forms of the protein precursor **thyroglobulin**, from which thyroid hormones are generated (see Sec. 3). Depending on the functional state of the thyroid (i.e., if it is normal, hyperactive, or hypoactive), both the cells and the colloid take on a distinctive appearance. Thus, normally the single layer of epithelial cells lining the follicle are cuboidal (about as wide as they are tall), and the lumen is largely filled with colloid (Figure 12.2A).

In pathological hyperactive states, to be discussed in Sec. 4 and 8, the epithelium is tall, the amount of colloid is diminished, and there is a peculiar vacuolation seen between the cells and the colloid substance that reflects the tremendous rate at which colloid is being taken up by the cells for conversion to thyroid hormone (Figure 12.2B).

Finally, the pathologically hypoactive thyroid displays a low, flat epithelium surrounding follicles packed with colloid (Figure 12.2C).

In addition to the epithelial cells surrounding the follicles, a distinctive type of cells can be seen under special stains in the spaces between follicles. Termed **parafollicu-**

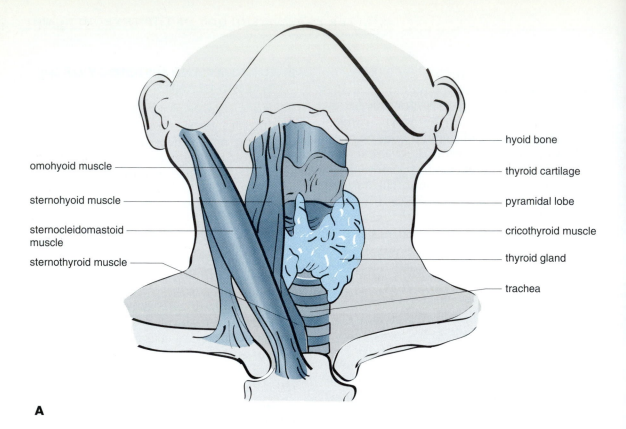

A

omohyoid muscle

sternohyoid muscle

sternocleidomastoid muscle

sternothyroid muscle

hyoid bone

thyroid cartilage

pyramidal lobe

cricothyroid muscle

thyroid gland

trachea

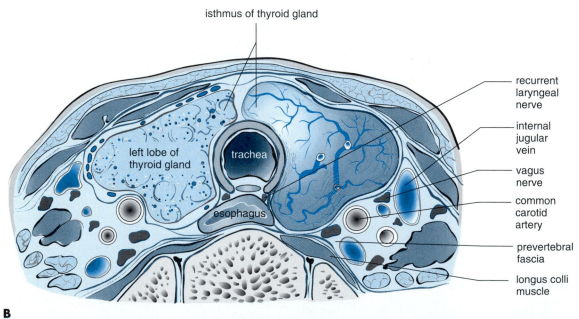

isthmus of thyroid gland

left lobe of thyroid gland

trachea

esophagus

recurrent laryngeal nerve

internal jugular vein

vagus nerve

common carotid artery

prevertebral fascia

longus colli muscle

B

FIGURE 12.1. Location of the thyroid gland. *A.* Gross anatomy of the thyroid gland, anterior view. *B.* Cross-sectional view displaying the structures in the neighborhood of the thyroid gland. *(Adapted, with permission, from Linder HH (1989). Clinical Anatomy. Norwalk, CT, Appleton & Lange, pp 134–135.)*

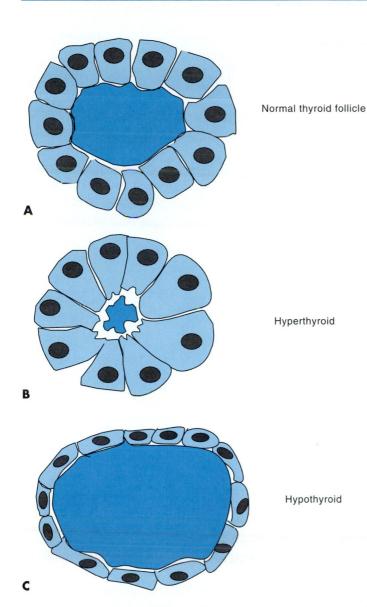

Normal thyroid follicle

Hyperthyroid

Hypothyroid

FIGURE 12.2. Thyroid histology. Schematic diagram of (A) a normal thyroid follicle, (B) a follicle from a hyperactive gland, and (C) a follicle from a hypoactive gland. Note that at lower magnification, thyroid tissue consists of numerous such follicles packed together in a minimal connective tissue matrix. Normal thyroid cells are roughly cuboidal, with ample colloid within the follicular lumen. The hyperthyroid gland has enlarged cells and scant colloid because of the rapid rate of colloid uptake and thyroid hormone release. The hypothyroid gland displays flat, inactive follicular epithelial cells surrounding a large lake of colloid.

lar cells, they secrete calcitonin, a hormone involved in calcium homeostasis that has nothing to do with the thyroid gland's functions (see Chap. 14).

Clinical Pearls

○ The normal thyroid gland is barely palpable. Hence physical examination is a good way to detect thyroid gland enlargement, as would occur either in hyperthyroidism (up to 3 to 4 × normal), or in those forms of hypothyroidism characterized by thyroid enlargement (e.g., iodine deficiency with goiter formation or autoimmune disorders with lymphocyte infiltration of the thyroid gland).

○ In hyperthyroidism, blood supply and flow increase with the enlargement of the gland, often resulting in turbulent blood flow that gives rise to an audible whistling sound termed a *bruit*. Sometimes this turbulence is even palpable, in which case it is termed a *thrill*.

Review Questions

3. How does thyroid histology change with alterations in the activity of the gland?

4. What hormone unrelated to thyroid function is made in the thyroid parafollicular cells?

3. STRUCTURE, BIOSYNTHESIS, AND SECRETION OF THYROID HORMONES

Structure

Thyroid hormone comes in two active forms, **triiodothyronine (T₃)** and **thyroxine (T₄)**, both of which are iodinated derivatives of the amino acid tyrosine (see Figure 12.3). T₃ is roughly ten times more active as a transcriptional activator than T₄, and most T₃ is generated by conversion from T₄. Thus, in most ways, T₄ can be thought of as a precursor to T₃.

Thyroid hormone is metabolized by enzymes called **deiodinases**, which are found in various tissues. Removal of the 5 rather than the 5' iodine from T₄ results in the formation of **reverse T₃**, a molecule with no biologic activity (see Sec. 6).

Biogenesis

The biogenesis of thyroid hormone involves a unique variation on the common biosynthetic themes of protein secretion and protease activation (see Figure 12.4).

The initial precursor of thyroid hormone is thyroglobulin, a huge secretory protein

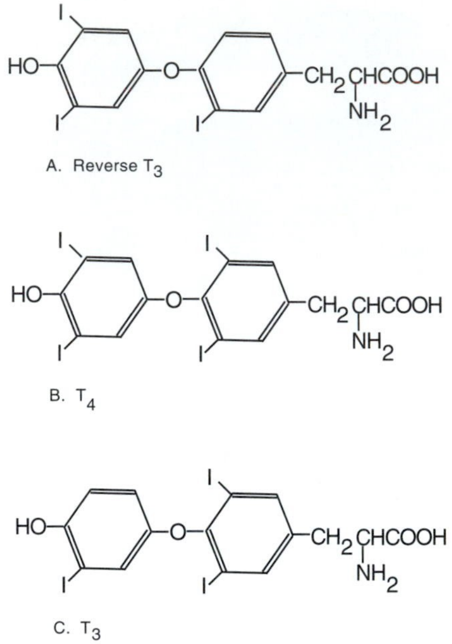

FIGURE 12.3. Structure of thyroid hormones. *A.* Reverse T₃ (inactive). *B.* Thyroxine (T₄) with 1× activity. *C.* Triiodothyronine (T₃) with 10× activity compared to T₄. By convention the rings are numbered such that the upper iodinated position is 5 and the lower iodinated position is 3. The outer ring (left) is the prime (') ring.

(330,000 Da in molecular mass, nearly 2800 amino-acid residues in length). Thyroglobulin is synthesized on membrane-bound ribosomes of the rough endoplasmic reticulum (ER) in thyroid follicular epithelial cells.

After synthesis and translocation to the ER lumen, two copies of thyroglobulin assemble as a dimer and are transported through the secretory pathway for export apically into the follicular lumen as colloid. Iodination of specific tyrosines in thyroglobulin is carried out by the enzyme **thyroid peroxidase** and most likely occurs during intracellular transport or on the apical plasma membrane at the cell–colloid interface.

Pairs of iodinated tyrosines within thyroglobulin are linked by a unique covalent **thy-**

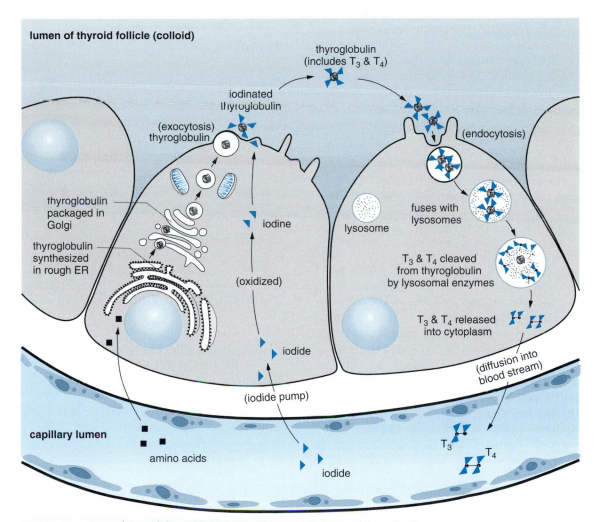

lumen of thyroid follicle (colloid)

thyroglobulin
(includes T₃ & T₄)

iodinated
thyroglobulin

(exocytosis)
thyroglobulin

(endocytosis)

thyroglobulin
packaged in
Golgi

thyroglobulin
synthesized
in rough ER

iodine

lysosome

fuses with
lysosomes

(oxidized)

T₃ & T₄ cleaved
from thyroglobulin
by lysosomal enzymes

T₃ & T₄ released
into cytoplasm

iodide

(diffusion into
blood stream)

(iodide pump)

capillary lumen

amino acids

T₃

T₄

iodide

FIGURE 12.4. Biosynthesis of thyroid hormone. Schematic diagram of thyroid cell ultrastructure. Thyroid follicular epithelial cell depicted on left side shows pathway of amino-acid and iodine uptake from the bloodstream, thyroglobulin synthesis, iodination, and colloid formation; adjacent cell on right side shows pathway of colloid uptake, transport, and proteolysis, with release of thyroid hormones into the bloodstream. In real life, both pathways normally occur simultaneously in all follicular epithelial cells.

ronine linkage. After secretion into the follicle lumen, the modified thyroglobulin is stored until stimuli for thyroid hormone secretion are received. Upon stimulation, colloid is taken up by endocytosis and cleaved by proteases, which release approximately three molecules of thyroid hormone from each 660,000-Da thyroglobulin dimer.

These newly generated molecules of thyroid hormone then leave the thyroid gland and enter the bloodstream. Historically, export from thyroid cells has been assumed to be by diffusion, as the thyroid hormone molecule is small enough and lipophilic enough to pass through membranes spontaneously. Recent studies, however, raise the possibility that thyroid hormone may, in some cases, be actively transported either into or out of cells. There is no known function for the other 99.9% of the mass of thyroglobulin left over after proteolytic release of thyroid hormone.

Organification of dietary iodide

Iodine is an element (see Chap. 10). **Iodide** is a specific molecular form of iodine in which the inorganic iodine molecule is charged (I^-). When iodine is covalently attached to carbon-containing compounds, it is said to be **organified.** Dietary iodine is absorbed in the upper gastrointestinal (GI) tract and enters the bloodstream as iodide. Inorganic iodide in blood is taken up by an active transport system in the basal surface of follicular cells of the thyroid gland. This active transport is actually a sodium/iodide co-transporter. Movement of sodium down the concentration gradient established by Na^+/K^+-ATPase (high sodium concentration outside of cells, low sodium concentration inside) drives the uptake of iodine to a concentration 40 times that found in plasma. Some iodide is also taken up by salivary, breast, and gastric tissue, but it is not organified and its significance is not known.

In the thyroid follicular cell, iodide is converted to a reactive intermediate by the enzyme thyroid peroxidase. This unstable intermediate rapidly reacts with selected tyrosines in newly synthesized thyroglobulin, resulting in organification. Secreted thyroid hormone has either three or four iodines. Precisely *which* iodines are present is extremely important: While T_3 is 10 times as active as T_4 as a regulator of transcription (the major mode of thyroid hormone action; see Sec. 4), rT_3

has no transcription-regulating activity at all (see Figure 12.3).

Review Questions

5. What fraction of the mass of the thyroglobulin precursor ends up as thyroid hormone?
6. What happens to the rest, as far as is known?
7. Briefly outline the pathway of thyroid hormone biogenesis, beginning with a molecule of iodine in the bloodstream and a molecule of thyroglobulin starting to be made on a ribosome.
8. In which cells is thyroglobulin made?
9. What is the difference in biologic activity between T_4, T_3, and rT_3?

4. THYROID HORMONE ACTION

Effects on development

The fetal thyroid does not function significantly before the second trimester. Thus, until that point, the fetus is dependent on maternal thyroid hormone; however, placental transfer of thyroid hormone is poor, and the degree of dependence of early pregnancy on thyroid hormone is not entirely clear. A higher rate of loss of pregnancies has been observed in women with mild to moderate hypothyroidism, but that may reflect the needs of maternal systems rather than those of the fetus.

There is, however, no ambiguity about the effect of thyroid hormone lack in early infancy. Thyroid hormone deficiency in early infancy results in profound mental retardation and small stature, as a result of effects on neural and skeletal development.

The critical period of thyroid hormone's influence on brain development encompasses the last month of fetal life and the first postnatal year. During this time, rapid myelinization and proliferation of dendritic and axonal processes, glial cells, and neuroblasts occur. Impairment of these events may not be fully evident until the child is older. No amount of thyroid hormone replacement therapy will restore normal mental development if thyroid hormone is lacking in the first 6 months post-birth. The extent of mental retardation depends on how early replacement therapy is begun. For this reason, the importance of recognizing and treating neonatal hypothyroidism cannot be overemphasized. Infants born in the United States and many other countries are routinely screened for the disorder at birth.

The window of time for thyroid hormone action on skeletal development is longer than that for the brain. Thus, the skeletal effects predominate if hypothyroidism develops later in childhood, when, presumably, the critical thyroid hormone–dependent aspects of brain development have already occurred. Likewise, deficient skeletal development due to thyroid insufficiency can be corrected by thyroid hormone replacement even well into early childhood.

Clinical Pearls

○ Significant maternal hypothyroidism is likely to prevent the mother from getting pregnant in the first place or from carrying the pregnancy to term. Given enough thyroid hormone to establish and maintain a successful pregnancy, mild hypothyroidism on the part of the mother does not appear to have much clinical consequence for the baby.

○ The fetal pituitary begins to function around week 11 of gestation; the thyroid, by week 20. Very little maternal thyroid hormone survives placental deiodinase activity, but this small amount may be crucial for early brain development. Antithyroid drugs like propylthiouracil (PTU) and methimazole *do* cross the placenta and in large doses will inhibit fetal thyroid function.

Effects on energy substrates, metabolism, and thermogenesis

Since normal levels of thyroid hormone are typically needed for optimum function of many organ systems, it is often easiest to identify effects of thyroid hormone by noting the consequences of *excess* or *deficiency* of thyroid hormone for various systems.

Thyroid hormone has effects on specific enzymes in a broad range of tissues that increase the metabolic rate. One of the most striking effects of thyroid hormone on many tissues is to increase the activity of Na^+/K^+-ATPase. The increased ATP consumption results in a compensatory increase in ATP production. This effect is probably responsible for the observation of a general increase in oxygen consumption in most tissues in the presence of excess thyroid hormone.

Another effect of an increase in thyroid hormone on many tissues is to increase the turnover (i.e., both synthesis and degradation) of carbohydrate, fat, and protein. Depending on the circumstances, the balance may shift in favor of synthesis or degradation.

With regard to protein metabolism, the growth-promoting effects generally predominate at normal levels of thyroid hormone, but protein degradation and hence muscle wasting is seen in hyperthyroidism.

Thyroid hormone deficiency potentiates insulin action, resulting in increased glycogen synthesis. Conversely, when thyroid hormone levels are high, epinephrine-induced glycogenolysis predominates.

In lipid metabolism, thyroid hormone generally stimulates cholesterol degradation more than synthesis, and thus serum concentration of cholesterol tends to be elevated in patients with thyroid hormone deficiency.

Overall, thyroid hormone effects include stimulation of various "futile cycles." As their activity increases, heat is generated. This is believed to be important in regulation of body temperature in homeothermic animals (e.g., like us; see Chap. 11).

Clinical Pearls

○ Apathetic thyrotoxicosis refers to the subset of hyperthyroid patients in whom weakness and fatigue rather than hyperactivity predominates. This subset of patients may be more sensitive to the potential for muscle wasting in the hyperthyroid state. The classical presentation would be an elderly patient with the "dwindles" (weight loss, no longer able to care for himself or herself alone at home) who is noted to have atrial fibrillation or some other form of supraventricular tachycardia and proximal muscle weakness when admitted to the hospital for "failure to thrive."

○ Hyperthyroidism exacerbates diabetes mellitus as a result of increased glucose absorption and increased glycogenolysis. It also increases the turnover of various vitamins, and therefore can result in vitamin deficiency syndromes.

○ Hypothyroidism tends to exacerbate hypercholesterolemia as a result of decreased lipid metabolism. Likewise, the accumulation of carotene as a consequence of decreased metabolism of carotene to vitamin A can give a mild yellowish tint to the skin in hypothyroidism (but unlike in jaundice, the sclera are *not* yellow).

○ Sensitivity to hot and cold environments is seen in hyper- and hypothyroidism, respectively. That is, the hyperthyroid patient often feels too hot in a room that others find comfortable, while the hypothyroid patient typically feels too cold.

This is due to the effects of thyroid hormone to promote futile cycles and thermogenesis.

Drug metabolism

In the presence of higher than normal levels of thyroid hormone, the metabolism of various substances (including drugs, adrenal steroids, etc.) is increased; therefore, the half-life typically decreases. Thus, the usual dose of many drugs may be inadequate in the hyperthyroid patient.

Some drugs, however, may appear to have increased activity in hyperthyroidism, despite the decrease in their half-life. These drugs may also appear ineffective in hypothyroidism. Often, these are drugs that need to be metabolized to form the active intermediates. In other cases, insensitivity to a particular drug may be due to receptor down-regulation in hypothyroidism. Conversely, if a receptor is disproportionately upregulated in a particular hyperthyroid patient, the patient may become more sensitive to the drug than he or she was in the euthyroid state.

Clinical Pearls

○ Thyroid hormone decreases the activity of the enzyme **superoxide dismutase**, which is involved in free radical detoxification. Hence there is increased exposure to damaging free radicals in untreated hyperthyroidism.

○ Hypothyroidism should be considered in a patient found to have toxic blood levels of a drug without an alternative explanation (e.g., a history of excessive ingestion, renal failure, etc.).

○ The body treats hormones as it does drugs. Thus, hormone turnover generally increases with hyperthyroidism. A patient with mild adrenal insufficiency may develop severe, life-threatening adrenal insufficiency in the face of new hyperthyroidism, as the combination of increased stress and decreased half-life overwhelms the synthetic capacity of a failing adrenal gland (see Chap. 8).

○ A key point to remember is that normal function (of organ systems, of drug metabolism, of hormone and drug effects, etc.) will be deranged in thyroid disease, although the precise consequence and direction of the derangement may be unpredictable, varying from patient to patient depending on the extent of thyroid dysfunction and the status of other organ systems in any given patient.

Effects on various specific organ systems

Although many of thyroid hormone's actions are general, multitissue, and system effects, some have distinctive manifestations in particular organ systems.

Effects on the heart

Thyroid hormone has a marked chronotropic (increasing the heart rate) and ionotropic (increasing the force of myocardial contraction) effect on the heart. This is due to a number of effects at the molecular level. Increased Ca^{2+}/ATPase in the sarcoplasmic reticulum, resulting in diminished diastolic relaxation, alteration in the isoforms of Na^+/K^+-ATPase synthesized, and increased concentration of G proteins inside cardiac myocytes, has been observed in humans.

Clinical Pearls

○ The general effect of thyroid hormone of increasing the metabolic rate in all tissues has important implications for a patient with coronary artery disease. In such patients, the heart may be barely able to get enough oxygen to meet its needs at rest. The recognition and treatment of hypothyroidism will result in increased thyroid hormone, and therefore increased oxygen consumption by the heart, at any given level of myocardial workload. Thus, even if heart rate or contractility stayed the same, there would be a substantial risk that myocardial ischemia (insufficiency of oxygen) would become severe enough to cause myocardial infarction (death of heart muscle cells).

This situation is further exacerbated by the effect of thyroid hormone of increasing the metabolic rate in the periphery. This will result in a demand for increased oxygen to the periphery, and hence increased heart rate and/or contractility to supply more blood to peripheral tissues.

For both of these reasons, the intrinsic effects on the heart and the response to demands of the periphery, thyroid disease and coronary artery disease are a dangerous combination. Treatment of the newly diagnosed hypothyroid patient who is suspected of having heart disease must be carried out extremely gradually, with close monitoring of the patient's symptoms of cardiac ischemia in response to thyroid hormone therapy.

○ Excess thyroid hormone can cause tachyarrhythmias; insufficient thyroid hormone can result in heart block (as a result of impaired conduction through the atrioventricular node) or pump failure. Hypothyroidism should always be considered in the patient who is hypotensive and responding poorly to catecholamine-related pressor drugs such as dopamine or norepinephrine. This is probably due to receptor down-regulation or desensitization.

Effects on the nervous system

In addition to its profound effects on early development of the nervous system, as discussed earlier, thyroid hormone also has important effects in adults.

Profound effects of thyroid hormone on the sympathetic nervous system are seen. The concentration of β-adrenergic receptors on the cell surface of heart, skeletal muscle, adipose tissue, and lymphocytes increases, while the concentration of myocardial α receptors decreases. Overall, the effect of thyroid hormone on adrenergic receptors is to cause an increased sensitivity to catecholamines.

Thyroid hormone excess or deficiency can have a range of effects on the mood and mental status of patients. In general, the hyperthyroid patient is more emotional, has difficulty concentrating on one task, and has a more "manic" presentation. Conversely, in general, the patient who becomes hypothyroid as an adult manifests a general slowing in neurologic function, with difficulty in thinking and depression.

Clinical Pearls

○ Slowed reflexes in hypothyroidism and hyperreflexia in hyperthyroidism probably reflect altered neural conduction and muscle contraction as a result of changes in transcription of various genes (e.g., myosin isoforms, channel proteins, etc.) in the altered thyroid hormone environment.

○ The neurologic manifestations of thyroid disease can be extremely variable. Despite the generalizations noted above, sometimes a hypothyroid patient, rather than being slow and quiet, manifests irritability, paranoia, and agitation. Conversely, sometimes a hyperthyroid patient can be depressed and withdrawn.

○ Excess thyroid hormone can cause respiratory muscle fatigue, making it difficult to wean an intubated patient from mechanical ventilation (see Chap. 8).

○ Thyroid hormone is necessary for normal functioning of the brain centers controlling hypoxic and hypercapneic respiratory drive. Thus, profound hypothyroidism can result in respiratory failure, especially in a patient with severe underlying lung disease such as emphysema, primarily by affecting the brain centers controlling hypoxic and hypercapneic drive.

Effects on hematopoiesis

Thyroid hormone can increase hematopoiesis (red blood cell formation). The most likely mechanism is that increased oxygen consumption in the presence of thyroid hormone results in increased production of erythropoietin, the renal hormone that regulates red blood cell production by the bone marrow.

Thyroid hormone also increases the 2,3-diphosphoglycerate concentration in erythrocytes (red blood cells). This allows increased oxygen dissociation from hemoglobin in response to tissue hypoxia.

Clinical Pearl

○ The effect of thyroid hormone of increasing 2,3-diphosphoglycerate means that in some patients with hypothyroidism, there may be a "physiologic anemia" due to decreased oxygen dissociation as a result of the fall in 2,3-diphosphoglycerate, causing a net decrease in effective oxygen-carrying capacity at any given hematocrit (red blood cell concentration). This is not a true anemia, since the supply of red blood cells and hemoglobin is adequate; however, because the ability of the red blood cells to release oxygen is impaired, tissues may suffer the same consequence of inadequate oxygenation in hypothyroidism that would occur in true anemia.

Note that this effect is counter to that described earlier, in which hypothyroidism, by decreasing tissue oxygen needs, can actually *protect* the heart from working harder than its oxygen supply will safely allow, so that the overly aggressive correction of hypothyroidism can cause harm. This emphasizes the point that the precise consequences of hypo- or hyperthyroidism are complex, are not easily predicted, and can be different from patient to patient, depending on variables that cannot easily be assessed.

Effects on the gastrointestinal system

Thyroid hormone stimulates GI motility. Thus, excess thyroid hormone causes increased GI motility, which can manifest as diarrhea and contribute to weight loss. Conversely, decreased GI motility causes the constipation and contributes to some of the weight gain typically observed in hypothyroid patients.

Effects on the skeletal system

The important effect of thyroid hormone on the skeletal system during development has already been discussed.

In addition, in adults, thyroid hormone stimulates bone turnover, with resorption being somewhat more prominent than bone formation in the presence of high levels of thyroid hormone. This can result in significant bone loss over time, and sometimes even in hypercalcemia in the severest cases.

Clinical Pearl

○ It is important to be sure that hypothyroid women are not taking too much thyroid hormone [as manifested by a subnormal thyroid-stimulating hormone (TSH)], as it will result in decreased bone density and increase their risk for significant osteoporosis and fractures in the future.

This poses difficulties in clinical management because often the level of thyroid hormone replacement at which the patient "feels best" results in excessive suppression of TSH.

Review Questions

10. What are the effects of thyroid hormone on development?
11. How does thyroid hormone increase the metabolic rate?
12. What are the effects of thyroid hormone deficiency on the GI tract and the respiratory system?
13. What is the effect of thyroid hormone excess on the brain and the skeletal system in adults?

Molecular mechanisms of thyroid hormone action

The best understood of thyroid hormone's effects are on gene transcription and hence take hours to days to be manifest.

In molecular mechanism, thyroid hormones work in a manner similar to that of steroid hormones. The best understood actions of thyroid hormone involve binding of thyroid hormone to its receptor, which is homologous in overall structure to steroid hormone receptors (see Chap. 3). As in the case of steroid hormones, binding of the activated hormone-receptor complex (in conjunction with other proteins) to specific regions of DNA results in enhanced or diminished transcription at those sites. The resulting change in mRNA composition (and therefore proteins translated) in specific tissues is believed to be the basis for most of the actions of thyroid hormone.

Whereas some steroid hormone receptors reside in the cytoplasm and are transported into the nucleus only upon binding of their ligand, the receptors for thyroid hormone are found in the nucleus all the time.

There are two thyroid hormone receptor genes, α and β, each of which generates two different alternatively spliced isoforms, α_1, α_2, β_1, and β_2. The receptors are differentially expressed in different tissues, and each is activated by different concentrations of thyroid hormone, with the α_2 variant not binding thyroid hormone at all. It may be that the α_2 variant of thyroid hormone receptor plays an important role in inhibiting thyroid hormone activation of certain genes.

The regulation of gene expression by thyroid hormone is greatly complicated by the recent discovery that thyroid hormone receptors can form homo- and heterodimers (see Chap. 2). The other protein, in the case of the heterodimers, is often a subtype of **retinoic acid receptor**. Each of these homo- and heterodimers activates a different pattern of gene expression.

Thus, the combinatorial possibilities are immense for activating different programs of gene expression in various tissues in response to thyroid hormone, as a function of the concentration of other hormones.

A mitochondrial binding site to account for thyroid hormone effects on ATP production and metabolic rate remains a controversial hypothesis. Other nongenomic effects of thyroid hormone, including effects of T_4 and rT_3 that are not observed with T_3, have been proposed but also remain controversial (see Sec. 9, Frontiers).

Review Question

14. What are the similarities and differences in mechanism between the action of steroids and thyroid hormone?

5. REGULATION OF THYROID FUNCTION

TRH and TSH

Thyrotropin-releasing hormone (TRH) is secreted in pulsatile fashion by a subset of neurons in the median eminence of the hypothalamus. Traveling through the pituitary portal circulation, it stimulates secretion of TSH (also called thyrotropin) from specialized cells (thyrotropes) of the anterior pituitary.

TSH is the primary stimulus for thyroid hormone secretion; it acts by binding to specific receptors on the surface of the thyroid follicular cell. The activated TSH receptor results in an elevation of intracellular cyclic AMP, which stimulates all aspects of thyroid function (thyroglobulin synthesis, secretion, endocytosis, proteolysis, and release of mature thyroid hormone as well as follicular cell growth). Thyroid hormones, in turn, feed back to inhibit TSH secretion (see Figure 12.5).

Most of TSH's effects of increasing thyroid hormone biosynthesis and secretion are mediated via cyclic AMP elevation. However, some effects (e.g., stimulation of thyroid peroxidase) are mediated via the inositol triphosphate and calcium signaling pathways.

A delayed effect of TSH is to stimulate growth and proliferation of thyroid follicular cells. This is why the thyroid gland enlarges upon prolonged TSH stimulation.

Clinical Pearls

◯ In Graves' disease, the commonest form of hyperthyroidism, the immune system makes an antibody that binds to and activates the patient's own TSH receptor (mimicking the action of TSH), thereby stimulating excessive thyroid hormone secretion. This does not respond to negative feedback, however, since it is an antibody-producing cell, rather than the hypothala-

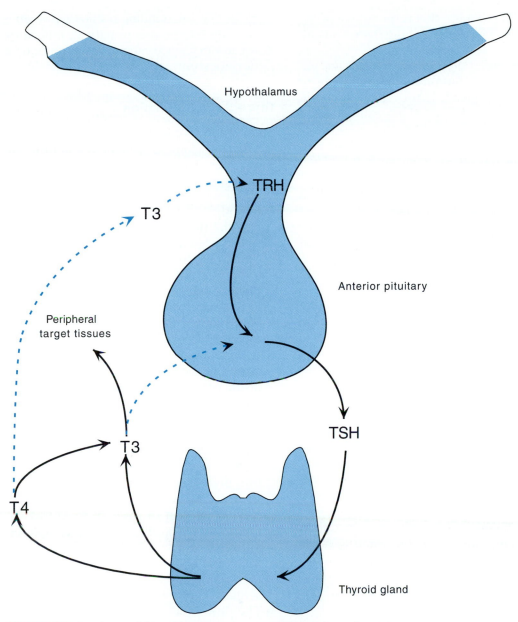

FIGURE 12.5. Regulation of thyroid hormone secretion. TRH travels via the pituitary portal system from the hypothalamus and triggers TSH secretion from the anterior pituitary thyrotrophs. TSH, entering the systemic circulation, in turn stimulates the thyroid to synthesize and secrete more thyroid hormones (mainly T_4, but also some T_3). Most T_3 comes from conversion of T_4 to T_3 in the bloodstream or in tissues, including upon negative feedback (dashed lines). *(Adapted, with permission, from Greenspan FS (1996). The thyroid gland, in Greenspan, FS and Strewler, GJ eds. Basic and Clinical Endocrinology, 5th ed. Stamford, CT, Appleton & Lange.)*

mus and pituitary, that is the source of the excessive stimulation of the thyroid gland. Thus, the TSH is suppressed.

○ Hashimoto's thyroiditis is also an extremely common autoimmune disease of the thyroid gland. However, in this case, the gland is destroyed by cell-mediated immune attack, resulting in hypothyroidism, whereas in Graves' disease, the autoimmune response is humoral, with production of antibodies that stimulate the TSH receptor, resulting in hyperthyroidism rather than destroying the gland.

○ Because these are both autoimmune disorders, and because antibody titers can change over time, sometimes a patient can switch from having Graves' disease to having Hashimoto's disease.

○ A goiter (enlarged thyroid gland) can occur for many different reasons:

• In iodine deficiency, goiter develops as a result of excess stimulation by TSH in an unsuccessful physiological attempt to boost thyroid hormone production.

• In Graves' disease, goiter develops because of the antibody mimicking TSH.

• In Hashimoto's disease, goiter is caused by a combination of lymphocytic infiltration and inflammation of the thyroid tissue as well as the trophic effects of high blood levels of TSH.

• In nodular disease, goiter can be due to a small focus within the gland that has become autonomous — i.e., does not respond to the usual controls — and either does or does not secrete thyroid hormone. The cases in which thyroid hormone is secreted include so-called toxic nodular goiter and some differentiated cancers, while those in which it is not, include "cold nodules" (so named because they fail to take up radioactive iodine used as a tracer in diagnostic testing for thyroid disease) and undifferentiated cancers. A cold nodule stands out be-

cause the surrounding normal tissue does take up iodine; it is usually an indication for surgery, since cancer, or its subsequent development, is a concern.

Thyroid autoregulation

Some distinctive features of the regulation of the thyroid gland involve iodine in different ways. These have been termed forms of **autoregulation**:

1. In iodide deficiency, transport of iodide into the thyroid gland is enhanced.

2. In the presence of excess iodide, *organification* of iodine is inhibited, a phenomenon termed **Wolff-Chaikoff block**. Generally this is a transient phenomenon, overcome in about a week's time by negative-feedback loops involving iodide transport within the thyroid.

3. A rapid and transient inhibition of thyroid hormone *secretion* by iodine is observed, distinct from Wolff-Chaikoff block. While the Wolff-Chaikoff effect can take a long time to be manifest (because of the large pool of intrathyroid organified precursor), this ability of iodine to block hormone secretion is very rapid, quickly decreasing free thyroid hormone levels in the bloodstream. Thus iodine is actually used as an *acute* treatment in cases of severe hyperthyroidism. Note that this is a completely different mechanism of action from the treatment of *chronic* hyperthyroidism with *radioactive* iodine (^{131}I) for the purpose of actually *killing* thyroid follicular cells.

4. The ratio of T_3 to T_4 synthesis by the thyroid gland is increased or decreased in the setting of iodine deficiency or plenty. Thus, when it has trouble making thyroid hormone as a result of iodine deficiency, the body secretes the more active form, T_3, directly.

5. The thyroid's set point for response to TSH can be altered by its organified iodide con-

tent. Thus, iodide-deficient animals develop bigger goiters (enlargement of the thyroid gland due to hypertrophy and hyperplasia in response to stimulation) in response to TSH than do iodide-sufficient animals injected with the same amount of TSH.

Extrathyroidal (peripheral) regulation

Several different deiodinases present in various tissues of the body can modify the structure and hence the activity of thyroid hormones, as will be discussed in Sec. 6.

Clinical Pearls

○ It might be expected that under certain circumstances, iodine, as a component of thyroid hormone, could cause hyperthyroidism (and this can sometimes be true; see Sec. 6). However, in most individuals, high doses of iodine actually are a good treatment for hyperthyroidism because of the inhibitory effect of high-dose iodine on thyroid hormone secretion.

○ Some individuals (particularly patients with autoimmune disorders such as Hashimoto's thyroiditis) are apparently unable to overcome Wolff-Chaikoff block, and hence, chronic exposure to large doses of iodide can induce hypothyroidism in these individuals.

○ Suddenly providing iodine to a population that has been chronically iodine-deficient can result in hyperthyroidism, as all of those revved-up thyroid epithelial cells suddenly have lots of iodine available. In most individuals this effect would be transient, as the inhibitory effects of iodine and feedback inhibition of TSH secretion by newly formed thyroid hormone would bring the system back into balance. However, in individuals with defects in auto-

regulation (e.g., a patient with an autonomously functioning nodule), the hyperthyroidism may be longer-lasting.

Review Questions

15. Describe five manifestations of thyroid autoregulation.

16. Compare and contrast the use of iodine acutely versus chronically in the treatment of hyperthyroidism.

6. IODIDE AND THYROID HORMONE

Iodide metabolism

Because thyroid hormones are the only iodinated products made by the body, iodine balance is a central feature of their metabolism and biogenesis. The total iodine content of the body is approximately 8 mg, most of it in the thyroid in organified form (thyroid hormone and thyroglobulin). The minimum daily requirement for iodine balance is about 50 to 75 μg, reflecting the approximately 1% turnover per day. Most Americans take in about 500 μg/d, thanks to the availability of iodized bread and salt. Renal excretion is the most important means of excretion of iodine in excess of daily needs. Figure 12.6 summarizes iodine balance and distribution throughout the body. From these numbers, it is easy to see why hypothyroidism often develops gradually and can be difficult to recognize in its early stages: The reservoir in the thyroid gland and in the bloodstream is large compared to the daily needs.

Plasma binding

Three proteins regulate the free hormone concentration in plasma: thyroid-binding globulin (TBG), thyroid-binding prealbumin (TBPA), and albumin. Both TBG and TBPA

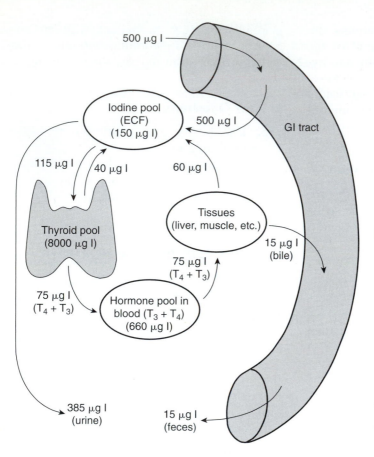

FIGURE 12.6. Idealized iodine metabolism. Approximately 500 μg of iodine is taken in by mouth daily and absorbed from the GI tract. Of this, 385 μg is promptly lost in the urine, while 75 μg is taken up and concentrated (organified) in the thyroid gland, just offsetting the net secretion of 75 μg of I in the form of T_4 and T_3. The balance sheet by which the initial 500-μg intake is offset by 500 μg of excretion in the urine and feces is indicated. (Adapted, with permission, from Ganong WF (1997). Review of Medical Physiology, 18th ed. Stamford, CT, Appleton & Lange.)

are specific, high-affinity binding proteins for the thyroid hormones. Only 0.03% of T_4 and 0.3% of T_3 is actually free hormone; the rest is protein-bound. The bioavailable fraction approximates the free hormone concentration, and thus the tightly protein-bound fraction serves as a reservoir by which free hormone levels can be maintained in equilibrium without transient fluctuations. There is enough thyroid hormone bound to plasma proteins to maintain adequate free thyroid hormone levels for about a week. The supply present in the form of colloid in the thyroid gland is much larger and is enough to meet body thyroid hormone needs for several months.

Some recent data suggest that part of the protein-bound fraction is indeed available to tissues. Nevertheless, the assumption that the free hormone is the active fraction provides a reasonable first approximation and serves as the basis for clinical testing.

Peripheral conversion of thyroid hormone

The most active thyroid hormone is T_3, yet most thyroid hormone is secreted in the form of T_4. T_4 can be thought of as a precursor in that its spectrum of actions is the same as that of T_3, but it has only one-tenth the biologic potency of T_3. About one-third of the daily output of T_4 (80 μg) is converted to T_3 each day by peripheral deiodination.

There are two forms of 5'-deiodinase involved in conversion of T_4 to T_3 (see Table 12.1). One form is found in the liver, the kidney, and the thyroid itself. Called type I 5'-deiodinase, its activity is typically increased in hyperthyroidism and decreased in hypothyroidism. It is sensitive to the drug PTU, which therefore can be used to treat hyperthyroidism. This deiodinase contains the rare amino acid selenocysteine, in which sulfur is replaced by selenium.

The other form of 5'-deiodinase, termed type II, is insensitive to PTU and is found in the brain and pituitary gland. By mediating local conversion of T_4 to T_3, type II 5'-deiodinase may be involved in the feedback regulation of thyroid hormone synthesis at the level of the thyrotrope and in maintaining preferential saturation of nuclear T_3 receptors in the central nervous system (90% nuclear receptor saturation in the brain versus approximately 50% for other tissues) under normal conditions.

Unlike that of the type I enzyme, the level of type II goes down in hyperthyroidism and up in hypothyroidism, consistent with its proposed role in regulating local tissue thyroid hormone concentrations. The action of the type II 5'-deiodinase can be thought of as buffering the brain from the effects of thyroid hormone deficiency.

Conversion of T_4 to rT_3 is controlled by a 5-deiodinase that is very different from the two forms of 5'-deiodinase discussed previously. Its importance is due to the fact that rT_3 has no thyroid hormone activity. Furthermore, increased formation of rT_3 via this deiodinase is an important basis for the euthyroid sick syndrome.

During various forms of systemic illness not directly involving the thyroid gland, as well as in starvation, the activity of this 5'-deiodinase is decreased. Thus, T_4-to-T_3 conversion is impaired, and hence the level of rT_3 rises and the T_3 level falls. However, there is often no compensatory rise in thyroid hormone production. Thus, seriously ill patients seem to be functionally slightly hypothyroid, but with no intrinsic thyroid lesion. This is termed the euthyroid sick syndrome and probably has the beneficial adaptive response of decreasing metabolic rate and catabolism in response to stress. This syndrome should *not* be treated with thyroid hormone.

With more severe systemic illness, both T_3 and T_4 can fall, although generally TSH remains normal. The reasons for the lack of an increase in TSH to stimulate more T_3 and T_4 production are unclear. Illness apparently inhibits TSH secretion by the pituitary, through unknown mechanisms. During recovery from illness, both T_4 and TSH rise and can transiently overshoot the normal range.

TABLE 12.1 PROPERTIES OF THE DEIODINASES

	Type I 5'-deiodinase	Type II 5'-deiodinase
Location	Liver, kidney, thyroid	Brain and pituitary
Increased activity in	Hyperthyroidism	Hypothyroidism
Decreased activity in	Hypothyroidism	Hyperthyroidism
Affinity for thyroid hormones (K_m)	Low	High
Sensitive to PTU	Yes	No

NOTE: K_m is a measure of the affinity of the deiodinase for thyroid hormones.

Clinical Pearl

○ Pregnancy is a physiologically hyperthyroid state in which the metabolic rate of the mother must increase to meet the needs of the fetus as well.

At least one molecular basis for this effect is through the high levels of human chorionic gonadotropin (HCG) that are generated during the first trimester of pregnancy. HCG, like TSH, is a glycopro-tein hormone consisting of two subunits, one of which is identical to the α subunit of TSH, the other of which is distinctive (and closely resembles the β subunit of LH). However, HCG does have some small binding capacity for the TSH recep-tor, and because it reaches such high con-centrations during early pregnancy, it is able to occupy and stimulate TSH recep-tors and thereby drive increased thyroid hormone secretion.

Review Questions

17. What is the daily turnover of iodine?
18. What are the plasma proteins that de-termine the free concentration of thy-roid hormone?
19. How does peripheral conversion of thyroid hormone serve as another level of regulation of thyroid status?

7. MEASUREMENT OF THYROID HORMONES

Initial considerations

It is important to distinguish between pro-tein-bound and free thyroid hormone, since only the free hormone is seen by tissues (both in the periphery and at the pituitary). Like-wise, it is important to consider whether the patient's condition is one in which changes in the level of plasma TBG are likely (e.g., increased in pregnancy, decreased in patients with liver disease or on glucocorticoids or androgens). In such conditions, total thyroid hormone levels will change to reflect the al-teration in the fraction that is protein-bound and hence not participating directly in feed-back inhibition at the level of the hypothala-mus and pituitary. Steady state will again be reached when the increase in total thyroid

hormone is sufficient to reestablish the nor-mal amount of *free* thyroid hormone.

An increase in *total* thyroid hormone levels in a patient with elevated TBG is *not* indica-tive of hyperthyroidism, because the excess thyroid hormone is all protein-bound (to TBG). Conversely, the patient with congeni-tally low TBG levels, or with liver disease, will achieve the appropriate free thyroid hor-mone levels at a lower-than-normal total thy-roid hormone concentration. Measuring only total thyroid hormone level might lead to the erroneous conclusion that the patient is hypo-thyroid.

Resin uptake tests, which measure only the free hormone, were developed for precisely these reasons. Now, more sophisticated anti-body tests that recognize only free thyroid hormone have been developed.

A rational approach to ordering thyroid function tests

If you suspect thyroid disease, either hypo- or hyperthyroidism, a TSH is the first blood test to order (after physical examination of the patient, of course). The currently avail-able TSH tests can distinguish either eleva-tion or suppression of TSH from the normal level and hence are good monitors for what is going on with the gland.

If the TSH comes back low, the patient could have either hyperthyroidism (e.g., Graves' disease) with pituitary suppression or hypothyroidism due to hypothalamic or pituitary failure (rare). A free T_4 test would distinguish between these possibilities: If free T_4 is elevated, the patient has true hyperthy-roidism; if is is low, the patient has hypothy-roidism due to hypothalamic/pituitary fail-ure. A serologic test for thyroid-stimulating antibody titer would confirm Graves' disease in a patient with elevated serum free T_4. An ^{125}I uptake study would identify a palpable thyroid nodule as either "hot" (hyperfunc-tioning) or "cold" (nonfunctioning, with high risk of being a cancer).

If the TSH is elevated, the patient could have either hypothyroidism (e.g., Hashimoto's thyroiditis) with lack of feedback inhibition of pituitary TSH secretion (very common) or hyperthyroidism due to a hypothalamic or pituitary tumor resulting in oversecretion of TSH (extremely rare). A free T_4 test would distinguish between these possibilities: If free T_4 is low, the patient has hypothyroidism, which could be shown to be Hashimoto's disease by demonstrating elevated antithyroid microsomal antibodies; if the free T_4 is high, consider the possibility of a TRH- or TSH-secreting tumor.

Remember that the free T_4 level tells you about the amount of thyroid hormone that the patient's tissues actually see (e.g., corrected for changes in binding globulins, etc., that would make total blood thyroid hormone level misleading). The TSH level normally tells you what the pituitary thinks is going on with the thyroid gland — and hence, the isolated TSH result may be misleading if the patient's neuroendocrine axis is disordered at the level of the pituitary or higher. Also, one has to be alert to the possibility that mild abnormality may reflect not intrinsic thyroid disease, but rather may be a response to severe systemic illness (see Sec. 6).

It should now be clear to you why we generally want to know the *free* rather than the total thyroid hormone level. But do we want to determine the free T_4, the free T_3, or both? Usually, the free T_4 alone is good enough, since most circulating thyroid hormone is T_4 and it should be in equilibrium with T_3. Rarely, a patient will have an unusual disorder that requires the determination of T_3 (or total thyroid hormone) level to make a clear-cut diagnosis.

Determination of TSH level

Although the TSH level is only an indirect reflection of the body's thyroid hormone status, it is generally viewed as the single best screening test for thyroid disease. It is a good test for hypothyroidism due to thyroid gland failure (far and away the most common cause of hypothyroidism), in which case the TSH level in the bloodstream is elevated.

Newer "supersensitive" TSH assays are now widely available and are also good for detecting hyperthyroidism (where TSH should be below normal). Note that the older assay (which may still be employed in some hospitals) is only sensitive enough to detect *elevations* in TSH.

Finally, in principle, a TRH stimulation test could physiologically distinguish a primary hypothalamic from a pituitary cause of hypothyroidism. In practice, these are extremely rare disorders that would probably be detected by imaging the brain rather than by their physiological responsiveness. Lack of an increase in an already high TSH in response to TRH has been used by some as a test for Graves' disease, but such extreme measures are rarely needed to make the diagnosis.

Review Questions

20. In what conditions might measurement of total thyroid hormone be misleading?
21. What single test would indicate destruction of the thyroid gland most reliably?
22. Why might the results of the above test be misleading in a patient with hypothyroidism due to pituitary disease?

8. A PHYSIOLOGICAL APPROACH TO DISORDERS OF THE THYROID GLAND

Patients with thyroid disease typically come to medical attention either because of symptoms that are manifestations of thyroid malfunction, or because of asymptomatic abnormalities discovered on physical examination or laboratory investigation (see Table 12.2). Furthermore, various drugs used to treat non-thyroid-related disease can influence thyroid status in subtle or dramatic ways (see Table 12.3). Your challenge as a clinician will be to:

1. Make the connection between the patient's presentation and thyroid disease.
2. Decide how to evaluate this possibility.
3. Determine the cause.
4. Initiate appropriate therapy.
5. Anticipate potential complications.

TABLE 12.2   SYMPTOMS AND PHYSICAL AND LABORATORY FINDINGS IN THYROID DISEASE

Symptoms of Thyroid Disease	Physical Findings and Laboratory Studies Suggesting Thyroid Disease
Typical for hyperthyroidism:	Typical for hyperthyroidism:
Heat intolerance	Tremor
Diarrhea	Atrial fibrillation
Emotional lability	Hyperactive reflexes
Hyperactivity or fatigue	Low serum cholesterol
Anxiety or irritability	Abnormal thyroid function
Heart palpitations and fast	tests (high free T_4, low
pulse	TSH)
Weight loss	
Menstrual abnormalities	
Typical for hypothyroidism:	Typical for hypothyroidism:
Cold intolerance	Thick, rough skin
Constipation	Delayed reflexes
Fatigue	High serum cholesterol
Altered mentation, including	Low serum sodium
agitation	Bradycardia or heart block
Weight gain	Abnormal thyroid function
Menstrual abnormalities	tests (low free T_4, high
	TSH)

NOTE: Not every patient with hyper- or hypothyroidism will demonstrate all or even most of the "typical" symptoms. Also, there is significant overlap in the manifestations of hyper- and hypothyroidism (e.g., menstrual irregularities are manifestations of both). Finally, symptoms can sometimes be paradoxical (e.g., agitation in a hypothyroid patient; the weakness and fatigue of apathetic thyrotoxicosis in the elderly).

TABLE 12.3   DRUG INTERACTIONS INVOLVING THYROID HORMONE

Inhibition of TSH release: dopamine, somatostatin, glucocorticoids

Stimulation of TSH release: metoclopramide

Raising of TBG levels and hence total T_3 and T_4: estrogen, pregnancy, narcotics, perphenazine, clofibrate

Lowering of TBG levels and hence total T_3 and T_4: androgens, glucocorticoids, L-asparaginase

Inhibition of T_4 binding to TBG: salicylate, phenylbutazone, phenytoin, furosemide, heparin (by activating lipoprotein lipase, which raises free fatty acid levels)

Acceleration of T_4 disposal due to increased hepatic conjugation: phenytoin (increasing the T_4 replacement requirement in some hypothyroid patients)

Block of peripheral conversion of T_4 to T_3, thus reducing serum T_3 and increasing serum T_4: propranolol, amiodarone, glucocorticoids, cholecystographic agents (Oragrafin, Telepaque)

Inhibition of oral absorption of T_4: cholestyramine

Block of release of T_4 and T_3 from the thyroid gland: lithium and iodine-containing drugs

Inhibition of the biosynthesis of thyroid hormone due to chronic ingestion of iodine, resulting in hypothyroidism: amiodarone

Adapted from Braverman, LE and Utiger RD (eds.) (1991), in *Werner and Ingbar's The Thyroid: A Fundamental and Clinical Text*, 7th ed. Philadelphia, Lippincott-Raven.

Clinical Pearls

There are several classes of antithyroid drugs:

○ Various monovalent anions such as perchlorate compete with iodine for uptake by the Na/I transporter. If ingested in excess, these compounds can prevent formation of thyroid hormone.
○ Thiocyanate inhibits the Na/I transporter, but is not itself concentrated in the thyroid gland. A number of foods in the brassica family (e.g., cabbage) contain thiocyanate derivatives and can cause goiter if eaten in excess.

○ The thiocarbamates (including the clinically useful drugs propylthiouracil and methimazole) are inhibitors of thyroid peroxidase. They also block the coupling reaction necessary to form thyroid hormones, and at higher doses compete for iodination with tyrosines and hence can block organification of iodine. In addition, they may have effects on thyroglobulin biosynthesis and structure. Finally, this class of drugs is immunosuppressive, which may contribute to its beneficial effect in Graves' disease, where patients have a high titer of a TSH receptor–stimulating antibody. A rare but serious reaction to these drugs can be agranulocytosis (lack of formation of white blood cells), which is very serious and requires that the drug be stopped. So ask the patient to report high fevers and sore throats and check the white blood cell count should those happen.

PTU (but not methimazole) also blocks 5'-deiodinase, thereby preventing conversion of T_4 to T_3 in the periphery.

○ β-Adrenergic blockers are useful agents for the treatment of the most unpleasant cardiovascular effects of hyperthyroidism in the short term (until the effect of thiocarbamizides is manifest). They also have some limited 5'-deiodinase inhibitory activity, thereby preventing conversion of T_4 to the more active T_3.

○ The selective and specific uptake of iodine by thyroid follicular cells can be used in another way. Patients can be treated with radioactive iodine, which will quickly concentrate in the thyroid, thereby preventing substantial exposure of other cells to ionizing radiation. Depending on the isotope of iodine used, this technique allows imaging of the thyroid (^{125}I) or destruction of thyroid tissue (^{131}I). Imaging is important if you want to determine whether a palpable nodule is cold — in which case it is more likely to be a cancer. Destruction of the thyroid with higher-energy iodine isotopes (^{131}I), with the patient placed on thyroid hormone replacement pills for the rest of his or her life, is one of the best ways of definitively treating Graves' disease. While this may seem an extreme course of action at first, when you consider the risks of the drugs and of recurrence of hyperthyroidism as the patient becomes older, and also the high degree of safety documented for thyroid ablation by ingested radioiodine, it is often the preferred approach to treatment.

○ Surgery remains an available alternative for thyroid ablation. However, it is generally reserved for patients unwilling to undergo radioactive iodine ablation and who are allergic to, or having side effects from, the available antithyroid drugs. A key issue is the skill of the surgeon. One who is very experienced will have a substantially lower complication rate.

9. FRONTIERS IN THYROID PHYSIOLOGY

Crosstalk, receptor heterogeneity, and tissue specificity of thyroid hormone effects

The "big picture" of gene expression in different tissues in response to thyroid hormone is quite complex (see Refs. 2–4). Recent studies suggest that some homologues of thyroid hormone receptor inhibit estrogen-mediated signaling in bone-derived cells but not in other tissues (see Ref. 5). Presumably developing a detailed understanding of the "code" by which specific factors activate or inhibit transcription in one tissue or another is just a matter of more work. However, along the way, some new and amazing concepts connecting myriad signaling pathways are likely to be discovered.

Apoptosis and the pathophysiology of Hashimoto's thyroiditis

Apoptosis, or programmed cell death, is one way that organs can physiologically control the number of their cells. One of many triggers of apoptosis is a pair of proteins known as fas (a receptor) and fas ligand (the protein that binds to fas).

Recently it was discovered that normal thyroid follicular cells constitutively express fas ligand, but not fas. Hashimoto's thyroiditis, the most common form of hypothyroidism, is a disorder in which autoimmune attack results in immune cell infiltration and inflammation of the thyroid gland. It seems that the cytokine interleukin 1β, released by macrophages and monocytes, during this process induces fas expression in thyroid follicular cells. The resulting interaction of fas with fas ligand triggers cell death (see Ref. 6).

Unorthodox actions of thyroid hormone: direct effects of T_3 on vascular smooth muscle relaxation

Most of the effects of thyroid hormone occur on a time scale of hours to days, consistent with an effect on transcription that is manifest only after synthesis, export, and translation of mRNA and intracellular trafficking of the encoded proteins. However, some effects occur rapidly, within minutes of exposure to thyroid hormone, which would be far too fast to be mediated via transcription. Relaxation of vascular smooth muscle is just such an example (see Ref. 7). Perhaps there are receptors for T_3 that prevent smooth muscle contraction. This may explain why patients with mild hypothyroidism are often hypertensive due to increased peripheral vascular resistance.

Unorthodox actions of thyroid hormone: regulation of actin polymerization in the brain by T_4

Moving from the unorthodox to the downright heretical, some workers argue for effects of thyroid hormone that not only are nongenomic but are mediated by T_4 and rT_3, but not T_3. Here is an example.

Recent studies have implicated integrins, "sticky" transmembrane proteins on the surface of neurons, in the molecular basis for short-term memory (see Ref. 8). Integrins themselves are regulated in many ways, including perhaps by interaction with cytoskeletal proteins such as actin. Some studies have suggested that actin polymerization may be affected by thyroid hormone acting by means of a non-transcription-mediated mechanism (see Ref. 9). Since actin polymerization is one way of regulating integrins, it is possible that at least some of the effects of thyroid hormone on the brain are mediated in such a fashion. Furthermore, it has been argued that T_4 rather than T_3 is the active form of thyroid hormone triggering these events. Whether or not these particular claims prove valid, it is important to recognize that a detailed understanding of *some* of thyroid hormone's actions (e.g., modulation of transcription) does not rule out the possibility of *other* kinds of actions. Only time (and further experimentation) will tell whether these observations are valid.

The effect of free radicals in thyroid disease

In Section 4, it was mentioned that T_3 has the effect of *decreasing* transcription of mRNA encoding the free-radical scavenging enzyme superoxide dismutase. Given this effect, free radicals have been long suspected as a culprit in hyperthyroidism. Recently, workers have reported that the effect of high T_3 on the electrical activity of the heart, which is accompanied by an increase in lipid peroxidation (a sign of free-radical generation), can be countered in rats by treatment with vitamin E, a potent antioxidant (see Ref. 10). This treatment is accompanied by a fall in lipid peroxidation. Perhaps antioxidants like vitamin C and E will someday be a part of the standard therapy for patients with hyperthyroidism.

10. HOW DOES UNDERSTANDING NORMAL PHYSIOLOGY PROVIDE INSIGHT INTO THE INITIAL CASE?

Ms F. has a common and serious medical condition (atrial fibrillation) that has a number of causes. One of the less common causes is thyroid disease. The more common causes are coronary artery disease and pulmonary emboli. Since the possibility of thyroid disease should have been suggested by the history and physical exam findings of this case, and can be ruled out less expensively and less invasively, it probably should have been ruled out first.

On testing, Ms. F. proved to be profoundly hyperthyroid. Treatment of her thyroid disease with medication eliminated the atrial fibrillation. Her heat intolerance, tremor, and falling cholesterol are all classic findings in *hyperthyroidism.* Had her other physician approached her illness from the perspective of *abnormal physiology*, he or she would have keyed in on the correct picture a lot sooner. Luckily, the physiological thinking of the resident spared the patient from being subjected to yet another expensive, high-risk procedure for no benefit.

SUMMARY AND REVIEW OF KEY CONCEPTS

1. The thyroid gland is located in the anterior neck, just below and adjacent to the thyroid cartilage. Normally barely papable, it en-

larges and atrophies in response to stimulation. Histologically, the thyroid gland is organized into epithelial follicles surrounding a lumen.

2. Thyroxine (T_4), the major secreted form of thyroid hormone, is a tetraiodinated derivative of two tyrosine amino-acid residues. It is derived from a large precursor protein called thyroglobulin that is exported via the secretory pathway into the follicular lumen, where it is called colloid. Along the way, it is iodinated through the action of the enzyme thyroid peroxidase. Upon demand, colloid is taken up and three molecules of thyroid hormone are released per molecule of thyroglobulin dimer.

3. Triiodothyronine (T_3) comes from two sources, the thyroid gland and peripheral conversion from T_4. T_3 is 10 times more active than T_4 and is probably generated in tissues by conversion of T_4. Deiodinases are enzymes that remove selective iodine residues from T_4. Different tissues have different forms of deiodinase. One form generates reverse T_3 (rT_3) by removal of the opposite iodine from T_3. rT_3 has no thyroid hormone activity.

4. Dietary iodine enters the bloodstream from the upper GI tract and is concentrated in the thyroid gland through action of an active Na/I transporter.

5. Thyroid hormone has effects on virtually all tissues during development. Most of its effects are permissive and facilitatory of particular subsets of the actions of other hormones. Some of its effects on particular organ systems are striking — e.g., on heart, bone, and brain. In addition, thyroid hormone controls the metabolic rate and heat generation in tissues.

6. The molecular mechanism of thyroid hormone's best understood actions is stimulation of transcription upon hormone binding to nuclear localized receptors. Complex patterns of gene expression are generated in different tissues and at different times through the interplay of thyroid hormone

with other nuclear hormone receptors and accessory transcription factors.

7. Thyroid hormone is regulated as part of a neuroendocrine feedback loop by TRH made in the hypothalamus, which stimulates release of TSH by the thyrotropes of the pituitary gland, which stimulates thyroid hormone synthesis and secretion by the thyroid gland. Thyroid hormone feeds back and inhibits further release of TRH and TSH.

8. Another level of regulation is the ability of iodine to inhibit or stimulate thyroid hormone synthesis, depending on the circumstances.

9. Thyroid hormone is regulated by the effects of deiodinases that can activate (T_4 to T_3) or inactivate (T_4 to rT_3) the hormone. While the active fraction is the free hormone, in equilibrium most thyroid hormone is largely bound to plasma proteins. Thus, measurement of free T_4 or T_3 is clinically more relevant than the absolute hormone level. Measurement of TSH level reveals the pituitary gland's assessment of thyroid status.

A CASE OF PHYSIOLOGICAL MEDICINE

K.B. is a 50-year-old librarian seen in the emergency room with pneumonia. The examining physician incidentally noted the classic "stare" of Graves' disease with a resting tachycardia of 150, and a closer history and physical examination elicited a wealth of findings that suggested hyperthyroidism.

Ms. B. was admitted to the hospital with the diagnosis of "complicated" pneumonia, and blood testing was done, which confirmed the clinical diagnosis of hyperthyroidism. This was initially treated with a β-adrenergic receptor blocker and PTU, an antithyroid drug. She was discharged a few days later.

However, Ms. B. quickly developed complications from taking PTU, requiring therapy with other drugs, to which she had other adverse reactions, including cholestatic jaundice. Her physician has discussed the therapeutic options, which include radioiodine ablation of her thyroid with subsequent daily thyroxine replacement or surgical removal of her thyroid. Ms. B. is having a hard time deciding what to do. Despite her physician's assurances, the thought of radiation terrifies her, as does the prospect of neck surgery.

QUESTIONS

1. What are some additional findings from a history and physical exam that would be most consistent with hyperthyroidism?
2. If only a subset of these findings were made in another patient, would that lead you to conclude that the patient was unlikely to have thyroid disease? Why or why not?
3. What blood studies would you order to make the diagnosis of Graves' disease?
4. How would you monitor Ms. B.'s thyroid status in the long run, regardless of whether her hyperthyroidism was controlled with medicines or resolved by radiation or surgical ablation of her thyroid, followed by lifelong thyroxine replacement?
5. How does radioiodine-induced thyroid ablation work? Why is drinking a millicurie (a measure of radioactivity) of ^{131}I different from drinking a millicurie of ^{32}P?
6. What are the different autoregulatory roles that iodine can play in thyroid physiology?

ANSWERS

1. Tremor, diarrhea, heat intolerance, emotional lability and anxiety, hyperactive reflexes.
2. No; for many reasons, different patients may display different subsets of clinical signs.

3. TSH or free T_4 and thyroid-stimulating antibody titers.
4. Follow the TSH and make sure it is in the normal range.
5. ^{131}I, which gives off ionizing radiation, is taken up by thyroid cells and destroys them. Iodine is rapidly concentrated in the thyroid gland or excreted and is used metabolically only to make thyroid hormone, whereas phosphorus is widely metabolized in all tissues and is incorporated into DNA and energy metabolites.
6. Acutely, iodine can shut off thyroid hormone secretion. On a slightly more delayed time scale, patients develop a block in synthesis, iodination, and proteolysis of thyroid hormone in the face of iodine excess (Wolff-Chaikoff block), but later escape from that effect. In the face of limiting iodine concentrations, T_3 (which is more active) rather than T_4 will be secreted, thereby self-correcting in activity for any lack of secretion due to iodine deficiency.

References and suggested readings

GENERAL REFERENCES

1. Greenspan FS (1996). The thyroid gland, in Greenspan FS, Strewler GJ (eds), *Basic and Clinical Endocrinology,* 5th ed. Stamford, CT, Appleton & Lange.
2. Brent GA (1994). The molecular basis of thyroid hormone action. *N Eng J Med* 331: 847–853.

FRONTIERS REFERENCES

3. Mangelsdorf DJ, et al. (1995). The nuclear receptor superfamily: The second decade. *Cell* 83:835–840.
4. Mangelsdorf DJ, Evans RM (1995). The RXR heterodimers and orphan receptors. *Cell* 83:841–850.
5. Harada H, et al. (1998). Cloning of rabbit TR4 and its bone cell-specific activity to suppress estrogen receptor-mediated transactivation. *Endocrinology* 139:204–212
6. Giordano C, et al. (1997). Potential involvement of Fas and its ligand in the pathogenesis of Hashimoto's thyroiditis. *Science* 275, 960–962.
7. Ojamaa K, et al. (1997). Acute effects of thyroid hormone on vascular smooth muscle. *Thyroid* 6:505–512.
8. Grotewiel MS, et al. (1998). Integrin-mediated short-term memory in *Drosophila. Nature* 391:455–460.
9. Leonard JL, Farwell AP (1997). Thyroid hormone-regulated actin polymerization in brain. *Thyroid* 7:147–155
10. Venditti P, et al. (1997). Vitamin E administration attenuates the T3-induced modification of heart electrical activity in the rat. *J Exp Biol* 200:909–914.

ADRENAL PHYSIOLOGY

13

1. INTRODUCTION TO THE ADRENAL GLAND

The role of the adrenal gland

The adrenal gland plays two broad physiological roles:

- Certain hormones made by the adrenal gland coordinate the body's response to various kinds of stress, in order to protect the body during deviations from the optimal baseline state.
- Some adrenal hormones dampen the actions of the immune system, thereby preventing an excessive immune response, which might otherwise do more harm than good.

Why is understanding adrenal physiology clinically important?

Three fundamental reasons for learning the nuances of adrenal physiology are that:

- Adrenal disease, like disorders of the thyroid gland, can be subtle. Often, adrenal disorders manifest as various nonspecific complaints and findings. Thus, if you do not explicitly think of the possibility of adrenal disease, you run a real risk of missing a key feature of the pathophysiology of your patient's illness — and thereby doing him or her great harm.
- Adrenal steroids are among the most valuable and potent medicines available, thanks largely to their powerful immunosuppressive effects. But if they are misused or overused, the treatment can be worse than the initial disease. In excess, or when given in large doses chronically rather than being given for brief periods of time, adrenal hormones can cause many different disorders affecting the brain, bones, eyes, blood sugar, and gastrointestinal (GI) tract, to name just a few. An understanding of normal adrenal physiology helps to explain why these com-

plications occur and how to avoid them when treating patients.
- Adrenal disease comprises a number of classic endocrinologic syndromes, including adrenal insufficiency (Addison's disease) and adrenocorticosteroid excess (such as Cushing's disease and Cushing's syndrome), and presents difficult management issues such as weaning patients off dependence on exogenous glucocorticoids.

Case Presentation

L.G. is a 40-year-old homeless panhandler who comes to medical attention after a syncopal episode downtown. In the emergency room, he describes vague abdominal pain, nausea, vomiting, and anorexia. On examination, he is notably tanned, and his tongue and gums have substantial pigmentation. He has marked orthostatic hypotension, but the physical exam is otherwise normal. Laboratory studies reveal a low serum sodium of 126 meq/L (normal 135 to 150 meq/L) and a high serum potassium of 5.7 meq/L (normal 3.5 to 5.0 meq/L).

Initially, Mr. G. was assumed to be dehydrated from alcohol ingestion and exposure. He was given intravenous fluids and sent back out onto the street. However, he was brought back with similar symptoms a few days later, and then again a week after that. On the fifth such episode, a clinician stepped back, looked at the big picture, and thought of adrenal failure as an explanation for the patient's recurring presentation. This was quickly confirmed with simple blood tests.

Looking for an underlying explanation for the adrenal insufficiency, the clinician ordered a chest x-ray and discovered a pattern suggestive of miliary tuberculosis, a diagnosis finally confirmed by bone marrow cultures. CT scan of the abdomen confirmed adrenal destruction, probably as a consequence of the disseminated infection. Unfortunately, Mr.

G.'s homelessness and poverty complicate the appropriate management of his medical condition.

The presentation of adrenal disease can be subtle and elusive even when it is screaming at you. If you do not remember adrenal physiology and consider adrenal disease when the characteristic constellation of nonspecific pathophysiological associations are observed, you will miss the diagnosis — and your patient may get worse until the correct diagnosis is made.

Review Questions

1. Name two roles of the adrenal gland.
2. Give three reasons why understanding the adrenal gland is clinically important.

2. ANATOMY AND HISTOLOGY OF THE ADRENAL GLAND

Anatomy and blood supply

The adrenals are a pair of glands located just above the kidneys, approximately 4 to 5 g each in size (see Figure 13.1A). The outer 80–90% of the adrenal gland, the **cortex**, is involved in the synthesis and secretion of **steroids**. The innermost 10–20% of the adrenal gland, the **medulla**, is involved in the synthesis and secretion into the bloodstream of **catecholamines** (see Figure 13.1).

Two sets of arteries provide a rich blood supply and converge to a single venous drainage. One of these sources, the subcapsular cortical arteries, sequentially supplies the outer to inner zones of the cortex; the other arterial blood supply penetrates directly to the medulla. Because of this arrangement, the venous drainage of the steroid-producing cortex bathes the catecholamine-producing medulla in high concentrations of cortical steroids, an arrangement that makes physiological sense (see the following).

The adrenal cortex enlarges (increases in both cell size and number of cells) in response to long-term stimulation and atrophies in response to long-term *lack* of stimulation, features that have important clinical implications (see Secs. 5 and 8).

Adrenal cortex

The adult adrenal cortex, embryologically derived from mesoderm, displays histologic and functional *zonation* (see Figure 13.1B). This means that, on cross section, different regions of the adrenal cortex look different and make different products. The outermost rim, the *glomerulosa,* consists of spherical clusters of cells just under the capsule that encases the adrenal gland. The glomerulosa produces the hormone **aldosterone**. The next layer, the *fasciculata,* appears as straight rows of cells surrounded by sinusoidal capillaries. The cells of the fasciculata produce predominantly the hormone **cortisol** but also some **androgens**. The innermost layer of the cortex, the *reticularis,* appears as cords of cells and produces primarily androgens but also some cortisol. The fasciculata and reticularis are a functional unit; excessive stimulation causes them to hypertrophy together, and lack of stimulation causes them to atrophy together (see Figure 13.2A–D). Whether these are indeed two distinct zones or a spectrum of cell types and how they are maintained, are points of controversy.

Histologically, large lipid droplets in organized arrays of cells are a prominent feature of the fasciculata. Cells of the reticularis are more irregular in organization, contain less lipid, and have prominent lipofuscin pigment granules (an indication of cellular aging). The blood supply arriving at each zone is rich in the steroid secretions of the outer zone(s). The effects of these products on the enzymes

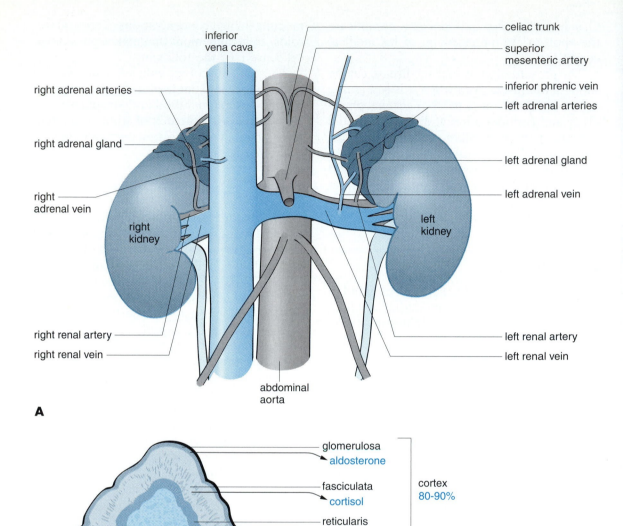

A

B

FIGURE 13.1. *A.* Location of the adrenal gland. Schematic of the position of the adrenal glands adjacent to the superior pole of the kidneys. *B.* Structure of the adrenal gland. Schematic diagram indicating the histologic layers, their products, and the relative contribution of cortex and medulla to the mass of the gland. *(B adapted, with permission, from Guyton AC (1986). Textbook of Medical Physiology. Philadelphia, Saunders, p. 909.)*

A. Normal

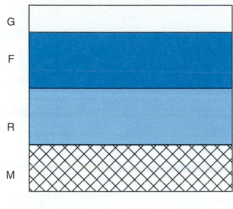

B. After ACTH stimulation

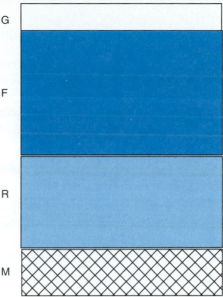

C. After prolonged glucocorticoid therapy

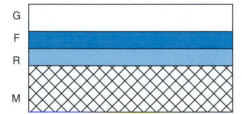

D. After hypophysectomy

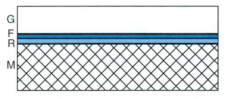

FIGURE 13.2. Functional zonation of the adrenal cortex. Schematic description of a hypothetical slice through part of the adrenal gland, illustrating the response of the layers of the adrenal cortex to stimulation and suppression. G = zona glomerulosa; F = zona fasciculata; R = zona reticularis; M = medulla. Note that atrophy of F and R is more profound in the case of hypophysectomy than after prolonged glucocorticoid therapy. A, normal, is intended as a comparison for the conditions described in B, C, and D. In B, the trophic effect of high-dose ACTH stimulation results in hypertrophy of the fasciculata and reticularis, with no response on the part of the glomerulosa or medulla. In C, prolonged glucocorticoid therapy results in inhibition of endogenous ACTH secretion and therefore atrophy of the fasciculata and reticularis. In D, hypophysectomy results in an even more profound atrophy, again limited to the ACTH-responsive fasciculata and reticularis. Perhaps this is because in C, a small amount of ACTH secretion occurs even in the presence of maximal suppression with ACTH (e.g., mediated by vasopressin), whereas in D, all ACTH-secreting cells are gone upon surgical removal of the pituitary gland, leading to complete atrophy of the adrenal gland.

involved in steroid synthesis play a role in maintaining zonation. In the fetus, an innermost *fetal zone* of the cortex is observed; it secretes large amounts of precursors that are converted to estrogen in the placenta (see Chap. 17). Upon parturition, loss of trophic actions involving the placenta results in involution of the fetal zone and the development of adult-type zonation.

Adrenal medulla

The adrenal medulla comprises irregular cords of cells surrounded by sinusoidal capillaries. In histologic preparations, the catecholamines in the medullary tissue react with chromium salts to give the distinctive appearance seen with "chromaffin tissue" of the sympathetic nervous system in other parts of the body. The chromaffin cells of the adrenal medulla are derived embryologically from epithelial cells of the neural crest. Hence, they can be considered to be modified postsynaptic cells of a sympathetic ganglion except that, instead of secreting its products at a neuromuscular junction (as do neurons that comprise the postsynaptic cells of the rest of the sympathetic nervous system), they release catecholamines into the bloodstream to engage adrenergic receptors at a distance.

Review Questions

3. What are the major secretory products of the adrenal gland?
4. Describe the adrenal gland's structural and functional organization.

3. STRUCTURE AND BIOGENESIS OF THE ADRENAL HORMONES

Although the adrenal cortical and medullary products are both involved in the response to stress, they are structurally and functionally quite different. The various regions of the adrenal cortex make different steroids as a result of the action of different enzymes present in the cells of the glomerulosa, fasciculata, and reticularis layers (see Figure 13.3). In contrast, the adrenal medulla makes only catecholamines.

Adrenal cortical hormones

The best way to approach the adrenal cortical hormones is in terms of their effects. These, in turn, are a consequence of which receptors they occupy. Thus, the glucocorticoid cortisol has the highest affinity for receptors regulating key features of carbohydrate metabolism, while the mineralocorticoid aldosterone has the highest affinity for receptors regulating electrolyte balance. Nevertheless, both cortisol and aldosterone can bind mineralocorticoid receptors in vitro. This overlap in receptor recognition, while normally not clinically significant for reasons to be described, can take on importance in certain overproduction syndromes.

In humans, the primary glucocorticoid is **cortisol**, although minor amounts of the considerably weaker glucocorticoid corticosterone are also secreted.

The primary mineralocorticoid is **aldosterone**, although minor amounts of deoxycorticosterone (DOC), an active mineralocorticoid, are also secreted. In 11-hydroxylase deficiency and 17-hydroxylase deficiency, secretion of DOC is significantly elevated.

The primary androgen secreted by the adrenal cortex is **dehydroepiandrosterone** (DHEA), a major fraction of which occurs in a sulfated form. The physiological role of DHEA is largely unknown.

Catecholamines of the adrenal medulla

Catecholamines are derivatives of the amino acid tyrosine. The biologically most relevant are epinephrine, norepinephrine, and dopa-

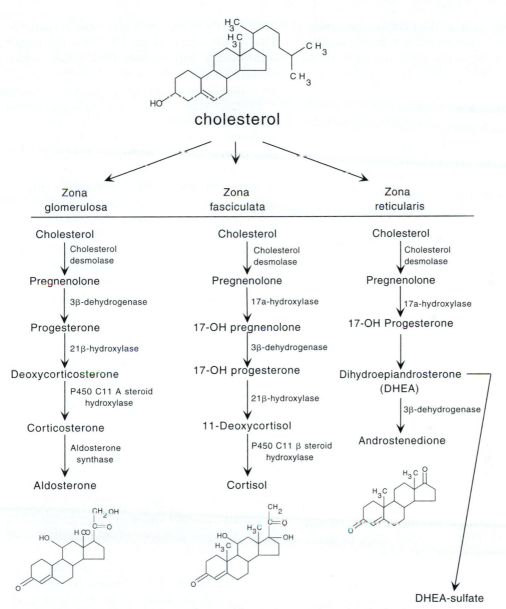

cholesterol

FIGURE 13.3. Simplified pathways of steroid biosynthesis in the adrenal gland. Note the differences in enzymes and order of enzymatic reactions in the different zones. The major product from the zona reticularis is actually DHEA sulfate, formed by modification of DHEA, as indicated. The physiological significance of DHEA has yet to be determined. (*Adapted, with permission, from McPhee S (1997), in McPhee S, et al. (eds): Pathophysiology of Disease, 2d ed. Stamford, CT, Appleton & Lange.*)

mine. Epinephrine is the primary catecholamine of the adrenal medulla, whereas norepinephrine is that of the sympathetic nervous system.

Review Questions

5. What are the secretory products of each region of the adrenal gland?
6. What is the effect of stimulation versus lack of stimulation on different regions of the adrenal gland?

Biogenesis of the adrenal hormones

Adrenal cortical steroid biogenesis

All of the adrenal cortical steroids are synthesized from cholesterol, which is itself either synthesized from acetate or taken up from the bloodstream via low-density lipoprotein particle (LDL) receptors. Cholesterol from either source is stored in intracellular lipid droplets covalently attached to triglycerides by an **ester linkage** (see Figure 13.3). The various intermediates in steroid biosynthesis must somehow shuttle rapidly between the mitochondrion and the endoplasmic reticulum, since the enzymes involved in biosynthesis are distributed between these organelles (see Chap. 2).

Upon stimulation by **adrenocorticotropic hormone (ACTH)**, the **steroidogenic acute regulatory protein (StAR)** somehow moves a pool of cholesterol from the outer to the inner mitochondrial membrane. The very first step, conversion of cholesterol to **pregnenolone** [through side-chain cleavage (scc)], occurs in mitochondria, catalyzed by the enzyme P450scc. This is the rate-limiting step for steroid biogenesis in the absence of stress. In stimulated steroidogenesis, access of cholesterol to P450scc, mediated by StAR, is the rate-limiting step. The activity of P450scc is controlled by ACTH, **angiotensin II**, and potassium ions in the glomerulosa and by

ACTH only in the fasciculata and reticularis. This makes sense, since ACTH is the major stimulus for cortisol secretion, while angiotensin II and potassium are the major stimuli for aldosterone secretion.

Pregnenolone leaves the mitochondrion and is rapidly converted to subsequent intermediates by P450-type enzymes organized into three different pathways for biogenesis of aldosterone, cortisol, or androgens, depending on the cortical zone (see Figure 13.3).

Unlike the packaged secretion of both proteins and catecholamines, which are stored in membrane vesicles and released by exocytosis, secretion of cortocosteroids is generally believed to require only synthesis, with export occurring via simple diffusion out of the producing cells. Thus, there is no stored pool of already synthesized adrenal cortical hormones to be discharged upon demand. Instead, synthesis must start from cholesterol. Nevertheless, the adrenal cortex responds to ACTH with cortisol secretion within minutes, owing to the activity of the StAR protein.

Clinical Pearls

○ As a consequence of this organization of biosynthetic enzymes, with a single precursor shunted down three different but interlocked cascades of intermediates, an enzymatic defect can have profound consequences. For example, deficiency of 21-hydroxylase (also known as P450c21) results in the inability to make cortisol, without whose negative feedback to the hypothalamus and pituitary gland more and more ACTH will be made. The ACTH pushes the adrenal gland to make cortisol, which it cannot do because of the enzyme defect. Instead, precursors accumulate and back up into the only pathway in which 21-hydroxylase does not occur, that of androgen production. As a result,

DHEA and androgens are overproduced when 21 hydroxylase is absent. This excess of androgens results in virilization of female fetuses and causes precocious puberty in male infants lacking the enzyme.
○ Although the size of the adrenal gland is roughly similar from one normal person to another, the actual rate of cortisol secretion correlates with body mass, approximately 8 to 12 mg/d for an average adult.

Adrenal medullary catecholamine biogenesis

The enzymes responsible for epinephrine synthesis are induced by cortisol (see Figure 13.4). Hence, when stress (such as an injury or infection) induces cortisol secretion, it also prepares the animal for production of catecholamines (e.g., for the "fight or flight" response), for which a sick or injured animal might have particular need if it is to survive.

Catecholamines are synthesized in the cytoplasm, pumped into vesicles for storage, and secreted by calcium-dependent exocytosis (see Figure 13.5). This process is similar to protein secretion in its final exocytosis step, but is very different in earlier steps. The secretory granules for catecholamines are "reloaded" by direct uptake from the cytoplasm, whereas secretory proteins can enter their secretory granules only after synthesis on membrane-bound ribosomes, translocation into the lumen of the endoplasmic reticulum, and transport via the Golgi apparatus (see Chap. 2).

Review Questions

7. From what starting material are all of the adrenal steroids made?
8. What are the distinctive structural features of each member of the family of adrenal hormones?
9. What is the rate-limiting step in adrenal steroid biogenesis?
10. How is the enzyme that makes pregnenolone controlled, and why does this make physiological sense?
11. How quickly after seeing ACTH does the adrenal cortex respond with a bolus of steroid secretion? What is the mechanism?
12. With what parameter does adrenal cortical secretion correlate?
13. What hormones induce the enzymes involved in catecholamine biosynthesis?
14. How does catecholamine biosynthesis and secretion differ from that of polypeptide hormones?
15. How does catecholamine biosynthesis and secretion differ from that of the adrenal cortical steroids?
16. Why does lack of the enzyme 21-hydroxylase, which is necessary to make cortisol, result in androgen excess?

4. MOLECULAR MECHANISMS OF ADRENAL HORMONE ACTION

Glucocorticoids

Glucocorticoids diffuse into cells and bind to receptor proteins located in either nucleus or cytosol. The receptor proteins are maintained in a relatively unfolded state in the cytosol by other cellular proteins, including members of the family of **molecular chaperones** (see Chaps. 2 and 19), to which they are bound. When the glucocorticoid comes along, it binds to the hormone, displaces some of the cellular binding proteins, and translocates through the nuclear pore complexes into the nucleus (see Figure 13.6).

The steroid hormone–receptor complex can then bind to regions of DNA that alter the transcription of sets of genes, thereby generating a new population of mRNAs. These mRNAs are transported into the cytoplasm for translation into proteins, which pre-

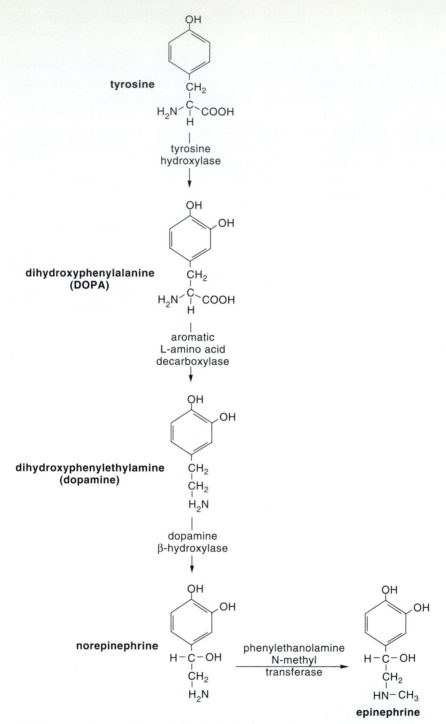

FIGURE 13.4. Enzymes of catecholamine biosynthesis. The amino acid tyrosine is modified by sequential hydroxylation and decarboxylation steps to form dopamine, the first of the three physiological catecholamines. In the sympathetic nervous system, the action of dopamine β-hydroxylase converts dopamine into norepinephrine, which is subsequently modified to form epinephrine, the major product of the adrenal medulla. These catecholamines differ in their relative affinity for various receptors and their half-lives (see Chap. 10).

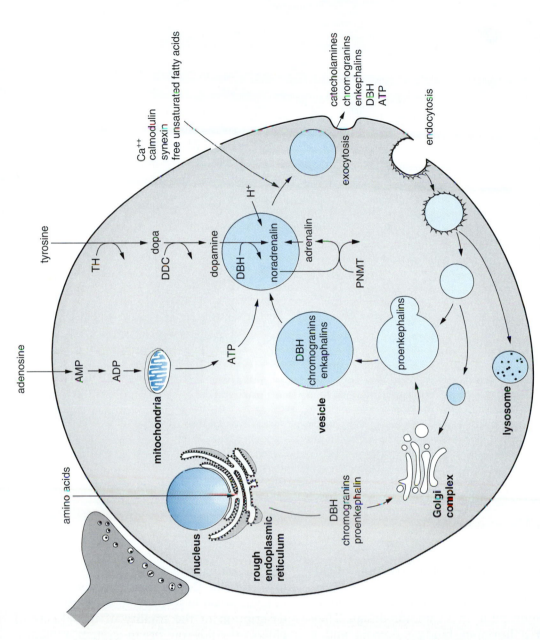

FIGURE 13.5. Pathway of catecholamine secretion. Schematic description of the pathways by which various substances needed for catecholamine biosynthesis are taken up and modified in the cytosol or in other compartments. Once catecholamines are generated in the cytoplasm, they are transported into vesicles and released upon regulated exocytosis, with recycling of the vesicle membrane. (Adapted, with permission, from Carmichael SW, Winkler H [1985]. Sci Am 253:45.)

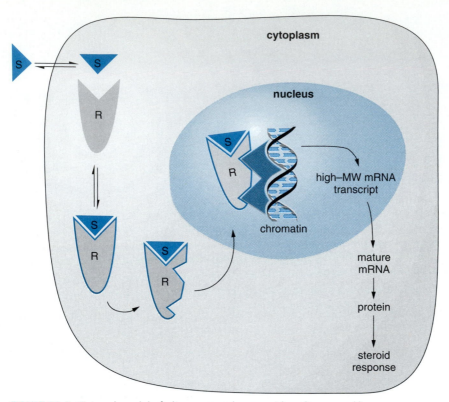

FIGURE 13.6. General model of glucocorticoid action. Like other steroid hormones, glucocorticoids are believed to diffuse across the plasma membrane and bind to receptors in the cytoplasm. The hormone-receptor complex then moves to the nucleus, where it binds to specific regions of DNA, resulting in initiation of transcription, splicing, and export of mRNA and translation of the encoded proteins that are the actual effectors of the response to the steroid. Modification, degradation, and elimination of the steroid hormone (S), or its receptor (R), regulate the extent and time course of hormone action. *(Adapted, with permission, from Catt KJ and Dafau ML. Hormone action: Control of target-cell function by peptide, thyroid, and steroid hormones. In Felig P et al. (eds) (1995).* Endocrinology and Metabolism, *3d ed. New York, McGraw-Hill.)*

sumably mediate the observed actions of glucocorticoids.

The steroid hormone receptors are modular proteins built on a common design. They contain a hormone-binding domain and a DNA-binding domain. Binding of hormone results in dimerization and association with other proteins that regulate transcription by increasing the affinity of the hormone-receptor complex for particular DNA sequences.

Despite enormous recent progress, includ-

ing the cloning of these receptors and the dissection of the mechanism of action, it is not yet possible to provide a full molecular description of the totality of the effects of glucocorticoids on organ system structure and function.

Based on our current understanding, there are three levels of complexity that go beyond the simple paradigm of glucocorticoid action just summarized.

First, recent data suggest that molecular

chaperones are doing more than just holding the glucocorticoid receptor in the cytoplasm while waiting for the arrival of hormone (see Figure 13.7). Rather, there appears to be a complex level of regulation based on the presence of various members of the molecular chaperone family and the effect of signaling pathways on glucocorticoid receptor activation (see Ref. 3).

Second, once the hormone has bound the receptor, association can take place in the nucleus with other hormone receptors, in particular with members of the retinoic acid receptor family. Different receptor dimers are, in turn, capable of binding different DNA sequences. Since different tissues express different members of the retinoic acid receptor family, this provides a mechanism for tissue specificity of glucocorticoid action.

Third, a large number of transcription factors are expressed in some tissues but not others. They can bind to the activated hormone-receptor complex, further expanding the possibilities for tissue-specific gene expression.

Catecholamines

Catecholamines function much like polypeptide hormones. They bind cell-surface receptors from the outside of the cell and trigger signaling events mediated by second messengers. There are three broad classes of adrenergic receptors. Their mechanism of action is discussed in greater detail in Chapter 10.

5. HYPOTHALAMIC–PITUITARY–ADRENAL AXIS

Control of the adrenal gland can be viewed in two ways. The simple view is that of a classical hypothalamic–pituitary–end organ axis (see Chap. 11). While that view accounts for the major clinically relevant features to-

day, it is inadequate to appreciate aspects of adrenal function that are likely to be clinically relevant in the not-too-distant future. For this, a more complex regulation must be considered.

A simple view of the adrenal neuroendocrine feedback loop

Let us start with the simple view of the adrenal gland controlled by a classical neuroendocrine feedback loop (see Figure 13.8). As described in Chapter 11, neurons of the paraventricular nucleus of the hypothalamus secrete a peptide hormone, **corticotropin-releasing hormone (CRH)**, into the pituitary portal venous system. CRH stimulates specific cells in the anterior pituitary to secrete ACTH into the pituitary portal blood. Upon its secretion, ACTH enters the systemic circulation, where it stimulates the adrenal cortex. In response to ACTH, the appropriate layers of the adrenal cortex secrete cortisol (and androgens), which has various effects on tissues throughout the body, including negative feedback on the pituitary and hypothalamus. This turns off further secretion of CRH and ACTH until either the cortisol level falls sufficiently low or some other stimulus (stress) results in a bolus of CRH and ACTH ease. Both CRH and ACTH work by raising levels of cyclic AMP.

A more complex view of the adrenal neuroendocrine feedback loop

A number of lines of evidence suggest that the adrenal neuroendocrine axis is far more complex than the above simple description. Consider these additional features:

1. The contribution from and output to higher centers that affect CRH release from the hypothalamus.
2. Stimulation of ACTH secretion by vasopressin released into the systemic circula-

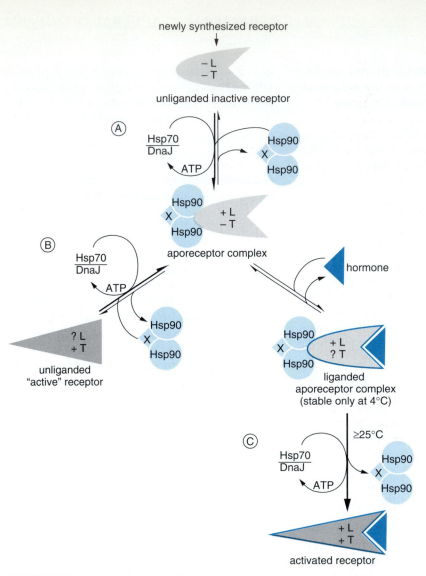

FIGURE 13.7. Complex regulation of glucocorticoid action. Molecular chaperones may assist in the assembly and maintenance of a poised, ligand-sensitive receptor complex (steps A and B) in the absence of ligand, but in the presence or absence of other associated proteins, and in the folding of the activated receptor to a transcriptionally active state (step C). Thus, association with various proteins in the cytoplasm, including molecular chaperone proteins that assist in folding of glucocorticoid receptor, is a newly appreciated level of regulation of glucocorticoid action. Perhaps the most remarkable implication is that under certain conditions, glucocorticoid action can occur in the *absence* of glucocorticoids, e.g., by activation of the receptor by an alternative pathway (B). *Binding* refers to a receptor capable of binding hormone; − or + L refers to a receptor incapable or capable of binding the steroid ligand, − or + T refers to a receptor incapable or capable of initiating specific transcription respectively. (*Adapted, with permission, from Bohen SP et al. (1995). Hold 'em and fold 'em: Chaperones and signal transduction. Science 268:1303.*)

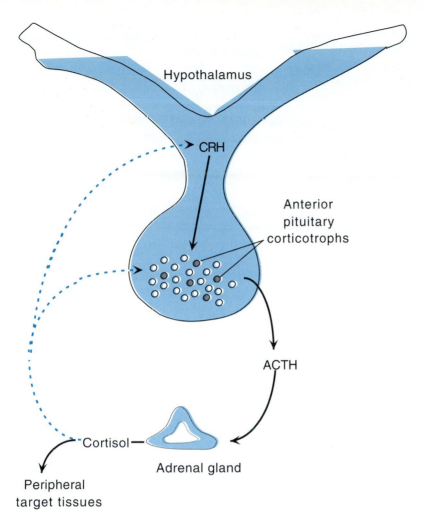

FIGURE 13.8. A simple view of the hypothalamic–pituitary–adrenal neuroendocrine axis. CRH, made in the hypothalamus, reaches the anterior pituitary via the pituitary portal system, where it stimulates proopiomelanocortin synthesis, processing to ACTH and other peptides, and secretion. This occurs in specific cells termed corticotrophs. Note that the corticotrophs (dark circles) are interspersed among other cells (white circles) of the pituitary gland that secrete various other hormones (see Chap. 11). ACTH leaves the pituitary gland in the venous drainage to the systemic circulation and travels to the adrenal gland, where it triggers cortisol synthesis and secretion. Cortisol has effects on peripheral target tissues as well as feeding back to the hypothalamus and pituitary gland to inhibit further CRH and ACTH secretion, respectively. (Adapted, with permission, from Junqueira LC, et al. (1995). Basic Histology, 8th ed. Stamford, CT, Appleton & Lange.)

tion from the posterior pituitary (see Chap. 11). This is one reason why hypophysectomy causes a more severe form of adrenal atrophy than suppression by long-term, high-dose glucocorticoid use (see Figure 13.2).

3. The many effects of cytokines and other products secreted from immune cells that stimulate CRH secretion from the hypothalamus and ACTH secretion from the anterior pituitary. The inhibitory effect of cortisol on the immune system closes a separate negative-feedback regulatory loop of immune function (see Figure 13.9).

4. Effect of the adrenal cortical hormones on the adrenal medulla constitutes another

potential level of complexity of adrenal responses to stress.

Regardless of whether one thinks in terms of the simple or the complex feedback loop, the stimulatory effects of ACTH on the adrenal cortex are myriad:

• Blood flow to the adrenals is increased.
• Conversion of cholesterol to pregnenolone increases (largely as a consequence of increased transport of cholesterol from the outer to the inner membrane of mitochondria).
• Steroid synthesis and secretion increase.

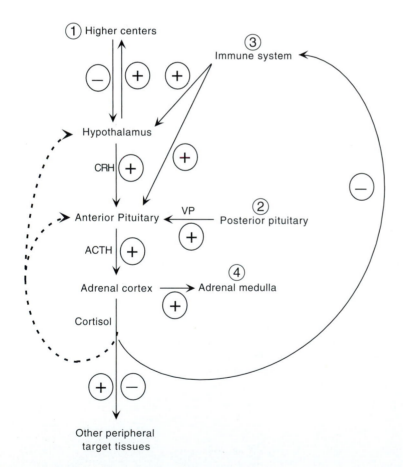

FIGURE 13.9. A more complex view of the hypothalamic–pituitary–adrenal neuroendocrine axis. The simpler scheme of Figure 13.8 is elaborated with indication of (1) contributions from higher centers of the brain; (2) contributions from vasopressin secretion from the posterior pituitary (VP); (3) the negative-feedback loop involving the immune system and secretion of cytokines such as interleukin 1, and (4) effects of the adrenal cortical hormones on the enzyme activities in the catecholamine-secreting medulla. Stimulatory interactions are indicated with a +, inhibitory ones with a −.

• Ultimately, with continued ACTH stimulation, the adrenal tissue itself undergoes hypertrophy and hyperplasia.

The magnitude of the basal swings in cortisol secretion by the adrenal may be regulated by the innervation of the adrenal glands, by chronic disease, or by other hormones.

Vasopressin is also a stimulus to ACTH secretion (see Chap. 6), which makes physiological sense in that substantial deviations from normal set points for osmolarity or volume that trigger vasopressin secretion also constitute a severe stress on the body for which glucocorticoid secretion is appropriate.

Recent findings (see Sec. 9, Frontiers) make it abundantly clear that even more complexity will need to be built into our thinking about adrenal steroid feedback control in the not-very-distant future.

Clinical Pearls

○ The circadian rhythm of basal cortisol secretion is actually quite reliable, but the peak is very early in the morning (like about 5 A.M.). Thus, the ACTH stimulation test is a more convenient way of testing for adrenal cortical function. This involves drawing a baseline blood sample, injecting 0.5 mg of ACTH intravenously, and drawing a subsequent blood sample 60 min later. Regardless of where a person is in the circadian cortisol rhythm, he or she will respond to an acute injection of ACTH with a burst of cortisol secretion if the pituitary corticotrophs are intact and functioning. Lack of response indicates adrenal disease or atrophy. A good cortisol response to injected ACTH does not rule out a hypothalamic or pituitary disorder, but it would have to be a disorder of recent onset, since the adrenal glands have not yet atrophied. A typical clinical situation in which this test might be used would be a patient who is severely ill, perhaps in shock, whose ability to mount the normal stress response was in question. After drawing the requisite pre- and post-ACTH injection blood samples, the patient would be treated with a high dose of glucocorticoids intravenously, just in case, pending return of the blood test results later that day.

○ The basal cortisol circadian rhythm can be changed by

1. Physical stress, such as major illness, surgery, trauma, or starvation
2. Psychological stress, including anxiety, endogenous depression, and manic-depressive illness
3. Central nervous system and pituitary disorders
4. Cushing's syndrome (pituitary ACTH-secreting adenoma)
5. Liver disease and alcoholism (affecting cortisol metabolism)
6. Chronic renal failure

○ The circadian rhythm of cortisol production first develops at the age of about 1 year.

Control of ACTH release

CRH (and vasopressin) stimulation of ACTH release is controlled in three ways:

1. Endogenous mechanisms in the brain, resulting in basal pulsatile secretion and episodic circadian and meal-stimulated rhythms.
2. Physical and emotional excitatory factors that stimulate ACTH secretion above the spontaneous baseline. These include such factors as trauma, major surgery, burns, hypoglycemia, fever, exposure to cold, irradiation, hypotension, dehydration, exer-

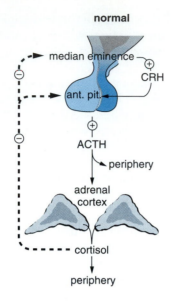

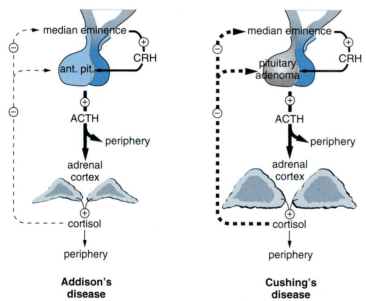

FIGURE 13.10. Hypothalamic–pituitary–adrenal relationships in disease. Solid arrows indicate stimulation; dashed arrows indicate inhibition. *Normal:* Standard axis as described in Figure 13.8. *Addison's disease* (primary destructive disease of the adrenal cortex): The level of plasma cortisol is very low, and the effect of CRH on the anterior pituitary proceeds without inhibition, resulting in high levels of ACTH, whose precursor also gives rise to melanocyte-stimulating hormone (MSH), resulting in tanning of the skin. *Cushing's disease:* Unregulated overproduction of CRH or ACTH due to a hypothalamic or pituitary adenoma, resulting in excess cortisol, bilateral adrenal hyperplasia, and manifestations of hypercortisolism.

cise, or any kind of "stress." For example, in response to major surgery, cortisol secretion may increase up to sixfold.

3. Finally, the negative-feedback inhibition of secretion by cortisol, which we have already mentioned.

A break in the hypothalamic–pituitary–adrenal (HPA) feedback loop, either as a result of excessive or deficient secretion or as a consequence of treatment for other medical problems, can result in disease (see Figure 13.10).

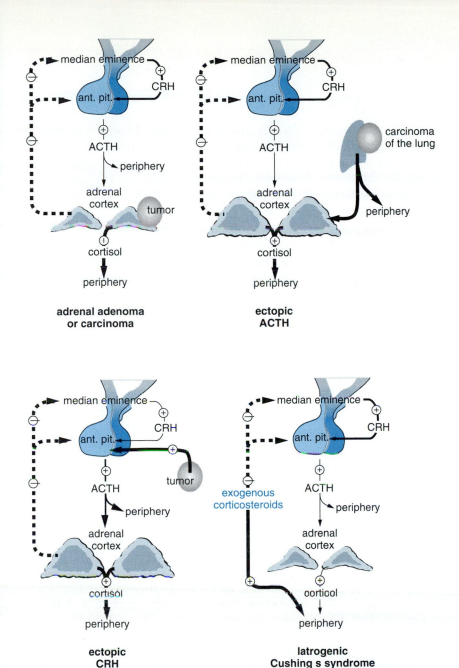

**adrenal adenoma
or carcinoma**

**ectopic
ACTH**

**ectopic
CRH**

**Iatrogenic
Cushing s syndrome**

FIGURE 13.10 — *(continued) Adrenal adenoma or carcinoma:* May produce cortisol autonomously, giving rise to Cushing's syndrome. *Ectopic ACTH:* ACTH or an ACTH-like substance is elaborated by a tumor, often in the lung. Endogenous CRH and ACTH secretion is inhibited by the tumor product, but the adrenals are stimulated. *Ectopic CRH:* Also from a tumor. Has effects only on the corticotrophs of the anterior pituitary, with no direct effects on the adrenal gland itself. *Iatrogenic Cushing's syndrome:* Results in hypercortisolism due to the effects of oral or intravenous steroids for a number of days. Also results in inhibition of endogenous CRH and ACTH secretion and atrophy of the adrenal glands and corticotrophs due to lack of stimulation by CRH and ACTH, respectively. *(Adapted, with permission, from Burns TW, Carlson HE (1985), in Soderman WA, Soderman TM (eds): Pathologic Physiology: Mechanisms of Disease. Philadelphia, PA, W. B. Saunders.)*

Clinical Pearls

○ A prolonged course of steroid treatment, which might occur, for example, in the treatment of severe asthma, results in suppression of endogenous ACTH secretion, leading to suppression of endogenous cortisol secretion and ultimately atrophy of the adrenal glands. If steroid therapy were abruptly discontinued, or if the individual were to face a major stress (see the preceding discussion), the atrophied adrenals would not be able to provide the necessary cortisol, and the individual might succumb. Therefore, these patients need extra doses of cortisol if they are critically ill or undergoing surgery.

○ CRH is also secreted locally by certain immune cells as a pro-inflammatory mediator (see Chap. 19). This CRH production is suppressed at doses of prednisone too small to completely suppress CRH production by the hypothalamus. This may explain why some patients with rheumatoid arthritis can sometimes get relief with as little as 1 mg of prednisone three times a day, a dose that does not fully suppress the hypothalamic–pituitary–adrenal axis.

Review Questions

17. What are the three mechanisms by which ACTH release is controlled?
18. What is the effect of exogenous cortisol treatment on the adrenal gland?
19. Describe the components of the neuroendocrine feedback loop involving the adrenal cortex.
20. What parameters can regulate the magnitude of the basal swings in cortisol secretion by the adrenal gland?
21. What parameters can regulate the magnitude of cortisol swings above basal levels?

6. ACTIONS OF GLUCOCORTICOIDS

Where thyroid hormone plays a key role in making many different systems function well at baseline conditions, glucocorticoids are involved physiologically in making various organ systems work as well as possible under stress.

In acute stress, glucocorticoids help to maintain vascular tone, endothelial integrity, and vascular permeability. They also help to maintain sensitivity to the vasoconstrictive effects of catecholamines and to prevent overreaction on the part of the immune system. In more chronically stressful situations, the corticosteroids work to maintain both the supply of glucose and body fluid content and distribution, thereby preserving vital organ functions.

In terms of fuel homeostasis, at first glance, glucocorticoids appear to be generally catabolic hormones, breaking down energy stores and making them available to vital systems. However, on closer inspection, their effects are far more complex. For example, while glucocorticoids promote lipolysis in the extremities, they also promote fat deposition in the abdomen, thus effecting a net redistribution of fat from the periphery to the center.

The actions of glucocorticoids are myriad. Most are so-called permissive or facilitory, meaning that they help other tissues to respond to various hormones optimally. By inducing the transcription of mRNA for various enzymes, etc., glucocorticoids prepare their target tissues for response to the signals from other hormones or effectors, e.g., glucagon and calcium.

Glucocorticoids are made with a diurnal basal variation, on which is superimposed the response to specific stresses. It is not clear whether the diurnal variation itself reflects a mild form of stress response or serves a function distinct from the response to specific stresses. Thus, the effects of normal levels of glucocorticoids on functions of various organ systems are not fully resolved. It is more instructive to consider the consequences of extremes of glucocorticoid excess or deficiency on the functions of various organs and systems.

Effects on intermediary metabolism: protection against glucose deprivation

The integrated action of glucocorticoids on intermediary metabolism is to protect the body against glucose deprivation during times of acute or chronic stress. Thus, glucocorticoids

- Increase glucose production by the liver.
- Decrease glucose uptake and utilization in the periphery.
- Increase protein breakdown.
- Decrease protein synthesis in the periphery.
- Increase lipolysis in the periphery.
- Redistribute fat stores.
- Elevate free fatty acid levels.

Many of the effects of glucocorticoids in the periphery serve to generate high levels of precursors for hepatic gluconeogenesis. Teleologically speaking, this all makes great sense as a protective response in the face of stress.

However, this also means that glucocorticoids confer a tendency to hyperglycemia and decreased carbohydrate tolerance, which can cause problems, e.g., for patients with diabetes mellitus who are placed on high doses of glucocorticoids. Despite their anti-insulin-like effects on most of glucose metabolism, glucocorticoids promote glycogen storage in the liver, an insulin-like action.

Conversely, lack of glucocorticoids results in increased sensitivity to insulin and a poor capacity to generate substrates for gluconeogenesis and hence, a tendency to hypoglyce-

mia. These effects are greatly magnified or diminished depending on the individual's food intake and insulin status.

The integration of glucocorticoid actions with those of other hormones is seen in the observation that adrenalectomized animals have normal baseline levels of gluconeogenesis but an impaired response of gluconeogenesis during the stress of fasting or in insulin deficiency. This is also why some patients can have profound adrenal insufficiency but only vague complaints — until a serious stress comes along, to which their adrenal glands are unable to respond appropriately.

Glucocorticoids stimulate an increase in lipolysis, resulting in elevated plasma free fatty acid levels, an action that is antagonistic to that of insulin on lipid metabolism. Importantly, tissues differ as to their relative sensitivity to glucocorticoids and to insulin. Thus, the net effect of glucocorticoid excess is not just fat mobilization but *redistribution* of fat from the extremities to the neck, face, and trunk.

Effects on protein and nucleic acid metabolism

Whereas the predominant effect of glucocorticoids on the periphery is to inhibit DNA, RNA, and protein synthesis, in particular tissues they can have specific opposite effects. Thus, for example, cortisol stimulates liver protein synthesis (induces enzymes for gluconeogenesis, etc.).

Immunologic effects

The effects of basal levels of glucocorticoids on the immune system are unresolved. However, in larger doses, glucocorticoids suppress the immune system, blocking cellular immunity more than humoral immunity (see Chap. 19).

More specific effects of glucocorticoids on the immune system include:

- A negative-feedback loop with cytokines (immunologic growth factors). Cytokines such as interleukin 1 (IL-1) stimulate hypothalamic CRH and therefore pituitary ACTH secretion. The resulting burst of glucocorticoids from the adrenal gland kills certain mature, fully differentiated immune cells and inhibits further IL-1 production.
- Note that this feedback loop is distinct from the local effects of CRH secreted from a subpopulation of immune cells, mentioned previously, which is also suppressed by low-dose glucocorticoids. The possible coordination or interaction between the two distinct sources of CRH (i.e., hypothalamus and immune cells) is not known.
- Immature, less fully differentiated immune cell progenitors are largely resistant to the toxic effects of glucocorticoids on the immune system. This is why the effects of glucocorticoids on the human immune system are generally reversible upon discontinuation of glucocorticoid therapy.
- Inhibition of eicosanoid and prostaglandin production and metabolism. Glucocorticoids do this far more broadly than aspirin or other nonsteroidal anti-inflammatory drugs (NSAIDs). The NSAIDS inhibit enzymes such as prostaglandin synthase that convert arachidonic acid into various active mediators such as the prostaglandins. However, glucocorticoids act earlier in the pathway, blocking the production of arachidonic acid itself, and thus have a much stronger anti-inflammatory effect than the NSAIDs (see Chap. 3). The anti-inflammatory action of glucocorticoids is believed to be mediated by **lipocortin**, a calcium-binding protein that is a phospholipase A_2 inhibitor.
- Impairment of antigen processing and antibody production and clearance (see Chap. 19).

Clinical Pearls

- ○ Patients on steroid inhalers can develop oral thrush (infection with the common fungus *Candida albicans*) and other signs of local cell-mediated immunosuppression.
- ○ Patients on long-term systemic high-dose steroids are at increased risk of dissemination throughout the body of infections that were being held in check by the immune system, including bacterial (tuberculosis), fungal (aspergillosis), and parasitic (strongyloidiasis) infections. Thus you should always perform a skin test for TB, check a chest x-ray and send a stool sample to rule out parasites before initiating this therapy.

Effects on bone metabolism

In excess, glucocorticoids have a number of effects on bone metabolism that chronically will contribute to accelerated osteoporosis (see Chap. 14). In particular, excess glucocorticoids:

1. Suppress the activity of osteoblasts.
2. Increase the activity of bone-destroying osteoclasts. The resulting unopposed osteoclast activity results in increased bone resorption and, consequently, increased renal calcium filtration.
3. Decrease renal reabsorption of calcium.
4. Stimulate a reflex increase in parathyroid hormone activity secondary to hypocalcemia as a result of renal calcium loss.
5. Partially block intestinal calcium absorption.
6. Inhibit collagen synthesis and proliferation of fibroblasts, a necessary early step for bone matrix formation.
7. Inhibit bone growth by decreasing synthesis (and serum levels) of matrix proteins.

Effects on growth and development

Systemic excess of glucocorticoids inhibits linear growth while accelerating developmental events by multiple mechanisms (which limits the therapeutic utility of glucocorticoids in children).

Clinical Pearls

○ The effects of too much glucocorticoid on bone and connective tissue accounts for the easy bruising, abdominal striae formation (wide purple stretch marks on the sides of the abdomen), osteoporosis, muscle weakness, and poor wound healing observed in patients with a pituitary tumor that is overproducing ACTH (termed Cushing's disease) or other syndromes of glucocorticoid excess, including patients treated with high-dose steroids for severe asthma, emphysema, or rheumatoid arthritis and other immunologic diseases.

○ Although individuals on glucocorticoids often have central obesity, the risk of osteoporosis from glucocorticoids is not related to obesity per se. Equally obese individuals with normal adrenal steroid levels are *not* at increased risk for osteoporosis or the other long-term effects of excess glucocorticoids.

○ A decline in growth rate is often the earliest sign of Cushing's disease in children.

Effects on reproduction

In general, glucocorticoids have inhibitory effects on both male and female reproductive functions, which can be viewed as an attempt to delay these processes in times of stress. Both luteinizing hormone (LH) levels and the response to LH are inhibited by increased levels of glucocorticoids.

Effects on fluid, electrolytes, and blood pressure

Because of their partial mineralocorticoid agonist effects (approximately one-tenth the affinity for the mineralocorticoid receptor displayed by aldosterone) and because cortisol is present in such high amounts compared to the primary mineralocorticoid aldosterone (approximately 1000 to 1), glucocorticoids ought to contribute nearly one-half of the overall mineralocorticoid effects normally present. In fact, their contribution to mineralocorticoid effects, while not negligible, is considerably less than that, under normal circumstances. This is probably because of the following:

1. Cortisol's high-affinity binding proteins, which effectively limit free cortisol to a few percent of the total cortisol present
2. The presence of 11-β-hydroxysteroid dehydrogenase, an enzyme that inactivates cortisol but not aldosterone, in mineralocorticoid receptor–containing tissues.

In excess, glucocorticoids result in expansion of intravascular volume, probably in part by "spillover" onto mineralocorticoid receptors.

Glucocorticoid deficiency (e.g., due to adrenal destruction, called **Addison's disease**) results in lowered serum sodium concentration, elevated serum potassium concentration, low blood pressure, and pigmentation.

The fall in serum sodium in Addison's disease is probably a consequence of a combination of three effects:

1. Increased ADH secretion as the body tries to compensate for a sluggish sensitivity to vasoconstrictors (whose actions are normally potentiated by glucocorticoids)
2. Impaired ability to excrete water (see Chaps. 9 and 10)
3. Loss of aldosterone action, whose net ef-

fect is to reclaim sodium in the renal filtrate in exchange for potassium in blood

The elevated potassium in adrenal destruction is due to aldosterone deficiency. Thus, it is not observed when adrenal failure occurs as a result of hypothalamic or pituitary disease or as a result of adrenal atrophy following a long course of exogenous glucocorticoids. This is because the zona glomerulosa, which makes aldosterone, does not depend on ACTH for its maintenance (see Chap. 10), unlike the rest of the adrenal cortex. Hence aldosterone synthesis and effects continue to function even when cortisol and androgen production is deficient as a result of lack of ACTH and adrenal atrophy.

The low blood pressure reflects intravascular volume depletion due to loss of sodium as well as loss of whatever fraction of mineralocorticoid-like action is due to glucocorticoids.

The pigmentation is a reflection of overproduction of melanocyte-stimulating hormone (MSH). MSH is a by-product of proopiomelanocortin precursor cleavage during the biogenesis of ACTH. ACTH is being overproduced because the failing adrenal gland is being hyperstimulated by the pituitary gland, whose ACTH production is no longer being feedback-inhibited by cortisol (see Figure 13.10).

Clinical Pearls

○ Patients with adrenal insufficiency may either be asymptomatic or have only minor, nonspecific complaints — until they are subjected to a sudden stress (e.g., illness, infection, accident, surgery). Then they may develop refractory shock. In part this is because basal levels of glucocorticoids are necessary for proper expression of adrenergic receptors on blood vessels that mediate the vascular response to stress.

○ Hypotension in a patient with adrenal insufficiency may mimic either hypovolemic shock (decreased preload, depressed myocardial contractility, and increased systemic vascular resistance) or septic shock (high cardiac output and decreased systemic vascular resistance). Hence the diagnosis must be considered in patients with either presentation.

○ A hypotensive patient who is unresponsive to pressor drugs that would normally be expected to elevate blood pressure should be assumed to have adrenal insufficiency until proven otherwise. A "stress dose" of glucocorticoid (e.g., hydrocortisone or methyl prednisolone) should be given immediately upon drawing blood for a serum cortisol determination before and 1 h after a dose of ACTH. The intravenous glucocorticoid will protect the patient pending the results of the ACTH stimulation test, which is necessary to confirm the diagnosis (see Sec. 8).

○ The manifestations of Addison's disease and other syndromes of adrenal insufficiency are highly variable. Not all patients will necessarily manifest hyponatremia, hyperkalemia, or any other particular finding. Hence, while the *presence* of these findings in a patient may lead you to consider the diagnosis, their *absence* does not help you rule out adrenal insufficiency. Thus, provocative testing is extremely important (see Sec. 8).

Effects on the central nervous system

Acute glucocorticoid excess typically has manifestations in the central nervous system ranging from mild euphoria to full-blown psychosis.

Chronic glucocorticoid excess probably results in atrophy of the hippocampus, a region of the brain crucial for memory and learning that has a high concentration of glucocorticoid receptors (see Ref. 4).

Glucocorticoid deficiency typically produces depression.

Clinical Pearl

○ Effects of glucocorticoids on the brain are highly unpredictable. Excess glucocorticoids, which usually cause euphoria acutely, can result in depression over time. Many patients also display cognitive impairment, especially in memory and concentration. Increased appetite, decreased libido, and insomnia with decreased REM sleep are also commonly noted.

Effects on the GI tract

In the GI tract, excess glucocorticoids decrease the protective mucosal barrier by blocking prostaglandin synthesis and mucus secretion.

Clinical Pearls

○ Patients on high-dose glucocorticoids are at increased risk of developing peptic or gastric ulcers, presumably because of the combination of increased stomach acid secretion in the absence of prostaglandins and a decreased mucosal barrier due to the effects on mucus-secreting cells.

○ Patients who have or develop ulcers on glucocorticoids are at higher risk of having these ulcers perforate through the wall of the stomach or duodenum, perhaps because of the effects on thinning of muscle and connective tissue. GI perforation is a surgical emergency. Without appropriate intervention and repair, peritonitis and death will follow quickly.

Effects on the eye

In the eye, excess glucocorticoids may cause development of cataracts or increased intraocular pressure, leading to glaucoma in some patients.

Clinical Pearl

○ Accelerated cataract formation is seen only in patients with exogenous glucocorticoid excess, not in those with endogenous glucocorticoid excess, for unknown reasons.

Table 13.1 summarizes the major effects of glucocorticoids at normal levels, excess, and deficiency.

Review Questions

22. How does an outpouring of glucocorticoids in response to stress normally protect the body against glucose deprivation?
23. What is the effect of excess glucocorticoids on reproductive function?
24. Summarize the effects of excess glucocorticoids on the immune system.
25. Summarize the effects of excess glucocorticoids on bone.
26. Summarize the effects of glucocorticoid excess and deficiency on fluid and electrolyte homeostasis.

7. TRANSPORT AND METABOLISM

Cortisol, the major glucocorticoid, is normally over 95% bound to proteins. It has a high affinity for cortisol-binding globulin (CBG), to which approximately 90% is bound, and a low affinity for serum albumin,

TABLE 13.1   MAJOR EFFECTS OF GLUCOCORTICOIDS AT NORMAL LEVELS, IN EXCESS, AND IN DEFICIENCY

Target tissue	Effect	Mechanism
Muscle	Catabolic	Inhibit glucose uptake and metabolism Decrease protein synthesis Increase release of amino acids, lactate
Fat	Lipolytic	Stimulate lipolysis Increase release of FFAs and glycerol
Liver	Synthetic	Increase gluconeogenesis Increase glycogen synthesis, storage Increase glucose-6-phosphatase activity Increase blood glucose
Immune System	Suppression	Reduce number of circulating lymphocytes, monocytes, eosinophils, basophils Inhibit T lymphocyte production of interleukin 2 Interfere with antigen processing, antibody production and clearance
	Anti-inflammatory	Decrease migration of neutrophils, monocytes, lymphocytes to sites of injury
	Other	Stimulate release of neutrophils from marrow Interfere with neutrophil migration out of vascular compartment
Cardiovascular	Increase cardiac output Increase peripheral vascular tone	
Renal	Increase glomerular filtration rate Aid in regulating water, electrolyte balance	
Other	Permissive action Resistance to stress Insulin antagonism	Increase blood glucose

FFA, free fatty acids.
Adapted from McPhee S (1997), in McPhee S et al. (eds): *Pathophysiology of Disease*, 2nd ed. Stamford, CT, Appleton & Lange, and Greenspan PS, Strewler GS (eds): (1997). *Basic and Clinical Endocrinology*, 5th ed. Stamford, CT, Appleton & Lange.

to which approximately 5% is bound. Because of protein binding, cortisol has a half-life in the bloodstream of 60 to 120 min.

Aldosterone, the major mineralocorticoid, has no high-affinity binding proteins, and only about 60% of it is found even weakly bound to proteins. Since protein binding is an important mechanism by which the half-life of many hormones in the bloodstream is maintained (see Chap. 3), it is not surprising that the half-life of aldosterone is less than 15 min.

Although it is the free hormone that is generally regarded as being directly active, the bound steroid serves as a readily available reservoir, since it is generally in equilibrium with the free hormone.

Metabolism of most corticosteroids is in the liver via conjugation to soluble metabolites excreted in the urine.

Clinical Pearls

○ As might be expected from their powerful, widespread, and poorly understood ac-

TABLE 13.2   RELATIVE POTENCIES OF SOME COMMONLY USED GLUCOCORTICOIDS

Steroid	Half-time (min)	Relative potency (glucocorticoid)	Relative potency (mineralocorticoid)
Cortisol	80–120	1.0	1.0
Cortisone		0.8	0.8
Prednisone	200–210	3.5–4.0	
Prednisolone	120–300	4.0	0.8
Methylprednisolone	120–180	5.0	0.5
Triamcinolone		5.0	0
Dexamethasone	150–270	30–150	0
Betamethasone	130–330	25–30	0

Modified from Greenspan FS, Strewler GS (eds.) (1997). *Basic and Clinical Endocrinology*, 5th ed. Stamford, CT, Appleton & Lange.

tions, glucocorticoids are both valuable therapeutic agents and the cause of terrible complications. Glucocorticoids are required for replacement therapy in adrenal insufficiency. They also are used as anti-inflammatory and immunosuppressive agents in treating a wide variety of diseases, sometimes in supraphysiologic doses. Their actions in these settings are often difficult to predict or control; this constitutes an important frontier for advancement of our knowledge of medical physiology. Table 13.2 indicates the potencies of various pharmacologic glucocorticoids relative to that of cortisol. However, when using steroids as therapeutic agents, it is important to consider the longer-term complications along with the short-term benefits (Table 13.3).

○ When stopping high-dose glucocorticoid therapy after a prolonged course (i.e., greater than 2 weeks), it is important to taper the dose slowly to avoid adrenal insufficiency as a consequence of adrenal atrophy, which developed during the course of therapy. These patients must be instructed to increase their glucocorticoid therapy in times of stress (e.g., accidents, infections, etc.), since their adrenal glands may be too atrophied to respond appropriately on their own.

○ In patients who probably have developed adrenal atrophy as a result of the need for prolonged high-dose glucocorticoid therapy (e.g., patients with autoimmune diseases such as systemic lupus erythemato-

TABLE 13.3   SOME COMPLICATIONS OF LONG-TERM PHARMACOLOGIC USE OF GLUCOCORTICOIDS

Fluid retention and hypervolemia
Hypertension
Electrolyte disorders (hypernatremia and hypokalemia)
Hyperglycemia and insulin resistance
Increased susceptibility to infections (including tuberculosis)
Increased risk of peptic ulcer disease
Increased risk of bleeding and/or perforation of peptic ulcers
Osteoporosis
Decreased protein content of bone, skin, and muscle
Myopathy with proximal muscle weakness
Behavioral and psychiatric disturbances (including euphoria, mania, nervousness, depression, schizophrenia)
Cataracts
Growth arrest in children
Fat redistribution (buffalo hump, moon facies, central obesity)
Ecchymoses and striae
Acne
Hirsutism
Hyperlipidemia
Erythrocytosis
Leukocytosis
Hypothalamic and pituitary suppression

From Baxter JD (1995) in Felig P, et al (eds.): *Endocrinology and Metabolism*, 3rd ed. New York, McGraw-Hill.

sus or severe end-stage lung disease), the time to recovery from adrenal suppression can be highly variable, is impossible to predict, and can be assessed only by provocative testing (see Sec. 8). A clinical rule of thumb is that full recovery from atrophy may take as long as the period of time during which the patient was being treated with high-dose glucocorticoids, often months, over which time glucocorticoids are tapered slowly.

○ Clinically, free cortisol measurement in a 24-h urine collection provides a reliable, integrated assessment of overall adrenal function.

Review Questions

27. How is protein binding of cortisol different from that of aldosterone, and what are the implications of this difference?

28. Where are most corticosteroids metabolized, and how are they excreted?

8. DIAGNOSIS OF ADRENAL CORTICAL DYSFUNCTION: A PHYSIOLOGICAL APPROACH

The fundamental principle of clinical diagnostic endocrinology is:

If you think it is low, try to stimulate it.
If you think it is high, try to suppress it.

This approach is termed *provocative testing*. It is extremely useful in the diagnosis of adrenal disorders.

Because the normal range for cortisol in the blood varies among individuals as well as with time of day, a random measurement is not always reliable for the exclusion (or localization) of disease within the hypothalamic–pituitary–adrenal axis.

• If the primary problem is lack of adrenal function (adrenal insufficiency), cortisol levels in the blood should be low, ACTH levels should be high, and the high ACTH should be suppressible by a low dose of dexamethasone (a powerful glucocorticoid approximately 100 times as active as cortisol).

• The simplest approach to proving adrenal insufficiency is to demonstrate a failure of plasma cortisol to increase (e.g., to >20 $\mu g/$ dL) in response to injected synthetic ACTH (also known as a Cortrosyn stimulation test).

• Insulin-induced hypoglycemia can be used under controlled circumstances to assess the ability to respond to a stress as measured by a resulting elevation of ACTH and cortisol.

• If the primary problem is suspected to be adrenal hyperfunction due to an ACTH-secreting tumor of the anterior pituitary, termed Cushing's disease, then cortisol should be high and ACTH should be high. The high ACTH should be suppressible with low doses of dexamethasone if there is pituitary tumor, or with high doses of dexamethasone if there is an ACTH-secreting tumor outside of the pituitary. These are termed the low-dose and high-dose dexamethasone suppression tests. This reflects the fact that an ACTH-secreting tumor in the pituitary is more "pituitary-like" than one outside, and that almost all ACTH-secreting tumors have some capacity to be feedback-inhibited by glucocorticoids, even if it takes enormous doses.

So, first measure 24-h urinary free cortisol, which should be high in the case of either pituitary or adrenal hyperfunction, and ACTH, which should also be high in pituitary but *not* in primary adrenal hyperfunction. If the ACTH is high, then determine whether the high ACTH can be suppressed by low-dose dexamethasone, thereby indicating a pituitary source. If the ACTH is *low* rather than high, the likely diagnosis is an adrenal tumor or adrenal hyperplasia.

Treatment of the patient with *metyrapone*, a P450c11 β inhibitor, should block cortisol production, relieve the feedback suppression of the pituitary, and result in a rise in plasma ACTH, demonstrating that the problem was not in the hypothalamic pituitary axis, but rather was due to cortisol overproduction by the adrenal end organ.

Clinical Pearls

○ Chronically ill patients may have impaired adrenal responses due to hypothalamic or pituitary disease, adrenal hemorrhage, metastases, or certain drugs.

○ In the real world, clinical presentations are often various shades of gray rather than black or white. Thus, the *really* tough diagnosis to make is identifying the *relatively* adrenally insufficient patient — one who has enough adrenal function to maintain basal glucocorticoid levels, and perhaps even to manifest a marginally positive ACTH stimulation test, but is unable to mount a full response and, because of the incompleteness of his or her stress response, has a worse clinical outcome. Recent clinical epidemiologic studies suggest that failure to mount a sufficiently strong response to corticotropin (an increase of less than 9 μg/dL cortisol in response to a standard dose of ACTH given intravenously) is associated with much higher mortality (see Ref. 11). There is a growing suspicion that often a poor response to corticotropin is the *cause* rather than the *consequence* of severe illness.

Review Questions

When would you use:
29. The Cortrosyn stimulation test?
30. The metyrapone test?
31. The dexamethasone suppression test?

9. FRONTIERS IN ADRENAL PHYSIOLOGY

The immune–hypothalamic–pituitary–adrenal axis

There is a growing appreciation of the bidirectional interactions between the adrenal neuroendocrine feedback loop and the immune system. Cytokines appear to be involved at every level. A rat model system has been developed in which genetic defects in CRH production are associated with the development of arthritis in response to inflammatory stimuli. Defects in the adrenal axis (e.g., in hypothalamic response to immune stimulation, resulting in inadequate cortisol production) may result in excessive inflammatory reaction, contributing to the development of disorders such as rheumatoid arthritis (see Refs. 5 to 7).

Why do glucocorticoids worsen glucose tolerance?

The pathogenesis of non-insulin-dependent diabetes mellitus is known to include impaired β-cell insulin secretion, insulin resistance in the periphery, and hepatic glucose overproduction (see Chap. 4). Until recently, it was thought that the glucocorticoids contribute to worsening glucose tolerance through effects on the latter two of these three parameters. Recent work suggests that glucocorticoids also have a direct effect of inhibiting insulin secretion from the pancreatic beta cell. The experiments involved the use of transgenic mice whose β cells were made hypersensitive to glucocorticoids by overexpression of glucocorticoid receptor behind the insulin promoter (see Ref. 8).

A new level of regulation of glucocorticoids?

Steroid hormones have long been thought to enter into and exit from cells by simple diffusion across the plasma membrane. Recent studies, however, suggest that members of the ATP-binding cassette family of transporters are involved in selective export of particular glucocorticoids out of cells. Thus, modulation of transport provides a new level of regulation by which the sensitivity of particular cells to particular glucocorticoids can be controlled (see Ref. 9).

Why does cortisol rise abruptly in response to ACTH?

The StAR protein, which moves cholesterol from the outer to thee inner mitochondrial membrane, where P450scc resides, is responsible for this phenomenon. Patients with mutations in this protein have the most severe form of adrenal insufficiency, termed *lipoid congenital adrenal hypertrophy,* and make no steroids postnatally. The study of the regulation of this important protein is an important frontier of adrenal research (see Refs. 10 and 11).

Adrenal function and immunity: newer aspects

In the adrenal, as just about everywhere else, the simple picture does not tell the whole story. So it is with the issue of the effect of adrenal hormones on the immune system, generally viewed as inhibitory. Recently workers have found that in mice, low-dose glucocorticoids and epinephrine actually stimulate delayed hypersensitivity reactions (see Chap. 19), a form of host defense against

certain microbes (see Ref. 13). This is likely to occur through a stress hormone–induced enhancement of white blood cell movement to the skin and suggests a role for stress hormones, at physiological doses, in mediating immune defenses. On the other hand, at high (pharmacologic) concentrations, these hormones did suppress delayed hypersensitivity in the skin. Thus, adrenal–immune interactions depend not only on dose, but also on the parameter of immune function you choose to measure. These features remain to be demonstrated and characterized in humans.

In another development, the power of modern molecular genetics is illustrated by a study of the immune system in mice that lack the enzyme dopamine β-hydroxylase and therefore cannot produce either epinephrine or norepinephrine, the principal catecholamine mediators of the adrenal medulla and sympathetic nervous systems, respectively. These catecholamines proved unnecessary for normal development of the immune system, as these animals, raised under germ-free conditions, had normal numbers of white blood cells and normal T-cell functions, including cytokine production, when measured in isolated immune cells. However, when subjected to inoculation with two different intracellular pathogens, the bacteria *Listeria monocytogenes* and *Mycobacterium tuberculosis,* these catecholamine-deficient animals were found to be much more susceptible to infection and to have impaired cytokine production (see Ref. 14). Thus, catecholamines play a crucial role in marshalling the immune system, but apparently not in its development.

Social stress, glucocorticoid regulation, and survival in AIDS

We always make a point of indicating the connection of the hypothalamus to "higher centers" in the brain. But how do these connections actually manifest themselves in real life? A recent study of rhesus monkeys infected with a monkey-specific form of the AIDS virus is provocative in this regard. The authors show that animals subjected to psychosocial stress had higher loads of virus in their bloodstream and shorter survival time than control infected monkeys (see Ref. 15). The viral titer differences were seen before the subsequent appearance of differences in basal concentrations of plasma cortisol, with the stressed animals showing higher concentrations than the animals in a more friendly, supportive environment. This study hints at the likely importance of social supports for immune system function, an aspect that clinicians must never forget in applying the more technical aspects of their training to the care of patients.

10. HOW DOES UNDERSTANDING NORMAL PHYSIOLOGY PROVIDE INSIGHT INTO THE INITIAL CASE?

In this case, these various nonspecific symptoms were probably due to adrenal destruction by the tuberculosis infection.

A patient who lacks the ability to increase adrenal steroid production in the event of stress is at great risk of dying of complications when a stress occurs. Mr. G.'s homelessness not only makes it more likely that he will suffer such a stress in the near future, it also greatly complicates his ability to take the life-long maintenance glucocorticoids and mineralocorticoid replacement he requires and his ability to increase his therapy in response to stressors such as accidents and infections. In addition, it makes very difficult the treatment of his tuberculosis, which can require up to four medications for 6 to 12 months.

Access to health care, which Mr. G. has but many others do not, is of limited usefulness when a social situation such as homelessness make adherence to treatment nearly impossible.

Pigmentation and electrolyte abnormalities are the key clues to adrenal insufficiency in this case and are a direct result of aberrant adrenal physiology. The suspicion of adrenal failure can be confirmed by provocative testing.

SUMMARY AND REVIEW OF KEY CONCEPTS OF ADRENAL PHYSIOLOGY

1. The clinical presentation of adrenal disease can be subtle and it cannot be reliably diagnosed without specific testing.
2. Adrenal steroids are potent pharmacologic agents as well as important endogenous products.
3. The cortex makes steroids; the medulla makes catecholamines.
4. The cortex displays functional zonation.
5. Adrenal cortical steroids are cholesterol derivatives synthesized by enzymes localized predominantly in the mitochondrion and the endoplasmic reticulum.
6. The major molecular mechanism of glucocorticoids involves binding of hormone to a cytoplasmic receptor protein complex. When this occurs, the receptor dissociates from various molecular chaperone proteins and translocates to the nucleus. In the nucleus, the activated receptor forms a dimer with another copy of itself and/or with other proteins. The resulting protein complex binds specific regions of DNA to activate or repress transcription of various genes.
7. Tissue-specific effects of glucocorticoids arise from (1) the ability of tissue-specific signaling pathways to regulate molecular chaperone–mediated receptor activation; (2) the tissue-specific dimerization of glucocorticoid receptors with receptors for other hormones, including retinoic acid receptors; and (3) tissue-specific transcription factors that can alter the ability

of the activated hormone-receptor complex to bind to particular regions of DNA and thereby turn on or off the transcription of those genes.

8. The role of adrenal steroids is to prepare the body for stress acutely and chronically, including suppressive effects on the immune system.

9. The effects of excess glucocorticoids include effects on intermediary metabolism (worsened glucose tolerance), the immune system (suppression), bone (osteoporosis), and fluids and electrolytes (hypertension and fluid overload).

10. Effects of adrenal insufficiency can (but not necessarily always) include pigmentation (due to overproduction of MSH in primary adrenal failure), hyperkalemia (due to lack of mineralocorticoids), hyponatremia (due to lack of glucocorticoids and mineralocorticoids), vague abdominal pains, and hypotension progressing to cardiovascular collapse (due to glucocorticoid and mineralocorticoid deficiency).

11. The zona fasciculata and reticularis of the adrenal cortex, which are involved in cortisol and androgen production, are controlled by a classical neuroendocrine feedback loop involving CRH, ACTH, and cortisol. Aldosterone production by the zona glomerulosa is largely ACTH-independent.

12. The proper approach to diagnosis and treatment of adrenal disease involves provocative tests to stimulate (ACTH test) or suppress (dexamethasone and metyrapone tests) the adrenal gland, depending on whether you think the problem is one of glucocorticoid excess or deficiency.

A CASE OF
PHYSIOLOGICAL MEDICINE

M.J. is a 54-year-old nurse with a 40-year history of one-pack-per-day cigarette use. For the past 5 years she has had progressively worsening shortness of breath that has been diagnosed as emphysema (destruction of the terminal air spaces of the lung; see Chap. 8), a common long-term complication of cigarette smoking. Her chronic obstructive lung disease also has a reversible bronchospastic and inflammatory component. She has required numerous hospitalizations. The only treatment that seems to keep her out of the hospital is prednisone. She has been taking 20 mg of prednisone a day more or less continuously for the last year. Every time she tries to get off the steroids by stopping them abruptly, she develops an exacerbation of her lung disease, requiring that they be restarted.

QUESTIONS

1. What findings in the history and physical exam might you expect in someone who has been taking high-dose glucocorticoid therapy for a long time?

2. Suppose Ms. J. was prescribed glucocorticoids for physiological treatment of a defect in her hypothalamic–pituitary–adrenal axis rather than as a pharmacologic treatment of her lung disease. In what way would her prednisone treatment be different from what she is on now?

3. Describe the expected histology of Ms. J.'s adrenal cortex in contrast to normal.

4. Would you be comfortable stopping the prednisone abruptly? Why or why not? What might happen if you did? How would you proceed to manage Ms. J.'s medical condition?

ANSWERS

1. Thinning of the skin with easy bruising, resulting in ecchymoses; physical evidence

of fat redistribution, including "moon facies" and "buffalo hump"; frequent skin infections; back and joint pains and compression fractures of the spine from osteoporosis; proximal muscle weakness; edema; hypertension; hyperglycemia symptoms (including frequent urination, polydipsia, and polyphagia).

2. She would be on lower doses (about 1 or 2 mg of prednisone per day) with instructions to increase the dose in the event of significant stress and instructions to avoid missing meals and other contributors to stress.

3. The fasciculata and reticularis of her adrenal cortex would be atrophied, although not as severely as in someone who has had hypophysectomy (removal of the pituitary gland). The medulla and glomerulosa would be largely unaffected, as they do not depend on ACTH for maintenance.

4. No. Abrupt stopping of glucocorticoids might cause an acute adrenal insufficiency crisis, especially in the setting of stress, when it could result in cardiovascular collapse, hypotension, and even death. Instead, you need to carry out a program of gradual, slight, controlled adrenal insufficiency to give her hypothalamus, pituitary, and adrenal a chance to awake from their atrophied state. The problems are that (1) Ms. J. may feel miserable and depressed as a consequence of the deprivation of glucocorticoids, which her brain has gotten used to; (2) it will take a long time (rule of thumb: as long as her period of high-dose therapy) for her to fully recover from the profound degree of atrophy her adrenal glands have undergone; and (3) she is at risk to have a stressful event (e.g., a respiratory infection, an accident, etc.) that will require her to take stress doses of glucocorticoids, which will send you tumbling back to square one of your attempt to wean her off of these powerful but toxic medicines.

References and suggested readings

GENERAL REFERENCES

1. Findling JW, et al. (1997). Glucocorticoids and adrenal androgens, in Greenspan FS, Strewler GW (eds): *Basic and Clinical Endocrinology,* 5th ed. Stamford, CT, Appleton & Lange.
2. Lamberts SWJ, et al. (1997). Corticosteroid therapy in severe illness. *N Engl J Med* 337:1285–1290.
3. Bohen SP, et al. (1995). Hold 'em and fold 'em: Chaperones and signal transduction. *Science* 268:1303–1304.
4. Sapolsky RM (1996). Why stress is bad for your brain. *Science* 273: 749–751.

FRONTIERS REFERENCES

5. Sternberg E, et al. (1989). A CNS defect in biosynthesis of CRH is associated with susceptibility of streptococcal cell wall–induced arthritis in Lewis rats. *Proc Natl Acad Sci USA* 86:4771–4775.
6. Chikanza IC, et al. (1992). Defective hypothalamic response to immune and inflammatory stimuli in patients with rheumatoid arthritis. *Arthritis Rheum* 35:1281–1288.
7. Gaillard RC (1994). Neuroendocrine-immune system interactions. *Trends in Endocrinology and Metabolism* 5:303–308.
8. Delaunay F, et al. (1997). Pancreatic beta cells are important targets for the diabetogenic effects of glucocorticoids. *J Clin Invest* 100:2094–2100.
9. Kralli A, et al. (1995). LEM1, an ATP-binding-cassette transporter, selectively modulates the biological potency of steroid hormones. *Proc Natl Acad Sci USA* 92:4701–4705.
10. Miller WL (1997). Congenital lipoid adrenal hyperplasia: The human gene knockout for the steroidogenic acute regulatory protein. *J Mol Endocrinol* 19:227–240.
11. Rothwell PM, et al. (1991). Cortisol response to corticotropin and survival in septic shock. *Lancet* 337:582–583.

12. Gething MJ, Sambrook J (1992). Protein folding in the cell. *Nature* 355:33–45.
13. Dhabhar FS, McEwen BS (1999). Enhancing versus suppressive effects of stress hormones on skin immune function. *Proc Natl Acad Sci USA* 96:1059–1064.
14. Alaniz RC, et al. (1999). Dopamine beta hydroxylates deficiency impairs cellular immunity. *Proc Natl Acad Sci USA* 96:2274–2278.
15. Capitanio JP, et al. (1998). Social stress results in altered glucocorticoid regulation and shorter survival in simian acquired immune deficiency syndrome. *Proc Natl Acad Sci USA* 95:4714–4719.

CALCIUM AND MINERAL METABOLISM

14

1. INTRODUCTION TO MINERALS

Elements are substances that cannot be broken down without changing their fundamental chemical properties. Substances that do not meet this criterion and can be broken down into simpler chemical constituents are termed **compounds**. Well over 100 elements are represented in the diverse forms of matter on earth.

Carbon, hydrogen, and oxygen are the most abundant elements in the human body, but many others are used in the course of life, some in extremely minute quantities, others in more substantial amounts. Some of these other elements are used to modify **organic** compounds (those that contain carbon) and are tightly bound. For example, some enzymes incorporate a single atom of the element **selenium**, without which they will not function. Similarly, a molecule of **iron** is at the core of hemoglobin and is necessary for normal oxygen–hemoglobin dynamics. Other elements are loosely associated with enzymes and other proteins, but are nevertheless essential for some aspect of function or regulation. Without these **trace elements**, one physiological process or another would not function properly (see Table 14.1). In their nonorganified state, that is, not bound tightly to carbon-containing molecules, elements present in the body are termed **minerals**. The most abundant minerals in the body are calcium, phosphate, and magnesium.

Why is understanding calcium homeostasis important for clinicians?

Disorders of calcium homeostasis are responsible for serious complications of some common diseases.

- Patients with many different forms of cancer can present with elevated blood calcium concentrations, called **hypercalcemia**. The hypercalcemia of malignancy (cancer) can occur for two very different reasons. Cancer cells sometimes make a hormone that raises blood calcium. Alternatively, cancer cells can invade bone, leading to bone breakdown, which releases calcium. In the extreme, hypercalcemia can cause kidney failure, put a patient in a coma, and be life-threatening.

- **Osteoporosis**, the thinning of bones after menopause and with advancing age as a result of calcium loss, is a disorder of epidemic proportions in modern industrial societies. The estimated yearly cost of this disorder in the United States alone, largely as a consequence of falls and resulting hip fractures on the part of elderly women with osteoporosis, is approximately $14 billion. Often, an osteoporosis-related fracture makes it impossible for a patient to care for herself alone at home, and therefore is associated with transfer to a long-term care facility and a diminished quality of life. Often, a hip fracture is "the beginning of the end," setting the patient up for multiple subsequent medical complications and setbacks, which can eventually result in the patient's death. It is also clear that the pain and suffering associated with this disease of calcium homeostasis goes far beyond the already staggering dollar figure indicated.

- **Renal stones** composed of calcium salts occur commonly, often in young people. Certain disorders predispose to development of renal stones. Besides subjecting the patient to repeated expensive and painful episodes, failure to recognize the presence of a disorder of calcium homeostasis as the underlying cause of renal stones can result in serious cases of ureteral obstruction, infection, irreversible renal injury, and, ultimately, renal failure.

- **Diet and lifestyle factors** have an enormous impact on calcium homeostasis over the long term. Certain diets and lifestyles interfere with, while other diets and lifestyles facilitate, an individual's reaching and maintaining the maximum bone mass possible with his or her particular genetic background. This is important because the higher an individual's bone mass, the longer the individual can go with a constant degree of bone loss (e.g., postmenopause) before reaching the threshold for increased fracture risk. By exhorting patients to change those aspects of their diet and lifestyle that are not conducive to bone health and maximizing bone mass, health care providers can have a major impact on morbidity and mortality in the distant future.

For these and other reasons, an understanding of calcium homeostasis is crucial for good medical practice.

Case Presentation

D.Y. is a 56-year-old musician who presented to medical attention in coma. She had been diagnosed with breast cancer 3 years ago. Unfortunately, at surgery, metastases to the axillary lymph nodes were found. After removal of the primary tumor, she was treated with radiation therapy and several cycles of chemotherapy and did reasonably well for over 2 years. Six weeks ago she was found to have widespread new metastases to bone and lung. Several features of the recurrent cancer suggested that it would be resistant to additional chemotherapy. Knowing that her remaining life span was short, Ms. Y. opted to forgo additional anticancer treatments and, instead, to spend her remaining time traveling.

Ms. Y. recognized that the likelihood that she will die relatively soon from this disease is extremely high. Her goal shifted from "beating this disease," which it was during her first 3 years as a patient with cancer, to "optimizing the quality of her remaining period of life." Her reasoning was that, if given a choice between living another 4 months but spending 3 of those 4 months in the hospital, and living for 2 to 3 months with most of her time spent out of the hospital doing what she most enjoyed doing, she would choose the latter.

This is one of the most difficult and personal decisions in medicine. The role of the clinician is neither exclusively that of providing technical assistance nor that of trying to convince the patient to accept the clinician's own values regarding when to accept the inevitability of one's imminent death and focus on quality of the remaining time of life. Rather, the clinician's first and foremost role must be to serve as the patient's advocate, providing information, interpreting what it means in a way that the patient can understand, and supporting the patient in using the information to make choices based on his or her own values.

The previous night, Ms. Y. had complained to her traveling companion of some nausea and vomiting and was noted to be slightly confused. In the morning she was unarousable and was taken to a local emergency room, where she was found to have an elevated total blood calcium of 12.1 mg/dL (normal being 8.5 to 10 mg/dL), with a mild metabolic alkalosis and a low serum albumin of 2.5 g/dL (normal 3.1 to 4.3 g/dL). Her renal function was normal. Based on the medical records she carried with her, it appeared that just 2 months ago, her calcium had been 9.6 mg/dL, with a serum albumin and blood pH in the normal range.

Anticipating that complications of her terminal disease might occur, Ms. Y. had arranged for her traveling companion to be empowered to make decisions regarding medical care on her behalf, should she not be able to make decisions for herself. Furthermore, she had expressed her wishes not to receive heroic measures such as mechanical ventilation or electric shock to restart her heart, in the event that those interventions would be necessary to keep her alive. However, as her quality of life was still good, she did wish to receive short-term medical intervention that would allow her to continue to travel and visit friends.

TABLE 14.1 TRACE ELEMENTS

Element	Requirements, mg/d[a]	Amount[b] Serum μmol/L	Selected biochemical functions	Enzyme and protein Classes	Examples	Disorders of metal metabolism Deficiency	Toxicity[c]
Fe	10–20	18	Oxygen transport	Oxidoreductases	Cytochrome oxidase	Anemia	Hepatic failure, diabetes, testicular atrophy, arthritis, cardiomyopathy, peripheral neuropathy, hyperpigmentation
Zn	15–20	15	Nucleic acid and protein synthesis and degradation, alcohol metabolism	Transferases, hydrolases, lyases, isomerases, ligases, oxidoreductases, transcription factors	RNA polymerases, alcohol dehydrogenases, glucocorticoid receptor	Growth retardation, alopecia, dermatitis, diarrhea, immunologic dysfunction, failure to thrive, psychological disturbances, gonadal atrophy, impaired spermatogenesis, congenital malformations	Gastric ulcer, pancreatitis, lethargy, anemia, fever, nausea, vomiting, respiratory distress, pulmonary fibrosis
Cu	2–6	16	Hemoglobin synthesis, connective tissue metabolism, bone development	Oxidoreductases	Superoxide dismutase, ferroxidase (ceruloplasmin)	Anemia, growth retardation, defective keratinization and pigmentation of hair, hypothermia, degenerative changes in aortic elastin, mental deterioration, scurvy-like changes in skeleton	Hepatitis, cirrhosis, tremor, mental deterioration, Kayser-Fleischer rings, hemolytic anemia, renal dysfunction (Fanconi-like syndrome)
Co	0.0001	0.0001	Methionine metabolism	Transferases	Homocysteine methyltransferase	Anemia (B_{12} deficiency)	Cardiomyopathy, goiter
Mn	2–5	0.001	Oxidative phosphorylation; fatty acid, mucopolysaccharide, and cholesterol metabolism	Oxidoreductases, hydrolases, ligases	Diamine oxidase, pyruvate carboxylase	Bleeding disorder (increased prothrombin time)	Encephalitis-like syndrome, Parkinson-like syndrome, psychosis, pneumoconiosis
Mo	0.15–0.5	0.007	Xanthine metabolism	Oxidoreductases	Xanthine oxidase	?Esophageal cancer	?Hyperuricemia

616

Element			Function	Enzyme	Consequences of deficiency	Consequences of excess/toxicity
Se	0.05–0.2	1.6	Antioxidant	Glutathione peroxidase	Cardiomyopathy, congestive heart failure, stricted muscle degeneration	Alopecia, abnormal nails, emotional lability, lassitude, garlic odor to breath
Ni	(−)	0.02	?Stabilizing RNA structure	Urease	?	Dermatitis (occupational), lung and nasal carcinomas, liver necrosis, pulmonary inflammation
Cr	0.005–0.2	0.004	?Binding of insulin to cells, glucose metabolism		?Impairment of glucose tolerance	Renal failure, dermatitis (occupational), pulmonary cancer
Si					?Impaired early bone development	Pulmonary inflammation, granuloma, fibrosis
F					?Impaired bone and dental structure	Mottled dental enamel, nausea, abdominal pain, vomiting, diarrhea, tetany, cardiovascular collapse

[a] Requirements may differ for different age groups and physiologic states, e.g. pregnancy.

[b] Reported normal values vary owing to differences in sample preparation, analytical instructments, and small quantities present in biologic materials.

[c] Symptoms are dependent on route of entry and tissue distribution.

NOTE: (−), Reported values variable or not available.

Adapted, with permission, from Falchuk, K.H., Disturbances in trace elements. in Fauci, A. et al. (eds): *Harrison's Principles of Internal Medicine*, 14th ed. New York, McGraw-Hill, 1997, pp 490-491.

The clinician, noting Ms. Y.'s nonfocal neurologic exam, her normal renal function, and the constellation of blood test abnormalities, expressed the opinion that hypercalcemia related to the malignancy might account for all of the patient's clinical presentation. He suggested a treatment plan involving nothing more invasive than intravenous fluids and injectible medicines, which he felt might quickly return the patient to a functional level. Ms. Y.'s surrogate decision maker had some concerns and asked a number of questions, including: Why would Ms. Y.'s malignancy result in elevation of her blood calcium? Why did the physician expect the medicines to work so quickly? Would transfer to a hospice with only medicines for comfort be more appropriate? Hypercalcemia is, after all, a pretty painless way to go. Suppose the treatment did not work — what then? Satisfied with the answers, the companion approved the plan.

Next, the clinician had to respond to questions from representatives of the patient's HMO. The questions were much the same — but perhaps the motivations were different. Given the compelling rationale for the clinician's therapeutic recommendations, the HMO authorized the care.

Treatment was instituted, and Ms. Y. had a remarkable short-term clinical response. Awake and talking within 24 h, she was discharged from the hospital a day later.

Ms. Y. completed her trip and lived long enough to take two additional adventures. She needed medical intervention for hypercalcemia one additional time, and finally died peacefully at home, about 3 months after the first episode of hypercalcemia.

Review Questions

1. What is the difference among elements, compounds, and minerals?

2. Suggest four reasons why calcium homeostasis is important for medical practice.

2. THE ROLES OF CALCIUM, PHOSPHATE, AND MAGNESIUM IN HOMEOSTASIS

Physiological roles of calcium

Calcium has a myriad of physiological roles. Calcium salts in bone, such as calcium chloride, calcium phosphate, and hydroxyapatite, provide the structural integrity of the skeleton. Calcium ions, both intracellular and extracellular, are required for a range of biochemical activities, including:

- Neuromuscular excitation
- Blood coagulation
- Membrane dynamics (such as vesicle fusion, including hormone secretion)
- Second messenger in signal transduction (including hormone action in target cells)

Amount and distribution of total body calcium

Approximately 99% of total body calcium is in bone. Less than 1% (about 10 g out of the total of 1 to 2 kg) is present in soft tissues and body fluids.

Calcium enters the body from the gastrointestinal (GI) tract. This requires not only calcium intake in foods, but also calcium absorption, an important step in calcium homeostasis.

Calcium leaves the body by excretion either in the urine or in the stool. Calcium in the stool is due to either failure of ingested calcium to be absorbed or excretion of calcium in bile. Figure 14.1 indicates the major organs involved in calcium homeostasis.

The concentration of calcium in extracellular fluids is approximately 10,000 times higher

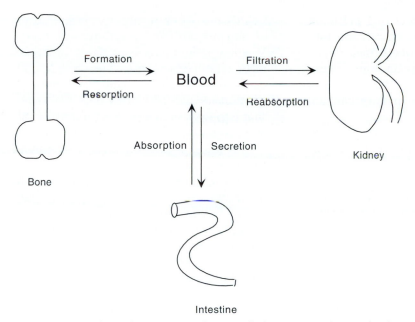

FIGURE 14.1. Calcium homeostasis. The overall short-term regulation of calcium homeostasis can be understood in terms of interactions between blood and bone, GI tract, and kidney. Changes in calcium concentration in the blood are monitored by the parathyroid glands. When calcium falls below the normal homeostatic range, PTH secretion by the parathyroid glands signals immediate effects on bone and kidney and delayed (indirect) effects on the GI tract. Together these effects reinforce one another and help maintain long-term homeostasis (see text). *(Adapted with permission, from Griffin JE, Ojeda SR: Textbook of Endocrine Physiology, 3d ed. New York, Oxford, 1996, p 316.)*

than the level of free calcium inside cells, which is about 10^{-7} M on average. The opening of calcium channels (e.g., during muscle contraction or transmission of action potentials) may briefly raise the intracellular free calcium concentration 10- to 100fold. But calcium that enters the cytoplasm in this way is quickly swept back out or bound up by proteins. In addition to the free calcium pool, about 40 to 50 times more calcium is found inside cells, bound to proteins, in reservoirs such as the endoplasmic reticulum and the mitochondria, and at the plasma membrane.

The total blood calcium concentration is 8.6 to 10.6 mg/dL (= 2.15 to 2.65 mM). Approximately half is free ionized calcium, with most of the rest bound to **albumin**, except for a small amount that is complexed in the form of phosphate or citrate salts.

Components of calcium homeostatic control

Hormonal, physiological, and physicochemical homeostatic control mechanisms operate to maintain the ionized free calcium at approximately 1.2 mM.

When the ionized free calcium concentration in blood falls even slightly below this concentration, **hormones** [primarily **parathyroid hormone (PTH)** and **vitamin D**, discussed in Sec. 4] are released.

The most immediate effect of PTH is on the kidney, causing it to retain calcium that would otherwise be lost in the urine.

Another effect of PTH is on bone. There is a rapidly releasable pool of bone calcium that leads to a quick increase in blood calcium in response to PTH.

On a more delayed time scale of hours to days, true **bone resorption** occurs, further increasing calcium release to correct the deficit.

If the stimulus to calcium release from bone persists, vitamin D, acting on a somewhat delayed time scale, has actions that increase the efficiency of calcium absorption from the GI tract.

Physiological mechanisms of control of acid–base balance and blood pressure regulation also have an important effect on calcium homeostasis:

- The increased glomerular filtration rate (GFR), occurring in response to a sodium load, results in increased calcium loss in the urine.
- Bone minerals (calcium and phosphate) serve as a buffer for fixed acids produced from ingested foods, resulting in their loss in the urine and further resorption of bone.
- Acidosis is also a stimulus to action of cells called **osteoclasts**, that break down bone, tilting the cycle of **bone remodeling** in favor of bone resorption.
- Calcium binding to albumin is increased in alkalosis, resulting in symptoms and signs of **hypocalcemia** even when total serum calcium is in the normal range.

Clinical Pearls

○ When the product of calcium (mg/dL) and phosphate (mg/dL) is greater than 60 to 70, painful deposition of calcium phosphate precipitates may occur in various soft tissues, often resulting in ischemic necrosis and cardiac dysrrythmias.

○ When a patient hyperventilates, he or she often eliminates more carbon dioxide than usual and therefore raises blood pH — a respiratory alkalosis (see Chap. 10). When that happens, the increased binding of calcium to albumin can transiently lower the serum ionized calcium level low enough to cause carpal and pedal spasm. This, of course, will only panic the patient even more, making him or her hyperventilate more and worsening the problem. Calming patients down and having them breathe into a paper bag to raise their blood carbon dioxide level, and therefore raise their blood pH, back toward normal shifts calcium back to the ionized free state and resolves the muscle spasms.

○ Mild hypercalcemia may be asymptomatic. However, in severe hypercalcemia (total serum calcium above 12 mg/dL with a normal serum albumin and blood pH), patients can develop a range of signs and symptoms. These include decreased neuromuscular excitability, cardiac dysrrythmias, dehydration, gastrointestinal symptoms related to constipation and exacerbation of peptic ulcer disease, depression, and disorientation (see Table 14.2).

○ Hypocalcemia produces increased neuromuscular excitability, including muscle spasms (see Table 14.3).

Phosphate

Like calcium, phosphate (PO_4^-) comes from the diet. About 85% of total body phosphate is found in crystalline (mineral) form in bone. The remaining 15% is in the form of phosphate esters and inorganic phosphate, which serve as critical intermediates in biochemical processes, including cellular energy generation and transfer. Phosphate is located largely in the intracellular compartment, at a concen-

TABLE 14.2   SIGNS AND SYMPTOMS OF HYPERCALCEMIA

Systemic
 Weakness
 Easy fatigue
 Weight loss
 Itching
 Ectopic calcifications

Neuropsychiatric
 Depression
 Poor concentration
 Memory deficits

Ocular
 Band keratopathy

Cardiac
 Shortened QT interval
 Hypertension

Renal
 Stones
 Polyuria, polydipsia
 Metabolic acidosis
 Concentrating defects
 Nephrocalcinosis

Gastrointestinal
 Peptic ulcer disease
 Pancreatitis
 Constipation
 Nausea
 Vomiting

Reproduced, with permission, from Shoback D, Strewler GS, in McPhee S et al. (1997). *Pathophysiology of Disease,* 2nd ed. Stamford, CT, Appleton & Lange.

tration of 100 μM. Thus, unlike calcium, the extraskeletal fraction of phosphate is largely intracellular. The normal phosphate concentration in the blood is 2.5 to 4.5 mg/dL (= 0.8 to 1.45 mM). Phosphate levels in the bloodstream are regulated primarily by renal tubular absorption and by 1,25-dihydroxyvitamin D. The effect of vitamin D is to promote intestinal phosphate absorption.

Magnesium and other minerals

Two-thirds of total body magnesium is also found in bone, associated with the mineral-ized matrix. Like that of phosphate, the extra-skeletal fraction of magnesium is primarily intracellular, where it is essential for nearly all ATP-driven processes.

A variety of other minerals are needed in minuscule quantities (see Table 14.1). In many cases, they serve as cofactors required for the function of specific enzymes. Either deficiency or excess of many of these so-called trace elements can result in human disease. Various binding proteins are involved in the uptake, distribution, and storage of these minerals. The mechanisms by which homeostasis is maintained for these minerals are not currently understood.

TABLE 14.3   SIGNS AND SYMPTOMS OF HYPOCALCEMIA

Systemic	Confusion
	Weakness
	Mental retardation
	Behavioral changes
Neuromuscular	Paresthesias
	Psychosis
	Seizures
	Carpopedal spasms
	Chvostek's and Trousseau's signs
	Depression
	Muscle cramping
	Parkinsonism
	Irritability
	Basal-ganglia calcifications
Cardiac	Prolonged QT interval
	T wave changes
	Congestive heart failure
Ocular	Cataracts
Dental	Enamel hypoplasia of teeth
	Defective root formation
	Failure of adult teeth to erupt
Respiratory	Laryngospasm
	Bronchospasm
	Stridor

Reproduced, with permission, from Shoback D, Strewler GS, in McPhee S et al. (1997). *Pathophysiology of Disease,* 2nd ed. Stamford, CT, Appleton & Lange.

Clinical Pearls

○ Phosphate depletion is often seen in seriously ill patients who are not eating, are dehydrated, and are receiving intravenous feedings with non-phosphate-containing solutions. Substantial phosphate may be lost during the osmotic diuresis that accompanies hyperglycemia in out-of-control diabetes mellitus, for example.

○ Phosphate depletion can result in muscle weakness (e.g., leading to respiratory failure, low cardiac output, or inability to walk). In severe cases, hemolysis (breakage of red blood cells) and defective bone mineralization (i.e., osteomalacia) can also be observed.

Review Questions

3. What are the two general physiological roles of calcium?
4. What is the level of ionized free calcium that homeostatic mechanisms work to maintain in the bloodstream?
5. What are some hormonal, physiological, and physiochemical mechanisms of calcium homeostasis?
6. What are the physiological roles of extraskeletal phosphate?
7. Typically, how much calcium and phosphate are absorbed and excreted daily?

3. PHYSIOLOGY OF BONE AND MINERAL HOMEOSTASIS

Bone consists of a matrix of collagen fibrils and other proteins secreted by cells called **osteoblasts**. Calcium and phosphate salts are deposited within this matrix in the form of hydroxyapatite crystals.

The epiphyseal plate is a layer of cartilage toward either end of long bones at which continued bone growth can occur (see Figure 14.2A). With maturation, this layer of cells disappears, and the ends of long bones fuse with the shaft (called closure of the epiphyses, see Figure 14.2). After that point, further increase in the length of long bones is not possible. However, remodeling of existing bone is an ongoing process that continues throughout life (see the following).

The adult skeleton has two types of bone:

1. **Cortical**, also known as compact or Haversian, **bone**, which makes up the shafts of long bones and flat bony surfaces and accounts for about 80% of the mass of the skeleton.
2. **Trabecular** or cancellous **bone**, which is a spongy network with a large surface area that makes up the center of bones. Although making up only 20% of skeletal mass, trabecular bone has five times the surface area of cortical bone, and therefore is the site of most active bone turnover (remodeling). Figure 14.2B summarizes some concepts of bone structure.

Bone cells

Two principal types of cells are found in bone and are central to understanding of the processes of bone formation and resorption.

Osteoclasts are multinucleated giant cells specialized for the resorption of bone. They are terminally differentiated and nondividing cells derived from granulocyte-macrophage stem cells in the bone marrow under the influence of various hematopoietic growth factors and cytokines, including macrophage colony-stimulating factor (M-CSF) and interleukin 6, and hormones such as PTH and vitamin D, to be discussed in Section 4 (see Figure 14.3).

When activated, osteoclasts isolate a region of bone by forming an adhesive ring of integrins (adhesive, largely extracellular, transmembrane receptor proteins on the cell

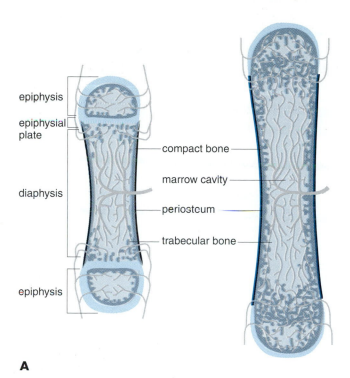

epiphysis

epiphysial plate

compact bone

marrow cavity

diaphysis

periosteum

trabecular bone

epiphysis

A

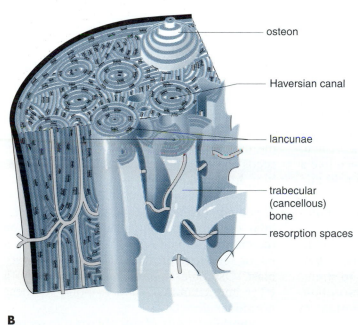

osteon

Haversian canal

lancunae

trabecular (cancellous) bone

resorption spaces

B

FIGURE 14.2. *A.* Long bone before and after fusion of the epiphyses. Schematic diagram of the structure of a typical long bone before (left) and after (right) closure of the epiphyses. *B.* Cortical versus trabecular bone. Diagram of features of bone structure seen in both transverse (top) and longitudinal sections. Areas of cortical (compact) and trabecular (cancellous) bone are included. *(A. Adapted, with permission, from Junquiera LC, Carniero J, Kelley RO (1995). Basic Histology, 8th ed. Stamford, CT, Appleton & Lange. B. Adapted, with permission, from Gray's Anatomy, 35th ed. Warwick R, Williams PL, eds. (1973). Longmans.)*

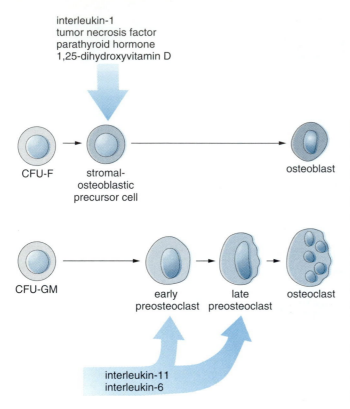

interleukin-1
tumor necrosis factor
parathyroid hormone
1,25-dihydroxyvitamin D

CFU-F

stromal-
osteoblastic
precursor cell

osteoblast

CFU-GM

early
preosteoclast

late
preosteoclast

osteoclast

interleukin-11
interleukin-6

FIGURE 14.3. Differentiation of osteoclasts and osteoblasts. Oseoclasts arise from precursor cells of the granulocyte-macrophage lineage (CFU-GM). Osteoblasts arise from precursor cells of mesenchymal-fibroblast origin (CFU-F). The development of osteoclasts is controlled by osteoblastic cells that produce cytokines, including interleukin 6 and 11, which regulate the pathway of osteoclastic differentiation. Hormones such as PTH and $1,25(OH)_2D_3$ and local factors such as interleukin 1 and tumor necrosis factor promote osteoclast differentiation indirectly, through their effects of stimulating IL-6 and IL-11 production. (Adapted, with permission, from Manolagas SC, Jilka RL, N Engl J Med 332:305–311, as adapted by Breslau NA, in Griffin JE, Ojeda SR, Textbook of Endocrine Physiology, 3d ed. New York, Oxford, 1996, p. 332.)

surface). The ligands that allow the integrins to bind tightly are amino-acid residues within bone matrix proteins. Within the isolated region of bone, a specialized membrane structure called the **ruffled membrane** is formed. The ruffled membrane functions much like a lysosome (see Chap. 2), containing acid and acid-activated enzymes that dissolve the isolated bone surface and degrade its component proteins.

It is thought that osteoclasts respond indirectly to PTH and vitamin D because osteoblasts are needed in order for PTH to stimulate osteoclast-mediated bone resorption. Thus, cell-cell interactions are important in bone physiology.

Osteoblasts are bone-forming cells that arise from mesenchymal stem cells (which also give rise to fibroblasts) in the bone marrow stroma. The osteocyte is a terminally differentiated osteoblast that resides in bone. Once an osteoblast has been activated and has laid down (secreted) bone matrix, it proceeds to mineralize its secretions by depositing **hydroxyapatite** crystals onto the collagen fibrils. This poorly understood process is dependent on an adequate supply of extracellular calcium and phosphate as well as on the enzyme alkaline phosphatase, which is a major secretory product of the active osteoblast. Osteoblasts have receptors for both PTH and vitamin D and respond to these hormones directly.

Another activity of osteoblasts is to secrete a variety of cytokines that regulate the differentiation of osteoclasts.

Bone remodeling

Bone is not an inert substance; rather, it is a tissue that is metabolically active and in a state of continuous remodeling, through the actions of these cells and their products, under the influence of hormones and other factors (see Figures 14.4A and B).

Cortical bone is remodeled from within by groups of osteoclasts, called *cutting cones*, that cut tunnels through the compact bone. They are followed by trailing osteoblasts, which lay down a cylinder of new bone on the walls until all that is left are the small spaces called the Haversian canals, channels through which the resident bone cells (called osteocytes) can be fed.

In trabecular bone, the remodeling occurs at the surface rather than within the bone. There, osteoclasts excavate a pit and osteoblasts fill it in with new bone and mineralize it. This cycle takes about 200 days and must be well balanced in order to maintain calcium homeostasis and prevent net bone loss, as occurs in osteoporosis.

Other hormones, including estrogens and glucocorticoids, play a facilitatory role in bone formation and resorption, both directly and indirectly.

Mechanical forces are probably also sensed by bone cells and can alter the balance between bone formation and resorption. Thus, complete bed rest or zero-gravity environments result in vastly accelerated bone loss, up to 1% of total bone mass per month. Conversely, weight-bearing exercise is associated with positive calcium balance and increased bone formation.

Another poorly understood variable in bone remodeling is the density of mineral deposition, which may vary from patient to patient on a genetic basis. The clearest role for heredity has been demonstrated for peak bone mass, a somewhat different measurement.

Clinical Pearl

○ African Americans (both men and women) are believed to have lower rates of osteoporosis and hip fractures, despite lower rates of bone formation, due to higher peak bone mineral content compared to Caucasian Americans and Asian Americans.

Bone physiology during childhood, adulthood, and old age

During childhood, linear bone growth occurs at the ends of long bones in specialized regions known as **epiphyseal plates** by replacement of cartilage with bone (see Figure 14.2). Bone width increases through addition of bone to the **periosteum**, at the outer surface of bones, just under the connective tissue layer.

When adulthood is reached, under the influence of sex steroid hormones (see Chaps. 15 and 16), the epiphyseal plates close and further linear growth is no longer possible. During adulthood, peak bone mass is maintained by the process of bone remodeling, assuming the absence of dietary and lifestyle factors that alter the balance in favor of bone loss. About 10% of bone mass normally turns over in the course of a year.

After about age 30 to 40 for females (but not males), bone resorption exceeds bone formation and total bone mass decreases slowly over time.

The increased risk for osteoporotic fractures in women is a function of:

1. On average, 25% lower peak bone density compared to men
2. An accelerated rate of bone loss, due to the fall in blood estrogen concentration, during the first few years after menopause

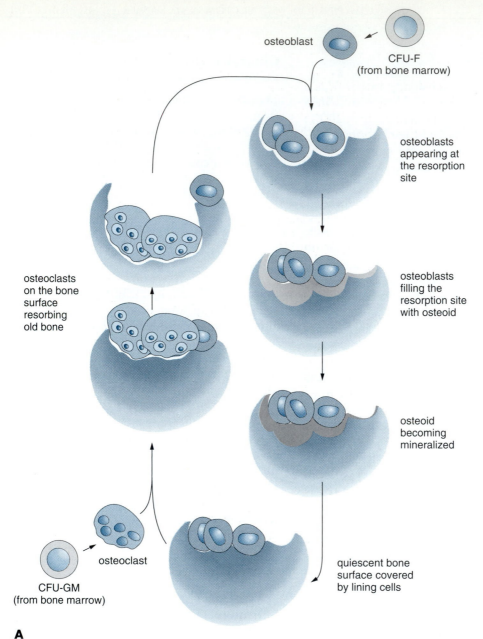

osteoblast

CFU-F
(from bone marrow)

osteoblasts
appearing at
the resorption
site

osteoblasts
filling the
resorption site
with osteoid

osteoid
becoming
mineralized

osteoclasts
on the bone
surface
resorbing
old bone

osteoclast

quiescent bone
surface covered
by lining cells

CFU-GM
(from bone marrow)

A

FIGURE 14.4. Bone remodeling. *A.* Remodeling is accomplished by cycles involving the resorption of old bone by osteoclasts and the subsequent formation of new bone by osteoblasts. The osteoclasts and osteoblasts are replenished from their progenitors in the bone marrow (CFU-GM and CFU-F, respectively). *B.* Osteoclast resorbing bone. The edges of the cell attach tightly to bone. Acid is pumped and lysosomal enzymes secreted from the ruffled membrane into the protected space along the surface of a region of bone, resulting in its resorption. *(A. Adapted, with permission, from Manolagas SC, Jilka RL. Bone marrow, cytokines, and bone remodeling: emerging insights into the pathophysiology of osteoporosis.* N Engl J Med *332:305–311, as adapted by Breslau NA (1996).* Calcium homeostasis, in Griffin JE and Ojeda SR. *Textbook of Endocrine Physiology, 3d ed. New York, Oxford, p. 331. B. Adapted, with permission, from Ganong WF. (1998).* Review of Medical Physiology, *19th ed. Stamford, CT, Appleton & Lange, p. 368.)*

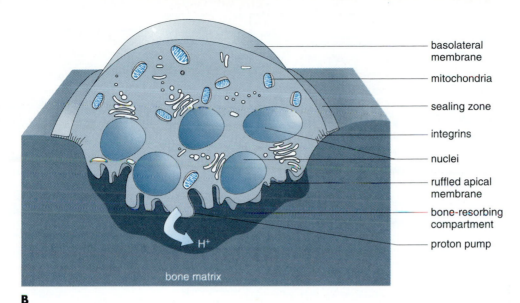

basolateral membrane

mitochondria

sealing zone

integrins

nuclei

ruffled apical membrane

bone-resorbing compartment

proton pump

H+

bone matrix

B

FIGURE 14.4 — (continued)

Subsequently, bone loss continues, but at a more gradual rate that is similar in both men and women, leading to a high risk of osteoporotic fractures in both genders above the age of 80.

Calcium and phosphate balance

Let us consider the actual magnitude of the flow of calcium and phosphate into and out of the body. Typical daily intake of calcium among Americans varies from about 500 to 1000 mg (see Table 14.4). Of this amount, the net absorption from the intestine (the sum of absorption and secretion) is about 200 mg daily. This amount of calcium must be excreted in urine daily to maintain calcium balance. If either urinary losses increase or GI absorption decreases, there will be a net loss of calcium, which must, inevitably, be balanced by resorption of bone.

Intake of phosphate is about 1400 mg daily, 900 mg of which is absorbed from the intestine, and hence must be cleared in the urine at steady state (see Figure 14.5).

The effects of the calcium and phosphate composition of foods on the absorption and elimination of these ions are very complex and still controversial. Net calcium absorption is affected not only by the amount of calcium taken in, but also by the amount of phosphorus present and the nature of the cal-

TABLE 14.4 CALCIUM REQUIREMENTS FOR HOMEOSTASIS

Calcium required to maintain balance	
Children	800 mg daily
Adolescents	1200 mg daily
Adults	800 mg daily
Pregnant/lactating women	1200–1500 mg daily
Elderly	1200–1500 mg daily
Average calcium intake in women under 65 in the United States	550 mg daily
Calcium sources	
Dairy product–free diet	400 mg
Cow's milk (8 oz)	300 mg
Calcium carbonate (500 mg)	200 mg

Reproduced, with permission, from Ganong WF. *Review of Medical Physiology* (1998). 19th ed. Stamford, CT, Appleton & Lange.

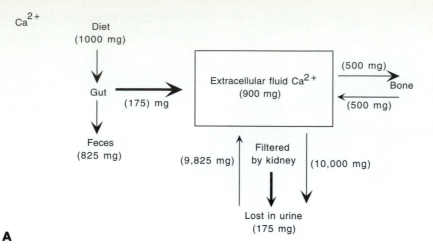

A

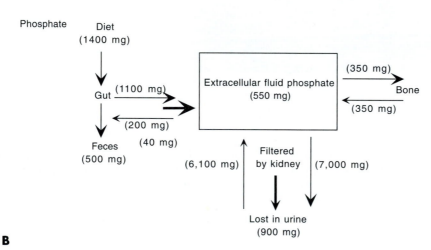

B

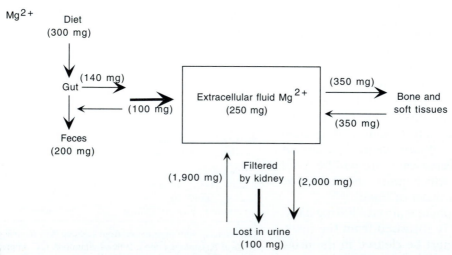

C

cium salts, which will affect parameters such as the absorption of calcium and phosphate from the GI tract, the excretion of calcium and phosphate in the urine, and the levels of hormones that control calcium and phosphate metabolism (e.g., PTH and vitamin D).

Clinical Pearls

○ The minimum daily recommendation for calcium intake is 800 mg for men and women.

○ Several important considerations support the idea that for most people, a much higher level of calcium intake may be more appropriate:

- The efficiency of absorption varies tremendously with the source of the calcium.
- Calcium associated with foods is, in general, more readily absorbed than tablet supplements (a property known as **bioavailability**).
- Of the supplements, calcium citrate appears to be superior to calcium carbonate.
- Calcium in milk is highly bioavailable, probably because of the ready absorption of the lactate with which the calcium is associated. Many people who are "lactose intolerant" can in fact drink up to one glass of milk or more, in small amounts over the course of the day, before developing symptoms such as bloating, gas, and diarrhea. Other individuals with lactose intolerance find that they can consume the equivalent of three glasses of milk daily in the form of yogurt, in which microbial action has broken down the lactose to lactate. Calcium in spinach is far less bioavailable than calcium in kale (5% vs. 40%) because of the presence of oxalic acid in spinach, which inhibits calcium absorption. As with most things in life, it is often more tolerable to work up to a goal (e.g., three glasses of milk, or its equivalent in yogurt, daily) over the course of, say, a month or two, than to attempt to make a major change in diet overnight.

○ For women, the maximal degree of bone density achieved during youth and young adulthood is believed to determine the ultimate risk of postmenopausal osteoporotic fractures. Thus, a higher calcium intake (e.g., 2000 mg daily) may promote maximal bone density, in conjunction with diminution of other risk factors such as alcohol intake, smoking, high meat consumption, and lack of exercise (see Sec. 5).

Review Questions

8. What is the difference between cortical and trabecular bone?

9. What are the major types of bone cells?

10. Describe the cycle of bone remodeling.

11. How does bone remodeling change from childhood to adulthood to old age?

12. What is the recommended minimum daily calcium intake? What percentage of the calcium ingested is actually absorbed?

FIGURE 14.5. Distribution and disposition of dietary calcium, phosphate and magnesium. *(Adapted, with permission, from Aurbach GD et al, in Wilson JD, Foster DW (eds): Williams Textbook of Endocrinology, 8th ed. Philadelphia, Saunders, 1992, p 1403.)*

4. HORMONAL CONTROL OF MINERAL METABOLISM

Overall plan of endocrine control of mineral metabolism

To fulfill their biochemical roles, calcium and phosphate must be maintained within a certain range in body fluids. The purpose of hormonal control is to prevent either excess or deficiency of these critical minerals by adjustments in either the bone reservoir, absorption from the gut, or loss in the urine.

To achieve mineral homeostasis, a hormonal axis consisting of **PTH** and **vitamin D** affects the target tissues of bone, intestine, and kidney and is controlled by short and long feedback loops involving ionized calcium (see Figure 14.6). However, other hormones (e.g., growth hormone) and other poorly understood factors are also important for mineral homeostasis (see Table 14.5). For example, if dietary phosphate is restricted, renal phosphate conservation becomes extremely efficient regardless of the presence or absence of PTH.

Clinical Pearls

Disorders of mineral homeostasis can lead to a wide range of symptoms, depending on how acute, severe, and prolonged is the development of the disorder. For example:

○ Hypocalcemia presents acutely with tetany, then muscle weakness, respiratory distress, seizures, and ultimately coma.
○ Anatomic deformities can develop over the long term. For example, compression fractures due to osteoporosis result in many elderly women having a hunchback-like appearance.

Parathyroid hormone

PTH is the major secretory protein product of **chief cells** found in the four parathyroid glands adjacent to the thyroid gland. Together, the parathyroid glands weigh a mere 150 mg.

The major regulator of PTH secretion is ionized calcium concentration in the blood. A calcium sensor in the chief cell responds to a fall in the ionized fraction of blood calcium by triggering PTH secretion. Through the actions of PTH, ionized blood calcium rises above the threshold for triggering calcium sensor activation, and thereby shuts off further PTH secretion (see Figure 14.6). Thus, the paramount goal of PTH is to maintain ionized blood calcium concentration at a set point, normally 1.2 mM.

PTH does this through a combination of effects that promote

1. Resorption of bone.
2. Calcium absorption from and phosphate loss in the renal filtrate.
3. Synthesis of the active vitamin D metabolite 1,25-dihydroxyvitamin D_3. On a somewhat delayed time scale, this results in increased calcium absorption from the GI tract (see the following discussion).

Although a very small fraction (about 10%) of PTH is secreted in a calcium-independent fashion, most PTH secretion is exquisitely sensitive to calcium ion level by negative feedback. Thus, increased serum calcium in the physiological range (8.5 to 10 mg/dL) inhibits PTH secretion; conversely, even an infinitesimally small fall in blood ionized calcium concentration below the physiological set point stimulates PTH secretion and sets in motion homeostatic corrective actions.

A secondary role of PTH is to maintain phosphate balance. It does this primarily by promoting phosphate excretion through inhibition of sodium-dependent phosphate transport in the renal tubule. Serum phosphate does not affect PTH secretion directly. Instead, it affects vitamin D metabolism, which in turn affects PTH (see the following discussion).

A tertiary role of PTH may be to promote urinary excretion of bicarbonate ions.

Clinical Pearl

○ The effect of magnesium on PTH secretion can seem paradoxical. As with calcium, low blood levels of Mg stimulate and high blood levels inhibit PTH secretion.

However, at *very* low Mg blood levels (e.g., less than 0.5 mM), the intracellular Mg level is sufficiently depleted to affect the very process of hormone secretion itself. As a result, further PTH secretion is blocked, despite what should be a strong stimulus for PTH secretion.

This is occasionally seen clinically in alcohol-intoxicated patients suffering from dehydration and exposure who have a combination of severe hypomagnesemia and persistent hypocalcemia, despite calcium therapy. The hypocalcemia will correct only after the magnesium deficit has been eliminated (e.g., by oral repletion or intramuscular injection), allowing resumption of PTH secretion.

PTH Actions on bone

The major effect of PTH on bone is to release calcium (and with it, phosphate). It does this through some rather complex rapid and delayed effects. Also, PTH generally causes more resorption of cortical bone than of trabecular bone.

The rapid effects (in minutes) of PTH include stimulation of bone resorption by pre-existing osteoclasts and inhibition of collagen synthesis in osteoblasts. The delayed effects include stimulation of the process of activation that converts quiescent precursor cells into mature osteoclasts and osteoblasts. This further enhances the process of bone remodeling, including *both* formation and resorption of bone.

Depending on conditions, increased PTH can stimulate either bone formation or bone resorption. Continuous exposure to PTH, as in a patient with hyperparathyroidism due to a parathyroid adenoma (a tumor secreting the hormone without regard to the ionized blood calcium), generally promotes bone loss in the manner just described. However, intermittent low-dose PTH administration can actually cause bone formation in humans. Several hypotheses have been proposed to explain this paradoxical effect. Perhaps under these conditions PTH stimulates the local production of insulin-like growth factor and other factors that promote bone formation.

The consequences of PTH action, in terms of bone formation versus bone loss, are also probably influenced by other factors such as mechanical stress; exercise; calcium, phosphate and vitamin D blood levels; and the blood levels of other hormones (see Table 14.5).

PTH Actions on renal ion transport

PTH has two principal effects on renal ion transport in the renal filtrate:

1. It increases calcium absorption.
2. It decreases phosphate absorption.

Approximately 60% of serum calcium is filtered at the glomerulus (the rest is not filtered

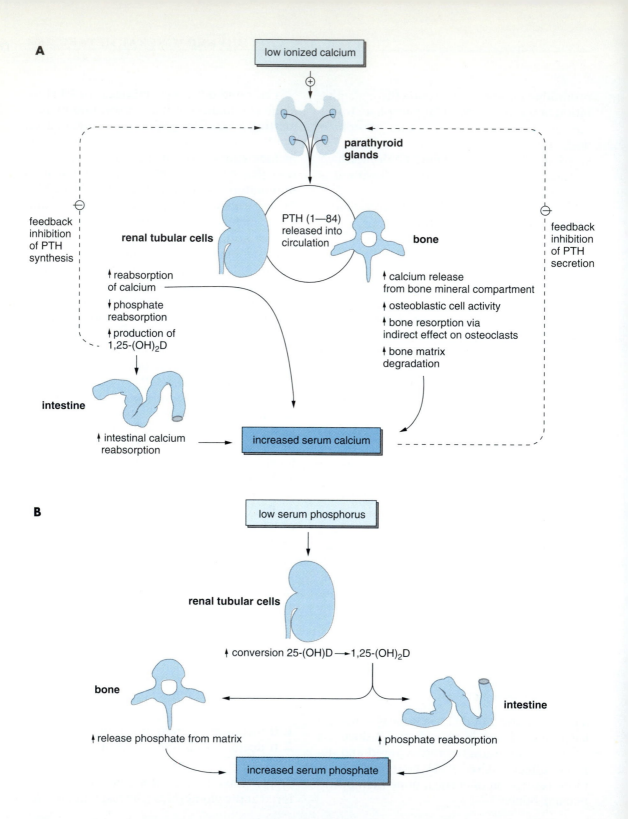

A

low ionized calcium

parathyroid glands

feedback inhibition of PTH synthesis

feedback inhibition of PTH secretion

renal tubular cells

PTH (1—84) released into circulation

bone

↑ reabsorption of calcium

↓ phosphate reabsorption

↑ production of 1,25-(OH)₂D

↑ calcium release from bone mineral compartment

↑ osteoblastic cell activity

↑ bone resorption via indirect effect on osteoclasts

↑ bone matrix degradation

intestine

↑ intestinal calcium reabsorption

increased serum calcium

B

low serum phosphorus

renal tubular cells

↑ conversion 25-(OH)D → 1,25-(OH)₂D

bone

intestine

↑ release phosphate from matrix

↑ phosphate reabsorption

increased serum phosphate

TABLE 14.5   OTHER HORMONES AFFECTING BONE

Bone formation	Bone resorption
Stimulated by	Stimulated by
Growth hormone (constant)	Parathyroid hormone
Insulin-like growth factors	(constant)
Insulin	Vitamin D
Estrogen	Cortisol
Androgen	Thyroid hormone
Vitamin D (mineralization)	Prostaglandins
Transforming growth factor β	Interleukin 1
Skeletal growth factor	Interleukin 6
Bone-derived growth factor	Tumor necrosis factor α
Platelet-derived growth factor	Tumor necrosis factor β
Calcitonin	
Parathyroid hormone	
(intermittent)	
Inhibited by	Inhibited by
Cortisol	Estrogen
	Androgen
	Calcitonin
	Transforming growth
	factor β
	γ-Interferon
	Nitric oxide

Reproduced, with permission, from Berne RM, Levy MN. (1998). *Physiology*, 4th ed. St. Louis, MO, Mosby, p. 854.

because it is tightly protein-bound). Most of this filtered calcium is reabsorbed in the proximal tubule and the loop of Henle, in a nonsaturable process linked to sodium reabsorption that is *insensitive* to PTH.

Only some 10% of the total filtered load of calcium reaches the distal tubule. However (as in the case of sodium and water, discussed in Chaps. 9 and 10), it is this relatively small distal fraction of filtered calcium, available for absorption at the distal tubule, that is under hormonal control and whose absorp-

tion or excretion can be manipulated by the receptor-mediated action of PTH. This constitutes the basis for the renal response to hypo- or hypercalcemia.

The PTH-sensitive distal tubular calcium transporter, located in the terminal segments of the distal convoluted tubule and in the collecting ducts, is completely independent of sodium transport and is saturable. Even though this fraction of calcium is small compared to total filtered calcium, it is five times greater in actual amount (1000 mg) than the amount of calcium absorbed daily (approximately 200 mg) from the intestine under normal conditions; thus, this degree of hormonal regulation is all that is needed to provide sensitive control of total body calcium balance.

Phosphate is also filtered at the glomerulus and reabsorbed largely in the proximal tubule by a sodium-phosphate co-transporter. The set point that defines the maximal rate of phosphate transport is decreased by a receptor-mediated action of PTH, thus allowing phosphate loss in the urine.

A logic for PTH's having opposite effects on calcium and phosphate in the renal tubular fluid is that bone resorption results in release of *both* calcium and phosphate. If uncorrected, this effect would elevate the calcium × phosphate product, perhaps to a point where calcium phosphate precipitation in important soft tissues might occur. By eliminating phosphate in the urine while absorbing calcium, the kidneys correct the fall in blood ionized free calcium without the undesired effect of concurrently elevating the blood phosphate.

Additional renal effects of PTH are to pro-

FIGURE 14.6. Overall plan of endocrine control of mineral metabolism. (Adapted, with permission, from Chandrasoma P, Taylor CE (1994). Concise Pathology. 2nd ed. Norwalk, CT, Appleton & Lange, as modified from Strewler GS, Shoback D. in McPhee S et al. (1997). Pathophysiology of Disease, 2nd ed. Norwalk, CT, Appleton & Lange, p. 401.)

mote magnesium absorption and to inhibit sodium and bicarbonate absorption.

PTH Actions on vitamin D synthesis

Another major effect of PTH on the kidney involves an increase in the activity of 1-hydroxylase, the enzyme involved in formation of active vitamin D from the 25-hydroxylated intermediate, which has little activity. The 1-hydroxylase enzyme has a short half-life (several hours). PTH both induces synthesis of this enzyme and stimulates its activity, although the induction of synthesis may generally predominate.

PTH Biosynthesis and secretion

PTH is a 84-amino-acid hormone, generated from a 115-amino-acid polypeptide precursor called preproparathyroid hormone by cleavage of first a signal sequence and then, subsequently, another peptide called a pro sequence (see Chaps. 2 and 3). After translocation to the lumen of the endoplasmic reticulum, PTH traverses the classical secretory pathway, during which time its proteolytic maturation is completed, and the mature hormone is stored in secretory granules. PTH-containing secretory granules are released by fusion to the plasma membrane in response to appropriate stimuli. PTH secretion is pulsatile, is greater at night than during the daytime, and increases with aging.

As would be expected from the general mechanisms of feedback control seen for other hormones (see Chap. 3), the stimulus for PTH secretion, hypocalcemia, if prolonged, also causes parathyroid gland **hyperplasia**. Conversely, hypercalcemia, which acutely shuts off PTH secretion from normal parathyroid tissue, will chronically result in metabolic inactivity and, eventually, **atrophy** of normal parathyroid tissue.

Review Questions

13. What are the effects of PTH on bone?
14. What are the effects of PTH on the kidney?
15. Describe the biosynthesis of PTH.
16. What is the effect of prolonged hypocalcemia on the parathyroid gland?

Vitamin D

Vitamin D and its metabolites are steroids, structural analogues of cholesterol. One of these, 1,25-dihydroxyvitamin D_3, a product of vitamin D metabolism in the liver and kidney, is the most active form of vitamin D. 1,25-dihydroxyvitamin D's role in mineral metabolism is a consequence of its effects on bone, kidney, and, most importantly, intestine, where it has a mechanism of action similar to that of steroid hormones (see Chap. 3).

Mechanism of vitamin D action

When we speak of vitamin D action, we are generally referring to the most active metabolite, 1,25-dihydroxyvitamin D, which results from conversion of precursors in the liver and kidney. 1,25-dihydroxyvitamin D diffuses into cells and binds to the vitamin D receptor, a protein found in both the cytoplasm and the nucleus. The hormone-receptor complex then binds to specific nuclear DNA sequences, turning on or off transcription of various genes. Thus, the vitamin D receptor can be thought of as a **ligand-dependent transcription factor** whose ligand is vitamin D. Binding of the vitamin D receptor to other proteins, including the retinoic acid receptor, allows more complex patterns of gene expression (e.g., different actions in different tissues) than would be possible owing to the binding of vitamin D to a single receptor protein alone.

As a result of these tissue-specific changes in transcription, there is a corresponding

TABLE 14.6 GENES ACTIVATED OR INHIBITED BY VITAMIN D

Gene	Transcription
Vitamin D receptor	Increased
Calcium-binding proteins	Increased
(calbindins)	Increased
Calcium pump	Increased
Osteocalcin	Increased
Alkaline phosphatase	Increased
24 Hydroxylase	Increased
Parathyroid hormone	Decreased
1 Hydroxylase	Decreased
Collagen	Decreased
Interleukin-2	Decreased
γ-Interferon	Decreased

Reproduced, with permission, from Berne RM, Levy MN (1998). *Physiology*, 4th ed. St. Louis, MO, Mosby, p. 858.

change in the amount of mRNA, and of protein synthesized from this mRNA, for various specific genes. These changes in gene expression constitute the primary activity of vitamin D (see Table 14.6).

Vitamin D effects that promote calcium absorption and bone mineralization

The net effect of many of these changes in transcription is to promote calcium absorption from the intestine. At low dietary calcium intake, the active calcium transport promoted by these gene products, provides for a greater efficiency of calcium absorption. These proteins are involved not only in calcium entry via the apical surface of the enterocyte, but also in the shuttling of calcium within the cell and its exit through the basolateral membrane via an ATP-driven calcium pump (Ca-ATPase).

Vitamin D also stimulates mineralization of bone. Without vitamin D, unmineralized osteoid accumulates as a result of lack of vitamin D–mediated repression of osteoblast collagen synthesis. Thus, the bone formed in the absence of adequate vitamin D is weak,

as is observed in children with the vitamin D–deficiency syndrome called rickets.

Vitamin D effects to promote bone resorption

The direct and indirect effects of vitamin D action on bone are complex. Under some circumstances, vitamin D can promote bone resorption. Osteoblasts, but not osteoclasts, have vitamin D receptors. However, vitamin D stimulates paracrine signaling from osteoblasts to osteoclasts, thereby promoting osteoclast action.

Vitamin D has a separate effect of stimulating the process of osteoclast precursor recruitment, differentiation, and fusion into multinucleated giant cells. PTH action on bone requires the presence of 1,25-dihydroxyvitamin D. Without it, PTH does not resorb bone properly.

Some other actions of vitamin D on mineral metabolism include facilitation of:

- Phosphate and magnesium absorption from the GI tract (independent of its effects on calcium uptake)
- Feedback repression of PTH synthesis
- Weak effects on renal tubular fluid calcium absorption and on uptake of calcium into skeletal and cardiac muscle

In vitro studies also show some other effects of vitamin D on metabolism (see Figure 14.7), although the in vivo significance of these remains unclear:

- Promotion of skin keratinocyte differentiation while inhibiting proliferation, thereby regulating 1,25-dihydroxyvitamin D formation
- Immune modulation by altering cytokine production by lymphocytes, macrophages, and monocytes
- Various effects on other tissues, such as the hypothalamus, pituitary, pancreatic islets,

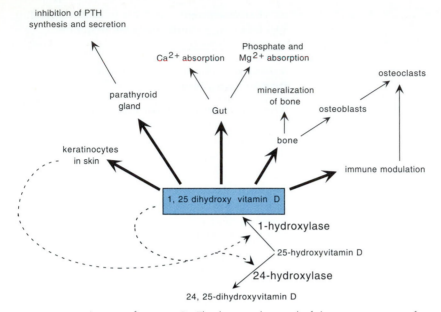

FIGURE 14.7. Actions of vitamin D. The best understood of the many actions of vitamin D are indicated by primary (heavy) arrows emanating from 1,25-dihydroxyvitamin D to skin, parathyroid, gut, bone, and immune system. Secondary (light) arrows indicate physiological consequences of vitamin D action on that organ system. Dashed line refers to inhibition of further 1,25-dihydroxyvitamin D formation by inhibition of 1-hydroxylase and stimulation of 24-hydroxylase. Vitamin D has distinct effects on bone to promote mineralization and to increase osteoblast-osteoclast signaling.

placenta, ovary, and aortic endothelium, including enhanced insulin and prolactin secretion in response to vitamin D

The complex interactions between various hormones, cytokines, and cell types of bone and the immune system have not been well elucidated. Thus, much of our use of vitamin D (e.g., orally to promote calcium uptake) is empirical. Paradoxically, in excess, vitamin D can promote excessive calcium uptake from the gut and renal calcium excretion, which may manifest with bone loss and formation of calcium-containing kidney stones.

Biosynthesis and metabolism

There are two ways to get vitamin D: through the diet and by the action of sunlight on cho-lesterol-derived precursors found in kera-tinocytes, specialized cells in skin. The product of UV irradiation of skin (termed vitamin D_3 or cholecalciferol) and the form obtained through the diet (termed D_2 or ergocalciferol, generated by UV irradiation of plant sterols) are stored in fat and muscle.

A high-affinity vitamin D–binding protein (DBP) is synthesized in and secreted from the liver. It carries the D_2 and D_3 precursors back to the liver, where the first of two hydroxylation reactions takes place. This generates 25-hydroxylvitamin D, the major circulating form in humans, which has a half-life of 2 weeks. Liver disease that results in a fall in DBP levels can alter the size of the reservoir of vitamin D metabolites, but frank signs of vitamin D deficiency will occur only if the free fraction of active metabolites is lacking. However, standard testing measures total vitamin D metabolites, not just the active free fraction.

Several dihydroxylated forms of vitamin D are generated from 25-hydroxyvitamin D by the action of specific hydroxylases, mostly concentrated in cells of the proximal tubule in the kidney. 1,25-hydroxyvitamin D is far more active than either the singly hydroxylated 25-hydroxyvitamin D or the other major doubly hydroxylated form, 24,25-dihydroxyvitamin D.

The activity of the two different hydroxylases that generate doubly hydroxylated vitamin D is reciprocally regulated, so that conditions favoring formation of $1,25(OH)_2D$ inhibit formation of $24,25(OH)_2D$, and vice versa.

The regulatory factors that determine the relative activity of 1-hydroxylase vs. 24-hydroxylase are blood levels of:

• PTH
• Phosphate
• 1,25-dihydroxyvitamin D itself
• Calcium ions

Thus, when plasma calcium or phosphate levels are low or PTH levels are high, the activity of the enzyme 1α-hydroxylase is high, resulting in more active vitamin D. Conversely, when plasma calcium, phosphate, or 1,25-dihydroxyvitamin D_3 levels are elevated, the activity of the enzyme 1α-hydroxylase is inhibited and that of 24α-hydroxylase is stimulated, resulting in a compensatory decrease in production of the active vitamin D metabolite.

Of the various vitamin D metabolites, 1,25-dihydroxyvitamin D has the shortest half-life, a few hours, while 24,25 dihydroxyvitamin D and 25 hydroxyvitamin D have half-lives of 2 weeks or more.

Figure 14.8 summarizes our current understanding of vitamin D biosynthesis.

Clinical Pearls

○ Along with changes in androgen and estrogen levels, a significant contributor to osteoporosis in the elderly is their decreased exposure to sunlight and therefore decreased synthesis of vitamin D. Only 10 to 20 min/week of exposure to direct sunlight is needed. But an elderly person who never leaves the house and never consumes dairy products (e.g., the "tea and toast" diet) may become vitamin D–deficient.

○ Normally, excess sun exposure does not result in vitamin D toxicity because excess sunlight causes degradation of the activated precursor, thereby limiting the amount of vitamin D produced.

Synthesis of the vitamin D receptor itself is increased by PTH, insulin-like growth factors, cortisol, and estrogen. Hyperphosphatemia resulting from excess vitamin D will also suppress PTH secretion.

Calcitonin

Calcitonin (CT) is a 32-amino-acid peptide secreted by the parafollicular C cells in the thyroid gland in response to hypercalcemia. Generally, the effects of CT on bone are reciprocal to those of PTH. Its primary action appears to be a profound inhibition of bone resorption through a direct action on osteoclasts. In response to CT, osteoclasts lose their ruffled membrane and detach from bony surfaces. Although CT is in many ways a PTH **antagonist** with respect to calcium, its net effect is to cause a decrease in blood phosphate concentration, similar to the effect observed for PTH.

However, CT does not appear to have any direct effect in promoting bone formation and, in general, does not seem to be an important contributor to overall mineral homeostasis in humans. Thus, total thyroidectomy with

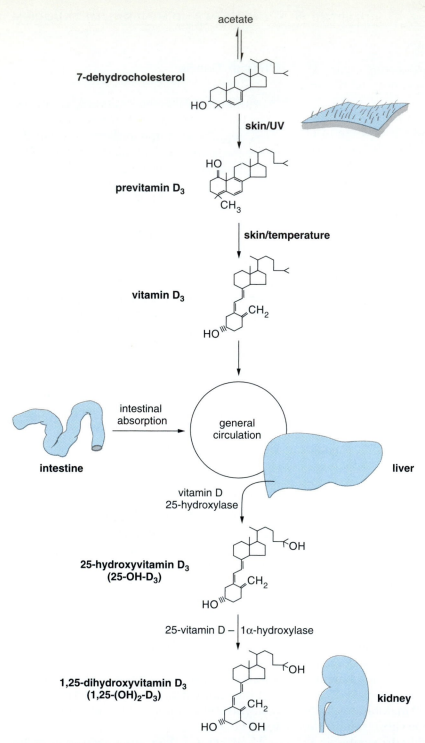

FIGURE 14.8. Vitamin D biosynthesis. Shown are the steps in vitamin D biosynthesis de novo and from dietary sources. *(Adapted with permission from Felig P et al., eds. (1995). Endocrinology and Metabolism, 3rd ed. New York, McGraw-Hill.)*

thyroid hormone replacement alone has no observed impact on calcium or mineral homeostasis. Conversely, patients with medullary carcinoma of the thyroid with a 20,000 fold elevation in serum calcitonin levels also display no clear abnormality in mineral metabolism. CT does have some pharmacologic value in treatment of hypercalcemia, but even this is limited by an escape phenomenon after large doses or prolonged treatment, as a result of receptor downregulation. Curiously, ingestion of food also is a stimulus to calcitonin secretion, with no resulting elevation in blood ionized calcium.

Parathyroid hormone–related protein

A 141-amino-acid protein that is homologous to PTH at the amino terminus, and hence is called parathyroid hormone–related protein (PTHrP), is also recognized by PTH receptors. Unlike PTH, which is synthesized only in the parathyroid gland, PTHrP is made in nearly every tissue in the body at one time or another in development or adult life. It functions mainly as a tissue growth and differentiation factor and paracrine mediator at the local level (e.g., in skin and in the conversion of cartilage to bone), and its circulating concentration is normally too low to have a significant systemic effect, except in cases of malignancy, in which large tumor masses making PTHrP can generate levels high enough to cause hypercalcemia by an endocrine mechanism.

The role of PTHrP in stimulating proliferation of chondrocytes and inhibiting mineralization of cartilage appears to be required for normal development, because embryos that lack it are nonviable and have various abnormalities of cartilage and bone. However, we do not yet have a clear picture of the role of PTHrP in normal physiology. Antibodies have now been developed that can distinguish PTH from PTHrP.

Clinical Pearl

○ PTHrP was first discovered as the cause of hypercalcemia in many patients with squamous cell cancers and was later found to be a factor involved in growth and differentiation of normal tissues.

Review Questions

17. What are the effects of vitamin D on the gut?
18. How does PTH control vitamin D synthesis?
19. What is the most biologically active form of vitamin D? How does its activity compare to that of the vitamin D precursors?
20. Where are active vitamin D metabolites produced, and how are they regulated?
21. Where is calcitonin made?
22. How can you distinguish hypercalcemia due to PTH from that due to PTHrP?

5. INTEGRATED CONTROL OF MINERAL HOMEOSTASIS

The full impact of a change in blood level of 1,25-dihydroxyvitamin D on the intestine takes 24 to 48 h to manifest; thus, the minute-to-minute control of calcium homeostasis is due to PTH effects on the acute phase of bone resorption and on the kidney. The net effect is that serum calcium normally varies by only 0.1 mg/dL during any given day.

Defense against hypo- and hypercalcemia

After a 12-h fast, a normal individual has an almost unmeasurable drop in serum calcium due to urinary calcium loss. This triggers a slight increase in PTH secretion, which corrects the change in serum calcium by acute resorptive effects on bone and by increased efficiency of calcium reclamation in the distal renal tubule.

A more severe hypocalcemic stimulus (e.g., decreased dietary intake of calcium and resulting diminished calcium absorption) triggers additional changes. These include:

1. Further increase in bone resorption (i.e., mobilization of both calcium and phosphate)
2. A change in tubular transport of phosphate, allowing excretion of the phosphate

load accompanying the calcium derived from bone (another PTH effect)
3. Increased efficiency of calcium absorption from the gut, due to the effect of increased levels of 1,25-dihydroxyvitamin D, which is manifest over the next 24–48 h

If the calcium deprivation were even more severe, e.g., complete calcium malabsorption, PTH and 1,25-dihydroxyvitamin D levels would rise even further, with skeletal loss by both acute and chronic PTH-mediated bone resorption as the body sacrificed skeletal homeostasis in order to maintain blood calcium concentration (see Figure 14.9).

FIGURE 14.9. Response to hypocalcemia. Immediate and delayed homeostatic mechanisms are triggered by a fall in plasma calcium. Each results in offsetting changes that normalize plasma calcium, initially at the expense of bone and through more efficient calcium recovery from urine, and later due to more efficient calcium absorption from the GI tract. Changes in plasma calcium that offset the initial hypocalcemic stimulus are indicated by double-headed arrows. Both immediate and delayed mechanisms also trigger negative-feedback loops (indicated by dashed lines) upon correction of the abnormality.

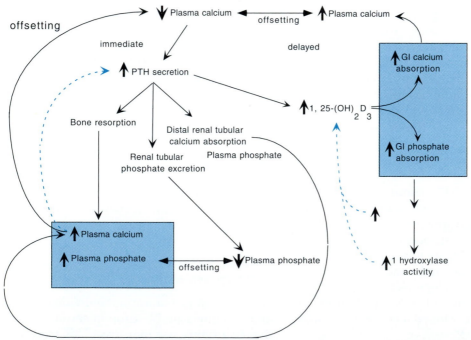

The response to hypercalcemia is largely a reversal of these processes. The weak link in this chain of homeostatic events is that the capacity for renal calcium excretion is limited, especially as the glomerular filtration rate drops. Thus, renal failure or dehydration can contribute significantly to hypercalcemia.

Defense against hypo- and hyperphosphatemia

Phosphate balance is largely controlled by the kidney. In the setting of hypophosphatemia, stimulation of 1,25-dihydroxyvitamin D synthesis occurs, which increases intestinal absorption of calcium and phosphate. As a consequence, PTH secretion is inhibited by the resulting increased calcium. This diminishes phosphate loss in urine with normalization of serum phosphate. Since the increased uptake of calcium from the intestine is offset by diminished calcium reclamation from the urine, there is no change in serum calcium, only correction of the phosphate deficit. The effects on the intestine eventually compensate for the effects on bone resorption, and thus the net increase in blood phosphate is due to increased intestinal absorption and decreased urine phosphate excretion (see Figure 14.10).

FIGURE 14.10. Response to hypophosphatemia. A fall in plasma phosphate triggers corrective measures involving 1,25-dihydroxyvitamin D synthesis, GI tract absorption of calcium and phosphate, diminished PTH secretion, and altered renal excretion of calcium and phosphate. Changes in plasma phosphate that offset the initial hypophosphatemic stimulus are indicated by double-headed arrows. Negative-feedback inhibition is indicated by dashed arrows.

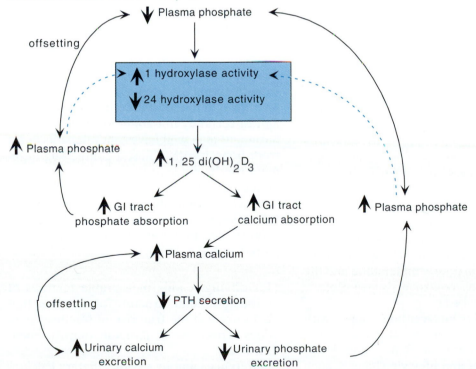

Clinical Pearls

○ The most common causes of hypercalcemia are hyperparathyroidism due to a tumor of the parathyroid gland (which is treated), production of PTHrP by a cancer (which is treated), and a benign condition called familial hypocalciuric hypercalcemia that is due to mutations in the calcium sensor (which is not treated).

○ Some drugs, such as lithium and thiazide diuretics, can stimulate PTH secretion and thereby elevate serum calcium. Both of these drugs also have renal effects and cause decreased urine calcium.

○ The most common cause of persistent hypocalcemia is parathyroid gland surgery.

Osteoporosis

An important issue in bone health is the effect of estrogen deficiency on calcium balance. The greater risk of fractures in elderly women compared to men is due to the fact that their peak bone mass is 25% less than that of men and that they have greater bone loss in the first several years after menopause as a result of the effect of lower blood estrogens. A hotly debated topic is whether clinicians should recommend estrogen replacement to their patients and, if so, to whom and in what form. The pros and cons of this question are considered in more detail in Chapter 16.

Clinical epidemiologic studies have revealed a host of risk factors contributing to the development of osteoporosis. The pathophysiological mechanisms by which these risks occur remain poorly understood and the source of ongoing controversy (see Refs. 1 and 2 and Table 14.7).

Pharmacologic intervention (e.g., with agents such as estrogen) is often considered as a way to modify bone remodeling. However, various diet and lifestyle changes, such

TABLE 14.7   RISK FACTORS FOR OSTEOPOROSIS

White and Asian women
Alcohol use
Tobacco use
Sedentary lifestyle
Family history of fractures and osteoporosis
Low bone mineral density
Advanced age
Early or surgical menopause
Thin body habitus
Drugs (glucocorticoids, thyroid hormone, anticonvulsants)
Habitual low calcium intake

Adapted from Ross PD (1998). *Endocrinol Metab Clin North Am* 27:290.

as encouraging the patient to stop smoking, decrease the consumption of alcohol, and increase weight-bearing exercise, (see Figure 14.11) should not be neglected as effective ways to affect calcium balance and get much of the same net effect on bone.

In addition to risk factors for bone loss that are supported by extensive studies, others can be identified based on theoretical risks or incomplete studies. These include high dietary consumption of meat, refined sugar, and sodium (see Figure 14.12). Changes in diet and lifestyle to modify these possible risks is almost certainly not going to cause a patient harm and may well have other benefits apart from bone health. Thus, a compelling argument can be made in favor of clinicians' recommending these changes to their patients now, even while awaiting further work to fully explore the mechanisms involved.

Variables that remain to be further explored include:

• Identifying readily measurable features of musculoskeletal structure or function that better reflect the true risk of fractures than does gross bone mineral density measurement
• Differences among various dietary calcium

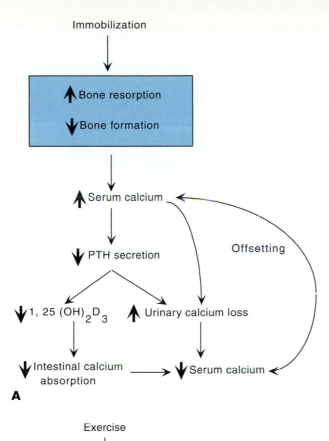

A

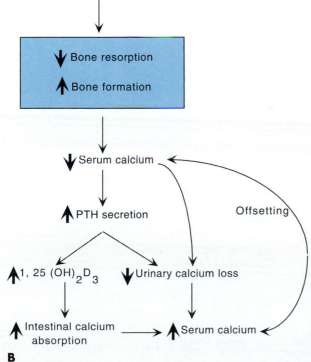

B

FIGURE 14.11. How immobilization might promote, and exercise prevent, bone loss. Diagram of ways in which immobilization and exercise could affect calcium balance. Note that a major unanswered question is how weight-bearing exercise actually influences bone formation and resorption and how immobilization versus exercise is integrated by the body with hormonal, dietary, and other factors. Effects on intestinal calcium absorption are a plausible final common pathway by which each of these factors is manifest. *(Adapted with permission, from Griffin JE, Ojeda SR (1996). Textbook of Endocrine Physiology, 3d ed. New York, Oxford, p. 335.)*

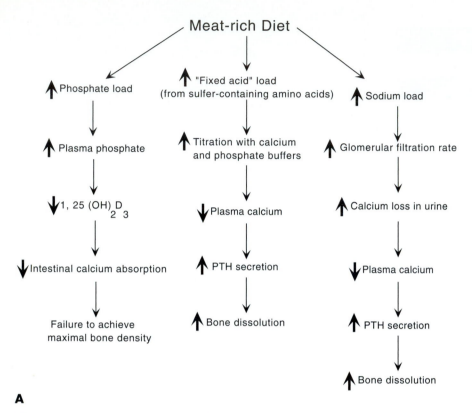

A

FIGURE 14.12. *A.* Possible mechanisms by which a high meat intake can promote osteoporosis. Meat consumption provides high concentrations of not only all amino acids but also sodium and phosphate, compared to equivalent calories obtained from most plant sources. Indicated are three possible mechanisms by which the amino acid, phosphate, and sodium load of a high-meat diet could contribute to bone dissolution and/or failure to achieve maximal bone density during early adulthood.

sources in terms of the efficiency of calcium absorption from the GI tract
- How the body integrates hormonal with mechanical, dietary, and other influences on calcium balance and bone health
- How factors that regulate calcium balance and bone health change with age and with the health of other organ systems (e.g., the kidney and the GI tract)
- Hereditary factors and where they affect bone density and bone strength

Review Questions

23. What are the body's responses to a small drop in blood ionized calcium below the normal range?
24. What are the body's responses to a small rise in blood-ionized calcium above the normal range?
25. What are the body's responses to a small drop in blood phosphate below the normal range?

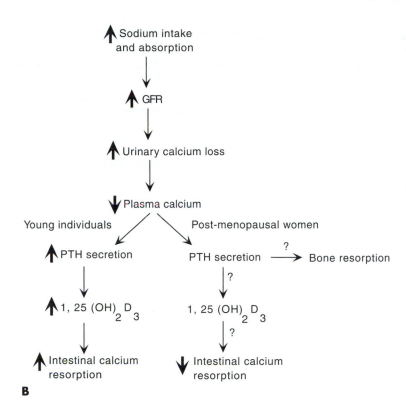

B

FIGURE 14.12 — *(continued)* *B.* Hypotheses on how high sodium intake might impair calcium absorption and how that effect might be different in young individuals versus postmenopausal women. Implied by the question marks (?) are that a consequence of aging is to impair either PTH or vitamin D secretion/action, resulting in diminished intestinal calcium absorption. Thus, good dietary habits developed early in life might be particularly valuable later (e.g., postmenopause), when protective mechanisms have been impaired.

26. What are the body's responses to a small rise in blood phosphate above the normal range?

27. What are some common risk factors for osteoporosis?

6. FRONTIERS IN CALCIUM AND MINERAL PHYSIOLOGY

Organ-specific features of physiology and development might be fully accounted for by differences in amounts of various known gene products. On the other hand, it is tempting to imagine that unique gene products will be found to be master regulators of organ-specific processes. The process of bone remodeling is a case in point. It requires participation of various cell types (e.g., osteoblasts and osteoclasts): their activation and differentiation, with accompanying changes in gene expression, in particular of various cytokines. Might there be some unifying theme that will make apparent the conceptual framework by which the whole system operates — and provide new therapeutic opportunities as well?

New insights into the mechanism of bone remodeling

Enter osteoprotegerin (OPG), a newly discovered secretory protein that is involved in the regulation of bone density (see Ref. 4). The OPG gene has been cloned, and its product has been overexpressed in transgenic mice. High blood levels of OPG cause the development of excessively dense bone, a disorder termed osteopetrosis. OPG was also demonstrated in vitro to block differentiation of osteoclasts and to reverse the loss of bone density normally associated with removal of the ovaries (resulting in estrogen deficiency) in rats.

OPG is a member of the tumor necrosis factor receptor family — but one that is secreted rather than integrated into the membrane. The recent work on OPG provides a new framework in which to understand regulation of bone density. It seems likely that this involves a complex network of interactions in which different proteins, including OPG, compete for binding to various as yet unknown membrane receptors. An understanding of factors that increase or diminish OPG synthesis will have great medical value — and not just for drug development. For example, it may allow more rapid identification of other risk factors for osteoporosis, as well as determination of the optimal mix of dietary and other influences that makes achievement of maximal bone density possible.

Calcium and hypertension: what is the connection?

A number of epidemiologic studies have demonstrated a relationship between low calcium intake and the presence of elevated blood pressure. Whether calcium supplementation ameliorates hypertension is less clear, with some outcome studies weighing in on each side of that conclusion. Given that calcium deficiency is a widespread nutritional problem in modern societies, the possibility that, at least for some patients, calcium deficiency and hypertension might be related is intriguing. It has been suggested that the calcium may ameliorate hypertension in a subset of patients with low plasma renin activity (see Table 14.8).

Based on studies in rats, it has recently been proposed that calcium deficiency sets in motion a vicious cycle by stimulating sodium intake. The resulting increase in body sodium is excreted by the kidneys in the urine. But with the sodium that leaves the kidney in the form of urine go also water and calcium, thereby exacerbating the original calcium deficiency. The physiological and pathophysiological mechanisms connecting a low-calcium diet with a craving for salt ingestion remains to be further explored. It appears that an adrenal factor may be a key determinant in this subset of calcium-sensitive essential hypertension (see Refs. 5 and 6).

The complex take-home message from calcium physiology

Could it be that substances such as calcium are involved in physiological regulation far too complex to study reliably by clinical epidemiologic correlations based on current understanding of calcium physiology? For example, a problem (e.g., hypertension) may be initiated by one factor (e.g., calcium deficiency), which then sets in motion dependence on a second factor. Until the second (unknown) factor is ameliorated, the system may not respond to correction of the calcium deficiency. Perhaps in some cases, the change caused by calcium deficiency, once established, is irreversible. Likewise, the consequences of calcium supplementation for blood pressure control may depend on other components of the diet or lifestyle whose relevance has not yet been identified. Figure 14.12 indicates how one effect on calcium balance (e.g., sodium-induced calcium loss) might become manifest as a result of changes in other aspects of human physiology (e.g., aging). Perhaps a more profound appreciation of the normal physiology of calcium will lead to identification of the additional features needed for productive study of dietary and other interventions designed to reinforce calcium homeostasis.

TABLE 14.8 COMPARISON OF HIGH-RENIN AND LOW-RENIN FORMS OF HYPERTENSION

Features/Treatments	High-renin	Low-renin
Plasma volume	Low	High
Peripheral resistance	High	Low
Cardiac output	Low	High
Aldosterone	High	Low–high

Prototypical models	Two-kidney, one-clip
	  adrenal regeneration
		One-kidney, one-clip
		  DOCA-salt

Most effective treatments	ACE inhibitors β-Adrenergic blockers (which block renin release)	Calcium channel blockers Diuretics α-adrenergic blockers
Calcium hormones		
Calcitonin	Normal	Low
PTH	Normal	High
1,25(OH)$_2$D	Normal	High
High-calcium diet		
Blood pressure	No effect/increased	Lowered
Plasma calcium	No effect	Normalized
Calcium hormones	No effect	Normalized
High-salt diet		
Blood pressure	No effect	Increased
Plasma calcium	No effect	Increased
Calcium hormones	No effect	Exacerbated

Note the difference in levels of calcium-regulating hormones and response to calcium supplementation.
Reproduced, with permission, from Tordoff MG. (1996). The importance of calcium in the control of salt intake. *Neurosci Biobehav Rev* 20:89–99.

Vitamin D analogues: new horizons for pharmacotherapy of disease

Although the best understood actions of vitamin D are those related to regulation of blood calcium, the presence of vitamin D receptors in many "nonclassical" tissues suggests a broader biologic role (see Table 14.9 and Ref. 7). Presumably variables such as dimerization of the vitamin D receptor with the retinoic acid receptor and the presence or absence of various cell type–specific transcription factors determine the specificity of vitamin D–dependent transcription in different tissues with vitamin D receptors.

Until now, the role of vitamin D receptors in these tissues and the consequences of their therapeutic manipulation were confounded by the effects on the classical tissues. That is, hypercalcemia or hypocalcemia would occur through classical pathways upon attempted manipulation of vitamin D receptors in nonclassical tissues.

However, vitamin D analogues have now been developed that have relatively little effect on calcium homeostasis and do not cause much hypercalcemia. With these tools in hand, and with the availability of knockout mice lacking the classical nuclear vitamin D receptor, it should be possible to explore the role of vitamin D receptors in specific tissues. A number of exciting frontiers for pharmaco-

TABLE 14.9   NONCLASSICAL TARGET TISSUES OF VITAMIN D

Classic targets	VDR	Functions	Nonclassic targets	VDR	Functions
Intestinal epithelium	✓	↑ Ca and P transport	Epidermis	✓	↓ 1,25(OH)$_2$D production, ↓ proliferation, ↑ differentiation
Osteoprogenitors	✓	↑ differentiation			
Osteoclast precursors	✓	↑ differentiation	Muscle	✓	↑ contractility, ↑ Ca uptake
Mature osteoclasts	—	↑ bone resorption	Brain	✓	↑ ↓ neurotransmitter production
Osteoblasts	✓	↑ bone formation	Liver	✓	↑ regeneration
Proximal renal tubule	✓	↓ 1,25(OH)$_2$D production	Prostate	✓	↓ proliferation
Distal renal tubule	✓	↑ calcium reabsorption	Testes	✓	↓ spermatogenesis, ↓ testosterone
			Breast	✓	↓ estrogen responses
			Lung	✓	↑ surfactant release
			Parathyroid gland	✓	↓ PTH production
			Pancreas	✓	↑ insulin secretion
			Pituitary	✓	↑ PRL secretion
			Monocytes, macrophages	✓	↑ differentiation, ↑ phagocytosis, ↓ 1,25(OH)$_2$D production
			Lymphocytes	✓	↓ proliferation, ↓ IL-2, IFN-γ secretion

Reproduced, with permission, from Bikle DD. (1995). A bright future for the sunshine hormone. *Sci Am* March/April, p. 59.

logic manipulation lie on the horizon, including use of vitamin D analogues to:

1. Inhibit proliferation and stimulate differentiation of a variety of cell types. It appears that 1,25-dihydroxyvitamin D inhibits proliferation and induces differentiation of normal skin keratinocytes, in part by reducing the level of *myc* mRNA (*myc* is an oncogene that is often associated with proliferation). Normally, local production of 1,25-dihydroxyvitamin D by keratinocytes may act as an autocrine regulatory mediator (that is, one that affects the cell that makes it, see Chap. 3) and does not contribute to systemic 1,25-dihydroxyvitamin D levels. Also, a number of cancers, including cancers of the breast, prostate, and colon, have vitamin D receptors, and, at least based on cell culture studies, 1,25-dihydroxyvitamin D$_3$ is often effective in blocking their proliferation. Whether these consequences will hold true in whole animals, including humans, remains to be explored.

2. Inhibit hormone secretion. 1,25-dihydroxyvitamin D is currently used in patients with renal failure to inhibit the secondary hyperparathyroidism that occurs as a result of renal failure (see Chap. 9). It generally is not possible to use this therapy to treat patients with primary hyperparathyroidism caused by a parathyroid gland adenoma because it would aggravate the hypercalcemia at doses that would be too low to get the desired effect of 1,25-dihydroxyvitamin D–mediated inhibition of PTH synthesis. However, 1,25-dihydroxyvitamin D analogues that selectively inhibit PTH synthesis but have no hypercalcemic effect might be effective.

3. Affect insulin secretion. It has been observed that the insulin-secreting beta cells of the endocrine pancreas also have vitamin D receptors. Perhaps therapy with nonhypercalcemic 1,25-dihydroxyvitamin

D analogues may be of value either for enhancing insulin secretion or for improving bone density in diabetic patients.

4. Regulate the immune response. Activated macrophages make 1,25-dihydroxyvitamin D, as occurs in diseases that cause formation of granulomas, such as tuberculosis and sarcoidosis.

7. HOW DOES AN UNDERSTANDING OF NORMAL PHYSIOLOGY PROVIDE INSIGHT INTO THE INITIAL CASE PRESENTATION?

Coma refers to a sleeplike state from which one cannot be awakened. It can have many different, unrelated causes. Of relevance to the topic of this chapter are the causes of coma called metabolic disturbances, which would include hypercalcemia. In evaluating a patient in coma, a physician uses clues from information provided by the patient's friends or family and from the physical examination to put the myriad possible causes of coma in order of likelihood. Thus, for example, the lack of empty pill bottles at the patient's bedside would make drug overdose, as would occur in a sucicide attempt, unlikely. Similarly, the lack of a history of trauma and lack of specific alterations in the neurologic examination localized to one side of the body or the other would make a stroke or bleeding inside the brain unlikely. The physician needs to be aware that these possibilities have not been excluded, but are unlikely. However, if additional relevant information comes to light, these possibilities should be reconsidered.

This is a common course for breast cancer, which remains one of the most challenging areas of cancer medicine.

Nausea and vomiting are early signs of hypercalcemia, which eventually progresses to altered mental status and coma. Not only Ms. Y.'s total calcium elevated, but the acidosis

and low albumin both tend to shift a greater fraction of the total from bound to ionized free calcium, magnifying the hypercalcemic effect.

The amount of undesired pain and suffering that people in the United States are subjected to because they did not make their end-of-life wishes clear is staggering. When a patient presents to the emergency room with a grave medical condition, as in this case, the clinician often feels obligated to intervene as much as his or her training allows. Sometimes this decision must be made in a vacuum, without even a full picture of the patient's past medical history. Sometimes a clinician who has not had a long-standing relationship with the patient must make medical decisions on the patient's behalf, with little guidance as to the patient's wishes. Knowing of her terminal illness, this patient has made excellent arrangements to assure that her end-of-life wishes will be followed. Far more often, patients have not made such arrangements with their clinicians and families, and the emergency treating clinician is without such crucial guidance.

There are two dilemmas here that must be recognized explicitly. One is the purely medical issues posed by having to decide where on the continuum from reasonable to heroic a particular treatment is likely to be and whether the patient would have opted for that intervention had she or he been able to express her or his wishes. A second is the insidious way in which reimbursement mechanisms can create a conflict of interest for the clinician. Thus, when the patient is in a capitated managed care plan, which reimburses health care providers per member per month regardless of services provided, the clinician often stands to gain financially by *not* providing expensive treatments. When a patient with fee-for-service insurance is being treated, the financial incentive is to provide all possible care — including care that is unlikely to be beneficial. How the conscious or unconscious motivations play out and whether an apparent conflict of interest is a real one or simply appears plausible to the patient or his or her loved ones is beyond the scope of this commentary. Suffice it to say that medical decisions are very difficult and complicated, and the ethical conflicts inherent in our health care reimbursement and delivery systems are making them increasingly so.

The clinician's thought process was as follows: The patient has a malignancy noted for production of products such as PTHrP that can cause hypercalcemia by mimicking the effect of PTH. As hypercalcemia proceeds, and the patient's mental status is progressively altered, she may become dehydrated, which exacerbates her hypercalcemia by decreasing renal excretion of calcium. Drugs that block osteoclast function (e.g., biphosphonates), together with intravenous hydration to correct her dehydration and flush more calcium out via her kidneys, typically resolve the hypercalcemia. Once awake, the patient may be able to leave the hospital quickly, although the grave prognosis of her underlying terminal illness remains the same.

A knowledge of physiology was used by the clinician in three ways in this case.

First, as an internal framework around which he organized his thinking, physiological knowledge allowed him to make the distinction between a short-term treatment plan that would facilitate achieving Ms. Y.'s wishes and the long-term consequences of the underlying disease, which in this case was beyond the clinician's ability to cure.

Second, told as a story, it allows him to convey the logic of his proposed treatment plan to Ms. Y.'s decision-making surrogate.

Finally, in an era of managed care, where financial incentives sometimes skew the decision in favor of *not* providing expensive care to patients, physiological reasoning provided rational grounds on which the clinician was able to argue the merits of the treatment plan to HMO representatives, who might otherwise be inclined to overrule clinical recommendations for financial reasons.

SUMMARY AND REVIEW OF KEY CONCEPTS

1. The body closely monitors the ionized free calcium concentration in the blood, using a calcium sensor on chief cells of the parathyroid glands. This system integrates calcium absorption or elimination by the GI tract and kidneys with deposition in bone and with the needs of the tissues.

2. The response to deviations from normal blood calcium involve hormonal, physiological, and physicochemical mechanisms.

   • Hormonal: Within minutes of a fall in ionized blood calcium, parathyroid hormone promotes bone resorption, renal calcium absorption, and phosphate loss. If the stimulus continues, PTH promotes vitamin D formation, which in turn increases calcium absorption from the GI tract.

   • Physiological: Acid–base status, sodium load and its enhancement of glomerular filtration rate, and phosphate load and its effect on 1,25 dihydroxyvitamin D synthesis all affect urinary calcium loss.

   • Physicochemical: Some 50% of blood calcium is bound to albumin. Alkalosis promotes binding of calcium to albumin, thereby lowering ionized free calcium. When the ionized calcium × phosphate product exceeds an upper limit of 60, calcium phosphate precipitates form in soft tissues.

3. Bone remodeling is a complex process that continues throughout life, in which resorption of bone by osteoclasts is offset by deposition of bone by osteoblasts. Complex

cytokine-mediated interactions between these two cell types are necessary for normal bone remodeling.

4. PTH is regulated primarily by ionized free calcium concentration. 1,25 dihydroxyvitamin D is regulated primarily by PTH. However, a host of other hormones, including estrogens, play significant supporting roles in calcium and phosphate homeostasis. The fall in blood estrogens is believed to be the major factor in accelerated loss of bone mass in women after menopause.

5. A range of common diet and lifestyle factors can promote calcium loss, including consumption of a diet low in absorbable forms of calcium and high in animal protein. Additional risk factors include alcohol consumption, smoking, and a sedentary lifestyle. Conversely, weight-bearing exercise and a high-calcium, low-phosphate diet are protective.

A CASE OF PHYSIOLOGICAL MEDICINE

D.Z. is a 50-year-old child care worker and foster mother who came to her health care provider for a checkup. Upon questioning, two points of history were noted. First, after witnessing an horrific traffic accident last year, the patient had an episode of hyperventilation associated with facial tingling and cramps in her hands and feet. The emergency room doctor ascribed these to "low blood calcium." However, Ms. Z.'s total blood calcium came back normal, and the doctor had no good explanation for this. Since by that time her symptoms had disappeared, she left the emergency room without further investigation or treatment.

Ms. Z. also noted a more recent history of occasional hot flashes and dizziness, and vaginal itching without a discharge. She had stopped menstruating 6 months ago. Based on this history, a physical examination, and a negative urine pregnancy test, the diagnosis of menopause was made.

Ms. Z. and her clinician discussed treatment options, and she was given some materials to read. A bone density study was ordered and found to show no signs of osteoporosis. Ms. Z. has been a lacto-vegetarian for the last 25 years, has never smoked or consumed alcohol in any significant quantity, and walks 2 to 4 miles daily. She considers the options of (1) continuation of her favorable diet and lifestyle habits without medical intervention or (2) adding exogenous estrogen and progesterone, and chooses option 1 with the approval of her health care provider.

QUESTIONS

1. How do you explain the normal calcium in the face of signs of hypocalcemia during Ms. Z.'s episode of hyperventilation 2 years ago?
2. Suppose the underlying physiological derangement that presented as hypocalcemic symptoms were to persist for a period of days. What would happen to the total blood calcium then, and why?
3. Should she have received any medical therapy during the hyperventilation episode?
4. Why do complaints of hot flashes, dizziness, and vaginal itching in a postmenopausal woman raise concerns regarding bone density and osteoporosis?
5. What aspects of the patient's current diet and lifestyle promote or detract from bone health?
6. Why has she opted not to take estrogen?

ANSWERS

1. The laboratory value was *total* calcium concentration; symptoms are determined by

free calcium concentration. Hyperventilation lowers blood pH and shifts calcium rapidly from ionized free to a protein-bound state.

2. Since the body monitors ionized free calcium, various physiological mechanisms involving PTH and 1,25-dihydroxyvitamin D would work to raise ionized free calcium to the normal range, thereby elevating total calcium.

3. She should have been asked to rebreathe into a paper bag to bring her P_{CO_2} up to normal, thereby normalizing her blood pH and reequilibrating her calcium between the ionized and protein-bound fractions.

4. Hot flashes, dizziness, and vaginal itching are signs of estrogen deficiency. Estrogen also promotes bone formation, so estrogen deficiency will be associated with bone loss, and therefore with an increased risk of osteoporosis and fractures.

5. Positive calcium balance is promoted by her high calcium intake, vegetarian diet (indirectly due to the effects of sodium and amino acids in meat on raising GFR and the effects of a high phosphate load on calcium absorption and excretion), lack of smoking or alcohol consumption, and excellent exercise habit, which have worked to optimize her bone density prior to onset of menopause, when she will, inevitably, lose bone density.

6. Because of the potential risks of estrogen therapy, including a definite increased risk of endometrial cancer (which is lowered substantially by also taking progesterone) and a possible but still controversial increased risk of breast cancer (effect of progesterone unknown. At higher doses than are generally used for postmenopausal hormone replacement, estrogens can cause an increased risk of pathologic blood clotting.

Because the other aspects of her diet and lifestyle are likely to be substantially protective against osteoporosis.

This remains an extremely controversial and rapidly changing area, in part because our understanding of the underlying physiology of bone and hormones that affect bone is inadequate.

References and suggested reading

1. Packard P, Heaney RP (1997). Reply to letters to the editor. *J Am Diet Assoc* 97:1370.
2. Calvo MA, Park YK (1996). Changing phosphorus content of the U.S. diet: Potential for adverse effects on bone. In Symposium on nutritional advances in human bone metabolism. *J Nutr* 126:1168S–1180S.
3. Strewler GS (1997). In Greenspan FS, Strewler GS (eds): *Basic and Clinical Endocrinology*, 5th ed. Stamford, CT, Appleton & Lange.
4. Simonet WS, et al. (1997). Osteoprotegerin: A novel secreted protein involved in the regulation of bone density. *Cell* 89:309–319.
5. Tordoff MG (1996). The importance of calcium in the control of salt intake. *Neurosci Biobehav Rev* 20:89–99.
6. Tordoff MG, Okiyama A (1996). Daily rhythm of NaCl intake in rats fed low-Ca_2^+ diet: Relation to plasma and urinary minerals and hormones. *Am J Physiol* 270:R505–R517.
7. Bikle DD (1995). A bright future for the sunshine hormone. *Sci Am* March/April, 58–67.

PHYSIOLOGY OF THE MALE REPRODUCTIVE SYSTEM

15

1. APPROACH TO MALE REPRODUCTIVE PHYSIOLOGY

Male reproduction involves four distinct physiological themes:

- Embryonic sexual differentiation and the development of **male external and internal genitalia**
- The many effects of **androgens**, the primary hormonal products of the testes, including appearance of **secondary sexual characteristics**
- Adequacy of **sexual function**, in terms of penile **erection** and **ejaculation**
- **Fertility**, defined as the ability to impregnate a female via sexual intercourse

Why is understanding male reproductive physiology important for medical practice?

- Disorders of sexual function are often perceived as significant impairments of quality of life, especially among aging male patients. **Impotence**, the inability to achieve and maintain an erection suitable for sexual intercourse, commonly occurs as a side effect of medicines such as antihypertensive drugs, with which older male patients are often being treated. Patients are sometimes too embarrassed to bring this complaint to the clinician's attention. Failure to inquire as to the adequacy of the patient's sexual functioning can result in the clinician's missing important information that affects other aspects of health care — such as the real reason the patient keeps "forgetting" to take his medicines.
- The availability of a pill (sildenafil or Viagra) and other therapies to treat impotence promises to cause a revolution in the generalist clinician's approach to these disorders — and raises difficult questions with regard to the cost of such coverage for health insurers. When does this therapy leave the realm of health care, an HMO's obligation, and enter the realm of recreation (generally not a covered service on most health plans)?
- *Androgen abuse* is a widespread problem, particularly among young athletes. The potential side effects of excessive, inappropriate androgen therapy include infertility and increased risk of heart disease and stroke.
- *Infertility* is a source of substantial distress to a subpopulation of male patients wishing to have children. The production of viable sperm is an intricate, sensitive process that takes over 2 months — and just one hot bath during that time could make it all for naught.
- Disorders of the **prostate gland**, including **prostatitis, benign prostatic hypertrophy (BPH)**, and **prostate cancer**, are extremely common. BPH and cancer both occur among men over the age of 50, with the latter increasing in incidence with age until, by age 90, almost all men will have at least a small focus of cancer within their prostate gland. However, the real mystery is why, in most men, the cancer remains latent in the gland, only found incidentally at autopsy, while in a small subset it becomes aggressive and spreads, contributing to their deaths.

Case Presentation

LR is a 38-year-old electrician who comes to you concerned about infertility and high cholesterol. He and his wife have been trying to have children for the last 4 years. Two years ago, a workup of his spouse suggested that she was fully fertile, and analysis of the patient's semen suggested normal sperm count and maturation. They were advised to "keep trying." One year ago, on the advice of his pals at the local gym, Mr. R started taking injectable androgens. He was led to believe that, in addition to augmenting his muscle mass, this therapy would make him "more of a man" and therefore, presumably, increase his chances of success at fathering a child. While the regimen did indeed result in substantial augmentation of his muscle mass and, in the opinion of his wife, has made him more aggressive, it has not resulted in a pregnancy. A recent repeat of Mr. R's sperm analysis came as quite a shock: Rather than demonstrating an increase, it appears that he now has defective sperm production and maturation. These abnormalities were not apparent at the prior analysis 2 years ago. Furthermore, his lipid profile, which had been normal then, is terrible now, with a substantial increase in his serum low-density lipoproteins (LDL) and a decrease in his high-density lipoproteins (HDL). Mr. R is quite distraught and wants an explanation and treatment for his current problem.

2. DEVELOPMENT AND ORGANIZATION OF THE REPRODUCTIVE SYSTEM

Most cells of the human body contain 23 pairs of chromosomes, one set inherited from each parent, and reproduce by duplicating all of their genetic material and then dividing. This process, called **mitosis**, allows the information within any given cell to be accurately transmitted to both of the two resulting cells. The main goal of cell division in mitosis is simply to make a faithful copy and let it be subject to the influence of hormones and other factors to guide its further development, differentiation, and function.

However, a different challenge is faced in sexual reproduction. The goal here is *not* to produce a carbon copy of the original cell or organism, but rather to combine a balanced selection of the genetic information from two individuals so that the resulting offspring will be a hybrid of the two. The advantage of this strategy, presumably, is that it introduces enough variability into the genetic information of the succeeding generation to allow a reasonable chance that at least some of the resulting offspring will have an improved chance of survival in a potentially changing environment.

The allocation of members of a species into two genetically determined sexes is but one of the ways in which this principle has been put into practice over the course of evolution. In some other species, environment rather than genes determines the sex of an individual member of a species. In yet others, there is plasticity between genetic and environmental determination of sex (see Ref. 2).

In the genetically programmed mode of sexual reproduction used by humans, specialized cells called **germ cells** are formed, in which the DNA complement is reduced by half. They contain a single set of 23 chromosomes, with each chromosome represented once rather than twice. The process of reduction division of the DNA to half the normal complement of genetic material, by which germ cells are made, is called **meiosis** (see Figure 15.1). Not only does meiosis result in random sorting of each pair of the 23 sets of homologous chromosomes, it allows a certain degree of **recombination** to occur. As a result of recombination, genetic information normally carried on one particular chromosome is relocated to another position on a different chromosome and is passed on to future generations in its new position (unless or until it is moved again by recombination). Upon joining of the germ cells of two members of the opposite sex, a full complement of DNA is reestablished and maintained in the form of somatic cells until the next generation of germ cells is formed. This approach solves the problem of propagating the species in a way that has worked quite nicely to avoid both insufficient and excessive genetic variation. Thus, each gener-

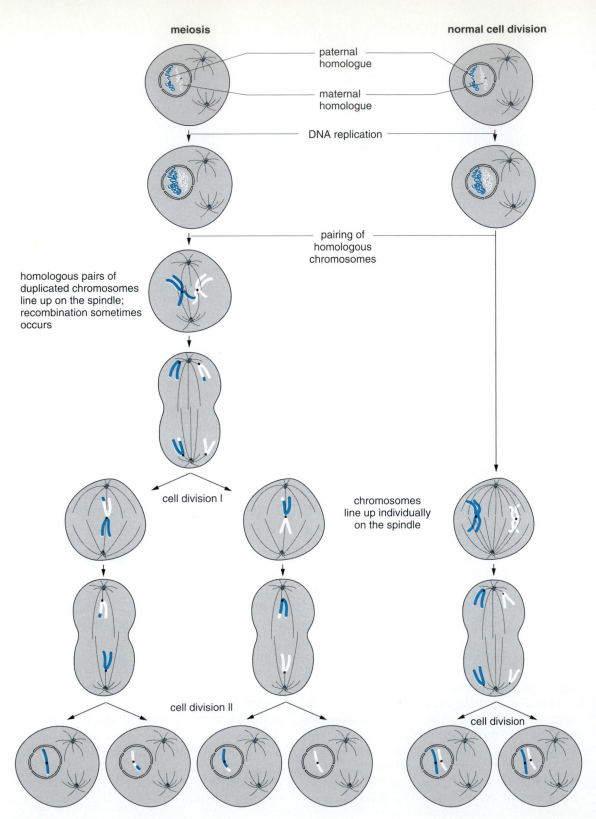

meiosis

normal cell division

paternal homologue

maternal homologue

DNA replication

pairing of homologous chromosomes

homologous pairs of duplicated chromosomes line up on the spindle; recombination sometimes occurs

cell division I

chromosomes line up individually on the spindle

cell division II

cell division

ation is neither a carbon copy clone of the previous one nor so different as to result in a high proportion of individuals with lethal changes.

Some definitions regarding sexuality

Four different topics need to be clearly distinguished. **Sexual differentiation** is the process by which specific gene products result in a gonad whose products make possible a male or female phenotype. **Sexual identity** refers to whether individuals consider themselves male or female and is distinct from the issue of what gonads they have. **Sexual preference** refers to whether an individual is sexually attracted to individuals of the same or the opposite sex and is also distinct from the simpler question of male versus female chromosomes, gonads, and phenotype. **Sexual functioning** refers to whether an individual has testes, ovaries, or gonads with both features (called *hermaphroditism*). Although this chapter will consider only sexual differentiation, the careful distinction between the meanings of these terms should be remembered.

Embryonic sexual differentiation

An individual's sex is determined by

1. The expression of particular **genes** in
2. A particular **cellular environment**, under
3. The influence of sufficient quantities of particular **hormones**.

Either gene defects or alterations in the cellular or hormonal environment within the developing embryo can alter aspects of sex determination (see Figure 15.2).

Normal human somatic cells have 46 chromosomes, including 2 sex chromosomes. One-half of these, including 1 sex chromosome, come from each parent. For females, the sex chromosomes received from both parents are X chromosomes. In the case of males, one sex chromosome is an X and the other is a Y chromosome. Thus, whether you inherit the X or the Y chromosome from your father determines your **chromosomal sex**.

Included on the Y chromosome is a gene termed *Sry* (sex-determining region of the Y chromosome), whose expression results in the development of male gonads (testes). In the absence of this gene, the individual will develop female gonads (ovaries). The presence of testes versus ovaries (normally a consequence of chromosomal sex) determines the **gonadal sex** of the individual.

The gonad is the source of hormones that normally determine the external and internal genitalia, called the **phenotypic sex** of an individual. The development of physiologically full phenotypic sex (a functioning male or female reproductive system) involves events set into motion during embryogenesis, some of which are not manifest until puberty (see Sec. 6). However, to what extent — or even whether — the *psychological* differences between males and females are genetically pro-

---

FIGURE 15.1. Comparison of meiosis to mitosis. Only one pair of homologous chromosomes is shown, although an actual human cell would have 23 such pairs. In meiosis (left), following DNA replication, two nuclear (and cell) divisions are required to produce the haploid germ cells. Each diploid cell that enters meiosis therefore produces four haploid cells, whereas each diploid cell that divides by mitosis (right) produces two diploid cells. Note that recombination has resulted in swap of a small piece of chromosome indicated by the small blue or white patches in the chromosomes of the final germ cells shown at the bottom left. *(Adapted, with permission, from Alberts B, et al. (1994). Molecular Biology of the Cell, 3d ed. New York, Garland, p. 1015.)*

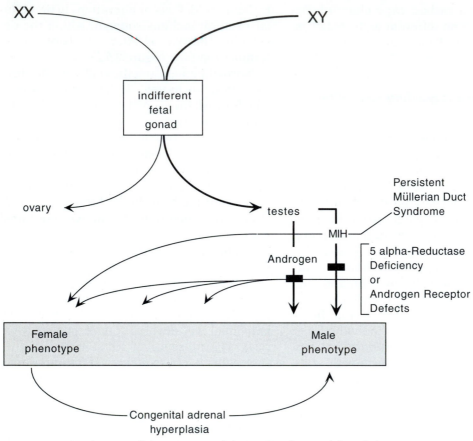

FIGURE 15.2. Mechanisms of determination of chromosomal, gonadal, and pheno-typic sex. The sex chromosome content (normally XX or XY, see top) determines whether the fetal gonad will be an ovary (in the absence of Y chromosome influence) or a testis (in the presence of Y chromosome products including the Sry gene). The testes produce androgens and müllerian inhibitory hormone (MIH), which results in the male phenotype (bottom right). Indicated are various genetic lesions that result in partial or complete failure of action of MIH or androgens, thereby giving various degrees of female phenotype even in the presence of testes. Conversely, congenital adrenal hyperplasia can result in varying degrees of virilization of a female fetus due to excessive androgens. *(Adapted, with permission, from Griffin JE, Ojeda SR (1996), Textbook of Endocrinology, 3d ed, New York, Oxford, p 162.)*

grammed as part of phenotypic sex or are the consequence of cues received during childhood and other social factors remains controversial.

Although the Sry gene is necessary for maleness, it is not sufficient. Thus a number of X chromosome genes, including those that encode the *androgen receptor*, are also necessary for an individual to develop as a phenotypic male. Lack of sufficient androgen results in defective or small (depending on the severity of the deficiency) male internal and external genitalia. Similarly, lack of estrogen results in female reproductive structures such as the uterus being poorly developed or too small.

Events in embryogenesis

By day 5 of embryogenesis, primordial germ cells have differentiated. Around day 22 to 24, they migrate from the yolk sac endoderm to the genital ridge, where they form a bipotential gonad that is not yet committed to being either male or female.

In the weeks of embryonic development that follow germ cell migration, secretions of the male gonads [**müllerian inhibitory hormone (MIH)**, **testosterone**, and **dihydrotestosterone (DHT)**] determine the development of male internal and external genitalia. In the absence of these secretions, female internal and external genitalia develop. Thus, the male represents an induced phenotype. In contrast, it is still unclear whether ovarian secretions are necessary for expression of the female phenotype.

Before the eighth week of gestation, the sex of the embryo cannot be recognized (see Figure 15.3). This period is termed the **indif-**

FIGURE 15.3. Embryonic sexual differentiation. Timing of key events in male and female sexual differentiation. First, second, and third trimester across the top and days along the bottom refer to time during pregnancy. Blue shading indicates testosterone synthesis in the male (top panel) and estrogen synthesis in the female (bottom panel). *(Adapted, with permission, from Griffin JE, Ojeda SR (1992). Textbook of Endocrine Physiology, 2d ed. New York, Oxford.)*

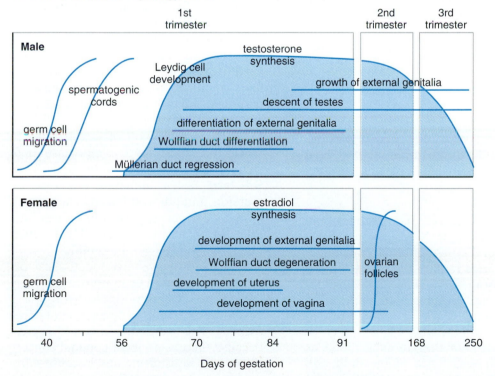

ferent phase of sexual development. The embryo acquires a dual genital duct system within the primitive kidney. The first to form is a structure called the **wolffian duct**. Subsequently, the *müllerian duct* forms, dependent on wolffian duct development. These two duct systems have different embryologic derivations.

After 8 weeks of gestation, the müllerian ducts regress in the male as a result of the production of MIH by **Sertoli cells** of the fetal testes, and the wolffian duct gives rise to various structures of the male reproductive system, including the **prostate**, **epididymis**, and **seminal vesicles**.

External genitalia of both males and females develop from common embryologic structures under different hormonal influences. Thus, *androgen exposure* results in a partial male phenotype in otherwise female embryos (a consequence that is called **virilization**), while *androgen failure* results in defective male development of otherwise male embryos (see Figure 15.2). Proper female development requires that androgens be converted to estrogens by the enzyme **aromatase**.

Clinical Pearls

A number of disorders of sexual differentiation can be understood within the paradigm of chromosomal, gonadal, and phenotypic sex described above:

○ Individuals with the XO chromosome karyotype (a single X sex chromosome) have neither ovaries nor testes. Fully functioning ovaries require the effects of two X chromosomes, not one, and development of testes requires both an X and a Y chromosome. Lacking MIH or testosterone, individuals with a single X chromosome have female external genitalia as a result of persistence of the müllerian duct and regression of the wolffian duct structures. This is also known as **Turner's syndrome**.

○ Individuals with **Klinefelter's syndrome** (XXY individuals) develop testes and normal male external genitalia as a result of the presence of the Y chromosome and normal gonadal androgens. However, seminiferous tubule development is abnormal for reasons that are not clear.

○ **Testicular feminization syndrome** occurs in XY individuals with a deficiency in the androgen receptor (located on the X chromosome), making them unable to respond to androgens. These individuals have testes and have regression of müllerian duct structures, but they lack the effects of testosterone and DHT, and therefore have no wolffian structure development and no masculinization of their external genitalia. Hence their external genitalia are female.

○ Defects in testosterone biosynthesis can occur in XY individuals. Because of the presence of the Y chromosome, they have testes and müllerian structure regression. Depending on the extent of the defect in testosterone biosynthesis, they will have partial or completely undeveloped wolffian structures (prostate, epididymis, vas deferens) and partial or completely female external genitalia.

○ Defects in conversion of testosterone to DHT (e.g., due to 5 α-reductase deficiency) can occur in XY individuals. They will have testes, müllerian structure regression, and full wolffian structure development. However, depending on the degree to which they lack DHT, their external genitalia will be female.

○ Adrenal androgen overproduction can occur in XX individuals in utero. The presence of two X chromosomes without a Y chromosome results in development of the ovaries. The wolffian structures regress because there is no local gonadal concentration of testosterone and because adrenal androgen overproduction occurs relatively later in development. However, depending on the severity of androgen excess, the individual will have varying degrees of virilization of the external genitalia.

A conceptual framework for organization of the reproductive system

Both male and female systems for generating mature germ cells work in ways that are, to some useful extent, roughly analogous. However, each uses distinctive variations on these common themes. Thus, both the male and the female contain primordial germ cells that were generated during embryogenesis (see the preceding discussion). But in the female the total number of germ cells (oocytes) to be produced in the individual's lifetime are already present at the time of that individual's birth (about one-half million per ovary). These oocytes are arrested in the middle of meiosis and remain dormant until adulthood, when they are called upon to complete their maturation (see Chap. 16). In contrast, in the male, the primordial cells are maintained throughout adult life and continue to divide, giving rise to cells that proceed down the pathway of **spermatogenesis** (sperm maturation) while maintaining the progenitor cells. In the course of a single individual's life, more than a trillion sperm may be produced. In any event, after puberty, mechanisms exist to recruit immature germ cells into the process of steroid-dependent maturation.

Another common feature of male and female reproductive systems is that in both, the germ cells mature under the influence of two different types of supporting cells, one that makes androgens (Leydig cells in the male, thecal cells in the female) and one that nurtures germ cells by direct and intimate contact (Sertoli cells in the male, granulosa cells in the female, see Table 15.1).

In both males and females, the androgens diffuse across the basement membrane that

TABLE 15.1   COMPARISON OF MALE VERSUS FEMALE REPRODUCTIVE PHYSIOLOGY

	Reproductive organ function		
Sex	Germ cell	Nurse cell	Steroid-producing cell
Male	Sperm	Sertoli cell	Leydig cell
Female	Egg	Granulosa cell	Thecal cell

separates them from the cells that directly "nurse" the primordial germ cells. In the female, the enzyme aromatase converts androgens, which would otherwise be toxic to oocytes, into estrogens, which support oocyte maturation. In the male, the androgens themselves appear to support sperm maturation, working in concert with a large number of other products made by Sertoli cells, including estrogens.

Review Questions

1. Summarize the events of male versus female embryonic sexual development.
2. What is the role of Sertoli cells versus Leydig cells?
3. What is aromatase?
4. In what way are germ cells and somatic cells different?

3. THE MALE REPRODUCTIVE NEUROENDOCRINE AXIS

The male reproductive neuroendocrine axis is a variation on the general theme of hypothalamic–pituitary neuroendocrine axes, as discussed in detail in Chapter 6 (see Figure 15.4).

Components of the male reproductive neuroendocrine axis

Selected neurons in the arcuate nucleus of the hypothalamus secrete the peptide **gonad-**

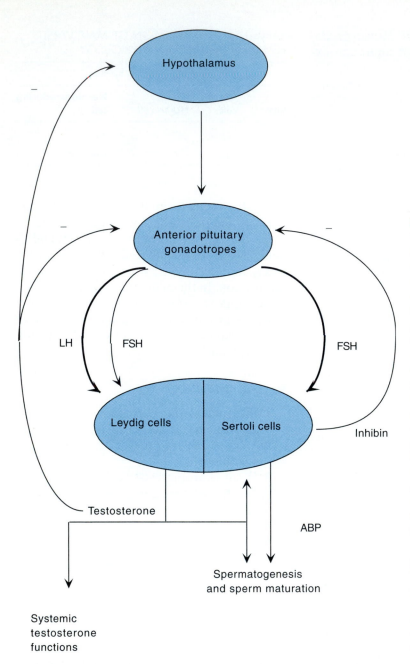

FIGURE 15.4. Male reproductive neuroendocrine axis. Schematic of key features of the male reproductive neuroendocrine axis. Pulsatile GnRH release from the hypothalamus results in pulsatile LH and FSH release from gonadotropes of the anterior pituitary. FSH stimulates Sertoli cells in the testes, while Leydig cells respond primarily to LH, with some effects of FSH. Testosterone produced by the Leydig cells drives both the systemic effects of androgens in the male and spermatogenesis, with androgen-binding protein (ABP) playing a crucial role in the latter process. Inhibin, made by Sertoli cells feedback, inhibits FSH secretion by gonadotropes, while testosterone from the Leydig cells feedback inhibits LH secretion at the level of both the hypothalamus and the anterior pituitary. The complex relationship of activin and inhibin is addressed in Figure 15.6. *(Adapted, with permission, from Speroff L, et al. (1994). Clinical Gynecologic Endocrinology and Infertility, 5th ed. Baltimore, MD, Williams & Wilkins, p 874.)*

otropin-releasing hormone (GnRH) into the pituitary portal bloodstream. The GnRH travels to the anterior pituitary, where specialized cells termed **gonadotropes** that have receptors for GnRH on their surface initiate signaling in response to GnRH binding. In response to GnRH-triggered signaling, gonadotropes synthesize and secrete the hormones **luteinizing hormone (LH)** and **follicle-stimulating hormone (FSH)**. These two pituitary hormones enter the systemic circulation and bind to LH and FSH receptors in the testes, triggering production and secretion of androgens, including **testosterone**, from Leydig cells and maturation of sperm by Sertoli cells.

In many ways testosterone can be consid-

ered a precursor, since it is converted into both DHT, through the action of the enzyme 5 α-reductase, and to estrogen, through the action of the aromatase complex (see Figure 15.5). However, testosterone is not an inac-

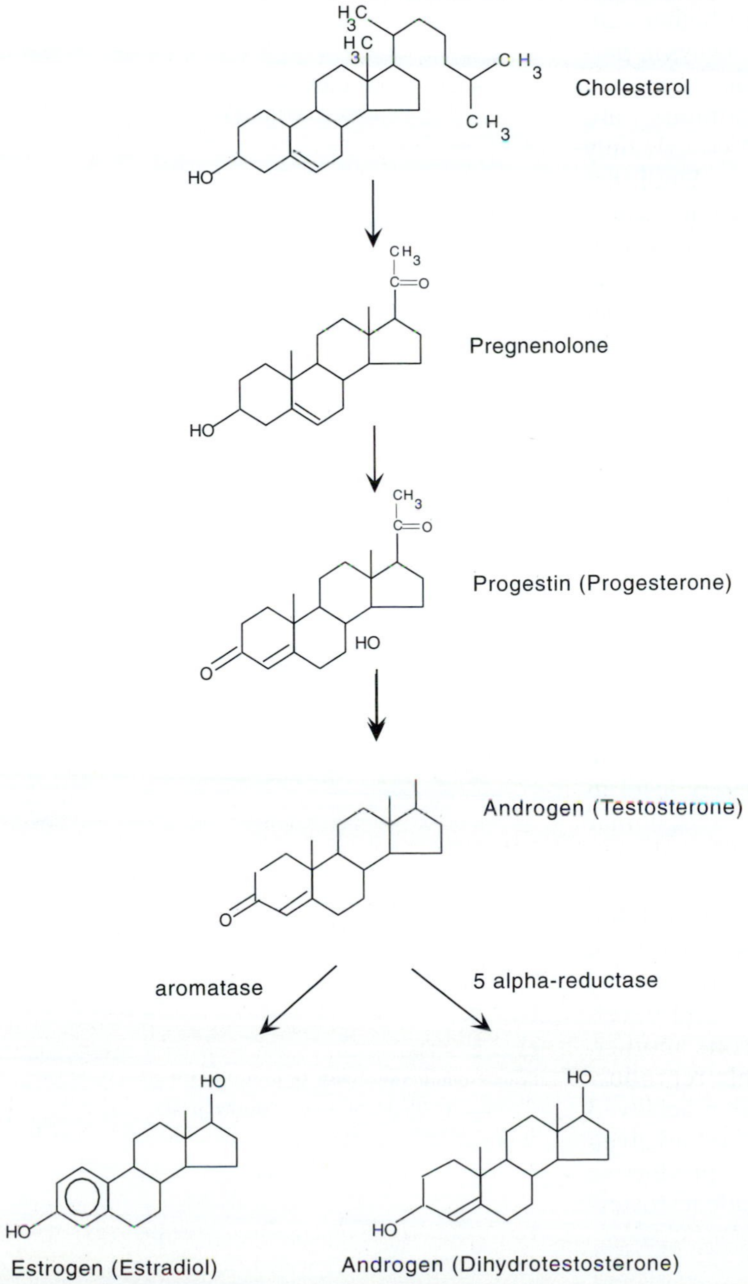

FIGURE 15.5. Structural relationship of testosterone to dihydrotestosterone and estrogen. Cholesterol is the common precursor from which all steroids are derived. It contains 27 carbons. Side-chain cleavage results in 21 carbon intermediates that give rise to progestins such as progesterone (see Chap. 17), which are converted to 19-carbon androgens such as testosterone, which can be "aromatized" to estrogens such as estradiol. Aromatization refers to the introduction of a third double bond in the first ring of the steroid nucleus, which makes a highly stable structure with unique chemical properties (depicted as a circle within the ring). Testosterone can also be subject to the action of the enzyme 5α-reductase to give dihydrotestosterone, an androgenic compound with higher affinity for the androgen receptor, which confers distinctive transcriptional activation properties (see text). (Adapted, with permission, from Genuth SM (1998), in Berne RM, Levy MN (eds): Physiology, 4th ed. St. Louis, MO, Mosby, p 971.)

tive precursor, as it causes most (but not all) of the effects of DHT (see Sec. 5).

Target tissues for androgens include external and internal genitalia (see Table 15.2), the larynx, hair, the musculoskeletal system, skin, and the brain (see Sec. 5).

GnRH secretion is affected both by negative feedback and by input from higher centers, with catecholaminergic pathways in particular playing a stimulatory role.

The hypothalamus and pituitary are needed for control of the fetal gonads only after the third month of gestation. Until that point, the production of androgen and estrogen from the early gonads required for embryonic sexual differentiation is driven solely by **human chorionic gonadotropin (HCG)**, an LH-like hormone made by the placenta (see Chap. 17). The placenta also converts cholesterol into pregnenolone for subsequent use by the fetal gonad as a precursor to androgen and estrogen. In the absence of the fetal pituitary gland, the fetal testes are unable to produce the amount of androgen needed for full development of the external male genitalia.

Feedback control of the male reproductive neuroendocrine axis

The male reproductive system is regulated in two ways. First, there is systemic control through negative feedback at every level in the reproductive neuroendocrine axis, similar to the regulation of thyroid, adrenal, and other endocrine gland functions (as discussed in Chaps. 11 to 13). Second, there is an elaborate and still largely mysterious program of local paracrine and autocrine interactions by which Leydig cells, Sertoli cells, and developing sperm communicate with one another.

Once full maturity of the male reproductive neuroendocrine axis has been achieved at puberty, a number of products are involved in feedback control of the male reproductive neuroendocrine axis. These include testosterone, inhibin, and estrogen.

TABLE 15.2   CLINICAL ACTIONS OF ANDROGENS

In utero
  External genital development
  Wolffian duct development

Prepubertal
  Possible male behavioral effects

Pubertal
  External genitalia
    Penis and scrotum increase in size and become pigmented
    Rugal folds appear in scrotal skin
  Hair growth
    Mustache and beard develop; scalp line undergoes recession
    Pubic hair develops
    Axillary, body, extremity, and perianal hair appears
  Linear growth
    Pubertal growth spurt
    Androgens interact with growth hormone to increase somatomedin C levels
  Accessory sex organs
    Prostate and seminal vesicles enlarge and secretion begins
  Voice
    Pitch is lowered because of enlargement of larynx and thickening of vocal cords
  Psyche
    More aggressive attitudes are manifest
    Sexual potential develops
  Muscle mass
    Muscle bulk increases
    Nitrogen balance is positive

Adult
  Hair growth
    Androgenic patterns are maintained
    Male pattern balding may be initiated
  Spermatogenesis
    Interaction with FSH modulates Sertoli cell function/stimulates spermatogenesis
  Hematopoiesis
    Erythropoietin stimulated
    Direct marrow effect exerted on erythropoiesis
  Psyche
    Behavioral attitudes and sexual potency are maintained
  Bone
    Bone loss and osteoporosis are prevented

From Genuth SM (1998), in Berne RM, Levy MN (eds): in *Physiology*, 4th ed. St. Louis, Mosby, p 985.

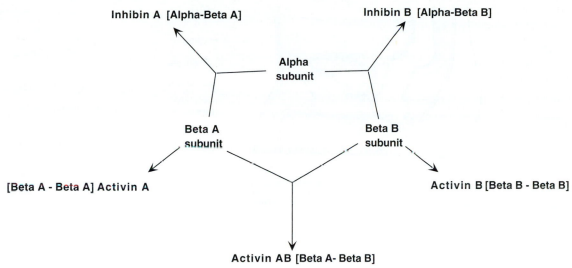

FIGURE 15.6. Activins and inhibins: local and systemic mediators of gonadal function. Inhibins A and B are synthesized from a common α subunit and two distinct β subunits. Activins are synthesized by combining the β subunits into homo- or heterodimers. *(Adapted, with permission, from Genuth SM (1998), in Berne RM, Levy MN (eds): Physiology, 4th ed. St. Louis, MO, Mosby, p 972.)*

Testosterone has its major feedback effect on the hypothalamus to inhibit GnRH pulsatile secretion (both rate and amplitude). It also has a smaller effect directly on the anterior pituitary.

Inhibins and **activins** are a family of proteins made by Sertoli cells (and granulosa cells in the female; see Chap. 16) in response to stimulation by FSH. These proteins are involved in complex systemic as well as local regulation of gonadal function and the neuroendocrine axis. The details of inhibin and activin action remain to be further explored (see Sec. 9, Frontiers). Three different protein subunits appear capable of coming together in five different ways to form functionally distinct protein complexes (see Figure 15.6).

Systemically, inhibin B has negative-feedback effects on FSH secretion, while inhibin A is believed to inhibit both LH and FSH.

Locally, inhibin increases while activin decreases Leydig cell testosterone secretion.

Although the testes do not secrete appreciable amounts of estrogen directly, testosterone itself can be converted to the estrogen **estradiol** by the action of the aromatase enzyme complex, which in the male is found in high levels in fat and hair follicles. Estrogen produced in the male by aromatase action is believed to play a role in feedback inhibition of LH and FSH secretion at the level of the anterior pituitary (see Figure 15.4).

4. THE MALE REPRODUCTIVE ORGANS

The male reproductive organs include the testes, the penis, the prostate gland, the epididymis, the vas deferens, seminal vesicles, and other accessory glands (see Figure 15.7). Sperm, made in the testes, are transported

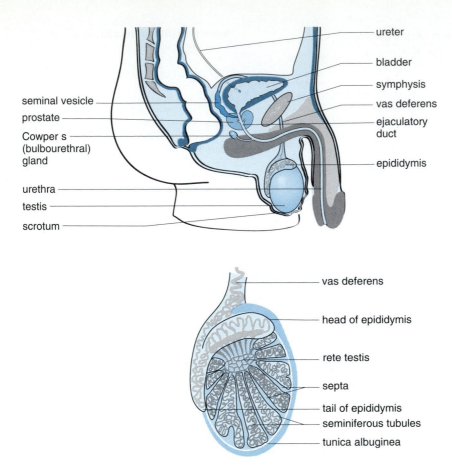

seminal vesicle
prostate
Cowper s
(bulbourethral)
gland

urethra
testis
scrotum

ureter
bladder
symphysis
vas deferens
ejaculatory
duct
epididymis

vas deferens

head of epididymis

rete testis

septa

tail of epididymis
seminiferous tubules
tunica albuginea

FIGURE 15.7. Male external and internal genitalia. Above, male reproductive system. Below, duct system of the testes.

and stored in the epididymis. During ejaculation, sperm move through the vas deferens, enter the urethra, and exit via the penis, mixing with fluids from various glands, including the prostate and the seminal vesicles, along the way.

Structure of the testes

The testes normally reside in the scrotum, outside the body. Their external location and the intertwining of the testicular arteries and veins makes possible efficient heat exchange, which allows testicular temperature to be 1 to 2 degrees below body temperature. This temperature difference is a necessary condition for optimal sperm production and viability.

As mentioned in Sec. 3, the testes contain three principal cell types: Leydig cells (which respond to LH by synthesizing testosterone), Sertoli cells, and sperm precursors in various stages of maturation. Testosterone influences both Sertoli cells and the developing sperm cells. Sertoli cells respond to FSH by induction of aromatase. Leydig cells also have FSH receptors, and one effect of FSH is to increase the amount of LH receptors on the Leydig

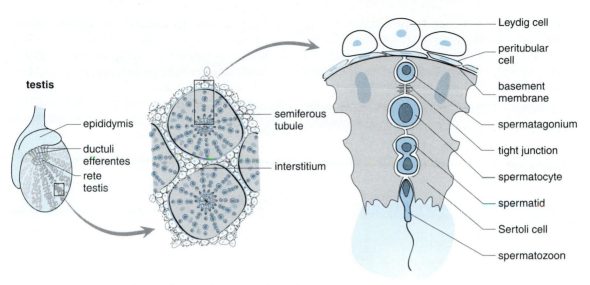

FIGURE 15.8. Structure of seminiferous tubules and their role in sperm maturation. Schematic representation of the architecture of the testes. Note that the Leydig cells are separated from the Sertoli cells by a basement membrane. Within the tubules, the germ cells are completely surrounded by Sertoli cell cytoplasm early in their development. Tight junctions between adjacent Sertoli cells separate ancestral spermatogonia from their descendents, including spermatocytes, spermatids, and spermatozoa, which represent different stages in sperm maturation. *(Adapted, with permission, from Skinner MK (1991). Cell-cell interactions in the testis. Endocr Rev 12:45–77. Copyright © 1993 by The Endocrine Society.)*

cell. A large number of growth factors and other products have been detected in the testes and are believed to be synthesized there. The functions of many of them may be as local paracrine mediators, but their precise role remains a mystery.

The Sertoli cells themselves are organized into so-called seminiferous tubules, which serve as specialized structures for maturation of sperm (Figure 15.8). The communication between Sertoli cells and developing sperm is complex and poorly understood. Sperm develop within endocytic vacuoles within Sertoli cells in an FSH-dependent fashion. Changes in morphology and gene expression of both the Sertoli cell and the developing spermatozoa occur during spermatogenesis.

Function of the testes

The testes perform three interrelated but distinctive functions.

1. The testes are a steroid factory, the source of most androgens in the male. Thus, the testes are necessary for the range of androgen-dependent functions, including male embryogenesis, development of secondary sexual characteristics, and various features of other physiological processes to be discussed in Sec. 5.
2. The testes are the site of germ cell production and maturation, necessary for propagation of the species.
3. The testes are the end organ of the male

reproductive neuroendocrine axis. Some of the same products that are responsible for the functions listed previously are also responsible for feedback inhibition of the hypothalamus and pituitary gland during the course of normal reproductive life. Late in life, or pathologically earlier, testicular function diminishes, and there is a corresponding elevation in blood levels of LH and FSH.

Physiology of penile erection and ejaculation

Effective male reproductive function requires not only the production of viable sperm in sufficient quantities to achieve fertilization, but also a means of delivering the sperm into the female genital tract. This occurs by the process of penile erection and ejaculation.

Erection occurs in five phases:

1. During the *flaccid phase*, sympathetic neural tone constricts smooth muscle of both the vasculature and the corpora cavernosa. As a result, blood flow to the penis is low, and the venous sinuses of the corpora cavernosa and spongiosa are empty.
2. The *filling phase* is initiated by parasympathetic stimulation, with decreased arteriolar constriction but no increase in corpus cavernosal pressure. This results in more blood flow to the penis, causing its elongation.
3. In the *tumescent phase*, the release of nitric oxide and production of prostaglandins relaxes the smooth muscle of the corpora cavernosa, allowing engorgement of the venous sinuses.
4. In the *full erection phase*, the cavernosa is engorged with blood and the cavernosal pressure is just under the systolic blood pressure.
5. In the *rigid phase*, the engorged cavernosa obstructs venous outflow, allowing caverno-

sal pressure to exceed the systolic blood pressure. This sets the stage for ejaculation, which is caused by sympathetic-mediated contraction of the ischiocavernous and bulbocavernous muscles via spinal reflexes.

In erection, there is eight times more blood content in the penis than there is in the flaccid state, and this can be mediated either by afferent sensory input from the penis via the *pudendal nerve* or via central signals from the brain.

Ejaculated fluid, called *semen*, normally contains 200 to 400 million sperm in a volume of approximately 5 mL; the fluid includes alkaline and fructose-rich prostatic and vas deferens secretions. Mature sperm can be stored in the epididymis for a period of several months. Sperm require interaction with the female genital tract, a process termed **capacitation** (see Chap. 17), before they are able to penetrate and fertilize an egg.

Clinical Pearl

○ Impotence can have many different causes, including psychological, neurological, hormonal, and vascular factors. A variety of therapeutic strategies have been developed to treat impotence:

- Instillation into the tip of the penis, or injection into the shaft, of prostaglandin or α-adrenergic antagonists to promote vasodilation and increased penile blood flow.
- External application of a vacuum suction device placed around the penis to enhance blood flow into the corpus cavernosa.
- Surgical implantation of an externally inflatable device into the penis.
- Taking a pill [sildenafil (Viagra)] that is an inhibitor of type 5 phosphodiesterase, an enzyme present on platelets, skeletal

muscle, and vascular and visceral smooth muscle, including that in the corpus cavernosum. Inhibition of this enzyme results in prolonged activity of nitric oxide and smooth muscle relaxation in various places, including the penis. This drug was developed originally for its potential value in enhancing blood flow to the heart, but the prominence of its effects on the penis were noticed and led to a completely different use. Given the nature of its mechanism of action, Viagra is contraindicated in patients being treated with nitrates because of the risk of **hypotension** (low blood pressure, see Chap. 7).

Physiology of the prostate and other accessory glands, vas deferens, and epididymis

Once sperm have fully matured, they are delivered to the epididymis, where they can be stored for a period of months unless or until they are either ejaculated or resorbed. During ejaculation, sperm move from the epididymis to the vas deferens, where they mix with fluid from various accessory structures, including the seminal vesicles and the prostate gland. The seminal vesicles provide a fructose-rich liquid that makes up approximately 60% of the volume of semen.

The prostate gland is a muscular, multilobed gland situated in the pelvis below the bladder, between the rectum and the base of the penis, surrounding the urethra (see Figure 15.7). The prostate provides an alkaline fluid that makes up about 20% of the volume of semen. From there, semen flows into the urethra for completion of ejaculation.

Starting from a size of a few grams at birth, the prostate enlarges at puberty to reach the adult size of approximately 20 g, under the influence of DHT. Prostate size then remains roughly constant until about age 50, when blood estrogen levels increase in males. The estrogen is believed to induce increased numbers of androgen receptors, thereby triggering renewed prostate growth, a condition known as benign prostatic hypertrophy (BPH). Whereas the pubertal prostatic growth was homogeneous, this later prostatic growth involves a histologically nodular proliferation of all cell types in the prostate: epithelial, stromal, and smooth muscle, which compresses the normal gland. In most older men, at least early on, the obstructive symptoms from glandular hypertrophy are offset by detrussor muscle hypertrophy, which assists in emptying the bladder. Later, the smooth muscle hypertrophy and spasm can actually worsen BPH symptoms.

Clinical Pearls

The clinical importance of the prostate is due largely to three entities:

○ Prostatitis: Both the urethra and the prostate can become infected with a variety of organisms, including the intracellular bacteria *Chlamydia* and the bacterium *Neisseria gonorrhoeae* (the cause of gonorrhea, also called gonoccocus). Spread through sexual intercourse with infected partners, these diseases typically give symptoms of burning on urination and purulent (pus-containing) discharge from the penis. When infection involves primarily the prostate, massage of this gland via a finger in the rectum can result in release of secretions from which the offending organism may be cultured.

○ BPH: A common treatment for BPH is with finasteride, a drug that inhibits 5 α-reductase and thereby removes the DHT needed to maintain the hypertrophied state. The prostate shrinks in about half of patients and probably just stops growing in the rest.

Another treatment for BPH takes advantage of the fact that in many patients the cause of obstructive symptoms is not the enlarged prostate per se, but rather the compensatory smooth muscle hypertrophy and constriction. Thus, α-adrenergic blockers (such as the drug terazosin) have been observed to increase urinary flow by relaxing this smooth muscle. Unlike finasteride, this treatment does not prevent the disorder from progressing as a result of continued prostatic hypertrophy.

○ Prostate cancer: This is the third most common cancer in males in the United States, behind lung and colon cancer; there are over 300,000 new cases and 40,000 deaths yearly. Whether BPH predisposes to prostate cancer is not known. Some cancers stay in the prostate, while others are more aggressive and metastasize, often to bone. What determines the characteristics of the cancer, and whether it can change with time in this regard, is not known. Pharmacologic (e.g., GnRH analogs) or surgical manipulation (e.g., orchiectomy) of androgens of early prostate cancer remains an important mainstay of therapy. Unfortunately, most prostate cancers eventually progress to a hormone-independent stage, presaging the demise of the patient.

Review Questions

5. What are the feedback controls in the male reproductive neuroendocrine axis?
6. Name two distinct actions of FSH on the testes.
7. For what testicular functions is a temperature 1 to 2 degrees below that of the rest of the body necessary?
8. What structural features facilitate achieving and maintaining testicular temperature below that of the rest of the body?

9. What are three distinct but interrelated functions of the testes?

5. ANDROGEN PHYSIOLOGY

Androgens are steroids whose best understood actions involve binding to the androgen receptor, with the hormone-receptor complex in turn binding to various regions of DNA to activate or repress transcription. Like other steroid hormones that fit this paradigm of gene expression (including the estrogens, progesterone, glucocorticoids, mineralocorticoids, vitamin D, and thyroid hormone), androgen actions are myriad.

In general terms, the effects of androgens can be thought of as either **anabolic actions** (because they promote growth of muscle, bone, etc.) or **androgenic actions** (because they promote maturation of structures involved in male secondary sexual characteristics). However, the molecular basis for this distinction remains obscure, and there is no such thing as a purely anabolic androgen (see Figure 15.9).

Although there is a single androgen receptor to which both testosterone and DHT bind, the binding of DHT is tighter than that of testosterone and causes a different spectrum of gene expression. One possible explanation for this is that the DHT–androgen receptor complex and the testosterone–androgen receptor complex associate with different accessory proteins and cofactors. Table 15.2 summarizes some of the documented and suggested actions of testosterone and DHT. It appears that DHT is required for certain androgen effects (beard growth and prostatic hypertrophy) but not others (stimulation of muscle, germ cell epithelium of the testes, and sexual potency), which are mediated by testosterone directly.

Like the other steroids, the androgens are products of cholesterol metabolism via P450 enzyme-mediated conversion, first in the mi-

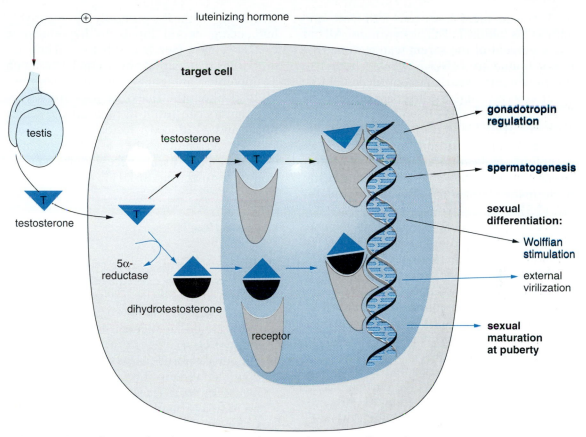

FIGURE 15.9. Mechanism of androgen action. Schematic description of steroid hormone action as it manifests in male reproductive system functions. Testosterone enters the target cells cytoplasm, where it may be converted to dihydrotestosterone by the action of 5α-reductase if that enzyme is present in the target cell. Upon entering the nucleus, DHT or testosterone binds the androgen receptor and, in conjunction with other proteins, binds to specific regions of DNA, resulting in specific patterns of transcriptional activation. These patterns of transcription differ from one target cell type to another and result in the actions indicated on the right. (*Adapted, with permission, from Wilson JD et al. (1993). Steroid 5 α-reductase deficiency. Endocrine Rev 14:577. Copyright © 1993 by The Endocrine Society.*)

tochondria and then in the endoplasmic reticulum, with diffusion of the final products (and some intermediates) out of the producing cells.

Some 7000 μg of testosterone is secreted daily in the adult male. About 300 μg of DHT is produced daily, 80% by conversion from testosterone. About 30 μg of estradiol is generated from testosterone daily in adult males, largely by peripheral aromatase activity.

The liver has an important role in testosterone metabolism. It makes **testosterone binding-globulin (TeBG)**, a polypeptide similar to androgen-binding globulin synthesized by Sertoli cells (see Sec. 7 below). About half of serum testosterone is tightly bound to TeBG in men. Estrogens stimulate and androgens inhibit TeBG biosynthesis. All but a few percent of the serum testosterone that is not bound to TeBG is weakly bound to serum albumin. Nearly 50% of the small free fraction is cleared in the first pass through the liver. Since the weakly bound testosterone is probably available to tissues and the half-life is short, total testosterone levels provide an acceptable indication of functional disturbance, except in those conditions that result in dramatic change in TeBG levels (see Table 15.3).

GnRH, LH and FSH, and testosterone are all secreted in a pulsatile fashion. However, despite pulsatile release, blood levels of LH, FSH, and testosterone are relatively steady in the male, without the huge range of variation observed during the course of the menstrual cycle in the female (see Chap. 16). However, there is a diurnal rhythm in the testosterone level, perhaps reflecting altered sensitivity of the testes to LH. Thus maximal levels of testosterone are achieved in the early morning, with minimum levels reached in the early evening; these levels differ from each other by about 30 percent.

The pituitary hormone prolactin has important effects on androgen production by the Leydig cell. A basal level of prolactin is required for testosterone biosynthesis. The physiological role of prolactin may also include an influence on tissue sensitivity to androgens. However, larger doses of prolactin exert a profound inhibitory effect on testosterone biosynthesis, primarily by negatively influencing neural inputs to hypothalamic GnRH release (see Sec. 8 below). Thus, either drugs that increase prolactin levels (such as dopamine antagonists like metoclopramide and phenothiazines) or prolactin-secreting tumors can result in reduced LH secretion and reduced testosterone levels. Prolactin also reduces the 5α-reductase activity in peripheral tissues necessary for conversion of testosterone to DHT.

Clinical Pearls

○ A negative consequence of the change in gene expression caused by androgens is to shift lipid profiles to a pattern associated with increased risk for cardiovascular disease, including increased LDL and decreased HDL.

○ Similarly, androgens favor visceral and abdominal fat deposition, which is also a risk factor for cardiovascular disease, perhaps because it promotes insulin resistance (see Chap. 6).

○ Epitestosterone is a testosterone metabolite, normally secreted from the testes, that has no known biologic activity and is not generated by peripheral metabolism of testosterone. Thus the ratio of testosterone to epitestosterone in the urine can be used to identify individuals who abuse androgens. The normal ratio is $1:1$. When exogenous testosterone is injected, it shifts that ratio. Greater than $6:1$ testosterone to epitestosterone in blood is considered indicative of androgen abuse.

TABLE 15.3   CONDITIONS THAT INCREASE OR DECREASE HEPATIC TeBG SYNTHESIS

Increased in
  Hyperthyroidism
  Estrogen therapy
  Androgen deficiency

Decreased in
  Hypothyroidism
  Obesity
  Acromegaly

Review Questions

10. What is the mechanism of action of androgens?
11. How many androgen receptors are there?

12. In which tissues are androgen-binding proteins made?

13. What is the difference in the spectrum of actions of testosterone and DHT?

6. AGE-DEPENDENT CHANGES IN TESTICULAR FUNCTION

Prepubertal

During fetal life, testosterone plays an important role in both wolffian duct development and (indirectly via DHT) differentiation of the external genitalia. The stimulating hormone during this period is probably placental HCG. As the fetus approaches term, pituitary LH contributes to stimulation of testosterone secretion.

A small peak of testosterone secretion is observed shortly after birth. The reason for this is not known; however, it may be important in priming subsequent development at puberty.

After this short time, the hypothalamic–pituitary–testicular axis becomes quiescent until puberty. Thus, despite the fact that testosterone levels are low, LH and FSH levels are also low. Presumably, a lack of maturation of the hypothalamic GnRH-secreting neurons accounts for this quiescence.

Pubertal

Puberty begins in males at approximately age 11 to 13. First, genetically programmed maturation of GnRH-secreting neurons results in increased pulsatility, triggering increased LH and FSH secretion and testicular enlargement.

Testicular enlargement, in turn, allows more testosterone to be made and blood testosterone levels to increase 20fold over about 2 years. This probably also involves both alterations in the set point at which testosterone negative feedback of LH secretions and a change in the balance of inhibitory and stim-

TABLE 15.4 MALE SECONDARY SEX CHARACTERISTICS

External genitalia: Penis increases in length and width. Scrotum becomes pigmented and rugose.

Internal genitalia: Seminal vesicles enlarge and secrete and begin to form fructose. Prostate and bulbourethral glands enlarge and secrete.

Voice: Larynx enlarges, vocal cords increase in length and thickness, and voice becomes deeper.

Hair growth: Beard appears. Hairline on scalp recedes anterolaterally. Pubic hair grows with male (triangle with apex up) pattern. Hair appears in axillas, on chest, and around anus; general body hair increases.

Mental: More aggressive, active attitude. Interest in opposite sex develops.

Body conformation: Shoulders broaden, muscles enlarge.

Skin: Sebaceous gland secretion thickens and increases (predisposing to acne).

Reproduced, with permission, from Ganong WF (1997). *Review of Medical Physiology*, 18th ed. Stamford, CT, Appleton & Lange, p 403.

ulatory neuronal pathways from the central nervous system to the hypothalamus.

Over the next 2 years or so, as blood levels of testosterone rise dramatically, secondary sexual characteristics develop (see Table 15.4). It appears that once maturation of the reproductive neuroendocrine axis has been achieved at puberty, some spermatogenesis can occur with either LH or FSH alone, although normal levels require both pituitary hormones.

Postpubertal

The hypothalamic–pituitary–testicular axis remains stable into the fourth decade, after which Leydig steroidogenesis may decline. However, effective spermatogenesis can be observed in some healthy elderly men into their eighties. As Leydig steroidogenesis and hence blood testosterone levels fall, LH and FSH levels rise, unlike the situation prior to onset of puberty (see Figure 15.10).

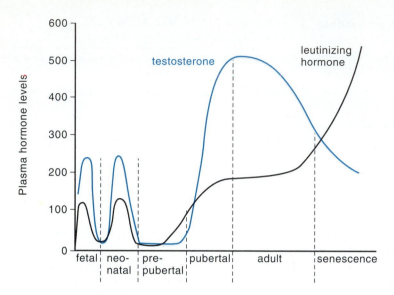

FIGURE 15.10. LH, FSH, and testosterone levels in males as a function of age. (Adapted, with permission, from Ganong, WF (1997). Review of Medical Physiology, 18th ed. Stamford, CT, Appleton & Lange, p. 403.)

7. SPERMATOGENESIS

The strategy selected through evolution involves production of enormous numbers of competent sperm to assure a single, occasional, successful fertilization. Thus, primordial germ cells, called **spermatogonia**, lie in the **basal compartment** abutting the Sertoli cells (see Figure 15.8). There they undergo many rounds of mitosis. Some spermatogonia remain as such, to provide a renewable source of germ cells. Others are induced, by mechanisms that are presently unclear, to start the long march to maturity (see Figure 15.11). The adult male's testes produce over 10^8 sperm daily. Morphologically this involves progression through a series of stages of spermatogenesis, culminating in development of a long cilium responsible for the ability of sperm to move (locomotion). Spermatogonia move from the basal to the lumenal side of the Sertoli cells via an endocytic vacuolar compartment. Cohorts of sperm appear to mature in waves, perhaps in communication with one another and with the Sertoli cells that nurture them. However, because there

is no synchrony between different waves of maturing sperm along the seminiferous tubule, actual sperm production and maturation manifests as to be a fairly continuous process, unlike the cyclical process observed in females (see Chap. 16).

Spermatogonia go through the process of reduction division (meiosis), which is completed before the appearance of the cilium.

After reaching maturity, a process taking approximately 90 days, sperm are ready for release by ejaculation together with prostatic and accessory gland secretions which together compose semen and provide the fructose and other requirements for sperm motility and sustenance.

Spermatogenesis requires extremely high concentrations of androgens in the testes. This is achieved by expression of an androgen-binding protein (ABP) by Sertoli cells. Testosterone and FSH are both required for ABP induction and for other steps in spermatogenesis. ABP is secreted into the fluid of the seminiferous tubule lumen, perhaps to create a reservoir of testosterone within the seminiferous tubule. In this way, the high con-

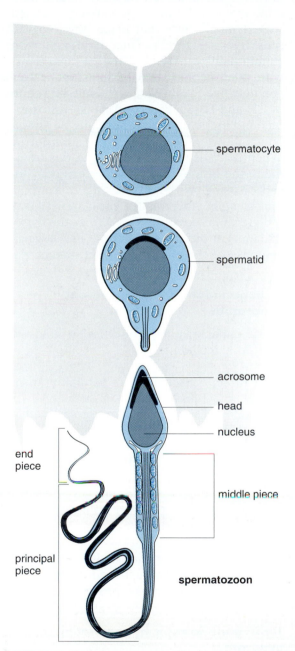

spermatocyte

spermatid

acrosome

head

nucleus

end
piece

middle piece

principal
piece

spermatozoon

centrations of testosterone in the epididymis necessary for the final steps in sperm maturation are maintained. These levels are approximately 50 to 100 times the concentration of testosterone in blood and are greater than can be achieved by exogenous peripheral injection of testosterone.

Tight junctions between the Sertoli cells form a *blood-testes barrier,* which also maintains distinct adlumenal (i.e., facing the lumen) and basal environments across the Sertoli cell through which the maturing sperm pass (see Figure 15.8). This means that the seminiferous tubules are essentially avascular, getting all of their nutritional needs, including oxygen, by diffusion across the basement membrane. As a result of this blood-testes barrier, sperm develop in an immune-privileged environment, devoid of exposure to cells of the immune system, which might otherwise attack them or result in the production of antisperm antibodies.

Clinical Pearls

○ Sperm are very immunogenic, and both male and female infertility can occur when the immune system is allowed to elicit an antibody response to sperm. Preventing this is believed to be one important role of the blood-testes barrier.

○ Vasectomy is a surgical procedure by which the vas deferens is ligated to render males infertile (e.g., for those who do not wish to father any or additional children). In principle, this procedure is reversible by religating the vas deferens. In practice, reversal of vasectomy, is effective only

FIGURE 15.11. Steps in spermatogenesis. Starting from spermatogonia on the basolateral side of the Sertoli cell, a number of morphologic stages in sperm development are apparent as the sperm moves through the Sertoli cell encased in a vacuole. During this time, the spermatogonium becomes a spermatocyte, which becomes a spermatid, which becomes a spermatozoon within the seminiferous tubule lumen. *(Adapted, with permission, from Genuth SM (1988), in RM Berne, MN Levy (eds): Physiology, 4th ed. St. Louis, MO, Mosby, p 978.)*

about half of the time. It has been observed that after vasectomy, a high titer of antisperm antibodies develops, which may contribute to the high rate of infertility after reversal of vasectomy.

Review Questions

14. How many days does it take for a newly produced sperm precursor cell to mature?
15. Describe the blood-testes barrier and one of its likely physiological roles.
16. How does the male reproductive neuroendocrine axis change over the course of infancy, puberty, adulthood, and old age?

8. CLINICAL DISORDERS AS DYSFUNCTION OF MALE REPRODUCTIVE PHYSIOLOGY

The majority of clinical problems involving male reproductive function are outside the scope of this book, as they involve genetic and structural disorders (e.g., chromosomal aberrations causing deficient puberty, vascular disorders causing impotence and infertility, etc). Nevertheless, a knowledge of male reproductive endocrinology provides a useful basis for investigating a significant number of patients whose complaints are due to endocrinologic disorders.

Assessment of male reproductive physiology

The episodic nature of GnRH secretion, and sometimes even of LH and FSH secretion, can make the measurement of these hormones in a single blood level relatively unreliable. If a random LH and FSH blood level is ambiguous (e.g., only slightly above or below

normal), the male reproductive neuroendocrine axis can be more definitively assessed with dynamic tests that make physiological sense (Figure 15.12). Thus, treatment with **clomiphene**, a strong estrogen antagonist with weak agonist activity, interrupts estrogen negative feedback. As a result, secretion of LH and FSH and secondarily of testosterone and estradiol would normally be stimulated, allowing evaluation of the entire axis. When the axis fails to respond to this treatment, the lesion can be more specifically localized using provocative testing. It is important to remember (as for the adrenal) that long-term failure at one level (e.g., the hypothalamus or pituitary) will result in a sluggish response of the atrophied target organs.

Hypogonadotropic hypogonadal syndromes

These encompass several different kinds of disorders, including

- The direct consequence of hypopituitarism (lack of LH and FSH)
- Hypogonadism due to hyperprolactinemia (which inhibits GnRH secretion)
- Specific genetic disorders that result in isolated gonadotropic deficiency (e.g., Kallman's syndrome, in which the GnRH-secreting neurons fail to migrate properly)
- Hypothalamic or pituitary failure as a consequence of a variety of chronic illnesses
- Physiological constitutional delayed puberty, in which individuals will ultimately develop normally, which needs to be distinguished from pathologic processes.

Hypergonadotropic hypogonadal syndromes

These are primary disorders of testicular function resulting in incomplete sexual maturation and hypogonadism with elevated go-

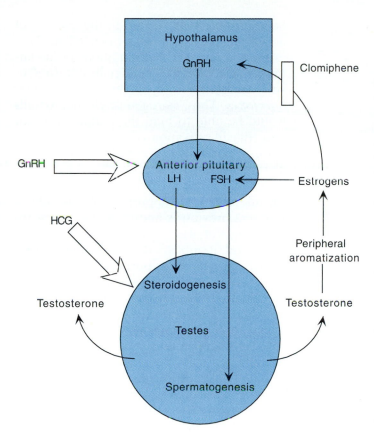

FIGURE 15.12. Testing of the male reproductive neuroendocrine axis. Intravenous boluses of GnRH and subsequently of HCG allow hypothalamic failure to be distinguished from testicular failure. In hypothalamic failure, GnRH would stimulate LH and testosterone secretion. In testicular failure, no testosterone production is observed in response to HCG. GnRH is gonadotropin-releasing hormone; LH is luteinizing hormone; FSH is follicle-stimulating hormone, HCG is human chorionic gonadotropin, clomiphene is an estrogen antagonist. Testosterone is depicted as being released from seminiferous tubules of the testes and undergoing peripheral aromatization to estrogen, whose actions are blocked by clomiphene. Open arrows are diagnostic interventions used by clinicians to probe the function of this neuroendocrine axis. Closed arrows describe the function of the axis. (Adapted, with permission, from Felig P et al. (1987). Endocrinology and Metabolism, 2d ed. New York, McGraw-Hill.)

nadotropin levels (due to a lack of feedback inhibition by testosterone).

Eugonadotropic germinal cell failure

Various causes of germ cell failure may have nothing to do with gonadotropin or testosterone levels; these include **varicoceles** (engorged veins that elevate the temperature in the testes), infections, and autoimmune processes.

Factors involved in male fertility

Factors involved in male infertility include a variety of endocrine disorders, anatomic abnormalities (such as a varicocele), and environmental insults that can cause abnormal sperm number, motility, or morphology. Table 15.5 summarizes these abnormalities.

Clinical Pearl

○ Some patients with neurologic dysfunction, as, for example, can occur as a complication of diabetes mellitus, can have retrograde ejaculation as an explanation for infertility. In this condition, ejaculate goes backward into the bladder, rather than forward out the end of the penis. In some of these cases, sperm has been collected by bladder irrigation and used for in vitro fertilization with success.

TABLE 15.5 FACTORS INVOLVED IN MALE INFERTILITY

Possible causes of abnormal semen analysis
  History of testicular injury or mumps
  Heat
  Severe allergic reactions
  Exposure to radiation or environmental toxins
  Heavy marijuana, tobacco, cocaine, or alcohol use
  Certain drugs (cimetidine, spironolactone, nitrofuran, sulfasalaz-
    ine, erythromycin, tetracycline, anabolic steroids, chemother-
    apeutic drugs)
  Excessive or insufficient coital frequency
  Exposure to diethylstilbestrol (DES) in utero
  Antisperm antibodies

Anatomical anomalies
  Hypospadias
  Vas deferens obstruction
  Retrograde ejaculation
  Varicocele

Endocrine disorders
  Thyroid disease (hyper or hypo)
  Gonadotropin or testosterone insufficiency
  Prolactin excess
  Diabetic neuropathy (resulting in impotence or retrograde ejac-
    ulation)

From Speroff L et al. (1994). *Clinical Gynecologic Endocrinology and Infertility*, 5th ed. Baltimore, Williams & Wilkins, pp. 882–890.

Review Questions

17. What are some factors involved in male infertility?
18. How can you use a knowledge of male reproductive physiology to assess the basis for apparent gonadal failure?

9. FRONTIERS IN MALE REPRODUCTIVE PHYSIOLOGY

Apoptosis, prostate cancer, and the multicellular contract

Why do prostate cancers start off androgen-dependent and later develop androgen independence? A number of mechanisms have been proposed, all related to the concept of genetic instability in cancer (see Chap. 2).

First, it appears that mutations in the androgen receptor may render it able to activate transcription upon binding by *other hormones*. Thus, estrogen or glucocorticoids would be able to bind the mutant receptor and trigger activation of the transcriptional pattern normally governed by androgens. This provides a molecular mechanism by which it becomes possible to bypass the need for androgens to support cellular proliferation in a previously androgen-dependent tumor (see Ref. 4).

Second, it appears that mutations that inactivate the tumor suppressor gene p53 are common in androgen-resistant tumors (see Ref. 5). This is likely to reflect the inactivation of a fundamental cellular defense mechanism against the development of cancer. As a result, cells survive that should have been destroyed.

Finally, some prostate cancers appear to have been selected to survive and proliferate by overexpression of Bcl-2, an antiapoptotic gene product (see Ref. 6).

In effect, these three mechanisms illustrate different ways in which a cancer can "cheat" in biological regulation. These observations have some profound evolutionary implications, with lessons for health care providers.

One interpretation of all this is that at the dawn of evolution of multicellular organisms, the ancestral cells in effect agreed to a *quid pro quo* in which the benefits of multicellularity were received — for a price. In exchange for joining a community of interacting cells (i.e., a multicellular organism), cells were wired to die if any of a large number of insults rendered them unable to make their contribution to the organism as a whole. Thus, a cancer cell, selected by virtue of the presence of antiapoptotic mutations, can be viewed as a doomed, rogue cell that refused to "live up to the contract" and was unwilling to die quietly for the benefit of the multicellular whole.

Recent work suggests that there are ways in which it may be possible to use the myriad pathways of apoptosis to re-establish control over cells that have chosen to disregard their apoptotic obligations. By triggering expression of other genetic loci encoding additional proapoptotic products, it may yet be possible to eliminate cancer cells that have insulated themselves from the standard means of activating apoptosis (see Ref. 7).

Androgens, estrogens, and more surprises in steroid hormone action

The conventional picture of steroid hormone action involves formation of a hormone-receptor complex and its activation of transcription of some genes and deactivation of others, in conjunction with tissue-specific cofactor proteins.

Several wrinkles in this simple picture have already been mentioned:

1. Steroid hormone receptors can sometimes be activated without their hormone (see Chap. 3).
2. Steroid hormone can be subject to peripheral metabolism that may result in its activation, inactivation, or transformation into a completely different steroid that engages a separate receptor with radically different actions (e.g., peripheral aromatization of androgen to estrogen).
3. Recent work has revealed the existence of a second estrogen receptor, which may account for the cardiovascular protective effects of estrogens. This estrogen receptor β, as it has been called, has a very different spectrum of effects from estrogen receptor α, the classic estrogen receptor (see Chap. 16).
4. Some steroid-type hormones (e.g., the vitamin D receptor) dimerize with other receptor proteins (e.g., the vitamin A receptor) and then display different functional properties (in terms of hormone binding, cofactor protein utilization, or transcriptional activation).

Recently, additional observations have related novel concepts of steroid hormone action to prostate cancer. It has long been known that antiandrogen therapy is initially effective at suppressing prostate cancer. However, after 1 to 3 years of good control, the cancer eventually becomes androgen-insensitive and more aggressive and rapidly causes the death of the patient. It has also been observed that when prostate cancer becomes resistant to antiandrogens, cessation of antiandrogen therapy actually slows tumor growth briefly, this is called the antiandrogen withdrawal syndrome.

Two recent papers suggest a remarkable explanation for this phenomenon (see Refs. 8 and 9). In the first paper, these workers present data that suggest that the induction of different cofactor proteins can completely change the transcriptional activity of an androgen *antagonist* into that of an androgen *agonist*. The working hypothesis is that steroid receptor–dependent transcription is a result of a three-way interaction among steroid, receptor, and cofactor proteins. Different cofactor proteins can dramatically change steroids that were receptor antagonists in the context of one cofactor into agonists in the context of another. In the second paper, the authors demonstrate a corollary of this notion: In the presence of specific cofactor proteins, some, but not all, estrogens can bind the androgen receptor and activate transcription.

The implications of this work, taken in the context of the earlier observations, are profound:

1. The mechanisms discussed previously, e.g., mutations in the androgen receptor or in signaling pathways of programmed cell

death and tumor suppression, are not the only ones by which androgen-resistant tumors can develop.

2. A bewildering array of permutations exists by which steroid action can be turned on and off physiologically. We need to establish a map of these actions and interactions in order to make sense of steroid responses in humans in health and disease. Until we have such a map of cofactors and their interactions with diverse hormones and receptors, we are "flying blind" in terms of understanding cause and effect in steroid hormone biology.

3. The effects of weak androgens and estrogens, derived from the diet or generated as minor metabolites in our bodies, have to be studied very seriously. They may hold the clue to why some patients do or do not develop prostate cancer, and why some prostate cancers are slow-growing tumors, while others are aggressive and metastatic.

4. Clinicians and scientists should have a little more humility when trying to understand and manipulate the product of a billion years of evolution. The reality is that our knowledge of vast stretches of molecular physiology is subrudimentary. We do not know all of the variables we should be looking at, nor the time frame over which they act. The effects of some variables may be cancelled out by the effects of other variables. Until we have a deeper understanding of biological systems, the practice of medicine, including the application of basic science to clinical care, is likely to remain largely an art.

5. Many conclusions from clinical epidemiology are dependent on a particular physiological frame of reference. When new paradigms for thinking about basic physiology emerge, the premises and variables on which any particular clinical epidemiologic study were carried out may be called into question. This is not a reflection on the quality of the clinical epidemiologic study, but rather on the fundamental feature of medical knowledge, namely, that it is in a state of flux (see Chap. 1).

Environmental toxins and reproductive health

Imprinting is the concept that exposure to a steroid hormone, such as androgen or estrogen, early in life has consequences that are not manifest until decades later. Normally this occurs as part of the paradigm of chromosomal sex leading to gonadal sex leading to phenotypic sex, and has been tailored by evolution to the particular environment in which humans evolved. Other work suggests that imprinting by estrogens during fetal life can predispose to the development of cancer years later (see Ref. 10). Might this concept have new implications? Consider the following:

It has long been observed that there are a host of estrogen-like compounds in the environment. Some are plant estrogens (called *phytoestrogens*; see Chap. 16) that have probably been present in our diets since the dawn of humankind but are now being lost as a result of industrial food preparation practices (e.g., as a consequence of removal of fiber, etc.). One can only wonder at present whether the modern diet might not be lacking in compounds such as phytoestrogens that have beneficial effects on physiological function.

Other estrogenic compounds are environmental pollutants introduced through human industrial activity recently in our history. Some have suggested that these are irrelevant because their biologic potency is low compared to that of the major estrogens in humans.

Doubtless the debate will continue to rage as to whether equal and opposite compounds that cancel out these effects exist in nature, etc. However, to the extent that any of these concerns ultimately prove to be justified, we may be poisoning ourselves through environmental pollution at a rate and to a degree never before seen in the history of our species (see Ref. 11). Health care providers have an obligation to let both patients and politicians understand the risks *to ourselves* when we alter the environment. Perhaps even more important is explaining that it will take a very long time before we can rule in or out certain potential effects with any confidence.

10. HOW DOES UNDERSTANDING NORMAL PHYSIOLOGY PROVIDE INSIGHT INTO THE INITIAL CASE?

Let us revisit the case of L.R., the 38-year-old electrician who came to you concerned about infertility and high cholesterol.

Infertility can have many causes. The only necessary component from the male is sufficient deliverable, viable sperm, whereas the female requires not only viable eggs, but also intact structures necessary for fertilization, implantation and development. About 40% of infertility is believed to be due to male factors.

Since the incidence of pregnancy as a result of sexual intercourse is statistically rather low, about 1 in 25, it is often not possible to identify a specific cause of infertility. Various means of augmenting the chances of success have been advocated, with the primary advice often being to "keep trying."

What Mr. R. did not understand is that the distribution and concentration of androgens in different parts of the body have an enormous impact on the consequences of androgen action. Fertility requires an extremely high *local* concentration of androgens in the testes to promote optimal spermatogenesis. Because of the intimate relationship of androgen-synthesizing Leydig cells to sperm-producing Sertoli cells in the seminiferous tubules, the needs of spermatogenesis for androgens normally are met first before andro-

gens spill over into the systemic circulation in high enough concentrations to inhibit the hypothalamic–pituitary–gonadal neuroendocrine axis. By taking high doses of exogenous androgens, *injected peripherally*, Mr. R. effectively shut down his neuroendocrine axis without ever achieving the 50 to 100 times higher than blood concentration of androgen needed locally in the testes for optimal support of sperm production and maturation. Thus, ironically, the very therapy that enhanced many male-specific peripheral characteristics was also responsible for worsening his ability to father a child.

An undesired effect of androgens is to worsen a patient's lipid profile, in terms of cardiovascular disease risk, as was demonstrated in the findings on this patient.

After a clear explanation, Mr. R. resolved to follow the advice of his health care provider. He stopped taking androgens. Three months later his lipid profile had returned to normal. Six months later a repeat sperm analysis was also back to normal. One year later he and his wife were overjoyed to discover that she was pregnant.

SUMMARY AND REVIEW OF KEY CONCEPTS

1. Sex determination during embryogenesis involves genetic, cellular, and hormonal factors. Genes on both the X and Y chromosomes are necessary for development of the full male phenotype. In normal development, these genes give rise to male gonads that produce hormones that direct development of external and internal male genitalia, a process that is not completed until puberty.
2. The mature male reproductive neuroendocrine axis involves pulsatile GnRH from the hypothalamus as a trigger of LH and FSH secretion by gonadotropes of the anterior pituitary, which directs maturation

of sperm in the seminiferous tubules and androgen production by the Leydig cells.

3. A blood-testes barrier creates an immune-privileged environment in which sperm develop.

4. At puberty, testosterone stimulates linear growth and development of secondary sexual characteristics in boys, as does estrogen in girls.

5. The most common medical problems involving the male reproductive physiology include impotence, infertility, prostatic hypertrophy, prostatic cancer, and androgen abuse.

6. Androgen actions can be categorized as either anabolic (promoting increased muscle mass) or androgenic (promoting male secondary sexual characteristics).

7. Testosterone and DHT are the two physiological androgens in males. Testosterone is responsible for gonadotropin feedback, spermatogenesis, and embryonic sexual differentiation. DHT is most important for external virilization and secondary sexual characteristics.

8. Sperm undergo a complex series of maturational events in seminiferous tubules that take about 90 days and require high concentrations of testosterone maintained by androgen-binding protein.

BPH, Mr. D. and his clinician elected to have the prostate removed surgically.

Pathologic analysis of the removed prostate specimen showed the presence of a focus of cancer in addition to benign nodules. A bone scan was negative. Mr. D. received several cycles of radiation therapy and was treated with antiandrogens, having refused surgical orchiectomy. Subsequently his PSA was noted to be normal, and he had no related symptoms for nearly 2 years.

About 20 months after his last radiation therapy treatment, Mr. D. noted leg and back pain. Another bone scan showed lytic lesions that suggested metastatic disease. His PSA had increased to 80. He was distraught that his cancer had recurred despite his careful adherence to his medical regimen, and he wondered whether orchiectomy now would do any good.

After much thought and discussion, Mr. D. opted for a course of palliative radiation for his bone metastases and no further therapy. Six months later he was noted to have an altered mental status. Head CT showed brain metastases. Blood studies suggested that he was in renal failure. As per his previously expressed wishes, he was transferred to a hospice for terminal care and died comfortably in his sleep 10 days later.

A CASE OF PHYSIOLOGICAL MEDICINE

A.D. is a 76-year-old former prize-fighter and avid gardener who presented to medical attention with a complaint of difficulty urinating. He had had this symptom for many years, but had not seen a health care provider previously. Physical examination showed an enlarged prostate gland. A serum PSA was elevated at 12 (normal <4), while renal function was normal. In view of the elevated PSA and the concern that this could reflect the presence of prostate cancer rather than simply

QUESTIONS

1. What is the explanation for Mr. D.'s difficulty urinating?

2. Suppose he had presented to medical attention several years earlier with the same symptoms, but with a normal PSA and an ultrasound examination of the prostate showing enlargement, but no sign of malignancy. How might he have been treated?

3. Why were the clinicians concerned about renal failure upon Mr. D.'s initial presentation?

4. What is the rationale for antiandrogen treatment of prostate cancer?

5. How would you answer Mr. D.'s questions as to why the cancer recurred despite his adherance to medical therapy and whether orchiectomy would do any good after his cancer had recurred and metastasized?

ANSWERS

1. The enlarged prostate gland is constricting the part of the urethra that traverses the prostate gland as a result of hyperplasia and hypertrophy of either epithelial or stromal (smooth muscle) components, dependent on both androgens and estrogens.

2. Treatments that either shrink the prostate (5α-reductase inhibitors like finasteride) or cause smooth muscle relaxation (α_1 receptor blockers like terazosin) can improve urinary flow. However, the latter does not treat the underlying problem, and therefore obstruction can return by the other mechanism, as the prostate continues to enlarge.

3. Because obstruction of urinary flow at the level of the prostate will eventually result in increased pressure back into the kidneys, which can destroy nephrons and lead to renal failure. Luckily, despite years of symptoms, Mr. D. did not have this development.

4. Most prostate cancers start out with androgen receptors. These malignancies are generally androgen-sensitive for growth. Thus, treatment with an antiandrogen blocks their growth and often results in death of a large number of cancer cells and a period of remission in the disease.

5. The therapy itself has resulted in selection pressure in favor of the emergence of a clone of cells that has lost its androgen dependence for growth. These tend to be less differentiated, more invasive and ag-gressive cells for which the antiandrogen therapy will do no good.

Because androgens are made by both the adrenal gland as well as the testes, some have suggested that treatment with an anti-androgen that would block the action of androgens from both sources may be superior to just orchiectomy or treatment with LHRH agonists that cause "chemical orchiectomy." However, there is no benefit the other way around, that is, from orchiectomy for a patient already being treated with antiandrogens.

Some patients who have ceased to respond to antiandrogens actually get a limited response to the subsequent withdrawal of antiandrogens. Perhaps this reflects selection of a subclone of tumor cells that actually is antiandrogen-dependent for its growth. However, the benefit of antiandrogen withdrawal in these cases is not very long-lasting.

References and suggested readings

GENERAL REFERENCES

1. Braunstein GD (1997). In Greenspan FS, Strewler GS (eds): *Basic and Clinical Endocrinology,* 5th ed. Stamford, CT, Appleton & Lange.

2. Gerhart JE, Kirschner MF (1997). *Cells, Embryos, and Evolution.* Malden, MA, Blackwell Science.

3. Mather JP, et al (1997). Activins, inhibins, and follistatins: Further thoughts on a growing family of regulators. *Proc Soc Exp Biol Med* 21:209-222.

FRONTIERS REFERENCES

4. Taplin ME, et al (1995). Mutation of the androgen-receptor gene in metastatic androgen-independent prostate cancer. *New Engl J Med* 332:1393-1400.

5. McDonnell TJ, et al (1992). Expression of the

protooncogene bcl-2 in the prostate and its association with emergence of androgen-independent prostate cancer. *Cancer Res* 52: 6940-6944.

6. Bookstein R, et al (1993). p53 is mutated in a subset of advanced-stage prostate cancers. *Cancer Res* 53:3369-3373.

7. Sanchez Y, et al (1996). Tumor suppression and apoptosis of human prostate carcinoma mediated by a genetic locus within human chromosome 10pter-q11. *Proc Natl Acad Sci USA* 93:2551-2556.

8. Yeh S, et al (1998). From estrogen to androgen receptor: A new pathway for sex hormones in prostate. *Proc Natl Acad Sci USA* 95:5527-5532.

9. Miyamoto H, et al (1998). Promotion of agonist activity of antiandrogens by the androgen receptor coactivator, ARA70, in human prostate cancer DU145 cells. *Proc Natl Acad Sci USA* 95:7379-7384.

10. McLachlan JA, et al (1998). Are estrogens carcinogenic during development of the testes? *APMIS* 106:240-242; discussion 243-244.

11. Colborn T, et al (1997). *Our Stolen Future.* Baltimore, Penguin Books.

PHYSIOLOGY OF THE FEMALE REPRODUCTIVE SYSTEM

16

1. INTRODUCTION TO PHYSIOLOGY OF THE FEMALE REPRODUCTIVE SYSTEM

The female does far more than just provide her "fair share" of the genetic material in the developing embryo. She also donates all of the initial cytoplasm (including cytoplasmic organelles such as mitochondria) and maintains the specialized environment within which the embryo will develop. This includes:

1. Storing germ cells, called **oocytes**, from early in fetal life through the end of the reproductive years. During adulthood, one oocyte will mature each month into an **egg**.
2. Preparing the **female reproductive tract lining** in ways that facilitate the fertilization of the single released egg by just one of the hundreds of millions of sperm present after insemination. At the same time, other features of the female reproductive tract prevent multiple fertilizations, infection, and other things bad for mother or fetus.
3. Sustaining the complex development of the **fetus** to term.

The hormones **estrogen** and **progesterone**, together with a host of other factors, work in concert on the primary organs of reproduction to achieve these tasks with extraordinary precision.

Why is understanding female reproductive physiology important for medical practice?

- Because embryos are carried to term within the human female, the possibility that a female patient anywhere close to the reproductive years *could be pregnant* must always be considered in any medical evaluation and before any medical treatment or procedure.
- Estrogens and progestins, the sex steroids that are necessary for female reproductive system function, also have major effects on the structure and/or function of many organ systems in the body, including organs whose primary function is not reproduction (e.g., brain, liver, kidney, bones, etc.). Thus, disorders affecting the levels of these hormones have widespread consequences.
- Disorders of the female reproductive system often present in ways that mimic disorders of other systems. Acute abdominal pain in a middle-aged man might lead one to consider disorders such as peptic ulcer disease, pancreatitis, diverticular disease, or appendicitis. When a woman in the reproductive years presents with the identical symptoms, all of these same diagnoses are possible. However, a range of additional possibilities, such as ectopic pregnancy, endometriosis, ovarian torsion, and pelvic inflammatory disease, must also be considered, because of the presence of specialized abdominal organs of reproduction in the female. Misdiagnosis of some of these female-specific disorders can rapidly be life-threatening or lead to lifelong infertility.
- The development of the birth control pill was one of the first and most dramatic examples of how knowledge of human physiology could increase individual freedom. The physiological thinking of those medical pioneers remains a cornerstone of modern medical practice today—tempered by a modern awareness that, in general, pharmacologic intervention should always be limited to those situations where more physiological means are not effective.
- Historically, the health of women has not received equal attention to that of men, corresponding to the discrimination against women in most human endeavors. Important aspects of this injustice persist today in our own society and, often more prominently, elsewhere around the world, affecting the health of women in major ways. Often the research on which current clinical teaching is based did not fully consider gen-

der-specific implications. Sometimes health care providers' training or socialization produces unconscious gender-related bias that affects interactions with patients or colleagues. Clinicians who are not sensitive to these possibilities and who do not strive to change such attitudes will never reach their full potential as healers. A physiological approach to the practice of medicine can aid in objectively recognizing the impact of gender on mechanisms of organ system function.

Case Presentation

A.V. is a 42-year-old businesswoman whose history demonstrates the complexity of the menstrual cycle. She has presented to medical attention concerned about cessation of menstrual periods three times over the past 20 years. Each time the cause has been different.

At the age of 20, just after initiating a vigorous daily exercise regimen accompanied by a 12-lb weight loss, Ms. V. noted cessation of her previously regular menstrual periods. Because she had a family history of thyroid disease, the physician directed the history and physical exam toward assessing this possibility, and blood studies were carried out to evaluate her thyroid function, which proved to be normal. The physician concluded that Ms. V. most likely had hypothalamic amenorrhea. In discussing the treatment options, the physician noted that various lifestyle and diet changes might work, as would a couple of different pharmacologic approaches. Opting for the diet and lifestyle changes, Ms. V. noted resumption of her menses 3 months later.

At the age of 35, Ms. V. again developed amenorrhea. For the prior 6 months or so she had suffered from severe depression. Her physician had tried her on several different psychotropic medicines, including a dopa-mine antagonist, trying to find one to which she demonstrated a good response without intolerable side effects. About 2 months prior to the onset of amenorrhea, she was involved in a serious car accident, in which she sustained a concussion and a fractured femur. A discussion with her physician of the array of possible causes of her amenorrhea left the patient frustrated and angry. She stopped taking the antidepressant and stopped seeing the physician, and the amenorrhea spontaneously resolved.

Now, at age 42, Ms. V. is quite anxious to get pregnant. She and her partner have been timing sexual intercourse in the hope of optimizing the likelihood of that outcome. Once again she is frustrated by the onset of amenorrhea and presents to medical attention for workup and some answers. A concern of her physician is that she may be running out of viable follicles — ovarian failure.

Ms. V. wonders whether the amenorrhea is related to recent headaches she has had. Partly to assuage her concerns, the clinician orders an MRI scan of the head, only to discover pituitary enlargement compared to the scan done after her car accident 7 years ago. What does this mean? What should be done now? What should the clinician tell the patient?

The clinician initially intended to approach the evaluation of amenorrhea systematically, starting a big workup with provocative testing to demonstrate the intactness of the uterus, its capacity to respond to progesterone followed by hormone withdrawal, the ability of the ovary to respond to appropriate stimulation, etc., however, remembering the sage words of her old physiology professor, the clinician considers the simplest physiological possibilities first and orders a pregnancy test. The result explains the amenorrhea and the MRI abnormality. The workup is canceled, prenatal care is scheduled, and Ms. V. and her partner are happy.

2. ANATOMY AND HISTOLOGY OF THE FEMALE REPRODUCTIVE ORGANS

The ovaries

The ovaries are a pair of structures, approximately 15 g each, attached by ligaments to the lateral pelvic wall and to the uterus (see Figure 16.1). Each ovary contains **germinal** **epithelium**, composed of follicles in which an individual oocyte is surrounded by a layer of cells called **granulosa cells** that are dedicated to its nourishment and protection. A basement membrane separates the granulosa cells from androgen-producing **thecal cells** (see Figure 16.2). An important activity of granulosa cells is to convert androgen from thecal cells into estrogen.

FIGURE 16.1. Anatomy of the female reproductive organs. Schematic diagram indicating anatomic landmarks of the uterus and adjacent organs.

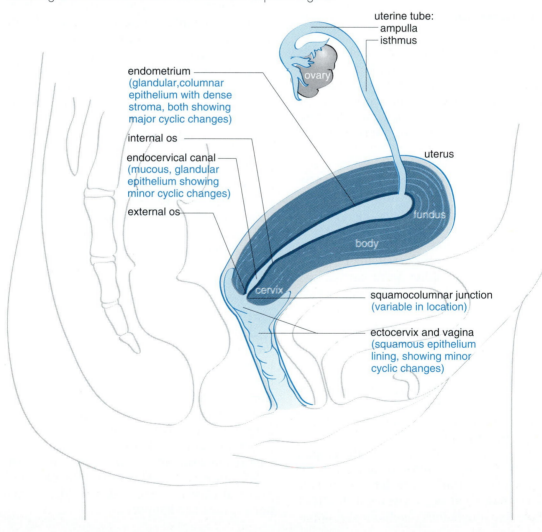

uterine tube:
- ampulla
- isthmus

ovary

endometrium
(glandular, columnar epithelium with dense stroma, both showing major cyclic changes)

uterus

internal os

endocervical canal
(mucous, glandular epithelium showing minor cyclic changes)

external os

fundus

body

cervix

squamocolumnar junction
(variable in location)

ectocervix and vagina
(squamous epithelium lining, showing minor cyclic changes)

Oocytes mature within the ovary in a monthly cycle. When the process of maturation is complete, the follicle ruptures, releasing the mature egg. The cells of the ruptured follicle that remain behind with the ovary form a short-lived endocrine structure called the **corpus luteum**. The corpus luteum is the primary source of progesterone prior to and through the first third of pregnancy and therefore is crucial for successful fertilization, implantation, and fetal survival (see Sec. 6).

In addition to estrogen and progesterone, the ovary is the source of a truly amazing array of secretory products, most of which are local mediators whose functions are poorly understood (see Table 16.1).

The uterus and fallopian tubes

The **uterus** is a muscular pelvic organ (see Figure 16.1) into whose hormone-responsive lining, called the **endometrium**, the fertilized egg must implant to create a successful pregnancy. Below the endometrium is a muscular layer called the **myometrium**, whose contraction is necessary to expel the mature fetus at the end of pregnancy (see Figure 16.1).

The endometrium undergoes a hormone-dependent cycle of proliferation and maturation (see Figure 16.3). At the end of this **proliferative phase**, conditions are optimum for sperm transport. This corresponds to the point in time when the mature egg has been released from the ovary. Later, during the **secretory phase**, conditions in the endometrium are optimal for implantation of a fertilized egg, but impede sperm transport. If no implantation and therefore no pregnancy occurs, the blood levels of estrogen and progesterone fall, removing the hormonal support needed to maintain the endometrium. As a result, most of the endometrium dies and is expelled in the form of menstrual bleeding.

The monthly process of preparing the endometrium for the possibility of implantation and then discarding it in the event that implantation does not occur is termed the **menstrual cycle**.

Attached to the uterus are two tubes, one on each side, that provide a conduit from the ovary (see Figure 16.1). At the far end of each **fallopian tube** are finger-like projections called **fimbriae**. The lining of the fallopian tube is composed of ciliated cells that beat in the direction of the uterus. Normally fertilization occurs within the fallopian tube, with subsequent transport of the fertilized egg to the uterus for implantation.

Like the ovary, the uterine endometrium is the site of production of a wide range of substances that probably serve as local mediators of signaling (see Table 16.2). However, their precise roles in endometrial development or implantation remain largely unknown.

The vagina

The **vagina** is a muscular tube connecting the vulva (external female genitalia) to the uterine cervix (see Figure 16.1). The vagina is lined with a squamous epithelium. Under the influence of estrogen, the vaginal epithelium accumulates glycogen, which is deposited in the vaginal lumen as epithelial cells **desquamate** (slough off). Fermentation of this glycogen to lactate by normal vaginal bacteria maintains a low-pH environment, which serves as a natural barrier to pathogenic microorganisms. Although the vagina lacks glands, fluid can extravasate into the lumen upon appropriate mechanical stimulation of the estrogen-primed epithelium.

Other estrogen-dependent tissues

The specialized organs of reproduction — the ovary, the uterus, and the breast — are

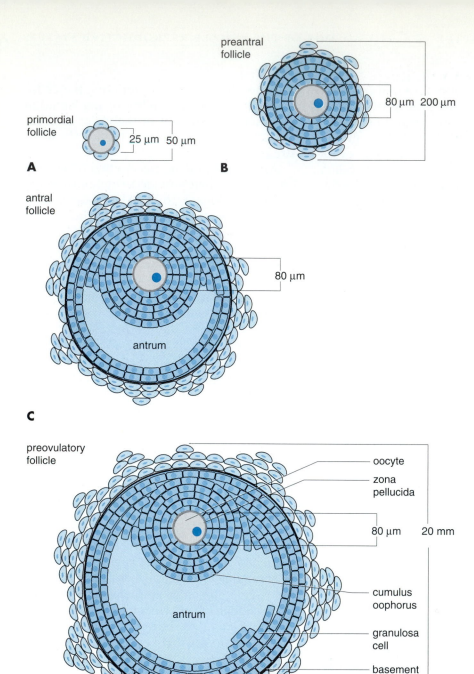

FIGURE 16.2. Histology of the ovarian follicle during the course of the follicular phase of the menstrual cycle. *A.* Primordial follicle. *B.* An activated follicle early in the follicular phase of the menstrual cycle. *C.* An antral follicle late in the follicular phase of the menstrual cycle. *D.* A nearly mature preovulatory follicle approaching mid-cycle.

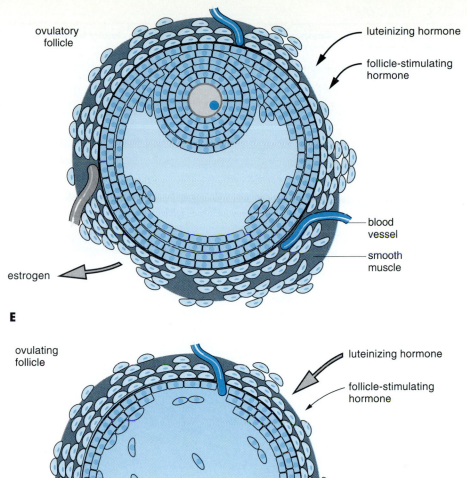

ovulatory
follicle

luteinizing hormone

follicle-stimulating
hormone

blood
vessel

smooth
muscle

estrogen

E

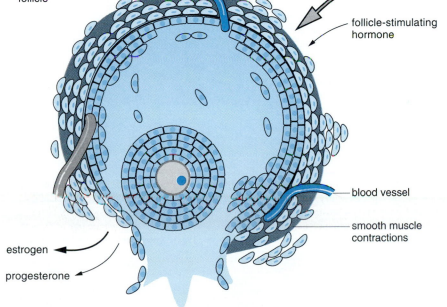

ovulating
follicle

luteinizing hormone

follicle-stimulating
hormone

blood vessel

smooth muscle
contractions

estrogen

progesterone

F

FIGURE 16.2 — (continued) *E*. Final maturation of the dominant follicle, with movement to the surface of the ovary setting the stage for follicular rupture. *F*. Rupture of a mature follicle at mid-cycle in response to the LH/FSH surge. The high levels of LH may also downregulate LH receptors on the thecal cells, resulting in a drop in androgen production, which may account for the transient spike and then fall in blood estrogen in response to the mid-cycle LH surge. (*Adapted, with permission, from Speroff L, et al. (1994). Clinical Gynecological Endocrinology and Infertility, 5th ed. Baltimore, MD, Williams & Wilkins.*)

TABLE 16.1 PRODUCTS OF THE OVARY

Products	Compartment	Regulatory factors
Inhibin	Granulosa, theca, corpus luteum	FSH, EGF, IGF-1, GnRH, VIP, TGF
Activin	Granulosa	FSH
Müllerian-inhibiting substance	Granulosa, cumulus oophorus	LH, FSH
Follistatin	Follicles	LH, FSH
Relaxin	Corpus luteum, theca	n.d.
	Placenta, uterus	?PRL, LH, oxytocin, PGs
Oocyte meiosis inhibitor	Follicular fluid	n.d.
Follicle regulatory protein	Follicular fluid, granulosa, luteal	FSH, GnRH
Plasminogen activator	Granulosa	n.d.
Extracellular membrane proteins	Granulosa, follicular fluid	FSH, GnRH
Insulin-like growth factor 1	Granulosa	LH, FSH, GH, EGF, TGF, PDGF, estrogen
Epidermal growth factor-like	Granulosa, theca	Gonadotropins
Transforming growth factor α	Theca, interstitial	FSH
Basic fibroblast growth factor	Corpus luteum	n.d.
Transforming growth factor β	Theca, interstitial, granulosa	Fibronectin, FSH, TGF-β
Platelet-derived growth factor	Granulosa	n.d.
Nerve growth factor	Ovary	n.d.
Proopiomelanocortin	Corpus luteum, interstitial, luteal, granulosa	n.d.
Enkephalin	Ovary	n.d.
Dynorphin	Ovary	n.d.
Gonadotropin-releasing hormone	Ovary, follicular fluid, ?granulosa	n.d.
Oxytocin	Corpus luteum, granulosa	LH, FSH, $PGF_{2\alpha}$
Vasopressin	Ovary, follicular fluid	n.d.
Renin	Follicular fluid, theca, luteal	LH, FSH
Angiotensin II	Follicular fluid	n.d.
Atrial natriuretic factor	Corpus luteum, ovary, follicular fluid	n.d.
Luteinization inhibitor and luteinization stimulator	Follicular fluid	n.d.
Gonadotropin surge-inhibiting factor	Granulosa	n.d.
Luteinizing hormone receptor-binding inhibitor	Corpus luteum	n.d.
Neuropeptide Y, calcitonin gene-related peptide, substance P, peptide histidine methionine, somatostatin	Nerve fibers	n.d.
Vasoactive intestinal peptide	Nerve fibers	n.d.
c-mos	Oocytes	Developmental

Key: EGF = epidermal growth factor; FSH = follicle-stimulating hormone; GH = growth hormone; GnRH = gonadotropin-releasing hormone; IGF = insulin-like growth factor; LH = luteinizing hormone; n.d. = not determined; PDGF = platelet-derived growth factor; PG = prostaglandin; PGF = prostaglandin F; PRL = prolactin; TGF = transforming growth factor; VIP = vasoactive intestinal peptide. Reproduced, with permission, from McPhee S, et al. (1997). *Pathophysiology of Disease*, 2d ed. Stamford, CT, Appleton & Lange, p. 516. Originally from Ackland JF, et al. (1992). Nonsteroidal signals originating from the gonads. *Physiol Rev* 72:731.

FIGURE 16.3. Hormone-dependent cycle of endometrial proliferation, maturation, and sloughing. The x axis displays the days of the menstrual cycle, indicating the proliferative and secretory phases and the onset of menses. The diagram shows changes in endometrial histology, with increase in thickness during the proliferative phase, maturation of the proliferated tissue in the secretory phase, with glands engorged with thick mucus, and sloughing of ischemic tissue upon withdrawal of estrogen and progesterone, manifest as onset of menses. Also indicated are the corresponding stages of ovarian follicular development. *(Adapted, with permission, from Chandrasoma P, Taylor CE (1994). Concise Pathology. Stamford, CT, Appleton & Lange.)*

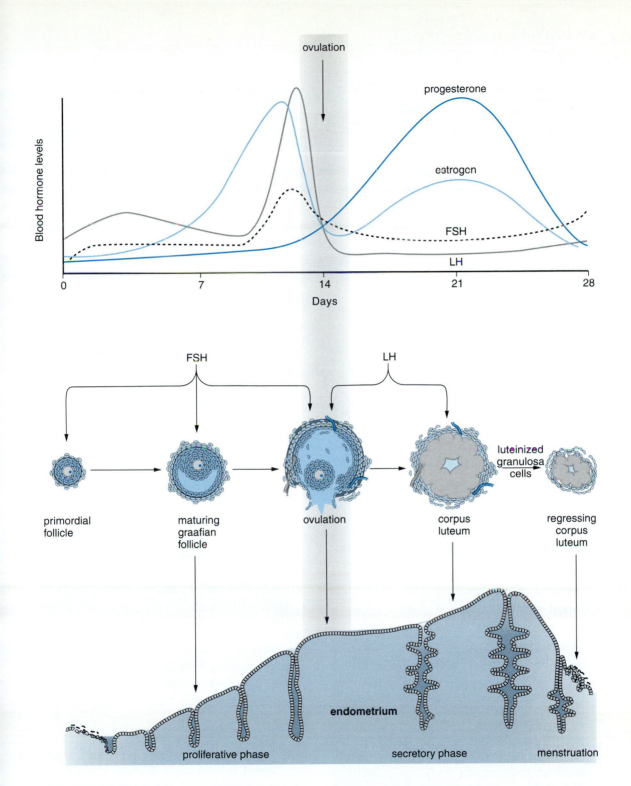

ovulation

progesterone

estrogen

FSH

LH

Blood hormone levels

Days

0   7   14   21   28

FSH

LH

primordial
follicle

maturing
graafian
follicle

ovulation

corpus
luteum

luteinized
granulosa
cells

regressing
corpus
luteum

endometrium

proliferative phase

secretory phase

menstruation

693

TABLE 16.2 PRODUCTS OF THE ENDOMETRIUM

Lipids	Cytokines	Peptides
Prostaglandins	Interleukin 1α	Prolactin
Thromboxanes	Interleukin 1β	Relaxin
Leukotrienes	Interleukin 6	Renin
	Interferon γ	Endorphin
	Colony-stimulating factor 1	Epidermal growth factor
		Insulin-like growth factors (IGFs)
		Fibroblast growth factor
		Platelet-derived growth factor
		Transforming growth factor
		IGF binding proteins
		Corticotropin-releasing hormone
		Fibronectin
		Tumor necrosis factor
		Parathyroid hormone-like peptide

From McPhee S, et al. (1997). *Pathophysiology of Disease*, 2d ed. Stamford, CT, Appleton & Lange, p. 516. Originally from Speroff L, et al. (1994). *Clinical Gynecologic Endocrinology and Infertility*, 5th ed. Baltimore, Williams & Wilkins.

TABLE 16.3 ESTROGEN AND PROGESTERONE-SENSITIVE TISSUES AND THEIR ROLE IN REPRODUCTION

Ovary	Location of oocytes; site of oocyte maturation
Uterus	Site of implantation of embryo
Fallopian tube	Transport of ovulated egg to the uterus; site of sperm-egg interaction
Brain Hypothalamus and pituitary	Control of reproductive neuroendocrine axis
Vagina	Avenue of entry of sperm and exit of fetus at term
Breasts	Ideal nutrition for the neonate
Adipose tissue	Site of peripheral aromatization; cause of insulin resistance; monitored centrally by the hypothalamus.
Bones	Pelvic outlet for newborn infant
Kidney	Increased metabolism, GFR, etc., in pregnancy
Liver	Alteration in SHBG etc.
Blood vessels	Vasodilation to optimize blood flow

GFR = glomerular filtration rate; SHBG = sex hormone-binding globulin.

not the only organs that are profoundly affected by estrogen. Table 16.3 summarizes the major estrogen- or progesterone-sensitive tissues and their relationship to reproduction.

Clinical Pearls

○ One of the signs of symptomatic estrogen deficiency is atrophy of the vaginal epithelium and loss of the natural protective barrier. As a result of these changes, some postmenopausal women have symptoms of vaginal dryness, itching, inflammation, and more frequent infections.

○ One of the consequences of pelvic infections and inflammation is the formation of scar tissue and adhesions between and within pelvic organs. Besides greatly increasing the difficulty in achieving effective sperm and egg transport, these complications increase the risk of an ectopic pregnancy, where implantation occurs inappropriately in the fallopian tube rather than in the endometrium. The patient has severe pain and, if she does not receive appropriate medical attention, may have tubal rupture, resulting in internal hemorrhage and sometimes death.

Review Questions

1. Give five reasons why an understanding of female reproductive physiology is important for clinicians outside the specialty of obstetrics and gynecology.

2. Which female reproductive organ houses germ cells prior to completion of their maturation?

3. What part of the uterus proliferates and differentiates in response to estrogen and progesterone?

4. The normal vaginal epithelium forms a line of defense against infection. Describe the role of estrogen in this process.

3. SEXUAL DEVELOPMENT

Embryonic events

The earliest cells committed to being germ cells migrate from the yolk sac to the genital ridge, which will form the ovary, at about 5 to 6 weeks of gestation. These cells form **oogonia**, primordial germ cells that are still capable of proliferating through mitosis. At 20 to 24 weeks of gestation, the embryo has about 7 million oogonia, and no more are ever produced (see Figure 16.4). From about the tenth week of gestation and continuing until shortly after birth, oogonia are converted to oocytes, a process that is dependent on the presence of two X chromosomes. The oocytes proceed to the diplotene stage of meiosis, reaching this stage by the time of birth, at which point their development is arrested until puberty (see Figure 16.5).

When they enter meiosis, individual oocytes develop a layer of spindle-shaped cells around them. These cells will eventually develop into the **granulosa cells** that directly

FIGURE 16.4. Age-dependent change in the female reproductive neuroendocrine axis. Shows the change in number of oogonia, which reaches a maximum of several million during early embryogenesis and then decreases inexorably throughout life. Note that FSH and LH levels in the fetus exceed the concentrations achieved during the mid-cycle surge in adulthood. After menopause, LH and FSH levels rise even higher due to lack of negative feedback from ovarian estrogens. *(Adapted, with permission, from Speroff L, et al. (1994). Clinical Gynecological Endocrinology and Infertility, 5th ed. Baltimore, Williams & Wilkins, pp. 102, 173.)*

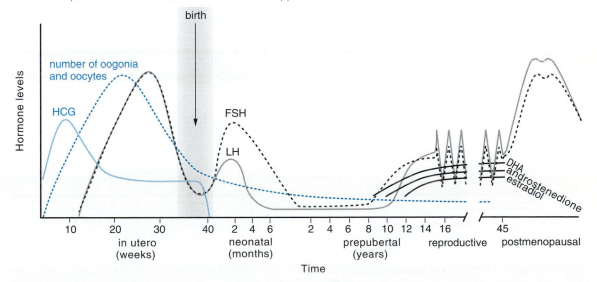

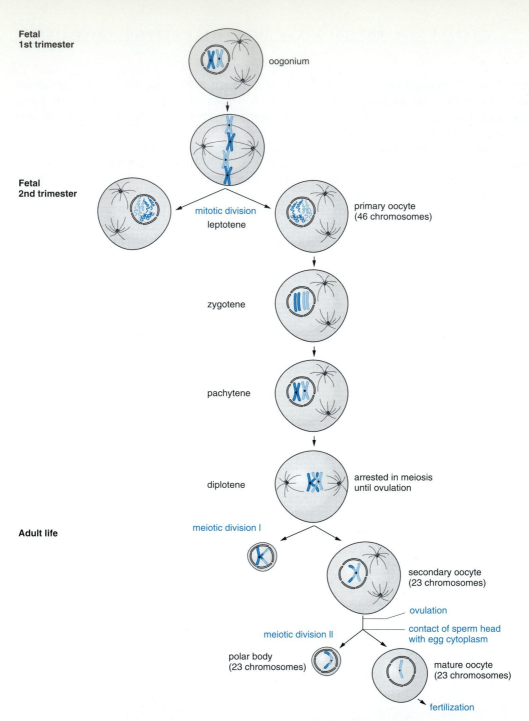

FIGURE 16.5. Oocyte meiosis. Primordial germ cells (oogonia) of the female fetus replicate early in pregnancy and enter meiosis late in the first trimester. Meiosis is arrested in the diplotene stage until ovulation, when the first meiotic division (reduction division) is completed, generating an oocyte with 23 chromosomes. The second meiotic division is completed after fertilization. A polar body accounting for the balance of replicated DNA not included in the oocyte is eliminated after each meiotic division. *(Adapted, with permission, from Speroff L, et al. (1994). Clinical Gynecological Endocrinology and Infertility, 5th ed. Baltimore, Williams & Wilkins, p. 990.)*

nourish the oocyte during its subsequent maturation in the adult, and probably play a role in arresting meiosis until ovulation. A basement membrane then develops, and another layer of spindle cells is recruited from the surrounding tissue. These cells will differentiate into the first of two layers of thecal cells, called the **theca interna**. The second layer of thecal cells, called the **theca externa**, will develop in adulthood. From birth to puberty there is a progressive loss of oocytes, so that by the time menstrual cycles start, only about 400,000 are left.

Puberty

From birth until puberty, the reproductive neuroendocrine axis is quiescent, with low levels of gonadotropins in the bloodstream (see Figure 16.4). Nevertheless, these low levels of luteinizing hormone (LH) and follicle-stimulating hormone (FSH) are necessary for subsequent proper adult reproductive function.

Puberty starts at approximately age 8 to 10 years in girls and 1 to 2 years later in boys. It is initiated by sufficient maturation of the hypothalamic gonadotropic releasing hormone (GnRH)–secreting neurons, which then display the characteristic adult pulsatile pattern of GnRH secretion. This pattern of GnRH secretion, in turn, activates the gonadotropes in the anterior pituitary to secrete more LH and FSH, with an increase in the LH-to-FSH ratio. In girls, the increased LH and FSH in turn activate the ovary, resulting in more estrogen production, which drives maturation of other tissues and development of secondary sexual characteristics. Breast development is one of the first signs of puberty. A growth spurt and, within 1 to 2 years, onset of menstrual cycles complete the transition to the adult pattern of reproductive axis function. The age at which the first menstrual period occurs is called **menarche**.

From puberty through the reproductive years, cohorts of 10 to 20 follicles are activated monthly by FSH. Whereas all oocytes that spontaneously activate prior to puberty are destined to degenerate and die, those that are activated at the start of the menstrual cycle have the potential to develop into a mature, fertilizable egg. This is a consequence of the hormonal environment of the adult female. Typically, only one follicle out of each monthly cohort will achieve this state of maturation. However, even in the follicle destined to form the mature egg, meiosis does not resume until ovulation, when the egg is released from the ovary. Whereas in the male, completion of meiosis results in four sperm, the product of one reduction division and one replication (see Figure 15.1), in the female, only one ovum is generated from each oocyte, with the excess genetic material extruded after each meiotic division and discarded (see Figure 16.5).

Clinical Pearls

○ It has been noted that the age of menarche has been falling over the last century in industrialized societies. Perhaps this is due to improved nutrition and earlier acquisition of adequate body fat stores. On the other hand, some argue that this is due to an effect of stress on hypothalamic maturation in the brain; others, that pollution of the environment with various toxins plays a role.

○ Chromosomal anomalies can accelerate the rate of oocyte loss. Thus, germ cell migration and mitosis is normal in patients with Turner's syndrome (45, X); however, meiosis does not occur, and accelerated oocyte loss results in a gonad that has no oocytes by birth and appears as nothing more than a fibrous streak.

Review Questions

5. Outline the female reproductive neuroendocrine axis.
6. What are the responses of the ovary to LH and FSH stimulation?
7. Approximately how many oocytes are present at the onset of puberty?
8. Approximately how many oocytes ovulate in total over a woman's 40-year reproductive lifetime?
9. Describe some changes that occur in the female with onset of puberty.

4. PHYSIOLOGY OF OVARIAN STEROIDS

Like the adrenal gland, the ovary is a massive steroid factory. The ovary secretes three types of steroids: some with 21 carbons, termed **progestins**; others with 19 carbons, termed the **androgens**; and some with 18 carbons, termed the **estrogens** (see Figure 16.6).

Steroid hormone synthesis occurs by conversion from cholesterol in a series of biochemical reactions catalyzed by enzymes in the mitochondrial membrane and in the endoplasmic reticulum. Generally, the rate-limiting step in steroid hormone production is side-chain cleavage of cholesterol within the mitochondrion to generate the basic steroid nucleus, which is further modified in the endoplasmic reticulum to generate the various steroid hormones. Because steroid hormones are synthesized by a cascade of enzyme reactions in various pathways, a block in one step (e.g., due to a congenital enzyme defect or due to inhibition by certain drugs) can result in lack of synthesis of one steroid and "spillover" of precursors into another. Conversely, induction of new enzyme activities can convert progestins to androgens or androgens to estrogens. Outside the ovary, it is possible to convert the 19-carbon androgens to 18-carbon estrogens by a process known as **peripheral aromatization**, but conversion in the reverse direction is not known to occur.

The major mechanism of estrogen action involves diffusion across the plasma membrane, binding to a receptor protein in the nucleus, and activation of transcription of specific genes by binding of the steroid-receptor complex to specific regions of DNA. The products of those genes, in turn, may activate or inhibit the transcription of yet other genes. In this way, the pattern of gene expression is changed in complex ways in the various steroid-responsive tissues (i.e., those that contain steroid hormone receptors).

Two different estrogen receptors have been identified. The classical estrogen receptor is called ER alpha. A newly discovered estrogen receptor, ER beta, has a different tissue distribution, and in at least some systems mediates the opposite effects on transcription to those observed for ER alpha. Most likely, this occurs because of differences in the transcription factors that the different estrogen receptors associate with when activated.

In addition, there may be membrane receptors for estrogen and for other steroids that work by other mechanisms, since some steroid hormone effects appear to be too rapid to be due to effects on transcription. These include feedback effects of estrogen on gonadotrophin secretion and some effects of estrogen on neuronal discharge in the brain.

Although steroids are physiological modulators of tissue phenotype through gene expression, modern medicine often uses them as pharmacologic agents. When they are used in this manner, certain of their effects are viewed as desirable, and others are considered undesirable side effects. Among the common pharmacologic uses of the ovarian steroids are **contraception** (prevention of

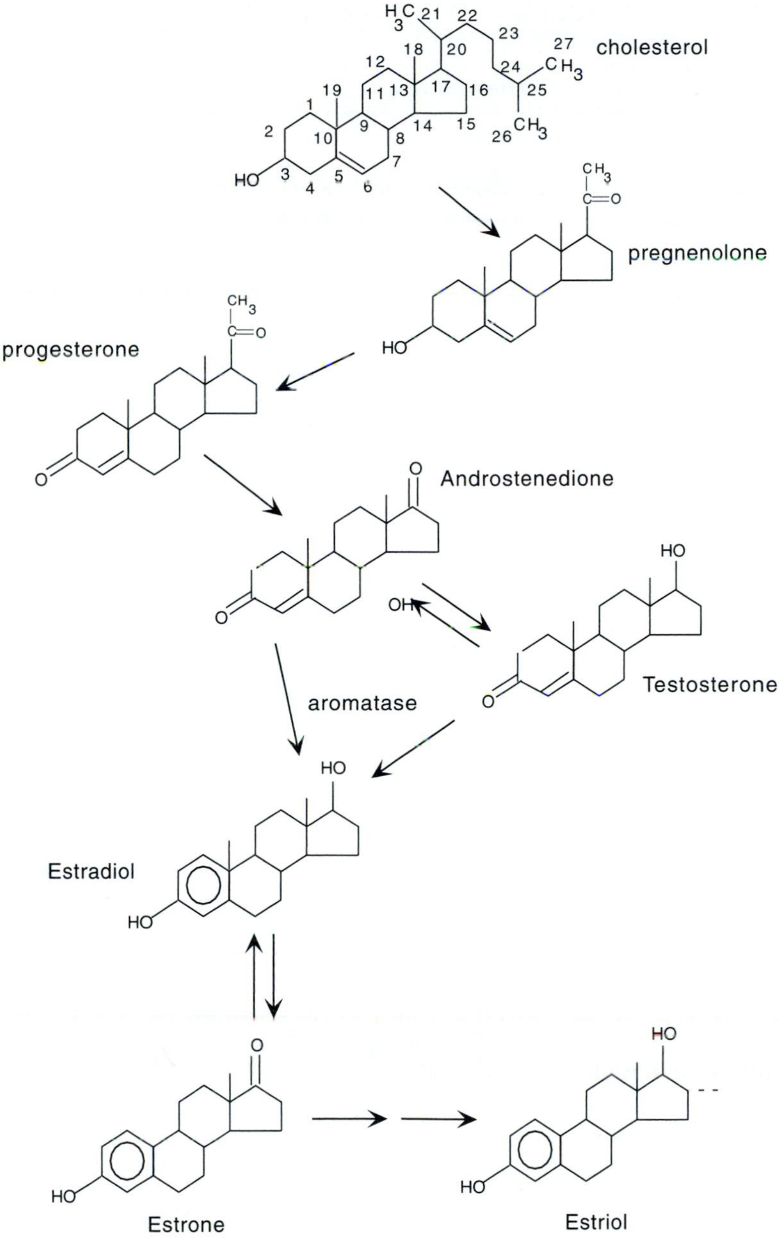

FIGURE 16.6. Steroid families of the female reproductive system. Note the numbering convention for the carbons in the cholesterol skeleton that is used for steroid synthesis. After side-chain cleavage to give pregnenolone in the mitochondria, subsequent steps in steroid biogenesis occur in the endoplasmic reticulum. How steroids shuttle between these two compartments of the cell is unknown. Androgens are converted to estrogens by the enzyme aromatase, involving two different pathways from androstenedione or testosterone. The latter pathway occurs largely in peripheral tissues (a process called peripheral aromatization) and is particularly significant in postmenopausal women and in men. Estradiol is the most active major estrogen secreted from the ovary. Estrone is less active. Estriol is a still less active metabolite of estrone. The full significance of the multiple pathways of steroid conversion to estrogen and antiestrogens has not yet been appreciated. (Adapted, with permission, from Speroff L, et al. (1994). Clinical Gynecological Endocrinology and Infertility, 5th ed. Baltimore, MD, Williams & Wilkins.)

pregnancy) and estrogen replacement after **menopause**, the point of cessation of menstrual periods. Estrogen replacement has some beneficial effects on estrogen-sensitive tissues, including augmentation of bone density. However, among the undesirable effects of estrogens is an increased risk of breast cancer. Table 16.4 summarizes the desired and undesired pharmacologic effects of estrogens and progestins.

TABLE 16.4　DESIRED AND UNDESIRED PHARMACOLOGIC EFFECTS OF ESTROGENS AND PROGESTINS

Estrogen	Progesterone
Desired	Desired
Maintenance of bone density	Contraception
Maintenance of health of estrogen-dependent tissues (e.g., vagina)	Cessation of dysfunctional uterine bleeding
Improved lipid profiles (increased HDL, decreased LDL)	Regression of endometrial cancer
Avoidance of menopausal symptoms (hot flashes, depression, etc.)	Undesired
Protection against dementia in the elderly	Possibly offsets beneficial effects of estrogen on cardiovascular system
Decreased autoimmune disease	Possible increased risk of breast cancer
Decreased ovarian cancer	Headache
Contraception	Weight gain
Undesired	Nausea
Thrombosis	Acne
Increased risk of breast and endometrial cancer	
Decreased breast milk production	

Estrogen action

The specific effects of estrogen on the hypothalamus and pituitary gland gonadotropes, the ovary, and the uterus will be discussed in Section 6, Menstrual Cycle. In addition, estrogen has profound effects on many other tissues. Some of these effects reinforce the goal of reproduction; others are more tangential. All are largely a consequence of estrogen versus testosterone predominance as the dominant sex steroid. These effects of estrogen on nonreproductive organs include:

- The development of almost all of the female secondary sexual characteristics, including breast development, pubic hair distribution in the typical female pattern, and enlargement of the labia majora and minora (external female genitalia).
- Linear growth. The earlier growth spurt of girls compared to boys is due to the greater sensitivity of the epiphysial plate to estrogen than to testosterone. But that also means that the epiphyses close sooner in the female, resulting in typically shorter final stature than in males. Also, the hips and pelvic inlet are enlarged in females, which facilitates future childbirth. Estrogens and androgens both inhibit bone resorption. Estrogens have both a direct action on osteoclasts and indirect effects suppressing cytokine production.
- Adipose tissue mass and distribution (e.g., in the hips). Adult females have about twice as much adipose tissue as adult males, but only two-thirds the muscle mass.
- Effects on blood lipids. For unclear reasons, estrogens elevate high-density lipoproteins (HDL) and lower low-density lipoproteins (LDL), thereby protecting against atherosclerosis.
- Effects on blood vessels. Estrogens are vasodilatory and antivasoconstrictive. In part this is an indirect effect that is due to promotion of nitric oxide and vasodilatory prostaglandins, and to a decrease in production of vasoconstrictors like endothelin 1.

Progesterone action

The actions of progesterone are less well understood than those of estrogen. Most important, progesterone is also believed to have immunosuppressive and muscle relaxant effects that are crucial for pregnancy (see Chap. 17).

Many of the effects of progesterone are on the central nervous system. Thus progesterone causes

- A 0.5°C rise in body temperature
- Increase in appetite
- Increase in sleepiness
- Increased sensitivity of the respiratory center to stimulation by carbon dioxide
- Feedback effects on LH and FSH secretion (in conjunction with the effects of estrogen; see Figure 16.7C).
- Antagonism of aldosterone action (and therefore promotion of natriuresis; see Chap. 10)

Peripheral metabolism of steroids

Within each class of steroids (see Figure 16.6) are molecules of a number of different specific structures. Many of these different forms of a given class of steroid have different spectra of activity, in terms of either affinity for the hormone receptor or being agonists versus antagonists of receptor binding. Sometimes different hormone-receptor complexes interact with different transcription factors, allowing them to turn on or off different sets of genes. Matters become further complicated by the fact that an activated estrogen receptor can bind different sequences with different affinities, depending on which steroid metabolite has activated the receptor and which accessory transcription factors (which differ from tissue to tissue) are bound. Thus it is possible for a given steroid to be an agonist of estrogen in one tissue and an antagonist of estrogen in another.

These observations have given rise to an entire industry of "designer" estrogen-like molecules that promise to allow a subset of desired effects of estrogen on one set of tissues without the undesired effects of estrogen on another set of tissues (see Ref. 12). Unfortunately, since there is an enormous amount we don't know or understand about steroids and their function, the full long-term implications of this pharmacologic approach for a diverse human population remain to be determined.

In some cases, particular modification enzymes allow particular forms to be made in particular tissues. Thus the presence of the enzyme **2-hydroxylase** allows the brain to make a class of compounds called **catecholestrogens** that are natural antiestrogens. They may have complex, tissue-specific effects — for example, interfering with negative feedback, thereby altering the sensitivity of the neuroendocrine axis at different points in the menstrual cycle.

Synthesis and activity of the modification enzymes and the transcription factors are independent of each other and of steroid production. Thus the possibilities for regulation of steroid hormone action are enormous and far beyond our current understanding of the potential for subtle differences in their action (see Sec. 9, Frontiers). In addition, many of these steroids undergo conjugation with sulfate and other molecules as part of their elimination.

Estradiol and estrone are weakly bound to steroid-binding globulin and albumin. Thus, the estrogens have shorter half-lives and a higher metabolic clearance rate than androgens such as testosterone, which are tightly bound to steroid-binding globulin.

Most of the estradiol in adult women in the reproductive years is derived from ovarian secretion, while the estrone is converted from estradiol by peripheral dehydrogenases. A small amount of estradiol comes from peripheral aromatization of testosterone in various sites, including adipose tissue and liver.

A major frontier for future work is understanding the physiological role of the mix of estrogen and progesterone metabolites generated in the body, which have various de-

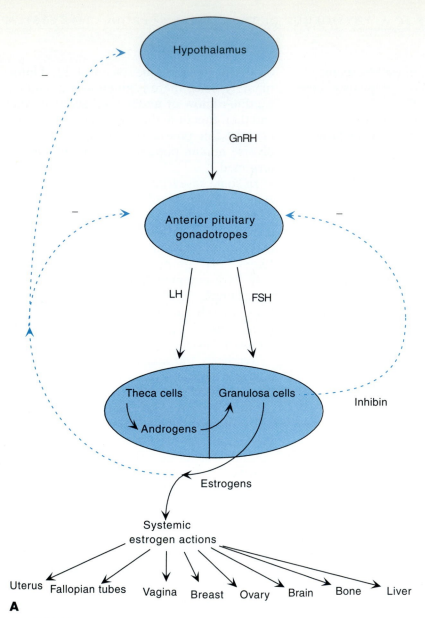

A

FIGURE 16.7. Female reproductive neuroendocrine feedback axis. *A.* The overall scheme of feedback regulation of the female reproductive neuroendocrine axis at the beginning of the menstrual cycle. Neurons in the arcuate nucleus of the hypothalamus make GnRH, which flows via the pituitary portal system to the anterior pituitary, where gonadotropes respond with LH and FSH secretion, which triggers androgen production in thecal cells and aromatase activity in granulosa cells, respectively. The androgens are aromatized to estrogens, which have effects on a myriad of peripheral tissues and also feedback-inhibit LH secretion by gonadotropes and GnRH secretion from the hypothalamus. Inhibin made by the granulosa cell feedback inhibits FSH production by the same gonodadotropes. Not shown in the diagram, FSH also activates a cohort of follicles (see text).

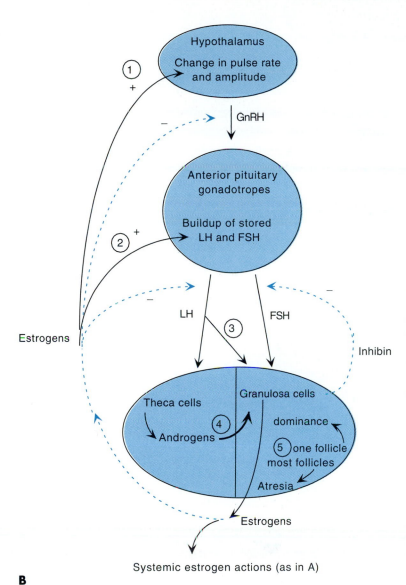

B

Systemic estrogen actions (as in A)

FIGURE 16.7 — (continued) B. The female reproductive neuroendocrine axis approaching mid-cycle. The axis is changed from that described in A in five ways (circled numbers). 1. Rising estrogen levels alter the pulse frequency and amplitude of GnRH secretion such that the pulse frequency goes down and the amplitude goes up. However, negative feedback over GnRH secretion is still maintained. 2. Rising estrogen levels promote a dissociation between gonadotropin synthesis and secretion, with synthesis (i.e., of LH and FSH) remaining at high levels although actual secretion is inhibited. As a result, LH and FSH levels build up within the pituitary. 3. Granulosa cells start to develop LH receptors. 4. Thecal androgen production increases (see text). 5. One follicle moves toward dominance while driving the other members of the cohort to atresia.

grees of activity. Likewise, the study of the effects of dietary intake of plant estrogenic compounds, called phytoestrogens, is an area of great current interest (see Ref. 13).

Clinical Pearls

○ Birth control pills are a pharmacologic means of inducing infertility by disrupting the precise timing of the hormone-directed events necessary for reproduction. Formulations include progestins alone and combinations of estrogens and progestins. Most preparations of estrogen and progesterone block the LH/FSH surge at mid-cycle, thereby preventing ovulation. However, their contraceptive actions also include effects on other estrogen- and progesterone-sensitive tissues, such as induc-

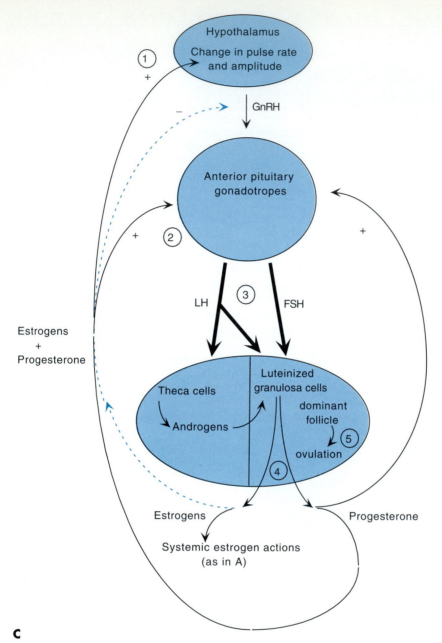

c

FIGURE 16.7 — (*continued*) *C.* Further change in the female reproductive neuroendocrine axis at mid-cycle. Circled numbers indicate five changes from the point depicted in *B.* 1. Continued estrogen effect plus the effect of progesterone on GnRH pulse frequency and amplitude. 2. Loss of the negative-feedback effect of estrogen, and its replacement by positive feedback effects. 3. Massive burst of LH and FSH secretion at mid-cycle. 4. As a consequence of the development of LH receptors, granulosa cells are said to be luteinized, meaning that they develop the ability to make the steroid progesterone. Granulosa cells continue to convert thecal androgen into estrogen. 5. With the mid-cycle surge, the final events of maturation of the dominant follicle are set in motion, culminating in ovulation (see text). The large rise in LH and FSH as a result of the events in *C* results in a correspondingly large burst of estrogen and progesterone secretion, which serves to reestablish negative feedback over the gonadotrope. With negative-feedback control reestablished, LH and FSH levels come crashing down, and the pattern described in *A* is reestablished. (*Adapted, with permission, from Ganong, WF (1997). Review of Medical Physiology, 18th ed. Stamford, CT, Appleton & Lange, p. 418.*)

ing changes in cervical mucus and the endometrial lining that are unfavorable to sperm transport and implantation. Over the years, the amount of estrogen contained in birth control pills has been decreased, and progestins have been added, in an attempt to mitigate unpleasant and dangerous side effects. Table 16.5 indicates the relative efficacy of various methods of contraception.

○ Recent powerful new pharmacologic contraceptives include mifepristone, also known as RU-486, a progesterone receptor antagonist, and methotrexate, an inhibitor of folate metabolism that blocks DNA synthesis and is particularly useful in termination of pregnancy either electively or when implantation has occurred in an inappropriate place, e.g., within the fallopian tubes (called an ectopic pregnancy).

TABLE 16.5 EFFICACY OF DIFFERENT METHODS OF CONTRACEPTION

Method	Failures per 100 woman-years
Vasectomy	0.02
Tubal ligation and similar procedures	0.13
Oral contraceptive	
>50 μg estrogen and progestin	0.32
<50 μg estrogen and progestin	0.27
Progestin only	1.2
IUD	
Copper 7	1.5
Loop D	1.3
Diaphragm	1.9
Condom	3.6
Withdrawal	6.7
Spermicide	11.9
Rhythm	15.5

From Ganong WF (1997). *Review of Medical Physiology,* 18th ed. Stamford, CT, Appleton & Lange, p. 418. Originally from Vessey M, et al. (1982). *Lancet* 1:841.

Review Questions

10. What is peripheral aromatization?
11. Name five estrogen-sensitive tissues and describe estrogen's effects.
12. Name five effects of progesterone on the central nervous system.
13. Which has higher affinity for steroid hormone-binding globulin, testosterone or estradiol?
14. What is the significance of 2-hydroxylase in the brain?

5. REPRODUCTIVE NEUROENDOCRINE AXIS

Normal female reproductive function involves a coordinated interaction of the hypothalamus, pituitary, ovary, and uterus under the influence of other organs, such as the liver (which makes steroid-binding globulin), adrenals, and thyroid gland. The functional anatomy of the female reproductive system is best approached as a neuroendocrine feedback axis (see Figure 16.7). The most striking feature of the female reproductive neuroendocrine axis is that it functions in an approximately monthly cyclic manner, as manifest by the menstrual cycle (see Sec. 6).

The peptide **gonadotropin-releasing hormone** is secreted in a particular pulsatile manner from the hypothalamus into the pituitary portal circulation. It stimulates certain cells in the anterior pituitary, termed **gonadotropes**. Gonadotropes respond to GnRH by secreting two polypeptide hormones known as gonadotropins, **luteinizing hormone** and **follicle-stimulating hormone**. The target tissues for LH and FSH are the ovaries, which make various steroids.

The basis for the cyclical character of ovarian function, in contrast to that of other neuroendocrine axes, is, in part, that the steroids produced by the ovaries do *more* than just feedback-inhibit secretion of the hormones higher up in the axis. They also promote changes in the expression of a number of genes over time within cells of the hypothalamus and anterior pituitary. This change in gene expression in response to ovarian steroids can be thought of as a kind of cyclical differentiation or maturation process. As a result of that process, the GnRH-secreting cells and the LH- and FSH-secreting gonadotropes respond to steroids differently from the way they did at the beginning of the cycle. As will be described in Sec. 6, several reinforcing mechanisms contribute to the cyclical nature of events in the hypothalamus, anterior pituitary, ovary, and uterus. Thus, for example, not only do the hypothalamus and the pituitary respond differently at different times in the cycle, the mix of hormones they see at those different times changes significantly, because maturation was also occuring in the ovary itself over the course of the cycle.

Because of these mechanisms, the female reproductive neuroendocrine axis, which starts off as described in Figure 16.7A, changes later to that described in Figure 16.7B, and then later to that described in Figure 16.7C, before returning to that of Figure 16.7A. These changes can best be understood by remembering that steroids induce not just one or two changes in gene expression, but rather a myriad of changes that affect many genes. As a result, both structure and function of various tissues are altered in a number of ways, as will be discussed in Sec. 6.

6. MENSTRUAL CYCLE

Complex interactions among the component organs of the female reproductive neuroendocrine axis (hypothalamus, pituitary, ovary, and uterus) give rise to the menstrual cycle.

Unlike in the other neuroendocrine axes, these interactions are not limited to those of a simple negative-feedback system. Two distinctive features are

1. The organs involved themselves undergo changes in response to the hormones released by the ovary. As a result, neither the structure nor the function of the hypothalamus, pituitary, ovary, or uterus at the middle of the menstrual cycle is the same as it is at the beginning.
2. In addition to blood-borne effects and feedback by hormones, important roles are played by local mediators, at least within the ovary, and probably within each of the other tissues as well. These local interactions reinforce the differentiation occurring in cells of the hypothalamus and pituitary, in response to the changing mix of ovarian steroids.

We will first consider each component of the axis and the ways in which the structure and function of that component change over the course of the menstrual cycle. Then we will survey over the course of one cycle how these changes relate to one another like a set of dominos falling in programmed sequence.

Hypothalamus and pituitary gland

At the beginning of a menstrual cycle, hypothalamic neurons manifest a particular pulse rate and amplitude of GnRH secretion, which translates into a particular pulse rate and amplitude of LH and FSH secretion. This triggers:

- Onset of maturation of a cohort of follicles
- Thecal cell androgen production
- Granulosa cell aromatase activity, and therefore conversion of thecal androgen to estrogen

• Secretion of inhibin. The estrogen and inhibin, in turn, feedback-inhibit both LH and FSH secretion, respectively, so their levels fall slightly over the course of the first half of the menstrual cycle.

Estrogen and progesterone affect the pulse rate and amplitude of GnRH secretion by neurons of the hypothalamus. The change from smaller, more frequent secretion of GnRH early in the cycle to larger, less frequent boluses later in the cycle, in turn, affects the gonadotropes of the anterior pituitary in two ways:

• Increased occupancy of the GnRH receptors in the presence of high concentrations of GnRH later in the cycle. As receptor occupancy increases, signaling from those receptors can change (e.g., first due to activation of additional signaling pathways, and later due to desensitization and other forms of adaptation that diminish signaling; see Chap. 3).
• Downregulation of receptors, like desensitization, is a form of adaptation that makes a cell resistant to subsequent stimulation.

Thus, late in the menstrual cycle, there is less effect of GnRH, even though there are higher levels of the hormone bathing the gonadotropes.

A result of estrogen action early in the menstrual cycle is that the gonadotropes start to make far more LH and FSH than they secrete. As a result, LH and FSH stores build up *within* the cells, reaching a peak at about mid-cycle (see Figure 16.7B).

At that point, the onset of progesterone secretion by the ovary transiently makes the gonadotrope less sensitive to negative feedback, and as a result there is a huge burst of LH and FSH secretion as the growing stored pool of LH and FSH is secreted en masse

(see Figure 16.7C). This is called the mid-cycle surge and serves as a trigger of ovulation. The subsequent large rise in estrogen production (as a consequence of the large burst of LH and FSH) reestablishes negative feedback over the gonadotropes (see Figure 16.7A), resulting in a fall in blood LH and FSH levels down to the low levels seen at the start of the cycle.

The preceding simple explanation largely accounts for what is observed in patients (see Figure 16.8), although our understanding and interpretation of the molecular mechanisms are likely to change in the future.

Ovary and follicular development

The events occurring in the ovary during the menstrual cycle are exceedingly complex. The function of most of the enormous range of products made by the ovary remains mysterious (see Table 16.1). What follows is a coherent story with which to make sense of the interactions occurring within the ovary; however, as was discussed in Chapter 1, scrutiny at deeper levels of detail reveals layer upon layer of additional complications.

The ovary responds to gonadotropins in several ways:

1. FSH promotes maturation of oocytes (see Figure 16.2). Under the influence of FSH, a cohort of follicles awaken from their quiescent state, and start to mature. Only one follicle in this cohort, called the **dominant follicle**, survives to complete the process, culminating in release of a fertilizable egg **(ovulation)**. The other activated follicles succumb along the way to a process of degeneration and death called **atresia**.
2. LH promotes androgen synthesis by thecal cells. The androgens then diffuse into the follicles, where they are converted into estrogens by the enzyme aromatase in granu-

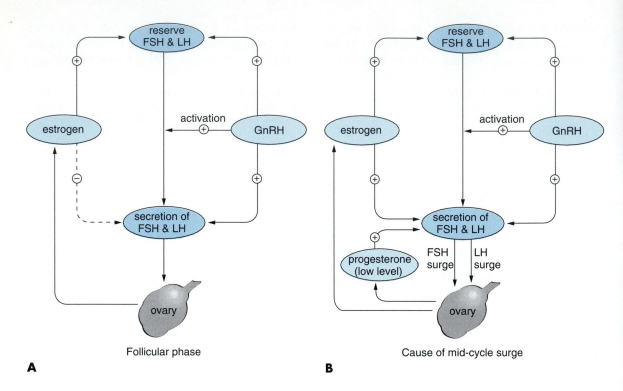

A

Follicular phase

B

Cause of mid-cycle surge

C

Self-limiting consequence of mid-cycle surge

FIGURE 16.8. Cycle of development in the hypothalamus and pituitary during the menstrual cycle. *A.* Schematic drawing indicating how estrogen from the ovary results in increased FSH and LH synthesis, even while it feedback-inhibits LH and FSH secretion. As a result, FSH and LH levels in the gonadotropes build up, so that a huge burst can be released when, in response to maturational changes induced by estrogen and progesterone, the gonadotropes are released from negative-feedback inhibition and secrete the large store of LH and FSH they have been accumulating (mid-cycle surge). *B.* This figure shows these interactions at mid-cycle, whereby estrogen and progesterone abrogate the negative-feedback response to estrogen (thereby allowing the surge in LH and FSH secretion). *C.* Subsequently, estrogen and progesterone at still higher doses have the effect of interrupting the previous effects of lower-dose estrogen and progesterone. As a result, reaccumulation of more intracellular LH and FSH in vesicles does not occur, thereby preventing another surge until reinitiation of a fresh cycle of follicular development. *(Adapted, with permission, from Speroff L, et al. (1994). Clinical Gynecological Endocrinology and Infertility, 5th ed. Baltimore, MD, Williams & Wilkins, pp. 166, 168, 169.)*

losa cells. The estrogen plays a key role in promoting maturation of the oocyte and diffuses out into the systemic circulation, where it has effects on many other target tissues, including feedback inhibition of LH secretion and other effects on the LH- and FSH-secreting cells in the pituitary gland.

3. FSH induces aromatase activity in granulosa cells, enhancing their ability to convert thecal androgens to estrogen. Another effect of FSH on granulosa cells, possibly due to estrogens, is the induction of more FSH receptors (the significance of which will be discussed in a later section).

4. The ovary initially responds to LH and FSH by feedback inhibition of further LH and FSH secretion at the level of both the hypothalamus and the pituitary gland. Two products made by the ovaries are primarily involved in feedback inhibition: the steroid estrogen, whose feedback inhibits primarily LH, and the protein inhibin, made by granulosa cells, whose feedback inhibits secretion of FSH.

response to estrogen and FSH) to maintain aromatase activity despite falling blood FSH levels. Thus, while the other follicles are driven to atresia, the dominant follicle stays ahead of the game and reaches maturity. Indeed, the dominant follicle actually *contributes* to driving the other follicles into atresia because the extra FSH receptors allow it to induce production of *more* inhibin, which further feedback-inhibits FSH, further starving the other follicles of the aromatase they need in order to convert androgen to estrogen (see Figure 16.9).

What allowed the dominant follicle to get the extra FSH receptors that allowed it to survive? It is not clear. Perhaps this is a case of survival of the fittest, where the most robust follicle is selected for ovulation. Alternatively, it may be dumb luck — whichever follicle happened to induce extra FSH receptors first, gets ahead of the others. In either event, once one follicle has a slight edge over the others, the consequence is predictable: The follicle with a slight edge proceeds to dominance; the others are driven into atresia. The rich get richer; the poor get poorer.

The struggle for dominance

A cycle starts with a small rise in FSH, which, like some kind of cellular alarm clock, triggers a cohort of follicles to awaken from decades-long dormancy and start to develop. The follicles enlarge, and secretions collect within a space called the **antrum** (see Figure 16.2).

A dramatic story unfolds within the ovary as each of the several follicles that have been activated struggles to become the dominant follicle that will achieve maturation and ovulate (Figure 16.9).

At some point, inhibin-mediated inhibition of FSH secretion starts to undermine the ability of most follicles to convert androgen to estrogen. At that point, only the dominant follicle has made enough FSH receptors (in

Luteinization

At the beginning of the cycle, granulosa cells have receptors only for FSH, while thecal cells have receptors for LH. One of the developmental changes that occurs in the ovary over the first half of the menstrual cycle is that granulosa cells, in response to estrogen, eventually develop LH receptors. Those LH receptors allow the granulosa cell to start making progesterone. This change in fundamental characteristics of the granulosa cell associated with onset of progesterone production, is termed **luteinization**.

Another effect of estrogen, progesterone, and innumerable local interactions occurring within the dominant follicle is the induction of new blood vessels. This has the effect of

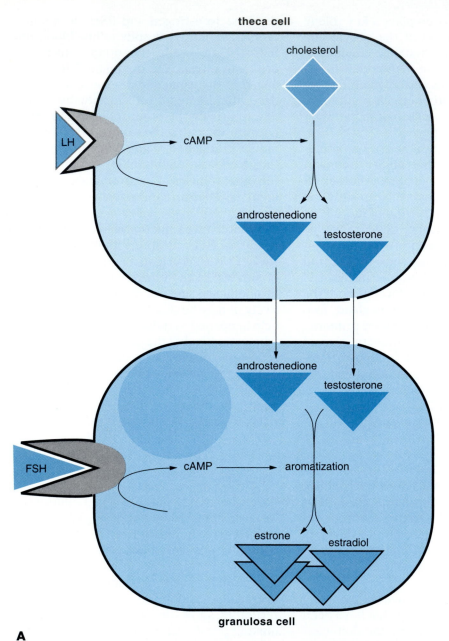

A

FIGURE 16.9. Struggle for dominance among activated ovarian follicles. Schematic of local interactions between thecal and granulosa cells that contribute to the emergence of one follicle as dominant while the others undergo atresia. A. The basic, initial interaction between thecal and granulosa cells. The thecal cells produce androgen in response to LH stimulation, and the granulosa cells respond to FSH by producing aromatase with which to convert thecal androgens into estrogens that support continued follicular development.

Early follicular phase

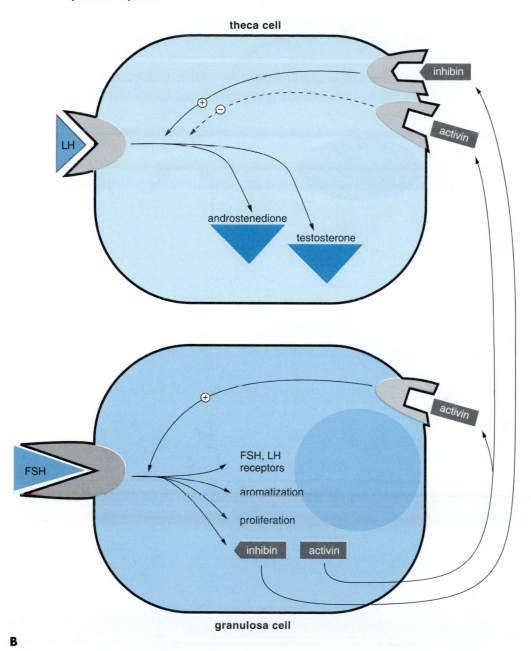

B

FIGURE 16.9 — (*continued*) *B.* An indication that the events in the early follicular phase are actually even more complex than was described in the text, and include opposing paracrine and autocrine actions of activin and inhibin. Since activin and inhibin come in multiple forms that are assembled from different combinations of common subunits, it is likely that their regulation is far more complicated than is described here.

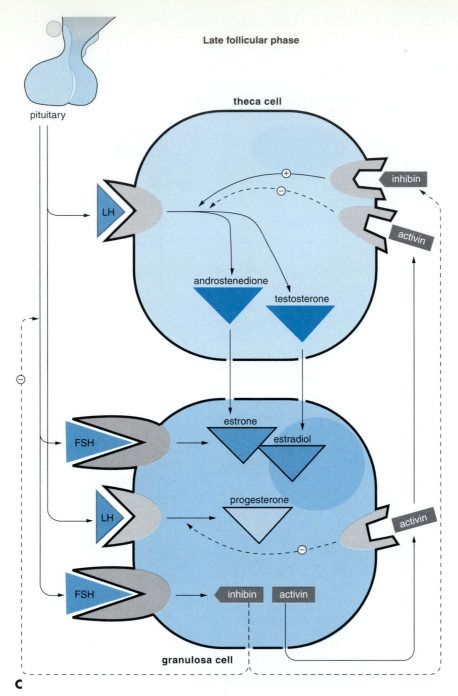

Late follicular phase

C

FIGURE 16.9 — (*continued*) C. The basis for emergence of the dominant follicle. Another effect of FSH on granulosa cells (besides induction of aromatase) is to induce more FSH receptors. These receptors allow the dominant follicle to maintain FSH stimulation of aromatase activity, even in the face of falling FSH concentration in the bloodstream, as a result of negative feedback by the rising estrogen concentration. Thus, the dominant follicle continues to grow, produce more estrogen, and further inhibit FSH secretion, while the other follicles are driven into atresia by thecal androgens and their inability to maintain enough aromatase activity because of falling FSH concentrations. (*Adapted, with permission, from Speroff L, et al. (1994). Clinical Gynecological Endocrinology and Infertility, 5th ed. Baltimore, MD, Williams & Wilkins, pp. 188, 204, 205.*)

changing the local environment within the oocyte, and efficiently transporting oocyte products into the systemic circulation.

Finally, the mid-cycle surge of LH and FSH may be important in triggering changes, including induction of proteases, necessary for rupture of the dominant follicle and release of the mature egg.

The onset of progesterone secretion, added to the high level of estrogen being secreted, is one of the cues to the hypothalamus and pituitary to be transiently released from negative feedback to carry out the mid-cycle surge (see the preceding section). The mid-cycle surge, in turn, provides the final push needed for release of the mature egg. Thus, luteinization links the cycle of development involving the hypothalamus and pituitary to that of the ovary in a way that allows both to move forward.

Formation of a corpus luteum

Ovulation occurs at mid-cycle, after which, probably in response to the LH surge, what is left of the dominant follicle (residual granulosa and thecal cells without their oocyte which has matured and been released) forms a new endocrine structure, the corpus luteum (see Figure 16.10). The corpus luteum is geared up for progesterone production in response to LH. It is the rising progesterone from the corpus luteum that drives subsequent changes in the uterus (see the following discussion). Figure 16.11 presents one view of how the complex interactions of autocrine and paracrine products such as the insulin-like growth factors (IGFs) may contribute to the story of ovarian follicular development.

In the absence of implantation, the fall in LH and FSH induced by reestablishment of negative feedback on the hypothalamus and pituitary removes the support for the corpus luteum, and it will degenerate after a 14-day

life span. However, if implantation and pregnancy do occur, the corpus luteum will be sustained by other means for an additional number of weeks, until the *placenta* is fully developed as a progesterone factory (see Chap. 17).

Uterus and endometrial development

The endometrium of the uterus is an estrogen-sensitive tissue. In response to estrogen, whose levels rise throughout the first half of the menstrual cycle, the endometrium proliferates. This involves not only hyperplasia of the tissue, but also growth of blood vessels to support that extra tissue. The blood vessels are peculiar in being extremely dependent on estrogen. Some of them are coiled (and hence called spiral arteries). In addition, the proliferated endometrium secretes thin, watery mucus from glands throughout its depth. These secretions facilitate sperm movement into the fallopian tubes. This is called the **proliferative phase** (see Figure 16.3).

With the onset of progesterone secretion, the proliferated endometrium undergoes a change in differentiated characteristics such that the secretions are thicker and more viscous. In the days following the mid-cycle surge, when progesterone levels reach their maximum, the glands become engorged and tortuous, filled with these thick secretions. These conditions now are a tremendous impediment to sperm movement, but are ideal for implantation of a fertilized egg. This is called the *secretory phase* (see Figure 16.3). As in the ovary, many complex actions and interactions of local mediators are involved in the cyclical function of the endometrium (see Table 16.2).

If implantation and pregnancy occur, the same events [i.e., production of human chorionic gonadotropin (hCG) by the developing placenta] that will intervene to maintain the corpus luteum will also maintain the endome-

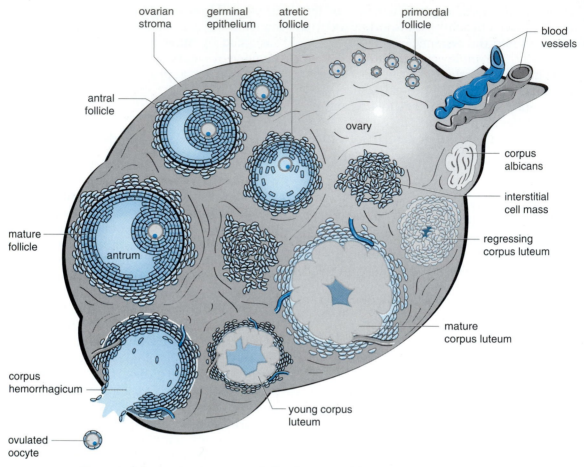

FIGURE 16.10. Stages in follicular development, including formation of the corpus luteum. Diagram of a mammalian ovary showing the sequential development of a follicle, formation of a corpus luteum, and follicular atresia. A section of the wall of a mature follicle is enlarged at the upper right. Note that all stages would not be seen at the same time; rather, a cohort of follicles would initiate as primordial follicles, with most being diverted to atresia prior to one follicle (the dominant one) reaching the stage of an antral follicle. The dominant follicle eventually ruptures at mid-cycle, releasing the mature egg and developing into a corpus luteum, which is optimized for progresterone production (see Fig. 16.9). *(Adapted, with permission, from Gorbman A, Bern H (1962). Textbook of Comparative Endocrinology. New York, Wiley.)*

trium. However, in the absence of implantation and pregnancy, the fall in pituitary LH that resulted in degeneration of the corpus luteum will remove the estrogen and progesterone support needed to maintain the endo-

metrium. In the absence of sufficient estrogen and progesterone, the spiral arteries undergo vasospasm and the endometrium becomes ischemic, necrotic, and finally sloughs, giving rise to menstrual bleeding.

Early follicular phase

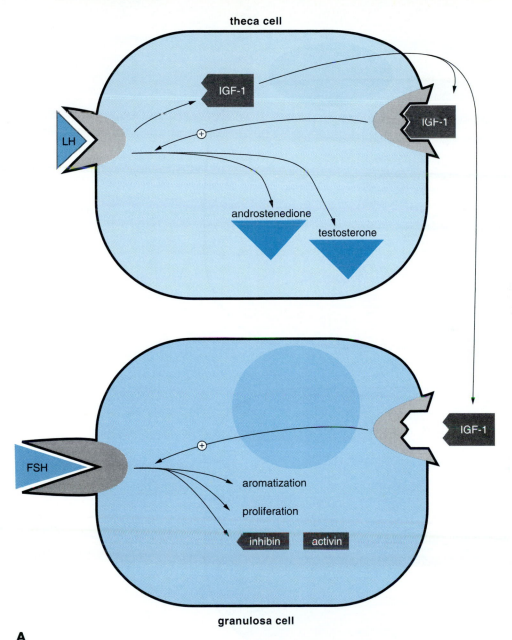

A

FIGURE 16.11. The role of IGFs in follicular development. Mechanisms can be viewed at many levels of complexity. The relatively simple story involving LH and FSH has already been complicated by local effects of activin and inhibin (see Figure 16.8). Here we see that it is further complicated by effects of IGFs. A. Schematic diagram of how IGF-1 reinforces the effect of LH on androgen production by thecal cells (an autocrine effect) and the effects of FSH on aromatase production by granulosa cells (a paracrine effect).

Preovulatory follicle

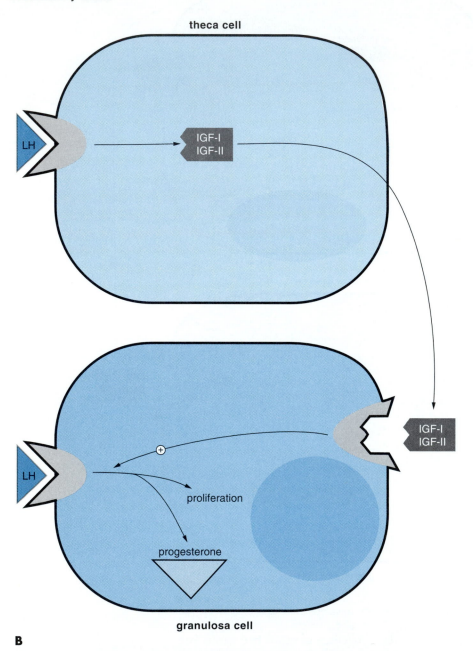

B

FIGURE 16.11 — (*continued*) *B.* Schematic diagram of how IGFs I and II act in a paracrine manner on granulosa cells late in the follicular phase (when the granulosa cells have started to express LH receptors) to stimulate the capacity for proliferation and progesterone production.

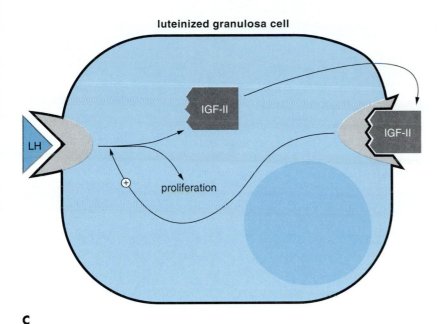

luteinized granulosa cell

C

FIGURE 16.11 — *(continued)* C. In the luteal phase, IGF-II acts in an autocrine manner to stimulate proliferation and maintain its own secretion. *(Adapted, with permission, from Speroff L, et al. (1994). Clinical Gynecological Endocrinology and Infertility, 5th ed. Baltimore, MD, Williams & Wilkins, p. 197.)*

Timing of hypothalamic–pituitary–ovarian–uterine interactions

In the preceding sections, the events in the menstrual cycle were considered from the point of view of each of the components of the female reproductive neuroendocrine axis. Here we will consider the menstrual cycle as a whole over time (see Figure 16.12). The menstrual cycle can be broken into three phases: a follicular phase from the point of activation of a cohort of follicles to the mid-cycle gonadotropin surge; a mid-cycle phase around the gonadotropin surge, culminating in ovulation; and a luteal phase from ovulation until onset of menses, when a new cohort of follicles is activated.

Follicular phase to mid-cycle

At the point of onset of menses, blood estrogen, progesterone, LH, FSH, and inhibin lev-els have reached their lowest point in the cycle. In response to the low levels of inhibin, blood levels of FSH increase (see 1 in Figure 16.12A). This rise in blood FSH concentration is believed to be the molecular basis for the alarm clock that triggers activation of a new cohort of follicles.

As the follicle develops, the augmentation of aromatase activity and FSH receptors discussed previously sets up a form of positive feedback that heightens follicular development. Many other ovarian follicular products are surely involved, and the details of autocrine, paracrine, and other local interactions in the ovary are likely to prove dauntingly complex (see Sec. 9, Frontiers).

Eventually, one follicle achieves dominance and in that process drives the other activated follicles into atresia. It does this by making more estrogen and inhibin than any other follicle. The estrogen induces FSH re-

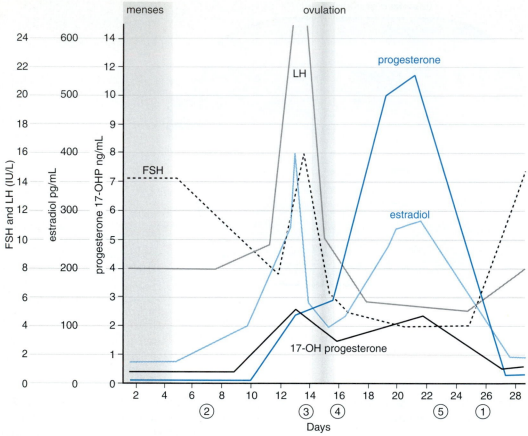

A

FIGURE 16.12. Hormonal changes over the menstrual cycle. A. Changes in hormone levels over the course of a menstrual cycle that does not culminate in pregnancy. Circled numbers at the bottom correspond to the numbers referred to in the text. B. Changes in hormone levels over the course of a menstrual cycle that culminates in pregnancy. Note that progesterone levels are maintained as a result of survival of the corpus luteum due to human chorionic gonadotropin (hCG), which replaces the supportive action of LH. LH has fallen as a result of reestablishment of negative feedback by the high levels of estrogen and progesterone being produced. hCG continues to maintain the corpus luteum for the first 6 to 10 weeks of pregnancy, until the placenta has matured as a progesterone production factory. The x axis shows days of the cycle in A and continues with weeks of pregnancy in B. C. Qualitative description of the events that occur in the polycystic ovary syndrome (PCO), in which the seesaw of oscillating LH/FSH and estrogen/progesterone is disrupted, presenting a picture of relatively high levels of androgens and low levels of estrogens (see text). (Adapted, with permission, from Speroff L, et al. (1994). Clinical Gynecological Endocrinology and Infertility, 5th ed. Baltimore, MD, Williams & Wilkins, pp. 191, 216, 463.)

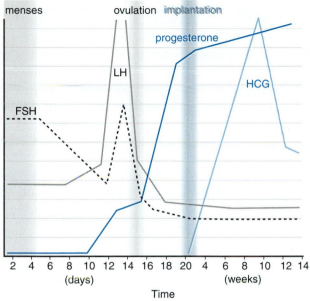

B

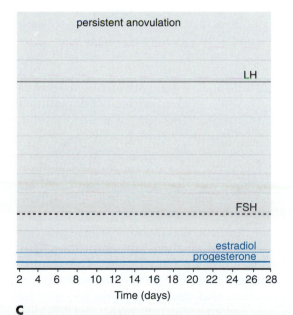

C

FIGURE 16.12 — (*continued*)

ceptors on the dominant follicle, and there-fore more of the enzyme aromatase. The in-hibin increases androgen production in thecal cells. The dominant follicle can survive the increased androgen production because of its increased aromatase activity, while the other follicles are driven into atresia by the rising androgen levels.

Inhibin also feedback-inhibits FSH pro-duction from the pituitary gland. As FSH falls in response to this feedback inhibition, the other follicles, which have fewer FSH recep-tors, than the dominant follicle are left with insufficient aromatase activity to convert the rising level of thecal androgen to estrogen. Only the dominant follicle has enough FSH receptors to continue to maintain aromatase activity and follicular development despite the falling blood FSH levels. Thus, the domi-nant follicle avoids the atresia to which the other follicles succumb. Moreover, the domi-nant follicle proceeds toward full maturation (see 2 in Figure 16.12A).

Once dominance is achieved, the granu-losa cells of the maturing dominant follicle start to display LH receptors, which were pre-viously found only on thecal cells. This is probably another effect of estrogen. The LH receptors, when activated, cause the granu-losa cells to make progesterone. The onset of progesterone secretion in the context of high blood estrogen triggers the mid-cycle surge of LH and FSH secretion from the pitu-itary, in conjunction with maturation of cells in the hypothalamus. This results in an al-tered GnRH pulse rate and amplitude (see Figure 16.7C).

The mid-cycle surge (see 3, Figure 16.12) is the exclamation point that follows the fol-licular phase, in that it triggers ovulation. The length of the follicular phase is somewhat variable, from 9 to 23 days, reflecting that it can take more or less time for follicular maturation and to synchronize events at the hypothalamus, pituitary, ovary, and uterus. Furthermore, the functions of the hypothala-mus and ovary are interconnected (e.g., by

LH, FSH, estrogen and progesterone) such that if one of them has not, for whatever reason, progressed to the appropriate level of development for that point in the cycle, further development of the other will be de-layed in order to allow "catch-up." When this proper feedback coordination is disordered or impaired, reproductive system dysfunc-tion, such as anovulatory cycles, occurs (see Sec. 8).

Mid-cycle phase to luteal phase

The mid-cycle phase lasts 1 to 3 days, culmi-nating in ovulation. After ovulation, the cor-pus luteum is formed, tremendously increas-ing the progesterone output of the ovary, which drives the maturation of the endome-trium (see 4 in Figure 16.12A). The huge burst of estrogen and progesterone synthesis in the wake of the mid-cycle LH and FSH surge also serves to reestablish negative feed-back on the hypothalamus and pituitary gland (whose stores of LH and FSH were depleted at the mid-cycle surge). As a result both of reestablishment of negative feedback by es-trogen and progesterone, and of depletion of LH (and FSH) stores, there is a sharp fall in LH (and FSH) secretion. But LH is necessary for the maintenance and survival of the cor-pus luteum (see 5 in Figure 16.12A). Without the support of LH or an LH-like hormone, the corpus luteum will degenerate, after a fairly precise 13-day life span. With degenera-tion of the corpus luteum, estrogen and pro-gesterone production fall, and the support for the endometrium is gone. The result is menstrual flow. The fall in estrogen and pro-gesterone that causes ischemia and necrosis of the endometrium (i.e., menstrual flow) also removes the negative-feedback inhibition on LH and FSH secretion. The resulting rise in LH and FSH marks the beginning of the next cycle of ovarian follicular development (see 1 on Figure 16.12A).

If implantation and pregnancy occur, a new hormone is produced by the early, developing placenta. Called human chorionic go-nadotropin (hCG), this protein is highly ho-mologous in structure to LH, and thus serves to replace LH in maintaining the corpus lu-teum. For nearly 3 months, the placenta makes hCG and thereby supports the corpus luteum until the placenta's own progester-one-secreting capacity is fully established (see Figure 16.12B and Chap. 17).

Review Questions

15. Describe the changes in the hypothala-mus and pituitary over the course of the menstrual cycle.
16. How does one follicle out of a cohort become dominant?
17. What is the fate of the nondominant follicles?
18. When during the menstrual cycle is the corpus luteum formed? What is its role?
19. Why is the follicular phase of the men-strual cycle more variable in length than the luteal phase?
20. What events of the menstrual cycle are responsible for menstrual bleeding?

7. MENOPAUSE

Menopause is the point in an adult female's life when menstrual cycles cease. It is likely that menopause represents not just the ex-haustion of follicles from the ovary, but also the aging of the various pacemakers in the brain and the ovary that normally regulate the menstrual cycle (see Sec. 6 and Ref. 3).

After approximately the age of 30, long before menopause, reproductive function starts to diminish. As age 50 is approached, there is decreased frequency of ovulation, with atrophy of the reproductive organs. Dur-ing this time, culminating in menopause, GnRH-stimulated LH and FSH secretion

does not result in as much estrogen secretion as in earlier reproductive years, in part be-cause of the relative paucity of follicles. Hence the cyclic changes in estrogen-depen-dent tissues diminish and estrogen-depen-dent tissues atrophy as a consequence of es-trogen deficiency. Also during this time, LH and FSH levels gradually rise, as a result of the decrease in negative feedback as blood estrogen and inhibin levels fall. This period of diminished reproductive function ap-proaching menopause is termed the **climac-teric period**. During the climacteric transition from the cyclic high-estrogen state to the low-estrogen postmenopausal state, **vasomotor symptoms** such as hot flashes, sweating, and chills and psychological symptoms such as ir-ritability, tension, anxiety, and depression can be observed.

Later, after the menopause, additional, more insidious changes occur. In addition to atrophy of various estrogen-dependent tis-sues such as the vaginal epithelium, these changes include a gradual loss in bone density called **osteoporosis**.

A significant degree of androgen produc-tion from thecal cells of the residual ovarian stroma continues even in the absence of folli-cles. Even in postmenopausal women, ovar-ian and adrenal androgens can be aromatized into estrogens by adipose tissue and hair folli-cles. The extent to which peripheral aromati-zation can affect the severity of symptoms of menopause remains to be determined. This may explain the variability of postmeno-pausal symptoms from one woman to an-other.

Review Questions

21. What are the symptoms of menopause?
22. What is the source of the estrogen found in the bloodstream of postmeno-pausal women who are not on estrogen replacement therapy?

23. What is the change in LH and FSH levels from before puberty to during the reproductive years to postmenopause?

8. CLINICAL PHYSIOLOGY OF FEMALE REPRODUCTIVE SYSTEM DISORDERS

A large number of female reproductive disorders can be traced back to a particular level of the neuroendocrine feedback axis, and thus can be categorized as resulting from central (pituitary, hypothalamus, or higher centers with influence over the hypothalamus), ovarian, or uterine dysfunction.

Presentation of female reproductive system disorders

Disorders of the female reproductive system occur as a result of pathology involving one of the reproductive organs (e.g., ovaries, uterus, fallopian tubes, vagina, breast) or involving organs whose function affects reproductive organs (e.g., brain, thyroid, adrenals, kidney, liver). Typically, many female reproductive system disorders present during reproductive years as *altered menstruation* or as *infertility* (i.e., inability to become pregnant) and can be either painful or painless.

Disorders of reproductive function that are a consequence of disease in nonreproductive organs (e.g., hypothyroidism) are typically painless. Intrinsic disease of the reproductive organs can present either painlessly or with pain. Often, pain does not occur until disease is far advanced, owing to the location and structure of reproductive organs. Some of these organs are deep and relatively inaccessible (e.g., ovary); others contain large amounts of adipose tissue (e.g., breast) or a paucity of sensory nerve endings (e.g., ovary, fallopian tubes). These features contribute

significantly, for example, to the high mortality and widespread metastases often associated with certain female reproductive system cancers, such as ovarian cancer. Whereas the introduction of the Papanicolaou smear as an early diagnostic test dramatically lowered the mortality from cervical cancer, the mortality from ovarian cancer has remained high.

Consequences and complications of disease

The reproductive system and its hormones are involved in other functions besides reproduction, including maintenance and health of various tissues. Thus, in addition to menstrual disorders and infertility, the consequences of reproductive system function disorder can include **osteoporosis** (loss of bone mass), atrophy and inflammation of estrogen-deprived tissues, an increased risk of some forms of **cancer**, and unique variants of systemic disorders such as **gestational diabetes mellitus** and the hypertensive syndrome of **preeclampsia** (see Chap. 17).

Disorders of central/hypothalamic/pituitary function

Any change in the precise rate and amplitude of GnRH secretion by the hypothalamus can result in altered pituitary responsiveness (e.g., downregulation of GnRH receptors or altered gonadotropin secretion), and hence altered ovarian functions (e.g., inadequate steroidogenesis with or without ovulation) and altered target tissue response (e.g., menstrual abnormalities).

Because many central and peripheral inputs affecting pulsatile GnRH release are integrated at the hypothalamus, amenorrhea due to altered GnRH release is extremely common in response to conditions ranging from psychogenic stress to low body fat content. The resulting low blood levels of

LH/ FSH, and therefore low estrogen, can result in clinically significant osteoporosis.

Disorders of the ovary

Proper ovarian function involves responsiveness to gonadotropins, intrinsic viability of follicles, and a host of paracrine interactions within and between individual follicles that are poorly understood.

If the level of estrogen produced is insufficient, the threshold needed to trigger the mid-cycle surge and ovulation may not be reached. The result is an **anovulatory cycle**, characterized by the lack of a luteal phase. This can also occur if the level of estrogen never fell low enough to release FSH from negative-feedback inhibition at the end of the previous cycle.

The **polycystic ovary syndrome (PCO)** is an example of anovulatory ovarian dysfunction caused by a self-perpetuating cycle of altered feedback relationships and altered ovarian structure. PCO is often triggered by weight gain or some other cause of increased insulin resistance (see Chap. 6). One possible mechanism is that the higher blood insulin levels that are present in an insulin-resistant state alter protein synthesis by the liver, so that blood levels of steroid hormone–binding globulin (SHBG) and insulin-like growth factor binding protein (IGFBP-1) decrease. These changes impinge on the ovary and the periphery (see Figure 16.13), resulting in increased local IGF-1 activity (in the absence of sufficient IGF-BP1). The increase in IGF-1 results in an increase in ovarian androgen production (see Figure 16.11A). The decrease in SHBG results in increased peripheral free (unbound) androgen levels. Together, these changes disorder the normal hormonal seesaw, giving constant high androgen levels, anovulation, hirsuitism (due to androgen effects, see Chap. 15), infertility, and either abnormal uterine bleeding or amenor-rhea characteristic of PCO syndrome (see Figure 16.13).

Sometimes anovulatory cycles can occur as a result of systemic endocrine disorders such as hyperprolactinemia or hypothyroidism. TRH can stimulate prolactin secretion, so hypothyroidism can sometimes manifest as hyperprolactinemia. Onset of these disorders can be slow and insidious, manifest as a continuum of conditions (see Figure 16.14).

Individuals who have anovulatory cycles frequently are at increased risk of endometrial cancer and possibly breast cancer.

Excessive atresia can result in exhaustion of the supply of oocytes before the expected time of menopause, a condition known as **premature ovarian failure**.

Figure 16.15 provides a comprehensive physiological approach to the evaluation of ammenorrhea.

Disorders of the uterus and fallopian tubes and the vagina

Since normal menstrual bleeding is most directly a function of the growth state of the uterine endometrium, disorders of the uterus — including fibroids, which are benign tumors of the underlying myometrium, and cancer of the endometrium itself — often present with abnormal vaginal bleeding.

Pelvic infections can produce adhesions and scarring of the uterus or fallopian tubes, which result in chronic pain and infertility.

Endometriosis often occurs when viable endometrial cells present in menstrual flow are seeded into the peritoneal space or elsewhere. These can generate foci of ectopic endometrial tissue, resulting in cycles of growth and necrosis with associated inflammation and pain.

Estrogen deficiency in postmenopausal women may present as dryness, irritation, and inflammation of estrogen-dependent tissues,

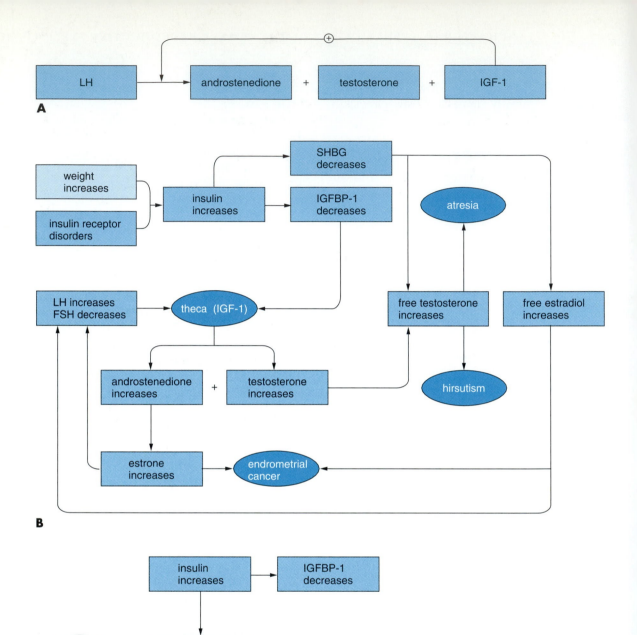

FIGURE 16.13. Pathophysiology of anovulation and polycystic ovary syndrome. The polycystic ovary syndrome is characterized by anovulation, infertility, hirsutism, and obesity. *A.* How IGF-1 stimulates thecal androgen production. *B.* How insulin resistance promotes more thecal IGF-1 and other features of hormone dysregulation in PCO syndrome. *C.* How hyperinsulinemia also affects the endometrium, increasing the risk of endometrial cancer. *(Adapted, with permission, from Speroff L, et al. (1994). Clinical Gynecological Endocrinology and Infertility, 5th ed. Baltimore, MD, Williams & Wilkins, pp. 470, 474–475.)*

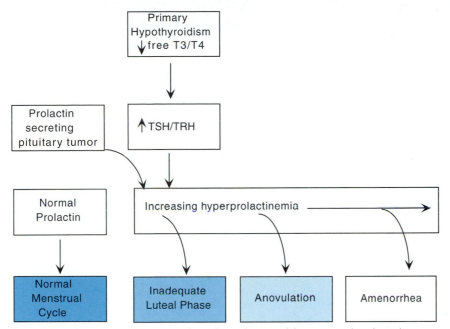

FIGURE 16.14. Hyperprolactinemia, hypothyroidism, and the menstrual cycle. Relationship of thyroid failure or pituitary prolactin-secreting tumor to menstrual disorders is presented. In primary hypothyroidism, $T_{3/4}$ levels are low and thyroid-stimulating hormone and thyroid-releasing hormone levels are high. Thyroid-releasing hormone is also a stimulus to prolactin secretion, so prolactin levels are high. Prolactin inhibits GnRH pulses, so depending on how high the prolactin is, you can see a continuum of menstrual disorders from shortened luteal phase to anovulation, or even frank amenorrhea. *(Adapted, with permission, from Speroff L, et al. (1994). Clinical Gynecological Endocrinology and Infertility, 5th ed. Baltimore, MD, Williams & Wilkins.)*

including the vagina, with increased susceptibility to infection.

In contrast, patients with estrogen excess, whether they are pre- or postmenopausal, may develop dysfunctional uterine bleeding, with increased risk of endometrial cancer.

Disorders of the breast

Intrinsic disorders of the breast are either malignant (i.e., breast cancer) or benign (e.g., fibroadenoma). Breast disease can also occur as a result of effects of other disorders or drug therapy, as in **galactorrhea** in either men or women and in **gynecomastia** in men.

The breast, like the uterus and other estrogen- and progesterone-responsive tissues, displays cyclic changes in concert with alterations in the level of ovarian steroids through the menstrual cycle. Subtle imbalances in the relative levels of estrogen and progesterone achieved have been considered a possible basis not only for endometrial dysfunction (infertility due to inadequate luteal phase progesterone support of the secretory endometrium), but for so-called benign breast "disease" as well. This term refers to abnormalities on a poorly defined continuum that has normal premenstrual breast tenderness relieved with menstruation at one extreme

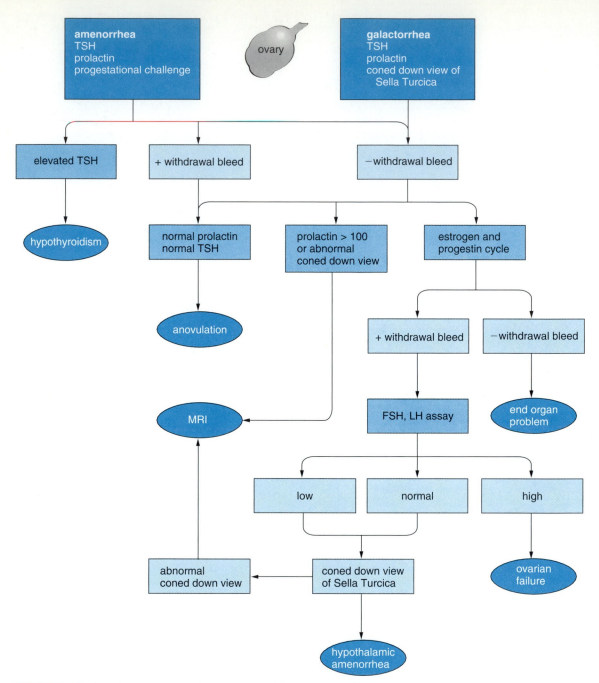

FIGURE 16.15. Physiological approach to evaluation of amenorrhea. If the patient presents with amenorrhea, the initial workup includes determination of serum TSH, prolactin, and response to several day treatments with progesterone. Outcome of those studies (and of head CT to rule out pituitary adenoma in a patient with galactorrhea) initiates a physiologically rational algorithm, as indicated, that culminates in a presumptive diagnosis. *(Adapted, with permission, from Speroff L, et al. (1994). Clinical Gynecological Endocrinology and Infertility, 5th ed. Baltimore, MD, Williams & Wilkins, p. 416.)*

and so-called **fibrocystic disease**, in which both fibrosis and cysts are present in association with mammary epithelial hyperplasia, at the other extreme. Normal tissue may have either fibrosis or cysts, but should not show epithelial cell hyperplasia. Thus, true fibrocystic disease with epithelial cell hyperplasia is a risk factor for breast cancer in much the same manner that endometrial hyperplasia due to unopposed estrogen action is a risk factor for endometrial cancer.

Review Questions

24. How do female reproductive system disorders present during reproductive years?
25. To what might you ascribe the lack of improvement in mortality from ovarian cancer in contrast to that from cervical cancer?
26. Why is a properly functioning reproductive system important even for women who never want to have children?
27. What are some central nervous system causes of menstrual disorders?
28. Are fibrocystic changes a risk factor for breast cancer?

Disorders of sexual differentiation

Under certain circumstances, aberrations can occur during embryogenesis that alter the normal course of events in chromosomal, gonadal, and phenotypic sexual development. Aberrations in chromosomal sex include **Klinefelter's syndrome** (47 XXY) and **Turner's syndrome** (45 X). Individuals with Klinefelter's syndrome have a male phenotype, but with infertility, breast enlargement, small testes, and decreased sperm as a result of incomplete virilization. Individuals with Turner's syndrome are phenotypic females with primary amenorrhea, lack of secondary sexual characteristics, short stature, multiple congenital anomalies and failure to develop gonads.

An example of altered gonadal sex is the syndrome of pure **gonadal dysgenesis**. These individuals do not develop gonads and have an immature female phenotype, but, unlike those with Turner's syndrome, they are of normal height, have no associated somatic defects, and have a normal male or female karyotype. Also unlike patients with Turner's syndrome, who have a single X chromosome, patients who have a normal karyotype, 46 XY, with gonadal dysgenesis are believed to have mutations in specific genes needed for male development.

Disorders of phenotypic sex include female and male **hermaphroditism**, where an individual has both ovarian and testicular tissue, either mixed or separate. **Pseudohermaphroditism** results from exposure of female embryos to excessive androgens during sexual differentiation or from defects in androgen synthesis or tissue sensitivity in male embryos, so that the external and internal genitalia are of different sexes.

Disorders of menopause

With the approach of menopause, the menstrual cycles become longer, reflecting an increase in the length of the follicular phase and a decrease in inhibin production, and resulting in decreased fertility. As follicles become completely depleted, estrogen levels fall and gonadotropin levels rise because of lack of feedback inhibition. Typically this results in symptoms of estrogen deficiency. Why some women have very mild perimenopausal symptoms while others find the symptoms debilitating is not known. One approach to managing disorders of menopause is hormone replacement therapy, which has both risks and benefits.

Clinical Pearls

Many patients presenting with a complaint of amenorrhea are best approached from a physiological perspective (see Figure 16.15):

○ If they have never had menstrual periods previously, then simple delayed puberty (which is not pathological) is likely in girls under the age of 15. Otherwise, genetic and developmental disorders would need to be considered (e.g., by karyotype analysis).

○ If they have had menstrual periods previously and are *not* currently pregnant (test to be sure!), take a careful history for evidence of excessive exercise, weight loss, or stress. In these cases, hypothalamic amenorrhea due to altered GnRH pulses is most likely. Simple diet and lifestyle changes that increase body fat and weight and decrease stress typically result in resumption of normal periods.

○ Because of the dependence of the menstrual cycle on precise coordination of cycles of development in different organs, excess or deficiency of thyroid hormone can result in either amenorrhea or excessive bleeding. Similarly, high prolactin levels (e.g., from dopaminergic-blocking medications such as metochlopramide or phenothiazines) can alter GnRH secretion and thereby disorder the axis. Conversely, a low blood prolactin level raises the possibility that the pituitary may have been invaded by some other process that has also destroyed the gonadotropes (e.g., a tumor).

○ Given a normal TSH and prolactin, the question is whether lack of menstrual periods is due to a uterine problem, an ovarian problem, or some other hypothalamic/pituitary factor. This is best approached by provocative testing to evaluate the function of one organ system in isolation.

Thus, if the endometrium is not diseased, it should bleed upon treatment with estrogen followed by progesterone and then withdrawal of both.

○ The ability of the endometrium to respond to a cycle of estrogen and progesterone treatment suggests that the uterus is functionally intact and that the problem is either at the ovary or higher in the axis. In the ovary, failure to ovulate would result in a constant high-estrogen state without progesterone or sloughing of the endometrium. If treatment of the patient with progesterone alone, followed by its withdrawal, results in menstrual bleeding, then failure to ovulate and the resulting lack of progesterone is the likely cause of amenorrhea.

○ Menstrual flow in response to a cycle of estrogen and progesterone, but not to progesterone alone, suggests either complete ovarian failure (e.g., lack of follicles) or hypothalamic/pituitary disease.

○ An LH or FSH level should confirm whether the problem is in the ovary or the central nervous system. An ovarian problem presents with high LH and FSH levels, since the lack of estrogen and inhibin should result in no feedback inhibition at the otherwise normal gonadotrope. If the LH and FSH levels are low, then the patient definitely has hypothalamic or pituitary dysfunction, since she lacks the response of a normal hypothalamus and pituitary to estrogen deficiency.

9. FRONTIERS IN FEMALE REPRODUCTIVE PHYSIOLOGY

Regulation of ovulation by human pheromones

It has been observed that women living together develop synchronization of their menstrual cycles. In rats, this behavior has been shown to be due to pheromones, airborne chemical signals released by an individual that alter the physiology of other members of the same species, without the recipient individual's being consciously aware of a particular smell. However, the mechanism for menstrual synchrony in humans has not been clear.

Recently, it was found that inhalation of odorless compounds from the armpits of women late in the follicular phase of the menstrual cycle is able to speed up the mid-cycle surge of LH and FSH and shorten the menstrual cycle in recipient women. The armpit secretions from the same women *after* ovulation had the opposite effect of delaying the mid-cycle surge and lengthening the menstrual cycle (see Ref. 4).

Thus, a whole paradigm of sensory experience not normally associated with human behavior appears to be at work in regulation of the menstrual cycle — literally, under our noses. Like most good research, this study raises far more questions than it answers. What are these compounds and how do they work? Will they lead to a major change in our understanding of the menstrual cycle or the way we treat menstrual or other disorders? What is the purpose of such a synchronization? Is it an evolutionary vestige? Or is it maintained—perhaps because of linkage to some other behavioral trait? What else in our lives is being regulated by pheromones (or dysregulated by environmental pollutants), unbeknownst to us?

Estrogen and cancer: new links

One reason why hormone replacement therapy (HRT) remains controversial despite its demonstrated ability to diminish postmenopausal osteoporosis is that it is associated with a small but significant risk of breast cancer. Until recently, the prevailing view on the mechanism by which estrogens increase the risk of breast cancer was that they were growth promoters. Thus, cells that were genetically damaged (e.g., by environmental causes, such as tobacco smoke) could more easily proliferate in the presence of higher estrogen concentrations.

New data suggest a very different and more disturbing view of estrogens (see Refs. 5 to 7). It appears that, in addition to their capacity to stimulate cell proliferation, estrogens are metabolized to compounds that are themselves capable of binding to and damaging DNA directly or generating free radicals that do so (see Figure 16.16). First, the risk of cancer caused by particular estrogen metabolites appears to be unconnected to their affinity for the estrogen receptor, the basis for their growth-promoting activity, suggesting an independent basis for their cancer risk. Second, the risk of cancer seems to correlate with high activity of enzymes that convert estrogens into metabolites suspected of mutagenicity.

Other workers remain skeptical of this hypothesis, in part because these compounds do not score as highly mutagenic on conventional mutagenesis assays, and in part because the reasoning from animal data to humans remains inferential (see Ref. 5). Nevertheless, this new line of thinking is being taken seriously by many researchers in the carcinogenesis field. Furthermore, it underscores the recognition that "facts" in biology and medicine are fluid in the face of new experiments, and that the significance of a given fact depends on the larger context in which that information is viewed (see Chap. 1).

It seems reasonable and prudent to acknowledge that estrogens may be far more dangerous than previously realized, and hence, pending further research, their pharmacologic use should perhaps be only a last report, carried out with great caution (see Ref. 8). Progestins too, are believed to con-

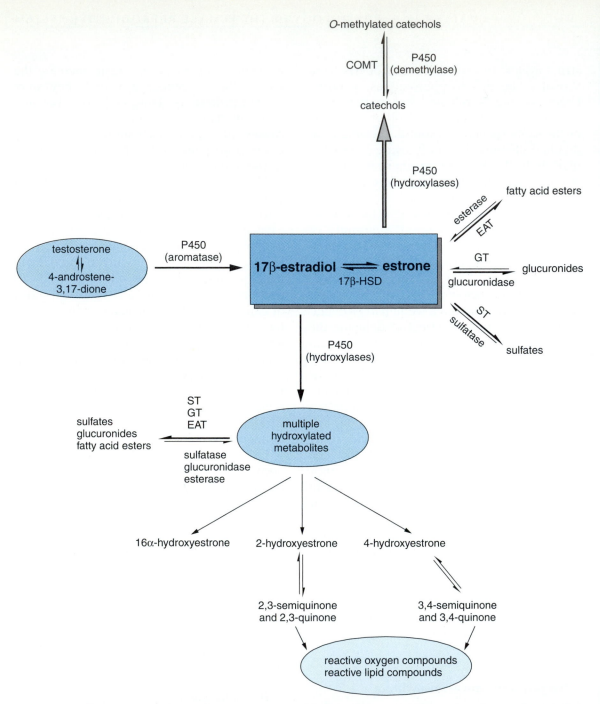

FIGURE 16.16. Estrogen metabolites with mutagenic potential. Indicated are some of the many pathways of metabolism of estrogens generating a range of different compounds whose physiological and pathophysiological roles remain to be explored. ST = sulfotransferase; GT = glucuronosyltransferase; EAT = estrogen acyltransferase (catalyses fatty acyl ester formation); COMT = catechol-o-methyltransferase; P450 = cytochrome P450. (*Adapted, with permission, from Service RF (1998). New role for estrogen in cancer?* Science *279:1631, and Zhu BT, Conney AH (1998). Functional role of estrogen metabolism in target cells: Review and perspectives.* Carcinogenesis *19:1–27.*)

tribute to the risk of breast cancer (see Ref. 9).

Estrogen and prevention of Alzheimer's disease

Recent data are by no means all bad for estrogen. Clinical epidemiologic studies have suggested that estrogen use is associated with a decreased incidence of one of the most dreaded afflictions of the modern age: Alzheimer's disease (AD), a rapidly progressive dementing illness of elderly patients (see Ref. 9). But what might be the molecular basis for estrogen's apparent protective effect?

Studies in mice, using a model that mimics some aspects of AD pathology, demonstrate that estrogen induces increased neuronal synapse formation in damaged areas of the brain (see Ref. 10). This effect of estrogen was dependent on apo E, a protein involved in carrying lipid in the bloodstream, because apo E knockout mice (see Chap. 2) do not demonstrate this effect.

It has long been known that one particular allele of apo E, termed apo E4, is an independent risk factor for development of AD. It had been previously hypothesized that apo E's protective effect was due to stimulation of choline transport and other steps in lipid synthesis. A study a few years ago demonstrated that synapse formation in cell culture is promoted by a non-AD-associated apo E but not by apo E4. Perhaps estrogen induces expression of key genes involved in lipid transport in a way that affects individuals differently, depending on which apo E allele they express (see Ref. 11). Thus, by one hypothesis, these two risk factors for AD may be mechanistically related.

Another line of research in AD has focused on abnormal metabolism of the amyloid precursor protein (APP), which in AD appears to generate a cleavage product called β-amyloid peptide. The β-amyloid peptide is a major component of the plaques that are noted throughout the brain of AD patients, along with neurofibrillary tangles and neuronal loss (see Chap. 18).

A recent paper demonstrates that estrogen reduces the formation of the AD-associated β-amyloid peptide (see Ref. 12), perhaps by stimulating the intracellular trafficking of APP and thereby diminishing the amount of protein available for conversion to the toxic fragments.

The confluence of biochemical with epidemiologic paradigms of AD pathogenesis is exciting because it suggests valuable future studies from each perspective. Might some individuals with genetic forms of AD be more or less protected by estrogen than the population at large (e.g., because their genetic lesion is in a gene that renders it noninduced by estrogen)? Might identification of estrogen-sensitive genes needed for apo E or APP trafficking in cells provide new targets for the development of more selective pharmacologic tools than estrogen for AD prevention?

On the other hand, there are hints that the linkage between estrogen, β amyloid, and AD may be more complex. Another recent study suggests that the protection from beta amyloid pathology conferred by estrogen is independent of cells having nuclear estrogen receptors, and thus may not be working through classical mechanisms of estrogen action (see Ref. 13). Furthermore, this study identified an important effect of antioxidants in greatly increasing the sensitivity of cells to this estrogen-protective mechanism. Both of these observations have significant potential to contribute to the prevention and perhaps even treatment of this dread disorder. Diet and lifestyle recommendations with at least some chance of improving the lives of patients may emerge from the answers to these questions in the near future. Perhaps these findings will also sow the seeds for a new pharmacologic growth industry offering treatment of this currently incurable disease.

10. HOW DOES AN UNDERSTANDING OF NORMAL PHYSIOLOGY PROVIDE INSIGHT INTO THE INITIAL CASE PRESENTATION?

One of the most difficult challenges of clinical medicine is that often disorders with very different pathophysiology present with common clinical signs and symptoms. Sometimes physiological thinking provides a clear understanding of what is going on and what should be done about it, even while the workup intended to make a precise diagnosis is still in progress.

During workup of the first episode of amenorrhea at age 20, blood studies would demonstrate low LH, FSH, and estrogen. The diagnostic question is, why? The history of vigorous exercise and weight loss strongly suggests hypothalamic amenorrhea due to stress, given the lack of other clinical signs or symptoms. For example, a tumor destroying the pituitary gland would probably present with headaches and double vision, given the densely packed, sensitive structures in the neighborhood of the hypothalamus and pituitary gland.

Leaving hypothalamic amenorrhea untreated for an extended period of time subjects the patient to an increased risk of osteoporosis. Treating it pharmacologically (for example, with GnRH pulses via a pump, injections of LH and FSH, or estrogen/progesterone replacement) is expensive and runs the small, but not insignificant, risk of complications of therapy. Changing the patient's diet and lifestyle would be the most effective intervention, solving the problem with little cost and without "medicalizing" the situation.

The second episode of amenorrhea at age 35 resulting in spontaneous resolution despite lack of specific treatment should remind us of just how common it is for symptoms to come and go for no clear reason. We often ascribe improvement to our treatments without recognizing that the treatment may have been irrelevant and the patient might have gotten better anyway. As long as the patient is getting better, we generally assume the best and move on. This is one reason why the treatment of individual patients (in contrast to a proper clinical trial) is rarely "scientific" — there is neither the opportunity nor the desire to carry out controls! Furthermore, even when the opportunity and inclination are present, the clinician has an ethical obligation to carry out treatments that are in the best interests of the individual patient. Finally, the variables are so many and so diverse and often unknown, as to make a truly controlled study virtually impossible.

It is plausible that this episode of amenorrhea was related to poorly understood effects of stress, which also may have contributed to Ms. V.'s depression. But subsequently, treatment of the depression (with the dopamine antagonist) might have elevated prolactin and downregulated her GnRH pulses, and thereby set in motion yet another mechanism for amenorrhea. By stopping her medicines, Ms. V. unknowingly may have removed the **iatrogenic** cause of her symptoms. Never forget to ask yourself: What is wrong with this picture? Could the problem be due to the attempted solution?

Regarding the 3rd episode of amenorrhea at age 42, sometimes patients raise concerns about possibilities that the clinician doesn't really think are likely. Often, the clinician orders testing to address those concerns and thereby reassure the patient. While this approach may sometimes be helpful, new concerns are generated when tests come back positive, as they sometimes do. First, is this a true or false positive? Even if true, does it represent real pathology (which the clinician did not really suspect in the first place), or is it a physiological finding, the proper interpretation of which may redirect the medical evaluation?

Never forget that amenorrhea could be due to pregnancy! During pregnancy, the pituitary hypertrophies substantially. There have even been cases where an unappreciated pregnancy has resulted in the patient's having her (normal) enlarged pituitary removed for a presumed tumor!

SUMMARY AND REVIEW OF KEY CONCEPTS

1. The female reproductive neuroendocrine axis controls the events that prepare the body for its role in human reproduction, in particular, maturation of germ cells and sequential optimization of the female reproductive tract for sperm transport, fertilization, implantation, and development.

2. The female reproductive organs include the ovaries, the uterus, and the fallopian tubes. In addition, the hypothalamus, pituitary gland gonadotropes, vagina, and breast play crucial roles in reproduction, and many tissues of the body are responsive to estrogen and/or progesterone, the primary female reproductive hormones.

3. The ovary consists of germ cells called oocytes, granulosa cells that surround and nourish the oocytes, and thecal cells that produce androgens. The oocytes and surrounding granulosa cells make up follicles. The androgens from the thecal cells diffuse across a basement membrane into the follicles. The enzyme aromatase in granulosa cells converts the thecal androgens, which are toxic to oocytes, into estrogens that promote maturation of activated oocytes.

4. Each month, in response to hormonal stimulation from the gonadotropes, a co-hort of follicles is activated for development. All except the dominant follicle will degenerate through a process called atresia.

5. Initially, granulosa cells have receptors for FSH and thecal cells have receptors for LH. Besides activating a cohort of follicles, FSH stimulates aromatase, the enzyme that converts androgen into estrogen, within granulosa cells. Estrogen, in turn, induces more FSH receptors on the granulosa cells, which results in increased estrogen production. Granulosa cells develop LH receptors approaching mid-cycle, which results in the capacity to produce progesterone.

6. The higher density of FSH receptors on the dominant follicle allows it to make enough aromatase to maintain estrogen production despite the fall in blood FSH levels caused by negative feedback by inhibin, a protein made by granulosa cells. LH is feedback-inhibited by estrogen.

7. Complex interactions between local mediators play a crucial role in maturation of the follicle.

8. The uterus contains a hormone-sensitive lining, the endometrium, which proliferates and develops copious mucus, in response to the rise in blood estrogen, that is optimized for sperm transport. Later, onset of progesterone results in changes in the endometrium that optimize it for implantation and impede sperm transport. Finally, if pregnancy does not occur, the fall in blood estrogen and progesterone removes the support from the proliferated and matured endometrium, which is then sloughed, resulting in menstrual bleeding.

9. Ovulation occurs as a result of a confluence of maturations occurring in the hypothalamus, pituitary gonadotropes, and follicle, which are also synchronized with the changes in the uterine endometrium. The dominant follicle ruptures, releasing

the mature egg into the peritoneal space, where it is taken up by a fallopian tube.

10. After ovulation, the residual granulosa cells of the follicle form an endocrine structure called the corpus luteum that is a progesterone factory. Progesterone and estrogen from the ovary maintain the endometrium for 14 days after ovulation.

11. The menstrual cycle consists of cycles of development in the hypothalamus and pituitary, the ovary, and the uterus, punctuated by ovulation and ending with the onset of menstrual flow. The follicular phase of the menstrual cycle is the time of development of the oocyte and preparation of the uterus; the mid-cycle surge is the phase that culminates in ovulation; the luteal phase is the period of high progesterone secretion when the endometrium is optimized for implantation.

12. During transit down the fallopian tube, the mature egg may be fertilized by sperm, followed by implantation of the embryo into the uterine endometrium.

13. After about 40 years of monthly periods, the ovary is exhausted of follicles, menstrual cycles cease, and blood estrogen levels fall. Some, but not all, women develop severe symptoms of estrogen deficiency, including vaginal dryness, hot flashes, vasomotor instability, and eventually osteoporosis.

strual periods for 6 months, and a recent pregnancy test was negative. On closer questioning, she reports intermittent "spotting" (small amounts of vaginal bleeding) between the time of expected menstrual periods. On physical examination, she is quite overweight, with prominent hirsutism.

The clinician suspects the polycystic ovary syndrome based on the confluence of overweight, insulin resistance, hirsutism, and amenorrhea. The diagnosis is confirmed by an ultrasound examination, which demonstrates the presence of polycystic ovaries, and by an elevated blood testosterone level with a low blood testosterone-binding globulin level and a high blood LH level.

Ms. J. and her clinician formulate a program designed to reduce insulin resistance, including a renewed focus on dietary goals, daily walking for exercise, and a decrease in job stress. She has decided not to work overtime, even though the pay is good. Ms. J. is also started on metformin, an oral hypoglycemic agent that works by decreasing insulin resistance (see Chap. 6).

Four months later, Ms. J. has lost 15 lb and feels a lot better. Her fasting blood glucose is down from 230 to 120 (normal 60 to 140). Blood testing confirms a fall in testosterone and LH and a rise in testosterone-binding globulin. She has had a return of normal menstrual periods.

A CASE OF PHYSIOLOGICAL MEDICINE

R.J. is a 38-year-old woman with diabetes mellitus who presents to medical attention with increasing blood glucose and cessation of menstrual periods. She has had diabetes for 6 years, treated effectively by watching her diet. In the last year, because of a less careful diet associated with the stress of her job as a paralegal assistant, she has gained about 25 lb, and her blood glucose is now much higher. She has not had regular men-

QUESTIONS

1. What is the significance of the small amounts of vaginal bleeding between the times of expected menstrual periods in a woman with probable polycystic ovary syndrome?

2. How might you explain the signs of androgen excess in Ms. J. (e.g., hirsuitism, polycystic ovaries)?

3. Is Ms. J. at risk for osteoporosis as a result

of the polycystic ovary syndrome? Why or why not?

4. For what other disorders was Ms. J. at risk?

5. Why do you think the treatment plan effectively resolved the amenorrhea?

6. Contrast the plan that was enacted to another physiological approach to treatment of this disorder, based on the abnormalities noted.

ANSWERS

1. The high-androgen state results in atresia of follicles and prevents ovulation. Without development of a corpus luteum, progesterone production fails to mature the endometrium. The result is a chronically excessively proliferated endometrium with occasional intermittent bleeding, but no cycles of complete endometrial sloughing.

2. High blood insulin levels result in decreased hepatic synthesis of testosterone-binding globulin, which results in a greater fraction of free androgen, therefore causing more androgen effect. High LH levels, due to the lack of sufficient estrogen to feedback-inhibit LH, result in overstimulation of thecal cells, excessive androgen production, excessive atresia of follicles, anovulation, polycystic ovaries, and persistence of this abnormal hormonal feedback condition. By binding to the receptor for insulin-like growth factor, high blood insulin levels may exacerbate this process. Many aspects of this syndrome remain unexplained (see Ref. 2).

3. No, because she has high rather than low blood levels of androgen and estrogen, which will protect her bones from osteoporosis.

4. She was at an increased risk of endometrial cancer because of the constant, unopposed effects of estrogen on the endometrium. Indeed, some clinicians would recommend endometrial biopsy in a patient with spotting, in order to rule out this possibility, prior to initiation of metformin therapy.

5. Perhaps by decreasing Ms. J.'s insulin resistance and thereby reversing the vicious cycle of effects of high blood insulin on the liver, pituitary, and ovary. In response to lower blood insulin levels for control of blood glucose upon diminution of her insulin resistance, the liver produced more testosterone-binding globulin. This resulted in less circulating free androgen and less LH. This allowed for the resumption of cyclical changes, ovulation, and resumption of a luteal phase.

6. Theoretically, Ms. J. could have been treated with an antiandrogen and an antiestrogen; her insulin resistance could have been treated with insulin injections. However, the therapy instituted, with its greater emphasis on diet, exercise, weight loss, and fewer drugs, was in some ways more "physiological." Pharmacologic intervention with metformin therapy, resulting in improvement of insulin resistance, may have also played a crucial role.

References and suggested readings

GENERAL REFERENCES

1. Speroff L, Glass RH, Kase NG (1994). *Clinical Gynecologic Endocrinology and Infertility,* 5th ed. Baltimore, Williams & Wilkins.

2. Utiger R (1996). Insulin and the polycystic ovary syndrome. *N Engl J Med* 335:657–658.

3. Wise PM, et al. (1996). Menopause: The aging of multiple pacemakers. *Science* 273:67–73.

FRONTIERS REFERENCES

4. Stern K, McClintock MK (1998). Regulation of ovulation by human pheromones. *Nature* 292:177–179.

5. Service RF (1998). New role for estrogen in cancer? *Science* 279:1631–1632.

6. Cavalieri EL, et al. (1997). Molecular origin

of cancer: Catechol estrogen-3,4-quinones as endogenous tumor initiators. *Proc Natl Acad Sci USA* 94:10937–10942.

7. Liehr JG (1997). Hormone-associated cancer: Mechanistic similarities between human breast cancer and estrogen-induced kidney carcinogenesis in hamsters. *Environ Health Perspect* 105(suppl 3):565–569.

8. Brinton LA, and Schairer C (1997). Postmenopausal hormone-replacement therapy — time for a reappraisal? *N Engl J Med* 336:1821–1822.

9. Schairer C, et al. (2000). Menopausal estrogen and estrogen-progestin replacement therapy and breast cancer risk. *JAMA* 263:485–491.

10. Paganini-Hill A, Henderson VW (1996). Estrogen replacement and risk of Alzheimer's disease. *Arch Intern Med* 156:2213–2217.

11. Stone DJ, et al (1998). Increased synaptic sprouting in response to estrogen via an apolipoprotein E-dependent mechanism: Implications for Alzheimer's disease. *J Neurosci* 18:3180–3186.

12. Xu H, et al. (1998). Estrogen reduces neuronal generation of Alzheimer beta amyloid peptides. *Nature Med* 4:447–451.

13. Green PS, et al. (1998). Nuclear estrogen receptor-independent neuroprotection by estratrienes: A novel interaction with glutathione. *Neuroscience* 84:7–10.

14. Spencer CP, et al. (1999). Selective estrogen receptor modulators: Women's panacea for the next millennium? *Am J Obstet Gynecol* 180:763–770.

15. Kurzer MS, Xu X (1997). Dietary phytoestrogens. *Annu Rev Nutr* 17:353–381.

PHYSIOLOGY OF PREGNANCY, THE NEONATE, AND GROWTH

17

1. INTRODUCTION TO THE PHYSIOLOGY OF PREGNANCY

Pregnancy is something of a physiological miracle in which an event that is normally forbidden, propagation of foreign tissue, is accommodated for a defined period of time by the immune system.

In evolutionary terms, early mammals branched off from reptiles some 250 million years ago; they were distinguished by lactation and nursing of their young. These behaviors set the stage for much more complex development of the young, who did not have to start foraging for food right after birth. Later, perhaps 120 million years ago, placentation and live birth emerged as distinguishing features of modern mammals. The development of a trophoblastic layer of cells (see Sec. 2) specialized for establishment of fetal-maternal interaction represented a major innovation in the physiology of pregnancy.

Why is understanding the physiology of pregnancy important for medical practice?

- Pregnancy is a time of tremendous stress on the body of the mother, involving a substantial increase in the workload of many different organs. Thus, disorders of other organ systems (e.g., heart disease and metabolic disease such as diabetes mellitus) that might be well controlled in the nonpregnant state can get out of control during pregnancy, with great potential for harm to either the mother or the fetus, or both.
- Pregnancy is a time of suppression of the immune system, rendering the mother vulnerable to a number of infectious diseases as a result of impairment of a subset of cell-mediated immunity. The availability of antibiotics masks the magnitude of this problem. For example, prior to the 1950s, tuberculosis was the single most common indication for therapeutic abortion.
- Certain disorders, such as rheumatoid arthritis, actually improve with pregnancy, as a consequence of the natural immune suppression that occurs during pregnancy.
- Many common drugs for problems unrelated to the reproductive system are contraindicated during pregnancy because of their damaging effects on the fetus.

Case Presentation

RZ is a 20-year-old immigrant who works as a farm laborer. Although she is a legal immigrant, the status of her husband is less clear. Seven months pregnant with her first child, for lack of health insurance and for fear of investigation of her husband's immigration status, she had not sought prenatal care.

One day, while working in the fields, she felt faint and subsequently lost consciousness. She was observed to have a seizure, and she was taken to the county hospital. There her blood pressure was measured at 180/110, she was noted to have pedal edema, and protein was detected in her urine.

Ms. Z had another seizure despite aggressive medical measures, and fetal distress was noted by fetal monitoring. An emergency cesarean section was performed, during which time the mother was hypertensive. Postoperatively, both mother and baby had difficulties and complications. The baby was sufficiently premature to require a ventilator in order to breathe. She also had a seizure within the first few hours of her life, a sign of damage caused by lack of oxygen to her brain, probably occurring during her mother's seizures. Ms. Z had signs of neurologic deficits, which are likely to impair her ability to work in the future.

Now Ms. Z and her family are fearful that her husband may be deported, since their situation has come to the attention of authorities. They ask you what the mother and child's capabilities and needs for the future are likely to be, and what could have been done differently. For lack of prenatal care costing relatively little, Ms. Z, her baby, her family, and society have paid, and will continue to pay, a high price. Preventable problems such as these contribute to the high cost of health care. They are part of a vicious cycle of real and imagined barriers that make health care more expensive, and hence less accessible to the very people who need it the most.

2. FERTILIZATION AND IMPLANTATION

After release from the ovary and uptake by one of the fallopian tubes, the mature egg is viable for a window of 12 to 24 h, during which time it can be fertilized. Sperm deposited in the female reproductive tract are viable for up to 48 h, during which time they must travel into the uterus and up the fallopian tube, and find the fertilizable egg. Contractions of the muscular wall of the fallopian tube serve a mixing and propulsion function that may facilitate egg-sperm interaction.

During the time that sperm reside in the female reproductive tract, a number of changes occur. Cholesterol is extracted from the sperm plasma membrane, proteins redistribute in the plane of the membrane, calcium is taken up, and the stage is set for fertilization to occur, possibly by removal or neutralization of fertilization-inhibiting substances. However, this process of **capacitation** seems relatively less important in humans than in some other species. Thus, in vitro fertilization works with sperm that have never resided in the female reproductive tract.

As sperm approach the egg, they undergo the **acrosomal reaction,** in which an internal compartment called the **acrosome** fuses with the sperm plasma membrane–releasing proteases, hyaluronases, and other substances that clear a path for fertilization to occur. Species-specific sperm receptors facilitate the binding of many sperm to the egg. The first sperm to penetrate the **zona pellucida** of the egg induces a calcium flux and depolarizes the plasma membrane, releasing proteases that alter the receptors so that they prevent rather than promote further sperm binding. In this way, **polyploidy,** the generation of a cell with more than two sets of homologous chromosomes, is effectively prevented.

The penetrating sperm's DNA is endocytosed by the egg, and the 46 chromosomes, two sets of 23 each from the mother and father, are arranged along a spindle, creating a new diploid individual called a **zygote**.

The embryo, now in the **blastocyst** stage of development (see Figure 17.1), takes about 3 days to make its way down the fallopian tube toward the uterus. Often the blastocyst lingers at the fallopian tube–uterine junction, perhaps waiting for progesterone-induced optimization of conditions for implantation into the uterine endometrium. Once the blastocyst is in the uterus, over the next 2 to 3 days, with the help of uterine factors, what is left of the zona pellucida is shed from the

FIGURE 17.1. The blastocyst. Schematic description of an early embryo. The blastocyst is the stage where a cavity develops, distinguishing an inner and outer cell mass. The inner cell mass will develop into the fetus. The outer cell mass will form the trophoblast, which is the embryo's contribution to formation of the placenta.

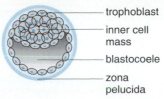

- trophoblast
- inner cell mass
- blastocoele
- zona pelucida

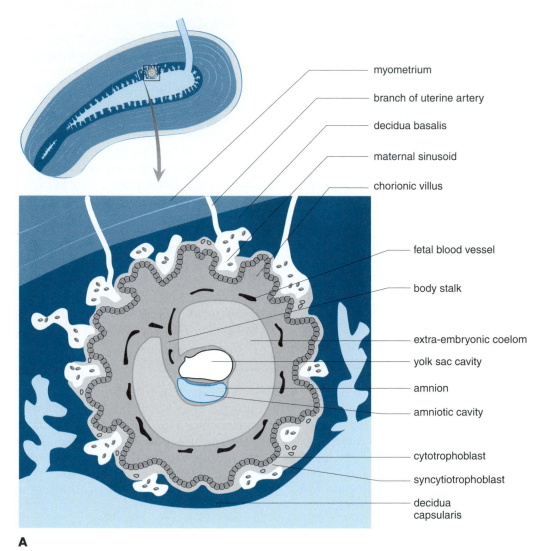

myometrium

branch of uterine artery

decidua basalis

maternal sinusoid

chorionic villus

fetal blood vessel

body stalk

extra-embryonic coelom

yolk sac cavity

amnion

amniotic cavity

cytotrophoblast

syncytiotrophoblast

decidua capsularis

A

FIGURE 17.2. Anatomy of implantation and early fetal development. *A.* Diagram of a coronal section through the uterus early in pregnancy and after formation of the intervillous spaces of the developing placenta (approximately week 3). Note an embryo at the blastocyst stage, embedded in the endometrium.

blastocyst, and implantation into the endometrium takes place in a three-step process involving:

1. Adhesion
2. Penetration
3. Invasion

A **trophoblast layer** separates from the remaining blastocyst cell mass and generates microvilli that interdigitate with cells of the endometrium (see Figure 17.2). **Histamine** and **prostaglandins** are believed to play a role as local mediators of this process, in conjunction with effects of **estradiol.** As the tropho-

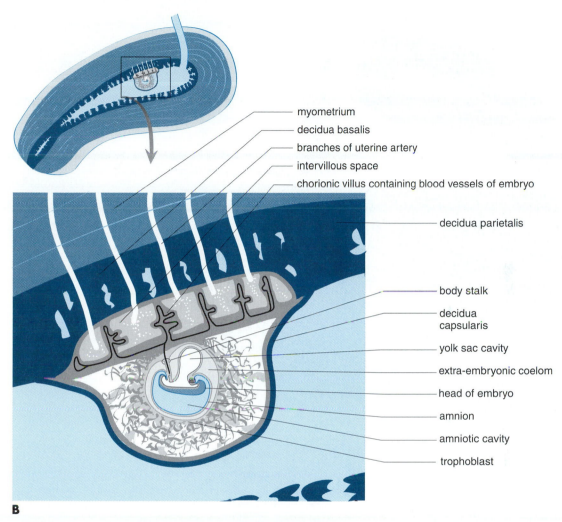

myometrium

decidua basalis

branches of uterine artery

intervillous space

chorionic villus containing blood vessels of embryo

decidua parietalis

body stalk

decidua capsularis

yolk sac cavity

extra-embryonic coelom

head of embryo

amnion

amniotic cavity

trophoblast

B

FIGURE 17.2 — (*continued*) B. Diagram of a coronal section through the uterus during the period of embryonic development (after week 4).

blastic layer invades the endometrium, it forms cavities termed **lacunae**. When the invading trophoblasts reach maternal arteries, these vessels rupture and fill the lacunae with blood, which drains via maternal veins.

At the same time, fibroblast-like cells of the stroma that underlies the endometrium change into **decidual cells**, which enlarge and accumulate glycogen and lipid, probably under the influence of estrogen and progester-

one. The decidual cells provide nutrition for the developing embryo until formation of connections to the mother's vascular supply has been induced.

Subsequently, the decidua may serve as a mechanical barrier to further invasion of the uterus by the developing embryo while protecting it from the maternal immune system. The decidua also plays an important endocrine role as a source of prolactin, relaxin,

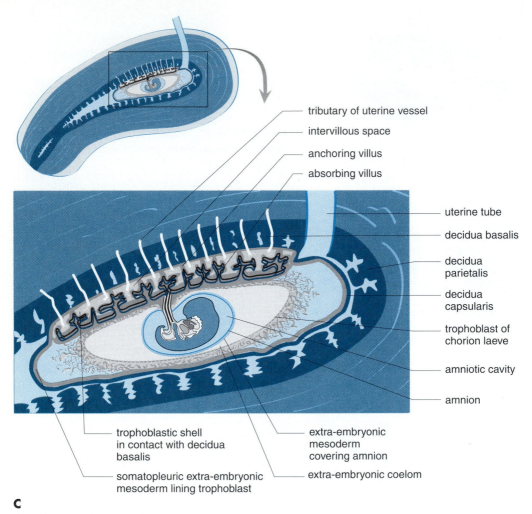

tributary of uterine vessel

intervillous space

anchoring villus

absorbing villus

uterine tube

decidua basalis

decidua parietalis

decidua capsularis

trophoblast of chorion laeve

amniotic cavity

amnion

trophoblastic shell in contact with decidua basalis

somatopleuric extra-embryonic mesoderm lining trophoblast

extra-embryonic mesoderm covering amnion

extra-embryonic coelom

C

FIGURE 17.2 — (continued) C. Diagram of a coronal section through the uterus after formation of the umbilical cord (after week 12). The uterine cavity is almost entirely obliterated.

and prostaglandins, which have a paracrine influence on uterine musculature and fetal membranes.

are lost during the first 14 days, probably as a result of failed or improper implantation.

Clinical Pearl

○ Implantation is a high-risk stage of pregnancy. Approximately 70% of fertilized eggs fail to develop to term. Most of these

Review Questions

1. For how long are released eggs and deposited sperm viable?
2. What is the acrosome reaction?

3. What are the time course and the steps from fertilization to completion of implantation?
4. What is the difference in origin of the trophoblast layer and the decidua?
5. What are the roles of the decidua?

3. STRUCTURE AND FUNCTION OF THE PLACENTA

Structure

The fetal trophoblasts that initiate implantation differentiate into two cell types. The outer layer (with respect to the fetus) is made up of fused cells that develop in response to **epidermal growth factor** and other paracrine influences and are called the **syncytiotrophoblasts.** They secrete proteins, peptides, and ever-larger quantities of steroids. The inner layer of trophoblastic cells is called the **cytotrophoblasts.** Among the many paracrine products produced by the cytotrophoblasts are hypothalamic peptides, including corticotropin-releasing hormone (CRH) and thyrotropin-releasing hormone (TRH), which regulate release of the corresponding pituitary-like hormones from the syncytiotrophoblasts.

The placenta is the only organ that consists of cells derived from two different individuals. The maternal part of the placenta, the **decidua basalis,** provides arterial blood to and venous drainage from the lacunae. The fetal part of the placenta consists of **chorionic villi** composed of connective tissue, syncytiotrophoblasts, and cytotrophoblasts and contains fetal blood vessels that grow into the lacunar spaces (see Figure 17.3). Exchange

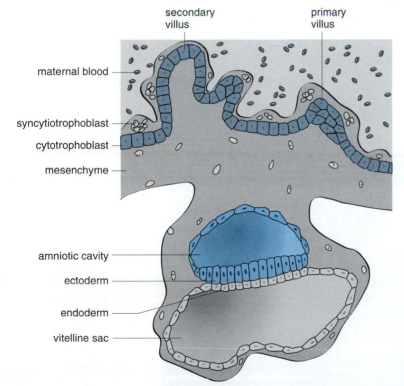

secondary villus

primary villus

maternal blood

syncytiotrophoblast

cytotrophoblast

mesenchyme

amniotic cavity

ectoderm

endoderm

vitelline sac

FIGURE 17.3. Histology of early placental formation. Human embryo at 15 days. At upper left is shown a chorionic villus protruding into a lacuna that contains maternal blood. (Adapted, with permission, from Junquiera LC, et al. (1989). Basic Histology, 6th ed. Norwalk, CT, Appleton & Lange, p. 455.)

of substances and gases between mother and fetus is possible because these villi containing fetal blood vessels are bathed in maternal blood in the lacunae. As the embryo develops, the vessels within the villi join the systemic circulation of the body of the embryo. Note that maternal and fetal blood rarely mix. Rather, most exchange takes place across the intact trophoblast layers. Eventually the lacunae form the intervillous spaces in the mature placenta (see Figure 17.4).

Functions

The placenta plays many different roles in the development of the fetus, some of which remain quite poorly understood. The most obvious functions are to:

- Procure nutrition from the mother.
- Exchange gases and remove wastes.
- Regulate fetal fluid and electrolyte composition.
- Synthesize peptides, proteins, and steroids, which serve a mind-boggling array of poorly understood paracrine and endocrine functions.

Some of the most evident functions of placental endocrine and paracrine products are to:

FIGURE 17.4. The mature placenta.

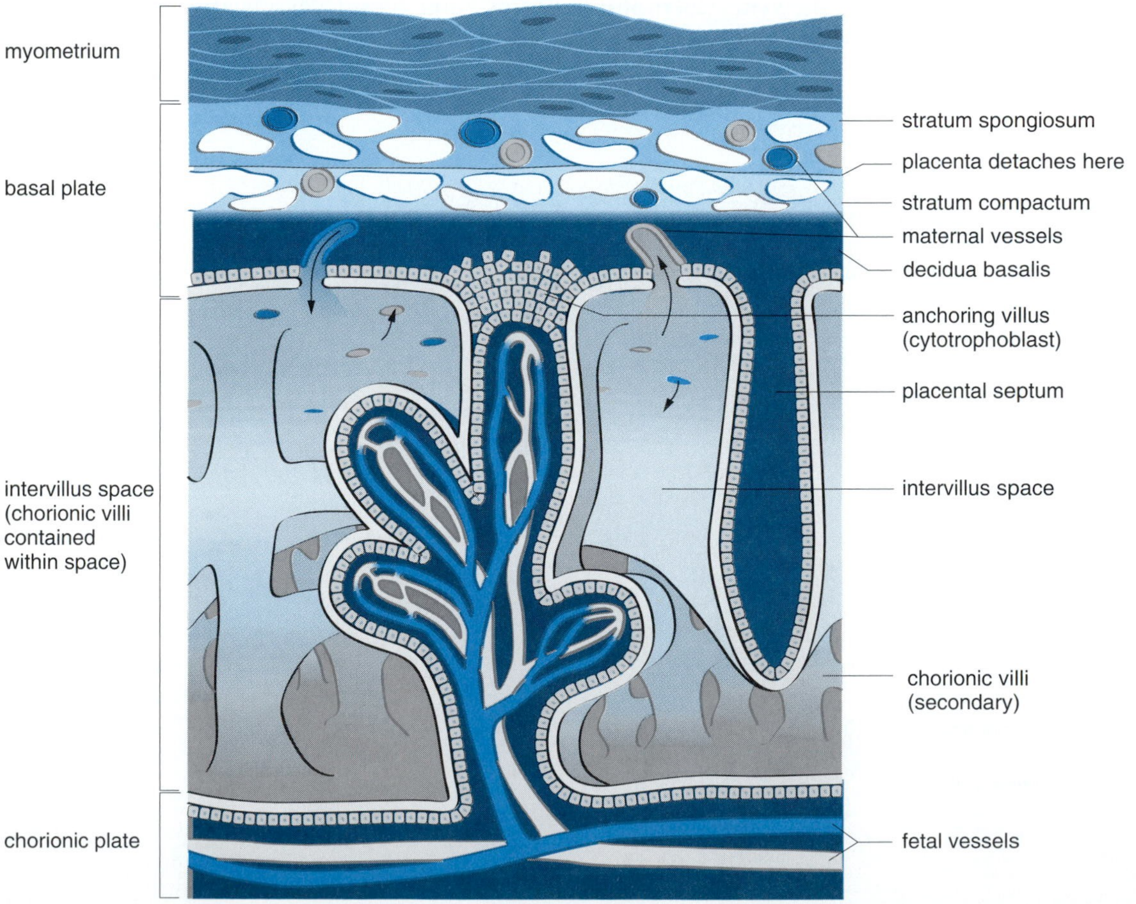

- Establish and maintain an immunoprivileged sanctuary for fetal development.
- Relax the uterine musculature so that it will not prematurely expel the developing fetus. At term, placental products may play a key role in exactly the opposite process: causing labor, in order to make possible the delivery and survival of the fetus.
- Ensure a steady supply of glucose and other energy substrates from the mother for fetal needs.
- Facilitate fetal osmoregulation.
- Contribute to proper fetal development.

Review Questions

6. Describe the differences between syncytiotrophoblasts and cytotrophoblasts.
7. What organs are composed of cells from two different individuals?
8. Name at least six categories of functions of the placenta.

4. HORMONES OF PREGNANCY: THEIR ROLES AND CONSEQUENCES

During pregnancy, the maternal metabolism undergoes tremendous changes that affect the underlying function of the cardiovascular system, lungs, kidneys, and gastrointestinal (GI) tract, to name a few. These changes are driven by hormones. During pregnancy, novel hormones (or new levels of preexisting hormones) are produced by the mother, placenta, and fetus (see Table 17.1). Moreover, the blood levels of those hormones change over the course of pregnancy, in some cases correlating with changes in maternal metabolism (see Sec. 7).

Novel placental and related hormones

Human chorionic gonadotropin

Pregnancy and the normal menstrual cycle part company when the corpus luteum survives beyond 14 days (see Chap. 16). When this happens, progesterone, made by the corpus luteum, remains at high levels (see Figure 17.5). This allows survival of the embryo.

Maintainance of the corpus luteum beyond day 14 is due to production of a luteinizing hormone (LH)–like hormone by the syncytiotrophoblast cells of the implanted blastocyst, under the influence of the cytotrophoblast cells. Called human chorionic gonadotropin (hCG), this LH-like hormone is a glycoprotein heterodimer that has the same alpha subunit as do LH, follicle-stimulating hormone (FSH), and thyroid-stimulating hormone (TSH), but contains a unique beta subunit that is different from, but highly homologous to, the beta subunit of LH. Like LH, hCG binds the LH receptor, a G protein–coupled receptor whose second messenger for hCG action is cyclic AMP.

hCG has a number of actions that promote pregnancy:

- hCG maintains the corpus luteum for an additional 10 to 12 weeks while the placenta is developing into an autonomous estrogen and progesterone factory. After this time, hCG levels decline about tenfold and maintain a low plateau throughout the remainder of the pregnancy.
- Some hCG enters the fetal circulation and stimulates fetal adrenal production of the androgen dehydroepiandrosterone sulfate (DHEA-S) and, in male fetuses, testosterone production by the testes.
- hCG may stimulate relaxin production by the endometrium, contributing to *uterine quiescence* (lack of contraction of the muscle that makes up the underlying myometrium of the body of the uterus) until the approach of term.
- hCG serves to feedback-inhibit hypothalamic gonadotropin-releasing hormone (GnRH) secretion and therefore, pituitary LH and FSH secretion.
- hCG resembles TSH, with which it shares the alpha subunit. Because hCG rises to ex-

TABLE 17.1 MATERNAL, PLACENTAL, AND FETAL PEPTIDE PRODUCTS

Fetal compartment	Placental compartment	Maternal compartment
Alpha-fetoprotein	Hypothalamic-like hormones	Decidual proteins
	GnRH	Prolactin
	CRH	Relaxin
	TRH	IGFBP-1
	Somatostatin	Interleukin 1
	Pituitary-like hormones	Colony-stimulating factor 1
	hCG	Progesterone-associated endometrial protein
	hCS	Corpus luteum proteins
	hGH	Relaxin
	hCT	Prorenin
	ACTH	
	Growth factors	
	IGF-1	
	Epidermal growth factor	
	Platelet-derived growth factor	
	Fibroblast growth factor	
	Transforming growth factor β	
	Inhibin	
	Activin	
	Cytokines	
	Interleukin 1	
	Interleukin 6	
	Colony-stimulating factor	
	Other	
	Opioids	
	Prorenin	
	Pregnancy-specific β-glycoprotein	
	Pregnancy-associated plasma protein A	

ABBREVIATIONS: GnRH = gonadotropin-releasing hormone; CRH = corticotropin-releasing hormone; TRH = thyrotropin-releasing hormone; hCG = human chorionic gonadotropin; hCS = human chorionic sommatotropin; hGH = human growth hormone; hCT = human chorionic thyrotropin; ACTH = adrenocorticotropic hormone; IGF-1 = insulin-like growth factor 1; IGFBP-1 = insulin-like growth factor 1 binding protein.
Reproduced, with permission, from Speroff L, Glass RH, Case NG (1994). *Clinical Gynecologic Endocrinology and Infertility*, 5th ed. Baltimore, Williams & Wilkins.

tremely high levels by the end of the first trimester of pregnancy, it "spills over" to some extent onto receptors in the mother nominally intended for TSH. The resulting increase in thyroid stimulation probably contributes to alteration of metabolism in pregnancy.

Human placental lactogen

Human placental lactogen (hPL), also known as **human chorionic somatomammotropin** (**hCS**), is a growth hormone–like protein hormone made by syncytiotrophoblasts of the placenta.

Production of hPL starts at about 4 weeks of gestation and increases steadily; a blood level of 6 μg/mL is reached at term. At that point, a pregnant woman's placenta makes as much as 2 g of hPL per day, the highest production of any polypeptide hormone in the body. After delivery of the placenta, hPL levels in maternal blood fall quickly, with a half-life of 20 min.

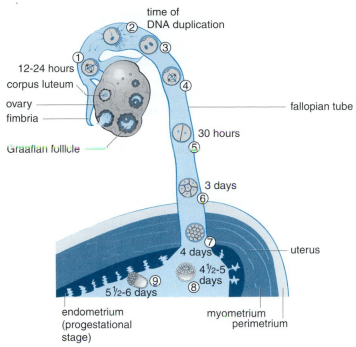

FIGURE 17.5. Early events in pregnancy. Timing of events after ovulation, culminating in implantation of the embryo. Schematic representation of events taking place during the first week of human development. 1. Oocyte immediately after ovulation. 2. Fertilization, approximately 12 to 24 h after ovulation. 3. Stage of male and female pronuclei. 4. Spindle of the first mitotic division. 5. Two-cell stage (approximately 30 h after formation of embryo). 6. Morula containing approximately 16 cells (approximately 3 days of age). 7. Advanced morula reaching the uterine lumen (approximately 4 days of age). 8. Early blastula (approximately 4½ days of age). 9. Early phase of implantation of blastula (approximately 6 days of age). Note the late secretory stage development of the uterine endometrium as a result of the influence of estrogen and progesterone. *(Adapted, with permission from Sadler JW (1995), in* Langman's Medical Embryology, *7th ed. Baltimore, MD, Williams & Wilkins, p. 36.)*

The amino acid sequence of hPL is extremely similar to that of growth hormone (GH) (>95% the same). Yet hPL has some very different effects because the differences in its structure allow it to bind to a unique receptor. Nevertheless, hPL's extremely high concentration in blood results in significant spillover onto GH receptors and therefore results in GH-like anabolic effects.

The major roles of hPL are believed to be to stimulate maternal lipolysis and antago-nize the effects of maternal insulin, whose secretion is increased in response to hPL. These effects result in the sparing of glucose utilization by the mother in order to make it available for the needs of the fetus (see Sec. 5).

Relaxin

Relaxin is a hormone with homology to pro-insulin that is made both by the corpus luteum (in response to hCG) and also by decidual cells of the endometrium. Its levels rise early in pregnancy, peak in the first trimester, and decline to some extent after that.

Relaxin's major role is believed to be suppression of uterine contractility. This is due, at least in part, to inhibition of myosin light-chain phosphorylation in the uterine myometrium. Relaxin also relaxes pelvic ligaments and promotes dilation of the uterine cervix, thereby possibly promoting delivery upon completion of fetal maturation.

Hormones produced elsewhere that are also made by the placenta

Progesterone

Made in large quantities initially by the corpus luteum and later by the placenta, progesterone is the central hormone of pregnancy. At term, progesterone production is approximately 250 mg/day, approximately ten times the highest level achieved during the luteal phase of the menstrual cycle. Yet it is remarkable how poorly the myriad roles of progesterone are understood:

- Early in pregnancy, progesterone stimulates fallopian tube and uterine endometrial production of substances that nourish the embryo until nourishment can be received via the placenta.
- Later in pregnancy, progesterone maintains the decidual cells on which the placenta, and hence the pregnancy, depends.
- Progesterone made by the placenta is the major substrate for androgen and glucocorticoid production by the fetal adrenal. The fetal adrenal lacks a key enzyme needed for progesterone synthesis, and therefore must work closely with the mother and the placenta (see Sec. 5).
- Uterine quiescence is at least partly maintained by progesterone.
- Regulation of hPL and hCG may also be

under the control, at least in part, of progesterone.
- Progesterone inhibits prostaglandin production and thereby reduces uterine contractions and the risk of premature labor. This effect is believed to be due, in part, to an effect of progesterone on sensitivity of the myometrium to oxytocin (see Sec. 10, Frontiers).
- Progesterone stimulates the maternal respiratory center, increasing ventilation to dispose of the extra carbon dioxide produced by the fetus.
- Progesterone promotes mammary gland development.
- Progesterone suppresses the maternal immune response in poorly understood ways.

Approximately 90% of progesterone production goes to the mother, while 10% goes to the fetus.

Estrogens

Like progesterone, estrogens have many different poorly understood roles in pregnancy:

- Estrogens stimulate continuous growth of the myometrium, preparing it for the eventual need to expel the fetus.
- Estrogens stimulate growth and development of the ducts and alveoli of the breast (see Sec. 7).
- Estrogens augment the effect of relaxin on pelvic ligament relaxation.
- Estrogens play paracrine roles in the placenta, increasing low-density lipoprotein (LDL) cholesterol uptake and cytochrome P450 activity (enzymes involved in conversion of steroid intermediates), and therefore promoting progesterone synthesis.
- By promoting placental inactivation of cortisol, estrogens may relieve feedback inhibition of the fetal pituitary corticotropin production, preparing the maturing fetus for the stress of birth.

Prolactin

Maternal prolactin levels rise linearly throughout pregnancy, reaching a value close to ten times that in the nonpregnant state. Prolactin is necessary for estrogen and progesterone's effects on the development of the mammary gland.

In addition to its synthesis by the pituitary gland during the nonpregnant state, prolactin is made by the decidual cells of the endometrium during pregnancy, and may contribute to maternal immune suppression.

Decidual prolactin also enters the amniotic fluid and may play a role in regulation of osmolarity in the fetus, as it does in fish and other evolutionarily more ancient vertebrates.

CRH and related peptides

Effects of pregnancy on the adrenal neuroendocrine axis are complex. First, total plasma cortisol is elevated during pregnancy. In part, this is because estrogen induces an increase in secretion of hepatic cortisol-binding globulin. However, in part, this is also due to an increase in ACTH and hence free cortisol levels (see Chaps. 11 and 13). The net effect of cortisol in pregnancy may be to stimulate maternal weight gain and mammary gland development.

The rise in ACTH is due, in large measure, to a large, protein-bound, nonpulsatile increase in *placental* CRH secretion, that is, distinct from pituitary ACTH production. The net effect of the increase in cortisol may be to prepare the mother for the stress of the last trimester of pregnancy, labor, and delivery.

Inhibin and related peptides

Inhibin A found during pregnancy comes from several sources. The corpus luteum produces inhibin A (in response to LH). Early in pregnancy, inhibin A is made by fetal trophoblasts (peaking by day 7 after conception). Placental production of inhibin A peaks at term.

A postulated role of inhibin A in pregnancy is to prevent FSH secretion and thereby conserve follicles that might otherwise be activated, which would be a waste, with a pregnancy in progress. In contrast, inhibin B levels remain low throughout pregnancy.

Activin A and follistatin are two additional members of the inhibin family of proteins, which have a complex and not well understood relationship in support of pregnancy. Activin A may stimulate, and follistatin inhibit, placental hCG and progesterone synthesis.

Effects of pregnancy on hormones produced elsewhere in the body

Insulin

Maternal insulin levels increase as a result of increased pancreatic beta cell insulin secretion. This effect partially compensates for the increased insulin resistance and elevated counterregulatory hormone level represented by the large increase in hPL, and probably explains why hyperglycemia is not observed in normal pregnancy.

Aldosterone

Aldosterone secretion increases throughout pregnancy, reaching 6 to 8 times the normal level by term. This is due to estrogen-mediated effects on renin and angiotensinogen production by the kidney and liver, respectively. A rationale for this effect is that a large amount of blood is sequestered in the placenta in advanced pregnancy, requiring an expansion of intravascular volume.

A large increase in the mineralocorticoid deoxycorticosterone is also seen. This is due exclusively to 21-hydroxylation of placental progesterone in the kidney.

Growth hormone and parathyroid hormone

Maternal production of both growth hormone and parathyroid hormone (PTH) is suppressed during pregnancy. Presumably the low growth-hormone secretion reflects the high level of hPL replacing the anabolic functions of growth hormone.

Calcium absorption from the diet increases during pregnancy, presumably to accommodate the needs of the fetal skeleton. This effect is largely mediated by increased levels of 1,25-dihydroxyvitamin D, synthesized in decidual cells and the placenta. These products, in turn, suppress maternal PTH secretion by 50% and maintain ionized free calcium levels in maternal blood.

Clinical Pearls

○ Measurement of hCG is the commonest form of pregnancy test. It is typically detectable in maternal plasma and urine by day 9 after conception.
○ The rise in maternal hCG should be exponential. A less than exponential rise suggests that the pregnancy is failing. In a patient with abdominal pain, this might be due to an ectopic pregnancy (implantation in the fallopian tube), which is nonviable and can be life-threatening for the mother if untreated (see Chap. 16).
○ HPL levels in maternal blood are a good measure of placental function during pregnancy.
○ Estriol is a form of estrogen in the body that is derived almost entirely from the fetal-placental unit. Thus maternal blood or urinary estriol is a good indicator of the health and well-being of the placenta and fetus.

○ Some patients may not be able to augment their pancreatic beta cell insulin secretion during pregnancy, as is normally observed, to compensate for increased hPL and other insulin-antagonizing hormones. As a result, they develop hyperglycemia, a condition termed **gestational diabetes mellitus**.

Review Questions

9. What are the major, novel placental-derived hormones?
10. What are nine possible roles for progesterone in pregnancy?
11. Production of which hormones actually diminishes in pregnancy?

5. MATERNAL–PLACENTAL–FETAL INTERACTION

The complexity of maternal–placental–fetal interaction is the fundamental distinguishing feature of placental mammals. To carry out its special role, the placenta makes a host of products, some of which interact with specialized products of the maternal and fetal compartments (see Table 17.1). Two examples of maternal-placental-fetal cooperation will be considered here.

Fuel homeostasis in pregnancy

During the first half of pregnancy, the mother is in an anabolic phase (see Chap. 6). Sensitivity to insulin is normal or slightly increased. Glucose, amino-acid, fatty-acid, and glycerol levels in the bloodstream are normal or slightly lower than normal. Protein synthesis is enhanced, and glycogen stores in liver and muscle are increased. These anabolic changes facilitate growth and development of the breasts and uterus and allow the mother to meet the substantial metabolic demands of the final trimester of pregnancy.

During the last half of pregnancy, maternal metabolism becomes catabolic (see Chap. 6). As a result, metabolism shifts to a mode that has been called "accelerated starvation." It is characterized by fasting hypoglycemia, as fuel substrates produced by the mother are sucked up by the growing fetus. Increased insulin resistance and decreased assimilation of dietary carbohydrate, protein, and fat make these substrates available to meet the needs of the fetus. The glucose gradient between mother and fetus does not have to be very large to ensure that the fetus gets all the glucose it needs. Thus, in a normal pregnancy, this effect is achieved without development of true hyperglycemia.

Very-low-density lipoprotein (VLDL) synthesis increases as a result of the effects of estrogen on the liver. The elevated VLDL promotes storage of triglycerides in the breast, in anticipation of milk production. Plasma cholesterol also rises to support the accelerated levels of steroidogenesis.

This change from anabolic to catabolic metabolism is believed to be driven largely by hPL, perhaps with contributions from other placental growth hormone–like products (besides hPL), and also by the rise in estrogen, cortisol, and progesterone.

HPL produced by the placenta in response to hypoglycemia serves to increase lipolysis in adipocytes, thereby raising free fatty acid and, ultimately, maternal blood glucose and ketone levels. This "diabetogenic" role of hPL is a major additional burden on the mother and contributes to the tendency for diabetes mellitus to first emerge during pregnancy. Normally, glucose is the major fuel source for the fetus. However, ketones provide a ready emergency fuel supply, just as they do in starvation, for both the mother and — transferred via the placenta — the fetus in the event of glucose deprivation.

Steroidogenesis in pregnancy

Few processes illustrate the intricate workings of maternal–placental–fetal cooperation better than steroidogenesis during pregnancy (see Figure 17.6). The mother is the source of the cholesterol from which estrogens, progesterone, androgens, and glucocorticoids are derived. This cholesterol is provided to the fetus via the placenta both directly and as pregnenolone, which is converted to androgens using the specialized fetal zone of the adrenal cortex (see Chap. 13).

The placenta is unable to make androgens or estrogens directly, but instead receives androgens from the fetus and converts them to estrogens, which flow into the maternal compartment. In this way, the pathways of steroidogenesis serve to link mother to placenta to fetus during pregnancy.

Clinical Pearls

○ During normal pregnancy, the average weight gain is 11 kg, half due to changes in maternal tissues and half due to the fetus and related structures.
○ Approximately 250 to 300 extra kcal of energy substrates must be consumed per day to achieve and support this weight gain.

Review Questions

12. What are some of the anabolic changes in early pregnancy?
13. What is the principal hormone of the maternal catabolic state during late pregnancy?
14. What are the roles of mother, placenta, and fetus in steroidogenesis during pregnancy?

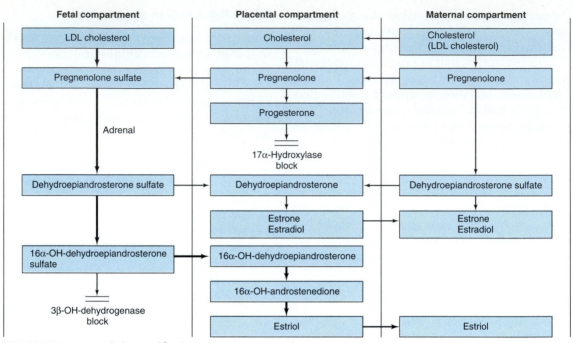

FIGURE 17.6. Maternal-placental-fetal cooperation in steroidogenesis during pregnancy. The mother is the source of cholesterol, which is converted to pregnenolone and made available to the fetus. The fetal adrenal gland converts pregnenolone into androgens, which are taken up by the placenta, converted into estrogen, and released to the mother. Note that, unlike that of estrogen, placental progesterone production is independent of the fetus. (*Reproduced, with permission, from Speroff L, Glass RH, & Case NG (1994).* Clinical gynecologic endocrinology and infertility, *5th ed. Baltimore, MD, Williams & Wilkins.*)

6. PARTURITION

A number of hormones, including cortisol, estrogen, progesterone, relaxin, CRH, oxytocin, and prostaglandins, have been implicated in maintaining uterine quiescence or initiating the onset of labor.

Once the fetus has reached a critical size, the muscles of the uterus are sufficiently stretched to stimulate their uncoordinated contraction. At least in some animals, a rise in fetal cortisol may play a role in initiating the concerted contractions of labor.

It has also been suggested that placental CRH, perhaps working through prostaglandins, plays a crucial role in onset of labor, as CRH levels in maternal blood rise dramatically in the third trimester, while CRH-binding protein levels fall sharply in the last month of gestation. The resulting increase in free CRH may occupy CRH receptors that are known to be in uterine muscle.

For these or other reasons, the uterine myometrium responds with strong contractions that ultimately expel the fetus and then the placenta. After separation of the placenta, oxytocin plays an important role in triggering uterine vasoconstriction in order to limit blood loss, which otherwise would be massive and fatal.

Review Questions

15. What are some of the hormones implicated in parturition?
16. What is the proposed role of CRH in parturition?

7. LACTATION

Structure and development of the breast

The mature adult female breast consists of a cluster of 15 to 25 lactiferous ducts, each emerging independently at the nipple (see Figure 17.7). The rudiments of breast development are established during embryonic development. During puberty, rising estrogen levels stimulate breast growth as one of a number of female secondary sexual characteristics. Finally, during pregnancy, the hormones progesterone, prolactin, and placental lactogen play a dominant role in stimulating breast growth and the capacity for milk synthesis. However, the presence of high levels of progesterone and estrogen during pregnancy blocks actual milk synthesis. Subsequent to delivery, with the fall in progesterone and estrogen levels, this block is removed. Both the pubertal and pregnant

FIGURE 17.7. Structure of the breast.

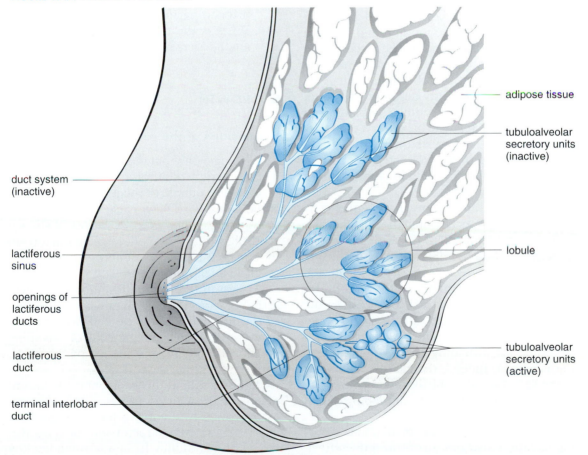

adipose tissue

tubuloalveolar secretory units (inactive)

duct system (inactive)

lactiferous sinus

openings of lactiferous ducts

lactiferous duct

terminal interlobar duct

lobule

tubuloalveolar secretory units (active)

phases of breast growth require the permissive influence of glucocorticoids, thyroxine, and insulin for full development, and their actions are potentiated by estrogen and progesterone.

Breast growth involves both proliferation and branching of lactiferous ducts and accumulation of adipose and connective tissue. In the mature breast, each terminal lactiferous duct drains clusters of tubuloalveolar secretory units lined by milk-secreting epithelial cells, and is suspended in connective and adipose tissue well populated with lymphocytes.

Initiation and maintenance of milk synthesis and secretion

Maintenance of milk secretion requires the joint action of both anterior and posterior pituitary factors in the mother, and also the interaction of infant and mother (see Figure 17.8). Suckling suppresses dopamine levels in the hypothalamus, thereby maintaining the high levels of prolactin necessary for milk synthesis. At the same time, suckling (and other stimuli such as the baby's cry, etc.) triggers an afferent sensory neural arc that stimulates synthesis, transport, and secretion of oxytocin, which is involved in contraction of mammary myoepithelial cells.

Toward the end of pregnancy, the IgA-secreting lymphocyte population in the vasculature and connective tissue of the breast increases. These lymphocytes secrete IgA into the local bloodstream, from which it is taken up by the mammary epithelial cells. By the process of transcytosis, IgA crosses the epithelial cell to be deposited into the lumenal secretion — milk. This mechanism is responsible for providing passive immunity to the newborn. Indeed, the earliest mammary gland secretion after birth, called colostrum, is particularly high in immunoglobulin content.

The high level of prolactin maintained during lactation also has a contraceptive effect, primarily by inhibition of pulsatile secretion of GnRH. The precise mechanism is not known but may involve a feedback loop by which prolactin stimulates endogenous opiates to inhibit GnRH secretion. There may also be effects of prolactin directly on the ovary that contribute to lactational amenorrhea and anovulation. However, it should be noted that this contraceptive influence is moderate and of low reliability, particularly when breast feeding is supplemented by bottle feeding.

Review Questions

17. Which hormones are involved in breast development?
18. Why is milk almost never secreted prior to parturition?
19. What is the mechanism of lactational amenorrhea?

8. GROWTH

Dimensions of the problem of growth

The biologic phenomenon of growth is manifest in a variety of different clinically relevant ways. One example of the problem of growth is the *continuum from* **cachexia** (*wasting*) *to obesity* (*excess body fat*). A variety of clinical syndromes of diverse etiology, characterized by negative or positive energy balance, can result in such outcomes.

A very different manifestation of growth is that of **cancer**: a cell that does not respond to the normal controls on cell division and hence proliferates out of control, invading the normal organs and tissues of the body, with devastating consequences.

Another side to this problem is the failure of cells to grow or proliferate. *Aging* in general appears to involve a loss of reparative and regenerative characteristics of cells. Removal of one kidney from a normal, healthy

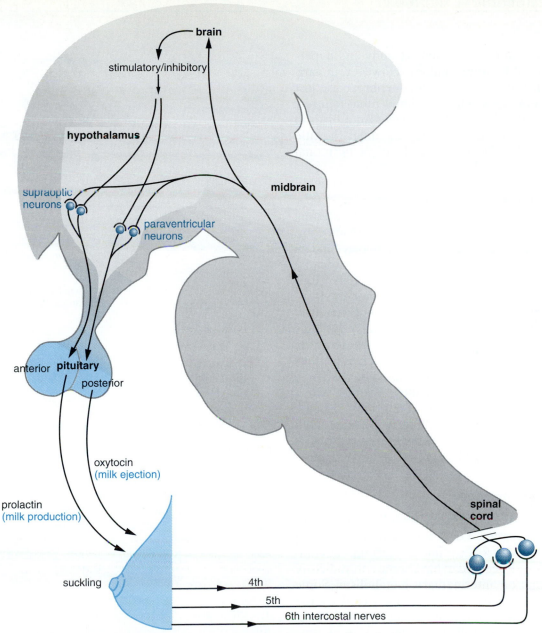

FIGURE 17.8. The role of anterior and posterior pituitary factors in milk synthesis and secretion. Prolactin plays many roles in pregnancy (see text), including a role in breast development and achieving the capacity for milk synthesis during pregnancy. However, the high levels of progesterone during pregnancy block actual milk formation. Upon expulsion of the placenta, progesterone levels fall and prolactin serves to promote milk synthesis. Suckling (nipple stimulation) results in afferent neural input to the hypothalamus, which triggers prolactin secretion from the anterior pituitary and oxytocin secretion from the posterior pituitary. Oxytocin causes contraction of myoepithelial cells to eject milk from the breast. *(Adapted, with permission, from Speroff L, Glass RH, Case NG. (1994). Clinical Gynecologic Endocrinology and Infertility, 5th ed. Baltimore, MD, Williams & Wilkins.)*

individual results in hypertrophy and hyperplasia of the other kidney. However, in various forms of renal disease, nephrons are lost and not replaced, resulting in renal failure.

Finally, *human development* from birth to adulthood can be considered under the title of growth. Development involves hormonal and other mechanisms that continue to operate to maintain homeostasis even in adulthood.

The mechanisms that underlie these different aspects of the problem of growth are complex and, in large measure, poorly understood. Moreover, they are inextricably intertwined with the problems of development and involve both genetic and environmental factors. Thus, kids are not just little people, cancer cells display bizarre biologic properties quite unrelated to proliferation, and obesity is not simply a problem of poor self-control. Whole books could be (and are) written on any one of these themes, which go far beyond the scope of this book. Instead, in this section, we will focus on one small dimension of this problem: the aspect involving **growth hormone**.

Growth hormone

Historically there has always been a discrepancy between GH's effects in vivo and in vitro. Moreover, under certain circumstances, it seemed to have some contradictory actions on intermediary metabolism. Some of this confusion has been clarified by the recognition of specific mediators of GH action (see the following) and different time courses of action (acute vs. delayed) in different tissues.

Direct actions of GH

It is necessary to separate the direct actions of GH from its indirect actions (see Figures 17.9 and 17.10). The direct actions of GH include several effects on carbohydrate and lipid metabolism that oppose the actions of

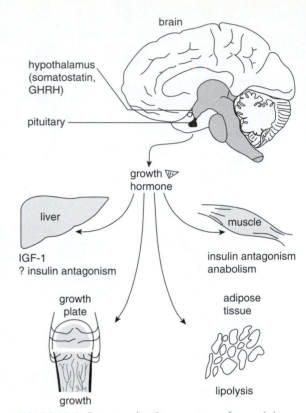

FIGURE 17.9. Direct and indirect actions of growth hormone. Under the control of growth hormone–releasing hormone (GHRH) as a positive stimulus and somatostatin as a negative regulator, growth hormone (GH) is released from the anterior pituitary and has direct and indirect effects. The direct effects on adipose tissue are antagonistic to insulin, promoting lypolysis. The direct effect on muscle is anabolic, promoting growth and anabolism. The direct effect on cartilage and the epiphyseal growth plate is to promote growth. The direct effect on the liver is to cause insulin-like growth factor 1 (IGF-1) synthesis and secretion. IGF-1 has negative-feedback effects on the anterior pituitary to suppress GH secretion. *(Adapted, with permission, from Thorner, MO, et al. (1992), in JD Wilson, DW Foster (eds): Williams Textbook of Endocrinology, 8th ed. Philadelphia, Saunders, 1992.)*

insulin; namely, it promotes lipolysis and hyperglycemia. The latter action may be caused by the blocking of the phosphorylation of glucose, which normally serves to retain it within cells. These actions of growth hor-

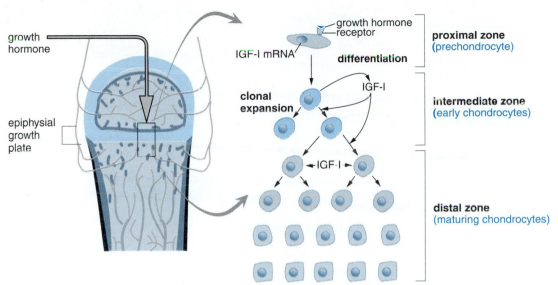

growth hormone

growth hormone receptor

IGF-I mRNA

proximal zone
(prechondrocyte)

differentiation

**clonal
expansion**

IGF-I

intermediate zone
(early chondrocytes)

epiphysial growth plate

◄IGF-I►

distal zone
(maturing chondrocytes)

FIGURE 17.10. Schematic diagram of growth hormone's effects on bone. GH acts directly at the epiphysial plate to stimulate linear growth by stimulating differentiation of prechondrocytres into early chondrocytes, which then secrete IGF-1. IGF-1 stimulates clonal expansion and maturation of chondrocytes. *(Adapted, with permission, from Thorner MO, et al. (1992), in Wilson JD, Foster DW (eds): Williams Textbook of Endocrinology, 8th ed. Philadelphia, Saunders.)*

mone are the ones that lead to its classification as a "counterregulatory hormone" in considering carbohydrate metabolism. Yet other direct actions of GH are anabolic: GH promotes the uptake of amino acids by both muscle and liver.

Indirect actions of GH

GH also has *indirect* actions, that is, effects that are the consequence not of GH itself, but of products secreted in response to GH. GH stimulates RNA and protein synthesis in a number of specific tissues, in particular the liver, where it induces the synthesis and secretion of a family of proteins termed the **somatomedins** or **insulin-like growth factors** (IGFs).

How do we make sense of these puzzling combinations of contradictory activities that are a consequence of growth hormone action? To understand what is going on here,

we must realize that multiple mechanisms of hormonal regulation, each triggered in response to different stimuli and having overlapping but not identical sets of actions, allow the body the maximum degree of fine-tuned control over physiological processes. Any seeming contradictions in a hormone's actions are likely to reflect our ignorance of the grand design of endocrinology and not a lack of elegance on the part of human physiology.

Regulation of GH secretion

Like its action, the regulation of GH secretion is complex (see Figure 17.11 and Table 17.2). As in the case of the other pituitary hormones mentioned (see Chap. 11), secretion is directly mediated by the pulsatile release of a hypothalamic releasing factor, growth hormone–releasing hormone (GHRH). Various neurotransmitters may stimulate GHRH release in response to dif-

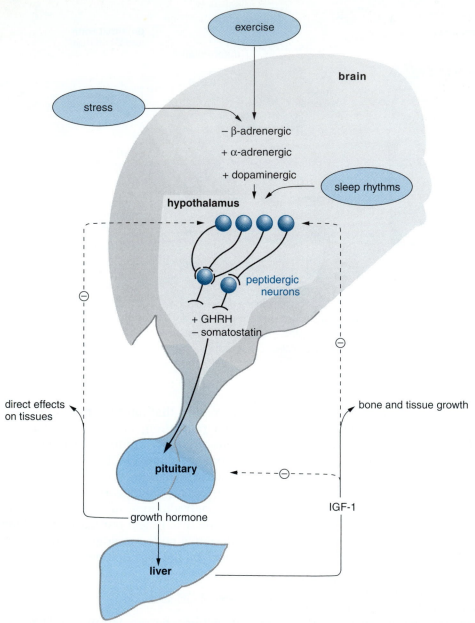

FIGURE 17.11. Schematic diagram of factors from higher centers that influence the hypothalamus, which in turn integrates various inputs to determine the magnitude of net stimulus or inhibition of GH secretion. *(Adapted, with permission, from Reichlin S (1992), in Wilson JD, Foster DW (eds): Williams Textbook of Endocrinology, 8th ed. Philadelphia, Saunders.)*

TABLE 17.2 REGULATION OF GROWTH HORMONE SECRETION

Factor	Augmented secretion	Inhibited secretion
Neurogenic	Stage III and stage IV sleep	REM sleep
	Stress (traumatic, surgical, inflammatory, psychic)	
	Alpha-adrenergic agonists	Alpha-adrenergic antagonists
	Beta-adrenergic antagonists	Beta-adrenergic agonists
	Dopamine agonists	
	Acetylcholine agonists	Acetylcholine antagonists
Metabolic	Hypoglycemia	Hyperglycemia
	Fasting	
	Falling fatty acid level	Rising fatty acid level
	Amino acids	
	Uncontrolled diabetes mellitus	Obesity
	Uremia	
	Hepatic cirrhosis	
Hormonal	GHRH	Somatostatin
	Low insulin-like growth factor level	High insulin-like growth factor level
	Estrogens	Hypothyroidism
	Glucagon	High glucocorticoid levels
	Arginine vasopressin	

GHRH = growth hormone releasing hormone.
Reproduced, with permission, from Thorner MO, et al. (1992), in Wilson JD, Foster DW (eds): *Williams Textbook of Endocrinology,* 8th ed. Philadelphia, Saunders.

ferent factors (e.g., seratonin mediates the observed sleep-related increase in growth hormone secretion, while catecholamines mediate the growth hormone secretory burst in response to hypoglycemia). Moreover, somatostatin, a peptide also secreted from the hypothalamus, serves as a primary inhibitor of GH secretion. Stress is a particularly confusing factor in that, while it is generally a stimulus of growth hormone secretion, sometimes it can inhibit growth hormone secretion. In most situations, stress increases growth hormone secretion because growth hormone is (like cortisol, glucagon, and epinephrine) a "stress hormone" that is counter-regulatory to the actions of insulin, that is, that serves to raise blood glucose (see Chap. 6). Presumably, different kinds and degrees of stress can do different things because they affect different combinations of neurotransmitters that are themselves stimuli or inhibitors of GH secretion.

Clinical Pearl

○ The clearest example of stress acting to inhibit growth hormone secretion occurs in the syndrome of psychosocial dwarfism. In this syndrome, children from emotionally deprived backgrounds or who have been subject to various forms of abuse, demonstrate a shutoff of GHRH and GH secretion. In addition, they may display bizarre behavior (e.g., eating from garbage cans, etc.). Sometimes only one of several siblings is affected, and the family history reveals the individual to have been selected for harsher discipline than siblings, etc. When removed from the source of the abuse, e.g., transferred to a nurturing foster environment, these children appear to reactivate their hypothalamic–pituitary growth hormone axis and can display amazing growth — 6 in. or more in a matter of a few months.

Review Question

20. Why is growth hormone called a "counterregulatory hormone" if its effect is, like that of insulin, to promote growth of tissues?

Somatomedins

The somatomedins, of which IGF-I and IGF-II predominate in human serum, share a strong homology to proinsulin, as do their receptors to the insulin receptor. These molecules serve to promote incorporation of proteoglycans by cartilage, increase cellular proliferation, and generally promote insulin-like actions in extraskeletal tissues. Although the liver is the primary systemic source, it appears that IGF-I is also synthesized by various other tissues (e.g., bone and cartilage), at which sites it serves growth-promoting autocrine or paracrine functions that are not well understood.

Serum levels of insulin and GH vary markedly in the course of the day as a consequence of the pulsatile and episodic nature of their secretion and their short half-life in plasma. However, IGFs are bound to large carrier proteins that maintain their serum concentration with less short-term fluctuation: No diurnal or circadian changes are observed in their levels, nor are they affected by daily activities such as eating. Normally, IGF-I levels are low at birth and gradually increase through puberty, after which there is a gradual decrease with age; the levels during puberty reach two to three times adult levels.

The major regulators of somatomedin secretion are GH and overall nutritional status. Thus, decreased levels are observed in hypothyroidism, malnutrition, and chronic disease.

Whereas both growth hormone and IGF-I stimulate somatostatin release from the hypothalamus, and thereby inhibit further growth hormone release, IGF-I also directly inhibits GH secretion from the anterior pituitary. The hormonal milieu modulates the magnitude of these influences. Thus, estrogen, testosterone, and thyroid hormone amplify the size of the GH response to any given regulatory influence, while glucocortcoids diminish it.

Because of the episodic nature of GH secretion, a single blood level is usually meaningless. The most reliable means of diagnosing a GH-related problem is with **provocative testing**. Thus, a vigorous growth hormone secretory response to insulin-induced hypoglycemia or to infusion of the amino acid arginine (another powerful stimulus, of growth hormone secretion for unclear reasons) reflects an intact hypothalamus-to-pituitary axis, etc.

Review Question

21. Describe the neuroendocrine feedback loop by which growth hormone has its effects and is controlled.

Other factors (besides growth hormone and IGF-1) involved in control of growth

Unusually short — or tall — stature is not necessarily a sign of pathology. If both parents are unusually tall or short, a similar outcome is likely for their offspring. Even if the parents are of normal stature, short stature in children can result from so-called constitutional delay of growth. Usually they will eventually catch up to expected growth curves.

Pathologic short stature may come about as a result of dysfunction of many different organ systems and does not necessarily reflect a disorder of the growth hormone neuroendocrine axis. The small for gestational age newborn may result from even moderate degrees of maternal alcohol consumption, smoking, malnutrition, or hypertension during pregnancy. Alcohol and smoking are directly toxic to the fetus. Hypertension damages the placenta, resulting in insufficient nutrient exchange to meet the growth needs of the fetus, irrespective of normal growth hormone levels.

Children whose short stature seems too severe, or otherwise unlikely to be accounted for by familial short stature or constitutional delay of growth (i.e., are far off the percentile growth curve), need to be evaluated for a broad range of occult medical problems, including

- Malnutrition
- Chronic illness (inflammatory disorders; GI tract malabsorption; renal failure; anemia of any cause; hypothyroidism; glucocorticoid excess; diabetes mellitus; congenital heart disease; chronic infections, including tuberculosis and syphilis)
- Psychosocial dwarfism (see the preceding Clinical Pearl)
- Genetic disorders
- Disorders of growth hormone secretion

Review Question

> 22. What are the broad causes of short stature, besides defective growth hormone secretion or action?

Clinical implications of altered GH secretion

A number of derangments of GH secretion/action are observed clinically. The most common abnormality is growth hormone deficiency due to a hypothalamic defect, resulting in lack of GHRH secretion. Less commonly, various forms of dwarfism have been observed.

- In the Pygmies of Zaire, there is a lack of synthesis of IGF-I by the liver, resulting in no prepubertal growth spurt.

- Defective growth hormone receptors in patients with Laron dwarfism
- Psychosocial dwarfism, in which emotional stress and malnutrition inhibit the hypothalamic–pituitary–end organ axis.

Deficient growth hormone secretion can now be treated with recombinant human growth hormone. However, the precise indications for this therapy remain controversial.

Excessive growth hormone secretion results in **gigantism** in children and **acromegaly** in adults (i.e., after epiphyseal closure, see Table 17.3). In such individuals, it is necessary to search for a GH-secreting tumor, typically in the anterior pituitary.

9. DISORDERS OF PREGNANCY

The normal events of pregnancy set the stage for a wide array of localized and systemic disorders:

- Abnormalities in the process of implantation appear to set in motion events leading to **preeclampsia**, a hypertensive syndrome associated with edema and proteinuria, occurring after 20 weeks of gestation. If untreated, preeclampsia can result in the development of **eclampsia**, involving seizures, with high risk to both mother and fetus.
- Inadequacy of the normal events of pregnancy (e.g., insufficient steroidogenesis by the placenta) will often result in spontaneous abortion or premature labor.
- Genetic predispositions to disease that might otherwise remain latent for decades may be manifest first, and often transiently, during pregnancy. A good example is the genetic predisposition to development of diabetes mellitus. As discussed, late pregnancy is a catabolic, counterregulatory state, with elevation of multiple blood glucose–elevating hormones, including hPL, estrogen, and progesterone. Because of

TABLE 17.3   EFFECTS OF GROWTH HORMONE EXCESS

Location	Symptoms	Signs
General	Fatigue Increased sweating Heat intolerance Weight gain Possible increased malignancy risk	Glucose intolerance Hypertriglyceridemia
Skin and subcutaneous tissue	Enlarging hands, feet Coarsening facial features Oily skin Hypertrichosis	Moist, warm, fleshy, doughy handshake Skin tags Acanthosis nigricans Increased heel pad
Head	Headaches	Parotid enlargement Frontal bossing
Eyes	Decreased vision	Visual field defects
Ears		Otoscope speculum cannot be inserted
Nose, throat, paranasal sinuses	Sinus congestion Increased tongue size Malocclusion Voice change	Enlarged furrowed tongue Tooth marks on tongue Widely spaced teeth Prognathism
Neck		Goiter Obstructive sleep apnea due to visceromegaly
Cardiorespiratory system	Congestive heart failure	Hypertension Cardiomegaly Left ventricular hypertrophy
Genitourinary system	Decreased libido Impotence Oligomenorrhea Infertility Renal colic	Urolithiasis
Neurologic system	Paresthesias Hypersomnolence	Carpal tunnel syndrome Nerve root compression due to bone and cartilage growth
Muscles	Weakness	Proximal myopathy
Skeletal system	Joint pains (shoulders, back, knees)	Osteoarthritis Increased 1,25-$(OH)_2D_3$ due to increased 1α-hydroxylase, resulting in increased Ca^{2+} absorption from gut and excretion in urine, increased bone density and turnover

Reproduced, with permission, from Daniels GH, Norton IB (1991), in Wilson JD et al. (eds): *Harrison's Principles of Internal Medicine,* 12th ed. New York, McGraw-Hill.

these counterregulatory features of pregnancy, blood glucose normalization in pregnant diabetics (pregestational diabetes mellitus) is more difficult than in those same individuals in the nonpregnant state. Moreover, many patients without known diabetes mellitus develop the disease during pregnancy (gestational diabetes mellitus). Gestational diabetes mellitus is six to ten times more common than pregestational diabetes mellitus, and involves 2 to 5% of all pregnancies in the United States.

Many individuals who will go on to develop non-insulin-dependent diabetes mellitus later in life will first manifest the disease during pregnancy.

High maternal blood glucose during pregnancy has prominent effects on the mother, the course of the pregnancy, and the fetus. **Retinopathy** and **nephropathy** may first appear in the mother with known diabetes during pregnancy, although the long-term severity of the mother's disease is probably not altered by pregnancy. There is a higher incidence of acute complications of diabetes, including ketoacidosis, hypoglycemia, and infections, during pregnancy. Patients with gestational and pregestational diabetes mellitus are at greater risk for preeclampsia. Since a long-term consequence of diabetes mellitus is small blood vessel damage, this observation is consistent with the hypothesis that preeclampsia results from endothelial cell injury as a consequence of ischemia. High maternal blood glucose, which results in excessive fetal weight gain, called **macrosomia**, also increases the rate and risk of cesarean section, with associated anesthetic and surgical morbidity, and the risk of complications from either cesarean section or birth trauma.

The effects of high maternal blood glucose on the fetus are even more profound than this discussion alone would suggest. Congenital anomalies are increased, as are unexplained fetal deaths and spontaneous abortions.

High maternal blood glucose triggers increased fetal insulin secretion and therefore results in a larger fetus. As the fetus becomes larger, it is more difficult for it to be expelled from the mother at birth. Called **fetopelvic disproportion**, this condition contributes to inability to deliver vaginally and is one reason for performing a **cesarean section** to remove the baby surgically. Neonatal morbidity due to hypoglycemia, hypocal-

cemia, polycythemia, and hyperbilirubinemia is also noted in the infants of diabetic mothers.

• Finally, the high levels of steroids and other products in the pregnant state can lead to a range of other serious medical complications. Thus, paradoxically, pregnancy is associated with both hemorrhage and thrombosis. Both are related to the unique structural and functional specializations of the placenta and compensatory adaptations in the course of mammalian evolution. On the one hand, separation of the placenta from the wall of the uterus at birth poses a threat of massive, life-threatening hemorrhage, given the intimate apposition of the placenta and the maternal blood supply. Perhaps as an adaptation to mitigate this risk, pregnancy has evolved as a hypercoagulable state.

Physiologically, this increased tendency to coagulation and decreased activity of the fibrinolytic system serves to control postpartum hemorrhage. Pathologically, these same factors pose a risk of inappropriate thrombosis and **disseminated intravascular coagulation**. It has been calculated that the risk of thrombophlebitis is increased nearly 50fold in the first month postpartum compared to before pregnancy. The risk of thromboembolism in pregnancy increases with age, the presence of hypertension, if the patient is at bed rest, and if delivery is by cesarean section. When thrombosis does occur, therapy is complicated by the fact that the standard treatment with the anticoagulant warfarin is contraindicated because of the risks of teratogenicity in early pregnancy and of fetal hemorrhage in the third trimester. Thus, pregnant patients with thrombosis are placed on subcutaneous heparin injection therapy.

One, but not the only, facet of the increased risk for thrombosis associated with pregnancy is the high estrogen state. Thus, an increased risk of thrombosis is also seen in pharmacologic estrogen use, as in oral contraceptives. The observation of enhanced cardiovascular mortality with high-dose birth control pills is probably due to these thrombogenic effects. The use of new low-dose estrogen combination pills reduces but does not eliminate this risk.

Spontaneous abortion and placental disorders

At least 15% of all implanted pregnancies terminate spontaneously (abort) as a result of genetic or environmental factors prior to the period when extrauterine life is possible (about 22 weeks of gestation and a mass of 500 g). When painless uterine bleeding occurs with a closed, long cervix, abortion is threatened. Heavy bleeding, pain, and dilatation of the cervix are signs of inevitable abortion. In patients presenting with these symptoms, spontaneous abortion must be distinguished from ectopic pregnancy (see Chap. 16), which typically is associated with more severe abdominal pain, and from hydatiform mole (see the following discussion). Making the correct diagnosis depends on the rate of rise of serum hCG over time and on **ultrasound examination** (the use of sound waves to image internal structures).

Third-trimester bleeding is sometimes caused by **placenta previa** (implantation of trophoblastic tissue on the lower uterine segment, obstructing all or part of the internal cervical os) or **placental abruption** (premature separation of a normally implanted placenta after more than 20 weeks of gestation).

Placenta previa is more prevalent in women who have had multiple prior pregnancies and is believed to be due to scar tissue formation from previous implantations. Placental abruption is due to hemorrhage into the decidual plate secondary to vascular rupture and is associated with hypertension, smoking, cocaine intoxication, trauma, and multiple pregnancies, all of which would be expected to affect the condition of the placental vasculature. Hemorrhage can be massive and life-threatening.

Trophoblastic malignancies

Molar pregnancies are abnormal growths due to trophoblastic proliferation (called a hydatiform mole), rarely, they are coexistent with a fetus (partial mole). The incidence in the United States is approximately 1 per 1500 pregnancies, but in certain areas of Asia the incidence is as high as 1 per 125 pregnancies. The tissue in complete moles has higher malignant potential and is purely of paternal origin, while that of partial moles is usually benign and may simply contain an excess of paternal chromosomes. Most moles present with vaginal bleeding and are diagnosed during evaluation of threatened abortion by the lack of a fetus and the presence of trophoblastic tissue by ultrasound. Particularly severe nausea of pregnancy and an extremely elevated hCG are suggestive but not diagnostic of molar pregnancy.

The complications of hydatiform mole include high risks of:

1. Developing **choriocarcinoma**, a highly malignant, trophoblastic neoplasm with high potential for metastasis, especially to lung and brain.
2. Coexisting hyperthyroidism, with a risk of thyroid storm during induction of anesthesia. The extremely high levels of hCG that occur with molar pregnancy and choriocarcinoma can result in cross-activation of the TSH receptor and trigger hyperthyroidism in some patients.
3. Severe hemorrhage or trophoblastic tissue pulmonary embolism during suction curettage procedure to remove the molar products.

Approximately 5% of women with hydatiform mole will subsequently be diagnosed with choriocarcinoma. The use of β-hCG as a sensitive monitor of the continued presence of malignant tissue and this tissue's exquisite sensitivity to chemotherapy have made choriocarcinoma readily curable if detected early.

Review Questions

23. What is preeclampsia? How does it differ from eclampsia?
24. What is the significance of third-trimester bleeding?
25. What is a molar pregnancy?

10. FRONTIERS IN THE PHYSIOLOGY OF PREGNANCY

How progesterone maintains uterine quiescence during pregnancy

In pregnancy, progesterone and oxytocin have somewhat opposite effects. Progesterone has long been suspected of a role in maintaining uterine quiescence, although its mechanism of action was not known. Oxytocin, on the other hand, stimulates contraction of uterine smooth muscle, and its rise late in pregnancy has been viewed as part of the mechanism by which labor is initiated.

Recent findings suggest a truly unexpected mechanism for the action of a progesterone metabolite (5 β-dihydroprogesterone) on uterine quiescence (see Ref. 6). It seems that the oxytocin receptor on the cell surface of uterine muscle cells has a binding site for this metabolite of progesterone. When the progesterone metabolite is bound, oxytocin cannot bind. Furthermore, progesterone metabolite binding causes a decrease in the number of oxytocin receptors present on the cell surface. Thus, higher concentrations of oxytocin are needed to occupy a given number of receptors and thereby carry out oxytocin effects (uterine muscle contraction). The progesterone metabolite antagonizes the effects of oxytocin in other ways as well: Production of inositol triphosphate second messengers is inhibited. The rise in intracellular calcium resulting from activation of oxytocin receptors is blocked.

With these remarkable findings, the authors add to the growing body of data suggesting that our understanding of steroid hormone action is fundamentally incomplete (see Chaps. 3, 15, and 16). These agents, conventionally thought to work through activation of transcription, are, in the present actions, working *directly* at the cell surface by effects on a polypeptide hormone receptor. The authors include elegant experiments that make other explanations for these effects unlikely.

Another pleasing derivative of this work is that it provides a rationale for the enormous amounts of progesterone made during pregnancy. The affinity constant (see Chap. 3) for the effects of progesterone derivatives on the oxytocin receptor is approximately 20 nM. In contrast, the effect of progesterone binding to the classical progesterone receptor for conventional steroid hormone action displays an affinity constant of <1 nM. Thus, vastly elevated levels of progesterone are needed for the effects on the oxytocin receptor to occur — just as is the case during pregnancy.

Molecular basis for maternal mammary gland insulin sensitivity in late pregnancy

Late pregnancy is a catabolic, relatively insulin-resistant state for the mother (see Sec. 5). Yet for some tissues, such as the mammary gland, which must prepare for its incipient role in providing nutrition for the newborn, late pregnancy is a time of substantial anabolic activity. How is this possible within the larger catabolic state occurring in the mother as a whole?

A recent study confirmed that the mammary gland is more insulin-sensitive in pregnant animals than in the nonpregnant (see Ref. 7). Furthermore, it provides a molecular explanation for this phenomenon.

The insulin receptor works in part by an intrinsic tyrosine kinase activity within the receptor molecule itself (see Chaps. 3 and 6). It appears that the increased sensitivity of mammary epithelial cells to insulin in late pregnancy is due to increased activity of the receptor tyrosine kinase. From other experiments, the authors suggest that there are mammary-specific mechanisms to inhibit insulin receptor kinase activity in the nonpregnant state. During pregnancy, these mechanisms are turned off to allow a differential increase in insulin sensitivity of the mammary gland, even while the mother is in a catabolic state. It would seem that, in the course of evolution, where there is a will, there is a way. Ingenious selective mechanisms have evolved to make opposites — in this case, anabolism within catabolism — work together for the best interests of the organism.

The molecular basis for neural tube defects in diabetes mellitus

One value of prenatal care is that it allows screening procedures for fetal defects to be performed. These procedures, which include **amniocentesis** (sampling of amniotic fluid, in which some fetal cells can be found) and chorionic villus biopsy, allow embryos with major congenital malformation to be identified so that either the family may be better prepared or the pregnant woman has the option of elective abortion early in the course of pregnancy.

Diabetic mothers have a two- to fivefold increased risk of congenital malformations even with optimal blood glucose control. An experimental system has recently been developed that allows this "embryopathy" associated with diabetes mellitus to be studied (see Ref. 6). Pregnant, diabetic mice whose blood glucose is maintained near the normal range are shown to have a threefold increased risk of congenital neural tube defects, similar to the increased risk of pregnant diabetic women.

Using this system, the authors show that expression of a gene called *pax-3,* required for neural tube closure, is significantly reduced in the embryos of the diabetic mice. As a result of *pax-3* underexpression, increased apoptosis was observed. Consistent with this observation, mice in which the *pax-3* has been knocked out (see Chap. 2) show similar neural tube defects in the absence of diabetes mellitus. The authors speculate on the role of disordered glucose metabolism, free radical generation, or disordered signaling pathways as the final common pathway by which *pax-3* underexpression leads to neural tube apoptosis.

Through this sort of work, a better understanding of what causes, and what can be done to prevent, the increased risk of birth defects associated with diabetes mellitus will continue to emerge. The benefit to all will be further improvements in prenatal care and the health and happiness of future generations.

11. HOW DOES AN UNDERSTANDING OF NORMAL PHYSIOLOGY PROVIDE INSIGHT INTO THE INITIAL CASE PRESENTATION?

Very serious problems in pregnancy can be anticipated and often avoided by monitoring various parameters of the health of the mother, the pregnancy, and the fetus.

Ms. Z appears to have had preeclampsia, an inflammatory vascular disorder (called a vasculitis) manifesting as increased blood pressure, edema, and protein in the urine, all of which would have been screened for during routine prenatal care. Undiagnosed and untreated, preeclampsia can progress to eclampsia, characterized by seizures in the mother. These disorders have grave consequences for both the mother and the fetus.

The hypertension and vasculitis associated with preeclampsia carry a significantly increased risk of stroke.

Cultural, economic, and political barriers to obtaining prenatal care need to be minimized in order to decrease the frequency of such tragic and expensive cases. With prenatal care, the high-risk features of this pregnancy could have been identified earlier and the mother and fetus monitored more closely, with a high likelihood that the outcome would have been better.

The future for both Ms. Z and her child is uncertain at this point. Depending on rehabilitation and luck, Ms. Z may recover fully or may be profoundly disabled. Likewise, the degree of disability of the baby will be manifest as she grows.

SUMMARY AND REVIEW OF KEY CONCEPTS

1. Fertilization takes place in the fallopian tube, with the resulting zygote starting to divide almost immediately. Over the course of the next 3 days, the fertilized egg travels to the uterus, and over the subsequent days, it proceeds to implant into the uterine endometrium.

2. The implanted embryo differentiates a trophoblastic layer committed to the enhancement of fetal-maternal cooperation and an inner cell mass that will give rise to the body.

3. The placenta consists of fetal and maternal parts. The fetal components are the syncytiotrophoblasts and the cytotrophoblasts, which give rise to chorionic villi. The maternal components are the decidual cells, which give rise to lacunae and later intervillous spaces in which exchange of nutrients and wastes with maternal blood occurs.

4. A number of hormones make pregnancy possible. The most important is probably progesterone, with estrogen, placental lactogen, relaxin, CRH, cortisol, and prolactin playing important roles ranging from suppression of the immune system to maintenance of uterine quiescence.

5. Special forms of maternal-placental-fetal interaction are observed, including use of hPL to preferentially siphon glucose and other substrates to the fetus, and compartmentalization of steps in steroidogenesis. Maternal cholesterol is converted in the placenta to pregnenolone and progesterone. The former provides the fetal adrenal with the substrate it needs for androgen synthesis. The placenta converts fetal adrenal androgens into estrogen for the maternal compartment.

6. Parturition is believed to be triggered by hormonal changes that end the quiescence of the uterine myometrium. Implicated hormones include CRH, cortisol, prostaglandins, and oxytocin.

7. Lactation requires development and maturation of the breast under the influence of a host of hormones, including insulin, estrogen and progesterone, and prolactin. However, actual milk synthesis cannot occur until blood estrogen and progesterone levels have fallen. This occurs shortly after expulsion of the placenta.

8. GH is part of a hypothalamic pituitary neuroendocrine axis whose end organs include both the liver and cartilage, which respond to growth hormone by synthesizing IGF-1. The liver secretes IGF-1 as a systemic hormone, while cartilage secretes IGF-1 as a local mediator.

9. GH secretion is enhanced by some, and suppressed by other, forms of stress. Measurement of GH requires provocative testing in response to insulin-induced hypoglyemia or arginine infusion.
10. Common problems during pregnancy include hypertensive syndromes, including preeclampsia and eclampsia; disorders of blood glucose regulation; abnormalities of placental location, function, structure, and viability; and malignancies related to trophoblastic tissue.

A CASE OF PHYSIOLOGICAL MEDICINE

MV is a 32-year-old woman with a healthy 10-year-old son and a family history of diabetes mellitus; she has had normal blood glucose on previous screening. During her previous pregnancy, she had received excellent prenatal care and was not noted to have any abnormalities of blood glucose. Her weight prior to her first pregnancy was 65 kg. Her blood pressure and blood glucose 1 year prior to the current pregnancy were both normal; however, her weight has risen gradually to 75 kg.

Ms. V is now in her second pregnancy. On routine prenatal screening at 5½ months, she was noted to have an abnormal glucose tolerance test. In this test, the blood glucose response to an oral load of glucose is determined. Normally, glucose will not rise above 140 mg/dL.

Unfortunately, Ms. V's husband had lost his job 1 week before. Her subsequent prenatal care fell between the cracks during the crisis posed by her husband's loss of employment and with it health care coverage for his family. The family moved to another state as the husband searched for employment. As a result, they could not be reached when the health care provider tried to refer the patient to the county hospital for follow-up care.

At 8 months into her pregnancy, Ms. V noted decreased movement of her fetus and sought care in an emergency room. Her blood pressure was noted to be elevated. There was protein in her urine. Her blood glucose was 280 mg/dL. After further evaluation, including ultrasound and fetal monitoring, Ms. V was informed that her baby had died, most likely due to placental insufficiency.

QUESTIONS

1. Why is late pregnancy called a state of "accelerated starvation"? How and why does this differ from early pregnancy?
2. What is the role of these metabolic changes in maintaining fetal energy needs?
3. Why did Ms. V have no history of hyperglycemia during or for 10 years after the first pregnancy but apparently develop gestational diabetes mellitus with the second pregnancy?
4. What are the possible consequences of maternal hyperglycemia in pregnancy for the fetus? For the mother?

ANSWERS

1. The rise of hPL, cortisol, and other counterregulatory hormones makes late pregnancy a high-stress state, resistant to storage of glucose in muscle and fat. Thus, glucose is available to meet the needs of the fetus.
2. Early in pregnancy, the needs of the fetus are very small. Hence it makes sense that insulin sensitivity would be closer to normal, as the body makes the structural and metabolic changes to prepare for the high-stress stage of late pregnancy.
3. She was last pregnant at age 22, when she not only was younger but also had a sub-

stantially lower weight. She may no longer have the insulin reserve to meet the high-stress needs of late pregnancy, although she had been able to maintain a normal blood glucose previously.

4. Consequences for the fetus include death, macrosomia, birth trauma, developmental anomalies, and hypoglycemia after delivery. Consequences for the mother include all types of end organ damage caused by hyperglycemia and increased risk of a traumatic delivery or a cesarean section, with its additional risk of anesthesia.

References and suggested readings

GENERAL REFERENCES

1. Taylor R, Martin M (1997). Endocrinology of pregnancy, in Greenspan FS, Strewler GS (eds.), *Basic and Clinical Endocrinology*, 5th ed. Stamford, CT, Appleton & Lange.
2. Speroff L, et al. (1994). *Clinical Gynecologic Endocrinology and Infertility*, 5th ed. Baltimore, Williams & Wilkins.
3. Keelan JA, et al. (1997). The molecular mechanisms of term and preterm labor: Recent progress and clinical implications. *Clin Obstet Gynecol* 40:460–478.
4. Styne DM (1996). Growth, in Greenspan FS, Strewler GJ (eds), *Basic and Clinical Endocrinology*, 5th ed. Stamford, CT, Appleton & Lange.
5. Rudolph AM, Hoffman JIE, Rudolph CD (1996). *Rudolph's Pediatrics*, 20th ed. Stamford, CT, Appleton & Lange, Chap. 26.

FRONTIERS REFERENCES

6. Grazzini E, et al. (1998). Inhibition of oxytocin receptor function by direct binding of progesterone. *Nature* 392:509–512.
7. Carrascosa JM, et al. (1998). Changes in the kinase activity of the insulin receptor account for an increased insulin sensitivity of mammary gland in late pregnancy. *Endocrinology* 139:520–526.
8. Phelan SA, et al. (1997). Neural tube defects in embryos of diabetic mice: Role of the pax-3 gene and apoptosis. *Diabetes* 46:1189–1197.

PHYSIOLOGY OF THE NERVOUS SYSTEM

18

1. INTRODUCTION TO THE PHYSIOLOGY OF THE NERVOUS SYSTEM

The nervous system comprises several trillion cells within our bodies that are specialized for recognizing, transmitting, and analyzing various kinds of information from other cells or from the environment. This immense system can be broken down into several component subsystems that can be understood as smaller pieces of the puzzle of neurologic function.

The *sensory system* is the means by which information from other cells and the environment is brought to, and decoded by, the nervous system. Input often comes in the form of environmental sensations such as pain, temperature, movement, and pressure. "Special senses," including vision (detecting light), hearing (detecting sound waves), smell, and taste, provide a means of detecting other forms of information in the environment.

The *motor system* is the means by which the nervous system carries out actions (e.g., in response to sensory information). Some of these actions are *voluntary* (e.g., those that involve most skeletal muscle); others are, to one degree or another, *involuntary* (e.g., the rate of heartbeat). Some involve simple reflex arcs, bypassing the brain. Others involve complex communication between various regions of the brain.

Decoding sensation, deciding on the appropriate motor response, and carrying out that motor response involve a tremendous amount of integration between motor and sensory nerve fibers and various other areas of the brain, including those responsible for memory, motivation, emotions, critical thinking, and judgment. Complex movements involve the brain regions known as the *cerebellum* and the *basal ganglia.* Judgment, memory, critical thinking, and other "higher" functions reside in the *cerebral cortex*. These

are the features that make us truly "human" — and about whose biological basis we have the least amount of insight.

There is a large gap between present knowledge and what is needed to answer the question, "What is the mechanistic basis for this patient's problem?" Nowhere in physiology is this question more challenging than as it applies to neurology. Nevertheless, there have been enormous advances in our understanding of the nervous system in recent years, and it is likely that a correspondingly great impact on clinical practice will soon follow.

Why understanding the nervous system is important for medical practice

Nervous system disorders are extremely common in the general population and hence are seen on a daily basis by the generalist clinician. Many patients have neurologic problems that, while not life-threatening, have a major negative impact on their quality of life (e.g., headaches, dizziness, peripheral neuropathy, etc.). Effective recognition of what they have, what is likely to have caused it, and simple (preferably nonpharmacologic) ways of preventing recurrence will do these patients tremendous good. For those patients who need pharmacologic intervention, recognizing potential side effects and limitations of the therapy, based on current insight into the physiology of the neurologic subsystem involved, is crucial to proper clinical care.

Some patients presenting with what at first glance seems to be a trivial problem in fact have an unstable and dangerous condition. How does one distinguish the rare condition with a common presentation? If this is the one person in a thousand whose focal neurologic finding was a harbinger of an impending but preventable neurologic catastrophe, it does little good for you to say that his or her condition was statistically unlikely. In at least some of these cases, a fairly simple understanding of normal neurologic anatomy and physiology may mean the difference between rapid diagnosis, treatment, and full recovery and life-long disability or even death. Understanding physiology is no panacea, but it can help — and good medical practice requires that we avail ourselves of all the help we can get.

A useful general approach to disorders referable to the nervous system is to always consider two questions. First, ask, "Where is the lesion?" — and use your understanding of normal anatomy and functional neurophysiology to determine the level and region within the nervous system at which there is a defect. Once a lesion has been localized, the next question the clinician generally asks is, "What is the cause of this lesion?" — with an emphasis on the possibilities that are treatable. To this we suggest be added a third question: "Why does this lesion cause this problem?" It seems likely that future insight into the physiology of the nervous system will elevate the third question to a prominence currently reserved for the other two, as new modalities of prevention and treatment become available.

Case Presentation

C.L. is a 24-year-old medical student who developed mild left third- and fourth-finger weakness and facial tingling while examining patients during his second-year preceptorship. He brought his symptoms to the attention of his attending physician, whose first reaction was that the student was imagining in himself the kinds of things he was looking for in the patients. On further questioning, the student reported playing "floor hockey" on the hospital ward while on call the night before and having been hit on the elbow by

whatever they were using as a puck. Hence the finger symptoms might simply be a mild traumatic ulnar **neuropathy** that would get better without any particular attention, and not something to worry about.

Nevertheless, one particular feature of his presentation was worrisome and led the student to suspect that something was terribly wrong — it might all be "in his head," but not in the way the attending physician seemed to think. He insisted on leaving the clinic and being evaluated in the emergency room. There, the neurologist on call noted a feature suggesting a central rather than a peripheral lesion and therefore inconsistent with an ulnar neuropathy, and ordered an emergency MRI scan — which revealed a leaking **cerebral aneurysm**.

The student, now a patient and quite distraught, was hospitalized and prepared for emergency surgery. The night before surgery, the surgeon met C.L. for the first time. He tersely uttered four words upon entering the room: "I can get it," and then left. The student-patient was tremendously relieved and had a restful night. The next day he came through the complex 4-h surgical procedure with flying colors. His postoperative course was complicated by the expected complications of transient inability to speak, **diabetes insipidus** (excessively dilute urine production; see Chap. 10) that lasted several days), and slow recovery from various **sensory and motor deficits** (lasting days to weeks). Likewise, he required treatment for a year with **antiseizure medications**. However, his long-term prognosis is excellent — and his sensitivity to the emotional state of his future patients has been substantially heightened. The experience of facing a potentially devastating medical problem that appeared out of the blue and the frustrations of a slow postoperative recovery have made him a better physician in more ways than he could have ever imagined.

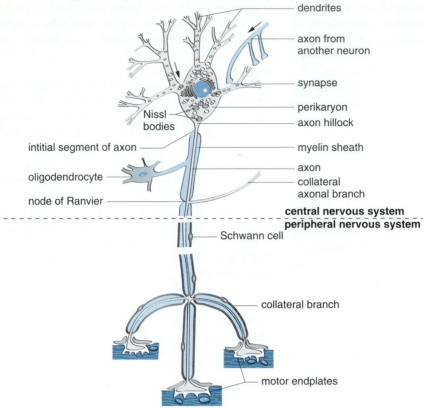

A

FIGURE 18.1. Structures of neurons and glia. *A*. Neuron with synapses and labeled parts; *B*. glial cells associated with vessel; *C*. myelinated and nonmyelinated neurons. Note that a myelinated neuron is one that has had a Schwann cell wrap itself around the axon. One Schwann cell can myelinate several neurons. *(A reproduced, with permission, from Jungueira LC, Carneiro J, Kelley RO (1995). Basic Histology, 8th ed. Stamford, CT, Appleton & Lange. C adapted, with permission, from Ganong WF (1997). Review of Medical Physiology, 18th ed. Stamford, CT, Appleton & Lange.)*

2. ANATOMY, CELL BIOLOGY, AND GENERAL PHYSIOLOGY OF THE NERVOUS SYSTEM

Anatomy

The nervous system consists of the **central nervous system** (CNS) and the **peripheral nervous system** (PNS). The brain and spinal cord make up the CNS. The PNS includes the nerves outside of the CNS that carry sensory information to the CNS and motor and other commands back from the CNS to muscles and glands. The **autonomic nervous system** (ANS) is a part of both the CNS and the PNS that has varying degrees of control over relatively automatic, largely involuntary functions (so-called visceral functions) of the body. These include gastrointestinal functions, blood pressure regulation, bladder

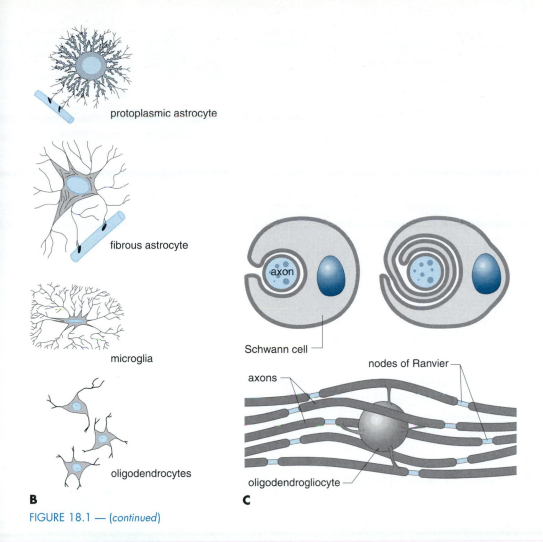

protoplasmic astrocyte

fibrous astrocyte

microglia

oligodendrocytes

B

axon

Schwann cell

axons

nodes of Ranvier

oligodendrogliocyte

C

FIGURE 18.1 — (*continued*)

emptying, sweating, and body temperature regulation. There is also an **enteric nervous system** (ENS) of neurons in the gastrointestinal tract that is partially independent and partially under ANS control. The ENS is discussed in detail in Chapter 5.

Cell biology

Two broad categories of cells make up the nervous system (see Figure 18.1): (1) **neurons**, cells specialized for communication through transmission of action potentials, and (2) **glial cells**, which play a wide range of supportive roles in maintaining neurons, facilitating their functions, protecting them from infection and injury, and responding to their dysfunction and death.

There are about 100 billion neurons in the body. Neurons themselves are extremely varied in structure. However, they have some basic features in common (see Figure 18.1A). **Dendrites** are structures through which neurons receive information, either from the environment via receptors or from other neurons. The **cell body** contains the nucleus of the neuron. The **axon** is the structure via which the neuron sends messages, in the form of electrical signals called **action potentials**, to other cells, including neurons, muscle cells, and endocrine glands. These messages are transmitted from a neuron to the next cell by **chemical signaling** across a structure called the **synapse** (see Figure 18.2). The chemical signals are **neurotransmitters** released from the presynaptic neuron that diffuse across the synapse and bind to receptors in the plasma membrane of the postsynaptic cell. Activation of a sufficient number of receptors on the postsynaptic cell membrane triggers various responses. If the postsynaptic cell is another neuron, another action potential may be triggered. If it is a muscle cell, a calcium flux and muscle contraction may be triggered. If it is an endocrine gland, hormone secretion may be triggered. Despite these common themes, individual neurons differ in terms of

- The number of dendrites they have
- The number of cells they contact with branches of their axon
- The number of other neurons from which they receive input in the form of axon branches
- The chemical nature of the neurotransmitter they release
- Whether the neuron is stimulatory or inhibitory in an electrophysiological sense (see the following discussion)
- The nature of their interactions with glial cells (see the following discussion)
- The type and direction of transport of membrane vesicles within the cytoplasm of the axon. Different forms of vesicular trafficking, called slow and fast **axonal transport** and **retrograde transport**, occur in neurons and are important for processes such as regeneration after injury.

The role of the synapse is not only to allow action potentials to travel from one neuron to another, but also to serve as a sort of filter,

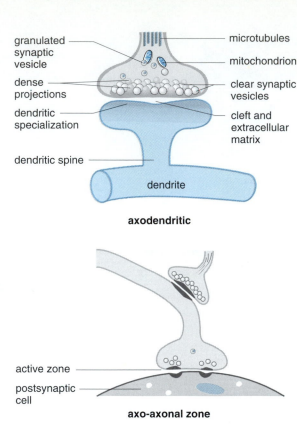

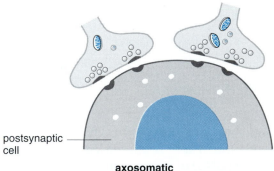

FIGURE 18.2. The synapse. Some examples of synapses formed (from top to bottom) between axons and dendrites, axons and axons, and axons and cell bodies of other neurons. *(Reproduced, with permission, from Ganong FW (1997). Textbook of Medical Physiology, 18th ed. Stamford, CT, Appleton & Lange, p 81.)*

preventing some weak signals from being propagated, while reinforcing, modifying, and sometimes redirecting other signals. Thus, the synapse is a crucial feature of information flow within the nervous system.

In addition to the neurons, there is a 10 to 50 times greater number of glial cells in the nervous system. A number of different types of glial cells exist in the CNS. **Astrocytes** are glial cells that have foot processes on blood vessels, allowing them to secrete various cytokines in response to CNS injury. Astrocytes also are involved in removing glutamate, a potentially toxic excitatory neurotransmitter, from the local brain environment. In addition, astrocytes respond to CNS injury by increasing in both size and number, a process called **reactive astrocytosis**.

Schwann cells and **oligodendrocytes** are glial cells in the peripheral and central nervous systems, respectively. They wrap themselves many times around certain neurons. This provides a form of electrical insulation that allows much faster propagation of action potentials along the neuron. The multiple layers of plasma membrane wrapping are called a **myelin sheath**. This name reflects the specialized enrichment of the protein myelin in the Schwann cell plasma membrane. Such myelinated neurons make up **white matter** within the CNS. The **nodes of Ranvier** are spaces between the myelin where sodium channels are concentrated on the neuronal plasma membrane, allowing the action potential to jump from node to node, called **saltatory conduction**. Unmyelinated neurons are able to conduct action potentials at speeds of 20 m/s. Because of saltatory conduction, myelinated neurons are able to conduct action potentials as much as 50 times faster.

Finally, **microglia** are macrophage-derived resident brain cells that provide a first line of defense against infection, injury, and neurodegeneration. When activated, they provide an inflammatory response, with release of cytokines, proteases, and reactive oxygen species. They are phagocytic cells that will consume invaders and dead tissue. Like other immune cells (see Chap. 20), however, they have the potential to mount an excessive response, and thereby cause harm to the host as well as the invader.

General neurophysiology

As already mentioned, signaling in the nervous system involves both electrical and chemical events. First, let us consider the electrical part. The plasma membrane of all cells has an **electrical potential**, determined by the steady-state distribution of ions across the plasma membrane, which is in turn a consequence of ion channels and transporter activity. Na^+/K^+-ATPase is the major transporter involved in maintaining the charge distribution that gives rise to this membrane potential. Most cells are normally highly impermeable to sodium ions but have a slight potassium ion leak that makes the inside of the cell slightly negative in charge compared to the outside, with the typical electrical potential being -70 MeV inside the cell.

In neurons, this general cellular property of an electrical potential difference across the plasma membrane is put to specialized use. Certain ion channels in the neuronal plasma membrane are triggered to open in response to chemical signals from specialized receptor cells or other neurons. When these so-called ligand-gated ion channels are opened, the flood of ions transiently reverses the electrical potential, a phenomenon called **depolarization**.

Depolarization results in a "spike" of electrical activity — the action potential. This action potential is transmitted down the axon through propagation of the transient ion flux caused by a wave of opening and subsequent closing of ion channels. When the action potential has propagated all the way to the end of the axon, it reaches the synapse, where it triggers release of stored neurotransmitters through a process called **regulated exocytosis** (see Chap. 2). This involves fusion of synaptic vesicles to the plasma membrane, releasing neurotransmitter into the space between the end of one neuron's axon and the beginning of the next neuron's dendrites. The neurotransmitter then diffuses across the synapse and binds receptor proteins on the plasma membrane of the **postsynaptic cell**.

Synaptic transmission, the effective propagation of a signal across a synapse, depends upon several variables:

First, the amount of neurotransmitter released has to exceed a given threshold. If this threshold is exceeded, a signal is transmitted to the postsynaptic cell. Whether signaling exceeds the threshold is in part determined by the sum total of other inputs (some inhibitory or hyperpolarizing, others stimulatory and depolarizing) to the postsynaptic cell.

Second, the nature of the postsynaptic cell affects the outcome:

- When the postsynaptic cell is a neuron, the signal generated by successful synaptic transmission is an action potential that travels down the axon of the post-synaptic cell.
- When the postsynaptic cell is a muscle cell, binding of the released neurotransmitter to a surface receptor triggers release of calcium, which in turn causes muscle contraction rather than another action potential.
- When the postsynaptic cell is an endocrine cell, release of calcium triggers hormone secretion rather than muscle contraction.

Let us consider events within a neuron in which an action potential has been generated. The membrane potential at any given point along the plasma membrane where depolarization has occurred quickly returns to baseline, as a result of closure of the ligand-gated channels that had triggered (or propagated) the depolarization. In addition, other channels and transporters remove the excess ions that had flooded in during the depolarization, thereby speeding the return to baseline. The duration of the spike of an action potential is determined by how long it takes to do this.

Immediately after a depolarization, there is a window of time called the *refractory period*, during which the cell is resistant to generating another action potential.

Myriad complexities can be built into the system by simply changing any one of many parameters, including the nature of the:

- Channels that are opened in response to stimuli
- Stimuli to which channels respond
- Transmitter that is ultimately released at the synapse
- Second messenger (within the cytoplasm of the target cell) that is triggered by receptor activation and channel opening
- Effector function to which the chemical second messenger is coupled (e.g., formation of another action potential vs. muscle contraction vs. hormone secretion)

Even the structure of the neurons themselves can change (e.g., increased or decreased density of receptors, induction of new receptors, downregulation or desensitization of receptors), contributing to the phenomenon of memory.

The chemical signaling across the synapse and how it is interpreted by the next cell depend upon the receptors available on the postsynaptic cell and the second messenger systems to which they are coupled (see Chap. 3). We have discussed the situation in which the neurotransmitter triggers an action potential in the postsynaptic cell. Often the neurotransmitter-receptor interaction is *inhibitory*. This means that the neurotransmitter either prevents opening of the ligand-gated ion channel that normally makes possible the ion flux to trigger an action potential, or opens a different channel to oppose that ion flux and thereby prevent the stimulus from being sufficient to depolarize the cell. Thus, the normal balance of output from a neuron is the complex summation of all the inhibitory and stimulatory synapses being made with myriad other neurons.

Clinical Pearl

○ There are many ways in which drugs, toxins, and even antibodies can interfere with transmission of chemical signals across a synapse. For example:

- In Lambert-Eaton syndrome, antibodies to the calcium channel inhibit calcium entry into the presynaptic nerve terminal and thereby slow down the vesicle fusion needed for neurotransmitter release. As a result, muscles are initially weak, but their power increases as contraction is maintained. This is because the amount of neurotransmitter released slowly reaches the needed threshold for muscle contraction, resulting in contraction of more and more muscle fibers over time. Aminoglycoside antibiotics can sometimes also interfere with calcium channel function and thereby cause a similar syndrome.
- In botulism food poisoning, ingestion of food contaminated with *Clostridium* toxins results in paralysis at cholinergic synapses. Botulinum toxin includes a protease that selectively cleaves presynaptic proteins necessary for neurotransmitter release.
- In myasthenia gravis, autoantibodies to the nicotinic acetylcholine receptor interfere with the ability of the neurotransmitter to trigger signaling in the post-synaptic plasma membrane, thereby causing muscle weakness.

- Some potent nerve gases used in biological warfare inhibit the enzyme acetylcholine esterase, which normally clears the synapse of acetylcholine after an action potential has been signaled. Without the action of this enzyme, it is not possible to send repetitive action potentials and maintain a certain level of neuronal activity.

Central nervous system

The brain

The brain is the part of the CNS that is housed in what neurologists call the **cranial vault** or **cranium** and what the rest of us just think of as the skull (see Figure 18.3). It consists of the **cerebral cortex**, the **brainstem**, and the **cerebellum**.

The cerebral cortex is the largest, most evolutionarily advanced, most complex, and least well understood part of the human brain. In overall organization, the cerebral cortex consists of left and right hemispheres, each of which consists of frontal, parietal, temporal, limbic, and occipital lobes. Each lobe is further organized into highly convoluted folds and ridges called **gyri**. The gyri are separated by grooves that are either shallow (called **sulci**) or deep (called **fissures**). The functions of the cerebral cortex are discussed in more detail in Section 7.

The brainstem is the more "ancient" part of the brain that carries out "automatic" functions such as breathing and blood pressure regulation. It consists of four regions (from front to back):

1. The **diencephalon** on either side of the third ventricle, including the **thalamus** and **hypothalamus**
2. The **midbrain**
3. The **pons**
4. The **medulla**

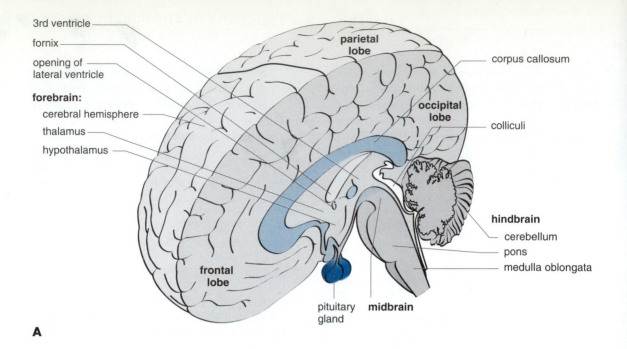

A

3rd ventricle
fornix
opening of lateral ventricle

forebrain:
cerebral hemisphere
thalamus
hypothalamus

parietal lobe

corpus callosum

occipital lobe

colliculi

hindbrain
cerebellum
pons
medulla oblongata

frontal lobe

pituitary gland

midbrain

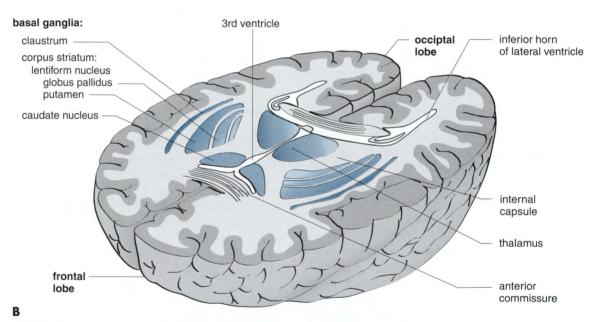

B

basal ganglia:
claustrum
corpus striatum:
    lentiform nucleus
        globus pallidus
        putamen
caudate nucleus

3rd ventricle

occipital lobe

inferior horn of lateral ventricle

internal capsule

thalamus

anterior commissure

frontal lobe

FIGURE 18.3. Anatomy of the brain. *A.* Vertical section through the longitudinal fissure separating the two cerebral hemispheres. Indicated is the corpus callosum, the tracts of fibers linking the two hemispheres. Also indicated are the forebrain (comprising the thalamus and hypothalamus, together with the cerebral cortex), the midbrain, and the hindbrain (including the pons, cerebellum, and medulla). *B.* Horizontal section through the brain showing surface gray matter (containing neuron cell bodies) and inner white matter (composed of nerve fibers). The basal ganglia make up additional masses of internal gray matter.

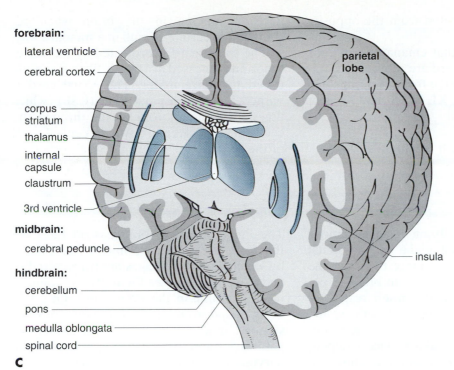

forebrain:
- lateral ventricle
- cerebral cortex
- corpus striatum
- thalamus
- internal capsule
- claustrum
- 3rd ventricle

midbrain:
- cerebral peduncle

hindbrain:
- cerebellum
- pons
- medulla oblongata
- spinal cord

parietal lobe

insula

C

FIGURE 18.3 — (*continued*) C. Coronal section through the central (transverse) sulcus. (*Reproduced, with permission, from Mackenna BR, Callendar R (1990). Illustrated Physiology, 5th ed. Edinburgh, Churchill Livingstone, pp 224, 223, 225.*)

Some important anatomic relationships of the brainstem are as follows:

- The **lateral ventricles** and **corpus callosum** lie superior to the diencephalon. The **internal capsule**, **caudate**, and **putamen** lie lateral to the diencepthalon. Caudally, the diencephalon joins the midbrain.
- The midbrain consists of the **tectum**, the **tegmentum** (just below the **cerebral aqueduct**, the **substantial nigra**, and the **crura cerebri**. Cranial nerves III and IV emerge from the midbrain.
- The pons contains many fiber bundles and nuclei and joins the **reticular formation** of the midbrain rostrally and the medulla caudally. The pons is where cranial nerves V, VI, VII, and parts of VIII emerge.

- The medulla goes from the **foramen magnum**, the opening at the base of the skull, to the caudal border of the pons.
- The **fourth ventricle** is a broad, shallow cavity just dorsal to the medulla and pons that extends from the central canal of the upper cervical spinal cord to the cerebral aqueduct of the midbrain. The roof of the fourth ventricle is the cerebellum. The **choroid plexus**, from which cerebrospinal fluid is made, projects into the caudal part of the fourth ventricle. The medulla is a region of transition from spinal cord to brainstem in which is found the major motor pathway (the **corticospinal** or **pyramidal tract**, see Sec. 4), which crosses over (**decussates**) from one side to the other in the medulla, so that signals to initiate movement on one side of

the body are generated from the opposite side of the brain.

- The spinal nerves that emanate from each level of the spinal cord are replaced by cranial nerves that emerge from the brainstem. Cranial nerves XII, XI, X, IX, and parts of VIII emerge from the medulla.

The cerebellum will be discussed in Section 4.

Spinal cord

Emanating from the brain is an enormous bundle of nerves that make up the spinal cord. The spinal cord is more than just the initial part of the conduit from brain to periphery. Certain automatic motor responses called **reflexes** can be triggered in the spinal cord. These reactions to certain forms of sensation are automatic, taking place independent of input from the brain, and allow the spinal cord to bypass the "bureaucracy" of

decision making in the brain when responding to certain stimuli in a standard way.

The spinal cord is protected by the vertebrae and is encased in a tough, fibrous capsule called the **dura mater**. The spinal cord is bathed in **cerebrospinal fluid** (CSF), which flows from the choroid plexus through the cerebral ventricles and down the central canal of the spinal cord, where it is reabsorbed by the **arachnoid villi** into the venous circulation.

Peripheral nervous system

The PNS consists of branches off the CNS that form a network covering the entire body, by which neural messages are transmitted to and from the CNS (see Figure 18.4). Communication traffic in the PNS is in both directions, to and from the CNS, and thus includes sensory, motor, integrative, and autonomic pathways, the functional components of the nervous system to be discussed below. Some peripheral nerves are *spinal nerves* that

FIGURE 18.4. Components of a typical peripheral nerve. There are two distinct functional categories of axons in a typical cutaneous (peripheral) nerve. The primary afferents have cell bodies in the dorsal root ganglia and sympathetic postganglionic fibers, with their cell bodies in the sympathetic ganglion. Primary afferents include those with large-diameter myelinated (Aβ), small-diameter myelinated (Aδ), and unmyelinated (C) axons. All sympathetic postganglionic fibers are unmyelinated.

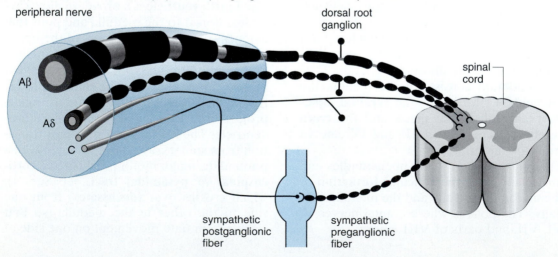

branch off from the spinal cord, while others are **cranial nerves** that exit directly from the brain.

The typical peripheral nerve contains three types of neurons:

- Primary sensory afferent neurons
- Motor neurons
- Sympathetic postganglionic neurons

The primary sensory afferent neurons detect stimuli in the environment and transmit that information back to the spinal cord. From the spinal cord, the information goes in two directions: back to the brain and over to the motor neurons. The motor neurons of the peripheral nerve respond to stimuli both from the CNS (after the information from the PNS has been interpreted and a motor decision made) and directly from the sensory afferent neuron (as part of a reflex arc; see Sec. 5). The cell bodies of the primary sensory afferent neurons lie in the dorsal root or cranial nerve ganglia, while those of the motor neurons lie in the spinal cord.

Primary sensory afferent neurons are of several different types, including

- Large-diameter, myelinated so-called Aβ neurons
- Small-diameter, myelinated so-called Aδ neurons
- Unmyelinated so-called type C neurons

The Aβ fibers mediate touch, while the Aδ and C type fibers include those that mediate painful stimuli.

Functional organization of the nervous system

Over the course of evolution, three levels of complexity of nervous systems have emerged:

- The simplest nervous response is that reflected in the simplest functions of the spinal cord, typified by reflexes (see Sec. 5).

- Lower brain (brainstem) functions are those that operate at a subconscious level; these include the workings of the medulla, pons, midbrain, cerebellum, basal ganglia, thalamus, and hypothalamus. Besides unconscious activities such as blood pressure regulation and balance, the lower brain is sufficient to carry out anger, excitement, sexual activity, pain and pleasure, feeding reflexes such as salivation, etc.
- For higher brain (cerebral cortex) functions, the cerebral cortex works in conjunction with the lower brain regions and the spinal cord. The lower brain is necessary for maintaining a *state of arousal* in which the information contained within the cerebral cortex can be used to modify sensory and motor pathways.

Clinical Pearls

○ Patients who are not arousable (e.g., with shaking, shouting, or even painful stimulation) are said to be comatose or in a coma. When a patient is brought to the hospital in a coma, it is crucial to determine the nature of the impairment. If the patient has a severe acidosis or a derangement in blood chemistry, correcting that abnormality will be crucial to regaining normal brain function. Delay in diagnosis and correction could be fatal to brain or body or both. For example, a patient who has received an insulin overdose may survive, but will suffer permanent brain damage after even very short periods (minutes) of severe hypoglycemia. Brainstem reflexes (see Sec. 5) can be used to determine whether a patient in coma has a lesion in the higher or lower brain (see later).

○ An important caveat in assessment of a comatose patient is that *no* prognosis (good or bad) can be made as long as depressant or sedative drugs (including illicit drugs that the patient may have taken before being brought to the hospital) are present in the bloodstream.

Review Questions

1. What are the major components of the nervous system?
2. Is the ANS part of the CNS or the PNS?
3. What are some of the specialized regions in a nerve cell?
4. What is an action potential?
5. How is information conveyed from one neuron to another?
6. What is the role of myelin?
7. Describe the major parts of the brain and what lies around them.
8. What is the anatomic distinction between the cranial and spinal nerves that make up the PNS?

3. SENSATION

Somatosensory pathways of the nervous system provide information about the body's experience of touch, pressure, temperature, pain, vibration, position, and movement. Some of these modalities of sensation are largely unconscious (such as those controlling blood pressure regulation and osmolality).

The brain has the ability to filter sensory information, ignoring up to 99% of the input from sensory receptors and changing its focus when necessary (Figure 18.5). This is why different patients or even the same patient under different circumstances can have markedly different sensations of pain. Unfortunately, we do not yet understand how the brain does this, and therefore we are unable to reliably manipulate the filter (e.g., to help patients deal with chronic pain).

Most of the sensory information that enters the central nervous system is relayed to nuclei in the *thalamus,* from which it is sent

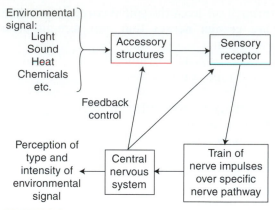

FIGURE 18.5. Flow of information in the pathway of sensory transduction by the nervous system. *(Reproduced, with permission, from Rhodes RA, Tanner GA (1996). Medical Physiology. Boston, Little, Brown, p 63.)*

on to the *sensory cortex* of the parietal lobes of the cerebral cortex (see Figure 18.6). There, conscious awareness of sensation occurs. Some fibers enter the midbrain and project to the *amygdala* and the *limbic cortex.* These inputs contribute to the emotions that we display in response to pain.

Innervation of the skin, muscles, and associated connective tissue is segmental. Thus the body can be divided into **dermatomes** that correspond to a surface map of sensory neurons (see Figure 18.7).

Clinical Pearl

○ The perception of pain is influenced by many learned features of behavior and accounts for much of the differences between the "stoic" patient and the "histrionic" one. There are cultural differences that affect how different patients respond to pain. Fore these reasons, bedside manner and the nature of the clinician-patient interaction are often important in de-

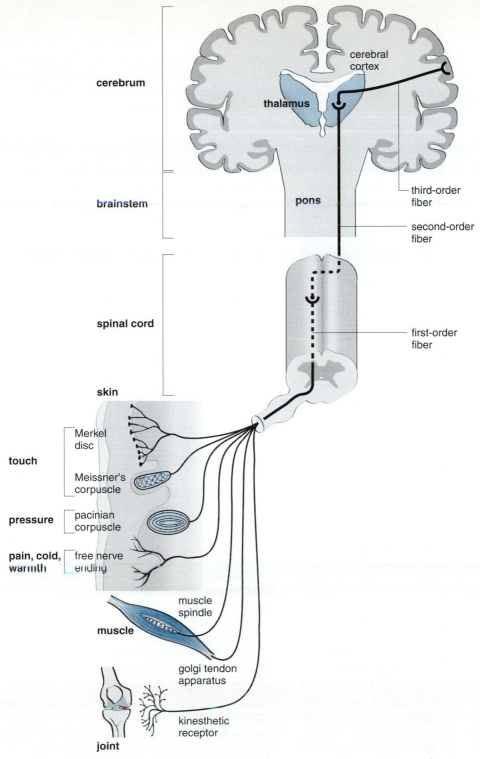

FIGURE 18.6. Organization of sensory pathways of the nervous system. Sensory input from various sorts of receptors travels up the spinal cord to various locations, including regions within the medulla and pons, bulboreticular formation, cerebellum, thalamus, somesthetic area, and motor cortex. Along the way, spinal and other reflexes allow the full path to be bypassed in situations or conditions where a programmed response can be anticipated.

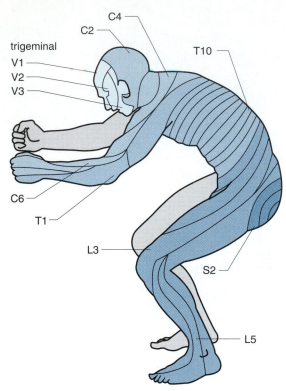

FIGURE 18.7. Dermatomes. Segmental distribution of the body dermatomes. V1, V2, and V3 refer to the divisions of cranial nerve V, the trigeminal nerve. Representative dermatomes of the cervical (C), thoracic (T), lumbar (L), and sacral (S) spinal nerves are indicated.

termining whether the patient gets better or fails to, in response to whatever therapy is initiated.

Sensory receptors

Sensation, in its simplest sense, is about detecting various forms of energy in the environment. The cells that do this are called **sensory receptors**. Note that this is a somewhat different use of the term *receptor* from that elsewhere in this book (e.g., see Chaps. 2 and 3). Previously, the term receptor has been used in reference to specific proteins in cells. Here we use the term to refer to the *cells themselves* that detect sensory information. In both uses of the word, information in the environment is being converted into a form that can be interpreted and used by the organism.

Once a sensory receptor has detected what it is designed to detect, it must generate a **receptor potential**, which in turn generates an action potential in the neuron(s) to which the sensory receptor is connected, which starts the pathway back to the sensory cortex (see Figure 18.6).

There are five classes of receptor cells that lead to sensory neural pathways (see Table 18.1).

Sensory receptors generate a receptor potential by opening ion channels that result in depolarization of the sensory receptor cell. The magnitude of the receptor potential depends on the intensity of the initial stimulus. Once the receptor potential reaches a certain threshold, it triggers an action potential in the sensory receptor cell. The more intense the initial stimulus, the greater the receptor potential and the greater the number of action potentials triggered (see Figure 18.8).

Sensory nerve receptors consist of many separate cells that innervate, for example, a patch of skin. Thus, there are two different ways to signify a large-magnitude stimulus: increasing the receptor potential and therefore the rate of action potential firing from one receptor cell (called **temporal summation**), or recruiting many receptor cells to fire (**spatial summation**). A combination of both of these modes is used to convey sensation of increasing intensity.

While the *magnitude* of the receptor potential increases in response to stronger and stronger stimuli, the *sensitivity* generally decreases. Thus, roughly 50% of the maximum response is elicited by a 25% maximal stimulus and 85% of the maximum response by a 50% stimulus, while only an additional 15% greater response (to 100%) is elicited by a further doubling of the stimulus. This is a

TABLE 18.1   MODALITIES OF SENSATION

Mechanoreceptors
  Skin tactile sensibilities
    (epidermis and dermis)
    Free nerve endings
    Expanded tip endings
      Merkel's discs
      Plus several other variants
    Spray endings
      Ruffini's endings
    Encapsulated endings
      Meissner's corpuscles
      Krause's corpuscles
    Hair end organs
  Deep tissue sensibilities
    Free nerve endings
    Expanded tip endings
    Spray endings
      Ruffini's endings
    Encapsulated endings
      Pacinian corpuscles
      Plus a few other variants
    Muscle endings
      Muscle spindles
      Golgi tendon receptors
  Hearing
    Sound receptors of cochlea
  Equilibrium
    Vestibular receptors

  Arterial pressure
    Baroreceptors of carotid sinuses and aorta
Thermoreceptors
  Cold
    Cold receptors
  Warmth
    Warm receptors
Nociceptors
  Pain
    Free nerve endings
Electromagnetic Receptors
  Vision
    Rods
    Cones
Chemoreceptors
  Taste
    Receptors of taste buds
  Smell
    Receptors of olfactory epithelium
  Arterial oxygen
    Receptors of aortic and carotid bodies
  Osmolality
    Probably neurons in or near supraoptic nuclei
  Blood CO_2
    Receptors in or on surface of medulla and in aortic and
      carotid bodies
  Blood glucose, amino acids, fatty acids
    Receptors in hypothalamus

Reproduced, with permission, from Guyton AC, Hall JE (1994). *Textbook of Medical Physiology*, 9th ed. Philadelphia, Saunders, p 584.

general principle that applies to many different biologic systems besides sensory signal transduction; in this case, it means that the sensory system is generally set up to be most sensitive to *weak* stimuli — because that is where an organism has to make the toughest decisions and hence needs the best information.

Another general principle of receptor biology that is of crucial importance to the sensory nervous system is **adaptation**, which is the decrease in magnitude of response over time in response to a constant degree of stimulation. There can be many molecular mechanisms of adaptation, including receptor downregulation through either internalization or degradation, phosphorylation, modification or loss of second messengers, etc., as discussed elsewhere (see Chap. 3).

Adaptation is a recurring theme in biologic systems, but it is not the only way in which cells can respond to repeated signaling. Memory, for example, involves various ways in which cells become *more* rather than less sensitive to recurrent stimuli.

How and why certain cells go from maintaining a system by simple negative feedback to either adaptations that *decrease* the sensitivity of the system or other changes that *increase* the sensitivity (e.g., positive feedback) is one of the more profound mysteries in biology.

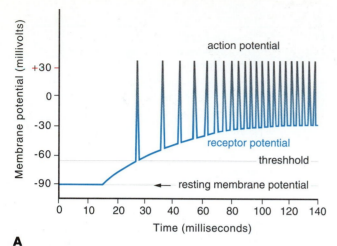

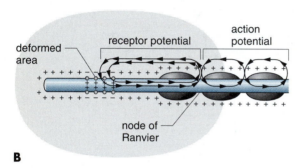

FIGURE 18.8. *A. Generation and propagation of a receptor potential. Note that above the threshold, the greater the stimulation of a sensory receptor, the greater the action potential frequency. B. Mechanism of excitation of a sensory nerve fiber by a receptor potential generated in a pacinian corpuscle, a type of touch-sensitive receptor. Pressure (from touch) results in a deformed area that initiates the receptor potential, which is transmitted as action potentials. (A adapted with permission, from Guyton AC, Hall JE (1997). Human Physiology and Mechanisms of Disease, 6th ed. Philadelphia, Saunders, p 377; B adapted, with permission, from Loëwenstein (1961). Ann NY Acad Sci 94:50.)*

Review Questions

9. What are the classes of sensory receptors?
10. What is a receptor potential?
11. What is the relationship of amplitude of receptor potential to intensity of stimulus?
12. Describe the frequency of action potentials in relation to receptor potential amplitude.
13. What is adaptation and what is its relevance to sensation?
14. What are spatial and temporal summation, and what role do they play in neurologic function?

Somatosensory pathways

While the nervous system connects the most peripheral sensory receptor to the highest parts of the cerebral cortex, it does not do so by using a single neuron. Rather, the neuron that synapses with the sensory receptor cell typically carries the action potential only back to the spinal cord. There the information is transmitted across a synapse to another neuron, which carries the message back to the brain. Within the brain, many layers of synapses must be crossed for the message to register appropriately in the **sensory cortex**.

The very fact that a synapse must be crossed places a certain threshold on the intensity of the stimulus that is necessary to send a message all the way back to the brain. Even above the minimum threshold, there are opportunities to interface with many other so-called **interneurons** that can reinforce or dampen the message through stimulatory or inhibitory signals.

Nerve fibers carrying sensation from the skin travel back to the CNS in sensory or mixed sensorimotor peripheral nerves:

- Some pain and temperature sensation is carried in small myelinated so-called *A δ fibers*.
- Position sense is carried in *large myelinated fibers*, and other pain and autonomic sensation is carried in *unmyelinated* C fibers. All of these go back to the spinal cord. The

cell bodies of all sensory neurons lie in the **dorsal root ganglia**. Sensation from skin, muscles, and related structures is organized regionally in a surface pattern called **dermatomes**, which can be useful in localizing a sensory or sensorimotor lesion (see Figure 18.7). The dorsal roots enter the spinal cord (see Figure 18.9), and individual fibers distribute to the various pathways described later.

- Sensation from the face is carried in fibers of *cranial nerve V*, the *trigeminal nerve*.

There are two major pathways that mediate somatic sensation, that is, sensations from various parts of the skin. One, the **dorsal column–medial lemniscal pathway**, is involved

FIGURE 18.9. Dorsal roots. A spinal cord segment is illustrated, with its dorsal root, ganglion cells, and sensory organs shown. The sensory organs shown (from top to bottom) are a pacinian corpuscle, a muscle spindle, a tendon organ, an encapsulated ending, and a free nerve ending. The organization of the different types of fibers within the dorsal columns, spinothalamic tract, and corticospinal tract is also shown. *(Adapted, with permission, from Waxman SG, DeGroot J (1995). Correlative Neuroanatomy, 22nd ed. Stamford, CT, Appleton & Lange.)*

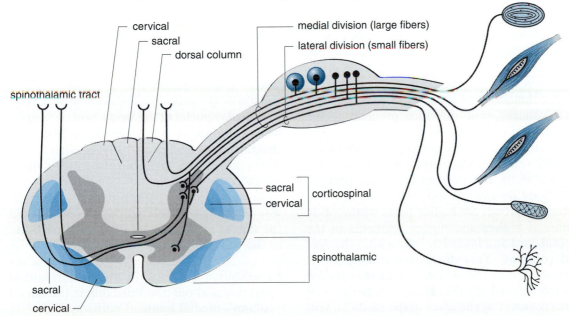

in sensations of *fine touch*, *vibration*, *position*, and *discrimination of fine gradations of pressure*.

The other major somatic sensory pathway is the **anterior lateral pathway**. It mediates *pain* and *temperature*, as well as *crude touch* and *pressure*, *tickle*, *itch* and *sexual sensations*.

These two pathways of somatic sensation are discussed in more detail in the following sections.

Dorsal columns — medial lemniscus

The signals for fine touch and pressure gradations and related sensations are generated through activation of specialized *mechanoreceptors*, resulting in action potentials in myelinated neurons that enter the spinal cord (see Figure 18.10).

Within the spinal cord, these neurons go to the lateral margin of the **dorsal white column.** There, the neurons divide into a medial branch that goes to the brain via the dorsal white column and a lateral branch that enters the **dorsal horn** of the spinal cord gray matter. This lateral branch divides many times and synapses with many different neurons, including those that are involved in various spinal reflexes. The medial branch goes up to the medulla, where it synapses with neurons of the dorsal column nuclei. These neurons cross over to the other side and continue up to the thalamus. Many more connections are made there, some of which proceed all the way to the somatosensory cortex.

Within the medial lemniscal pathway, a precise spacial orientation is maintained (see Figure 18.9). Fibers from the lower parts of the body lie toward the center, while those from progressively higher parts of the body enter at higher and higher segments of the spinal cord and layer laterally within the dorsal columns. This distinctive orientation is maintained in the thalamus and transmitted to the sensory cortex. However, because of the crossover at the level of the medulla, *sensory input from the left half of the body is represented in the thalamus and sensory cortex of the right half of the brain.*

The somatosensory cortex encodes exaggerated representation of the most sensitive areas of skin, such as the lips, face, and thumb, while the trunk and lower extremities are relatively underrepresented. The somatosensory cortex itself consists of six layers of neurons that perform different complex functions necessary for proper feedback and integration of sensory information.

The representation of the body in the somatosensory cortex is not fixed, but rather is subject to alteration as a function of training. This ability of the cortex to expand the area of a particular representation, in response either to training or to loss of other areas, is called **plasticity** and is the basis for learning in the nervous system. For example, violinists starting at age 3 have an increased area of representation of the right hand.

Anterolateral pathway

The fibers carrying pain, temperature, and related sensations enter the spinal cord and terminate in the dorsal horn. From there, fibers cross over to the opposite anterior and lateral white columns and ascend diffusely to the brain in the form of the **anterior and lateral spinothalamic tracts**. Upon reaching the brain, these neurons generally terminate in **reticular nuclei of the brainstem** or **ventrobasal complex** and **interlaminar nuclei of the thalamus** (see Figure 18.10). Together, these tracts and nuclei make up the anterolateral pathway.

Transmission via the anterolateral pathway (see Figure 18.11) differs from that via the dorsal column–medial lemiscal pathway in the following ways:

- Transmission speed in the anterolateral pathway is about one-third that in the dorsal column–medial lemiscal pathway.

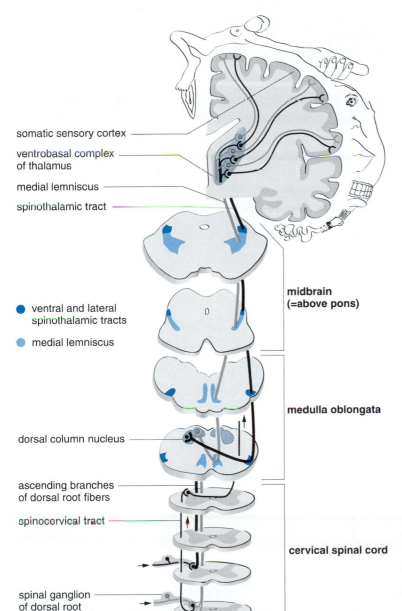

somatic sensory cortex

ventrobasal complex
of thalamus

medial lemniscus

spinothalamic tract

● ventral and lateral
spinothalamic tracts

● medial lemniscus

**midbrain
(=above pons)**

medulla oblongata

dorsal column nucleus

ascending branches
of dorsal root fibers

spinocervical tract

cervical spinal cord

spinal ganglion
of dorsal root

FIGURE 18.10. Dorsal column–medial lemniscal pathway. The overall pathway projecting first to the thalamus and then to the somatic sensory cortex is indicated.

- The degree of spatial localization of signals in the anterolateral pathway is poor compared to that in the dorsal column–medial lemiscal pathway.
- There are only 10 to 20 gradations of

strength of stimulation in the anterolateral pathway, whereas the dorsal column–medial lemiscal pathway has as many as 100.
- The anterolateral pathway transmits rapidly

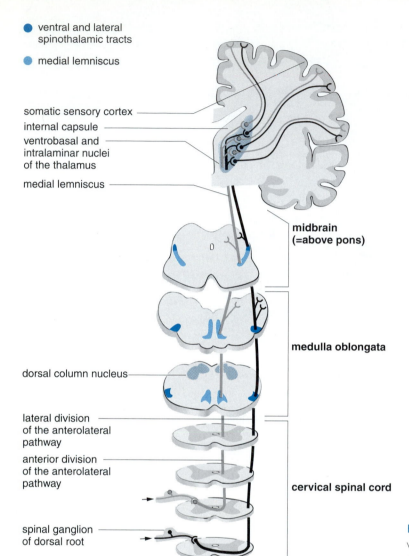

● ventral and lateral
  spinothalamic tracts

● medial lemniscus

somatic sensory cortex

internal capsule

ventrobasal and
intralaminar nuclei
of the thalamus

medial lemniscus

midbrain
(=above pons)

medulla oblongata

dorsal column nucleus

lateral division
of the anterolateral
pathway

anterior division
of the anterolateral
pathway

cervical spinal cord

spinal ganglion
of dorsal root

FIGURE 18.11. Anterior and lateral divisions of the anterolateral pain pathway.

repetitive signals poorly compared to the dorsal column–medial lemiscal pathway.

Clinical Pearls

○ When we sit or lie in one position, blood flow to those points of the body that bear the most weight is compromised. Normally we shift position unconsciously in response to pain sensations caused by lack of adequate oxygenation due to poor blood flow, and thereby prevent pressure necrosis of skin and other tissues. However, when a person is unable to make these fine unconscious adjustments, either because of a sensory or motor neurologic deficit or because of weakness, pressure ulcers develop, with skin breakdown. If not intensively treated, these will result in infection, a common cause of death in chronically ill, debilitated patients. Thus, frequent repositioning and careful attention to skin care is mandatory for patients who are bedbound.

○ Symmetrical distal loss of sensation in both extremities generally signifies a peripheral polyneuropathy, as occurs in diabetes mellitus, rather than a specific structural lesion.

○ Signs and symptoms limited to a dermatome suggest a spinal root lesion (radiculopathy).

○ Segregation of fiber tracts in the spinal cord gives rise to distinctive patterns of sensory loss:

○ In the *Brown-Séquard syndrome*, lesions of one-half of the spinal cord result in (1) loss of sensation on the side of the lesion in the immediate vicinity of the lesion, (2) loss of pain and temperature sensation on the opposite side below the level of the lesion, and (3) loss of proprioception, vibration, two-position discrimination, and joint and position sensation on the same side and below the level of the lesion (see Figure 18.12A).

○ Pain and temperature fibers that enter the spinal cord take a more central position in the ascending pathways. As a result, lesions such as *syringomyelia*, a condition in which the central cervical canal of the spinal cord is expanded, will produce loss of pain and temperature in the distribution of the shoulders and upper arms (see Figure 18.12B).

Review Questions

15. What are the two major pathways of somatic sensation?

16. Describe the pathway of the dorsal column–medial lemiscal system.

17. What sensory modalities does the dorsal column pathway subserve?

18. Describe the pathways of the spinothalamic tracts.

19. What sensory modalities does the anterior lateral pathway subserve?

20. What kinds of sensation are carried in the dorsal column–medial lemniscal pathway?

21. What is the role of the anterolateral pathway?

22. What are four differences between the dorsal column–medial lemiscal and anterolateral pathways, besides their mediation of different sensory modalities by different anatomic routes?

Pain

Pain receptors are free nerve endings distributed throughout the tissues of the body, designed to transmit the presence in the environment of so-called noxious stimuli — those that can damage tissue, including certain *mechanical*, *thermal*, and *chemical* stimuli. The most pain-sensitive tissues are those with the greatest density of pain fibers.

Some Aδ and type C neurons respond only to stimuli that are subjectively painful. These are called *primary afferent nocioreceptors*. In addition to transmitting painful sensations back to the CNS, these neurons have an effector function: They release various peptides such as **substance P** whose local effects in the surrounding tissues include:

• Vasodilation
• Mast cell degranulation
• Leukocyte chemoattraction
• Release of inflammatory mediators from the attracted leukocytes

Some nocioreceptors are entirely silent until the release of inflammatory mediators, at which point they respond maximally to stimuli to which they had previously been oblivious. Thus, an initial painful stimulus often

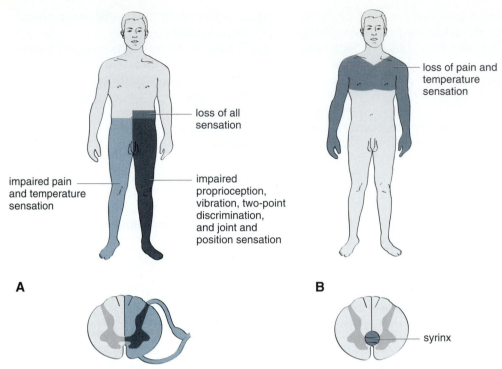

FIGURE 18.12. Classical spinal cord lesions and their effects on sensation, indicating the location of the sensory pathways within the spinal cord. A. Brown-Séquard's syndrome with lesion at the left tenth thoracic level (motor deficits not shown). B. Syringomyelia (the presence of a cavity in the spinal cord due to a degenerative neurologic disorder presenting clinically with pain and paresthesias followed by muscle atrophy of the hands) involving the cervicothoracic portion of the spinal cord. (Modified, with permission, from Waxman SG, DeGroot J (1995). Clinical Neuroanatomy, 22nd ed. Stamford, CT, Appleton & Lange.)

sensitizes a tissue to the perception of subsequent painful stimuli (see Figure 18.13). This is why normally nonpainful touch becomes exquisitely painful when one has a bad sunburn, for example.

Fast and slow pain

Pain consists of *fast pain* and *slow pain* (see Figure 18.14A). Fast pain tends to be a surface sensation that is sharp and well localized, occurring about 0.1 s after application of the painful stimulus. Slow pain tends to arise from poorly localizable deeper structures as

well as from the surface. It tends to be chronic, burning and aching in quality, and more indicative of tissue damage. Typically, slow pain takes a second or so to start and increases over seconds to minutes.

These two types of pain correspond to two different pathways of transmission. Fast pain is conducted by so-called small type Aδ fibers via the **neospinothalamic tract**. These fibers terminate in the dorsal horn of the spinal cord on neurons that almost immediately cross over in the anterior commissure and travel up to the brain in the anterior lateral pathway, terminating in the thalamus. From

A primary activation

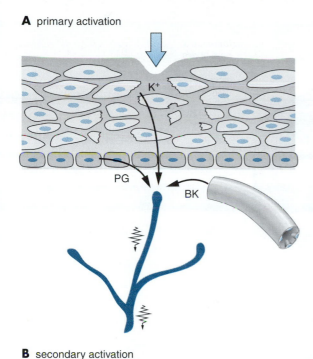

B secondary activation

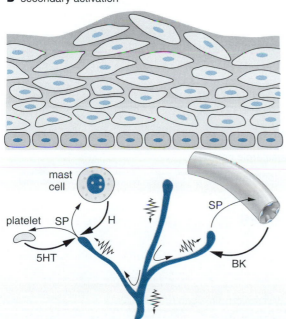

there, fibers pass to the somatosensory cortex and to other brain regions. Tactile fibers in the dorsal column–medial lemniscal pathway contribute to the fine degree of localization possible for this type of pain.

Slow pain is transmitted via even smaller C-type fibers in the **paleospinothalamic pathway**. After one or more short neurons within the dorsal horn, this pathway crosses over and joins the fast pathway traveling up to the brain. However, most of the fibers from this pathway terminate in the medulla, pons, and midbrain, with very few fibers going directly to the thalamus. The multisynaptic nature of this pathway probably contributes to the difficulty in localizing even very severe chronic, deep pain.

Pain-modulating networks of neurons also occur (see Figure 18.14B). Much of the effect of opiates in pain relief is believed to occur through these circuits that respond to pain via the cerbral cortex, hypothalamus, midbrain, and medulla.

Without a functioning cerebral cortex, an individual has the perception of pain, but without the ability to discriminate aspects of the quality of the pain. The reticular forma-

---

FIGURE 18.13. Neuroeffector functions of nocioceptors. Events leading to activation, sensitization, and spread of sensitization of primary afferent nociceptor terminals. *A.* Direct activation by intense pressure and consequent cell damage. Cell damage leads to release of potassium (K^+) and to synthesis of prostaglandins (PG) and bradykinin (BK). Prostaglandins increase the sensitivity of the terminal to bradykinin and other pain-producing substances. *B.* Secondary activation. Impulses generated in the stimulated terminal propagate not only to the spinal cord, but also into other terminal branches, where they induce the release of peptides, including substance P (SP). Substance P causes vasodilation and neurogenic edema with further accumulation of bradykinin. Substance P also causes the release of histamine (H) from mast cells and serotonin (5HT) from platelets. *(Reproduced, with permission, from Fields, H, in Fauci, A, et al. (eds): Harrison's Principles of Internal Medicine, 14th ed. New York, McGraw-Hill, p 54.)*

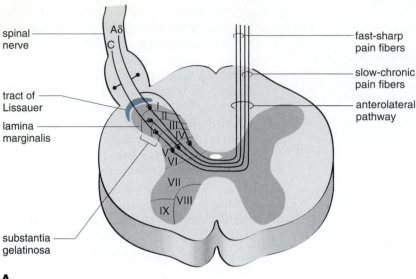

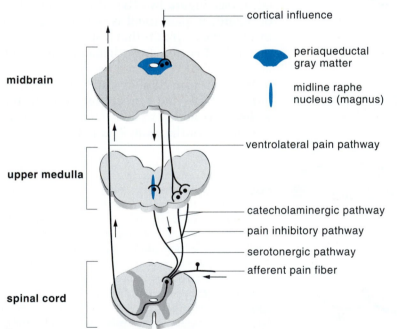

FIGURE 18.14. Pain pathways. *A*. Both fast-sharp and slow-chronic pain signals enter via a spinal nerve at the level of the spinal cord and proceed via the anterolateral pathway to the brainstem. *B*. Pain inhibitory pathways, including catecholaminergic and serotoninergic pathways, impinge on afferent pain fibers and modify the output that enters the anterolateral pathway. The pain inhibitory pathways are, in turn, influenced by pathways emanating from the cerebral cortex. *(B reproduced, with permission, from Waxman SG, DeGroot J (1995). Clinical Neuroanatomy, 22nd ed. Stamford, CT, Appleton & Lange.)*

tion involved in arousal is a major target of the pain pathways, perhaps accounting for the particular difficulty patients with severe or chronic pain often have in falling asleep.

Hyperalgesia

Unlike most other sensory receptors, pain receptors are generally nonadapting. Indeed, sometimes they display the opposite of adaptation, hyperalgesia — *increased* sensitivity with chronic stimulation. Hyperalgesia has both a local and a central component. It appears that factors are released locally that makes pain fibers in the neighborhood of a recent painful stimulus respond to stimuli (e.g., touch) that would not normally cause pain. At the same time, the spinothalamic tract appears to mediate an increased sensitivity to subsequent painful stimuli. The reticular formation, thalamus, and cortex function in awareness of pain, which has a general effect of arousing the nervous system.

Deep pain has the capacity to elicit reflex muscle contraction. Prolonged muscle contraction — spasm — results in ischemia, which causes more pain and sets up a vicious cycle of pain causing spasm and ischemia, causing more pain, which can continue even when the initial inciting painful stimulus has diminished.

Bradykinin is the most "painful" of the chemical stimuli to pain.

Sometimes, malfunction of the sympathetic, peripheral, or central nervous system can create a situation in which chronic pain is maintained by neural activity even in the absence of a sensory trigger.

Psychological depression can exacerbate the perception of pain, and, by unknown mechanisms, certain antidepressant medicines are observed to be effective in the treatment of pain.

Analgesic systems of the brain

The brain has two mechanisms by which it can provide relief from an ongoing painful stimulus.

First, there are *pain-suppressing neural pathways* that originate in the **periaqueductal gray** and periventricular areas of the third ventricle, a part of the hypothalamus. These pathways go to the **raphe magnus nucleus** of the pons and medulla. From there, signals go down the dorsal columns to a **pain inhibitory center** in the dorsal horn of the spinal cord. The neurotransmitters of this system include **serotonin** and **enkephalin**. These can serve to block pain signals at the spinal cord before they arrive at the brain.

Second, there are **endogenous opioid peptides** (e.g., β-endophin, the enkephalins, and dynorphin) that are released as *hormones* into the bloodstream or used as *local mediators* or *neurotransmitters*, both in peripheral tissues and in the brain. They can suppress either the entry of pain signals at the peripheral nerves or the appreciation of these signals in the brain.

Teleologically, this system may have been necessary in order to condition an organism to avoid painful stimuli — by appreciation of how much better it feels when the painful stimulus stops. Also, it may have allowed an injured organism to survive by being able to continue to function (e.g., to run away or to fight) in the face of otherwise disabling pain.

Opiates are the strongest medicines available for treatment of pain. The placebo effect (the ability of the expectation of relief to result in the subjective sensation of relief) probably has as its basis the release of endogenous opioids.

Often the effects of opiates are additive to that of nonsteroidal anti-inflammatory medicines.

Complications of opiate therapy include

- GI hypomotility, resulting in nausea and constipation
- Somnolence
- Tolerance, requiring higher and higer doses to achieve the same therapeutic efficacy

- Addiction (physical and psychological dependence upon long-term use)
- Respiratory depression due to effects of opiates on medullary centers that control respiration

Referred pain

Referred pain is the phenomenon in which injury to internal organs causes pain that localizes, in part, to surface structures or other organs clearly distinct from the site of primary injury (see Figure 18.15). Typically the pain is referred to other structures that have the same embryologic origin.

The basis for referred pain is that many different afferent sensory nocioceptive neurons synapse with the same ascending fibers in the spinal cord. These include nocioceptors both from surface structures (which are commonly activated from time to time in the course of daily living) and from deep structures (which are usually silent until some other underlying problem results in their activation). However, since nocioceptors from both locations synapse with the same neurons of the spinal cord, the CNS is unable to tell which of these sources is giving rise to the pain. Furthermore, since the CNS usually has more recent or frequent memory of pain from surface structures, it often erroneously interprets the pain from deeper structures as coming from the surface structures.

Clinical Pearls

○ Here are some examples of classical referred pain syndromes:

- Cardiac ischemia often results in pain being referred to the left arm or jaw.
- Irritation of the diaphragm results in pain at the tip of the shoulder.
- Irritation of the ureter (e.g., by a kidney stone) results in shooting pains in the testicle on the same side.

○ Often arthritic pain from the hip will be felt in the upper leg to the knee, whereas peripheral nerve–related pain typically involves the entire leg.
○ A good example of how different systems can interact to cause similar clinical manifestations is seen in headache.

- Migraine headache is an extremely common headache syndrome in which there is a unilateral, throbbing headache that is often preceded by visual or other neurologic symptoms. Migraine headache is believed to have one or more of three components: (1) excessive vascular constriction followed by excessive vasodilation, (2) a neural serotoninergic component related to the *dorsal nucleus of raphe* in the midbrain, and (3) activation of the trigeminal vascular system with release of vasoactive peptides. Since serotoninergic receptors are found in all of these locations, the efficacy of serotonin agonists in treatment of migraines does not distinguish among them. Such patients are recommended to avoid known precipitants such as alcohol and stress, and headaches can be effectively treated with drugs that are serotonin receptor agonists, such as ergotamine and sumatriptan.
- Cluster headaches are also serotoninergic in origin, but are notable for the clustering of attacks with a striking periodicity that has led some to implicate the circadian pacemakers of the anterior hypothalamus. Pain is often unilateral, periorbital, and associated with autonomic symptoms such as tearing and nasal stuffiness.
- Tension headaches manifest with a band-like head pain associated with stress and

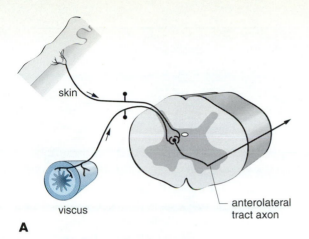

A

skin

viscus

anterolateral
tract axon

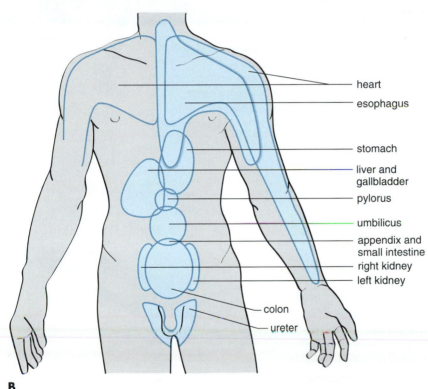

heart

esophagus

stomach

liver and
gallbladder

pylorus

umbilicus

appendix and
small intestine

right kidney

left kidney

colon

ureter

B

FIGURE 18.15. Pathways of referred pain. *A.* One hypothesis for the mechanism of referred pain in which visceral afferent nociceptors converge on the same pain-projection neurons as the afferents from the somatic structures in which the pain is perceived. The brain cannot distinguish the actual source of pain and erroneously attributes the sensation to the somatic structure rather than the visceral one. *B.* Syndromes of referred pain. Indicated in gray are surface areas to which pain from various indicated internal organs can sometimes be referred. *(A. Adapted, with permission, from Fields H. In Fauci, A, et al. (1998) (eds): Harrison's Principles of Internal Medicine, 14th ed. New York, McGraw-Hill, p 54. B. Adapted, with permission, from Guyton AC, Hall JE (1997). Human Physiology and Mechanisms of Disease, 6th ed. Philadelphia, Saunders, p 396.)*

depression lasting up to several days. Some investigators think that they too involve serotoninergic pathways.

- Migraine and tension headaches are the two most common headache syndromes.

Review Questions

23. What is the difference between so-called fast pain and slow pain?
24. What are the two general ways in which the nervous system can suppress the sensation of pain?
25. What is the strongest chemical stimulus for pain?
26. What is referred pain?

4. MOTOR PATHWAYS

The motor pathways of the brain are those neural pathways whose activation brings about movement (see Figure 18.16). Motor pathways start from regions in the cerebral cortex, where discrete groups of neurons, organized into vertical columns, control the contraction of individual muscles. The neurons that make up the **motor cortex**, like those of the sensory and visual cortex, are composed of columns six layers of cells deep and thousands of neurons across. Input arrives to the motor cortex largely in layers 2 and 4. The fifth layer gives rise to the pyramidal cells of the corticospinal or **pyramidal tract**. The sixth layer is largely involved in internal communication between areas of the cerebral cortex.

Motor responses, either voluntary or in response to sensory information, are actually triggered at many different levels. These include spinal reflexes (see Sec. 5) as well as feedback from the medulla, pons, midbrain, basal ganglia, cerebellum, and cerebral cortex. The "lower" responses (i.e., those involving neurons other than those of the cerebral

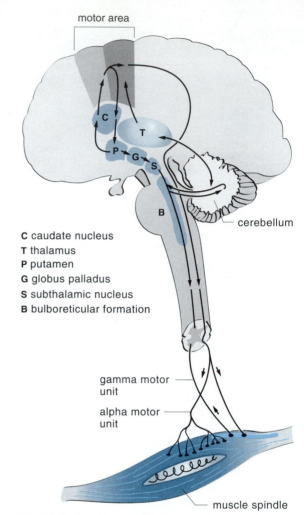

C caudate nucleus
T thalamus
P putamen
G globus palladus
S subthalamic nucleus
B bulboreticular formation

FIGURE 18.16. Flow of information in the motor system. The conceptual framework indicated is placed in the context of the structure of the motor system with emphasis on the distinction between voluntary motor activity (requiring input from the cerebral cortex) and reflex motor activity (e.g., gamma motor neurons activity is monitored by the muscle spindle which provides feedback to alpha motor neurons, which partly bypass and partly modify input from the cortex).

cortex) are involved in various automatic responses. Direct input from the cerebral cortex makes possible voluntary motor responses to sensory stimuli, that is, responses for which some thinking is involved.

While the cerebral cortex controls all voluntary movements, it often does so by directing lower centers such as the basal ganglia, cerebellum, and brainstem to send the actual messages for specific movements, often in the form of programmed responses. In other instances, however, the cerebral cortex takes direct control of motor neurons, bypassing other motor centers. This is particularly true for fine movements of the fingers and hands.

The motor cortex makes up the posterior third of the frontal lobes, just anterior to the central sulcus. The **primary motor cortex** contains a topographic representation of the muscles of the body. Nearly half of the human primary motor cortex is occupied with the muscles of the hands and those controlling speech, two areas that account for the most distinctly human of all of our motor activity. The Betz cells are heavily myelinated neurons of the primary motor cortex whose speed of transmission is 70 m/s, the fastest in the nervous system. These cells are the beginning of the **pyramidal tracts**, the major motor pathways of the body (see the following discussion).

Anterior to the primary motor cortex are the **premotor and supplementary motor areas**, which are also organized in roughly similar topographic orientation as the primary motor cortex. They control groups of muscles that set the stage for the finer control exerted by the primary motor cortex.

Within the premotor cortex are some specialized areas involved in control of specific motor functions. **Broca's area**, for example, controls word formation. Damage to it results in great difficulty in giving more than a simple yes or no answer to questions.

The motor cortex receives input not only from the somatic sensory cortex, but also from the pathways mediating other sensations, such as hearing and vision. Working in concert with the basal ganglia and cerebellum, the motor cortex triggers the appropriate actions.

Pyramidal tract

The **corticospinal (pyramidal) tract** is the major pathway of output from the motor cortex. It derives about 30% of its fibers from the primary motor cortex, 30% from the premotor and supplementary motor areas, and 40% from the sensory cortex posterior to the central sulcus.

The corticospinal tract passes through the brainstem and, upon reaching the medulla, crosses to the opposite side and descends as the **lateral corticospinal tract** in the spinal cord. At each level, some of these neurons synapse with motor neurons of the anterior horn which exit the spinal cord to form peripheral nerves. These are the actual neurons that innervate specific muscles and cause contraction upon stimulation.

The **extrapyramidal motor system** is important in controlling motor tone. It includes the basal ganglia, striatum, and substantia nigra, all of which help to provide input to the pyramidal system for muscle control. Disorders of this system give rise to tremor, spasticity, and other disorders of motor function.

The organization of the various motor pathways in the spinal cord and their convergence on anterior motor neurons is described in Figure 18.17.

Clinical Pearl

○ In clinical parlance, an important distinction is made between upper motor neurons and lower motor neurons. The upper motor neurons are those of the pyramidal tract, from the primary motor cortex down to the spinal cord. The lower motor neurons are those that travel from the anterior horn of the spinal cord to innervate specific muscles. Much of what we know about motor pathways in the brain comes from observation of patients who have

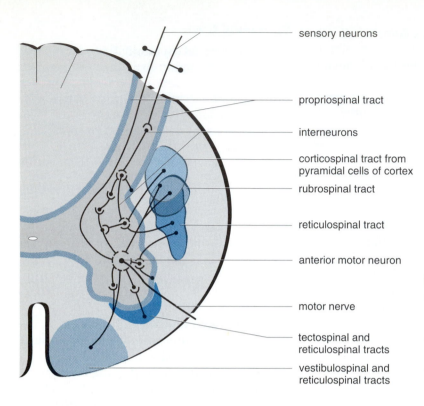

sensory neurons

propriospinal tract

interneurons

corticospinal tract from
pyramidal cells of cortex

rubrospinal tract

reticulospinal tract

anterior motor neuron

motor nerve

tectospinal and
reticulospinal tracts

vestibulospinal and
reticulospinal tracts

FIGURE 18.17. Convergence of various motor pathways on the anterior motor neurons. (Adapted, with permission, from Guyton AC, Hall JE (1997). Human Physiology and Mechanisms of Disease, 6th ed. Philadelphia, Saunders, p 458.)

brain damage. The most common forms of brain damage are those due to a stroke — which results in death of brain cells as a result of blood vessel rupture or of thrombosis and inadequate blood flow — or due to a discrete, localized, and specific traumatic injury, such as a gunshot wound.

- Damage to the primary motor cortex without involvement of deeper structures such as the caudate nucleus or surrounding structures such as the premotor cortex results in loss of fine motor control, but not the capacity for gross limb movement.
- Damage to areas adjacent to the primary motor cortex results in spasticity and hyperactive reflexes. This is because many of the damaged neurons were involved in inhibitory activities, without which neuronal messages either from the motor cortex for muscle contraction or via sensory neural reflex arcs are excessive. Many of these inhibitory neurons of the CNS are part of the extrapyramidal motor system. Hyperactive reflexes are often not seen acutely after a stroke. Rather, they take days to weeks to develop.
- Damage to the lower motor neurons results in flaccid paralysis and atrophy and loss of tone of the muscle. Deep tendon reflexes are also lost, since they depend on an intact lower motor neuron.

Review Questions

27. Describe the pathway of the pyramidal tract and identify the level at which its fibers cross over to the other side of the body.

28. From where do the inputs to the pyramidal tract derive?

29. What is the clinical significance of lesions of upper versus lower motor neurons?

Cerebellum

The cerebellum is the distinctive posterior part of the brain, responsible for the *coordination of motor functions.* Remarkably, electrical stimulation of the cerebellum fails to result in contraction of any muscles, in striking contrast to the motor cortex. Yet without the cerebellum, there is almost complete loss of motor coordination.

It appears that the cerebellum regulates the *order*, *timing*, and *sequence* of motor activity. The cerebellum constantly monitors neural activity between the cerebral cortex, basal ganglia, and muscles. When a discrepancy is noted between what the cerebral cortex intended and what the muscles are doing, the cerebellum instantaneously adjusts the neural activity so that what is supposed to be done is what gets done. But the cerebellum does not just monitor what has happened and adjust for it after the fact. Rather, part of its function is to anticipate the likely course of events and adjust the timing and rate of speed of movements so that the intended consequence of the motor activity is achieved without under- or overshooting the goal. The cerebellum is also concerned with equilibrium, balance, and posture.

Anatomically, the cerebellum consists of three parts:

The **flocculonodular lobe** of the cerebellum is connected to the vestibular nuclei and controls posture and coordination of eye movements.

The **anterior lobe** of the cerebellar hemispheres, which is *rostral* to the primary cerebellar fissure, receives proprioceptive sensory input from muscles and tendons and contributes to the control of posture, muscle tone, and gait.

The **posterior lobe** of the cerebellar hemispheres receives input from the cerebral cortex via the pons and middle cerebellar peduncles and plays an important role in the coordination and planning of voluntary skilled movements that are initiated by the cerebral cortex.

Clinical Pearls

○ Given the above discussion of the functions of the cerebellum, how might you expect cerebellar disease to be elicited on clinical examination of a patient?

- "Finger-nose-finger" testing. Having the patient move his or her finger rapidly from your finger to his or her nose and back again, with a change of your finger's position in space between attempts, is a way to assess whether the cerebellum is coordinating motor activity appropriately and is able to correct a discrepancy between intended and actual motor function. Patients with cerebellar disease typically have a delay in onset of movement and decreased rates of acceleration and deceleration, resulting in overshooting of the goal called **dysmetria**.
- Rapid alternating movements. Having the patient turn her or his hand over rapidly from palm up to palm down requires proper sequencing of the action of various muscle groups. Without proper cerebellar input, this action will be a jumble of incoherent movements.
- A patient who has no tremor at rest but develops severe tremor on attempting to carry out motor tasks. This is called an *intention tremor* and reflects the overshooting that would occur in the absence of cerebellar input into fine-tuning of motor actions.

○ Cerebellar lesions are often associated with a decrease in muscle tone due to depression of activity of α and γ motor neurons.

○ Unilateral cerebellar or cerebellar peduncle lesions result in poorly coordinated or irregular muscle movement on the same side. However, lesions that lie below the decussation of efferent cerebellar fibers in the midbrain manifest as limb ataxia on the opposite side.

Basal ganglia

The **basal ganglia** consist of the neuronal masses deep to the cerebral cortex and lateral to the thalamus. They include the *caudate nucleus*, the *putamen*, and the *globus pallidus* (collectively called the *corpus striatum*), the *substantia nigra*, and the *subthalamic nucleus* (see Figure 18.18).

Like the cerebellum, the basal ganglia function in close coordination with the cerebral cortex and are crucial for proper regulation of voluntary movement and normal posture. Almost all of the sensory and motor neurons that connect the cerebral cortex with the spinal cord pass through the basal ganglia. Almost all of the neural activity involving the basal ganglia is to and from the cerebral cortex. Input from the basal ganglia is crucial for complex motor skills, such as writing the alphabet, cutting paper with scissors, hitting a baseball, etc. Without input from the basal ganglia, these activities become crude, as if one were learning the alphabet, using scissors, or playing a game for the first time. In addition to the complex interplay between the cerebral cortex and the basal ganglia, there is tremendous communication within and between the nuclei of the basal ganglia.

The Acetylcholine, γ-aminobutyric acid (GABA), and dopamine are important neurotransmitters of the basal ganglia. Dopamine, synthesized by neurons of the substantia nigra, is released in the globus pallidus, where it inhibits the release of GABA, which is itself an inhibitory neurotransmitter. The proper balance of acetylcholine, GABA, and dopaminergic activity is necessary for normal movement.

Clinical Pearls

○ Let us consider some disorders of the basal ganglia and how they manifest:

• In Parkinson's disease, the dopamine-releasing neurons of the substantia nigra degenerate. As a result, there is excessive GABA activity (which would normally be inhibited by dopamine). The resulting imbalance leads to excessive inhibitory effects of GABA, which manifest as a peculiar difficulty in initiating movement, combined with a distinctive tremor.

• In Huntington's disease, an inherited autosomal dominant disorder, patients have degeneration of a subset of GABA-secreting neurons of the striatum. The net decrease in GABA-mediated inhibition results in involuntary hand and arm movements known as *chorea* (brisk, graceful, and complex involuntary movements of the distal extremities and muscles of facial expression) and *athetosis* (slow, writhing, involuntary movements of the distal extremities or muscles of facial expression). In addition, a poorly understood progressive dementia is observed.

• Isolated damage to the subthalamic nucleus results in violent, forceful, and persistent involuntary choreoid movements, called *hemiballism*, on the side opposite the lesion. The proximal muscles of the upper and lower extremities are usually involved, although facial and cervical muscles can be involved as well.

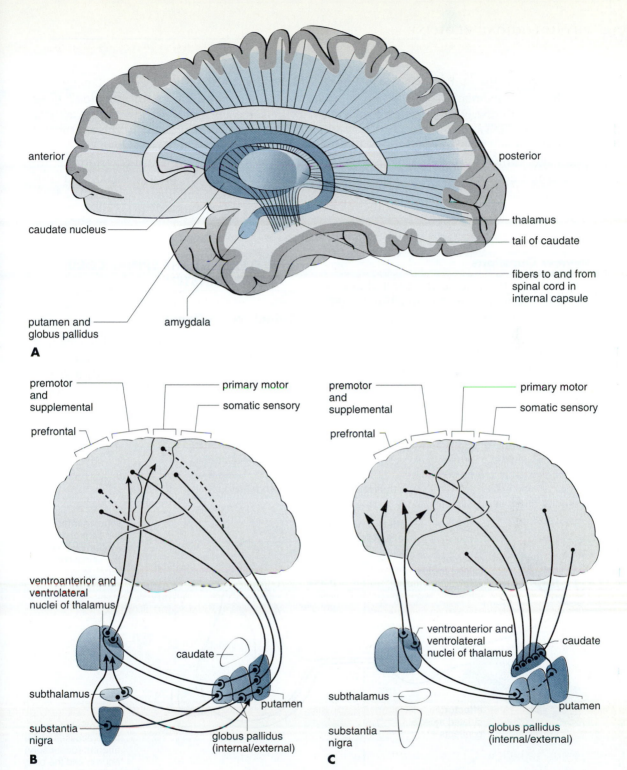

FIGURE 18.18. Basal ganglia. *A.* Anatomy of the basal ganglia. *B.* Putamen circuit through the basal ganglia for subconscious execution of learned patterns of movement. *C.* Caudate circuit through the basal ganglia for cognitive planning of sequential and parallel motor patterns to achieve specific conscious goals. *(B and C adapted, with permission, from Guyton AC, Hall JE (1997). Human Physiology and Mechanisms of Disease, 6th ed. Philadelphia, Saunders, pp 466–467.)*

○ Damage to the globus pallidus results in athetoid movements.

○ Parkinson's disease is an example of a disorder in which a specific therapy to replenish dopamine has been developed, based on the known importance of this neurotransmitter from the substantia nigra to the corpus striatum.

Review Questions

30. What is the role of the cerebellum in the control of motor function? Give some examples of how motor activity would be disordered in the absence of cerebellar input.

31. What are the components of the basal ganglia?

32. What is the role of the basal ganglia in the control of motor function? Give some examples of how motor activity would be disordered in the absence of input from the basal ganglia?

33. What are the neurotransmitters involved in the basal ganglia, and how does their imbalance result in the findings of Parkinson's disease?

5. REFLEXES OF THE SPINAL CORD AND BRAINSTEM

Spinal cord reflexes

Spinal cord reflexes are those for which the connection between the afferent and efferent limbs is made in the spinal cord, bypassing the brain (see Figure 18.19). The simplest

FIGURE 18.19. Spinal cord reflexes. A. Structural basis for the simplest reflex arc. A receptor receives a stimulus, which is conducted by an afferent nerve fiber to the spinal cord, where the afferent (sensory) neuron synapses with the body of an effector (motor) neuron whose stimulation triggers muscle contraction. Modifying pathways and pathways leading to the brain are not shown.

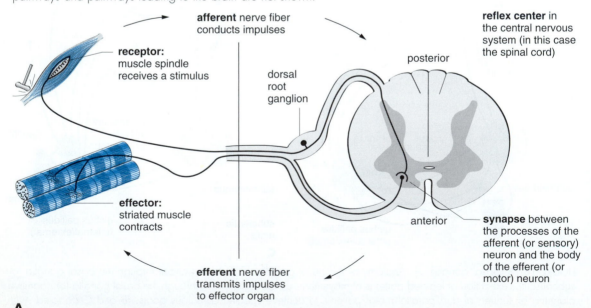

afferent nerve fiber conducts impulses

receptor: muscle spindle receives a stimulus

dorsal root ganglion

posterior

reflex center in the central nervous system (in this case the spinal cord)

effector: striated muscle contracts

anterior

synapse between the processes of the afferent (or sensory) neuron and the body of the efferent (or motor) neuron

efferent nerve fiber transmits impulses to effector organ

A

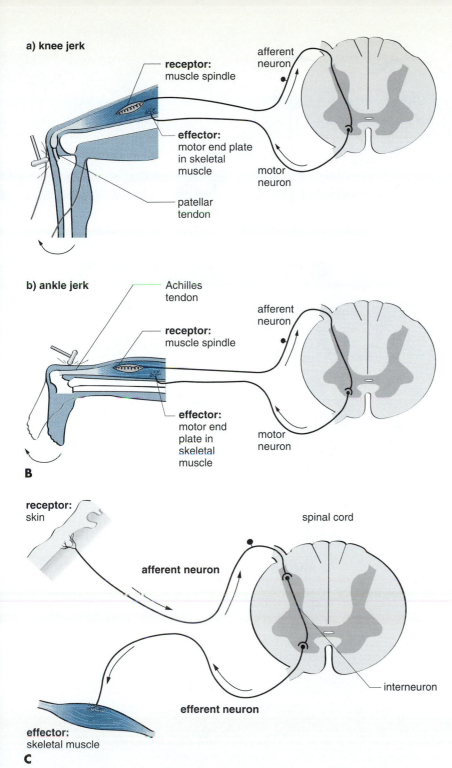

a) knee jerk

receptor:
muscle spindle

afferent
neuron

effector:
motor end plate
in skeletal
muscle

motor
neuron

patellar
tendon

b) ankle jerk

Achilles
tendon

receptor:
muscle spindle

afferent
neuron

effector:
motor end
plate in
skeletal
muscle

motor
neuron

B

receptor:
skin

spinal cord

afferent neuron

interneuron

efferent neuron

effector:
skeletal muscle

C

FIGURE 18.19 — (*continued*) *B.* The simplest reflex arcs involve just two neurons; these include the knee jerk and ankle jerk, commonly tested as part of the physical examination. *C.* Most reflex arcs are more complex involving one or more interneurons. (*Adapted, with permission, from Mackenna BR, Callendar R (1990). Illustrated Physiology, 5th ed. Edinburgh, Churchill Livingstone, pp 229–231.*)

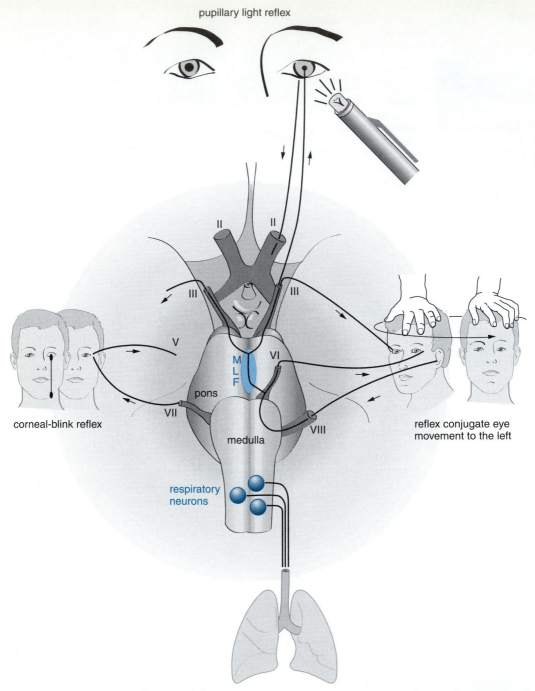

pupillary light reflex

II   II

III   III

V   VI

M
L
F

pons

VII

corneal-blink reflex

VIII

medulla

respiratory
neurons

reflex conjugate eye
movement to the left

FIGURE 18.20. Brainstem reflexes and their use in examining a patient in coma. The pupillary reaction to light tests the function of the midbrain and cranial nerve III. Spontaneous and reflex horizontal conjugate eye movements test for intactness of the pons. This is because the medial longitudinal fasciculus fiber tract that traverses the pons connects the nuclei of cranial nerves III and VI. Head movements or caloric stimulation trigger reflex eye movements that are normally suppressed in the conscious patient. Normally the eyes deviate in the direction of the side receiving cool-water irrigation of the external auditory canal. With head movement, the eyes look toward a hemispheric lesion and away from a brainstem lesion. Reflex blinking upon touching

spinal cord reflexes are monosynaptic: A single afferent neuron synapses with an efferent neuron to give an immediate motor response to sensation. A good example of this is the stretch reflex. When a muscle is stretched, it responds by contracting. The muscle spindle, a sensory receptor structure encased in connective tissue at the ends of the muscle, senses the stretch and transduces it into an action potential that stimulates a motor neuron to trigger contraction. This is why leg extension occurs, for example, when the patellar tendon is tapped with a reflex hammer.

In contrast to simple stretch reflexes, some spinal cord reflexes are complex, with multiple interneurons that provide input that affects the reflex. A good example is the withdrawal reflex. A mild noxious stimulus to a limb results in flexor muscle contraction and inhibition of extensor muscle contraction, so that the limb is withdrawn. However, if the noxious stimulus is of sufficient severity, not only is the limb withdrawn, but the other limb is extended. The stronger the stimulus, the more neurons are recruited into the reflex, eventually affecting all four extremities and triggering more and more neurons at other levels of the spinal cord. A typical motor neuron has about 10,000 synapses with other neurons providing stimulatory and inhibitory information to affect the final common pathway of motor activity.

Muscle spindles and golgi tendon organs

Muscle spindles and Golgi tendon organs are specialized receptors in muscle and tendons that provide the spinal cord with a constant input of information as to the rate of change in muscle length and tendon tension, respectively. Stretching a muscle spindle increases its rate of firing, whereas the rate of firing is decreased upon shortening.

Brainstem reflexes

A coma is a sleeplike state from which a patient cannot be aroused. There are a number of reflexes involving the *cranial nerves* that are clinically very useful in assessing the location of the lesion in a comatose patient (see Figure 18.20).

1. The **pupillary light reflex**. The size of the pupil is controlled by the amount of light reaching the retina. Fibers from each retina travel via the optic nerve to the pretectal nucleus of the midbrain, and from there to each **Edinger-Westphal nucleus**. Output from the Edinger-Westphal nuclei via **cranial nerve III**, the **oculomoter nerve**, mediates pupillary constriction in bright light. When light is dim, this reflex is inhibited and sympathetic innervation dominates, causing dilation of the pupils.
2. The **corneal blink reflex** (brief bilateral lid closure upon touching the cornea with a wisp of cotton). This depends on reflex connections between **cranial nerves V and VII** in the pons. Noxious stimuli are detected by cranial nerve V (trigeminal nerve), which then relays information to the motor

---

FIGURE 18.21 — (*continued*) the cornea with a wisp of cotton is another brainstem reflex indicative of pontine function involving cranial nerves V and VII. Respiratory patterns are controlled by the medulla. Shallow, slow, well-timed regular respirations suggest a drug-induced or metabolic cause of coma. Rapid deep breathing (called Kussmaul respirations) is seen in metabolic acidosis and pons and midbrain brainstem lesions. Cheyne-Stokes respiration, a cyclic pattern of increasingly rapid breaths punctuated by a brief period without breaths, usually signifies mild bilateral hemispheric damage or metabolic suppression and often occurs with relatively light coma. Intermittent gasps are called agonal respirations; they are seen in bilateral lower brainstem damage and usually indicate that death is imminent. (*Reproduced, with permission, from Fauci, A, et al. (eds) (1998). Harrison's Principles of Internal Medicine, 14th ed. New York, McGraw-Hill, p 129.*)

nucleus of cranial nerve VII (facial nerve) to effect a blink. CNS depressants diminish this response.

3. **Reflex conjugate eye movements** in response to certain stimuli. "Doll's eyes" are reflex movements of the eyes in the direction opposite to the direction of movement of the head from side to side. They are dependent on brainstem mechanisms that originate in the **labyrinths** (see Sec. 8), with input from cervical proprioceptors and are normally suppressed by visual fixation. However, when the cerebral hemispheres are suppressed or inactive, this reflex appears. Intact cranial nerves VI, III, and VIII are thus necessary for doll's eyes reflex horizontal eye movements.

Caloric stimulation (irrigation of the external auditory canal with cool water) is a stronger stimulus that tests similar pathways to those tested by the doll's eyes maneuver. An intact brainstem is indicated by tonic deviation of the eyes, following a brief latency, in the direction of the caloric stimulation and lasting for 30 to 120 s. If the cerebral hemispheres are functioning properly, there is an obligate rapid corrective movement of the eyes away from the side of tonic deviation. Loss of this quick corrective phase indicates cerebral hemisphere damage, while absence of the tonic deviation toward the stimulus indicates damage to one or more of the cranial nerves involved in this reflex.

4. **Respiratory patterns** (see legend to Figure 18.20).

Clinical Pearls

○ Light in one eye causes pupillary constriction in the other eye because the connections from each retina go to both pretectal and Edinger-Westphal nuclei. However, output from each Edinger-Westphal nucleus goes only to the pupillary constrictor muscle on the same side.

○ Symmetrically reactive pupils generally exclude midbrain damage as a cause of coma.

○ One enlarged and nonreactive or poorly reactive pupil suggests either compression of the third cranial nerve (e.g., by a mass) or an intrinsic midbrain lesion, usually on the same side. Oval or eccentric pupils are seen in early midbrain or third nerve compression syndromes.

○ Bilateral dilated and nonreactive pupils suggest severe midbrain damage or an overdose of drugs with anticholinergic activity. Be sure a previous examiner or the patient didn't use mydriatic (pupil-dilating) eyedrops in the recent past!

○ Reactive and bilaterally small but not pinpoint pupils are seen in metabolic encephalopathy and deep bilateral hemispheric lesions (hydrocephalus or thalamic hemorrhage).

○ Pinpoint but reactive pupils (look with a magnifying glass) suggest opiate or barbiturate overdose, or bilateral damage to the pons. Use the response to naloxone (an opiate antagonist) and reflex eye movements to distinguish between these possibilities.

○ Lid tone decreases as the depth of coma increases. Test this by resistance to opening of eyelids and speed of closure.

○ Horizontal deviation of the eyes occurs with drowsiness and disappears as either the patient wakes up or coma deepens.

○ An outwardly deviated eye suggests lateral rectus muscle weakness due to a sixth cranial nerve lesion. When bilateral, it suggests elevated intracranial pressure.

○ An externally deviated eye (so-called "down-and-out" eye), often accompanied by pupillary dilation on the same side, suggests third cranial nerve damage. This occurs because of the unopposed action of the lateral rectus muscle (cranial nerve VI).

○ Vertical separation of the axes of the eyes suggests cerebellar or pontine lesions.

○ Spontaneous, conjugate (both together), horizontal, roving eye movements in comatose patients suggest that the midbrain and pons are intact. Conversely, loss of horizontal eye movements is seen in particular syndromes. For example, brisk downward and slow upward eye movements, termed *ocular bobbing*, are seen in bilateral pontine lesions. Slower, arrhythmic downward movements followed by faster upward movement, in the presence of normal reflex horizontal gaze, is seen in diffuse anoxic damage to the cerebral cortex. Thalamic and upper midbrain lesions are associated with the eyes turning down and inward.

○ The ease with which the eyes move in the opposite direction to head movement in doll's eyes indicates the degree of cerebral hemisphere damage and the intactness of the brainstem pathways.

○ At rest, conjugate horizontal eye deviation is toward a hemispheric lesion and away from a brainstem lesion.

Review Questions

34. Describe the withdrawal reflex.
35. What is a Golgi tendon organ and what does it do?
36. Describe the reflex conjugate eye movements.

6. THE AUTONOMIC NERVOUS SYSTEM

The autonomic nervous system (ANS) is a reflex system analogous to the reflex arcs of the somatic sensory and motor systems. The difference between these systems and the ANS is that the sensory input to the ANS (afferent fibers) comes generally from internal organs and the responses (efferent fibers), after integration of central input, typically go to the smooth muscle of blood vessels and organs. Functions of the ANS include control of arterial pressure, gastrointestinal motility, secretion, emptying of the urinary bladder, and sweating.

The ANS has two major subdivisions, the **sympathetic nervous system** (SNS) and the **parasympathetic nervous system** (PsNS). The enteric nervous system (ENS) of the GI tract is sometimes considered a third subdivision of the ANS (see Chap. 5). Both the SNS and the PsNS are characterized by a two-neuron effector system in which ganglia are structures where the two neurons meet.

The ganglia of the SNS generally occur close to the spinal cord, whereas in the PsNS, the ganglia generally reside close to the target organ, often in the wall of the organ innervated.

Neurotransmitters work via receptors, and hence the effect of the ANS on any particular organ or tissue is dependent on the distribution of the various subtypes of adrenergic and cholinergic receptors from one organ to another (see Table 18.2).

Most preganglionic neurons of both the SNS and the PsNS release acetylcholine, although many different neurotransmitters are used by small subpopulations of preganglionic neurons, including peptides such as vasoactive intestinal peptide (VIP) and gonadotropin-releasing hormone (GnRH), which have completely different functions elsewhere in the body (see Chaps. 4 and 16, respectively). The acetylcholine released by the preganglionic fibers acts through a subtype of acetylcholine receptors known as **nicotinic receptors**.

The neurotransmitter used by the postganglionic neuron differs depending on whether the neuron is part of the SNS or the PsNS. In the SNS, norepinephrine is typically the postganglionic neurotransmitter, while in the PsNS, acetylcholine is the postganglionic

TABLE 18.2   DISTRIBUTION OF SUBTYPES OF RECEPTORS IN THE ANS

Effector organs	Cholinergic impulse response	Noradrenergic impulses	
		Receptor type[a]	Response
Eyes			
Radial muscle of iris	—	α_1	Contraction (mydriasis)
Sphincter muscle of iris	Contraction (miosis)		—
Ciliary muscle	Contraction for near vision	β_2	Relaxation for far vision
Heart			
S-A node	Decrease in heart rate, vagal arrest	β_1, β_2	Increase in heart rate
Atria	Decrease in contractility and (usually) increase in conduction velocity	β_1, β_2	Increase in contractility and conduction velocity
A-V node	Decrease in conduction velocity	β_1, β_2	Increase in conduction velocity
His-Purkinje system	Decrease in conduction velocity	β_1, β_2	Increase in conduction velocity
Ventricles	Decrease in contractility	β_1, β_2	Increase in contractility
Arterioles			
Coronary	Constriction	α_1, α_2	Constriction
		β_2	Dilation
Skin and mucosa	Dilation	α_1, α_2	Constriction
Skeletal muscle	Dilation	α_1	Constriction
		β_2	Dilation
Cerebral	Dilation	α_1	Constriction
Pulmonary	Dilation	α_1	Constriction
		β_2	Dilation
Abdominal viscera	—	α_1	Constriction
		β_2	Dilation
Salivary glands	Dilation	α_1, α_2	Constriction
Renal	—	α_1, α_2	Constriction
		β_1, β_2	Dilation
Systemic veins	—	α_1, α_2	Constriction
		β_2	Dilation
Lungs			
Bronchial muscle	Contraction	β_2	Relaxation
Bronchial glands	Stimulation	α_1	Inhibition
		β_2	Stimulation
Stomach			
Motility and tone	Increase	$\alpha_1, \alpha_2, \beta_2$	Decrease (usually)
Sphincters	Relaxation (usually)	α_1	Contraction (usually)
Secretion	Stimulation	α_2	Inhibition
Intestine			
Motility and tone	Increase	$\alpha_1, \alpha_2, \beta_1, \beta_2$	Decrease (usually)
Sphincters	Relaxation (usually)	α_1	Contraction (usually)
Secretion	Stimulation	α_2	Inhibition
Gallbladder and ducts	Contraction	β_2	Relaxation
Urinary bladder			
Detrusor	Contraction	β_2	Relaxation (usually)
Trigone and sphincter	Relaxation	α_1	Contraction

TABLE 18.2   DISTRIBUTION OF SUBTYPES OF RECEPTORS IN THE ANS (*Continued*)

Effector organs	Cholinergic impulse response	Noradrenergic impulses	
		Receptor type[a]	Response
Ureters			
Motility and tone	Increase (?)	α_1	Increase (usually)
Uterus	Variable[b]	α_1	Contraction (pregnant)
		β_2	Relaxation (pregnant and non-pregnant)
Male sex organs	Erection	α_1	Ejaculation
Skin			
Pilomotor muscles	—	α_1	Contraction
Sweat glands	Generalized secretion	α_1	Slight, localized secretion[c]
Spleen capsule	—	α_1	Contraction
		β_2	Relaxation
Adrenal medulla	Secretion of epinephrine and norepinephrine		—
Liver	—	α_1, β_2	Glycogenolysis
Pancreas			
Acini	Increased secretion	α	Decreased secretion
Islets	Increased insulin and glucagon secretion	α_2	Decreased insulin and glucagon secretion
		β_2	Increased insulin and glucagon secretion
Salivary glands	Profuse, watery secretion	α_1	Thick, viscous secretion
		β	Amylase secretion
Lacrimal glands	Secretion	α	Secretion
Nasopharyngeal glands	Secretion		—
Adipose tissue	—	α_1, β_1, β_3	Lipolysis
Juxtaglomerular cells	—	β_1	Increased renin secretion
Pineal gland	—	β	Increased melatonin synthesis and secretion

[a]Where a receptor subtype is not specified, data are as yet inadequate for characterization.
[b]Depends on stage of menstrual cycle, amount of circulating estrogen and progesterone, pregnancy, and other factors.
[c]On palms of hands and in some other locations ("adrenergic sweating").
Reproduced, with permission, from Ganong FW (1997). *Textbook of Medical Physiology.* Stamford, CT, Appleton & Lange, p 214, as modified from Hardman JG, et al. (eds) (1996). *Goodman and Gilman's The Pharmacological Basis of Therapeutics,* 9th ed. New York, McGraw-Hill.

neurotransmitter. One exception to this rule is that the postganglionic sympathetic nerve fibers that innervate the sweat glands, the piloerector muscles, and some blood vessels use acetylcholine. The acetylcholine released by postganglionic fibers carries out its effect through a different receptor subtype, called **muscarinic acetylcholine receptors**.

The ANS can be activated by centers in the spinal cord, brainstem, and hypothalamus, and is influenced by the cerebral cortex, especially the limbic cortex.

The ANS can also function through visceral reflexes without involving the cerebral cortex. In such autonomic reflexes, sensory signals enter the autonomic ganglia, spinal cord, brainstem, or hypothalamus and trigger reflex responses directly back to visceral organs to adjust their functions. Examples of autonomic reflexes are:

- The **baroreceptor reflex**, whereby elevated arterial pressures are sensed and trigger brainstem-mediated inhibition of sympathetic impulses to the heart and blood vessels, resulting in a compensatory drop in sympathetic tone and hence blood pressure.
- The **salivation reflex**, whereby the smell and taste of appealing foods trigger signals from the nose and mouth to activate vagal, glossopharyngeal, and salivary nuclei of the brainstem. These nuclei then use the PsNS to stimulate salivation in anticipation of eating.
- The **defecation reflex**, whereby stretching of the rectum by feces signals, via the sacral spinal cord to the PsNS, the triggering of peristaltic contractions that cause the urge to defecate.
- The **bladder-emptying reflex**, controlled in much the same way as the defecation reflex. In this case, the consequence of its activation is both bladder contraction and urinary sphincter relaxation, resulting in the flow of urine.
- **Sexual reflexes** involve a convergence of input from the cerebral cortex with stimulation of the sex organs. In males, penile erection is the result of PsNS innervation, while ejaculation involves the SNS.

In addition to responding to central input and to autonomic reflexes, the ANS is in a state of constant activity, called **sympathetic and parasympathetic tone**. This allows greater sensitivity in that signals via the brain or via reflexes can either increase or decrease the baseline ANS activity. Without sympathetic tone, the SNS could only raise blood pressure (e.g., by triggering vasoconstriction). The presence of a certain amount of sympathetic activity even at rest allows the SNS to also be able to contribute to a *decrease* in blood pressure by *inhibition* of the baseline sympathetic tone, when desired. Likewise, parasympathetic tone contributes to gastrointestinal tract motility, even in the absence of a specific program such as peristalsis. This allows alteration of PsNS activity to either increase or decrease gastrointestinal motility when so desired.

Clinical Pearls

○ Loss of autonomic innervation of the blood vessels impairs sympathetic tone and contributes to the dizziness upon standing (called *orthostatic hypotension*) that is often experienced by individuals with autonomic disorders or those treated with medications such as α-adrenergic blockers that can impair the sympathetic nervous system.

○ Absence of a compensatory increase in heart rate during a hypotensive episode implies a neurogenic process, whereas hypotension with compensatory tachycardia indicates intact baroreceptors and cardiovascular reflexes. Conversely, neurologic diseases that alter brainstem neurochemistry and sympathetic output, such as Parkinson's disease or Shy-Drager syndrome, cause orthostatic hypotension.

○ Loss of autonomic innervation of the GI tract, either due to surgical severing of branches of the vagus nerve or due to destruction of the nerves (for example, as a complication of diabetes mellitus) results in decreased parasympathetic tone. Decreased parasympathetic tone of the ANS in turn results in constipation, bloating, risk of obstruction, poor digestion, etc.

Review Questions

37. What is the difference between the ANS and other reflex systems?
38. What are the major subdivisions of the ANS, and what do they control?
39. What are the neurotransmitters generally used by the pre- and postganglionic fibers of the major subdivisions of the ANS?

7. HIGHER BRAIN FUNCTIONS AND CONSCIOUSNESS

As mentioned previously, the cerebral cortex is the seat of higher brain functions and is organized into a number of lobes. In addition to playing roles in integration with all other parts of the brain, each lobe subserves certain primary and specialized functions:

• The frontal lobe is important for motor behavior and for aspects of personality.
• The parietal lobe is most important for processing somatosensory information.
• The temporal lobe performs many different functions, including processing of information related to hearing and visual information necessary for recognition of images. The hippocampal formation of the temporal lobe is crucial for formation of memories (see the following discussion).
• The limbic lobe is involved principally in emotions and behavior.
• The occipital lobe is crucial for vision.

Beyond these generalizations as to the roles of the various lobes of the cerebral cortex (see Sec. 2), specific regions within each lobe have been recognized to perform specific functions. Thus, a primary motor cortex and a primary sensory cortex with precise correlation to particular muscles and regions of the body have been identified, as discussed previously.

The **secondary motor cortex** and **second-ary sensory cortex** are regions that are crucial to an individual's being able to correctly interpret and understand the information generated in the primary motor and sensory cortex, respectively.

A third type of area in the cerebral cortex is the so-called association areas. These are mixed sensory and motor regions that have particular categories of functions. For example, within a broad band of the cortex called the **parieto-occipitotemporal area** are subareas that are important for language comprehension, analysis of spatial coordinates of the body, reading, and naming objects. **Wernicke's area** within the parieto-occipitotemporal area is particularly important, as information from visual, auditory, and somatic interpretive areas flows to Wernicke's area as a necessary precondition for fluent speech.

Another crucial area within the cerebral cortex is the **prefrontal cortex**, which is the seat of thinking. Patients with lesions of the prefrontal cortex are able to go through the motions of life, but without any intellectual input or thought associated with their pleasantly demented existence.

In addition to recognizing functional regions within the various lobes of the cerebral cortex, it is important to appreciate that the entire cortex has *depth*, with six distinct layers of cells.

While symmetrical in gross structure, the two halves of the cerebral cortex are not identical. One side or the other is called **dominant**, meaning that the motor activities controlled by that side are capable of finer, more precise actions than those controlled by the other side. Wernicke's area in the dominant hemisphere is substantially larger than the same area on the other side.

Distinct from the issue of dominance of one hemisphere over another is the fact that language is typically a left-brain function. Thus 99% of right-handed people are left-hemisphere-dominant for language, while only about 20% of left-handed people are right-brain-dominant for language. On the other hand, the right hemisphere is generally dominant for interpreting music, drawing, and other nonverbal experiences.

The **corpus callosum** comprises myelinated fibers that connect the two cerebral hemispheres. Without it, the ability to coordinate between the two hemispheres is impaired. Thus, for example, the usually dominant left hemisphere loses control over the right motor cortex and, with it, voluntary control over the actions of the left hand.

Another aspect of higher brain function is awakefulness or **arousal**. The distinction between sleep and coma is that a person can be awakened from sleep by simple stimuli, whereas a patient in coma is not fully arousable, although he or she may respond partially to some degree of discomfort or other stimulation.

Arousal is generated by activity of neurons in the central midbrain, lateral hypothalamus, and various nuclei of the thalamus, which make up the **ascending reticular activating system**. Neurons whose cell bodies lie in these nuclei project to the cerebral cortex to trigger arousal. Other nuclei, particularly in the pontine reticular formation, play a crucial role in the active process of triggering sleep.

Memory involves short-term, intermediate, and long-term processes. For memory to occur, information must be registered in the **primary somatosensory**, **visual**, **or auditory cortex**. Immediate recall of written or spoken information requires posterior cortical areas involved in language comprehension.

The hippocampi and their connections to the dorsal medial nucleus of the thalamus and the mamillary nuclei of the hypothalamus make up a limbic system network needed for the processing of information for long-term storage (see Figure 18.21A). Damage in these areas impairs new learning and recall of information from the recent past, but not long-term memories. Learning seems to occur in the hippocampus and the cerebral cortical structures of the limbic system. However,

upon conversion to long-term memory, the information is transferred to association regions of the cortex, including the parietal association cortex, visual association cortex, and auditory cortex, depending upon whether the basis of the memory is motor, visual, or auditory, respectively. Thus, the capacity to remember new things can be impaired even when long-term memory is intact.

The molecular basis of memory is believed to involve long-lasting, use-dependent changes in the ease with which transmission occurs across particular synapses. Short-term memory might involve chemical changes that have this effect (e.g., elevation in intracellular calcium that facilitates neurotransmitter release at synapses made by particular neurons). Long-term memory seems more likely to involve structural changes, such as an increase in the number of presynaptic terminals. The study of the molecular basis of memory and learning is still in its infancy and is an area in a tremendous state of flux (see Sec. 10, Frontiers).

Clinical Pearl

○ Patients with disorders of arousal can fall into several categories.

- Coma is a failure of arousal. It can have structural or metabolic causes (see Table 18.3). Common structural causes include hemorrhage, ischemic infarction, abscess, tumors, or increased intracranial pressure for any reason. Expanding masses not only raise intracranial pressure but can result in herniation syndromes, in which regions of the brain are pushed from their usual location, with devastating outcomes.
- Metabolic causes of coma (e.g., drug overdoses) typically preserve pupillary light responses despite impaired ocu-

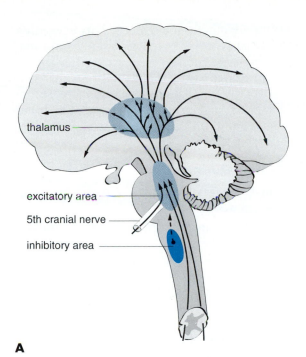

A

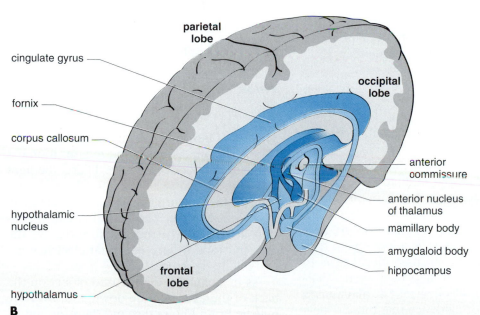

B

FIGURE 18.21. Arousal, motivation, and emotion. A. Various regions of the brain-stem activate higher centers of the brain. Other regions in the brainstem serve to inhibit the activation system. B. Anatomy of the limbic system, which provides the neuronal circuitry for motivational drives and emotional behavior. (Reproduced, with permission, from Guyton AC, Hall JE (1997). Physiology and Mechanisms of Disease, 6th ed. Philadelphia, Saunders, p 483.)

TABLE 18.3 NONSTRUCTURAL AND METABOLIC CAUSES OF COMA

Drugs (sedative-hypnotics, ethanol, opioids)
Global cerebral ischemia
Hepatic encephalopathy
Hypercalcemia
Hyperosmolar states
Hyperthermia
Hypoglycemia
Hyponatremia
Hypoxia
Hypothyroidism
Meningitis and encephalitis
Seizure or prolonged postictal state
Subarachnoid hemorrhage
Uremia
Wernicke's encephalopathy

Reproduced, with permission, from Messing RO (1997). In McPhee S et al. (eds): *Pathophysiology of Disease*, 2d ed Stamford, CT, Appleton & Lange, p 148.

lovestibular or even respiratory function (see Table 18.3 above).

• Uncal herniation (of the temporal lobe) often compresses the third cranial nerve on the same side, causing pupillary dilatation and impaired extraocular muscle function first. Further elevation of pressure distorts the midbrain, with coma, posturing of limbs, loss of oculovestibular responses, and eventually respiratory arrest.

• Central herniation due to hemispheric lesions closer to the midline causes coma before eye findings. Later, pupils dilate, limbs posture, and pontine vestibular and medullary respiratory functions are lost.

• A confusional state is a less severe dysfunction of the arousal mechanism in which perceptions may be distorted (hallucinations) or beliefs may be maintained in the face of evidence that these beliefs are false (delusions).

• Delirium is a confusional state characterized by heightened alertness, disordered perception, agitation, delusions, and hallucinations. Patients with delirium dis-

play autonomic hyperactivity (sweating, tachycardia, hypertension) and may have seizures.

• Lesions rostral to the midbrain must generally be bilateral or cause increased intracranial pressure affecting the brainstem in order to cause coma.

Review Questions

40. What is the difference between coma and sleep?
41. What are the roles of the primary motor/sensory, secondary motor/sensory, and association areas of the cerebral cortex?
42. What is dominance, and what structures are necessary for it to be manifest?
43. What is arousal, and how is it controlled?

8. SPECIAL SENSES

Vision

Optics of the eye

The eye is basically a camera that takes light reflected from an image and focuses it on the retina at the back of the eye. There, the light activates special receptor cells, the rods and cones, which in turn trigger electrical activity in the optic nerve. The neural circuit for vision leads back to the visual cortex in the occipital lobe, where neuronal electrical activity is interpreted.

As in a camera, the focused object on the back of the eye is upside down and inverted, but the brain knows this and therefore interprets the information in the correct way. Instead of a single lens as in a camera, the eye has a series of compartments through which light passes, each with a slightly different refractive index, which is what allows incoming light to be bent and focused. One of these compartments is the lens, which can change its shape and therefore adjust the degree of refraction, a process called **accommodation** (see Figure 18.22). Contraction of the ciliary muscle relaxes the ligaments of the lens capsule, allowing the lens to assume a more spherical shape. This increases the degree of refraction of light. The ciliary muscle is under parasympathetic control via cranial nerve III, whose nucleus lies in the brainstem. Thus, as an object moves closer, more and more parasympathetic activity is needed to keep the object in focus (by more and more contraction of the ciliary muscle).

By changing the diameter of the pupil from as little as 1.5 mm to a maximum of 8 mm, the **iris** is able to adjust the amount of light entering the eye 30fold to provide the optimal degree of illumination.

Defects in refraction

Ideally, the light rays from distant objects would be in sharp focus when the ciliary muscle was completely relaxed. That would allow the maximum capacity for adjustment (accommodation) to keep objects in focus as they get nearer and nearer. The (normal) condition in which eyes have this full dynamic

FIGURE 18.22. Mechanism of accommodation (see text). *(Adapted, with permission, from Guyton AC, Hall JE (1997). Human Physiology and Mechanisms of Disease, 6th ed. Philadelphia, Saunders, p 401.)*

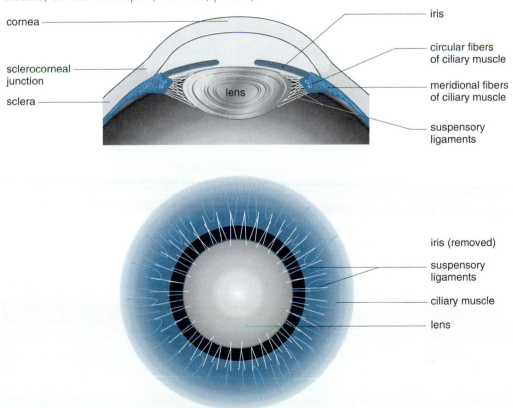

range is called **emmetropia**. However, the eyes of many individuals do not achieve this ideal.

In some people, when the ciliary muscle is relaxed, rays of light from distant objects have not been bent enough to be brought into focus. Thus, to bring them into focus, some degree of ciliary muscle contraction is necessary. In effect, these individuals have eyeballs that are too short (in the direction of the object being viewed) or ciliary muscles that are too weak. This condition will diminish the range of additional accommodation possible in order to look at nearer objects. Often, especially in the elderly, even maximal ciliary muscle contraction is insufficient to bring even distant objects completely into focus, let alone those that are close by. Such individuals are said to be farsighted or to have **hyperopia** and require corrective lenses. This condition is called **presbyopia** in the elderly because of its common occurrence.

Conversely, nearsightedness, called **myopia**, occurs when even the fully relaxed ciliary muscle brings objects into focus before the rays of light reach the retina. In effect, the eyes of these individuals are too long (in the direction of the object being viewed). Thus, accommodation cannot help bring the object into focus; instead, the eye must be closer to the object. At some point, the object is sufficiently close to the eye to be either exactly in focus on the retina or in the range where accommodation can bring it exactly into focus. However, to see distant objects, these individuals require corrective lenses. Figure 18.23A indicates the problem with hyperopia and myopia, and Figure 18.23B indicates how it is remedied by corrective lenses.

In **astigmatism**, the refractive error is found in one plane but not another. This is because the curvature of the lens is greater in one plane than in another (see Figure 18.24C). Combinations of spherical and cylindrical lenses can be used to determine the degree of correction needed in different planes, and then special lenses can be ground to those specifications.

Depth perception

There are two mechanisms by which we are able to discriminate the distance between two objects. First, the brain is able to unconsciously and automatically take into account what it knows from prior experience to be the size of an object. Thus, for example, cars viewed from the top of a 50-story building are understood to look tiny not because they are, but because they must be far away.

A second mechanism for discriminating distance and depth is binocular vision, or **stereopsis**. The closer an object is to the eyes (within the range where full accommodation is possible), the greater the degree to which the image of the object will be located in different parts of the retina in the left versus the right eye (see Figure 18.24). The more distant an object, the less the position of its image on the retina diverges from one eye to the other. Thus, the brain is able to interpret the difference in position on the retina of images of objects in each of the two eyes to correspond to differences in distance *from* the eyes.

Clinical Pearls

○ Patients who have an eye patched (e.g., because of a corneal abrasion) should be warned *not* to drive, because the loss of stereopsis will impair their ability to discriminate distance (e.g., from the car in front of them) and make them far more prone to accidents.

○ Refractive errors are eliminated when one looks through a pinhole (similar to the

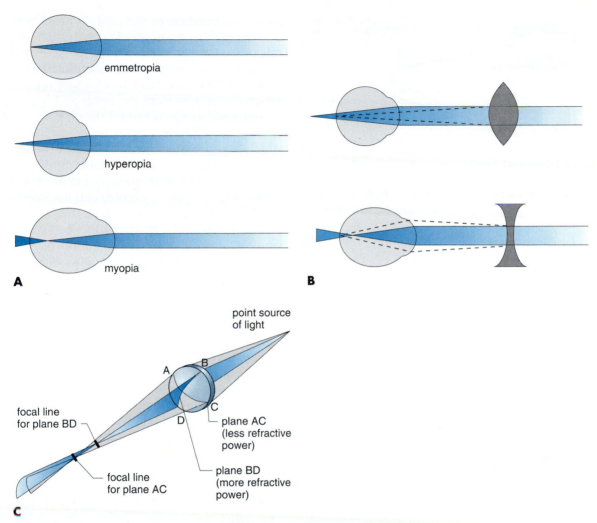

FIGURE 18.23. Errors of refraction and the use of corrective lenses. *A.* In emmetropia, parallel rays of light are focused exactly on the retina in perfect focus. In myopia, perfect focus is in front of the retina. In hyperopia, perfect focus is behind the retina. *B.* Correction of myopia with a concave lens, and correction of hyperopia with a convex lens. *C.* Illustration that astigmatism results from light rays that focus at different focal distances in different planes (plane AC vs. plane BD). *(Adapted, with permission, from Guyton AC, Hall JE (1997). Human Physiology and Mechanisms of Disease, 6th ed. Philadelphia, Saunders, pp 402, 403.)*

principle of closing the camera lens aperture down to gain depth of field, or as in a pinhole camera, which has no lens). This is also why people can improve their vision by squinting. Neurologists examine for lesions of the optic nerve by testing vision while the patient is looking through a pinhole. This removes the contribution of a lens or refractive problem in evaluating a patient's vision complaint.

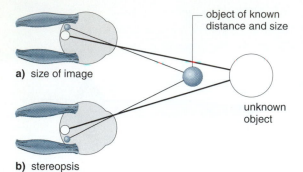

a) size of image

b) stereopsis

FIGURE 18.24. Perception of distance. As illustrated, distance is perceived in two ways: first, by the size of the image on the retina, and second, as a result of stereopsis in comparison to objects of known distance and size. (*Adapted, with permission, from Guyton AC, Hall JE (1997). Human Physiology and Mechanisms of Disease, 6th ed. Philadelphia, Saunders, p 405.*)

The retina

The retina is the part of the back of the eye that contains the photosensitive receptor cells called **rods** (responsible for vision in the dark) and **cones** (responsible for color vision). The retina itself consists of many layers of cells. The several-hundred-micrometer-thick inhomogeneous retina would be expected to severely impair visual acuity. However, a small area (1 mm square) in the middle of the retina, called the *macula*, and its central portion, the *fovea*, has the other cell layers pulled away so that, at that point, focused light lands directly on the photoreceptor cells. This region allows the formation of extremely detailed visual images, in contrast to those of the photoreceptors more peripherally.

Photochemistry of vision

Light focused by the lens and vitreous humor enters the retina and travels all the way back to the rods and cones. These photoreceptor cells contain a highly specialized form of plasma membrane packed with light-sensitive pigments. In the rods, the pigment is **rhodop-**

sin, a combination of the protein opsin with a carotenoid pigment, 11-*cis* retinal. In response to light, rhodopsin is activated through a complex pathway, resulting in conversion of 11-*cis* retinal to all *trans* retinal, which dissociates from the opsin and is converted back to 11-*cis* retinal through the action of the enzyme retinal isomerase, after which it recombines with opsin (see Figure 18.25A). One of the intermediates in this cycle, metarhodopsin II, triggers the electrical changes in the photoreceptor cell leading to a receptor potential (see Figure 18.25B).

The pathway of signal transduction leading from absorption of a single photon of light to the receptor potential involves multiple amplifying steps:

• The activated rhodopsin molecule in turn, activates a G protein homolog called **transducin**.
• Transducin activates many molecules of a phosphodiesterase.
• The activated phosphodiesterase hydrolyzes many molecules of cyclic GMP.
• The cyclic GMP had been holding a sodium channel open (called the **dark current**), so upon hydrolysis of the cyclic GMP, the channel closes.
• The diminished flow of sodium ions triggers the receptor potential in the photoreceptor cell.
• The excited photoreceptor cell transmits the potential to sequential layers of neurons of the retina, then to the optic nerve, and ultimately to the cerebral cortex, where the signals are interpreted as vision.

One unusual feature of photoreceptor function is that the receptor potential resulting from exposure of a rod to light is *hyperpolarizing*. Thus, the negative charges inside the cell increase rather than decrease, as is the case for most other sensory receptors.

The process is reversed instantly because an enzyme, rhodopsin kinase, inactivates the

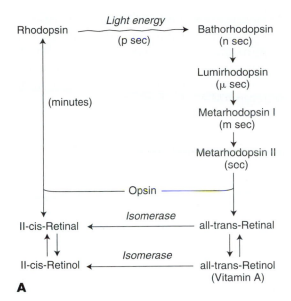

A

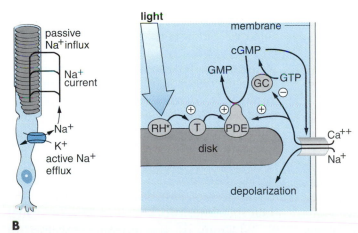

B

FIGURE 18.25. A. Rhodopsin-retinal visual cycle in the rod, involving rapid light-induced decomposition and slower chemical reformation of rhodopsin. B. Generation of a visual receptor potential (see text). (Reproduced, with permission, from Guyton AC, Hall JE (1997). Human Physiology and Mechanisms of Disease, 6th ed. Philadelphia, Saunders, pp 408–410. B. Reproduced, with permission, from Berne HM, levy MN (eds) (1997). Physiology, 4th ed. St. Louis, Mosby.)

metarhodopsin II and results in a cascade of changes that once again open the sodium channels.

This particular way of setting up the visual signaling system is responsible for its extraordinary sensitivity: Detection of a single photon results in the transient movement of millions of sodium ions.

Color vision involves the use of blue-, green-, and red-sensitive pigments that are activated by light of the appropriate wavelength. Most of the details of the subsequent signal transduction are essentially as described for rhodopsin.

Neurophysiology of vision

There are two pathways by which signals from the photoreceptors are sent back to the brain. The older, slower, "black-and-white" pathway is that of the rods. The newer, faster, color pathway is that of the cones.

Neural transmission of visual information is unique in that much of it involves a form of electrical conduction called **electrotonic conduction**, which is different from action potentials. Whereas action potentials are an "all or none" form of information flow, electrotonic conduction allows a fine gradation of signal strengths to be conducted. Thus, visual input to the brain is a direct function of intensity of illumination. The various layers of cells in the retina serve to process the information event before it has left the eye, allowing visual contrast between borders to be enhanced, for example.

Once impulses from the photoreceptors reach the ganglion cells, they revert to action potentials, a change necessitated perhaps by the longer distances that the information must travel. These neurons form fibers of the **optic nerve** that travel back to the **lateral geniculate nucleus** of the thalamus (see Figure 18.26A). Along the way, the fibers representing the nasal half of each retina cross over to the other side, joining the fibers from the temporal half of the other retina in their journey to the lateral geniculate nucleus. From the lateral geniculate nucleus, fibers travel as the optic radiation to the **primary visual cortex** of the occipital lobe of the cerebral cortex (see Figure 18.26B). Along the way, fibers pass from the optic tracts into older areas of the brain that allow control of eye movements and the pupillary light reflex (see the following discussion).

Because the optic chiasm is adjacent to the pituitary gland, expanding pituitary tumors often cause an early selective loss of crossed fibers, manifesting as loss of the outer visual field on both sides (called bitemporal hemianopsia).

Intraocular fluid and pressure

The portion of the eye in front of the lens is filled with fluid called **aqueous humor**, which is what keeps the eyeball distended. This fluid, which is constantly being formed and resorbed at the rate of 2 to 3 μL/min, is secreted by the **ciliary processes**. Formation of aqueous humor involves active transport of sodium, with passive movement of chloride, bicarbonate, and water to maintain electrical neutrality and iso-osmolality. Amino acids, glucose, and ascorbic acid are also transported specifically into aqueous humor.

Once secreted, aqueous humor flows into the angle between the cornea and the iris, through a trabecular meshwork, and into the **canal of Schlemm**, which leads to a thin-walled vein that empties into the extraocular venous drainage.

Normal intraocular pressure is 12 to 20 mmHg, determined mainly by the resistance to the flow of aqueous humor through the trabecular meshwork leading into the canal of Schlemm. If the pressure exceeds 15 mmHg, the openings in the trabeculae open up to allow more flow.

Clinical Pearl

○ The somewhat convoluted pathway of information from the retina to the visual cortex allows certain brain lesions to be localized based on their effects on *visual fields*. Shown in Figure 18.26A are various visual field defects resulting from lesions in particular regions of the visual pathway.

Clinical Pearls

○ Accommodation allows us to look at a close-up object, and then refocus our eyes to see something clearly in the distance. With age, this ability to accommodate is substantially lost as the ability to distend the lens diminishes, a condition called

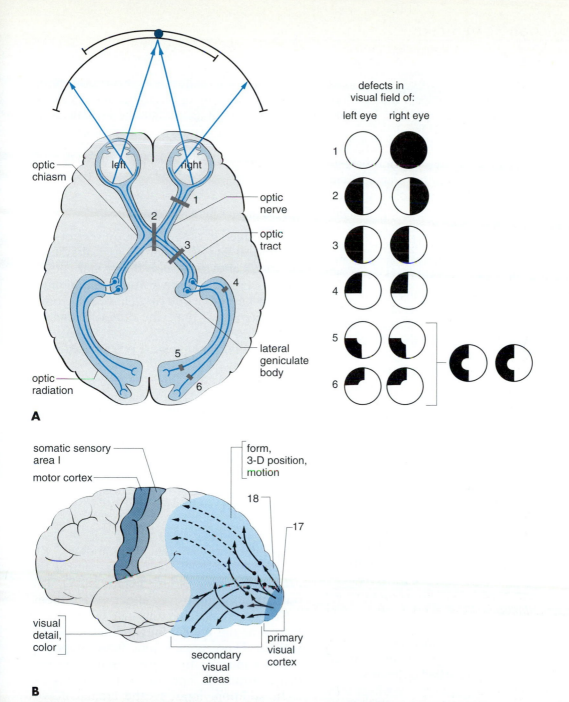

FIGURE 18.26. Neural visual pathways. A. Light on the retina stimulates the photoreceptor cells, whose receptor potentials are transmitted to the optic nerve, whose action potentials are transmitted to the lateral geniculate body, from which the visual cortex is stimulated via the optic radiations. Indicated are the distinct pathways of fibers from the nasal and temporal parts of the retina, which capture visual images from different visual fields. Thus lesions in different parts of the visual pathway (indicated by numbers) manifest as different patterns of visual field defects (see right of figure) on careful testing. B. Anatomy of the visual cortex. Signals received by the primary visual cortex are transmitted to the secondary visual areas, where details and color (anteroventral portion of the occipital lobe and ventral portion of the posterior temporal lobe) and form, motion, and three-dimensional position (posterior portions of the parietal lobe) are added. (Adapted, with permission, from Guyton AC, Hall JE (1997). Human Physiology and Mechanisms of Disease, 6th ed. Philadelphia, Saunders, p 419.)

presbyopia. As a result, by age 70, most people need bifocal glasses if they wish to both read easily (see up close in sharp focus) and see well at a distance.

○ A cataract is a clouding of the lens that results in reduced vision. Often a normal consequence of aging, cataracts occur more rapidly in patients with diabetes mellitus, eye trauma, or certain types of inflammation of the eye. Cataracts also occur in certain genetic diseases (myotonic dystrophy, neurofibromatosis type 2, and galactosemia) and are a side effect of radiation therapy and chronic high-dose glucocorticoid therapy. The cataracts seen with radiation and glucocorticoid excess are typically posterior subcapsular in location.

On physical examination, cataracts can be most readily detected by noting an impaired red reflex on viewing light reflected from the fundus of the retina through an ophthalmoscope.

The only treatment for cataracts is surgical extraction of the opacified lens. A million such procedures are performed in the United States yearly, with 95% resulting in improved vision.

○ Sometimes the trabeculae through which aqueous humor must percolate are clogged, either by inflammatory debris or by fibrosis, and intraocular pressures can build up to as high as 60 mmHg, a disorder called *glaucoma*. Over time, even pressures of 20 to 30 mmHg can result in blindness. Higher pressures can cause blindness in a matter of hours. The reason elevated intraocular pressure is bad is that it presses on the axons of the optic nerve where they leave the eyeball at the optic disk. This, in turn, blocks axoplasmic flow, starving the distal tips of the neurons that enter the brain. Eventually these neurons die and cannot be replaced, resulting in blindness. Treatments for glaucoma include eyedrops to block secretion of aqueous humor or to enhance its resorption, surgical opening up of the trabeculae, or diversion of the fluid outside the eyeball, all of which effectively reduce intraocular pressure.

Eye movements and their control

Proper function of the eyes requires not only the optical and electrophysiological systems described above, but also the proper coordination of *eye movements*. It doesn't do much good to know that you *could* have seen something coming — but you didn't bother to look.

There are three separate pairs of extraocular muscles:

- The **medial and lateral recti**, which move the eyeballs reciprocally from side to side
- The **superior and inferior recti**, which move the eyeballs reciprocally up and down
- The **superior and inferior obliques**, which rotate the eyeballs to keep visual fields in an upright position

Cranial nerves III (oculomotor), IV (trochlear), and VI (abducens) control the extraocular muscles (see Figure 18.27). The outputs from these cranial nerves are themselves interconnected through the pathway known as the **medial longitudinal fasciculus** (MLF). These connections allow opposing pairs of muscles to "know" that when one pair contract, the opposing pair should relax.

In addition, input to the cranial nerves comes from:

- The occipital visual areas
- The frontal cortex via the **frontal-tectal tract**
- The vestibular nuclei in the brainstem (via the MLF)

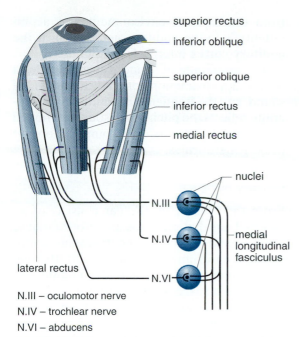

superior rectus
inferior oblique
superior oblique
inferior rectus
medial rectus
nuclei
N.III
N.IV
medial longitudinal fasciculus
lateral rectus
N.VI

N.III – oculomotor nerve
N.IV – trochlear nerve
N.VI – abducens

FIGURE 18.27. Extraocular muscles of the eye and their innervation. (Reproduced, with permission, from Guyton AC, Hall JE (1997). Human Physiology and Mechanisms of Disease, 6th ed. Philadelphia, Saunders, p 422.)

Fixation, accommodation, and control of pupillary aperture

An important feature of eye movements is the capacity for fixation — the ability to focus on an object as it or the observer moves. As the object starts to drift from the foveal portion of the retina, the secondary area of the visual cortex recognizes the problem and responds with rapid corrective eye movements.

The focal power of the lens is constantly being adjusted to maintain the highest degree of visual acuity possible. The brain is believed to utilize a number of different cues to make these adjustments:

• The message telling the eyes to converge occurs simultaneously with the message adjusting the strength of ciliary muscle contraction.

• Differences between the clarity and focus at the center and at the edges of the fovea allow comparison for in- and out-of-focus adjustments. Thus the brain takes advantage of the fact that the fovea is a hollowed-out depression in the retina whose focus will be distinctive.

• The degree of accommodation oscillates slightly at a frequency of approximately two times per second. This provides constant input concerning the direction in which changes need to be made in order to keep the eyes in optimal focus.

The eye is controlled by both parasympathetic and sympathetic autonomic innervation. The parasympathetic fibers arise in the Edinger-Westphal nucleus and enter cranial nerve III, by which they get to the ciliary ganglion behind the eye. The postganglionic fibers excite the ciliary muscle and also the sphincter of the iris, which mediates pupillary constriction, also called **miosis**. The sympathetic innervation originates from the intermediolateral horn cells of the first thoracic segment of the spinal cord. The sympathetic fibers enter the sympathetic chain and go to the **superior cervical ganglion**. There they synapse with postganglionic neurons, which spread along the arteries, starting with the carotid artery and then proceeding to smaller arteries to the eye. Stimulation of the sympathetic nerves causes pupillary dilatation or **mydriasis** by exciting the radial fibers of the iris.

Review Questions

44. What is the mechanism of accommodation?

45. What is the pathway by which aqueous humor is made and cleared?

46. What is the normal intraocular pressure?

47. What is the visual pigment of the rod cells, and how does it send a signal to the visual cortex?

48. What are the levels of signal amplification in the visual pathway by which a single photon causes movement of millions of sodium ions?

49. What is electrotonic conduction, where is it used, and what is its distinctive feature?

Hearing

General introduction to the auditory system

Sound is a form of sensation that occurs as a result of the motion of molecules in the external environment. Such motion travels in the form of **sound waves**, which travel through the air at speeds of about 344 m/s. The **ear** serves to convert such sound waves from the external environment into action potentials in the auditory nerves, which the **auditory cortex** interprets as sounds.

The **amplitude** of sound waves provides a rough approximation of the loudness of sound, and the **frequency** of sound waves generally reflects the pitch of the sound, although there are exceptions and complications to these general rules.

Anatomy of the ear

From the outside in, the ear consists of an **external ear** that serves as a sort of funnel to bring sound waves to the **tympanic membrane** or eardrum (see Figure 18.28). Beyond the tympanic membrane is the **middle ear**, an air-filled space in the temporal bone that opens to the nasopharynx intermittently (e.g., during chewing, swallowing, and yawning). When open, the middle ear serves to equalize the pressure on the two sides of the tympanic

FIGURE 18.28. Anatomy of the ear, including the tympanic membrane, the ossicular system of the middle ear, and the inner ear.

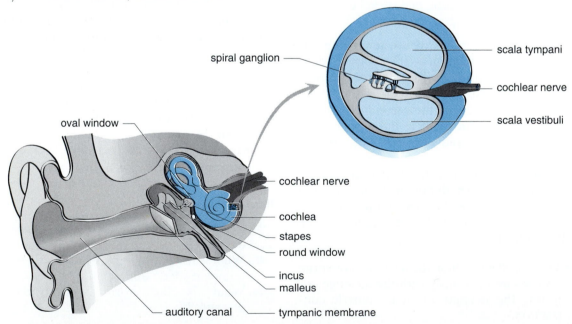

spiral ganglion

scala tympani

cochlear nerve

scala vestibuli

oval window

cochlear nerve

cochlea

stapes

round window

incus

malleus

auditory canal

tympanic membrane

membrane. The middle ear also contains the three **auditory ossicles**, small bones named the **malleus**, the **incus**, and the **stapes**. Beyond the middle ear lies the **inner ear**, which includes a fluid-filled structure also known as the **labyrinth**. The inner ear also includes the **cochlea**, a coiled tube that contains two membranes, the **basilar membrane** and **Reissner's membrane**. These membranes divide the cochlea into three chambers: the **scala vestibuli**, **scala tympani**, and **scala media**.

The **organ of Corti** is a structure on the basilar membrane that contains **hair cells**. Hair cells are the actual auditory receptors that transduce sound waves into action potentials in the sensory neurons of the auditory system. There are two types of hair cells in the organ of Corti: a single row of approximately 3500 individual internal hair cells, and three or four rows of external hair cells, totaling about 12,000 individual cells. Free nerve endings of the cochlear nerve synapse with the base and sides of the hair cells, predominantly the internal hair cells.

How hearing works

Noise sets off sound waves, which bounce off the tympanic membrane, displacing it slightly. This, in turn, causes sequential movement of the malleus, incus, and stapes to transmit that displacement. Movement of the stapes against the fluid-filled cochlea sets up waves in the fluid that produce distortions in the basilar membrane. The hair cells are sandwiched between the basilar membrane on which they sit and the tectorial membrane above them. Hair cells contain specialized bundles of actin filaments called **stereocilia**. It is the bending of these stereocilia that opens motion-sensitive channels that trigger receptor potentials in the hair cells. The movement of the basilar membrane results in a shear force being exerted by the **tectorial membrane** to bend the stereocilia. Bending in one direction depolarizes the hair cells while

bending in the other direction hyperpolarizes them. The receptor potentials generated in the hair cells in turn trigger action potentials in the cochlear nerve endings that ultimately travel back to the auditory cortex, where they are interpreted as sound (see Figure 18.29). These nerve fibers go to the spiral ganglion of Corti in the middle of the cochlea. From there, about 30,000 axons travel in the cochlear nerve and enter the CNS at the upper medulla.

Determination of loudness and the attenuation reflex

There are three principal determinants of loudness in the auditory system:

- The degree of movement of the basilar membrane. The more it moves, the louder the stimulus is perceived. Increasing amplitude of vibration results in activation of more hair cells. Spatial summation of the impulses then increases the number of nerve fibers in which an action potential is triggered.
- The outermost hair cells are much less sensitive to vibration than the innermost hair cells. Thus, their stimulation apprises the nervous system of the loudness of the sound.
- The attenuation reflex is the ability of the auditory system to reduce the intensity of the greatest stimuli. This occurs due to contraction of the stapedius and tensor tympani muscles, which makes the ossicular system more rigid and therefore less sensitive to stimulation.

The functions of the attenuation reflex are to:

- Protect the cochlea from damage
- Mask low-frequency background environmental noise

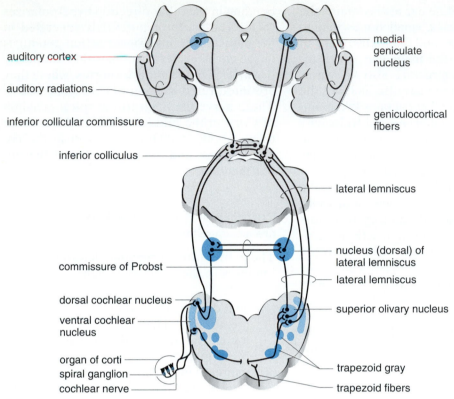

FIGURE 18.29 The neural pathway from the cochlear nerve to the auditory cortex.

- Decrease a speaker's sensitivity to his or her own voice

Clinical Pearls

○ The normal function of the cochlea involves air conduction — sound waves impinging on the tympanic membrane setting in motion a domino effect of movement of the ossicles, the oval window, the cochlear fluid, the basilar membrane, and finally the hair cells in the organ of Corti. However, much the same effect can be achieved by bone conduction — that is, by transmitting sound

waves to the cochlea via vibrations through bone, e.g., by a sound generator applied to the skull.

○ Deafness can be categorized as being due to either (1) damage to the cochlea or auditory nerve (also called nerve deafness) or (2) impairment of the mechanism for transmitting sound into the cochlea (also called conduction deafness). Nerve deafness is permanent and irreversible. However, conduction deafness can be ameliorated in various ways. In some cases it is due to fibrosis (e.g., due to chronic infection), so that sound waves are not easily transmitted from the tympanic membrane via the ossicles to the oval window. In this case, air conduction can be restored by replacing the fibrosed stapes with a more mobile Teflon or metal equivalent.

Review Questions

50. What is the difference between amplitude and frequency?
51. What is the organ of Corti and what does it contain?
52. Describe the pathway from sound wave to hearing.
53. What are the three determinants of loudness in the auditory system?
54. What is the attenuation reflex?

Movement, balance, and the vestibular system

Maintaining upright posture and balance of spindly creatures such as ourselves requires an intricate sensory mechanism for equilibrium that is able to detect linear and rotational acceleration. The role of the **vestibular system** is to provide the brain with input on the equilibrium state of the head.

Like the auditory system, to which it bears some structural resemblance, the vestibular system involves the detection by the brain of waves in the fluid (called **endolymph**) of specialized regions of the labyrinth that are adjacent to the cochlea, namely, the three **semicircular canals** and the associated chambers called the **utricle** and the **saccule**. The waves of endolymph are detected by the fact that they bend the stereocilia (and a larger cilia-like structure called the **kinocillum**, found at one end of each of these hair cells). The bending of these cilia opens pressure-sensitive ion channels that depolarize or hyperpolarize the hair cell, promoting or inhibiting the generation of receptor potentials. As a result, the rate of firing of the vestibular nerve fibers associated with the base of these hair cells increases or decreases.

The hair cells of the saccule and utricle are part of sensory organs called **maculae** that are responsible for the sensations of static equilibrium and linear acceleration. The hair cells of the semicircular canals are part of sensory organs called **cristae ampularis**, which are responsible for the sensation of rotational acceleration. The three semicircular canals are at right angles to one another and thereby represent the three planes of space. As the head begins to be rotated forward or backward or to one side or another, and when it stops, different hair cells in different semicircular canals are activated, thereby providing rotational information to the brain.

Balance of the body is far more complex than just maintaining the equilibrium of the head. In addition, proprioceptive receptors in the neck and elsewhere in the body provide input to the vestibular, cerebellar, and reticular nuclei, which respond with output to various muscle groups to maintain balance. It is, for example, input from the proprioceptive receptors in the neck that precisely opposes output from the vestibular system, to allow the head to be bent without creating a sense of dysequilibrium. Visual information also plays an important role in maintaining equilibrium. Even complete destruction of the vestibular system can be completely compensated for by visual information. However, balance in these cases is completely lost upon closing the eyes.

Clinical Pearls

○ *Dizziness* is complicated by the fact that patients often use the term to signify symptoms (e.g., weakness, nonspecific malaise, etc.) other than true *vertigo* (disorders of movement, such as the sensation that the room is spinning).
○ True vertigo can be due to disease of the labyrinth (central vertigo) or vestibular

nerve (peripheral vertigo) or to disease of the CNS, including the brainstem. Central vertigo is generally milder than peripheral vertigo, but it is more likely to be present on vertical or multiple directions of gaze, often with other signs of brainstem pathology. Central causes include brainstem ischemia, tumor, and multiple sclerosis.

○ The most common cause of peripheral vertigo, benign positional vertigo, is due to the presence of free-floating calcium carbonate crystals under the influence of gravity within the endolymph of the semicircular canals. This specific condition is also called canalithiasis. A 90% remission rate can be achieved by simple lateral head positioning (12 h lying down with the head turned to the healthy side).

Review Questions

55. Name some similarities and some differences between the vestibular and auditory systems.

56. How is balance achieved?

The chemical senses: taste and smell

Taste

Taste occurs largely through the action of a set of sensory receptors known as **taste buds**. However, smell contributes in a major way to the perception of taste.

There are four primary sensations of taste: **sour**, **salty**, **sweet**, and **bitter**.

Sour taste is caused by **acids** — the lower the pH, the stronger the sense of sourness.

Salty taste is caused by ionized salts.

Sweet taste is caused by various organic compounds, including sugars, alcohols, aldehydes, ketones, amino acids, esters, and amides.

Bitter taste is also caused by various organic compounds, particularly those with nitrogen substituents, and by alkaloids such as quinine, caffeine, strychnine, and nicotine. The adaptive value of the unpleasantness of bitterness is that it probably helped our ancestors avoid poisonous plants that contained dangerous alkaloids.

Each of the taste buds has different proportions of all four classes of receptors. Thus, intense stimulation by any particular compound is likely to trigger all of the four primary senses.

Most adults have 3,000 to 10,000 taste buds (see Figure 18.30). These complex sensory receptors each contain a set **taste hairs**. These are actually microvilli covered with specific receptors for the primary sensations. Binding of the taste substance to specific receptor proteins on the taste hairs opens sodium channels. The resulting influx of sodium depolarizes the cell, creating a receptor potential for that taste that is transmitted to fibers of the glossopharyngeal nerve. These sensory neurons converge on the **tractus solitarius** in the brainstem. From there, fibers travel to the thalamus and then on to the central gyrus of the cerebral cortex, terminating near the somatosensory area for the tongue.

Smell

Smell is an extremely primitive sense that is not terribly well developed in humans. It is estimated that there are 50 to 100 different primary odorant receptors.

Within the nostril is an olfactory membrane containing approximately 100 million olfactory cells, each of which bears 6 to 12 olfactory hairs enmeshed in a layer of mucus. So-called odorant molecules, the ones we can smell, must first dissolve in the mucus layer before they can bind to receptor proteins in the ciliary membrane. These receptor proteins are coupled to cytoplasmic G proteins. Activation results in dissociation of the alpha subunit of the G protein, activation of adenylate cyclase, and the production of cyclic

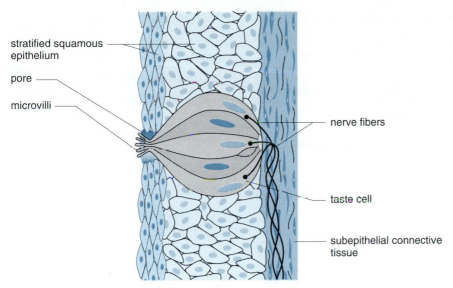

stratified squamous
epithelium

pore

microvilli

nerve fibers

taste cell

subepithelial connective
tissue

FIGURE 18.30. The structure of a taste bud.

AMP. The cyclic AMP, in turn, opens sodium channels, resulting in depolarization and a receptor potential. Because it is coupled to a G protein–based amplification system, the olfactory system is exquisitely sensitive, able to detect substances at a concentration of only one part per billion. In order to be sensed by the olfactory system, substances must be at least slightly water-soluble and slightly lipophilic.

There are three olfactory pathways leading to the CNS. The oldest pathway is that mediated by the **medial olfactory area**, a group of nuclei anterior to the hypothalamus.

A second, less old system is that of the **lateral olfactory area** of the **pyriform cortex**. It is this area that is involved in the development of aversions (e.g., with nausea and vomiting) to specific foods that have, in the past, made us sick.

The newest olfactory pathway passes through the thalamus and on to the latero-posterior quadrant of the orbitofrontal cortex. It appears to be important for the conscious analysis of smells.

Clinical Pearl

○ Taste preferences change, to some extent, with the physiological needs of the body. Thus, adrenalectomized animals have a craving for salt and will often choose salty water over fresh water, thereby preventing the life-threatening salt depletion that might otherwise occur in the absence of mineralocorticoids.

Review Questions

57. What are the four primary tastes?
58. What is the pathway involving taste from tongue to brain?
59. What are the three pathways of olfaction?

9. PATHOPHYSIOLOGY OF SOME NERVOUS SYSTEM DISORDERS

Table 18.4 indicates some features of certain chronic, debilitating neurologic disorders. In

TABLE 18.4   SUMMARY STATISTICS OF THE NEUROBIOLOGY OF DISEASES OF THE CNS

	Number of cases (in US)	Time course	Brain regions	Cellular pathology
Cerebrovascular disease	1.5 million new cases per year: third commonest cause of death	Acute, often persistent disability	Grey matter/ white matter	Ischemia/infarction; death of neurons; damage to axons
Epilepsy	~2.5 million cases	Paroxysmal	Neocortex, hippocampus, thalamus	Neuronal hyperexcitability
Alzheimer's disease	>5 million cases	Chronic, progressive	Neocortex, hippocampus, subcortical nuclei	Hyperphosphorylated tau in tangles; extracellular $A\beta$ deposits; degeneration of subsets of neurons in specific brain regions
Parkinson's disease	>500,000 cases	Chronic, progressive	Substantia nigra	Degeneration of dopaminergic neurons; α-synuclein inclusions (Lewy bodies)
Multiple sclerosis	300,000 cases	Acute, subacute, remitting, chronic	White matter	Demyelination; loss of oligodendroglial cells

Reproduced, with permission, from Price DL (1999). New order from neurological disorders. *Nature* 399:A1–5.

this section, we will summarize the current state of knowledge as to the contribution of physiology to the pathophysiology of these disorders.

Stroke

A stroke is the sudden loss of a subset of neurologic function as a result of occlusion or rupture of blood vessels in the brain. Stroke can manifest with a range of symptoms that differ from patient to patient, but that generally include some degree of weakness and paralysis, usually focal (affecting one part of the body but not another) in nature. The natural history of stroke is highly variable. In some patients, near-strokes, called transient ischemic attacks, in which vessel occlusion is temporary, precede the major event. Some-

times, after a major event, a patient will eventually recover most or all of the neurologic function that was acutely lost with the stroke. Other times, a patient may be left with subtle or major irreversible defects. Important determinants of where on the continuum of size, distribution, and likelihood of recovery any given patient lies are the nature of the lesion and the size and distribution of the occluded vessel.

Occlusion of blood vessels in the brain (or anywhere else, for that matter) can be due to a clot formed of platelets and activated clotting factors. Alternatively, in a patient with severe atherosclerotic disease, calcified, fatty debris from an atherosclerotic plaque can break off from its original site and float downstream until it lodges in a smaller vessel, occluding distal blood flow. Less commonly, vasospasm, dehydration, and other factors may trigger a stroke, especially when superimposed on vessels that were already abnormal, e.g., due to atherosclerotic disease.

When a blood vessel is occluded by a clot, this clot can, in principle, by dissolved by enzymes that break up fibrin strands, a process called **thrombolysis**. But this susceptibility to thrombolysis is limited in time — within a few hours after clot formation, the clot is invaded by epithelial cells that work to convert the clot into a **scar**, which will obliterate the blood vessel that used to exist there, making the loss of blood flow to that region of the brain permanent.

When a region of brain becomes suddenly ischemic as a result of occlusion of a vessel, several pathologic processes are believed to be set in motion. First, the lack of blood flow and therefore of oxygen results in a deficiency in ATP generation (see Chap. 2 for the difference in ATP generation in the presence of oxygen and under anaerobic conditions). With increased severity, the deficiency in ATP production impairs channel and transporter function and ionic balance in cells. Depolarization of these ischemic, dying cells can result in a massive release of neurotransmitters, which may be harmful to other cells in the neighborhood that were not directly made ischemic. Eventually, severe loss of plasma membrane and organelle function results in cell death through necrosis, a process in which inflammatory cells are activated to enter the region and phagocytose the dead cells and debris. In addition to the damage caused by cell necrosis, programmed forms of cell death (apoptosis) are also triggered. Many different processes may contribute to these forms of cell death. For example, deficient production of survival factors that normally work to suppress apoptosis could activate the process. Likewise, either apoptosis or necrosis could be triggered by altered concentrations of excitatory neurotransmitters such as glutamate or ions such as zinc or

calcium. At present, not enough is known about the normal function of various ion channels and their activators, and the consequences of their disregulation, to indicate specific physiological and pathophysiological pathways by which strokes cause damage. One appealing notion is that each of these factors can operate in different ways under different circumstances. For example, Figure 18.31 shows a currently appealing relationship between calcium and necrosis versus apoptosis in cell injury.

At present, therapies for acute stroke involve (1) in the case of fibrin thrombi, attempts to promote thrombolysis of the clot and reperfusion of the affected region of the brain, and (2) attempts to limit the amount of brain tissue that is damaged by ischemia through the infusion of neuroprotective agents. The neuroprotective agents that are currently being studied include calcium channel and glutamate channel blockers and growth factors. The logic for channel blockers is that glutamate efflux and calcium influx

FIGURE 18.31. Speculative relationship of necrosis versus apoptosis as a function of cytosolic free calcium $[Ca^{2+}]_i$ and injury in the brain. The hypothesis implied by this proposed relationship is that there is a homeostatic range of free calcium concentrations within a cell. Perturbations that alter this range lead to injury and death. Within a narrow range, injury triggers death by apoptosis. Beyond that range, either overwhelming injury or excessively elevated calcium concentration results in death by necrosis.

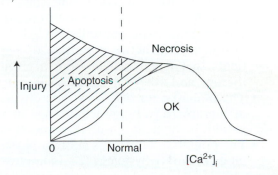

appear to be a key step occurring after ischemia that contributes to cell death in various model systems. Growth factor treatments are also being tried to promote regeneration and healing of damaged brain tissue. Whether these new approaches will help humans with strokes, and if so under what conditions, remains to be determined.

Prevention of stroke involves reduction of factors that lead to atherosclerotic damage to small or large blood vessel walls (such as hypertension, diabetes, and hypercholesterolemia). In patients who may already have developed atherosclerosis, partial anticoagulation decreases the risk of inappropriate clot formation. This can be achieved by treatment either with aspirin or other agents to make platelets less able to participate in clot formation or with the drug warfarin at sufficient doses to partially block vitamin K–dependent clotting factors (see Chap. 20).

Clinical Pearl

○ A number of therapies for acute ischemic stroke that appear effective at limiting stroke size in experimental animal models have yielded disappointing results in human clinical trials. Difficulties include

- Getting patients to medical attention within the brief window of time (hours) in which neuroprotection and thrombolysis might be expected to do any good
- Distinguishing between subsets of patients that might benefit from a given therapy and other subsets that will not
- The potential for disastrous side effects of therapy (e.g., brain hemorrhage in a patient being treated with thrombolysis)
- The potential differences in brain physiology or pathophysiology (e.g., complex-

ity of response to growth factors) between small animals and humans (see Ref. 1)

Epilepsy

A **seizure** is an episode of abnormal discharges from CNS neurons. About 5 to 10% of the population will have at least one seizure at some time in their life. Recurrent seizures due to an underlying brain disorder are called **epilepsy** and occur in 1 to 2% of the population.

There are many different syndromes of epilepsy. Some are limited to brief periods of abnormal motor or sensory activity (called **partial seizures**). Others are associated with altered consciousness. The most common epilepsy syndrome is that of **generalized, tonic-clonic seizures**. In these, the patient loses consciousness and has rhythmic contraction of various muscle groups in the body, typically lasting a minute or two. The patient is often incontinent of urine or stool. Typically, after conclusion of the seizure, the patient is sleepy and confused for a period of time, a condition called a **postictal state**.

Seizures are due to a shift in the balance of excitatory and inhibitory neural activity in the brain. This shift can occur for many different reasons. For example, in certain rare forms of inherited epilepsy, a mutation in an ion channel has been identified as the cause. In the far more common case of epilepsy following brain injury, one hypothesis is that in response to injury, certain cells sprout additional processes that increase their excitability to pathologic levels. Various factors normally regulate the balance between excitatory and inhibitory activity, providing lines of defense against the development of seizures. Under certain conditions, these lines of defense can be weakened, such that a seizure can sometimes occur (see Table 18.5).

Various forms of brain injury can lower

TABLE 18.5 CAUSES OF SEIZURES

Neonates (<1 month)	Perinatal hypoxia and ischemia Intracranial hemorrhage and trauma Acute CNS infection (bacterial and viral meningitis) Metabolic disturbances (hypoglycemia, hypocalcemia, hypomagnesemia, pyridoxine deficiency) Drug withdrawal Developmental disorders (acquired and genetic) Genetic disorders
Infants and children (>1 mo and <12 years)	Febrile seizures Genetic disorders (metabolic, degenerative, primary epilepsy syndromes) CNS infection Developmental disorders (acquired and genetic) Trauma Idiopathic
Adolescents (12–18 years)	Trauma Genetic disorders Infection Brain tumor Illicit drug use Idiopathic
Young adults (18–35 years)	Trauma Alcohol withdrawal Illicit drug use Brain tumor Idiopathic
Older adults (>35 years)	Cerebrovascular disease Brain tumor Alcohol withdrawal Metabolic disorders (uremia, hepatic failure, electrolyte abnormalities, hypoglycemia) Alzheimer's disease and other degenerative CNS diseases Idiopathic

Drugs and Other Substances That Can Cause Seizures

Antimicrobials
  β-lactam and related compounds
  Quinolones
  Isoniazid
  Ganciclovir
Anesthetic and antiarrhythmics
  Beta-adrenergic antagonists
  Local anesthetics
  Class 1B agents
Immunosuppressants
  Cyclosporine
  OKT3 (monoclonal antibodies to T cells)
Psychotropics
  Antidepressants
  Antipsychotics
  Lithium

Radiographic contrast agents
Theophylline
Sedative-hypnotic drug withdrawal
  Alcohol
  Barbiturates
  Benzodiazepines
Drugs of abuse
  Amphetamine
  Cocaine
  Phencyclidine
  Methylphenidate

Modified, with permission, from Lowenstein D (1998). In Fauci, A, et al. (eds): *Harrison's Principles of Internal Medicine*, 14th ed. New York, McGraw-Hill, p 2316.

the defenses against development of a seizure to the point where the patient develops epilepsy. Thus, the presence of epilepsy involves a combination of:

- Endogenous genetic factors (e.g., implied by a family history of epilepsy)
- Epileptogenic factors (e.g., penetrating head injury)
- Precipitating factors (e.g., sleep deprivation and other forms of stress, hormonal changes such as occur during the menstrual cycle, and certain drugs and metabolic conditions: see Table 18.5)

Together, these factors determine: i) whether a normal individual will develop a sporadic seizure, ii) pattern of seizures in any given patient with epilepsy.

Dementia

Dementia is the deterioration of cognitive abilities to the point of interference with activities of daily living. Memory is the most prominent of the cognitive abilities affected in dementia. While the incidence of dementia increases with age, dementia is not a necessary part of normal aging. Although most cases of dementia are irreversible and poorly, if at all, treatable at the present time, there are a few causes of dementia that can be effectively and simply treated and therefore should never be overlooked. Dementing disorders are variable in progression and range of characteristics. Some dementing disorders and some of their key characteristics are listed in Table 18.6.

The most common cause of dementia is **Alzheimer's disease** (AD). The prevailing hypothesis as to its cause proposes that altered processing and metabolism of a fragment of a brain glycoprotein, the **amyloid precursor protein** (APP), results in proteinaceous **amyloid deposits**, leading to the development of

neurofibrillary tangles and **neuritic plaques**. These plaques are extracellular accumulations of denatured proteins, of which the **amyloid beta peptide** (**A beta peptide**), a proteolytic fragment of APP, is a major component. Astrocytes, microglia, and dystrophic axons and dendrites are also found in the plaques. There is no correlation between disease severity and number of plaques, and the precise relationship among plaques, tangles, and disease continues to be hotly debated. Neurofibrillary tangles, while not specific for AD, correlate better with severity of disease than does plaque number.

The role of altered beta amyloid peptide (precursor) metabolism in the disease remains unclear. Some forms of A beta peptide appear toxic to neurons in culture and stimulate cytokine production by microglia, perhaps reflecting their ability to set off an inflammatory response in the brain. Whether this is the mechanism of neuropathology in AD remains to be proven.

In some cases of AD, the disorder is familial (see Figure 18.32). At least some of these cases appear to be due to mutations in the presenilins, endoplasmic reticulum glycoproteins of unknown function that are believed to be involved in intracellular processing of the beta amyloid precursor protein. Some workers believe that the presenilins themselves contain the "secretase" enzyme activity that cleaves APP to release the A beta peptide.

In other cases of AD, a particular isoform of apolipoprotein E (*apo* E4) has been identified as a risk factor. However, not everyone with apo E4 develops AD, and not everyone with AD has the *apo* E4 isoform. In contrast, the apo E2 isoform is associated with delayed onset of familial AD. There is currently no clinical utility in genotyping patients or their family members with regard to *apo* E.

Apo E is found in neuritic plaques, with *apo* E4 binding the A beta peptide more

TABLE 18.6   DEMENTING DISORDERS

Most common causes of dementia

Alzheimer's disease
Vascular dementia
  Multi-infarct
  Diffuse white matter disease (Binswanger's)

Alcoholism[a]
Parkinson's disease
Drug/medication intoxication[a]

Less common causes of dementia

Vitamin deficiencies
  Thiamine (B₁): Wernicke's encephalopathy[a]
  B₁₂ (Pernicious anemia)[a]
  Nicotinic acid (pellagra)[a]
Endocrine and other organ failure
  Hypothyroidism[a]
  Adrenal insufficiency and Cushing's syndrome[a]
  Hypo- and hyperparathyroidism[a]
  Renal failure[a]
  Liver failure[a]
  Pulmonary failure[a]
Chronic infections
  HIV
  Neurosyphilis[a]
  Papovavirus (progressive multifocal
    leukoencephalopathy)
  Prion (Creutzfeldt-Jakob and Gerstmann-Sträussler-Scheinker diseases)
  Tuberculosis, fungal, and protozoal[a]
  Sarcoidosis[a]
  Whipple's disease[a]
Head trauma and diffuse brain damage
  Dementia pugilistica
  Chronic subdural hematoma[a]
  Postanoxia
  Postencephalitis
  Normal-pressure hydrocephalus[a]
Neoplastic
  Primary brain tumor[a]
  Metastatic brain tumor[a]
  Paraneoplastic limbic encephalitis

Toxic disorders
  Drug, medication, and narcotic poisoning[a]
  Heavy metal intoxication[a]
  Dialysis dementia (aluminum)
  Organic toxins
Psychiatric
  Depression (pseudodementia)[a]
  Schizophrenia[a]
  Conversion reaction[a]
Degenerative disorders
  Huntington's disease
  Pick's disease
  Diffuse Lewy body disease
  Progressive supranuclear palsy (Steel-Richardson syndrome)
  Multisystem degeneration (Shy-Drager syndrome)
  Hereditary ataxias (some forms)
  Motor neuron disease [amyotrophic lateral sclerosis (ALS); some forms]
  Frontal lobe dementia
  Cortical basal degeneration
  Multiple sclerosis
  Adult Down's syndrome with Alzheimer's
  ALS–Parkinson's–Dementia complex of Guam
Miscellaneous
  Vasculitis[a]
  Acute intermittent porphyria[a]
  Recurrent nonconvulsive seizures[a]
Additional conditions in children or adolescents
  Hallervorden-Spatz disease
  Subacute sclerosing panencephalitis
  Metabolic disorders (e.g., Wilson's and Leigh's diseases, leukodystrophies, lipid storage diseases, mitochondrial mutations)

[a]Potentially treatable dementia.
Reproduced, with permission, from Bird TD (1998). In Fauci, A, et al. (eds): *Harrison's Principles of Internal Medicine*, 14th ed. New York, McGraw-Hill, p 145.

tightly than E3; hence, it is speculated that *apo* E4 may foster plaque formation. Conversely, the microtubule-associated protein tau, which is found in neurofibrillary tangles, binds more tightly to E3 than to E4. In this case, it has been argued that tau binding by

apo E3 *prevents* it from being available to form tangles. As these divergent hypotheses suggest, a clear understanding of the pathophysiology of AD has yet to emerge.

Another common cause of dementia is the occurrence of numerous small ischemic

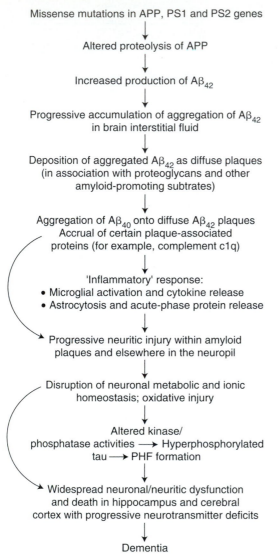

Missense mutations in APP, PS1 and PS2 genes

↓

Altered proteolysis of APP

↓

Increased production of $A\beta_{42}$

↓

Progressive accumulation of aggregation of $A\beta_{42}$
in brain interstitial fluid

↓

Deposition of aggregated $A\beta_{42}$ as diffuse plaques
(in association with proteoglycans and other
amyloid-promoting subtrates)

↓

Aggregation of $A\beta_{40}$ onto diffuse $A\beta_{42}$ plaques
Accrual of certain plaque-associated
proteins (for example, complement c1q)

↓

'Inflammatory' response:
• Microglial activation and cytokine release
• Astrocytosis and acute-phase protein release

↓

Progressive neuritic injury within amyloid
plaques and elsewhere in the neuropil

↓

Disruption of neuronal metabolic and ionic
homeostasis; oxidative injury

↓

Altered kinase/
phosphatase activities ⟶ Hyperphosphorylated
tau ⟶ PHF formation

↓

Widespread neuronal/neuritic dysfunction
and death in hippocampus and cerebral
cortex with progressive neurotransmitter deficits

↓

Dementia

FIGURE 18.32. Hypothetical sequence of events in familial Alzheimer's disease. A range of mutations in either the APP or the presenilin 1 or 2 genes results in aberrant proteolytic cleavage of APP with increased production of the pathogenic A β_{42} peptide. Accumulation, aggregation, and deposition results in the formation of plaques and activation of an inflammatory response that damages neurons and alters signaling pathways, resulting in further neuronal dysfunction and the progressive deficits that characterize dementia. *(Reproduced, with permission, from Lee J-M, et al. (1999). Nature 399: A7–14.)*

strokes. While no one such stroke is large enough to cause an obvious neurologic deficit, the sum total of many such small events over a period of years can be devastating to cognition.

Review Questions

60. What is the hypothesized role of glutamate in the pathophysiology of stroke?
61. What are some factors contributing to development of epilepsy?
62. What is the relevance of apolipoprotein E to dementia due to AD?

10. FRONTIERS IN NEUROLOGIC RESEARCH

Neurotrophic factors, neurite growth inhibitors, and nerve regeneration

An important set of mysteries of the nervous system is (1) how it gets assembled, (2) how it maintains itself, and (3) what makes nerve regeneration in the central nervous system so difficult. The first is particularly remarkable because the pathways that neurons follow seem quite convoluted, far from the shortest path to a particular target. If it were possible to regenerate CNS neurons, a wide range of currently irreversible neurodegenerative and traumatic disorders of the nervous system might be able to be treated.

Molecular neurobiology has provided insights into each of these issues. Neurotropins and neuregulins are a family of secreted proteins that form a gradient that can either attract or repel neurons. These proteins and their cognate receptors are believed to be extremely important in both the formation and the maintainance of the nervous system (see Refs. 6, 7). A recent complexity was the discovery that the same neurotropin can trigger opposite turning behavior of the same population of neurons, as a function of cyclic AMP–mediated signaling activity (see Ref. 8). This makes possible a mind-bogglingly complex combinatorial set of possibilities used in formation of the nervous system. The variables include many different neurotropins, each of which affects different populations of neurons differently, and each of which is able to be switched from attractive to repulsive movement by changes in signaling pathways. Each of these variables is in turn influenced by other properties of the nervous system, such as signaling by astrocytes or glial cells (see Ref. 9).

In at least some cases, neurite growth inhibitors have been directly shown to restrict the ability of neurons to regenerate following central nervous system injury (see Ref. 10). Perhaps equally remarkable are some recent observations on macrophages, a type of immune cell that is a known mediator of the inflammatory response (see Chap. 19). Normally, macrophages are prevented from entering the CNS by the blood–brain barrier. In at least one model system, when macrophages were relocated to sites of injury within the CNS, they were able to stimulate a remarkable degree of recovery of motor function (see Ref. 11).

Recent work has revealed other surprises involving signaling and regeneration in the central nervous system. For example, it appears that at least a subpopulation of a type of glial cell called **ependymal cells** has the potential to actually *become* neurons (see Ref. 12).

New insights into memory and learning

What is the molecular basis of learning? More than 25 years ago, the observation was made in the hippocampus of rabbits that synaptic transmission undergoes a long-term enhancement upon repeated electrical stimulation. This phenomenon is called **long-term potenti-**

ation (LTP) and is believed to be a key process involved in memory and learning.

In recent years, studies using gene knockout technology have shown that elimination of specific receptors (e.g., the N-methyl-D-aspartate or NMDA receptor) and specific signaling molecules (e.g., calcium-calmodulin–dependent protein kinase II) from the hippocampus disrupts both LTP and learning in mice (see Refs. 13, 14). However, the behaviors involved (e.g., in a mouse swimming in a water maze) are sufficiently complex that it has been hard to prove that the LTP is not involved in some feature of sensation or some feature of motor response, rather than in learning itself.

Recent work with the sea slug *Aplysia*, a marine invertebrate, has provided a more direct connection. *Aplysia* has been a favorite organism for study by neurobiologists for decades because of the large size of its neurons, the simplicity of its behaviors, and the relative simplicity of its nervous system. At one time, this was thought to be too simple to be a useful model for learning of the sort represented by LTP. However, from more recent work, it appears that there is a link between LTP and learning, in the form of the classical withdrawal response to painful stimuli, in this simple system: It is blocked by antagonists of the NMDA receptor (see Refs. 15, 16). Thus, mechanisms of learning may well be substantially conserved between invertebrates and mammals.

While LTP involves enhanced transmission across particular synapses, sometimes the opposite is seen: **long-term depression** (LTD) with diminished transmission across particular synapses. Both of these changes are believed to be examples of **synaptic plasticity** and the basis for learning. One of their characteristics has been that they are highly spatially restricted to particular synapses. However, recent work on neurons in culture (see Ref. 17) suggests that LTD can occur over enormous distances. It appears that the signal for LTD travels slowly and intracellularly retrograde up axons to dendrites and is able to cross synapses.

Bridging so-called "systems approaches" to learning (e.g., investigation of particular neural circuits in monkeys with particular neuroanatomic lesions) and "cellular approaches" to learning (e.g., changes in LTP and LTD in neuronal cell cultures from mice with gene knockouts) is an important challenge to be met for the future (see Refs. 18 to 21).

Molecular mechanisms of addiction

Drug addiction is a pathologic state that shares features with learning. In both cases, repeated exposure alters the functioning of neurons in ways that facilitate some circuits of synaptic transmission more than others, in various regions of the brain. These changes are manifest in the form of complex behaviors, including dependence, tolerance, sensitization, and craving, that characterize addiction.

Neurons in the **locus caeruleus** that normally mediate attention and regulate the autonomic nervous system have been implicated in addiction. It appears that the cyclic AMP signaling pathway is upregulated in these neurons during chronic opiate administration, as a result of upregulation of two forms of adenylyl cyclase (types I and VIII). The increase in type VIII adenylyl cyclase activity appears to be mediated by an increase in the amount of a particular transcription factor, called **cyclic AMP response element–binding protein (CREB)**. Thus, treatment with antisense oligonucleotides, which bind to a specific mRNA, block its translation, and promote its degradation, has been claimed to partially block the activation of the locus caeruleus that occurs during drug withdrawal. The severity of opiate withdrawal symptoms was also noted to be diminished. Conversely, mutant mice that are deficient in CREB have

an attenuated opiate withdrawal response (see Ref. 22).

Another mechanism that is believed to be important in tolerance is adaptation. Phosphorylation and other modifications that affect receptor–G protein coupling are examples of this mechanism (see Chap. 3). Recently it has been determined that agonist-bound opioid and dopamine receptors are phosphorylated by G protein receptor kinases. Furthermore, both the kinases and a family of associated proteins called arrestins that serve to sequester the phosphorylated receptors are found to be upregulated in specific regions of the brain during chronic opiate use.

Finally, a role for the neurotropins (see the preceding discussion) in addiction has also been suggested recently. It appears that infusion of neurotropins directly into specific brain regions prevents or reverses some chronic effects of cocaine and opiate abuse.

Taken together, the new insights are cause for great optimism. They suggest that specific, molecular-based therapies for various aspects of addiction may be one of the many fruitful products of the ongoing molecular revolution in neuroscience.

Multiple mechanisms and therapies for migraine syndromes

The drug sumatriptan, a serotonin receptor (subtype 1B/D) agonist, has represented a major addition to the pharmacologic options available in the treatment of migraine headaches. However, the mechanism by which sumatriptan relieves migraine remains controversial (see Ref. 23).

Three mechanisms have been proposed: (1) decreasing the sensitivity to pain in the CNS; (2) ameliorating neurogenic inflammation around cranial arteries, which would otherwise result in plasma protein leakage and other effects that are believed to cause pain; (3) blocking dilatation of the cranial arteries.

Clinical studies in the near future will reveal whether compounds that are selective for the proposed neurogenic component will be even more effective in treatment of migraine headaches (see Ref. 24).

There is, however, growing evidence that there may not necessarily be just one mechanism of migraine, but rather that all the above mechanisms — and possibly others — play a role in pathogenesis for various subsets of patients. For example, familial hemiplegic migraine has been shown to be due to a calcium channel defect, whereas a genetic basis for other migraine syndromes (e.g., migraines with and without associated sensory or motor neurologic findings) remains unproven. Indeed some data suggest that these different migraine syndromes have very different etiologies. For example, so-called migraine with aura (associated with premonitory sensory or visual symptoms), but not common migraine (without aura), is associated with a phenomenon of depolarization of neurons and glial cells that advances slowly across the surface of the cerebral cortex (see Ref. 25).

New directions in pain research

A number of long-standing issues in understanding pain are in the process of being clarified at present.

How do so many different stimuli (thermal, mechanical, chemical) activate pain receptors? It appears that changes in the cytoskeleton caused by mechanical stimulation open specific ion channels in mechanosensory receptor cells. Cytokines and other inflammatory mediators serve to lower the pain threshold by sensitizing these pain receptors. The mechanisms they use include prostaglandin-mediated suppression of outward potassium channels and increases in the number of sodium channels expressed.

After a pain receptor has been activated, it transmits its signal to the spinal cord. A number of novel observations, with potential clinical implications, have been made on this so-called first synapse in the pain pathway:

1. A form of long-term potentiation has been observed, whereby transmission of signals for painful stimuli is enhanced by **facilitation** of synaptic transmission across the first synapse.
2. After nerve injury, sprouting of axons from nonpain fibers is seen to invade regions of the dorsal horn of the spinal cord normally occupied exclusively by pain fibers. This may explain why pain can sometimes be induced by normally nonpainful stimuli, following nerve injury.
3. Conversely, there are pathways by which neurotransmitter release at the first synapse can be inhibited, thereby dampening the sensation of pain transmitted to the brain (see Ref. 26).

Pain is, in some sense, what the brain makes of it. Thus, it appears that, besides neuropathic and inflammatory pain, a third pain syndrome exists: that of general "not feeling well" and "hurting all over" due to heightened central sensation of pain (see Ref. 27).

Finally, in treatment of pain, it has long been observed that the combination of aspirin and opiates taken together is more powerful than the sum of these two analgesics taken separately. Recently a possible mechanism has become clear. It appears that activation of opioid receptors causes a presynaptic inhibition of transmitter release, mediated by arachidonic acid metabolites. Inhibition of cyclooxygenase by nonsteroidal anti-inflammatory agents such as aspirin allows arachidonic acid to be metabolized exclusively by the lipoxygenase pathway (see Chap. 3). This diminishes the pain-producing prostaglandins normally generated by cyclooxygenase, while increasing production of the pain-relieving lipoxygenase metabolites, which are activated by opioids (see Ref. 28).

11. HOW DOES AN UNDERSTANDING OF NORMAL PHYSIOLOGY PROVIDE INSIGHT INTO THE INITIAL CASE PRESENTATION?

The key to this case is to approach the patient's neurologic findings logically, asking the classic, all-important first question of neurology: Where is the lesion?

Only a central rather than a peripheral lesion would give the combination of facial tingling and finger numbness; hence the legitimate alarm over the combination of these two otherwise subtle findings. The miracle of modern imaging (the MRI scan) told the rest.

The brain is an extremely fragile structure. Postoperative edema and the trauma of gently moving sensitive structures to get to the aneurysm is sufficient to account for the diabetes insipidus, aphasia, and motor deficits. It is also why seizure prophylaxis (prevention by preemptive treatment with medications) is needed.

Nothing heightens a clinician's sensitivity to "bedside manner" more than becoming a patient oneself.

SUMMARY AND REVIEW OF KEY CONCEPTS

The physiology of the nervous system can be approached in many different ways at many different levels:

1. From a molecular physiological perspective, the basis for nervous system function is both electrical (action potentials) and chemical (neurotransmitters released to diffuse across a synapse). The neurotransmitters bind to receptors, which trigger the next action potential by opening various types of channels, resulting in depolarization of the neuron. An enormous range of substances, including amino acids, modified amines, peptides, and other substances serve as neurotransmitters in various pathways.

2. Cell biologically, the nervous system consists of neurons and glial cells, both of which play crucial roles in neurobiology. Myelin sheaths composed of Schwann cell plasma membrane serve as an insulator to greatly speed up the time it takes to send a neural transmission.

3. Anatomically, the nervous system consists of the central nervous system (brain and spinal cord) and the peripheral nervous system (spinal nerves). The organization of the brain itself includes the brainstem, which carries out older, more "automatic" functions; the cerebral cortex, responsible for the final steps of sensory discrimination and all "higher" functions, including the distinctly human features of language, judgment, and fine motor skills; and the cerebellum, which is involved in a range of anticipatory and coordination functions. The spinal cord is organized to allow both immediate (reflex) responses to sensory input and considered responses as a result of signaling back to the brain for decision making. Within both the CNS and the PNS are neural pathways that mediate sensation and motor function. Sensory systems detect signals in the environment and transmit them back to the brain. Within the sensory systems are the pain and temperature pathways and the vibration, balance, and position sense pathways, as well as seeing and hearing. Motor pathways consist of both voluntary pathways (e.g., to skeletal muscle) and involuntary pathways (e.g., the autonomic nervous system and its control of smooth muscle and various glands).

4. Physiologically, the enormous complexity of the nervous system is due to differences between (1) the trillions of cells that make up the nervous system, (2) the ion chan

nels and receptors that activate the cells, (3) the patterns of action potentials that are produced as a result of ion channel and receptor activation in individual neurons, (4) the various neurotransmitters used by different neurons, (5) the nature (stimulatory versus inhibitory) and number of synapses to other neurons, to name some of the currently appreciated variables.

5. Once various classes of receptor cells in the periphery have sensed what they have receptors to detect, this information is transmitted back, to the thalamus via pathways in the spinal cord, and finally is integrated in the parietal lobe of the cerebral cortex to give conscious sensation. Along the way, considerable complexity occurs. Signals are transmitted to the spinal cord, medulla, pons, midbrain, and cerebellum, and to just about every other area of the brain. Some of the ascending fibers that reach the brainstem, particularly those carrying painful sensations, go to the amygdala and limbic cortex, where they contribute to the emotional response to the sensation. Along the path back to the brain, sensory input can be tremendously modified by stimulatory and inhibitory fibers.

6. Pain is one important modality of sensory signaling that is mediated by multiple "slow" and "fast" pathways and can be modified by both neural input (inhibitory and stimulatory interneurons) and endogenous morphine-like products called endorphins.

7. Motor systems are the ways in which organisms respond to their environments. The pyramidal tract, a series of neurons running from the cerebral cortex to individual skeletal muscle groups, controls movement.

8. An important distinction within the motor pathway is that upper motor neuron lesions result in spasticity and muscle twitching, while the lower motor neuron lesions are associated with flaccid paralysis and atrophy. The difference is that the upper motor neuron lesions also affect inhibitory neurons that play important roles in regulation of synaptic transmission, while the lower motor neuron lesions simply affect the final common pathway, after factoring in all stimulatory and inhibitory inputs.

9. The basal ganglia and cerebellum play crucial roles in the coordination of different motor actions. The cerebral cortex adds the elements of thought, memory, emotion, and judgment to motor actions.

10. The cerebral cortex has regions that encode an exaggerated representation of the sensory and motor systems, proportional to their innervation rather than to their real-life sizes. Additionally, accessory regions of the cortex play roles in coordinating between different functions.

11. The special senses are vision, hearing, balance, taste, and smell; each of these is mediated by complex sensory receptors and intricate neural pathways to various regions of the brain. Vision, for example, is mediated by the eye, a structure that works much like a camera, from an optical point of view. The eye generates images that are detected by the retina and encoded into action potentials for transmission back to the vision-interpreting regions in the occipital cortex (and everywhere else that vision is an important component).

A CASE OF PHYSIOLOGICAL MEDICINE

L.L. is a 43-year-old chef who was in good health until 6 years ago, when she had a severe car accident. Her experiences related to this incident shed light on several aspects of pain. Immediately after the accident, she awoke to find her companion unconscious and badly injured and the car on fire. Somehow, she managed to extricate herself, extricate her companion, and get a safe distance away from the car before it exploded into flames. She subsequently lost consciousness herself. Only later was she aware of the fact that her arm was broken in three places. In addition she had received a severe concussion and a whiplash injury to the neck.

In the days following the accident, she had agonizing pain. A clinician without a lot of experience in treatment of pain had given her acetaminophen, but he hesitated to use opiates. Later, when informed of Ms. L.'s extreme discomfort, the provider gave her codeine (whose half-life is 3 to 4 h) and instructed her to take it no more frequently than twice daily. Fortunately, on her third visit to the hospital, she was seen by an experienced clinician who identified several errors in her pain management and adjusted her medicines, resulting in substantial relief.

Subsequently, Ms. L. developed headaches, confusion, and neck pain. She was unable to work and was placed on disability leave. She became frustrated and depressed at what she perceived to be a lack of appreciation of her situation by health care providers. Finally she was referred to a chronic pain clinic for treatment of her problems.

QUESTIONS

1. How can you explain Ms. L.'s ability to perform the remarkable feat of dragging her companion from the burning wreckage despite a broken arm and other injuries?
2. What were some of the errors in pain management during the acute post-injury period?
3. What are some complications of the use of opiates for pain management?
4. If you were the clinician at the pain clinic, what would be your approach to Ms. L.?

ANSWERS

1. Sympathetic and other pathways tremendously influence the perception of pain. It is likely that the release of endogenous opiates and sympathetic nervous system activation at the time of the accident combined to render her relatively unaware of her pain.
2. There is generally no reason to hesitate to use opiates in the acute setting. Short-term use of opiates to treat pain does not cause addiction.

   In treating acute pain, medicines should be given sufficiently frequently to prevent return of the pain. Autonomic responses to the returning pain make it more difficult to treat and cause the patient to suffer needlessly.
3. Acutely, the patient may have nausea, GI hypomotility, and constipation.

   Chronically, tolerance (the need for higher and higher doses to achieve a given effect), addiction (physical and psychological dependence on receiving the drug), and, at very high doses, respiratory depression (due to effects on medullary respiratory centers) are seen.
4. Listen to her. Nothing is more frustrating to the patient than to have a clinician pay no attention to the patient's own individual experience — which may include having tried without satisfaction whatever measures the clinician is considering. Even if you wish to try this same therapy again, it is important that you know details about how it was tried the first time (e.g., dose, compliance, etc.) that, if changed, might result in a better outcome.

   Recognizing the role of perception and individual variation in pain, involve the patient actively in identifying precipitants and sources of relief, and in treating the condition.

   Recognize the important role of depression in heightening the perception of pain.

Evaluate Ms. L. for neuropathic components of pain.

Consider physical therapy and rehabilitation, nerve blocks, behavioral modification, nonallopathic therapy, and surgery as alternatives when medical management is unsuccessful.

References and suggested readings

GENERAL REFERENCES

1. Fisher M, Bogousslavsky J (1998). Further evolution toward effective therapy for acute ischemic stroke. *JAMA* 279:1298–1303.
2. Carpenter MB (1972). *Core Text of Neuroanatomy*. Baltimore: Williams & Wilkins.
3. Messing RO (1997). Nervous system disorders, in S. McPhee, et al. (eds.). *Pathophysiology of Disease,* 2d ed. Stamford, CT, Appleton & Lange.
4. Price DL (1999). New order from neurological disorders. *Nature* 399 supplement:A3–A5.

FRONTIERS REFERENCES

5. Lempert T (1998). Vertigo. *Curr Opinion Neurol* 11:5–9.
6. Finkbeiner S, et al. (1997). CREB: A major mediator of neuronal neurotrophin responses. *Neuron* 19:1031–1047.
7. Burden S, Yarden Y (1997). Neuregulins and their receptors: A versatile signalling module in organogenesis and oncogenesis. *Neuron* 18:847–855.
8. Song H-J, et al. (1997). cAMP-induced switching in turning direction of nerve growth cones. *Nature* 388:275–279.
9. Riethmacher D, et al. (1997). Severe neuropathies in mice with targeted mutations of the erbB3 receptor. *Nature* 389:725–730.
10. Thallmair M, et al. (1998). Neurite growth inhibitors restrict plasticity and functional recovery following corticospinal tract lesions. *Nature Neuroscience* 1:124–130.
11. Rapalino O, et al. (1998). Implantation of stim-ulated homologous macrophages results in partial recovery of paraplegic rats. *Nature Medicine* 4:814–821.
12. Johansson CB, et al. (1999). Identification of a neural stem cell in the adult mammalian central nervous system. *Cell* 96:25–34.
13. Tsien JZ, et al. (1996). Subregion and all type-restricted gene knockout in mouse brain. *Cell* 87:1317–1320.
14. Rotenberg A, et al. (1996). Mice expressing activated CaMKII lack low frequency LTP and do not form stable place cells in the CA1 region of the hippocampus. *Cell* 87:1351–1352.
15. Lin XY, Glanzman DL (1994). Hebbian induction of long-term potentiation of Aplysia sensorimotor synapses: partial requirement for activation of an NMDA-related receptor. *Proc R Soc Lond* Ser. B 255:215.
16. Murphy GG, Glanzman DL (1997). Mediation of classical conditioning in Aplysia California by long-term potentiation of sensori-motor synapses. *Science* 278:467–471.
17. Fitzsimonds RM, et al. (1997). Propagation of activity-dependent synaptic depression in simple neural networks. *Nature* 388:439–448.
18. Lisberger SG (1998). Cerebellar LTD: A molecular mechanism of behavioral learning? *Cell* 92:701–704.
19. De Zeeuw CI, et al. (1998). Expression of a protein kinase C inhibitor in Purkinje cells blocks cerebellar LTD and adaptation of the vestibulo-ocular reflex. *Neuron* 20:495–508.
20. Mansuy IM, et al. (1998). Restricted and regulated overexpression reveals calcineurin as a key component in the transition from short-term to long-term memory. *Cell* 92:39–49.
21. Xu L, et al. (1997). Behavioural stress facilitates the induction of long-term depression in the hippocampus. *Nature* 387:497–501.
22. Nestler EJ, Aghajanian GK (1997). Molecular and cellular basis of addiction. *Science* 278:58–64.
23. Goadsby PJ (1997). Bench to bedside: What have we learnt recently about headache? *Curr Opinion Neuro* 10:215–220.
24. Olesen J (1994). Understanding the biological basis of migraine. *N Engl J Med* 331:1713–1714.
25. Ophoff RA, et al. (1996). Familial hemiplegic

migraine and episodic ataxia type-2 are caused by mutations in the Ca2+ channel gene CAC-NL1A4. *Cell* 87:543–553.

26. Levine JD (1998). New directions in pain research: Molecules to maladies. *Neuron* 20: 649–654.

27. Watkins LR, et al. (1994). Neurocircuitry of illness-induced hyperalgesia. *Brain Res.* 639: 327–331.

28. Vaughan CW, et al. (1997). How opioids inhibit GABA-mediated neurotransmission. *Nature* 390:611–614.

INTRODUCTION TO HOST DEFENSE

19

1. INTRODUCTION TO HOST DEFENSE

This chapter is about the physiological mechanisms by which we defend ourselves against potential causes of death. This topic is a huge one, part of which is typically the subject of a course in immunology. However, given the clinical orientation of this book, the topic of host defense is a necessary dimension of human physiology. The purpose of this chapter is to provide an introduction to this vast topic, placing host defense in the overall context of organ system function and dysfunction.

Through most of human history, survival beyond about age 50 was unusual, and death rates nearly kept up with birth rates. The development of agriculture made it possible for humans to live in large groups in fixed locations. But that same change from hunter-gatherer to village and city life rendered humans much more susceptible to infectious organisms transmitted from one individual to another. As a result, until recently, the earth's human population increased only gradually, subject periodically to massive episodes of depopulation due to wars, famine, and infectious epidemics. For example, during the fourteenth century, epidemics of bubonic plague killed off perhaps 25% of the entire human population of Europe in the space of a few years.

When subpopulations of humans separated by at most one hundred thousand years of evolution came into contact, the effects were sometimes disastrous. In part this was because one population had never been exposed to particular infectious diseases, whereas the other population had been selected for resistance and therefore had adequate defenses.

Because of a number of factors, including selection for host resistance, the elucidation and application of principles of public health, and the discovery and widespread use in the last century of vaccines and antibiotics, the death rate has plummetted — and the size of the human population has skyrocketed. As a result, we must now struggle with a new problem: global human overpopulation and consequent resource depletion and devastation of the environment. Meanwhile, the ominous phenomenon of widespread antibiotic resistance raises the possibility that the clear upper hand in the battle with pathogens may not belong to the human host forever. How we, as a species, will handle these new challenges posed by our "success" in the twentieth century in beating back the past scourges of humankind remains to be seen.

Response to a harsh and dangerous world

There are many forms of host defense. We will focus on five of the most important ones:

1. **Non-specific barriers** to invasion or to other forms of cell damage. These include mechanical, environmental, and anatomic features of the host that serve to prevent invasion by pathogens. We shall also include in this category features that have been built into potentially dangerous host biochemical pathways in the course of evolution that limit their potential for causing harm.

2. **Innate immunity** in the form of various mechanisms that actively counter an invader that has successfully breached the first lines of defense. These generally do not require prior exposure to the invader to be fully effective against a susceptible pathogen. In multicellular eukaryotes, many aspects of the innate immune system are directed against carbohydrate-containing structures, i.e., sugars (see Chap. 2). Thus, at one time, the innate immune system of multicellular eukaryotes apparently divided the world between those carbohydrates that are deemed benign and those that must be eliminated.

Presumably this reflects that fact that the carbohydrates of most microbes are distinctly different from those of the human host, providing a reliable means of discriminating between friend and foe.

3. **Acquired immunity**, by which the body learns to defend itself against specific outside invaders, predominantly infectious organisms in the environment, including particular **bacteria**, **viruses**, and **parasites**. This is the classic immune system, including both **humoral immunity** and **cell-mediated immunity**. Acquired immunity is based on **memory**: the ability of selected cells in the body to be sensitized by their first contact with a would-be invader so that upon repeat exposure, they are already primed to respond and do so more rapidly than they did on initial contact.

4. Mechanisms that protect the body from undesirable environmental conditions, including excessive heat, nutrient deprivation, irradiation, and toxic exposures that would otherwise damage individual proteins, kill cells, and, eventually, incapacitate the host. These mechanisms constitute the **stress response**, a fundamental feature of host defense from *Escherichia coli* to humans. This also includes biochemical pathways that have evolved to defend the body against potential enemies within. Examples include the signaling mechanisms that trigger apoptosis (programmed cell death) when a cell fails to respond to instructions or is damaged beyond hope of repair (see Chap. 2).

5. Mechanisms that exist to prevent damage to the host caused by its own ferocious defensive mechanisms, including the adrenal steroids, which kill activated, mature immune cells and serve to attenuate various aspects of the immune response (see Chap. 13).

The first three of these forms of host defense are discussed primarily in this chapter, while the others are covered primarily in Chapters 2 and 13.

The importance of host defense in health and disease

We are creatures with formidable lines of defense. Most of our internal organs and our internal environment are kept sterile most of the time. When this sterile environment is breached, the offense is usually transient, with homeostatic mechanisms quickly restoring a pristine state.

The history of host-microbe interactions is, in some respects (but not others; see Sec. 6, Frontiers), reminiscent of an arms race: As one side develops a new offensive or defensive capability, over the course of time, the other develops a mean of overcoming or circumventing it. All of these developments follow the principle of natural selection. Put simply, if individuals with the appropriate genes to counter one side's innovations do not exist, or do not develop through mutation or gene transfer from elsewhere, that species is doomed to extinction, or at least will be restricted as to the niche in the environment that it can occupy. For the human host, this applies to both genetic and pharmacologic defenses. Furthermore, all aspects of our world can influence the outcome of the battle between host and pathogen. Decisions to build dams and other human-made alterations of the environment, changes in cultural and corporate practices, and politics, as well as things further "out of our control," such as the weather, all affect the battle between human host and pathogens.

Typically, an invader needs a special strategy if it is to overcome the very first lines of host defenses and enter the body (see Figure 19.1). Thus, for example, many pathogens have evolved the ability to recognize components on the host cell surface and use those structures as **receptors** with which to bind tightly. Thus targeted to a specific host cell,

Direct Penetration

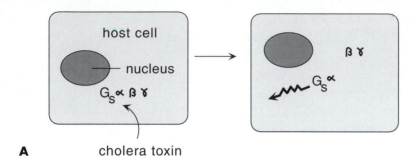

A   cholera toxin

Endocytocis and Membrane Fusion

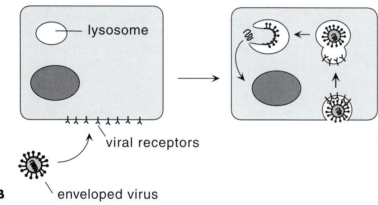

B   enveloped virus

FIGURE 19.1. Modes of entry of pathogens and their toxins into the host. *A.* Direct penetration, e.g., by cholera toxin. *B.* Endocytosis and membrane fusion.

the pathogen or its toxin is able to enter the cell by either direct penetration or endocytosis, followed by fusion or lysis of the endosomal membrane. If a pathogen cannot recognize any receptors on a cell's surface, usually it cannot infect that cell. By corollary, subpopulations of either host and pathogen that express genes that affect receptor binding will have an increased or decreased likelihood of infection. Sometimes these genetic differences affect the **severity** of infection instead of, or in addition to, the **incidence** of infection.

Once an invader has entered the body, a series of defenses are called into play. If those that arrive on the scene initially are unable to handle matters, a subsequent line of defense is called upon, and so on. Sometimes an invader overcomes these successive host defenses slowly. Other times, multiple lines of defense are overcome more rapidly. Should an invader achieve a sufficient foothold in the body to have ready access to the bloodstream, the situation becomes much more grave, as this essential conduit of the body becomes a means of spread. From the bloodstream, the invader can travel to any tissue, including crucial organs such as the heart or the lining of the brain, resulting in life-threatening infections such as **endocarditis** or **meningitis**, respectively. At that point, matters becomes more difficult for the immune system, which then has to track down intruders in many directions at once. Often seeding of organisms via the bloodstream results in their establishing footholds in the form of **abscesses**, walled-off pockets of infection, that are difficult for the body to eliminate. There, the intruder may lie in wait for the best opportunity to spread to other parts of the body.

Should a severe infection get beyond all lines of defense and overwhelm the host, multiorgan system failure often follows rapidly. At that point, even antibiotics that are effective against the invader and would have rapidly eliminated the infection, if they had been provided at the outset, are often too little, too late, and the host will succumb. Thus, when a patient who is sick with an infection comes to medical attention, a most important question to be answered is: What is the status of the host defenses in the battle with an invader? If the host is holding his or her own, or giving ground only slowly, fighting every step of the way, then appropriate antibiotics are typically effective at turning the tide of battle in the host's favor. If, on the other hand, defenses have collapsed, and multi-organ failure is imminent, then the patient's situation is grim. At best, the patient faces a stormy course — and will probably get worse before getting better. Patients in this latter category need far more intensive care than one might have otherwise expected, if they are to recover. The sooner the gravity of the situation is appreciated and appropriately intensive supportive measures are put into place, the greater the likelihood of survival.

Organs and tissues of host defense

A striking feature of host defense is that its components are not localized to a discrete position in the body. Like police officers in a tough part of town, they have to walk the beat, not just hang out at the station. Thus, while there are organs of cell proliferation related to host defense (the bone marrow), organs of cell education related to host defense (the thymus and lymph nodes), and organs of host defense function (the spleen and liver), at any given point in time, huge numbers of host defense cells and products are elsewhere. The "beat cops" and "shock troops" of host defense are the cells and proteins that search for and attack intruders, where ever they may be. Many of these cells derive from the bone marrow (see Figure 19.2). Many of their specific functions will be described in Section 3.

Case Presentation

A.F. is a 66-year-old designer with multiple sclerosis who has not had the use of muscles below the neck for nearly two decades. Lack of muscle tone has resulted in a loss of ability to control urinary bladder emptying. As a result, he has needed frequent catheterization (three times daily) to empty his bladder.

At one point, difficulty in providing adequate nursing staff to perform the catheterizations, because of budget cutbacks, resulted in the placement of an indwelling catheter, which continually drains urine from the bladder.

Shortly after its placement Mr. F. developed the first of a series of urinary tract infections (UTI), despite meticulous handling by the staff. After the fourth UTI, cultures suggest that he is now colonized by a resistant organism.

Frustrated at the recent development of recurrent urinary tract infections after having gone many years with only occasional (approximately twice a year) infections, Mr. F. asks your advice as to (1) why he is developing more frequent infections, (2) the significance of the colonization by resistant organisms, and (3) recommendations as to how the colonization with resistant organisms might be eliminated in an attempt at diminishing the recurrence of future UTIs.

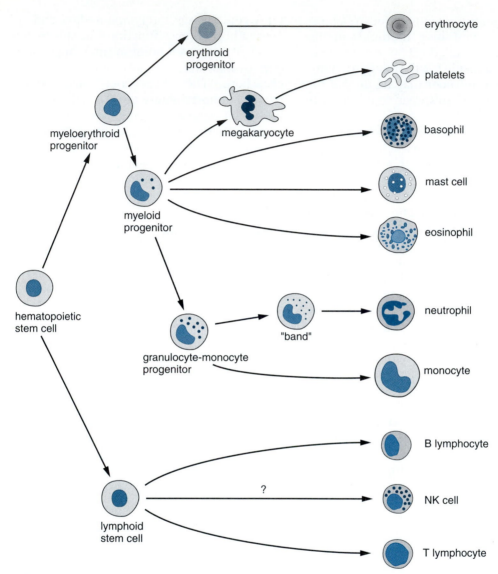

FIGURE 19.2. Overview of hematopoiesis, illustrating the derivation of erythroid, myeloid, and lymphoid cellular lineage from a common hematopoietic stem cell precursor. Not shown in this simplified scheme are many intermediate cell types in each final pathway. Normally, all the cells develop to maturity in the bone marrow except for T lymphocytes, whose marrow-derived progenitors migrate to the thymus for maturation. The relationship of natural killer (NK) cells to other classes of lymphocytes is not currently known. *(Reproduced, with permission, from Stites DP, et al. (1997). Medical Immunology, 9th ed. Stamford, CT, Appleton & Lange. p. 10.)*

Clinical Pearls

○ In addition to the CD4 antigen that is its primary receptor, human immunodeficiency virus (HIV) infection is greatly facilitated by a coreceptor, which happens to be the receptor that normally binds a cytokine (see Sec. 3). Individuals who lack the coreceptor are much less likely to be infected by HIV. Currently, these individuals represent approximately 1% of the population. Particularly in areas of the world where HIV infection proceeds unchecked by drugs (e.g., the Third World), it can be expected that preferential death of susceptible individuals will result in the percentage of the population made up of resistant individuals increasing — until forms of HIV that utilize a different coreceptor or dispense with this need develop.

○ The mortality from pneumococcal sepsis (systemic infection by the bacterial species *Streptococcus pneumoniae*) remains extremely high (approximately 50%), even when the organism is sensitive to penicillin and the patient is in an intensive care unit. The cause of death in these cases is usually multiorgan failure.

○ There are numerous hints to the health care provider that a desperately ill patient's defenses may be in the process of being overwhelmed:

• Most infections are accompanied by fever. When the opposite happens — that is, hypothermia — it can indicate either that the patient is too debilitated to mount a fever or that the normal mechanisms that regulate temperature are in collapse, and multiorgan system failure may soon follow.
• Most bacterial infections are accompanied by a high white blood count. When a patient who has signs of infection has a low white blood count, this suggests either that the infection is caused by a virus (which often suppresses the immune response) or — and this is the worrisome sign — that the bone marrow is failing and the immune system is in a state of impending collapse in the face of overwhelming infection.
• Most patients with systemic infection are able to maintain their blood pressure despite a fall in peripheral vascular resistance by increasing their heart rate and cardiac output (see Chap. 10). When a patient with an infection manifests a drop in blood pressure, the possibility of sepsis syndrome (due to overwhelming systemic infection and excessive cytokine response) and subsequent cardiovascular collapse must be considered.

Review Questions

1. What are some of the changes that have resulted in falling death rates and a skyrocketing human population?
2. What are some of the challenges faced by humans that, if not met, may change these demographic characteristics in the coming century?
3. Name five types of host defenses in the body.
4. What is generally necessary for an invader to pose a threat to a cell?
5. What is an abscess, and what is its significance for host defense?

2. NON-SPECIFIC MECHANISMS OF HOST DEFENSE

Mechanical, environmental, and anatomic barriers as host defense

Before they can infect us, pathogenic organisms must gain access to our internal environment. We have a tough external skin that is largely impervious to would-be invaders, barring injury. Such invaders have a better chance of breaching our defenses at the mucous membranes of the gastrointestinal (GI), respiratory, and urogenital tracts. These regions of our surface are wet and slippery; lack a reinforced external layer of dead, keratinized cells; and are often a single cell away from access to the bloodstream. Thus, these potential portals of pathogen entry must be highly guarded in other ways. As a result of our defenses, we are usually able to prevent invasion even at these potentially vulnerable sites. Even when infection does occur, host defenses are usually sufficiently powerful to successfully beat it back, except in the compromised host (i.e., one with a defect in some aspect of host defense).

An important first line of defense is mechanical, environmental, and anatomic barriers to invasion:

- Cilia, which are hair-like structures on the surface of epithelial cells, provide mechanical force for movement (see Chap. 2). Mucus, a glycoprotein polymer secreted by cells in mucus membrane linings, traps bacteria and other sources of infection and allows them to be swept out of the body by the cilia. Thus, the respiratory epithelium is able to move mucus against gravity and, with the help of the cough reflex, to eliminate potentially infectious material from the body.
- Production of a low-pH environment rich in substances that are toxic to pathogens but not to the host. For example, glycogen is produced in abundance by epithelial cells of the vagina. The normal turnover and sloughing of epithelial cells results in a constant release of this glycogen into the urogenital tract, where its fermentation by beneficial microbes results in production of acidic products that create an environment unfavorable for the proliferation of most pathogens.

- Production of a high-temperature environment (fever) impairs invaders more than it does the host, and hence promotes host defense (see Chap. 11).
- Rapid turnover of cells is a formidable line of defense simply because, by the time an invader succeeds in entering an exposed epithelial cell, it is sloughed and replaced by a "fresh" cell, whose defenses are intact. Thus, for example, in the intestine, immature cells rapidly proliferate in the crypts between villi and move up to the villus tip, from which they are sloughed, with a total lifespan of a few days (see Chap. 5).
- Other structural features that make invasion difficult. For example, the increased frequency of middle ear infection in children compared to adults is believed to be due to the fact that the eustacian tubes are nearly horizontal in children, and are more "floppy" because of lack of connective tissue support. Both of these features impede their drainage, predisposing to infection. With normal growth and development, the eustachian tubes become more steeply inclined and more rigid. As a result of these age-related changes, drainage is better and the chance of infection diminishes.

In cases where the host cannot effectively eliminate a pathogen immediately, attempts are made to mechanically wall the invader off through the formation of fibrin, cellular, and then connective tissue boundaries that are difficult to cross. This gives the host more time to develop a more successful immune response. The **granuloma** formed in diseases such as tuberculosis (TB) are an example of the host's throwing up a makeshift mechanical barrier to disease spread. In that case, a stalemate often occurs, in which the organisms are held in check but remain alive for decades. Later, when other illness or poor nutrition weakens the host, the TB bacillus can break out and start to spread. Antibiotics are recommended for months in young patients with a new positive skin test for TB exposure, to be sure of eradicating the invader and preventing this scenario from unfolding years later.

To counter these efforts, microbes often actively participate in overcoming mechanical and anatomic barriers to their spread by secreting **hydrolases**, enzymes that break down host products (e.g., fibrin in clots, hyaluronic acid of connective tissue, etc.) that would otherwise tend to keep the microbes localized. This is an important distinguishing feature of more aggressively invasive strains of certain pathogens.

Clinical Pearls

○ Low pH is only one of the many environmental mechanisms by which invaders are deterred from colonizing (living in a host without deep tissue penetration or serious symptoms) or invading a host. Others include:

  • Peptide antibiotics that work in an environmentally tailored way. Human respiratory epithelium includes a family of small peptide gene products called defensins, which are toxic to microbes. The increased susceptibility of patients with cystic fibrosis to infections is in large part due to the inactivation of defensins by the high-salt environment occurring in the absence of functional fibrosis transmembrane regulator (CFTR; see Chap. 8).
  • Beneficial bacterial metabolism includes the production of short-chain fatty acids that can be used by the GI tract both as nutritional sources and as a line of defense (see Chap. 5).
  • Crowding of surfaces with beneficial, nonpathogenic bacteria serves as an important barrier to invaders. The combination of competition for resources and an acidic, fermentative environment created by a high concentration of beneficial bacteria is just too much for most pathogens to handle.

○ The fungi that cause athlete's foot secrete keratin-hydrolysing enzymes that allow them to penetrate the formidible barrier posed by skin. Fortunately, their temperature requirements favor cooler, external regions of the body and generally prevent them from causing invasive disease.
○ In the particularly immunocompromised host, tuberculosis may manifest not as focal pulmonary disease, but instead in a disseminated form called "*miliary TB*," so named because the blood-borne form of TB infection seeds the lungs with many, many millet seed-like foci. In effect, these individuals' host defenses were incapable of putting up even partial resistance by walling off or slowing down the pathogen.

Review Questions

6. Give examples of mechanical, environmental, and anatomic first lines of host defense.
7. What is the role of cilia in host defense?

Inflammation

When the first lines of mechanical, environmental, and anatomic defenses are breached by a pathogen, several different emergency response teams are called rapidly into play. Together, the entire set of responses to tissue injury and infection is called **inflammation**. Inflammation can be categorized as acute or chronic. Acute inflammation occurs when the injury or infection is new and sudden. Chronic inflammation occurs when injury or infection is either ongoing or rapidly recurrent with failure of the host defense to achieve full healing and/or eradication of the offending pathogen. Both acute and chronic inflammation are powerful and valuable lines of host defense. However, if excessive, either can do harm to the host. Like the mechanical, environmental, and anatomic defenses, inflammation is **constitutive**. This means that no prior contact with the pathogen is necessary; these defenses are not tailored to the specific pathogen or injury but are a nonspecific host response to the existence of injury or signs of a pathogen.

Acute inflammation

Immediately after an acute injury or new infection, the affected area typically becomes red, hot, and swollen. This is because tissue cells, endothelial cells (that make up the walls of blood vessels), and marrow-derived resident immune cells have become **activated**. As a result of activation of both cells and biochemical pathways of blood coagulation and complement fixation (see the following discussion), local mediators have been released that cause local blood flow to increase, attract immune cells and fibroblasts to the area of injury, and make capillaries in the injured region more permeable. These changes, in turn, result in a leak of fluid from intravascular to extracellular space. In addition to this **extravasation** of fluid into the affected tissue, the ability of proteins to cross the capillary wall is increased. Certain white blood cells that were enticed to the region, work their way across the endothelium and into the affected tissues, a process called **diapedesis**. Fibroblasts attracted to the region contribute to the early phase of wound healing, including formation of **granulation tissue** (new blood vessels and extracellular matrix) that paves the way for repair of the injured tissue and either tissue remodeling to recreate the uninjured state, or formation of a scar (see Ref. 5).

When this **inflammatory response** is relatively mild, the extravasated fluid is relatively low in protein, lacks fibrinogen, and is called a **serous exudate**. However, should the inflammation be severe, fibrinogen is present and clotting eventually occurs, creating a **fibrinous exudate**.

One key effect of inflammation is to create a local low-pH environment that inhibits further microbial proliferation and helps tip the balance against most bacterial pathogens, for reasons discussed previously. Local oxygenation also changes with inflammation. First it increases, as a result of increased blood flow; later it may decrease if swelling impairs further blood flow into the region.

The local mediators, whose release upon injury results in the increased blood flow, extravasation of fluid, diapedesis, and pain, in-

TABLE 19.1   SOME LOCAL MEDIATORS OF INFLAMMATION

Mediator	Actions
Histamine	Smooth-muscle contraction, increased vascular permeability
Slow-reacting substance of anaphylaxis (SRSA) (leukotriene C_4, D_4, E_4)	Smooth-muscle contraction
Eosinophil chemotactic factor of anaphylaxis (ECF-A)	Chemotactic attraction of eosinophils
Platelet-activating factor	Activates platelets to secrete serotonin and other mediators; smooth-muscle contraction; induces vascular permeability
Neutrophil chemotactic factor (NCF)	Chemotactic attraction of neutrophils
Leukotactic activity (leukotriene B_4)	Chemotactic attraction of neutrophils
Heparin	Anticoagulant
Basophil kallikrein of anaphylaxis (BK-A)	Cleaves kininogen to form bradykinin

Reproduced, with permission, from Haynes BS, Fauci AS (1998). Introduction to the immune system. In Fauci AS, et al. (eds), *Harrison's Textbook of Internal Medicine*, 14th ed. New York, McGraw-Hill, p 1768.

clude histamine, bradykinin, and other products (see Table 19.1). Some of these products are precursors that get activated by proteases. Once activated, some of the products are themselves proteases that cleave other precursors to start other cascades. In this way, the inflammatory response can interlock multiple pathways of physical, cell biological, and biochemical events (see Figure 19.3). The acute-phase reactants, the clotting cascade, and the complement pathway are examples of aspects of the inflammatory response, which will be discussed later.

Chronic inflammation is largely mediated by immune cells and refers to situations in which acute inflammation is not self-limited, but instead continues beyond the time needed to clean up the mess and get on with repair. Sometimes this occurs because the cause of injury or invasion is unusually persistent or repetitive. Further discussion of chronic inflammation will be deferred until after presentation of the cellular immune system (see Sec. 3).

Whether acute or chronic, inflammation is sometimes inappropriate in that there is no

FIGURE 19.3. Interlocking pathways of acute inflammation. Products from the bone marrow, circulation, and tissue interact to give rise to the classic symptoms of inflammation (redness, edema, pain, and fever). *(Adapted, with permission, from Holland SM, Gallin JI (1998). Disorders of granulocytes and monocytes. In Fauci A, et al. (eds), Harrison's Textbook of Internal Medicine, 14th ed. New York, McGraw-Hill, p 351.)*

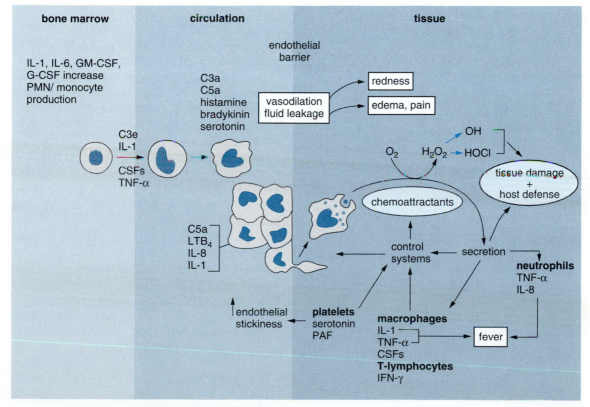

invader to defeat, or the invader is easily turned back and the major injury to be healed is caused by "friendly fire" from host defensive forces. These conditions are due to poorly understood disorders of immune cell function and interaction, including autoimmune and allergic disorders (see Sec. 4).

Acute-phase reactants

Acute-phase reactants are substances whose concentration in the bloodstream increases in response to infection, tissue injury, or other forms of stress (see Table 19.2). They include the cellular elements of blood clotting called **platelets** (see the following discussion) and a number of proteins. Most of the acute-phase proteins are specialized secretory products made by the liver, and hence, work outside of the cell. Various acute-phase reactants are induced to different extents. **Serum amyloid A protein**, for example, increases during inflammation 1000-fold over the non-inflam-

TABLE 19.2   ACUTE-PHASE REACTANTS

Inducible by IL-1, IL-6, or TNF
   Complement factors C3, C9, and B
   Mannose-binding protein
   Serum amyloid proteins A and P
   C-reactive protein
   Haptoglobin
   α_1-Acid glycoprotein

Regulated only by IL-6
   Albumin
   Prealbumin
   Fibrinogen
   Fibronectin
   Cysteine proteinase inhibitor
   α_1-Antichymotrypsin
   Ceruloplasmin
   Angiotensin

ABBREVIATIONS: IL = interleukin; TNF = tumor necrosis factor.
Reproduced, with permission, from Oppenheim, JJ, Ruschetti, FW (1997). Cytokines. In Stites DP, et al. (eds), *Medical Immunology*, 9th ed. Stamford, CT, Appleton & Lange, p 151.

matory state, while α_1 **antitrypsin** increases only two- to three-fold. Some of the acute-phase proteins, such as the hemoglobin-binding protein **haptoglobin**, are also antioxidants.

Many of the acute-phase reactants are induced by **cytokines**, small secreted soluble mediators released in response to a pathogen's breaching the first lines of defense. A number of acute-phase proteins, including **C-reactive protein**, not only are released in response to cytokines but also affect the immune system by themselves, regulating the secretion of cytokines (see Sec. 3). Other acute-phase reactant proteins have functions that are not, strictly speaking, immunologic but nevertheless make other crucial contributions to host defense. We will discuss two of these examples.

Iron-binding proteins

A key advantage of multicellularity is that no one cell has to take on specialization for all of the tasks of life. Rather, each can become expert in a limited repertoire of activities while relying on other cells to fulfill other functions. Host defense has evolved to take advantage of some implications of these relationships.

Iron is a crucial nutrient for survival of most organisms. When iron is not available, invaders that depend on "foraging off of the land" are at a significant disadvantage and have their ability to proliferate and invade significantly diminished (see Ref. 6). Thus, over the course of evolution, the liver has evolved to release various iron-binding proteins, including transferrin, haptoglobin, and hemopexin, into the bloodstream in times of potential infection or other stress. By binding free iron, these proteins fulfill three important functions:

• They keep iron from being accessible to the invaders, which generally lack receptors to recognize iron in these protein-bound forms. Thus, induction of haptoglobin during infection makes it that much more difficult for the pathogen. A similar function is ascribed to the protein **lactoferrin**, which is found in milk, in mucosal secretions, and in certain white blood cells called **polymorphonuclear leukocytes** or **neutrophils** (see the following discussion).

- As cells die and release their contents of valuable nutrients, such as iron, those nutrients can be salvaged rather than being lost, and can be prevented from doing oxidative damage, which might otherwise occur.
- The bound iron may be specifically taken up by host cells with appropriate receptors, allowing the host to better survive a protracted "war of attrition," should that be necessary to eliminate a stubborn invader.

Lipoproteins

In Chapter 4, lipoproteins were discussed as part of the solubilization function of the liver. As such, they play the key role of providing cholesterol and other lipids to cells of the body and removing them from those cells. Excess cholesterol beyond the needs of the body is returned to the liver for disposal in the form of bile.

A growing body of literature suggests that lipoproteins can also be thought of as making a significant contribution to host defense (see Ref. 7). The possible roles of lipoproteins in host defense include:

- Competition with viruses for entry into cells. Certain viruses use lipoprotein receptors to infect cells. Elevated lipoprotein levels may make this initial requisite step for infection more difficult.
- Redistribution of nutrients. By increasing triglyceride levels, the acute-phase response provides additional fuel for elevated metabolic needs to fight off infection. By decreasing the activity of the enzyme **lipoprotein lipase** that normally provides lipids for storage in adipose tissue, cytokines promote distribution of fuel to macrophages and other cells that will be particularly busy in the battle with the invader. By a change in the composition of high-density lipoprotein (HDL), cholesterol may be redirected away from the liver and to the peripheral tissues, where it may be needed for wound healing and tissue repair.
- Some lipoproteins have viral-neutralizing features. The composition of HDL particles changes as a result of the acute-phase response. A specific lipoprotein, apoprotein A-1, which has been implicated in such antiviral effects, is replaced by other proteins — perhaps freeing apoprotein A-1 to carry out its antiviral functions.
- Binding, oxidation, and lysis of invaders. Oxidation reactions are often used as defense mechanisms. Some lipoproteins that bind to invaders are subject to oxidation, while others have been shown to have a direct ability to lyse specific invaders.
- Titration of the host immune response. Cytokines released by immune and other cells in response to endotoxin found in the cell walls of certain bacterial pathogens serve to invoke an intense defensive reaction. Sometimes these defenses, rather than the invader, can be the cause of the host's demise. Lipoproteins are sinks in which endotoxin and other triggers of cytokine release can be trapped and sequestered from the immune system. Instead of triggering cytokine release, the lipoprotein-bound fraction of endotoxin is instead targeted to the liver, from there to bile, and finally excreted in stool. This way the host gets rid of the toxin — without triggering an excessive immunologic response.

Thus lipoproteins may serve as a limb of the innate immune system (see Ref. 8). Whether there are subtle aspects of lipoprotein structure that distinguish between molecules' functioning as purveyors of lipid in the bloodstream and as a line of defense against invaders is currently unknown.

Clinical Pearls

○ One of the many risks faced by patients in diabetic ketoacidosis (see Chap. 6) is fungal infections of the genus *Mucor*. One possible explanation for this is that the transferrin-iron complex dissociates in acid pH, releasing free iron and making it possible for this and other would-be pathogens to cause serious disease.

○ The affinity of lactoferrin for iron *increases* with fall in pH. Thus, at sites of infection and inflammation where the pH drops as a result of accumulation of products of anaerobic metabolism, a new line of defense springs up to deny the pathogen iron. Furthermore, macrophages (a form of white blood cell; see the following discussion), when activated to join the battle at a site of infection, display an increase in number of lactoferrin receptors, allowing them to further sequester iron from pathogens.

○ Degenerative joint disease is now recognized to have an inflammatory component. Thus, drugs that affect production of key stimulations of inflammation such as cytokines (see Sec. 3) are likely to be valuable modes of therapy in the future.

Review Questions

8. What are the acute-phase reactants?
9. What is the major iron-binding protein in the bloodstream? In milk?
10. What are possible roles for lipoproteins in host defense?

Self-limiting proteolytic cascades: the case of blood clotting

One form of host defense is to ensure that potentially damaging biochemical pathways are always well controlled. Blood clotting is a good case in point. Inappropriate clotting, when it occurs, can be an even more serious short-term problem than lack of adequate clotting. The body normally has mechanisms to ensure that clotting is instantly ready when we need it, but is strictly limited to appropriate locations. First, however, let us describe the composition of blood.

Blood consists of **red blood cells**, **white blood cells**, and **platelets** suspended in the fluid phase, called **plasma**. The main function of red blood cells is to carry oxygen (see Chap. 8). The main function of white blood cells is as components of the immune system (see the following discussion). Platelets are fragments of cells derived from large bone marrow cells called **megakaryocytes**. They are involved in the mechanism of blood clotting (to be discussed). They also release a host of products that contribute to attracting immune cells and other players in the process of wound healing to the site of an injury.

All of the different cell types found in blood are derived from stem cells in the bone marrow, which proliferate and differentiate into specific cellular lineages under the influence of various cytokines. This process of maturation of any particular type or types of blood cells can be stimulated by demand. Thus, typically, in response to inadequate oxygenation, the number of red blood cells goes up; in response to infection, the number of white blood cells goes up; and in response to blood loss or other signals, the number of platelets will increase. In each case, the pathway from physiological stimulus to cellular proliferation is only partly understood. Thus, for example, erythropoietin is the hormone, made by the kidney, that stimulates red blood cell proliferation and maturation. However, the precise intracellular signaling pathways by which erythropoietin does this is not yet known.

Plasma is more than just a vehicle for carrying blood cells. It contains a myriad of proteins, including albumin, growth factors, hormones, acute-phase reactants, and clotting factor precursors. Blood clotting involves a series of proteases that activate one another, culminating in clot formation around a platelet plug. Key defensive features are built into these pathways so that:

- Blood does not normally clot in the absence of injury.
- When an injury occurs, clot formation is activated almost immediately.
- Blood clot formation is extremely self-limited, so that clots form only where and when they are supposed to.
- Mechanisms to dissolve the clot and repair the underlying tissue whose injury activated clot formation are activated almost simultaneously with clot formation. However, they work on a slower time scale.

The net effect of these multiple mechanisms is that, normally, clots form, have a finite lifetime, and after a period of time are replaced by a scar.

Activation of the clotting cascade

Blood clotting starts with an injury that exposes collagen of the basement membrane below endothelial cells to platelets in the bloodstream. A receptor on the platelet cell surface binds the collagen and sticks to it. This interaction sets off a number of signaling pathways within the platelet, resulting in its **activation** (see Figure 19.4). Thus, within seconds of an injury, an activated platelet plug has formed at the site of injury. **Von Willebrand's factor** is a glycoprotein that adds strength to the platelet plug, preventing it

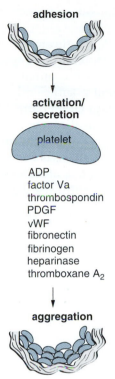

FIGURE 19.4. Products released upon platelet activation. The process of clot formation is initiated by adhesion of platelets and interaction with an activating surface such as vascular subendothelium that triggers platelet activation. Products secreted by platelets are indicated in the figure. The net effect of platelet activation is aggregation, which covers up the exposed subendothelial collagen and prevents further platelet activation. Abbreviations: ADP, adenosine diphosphate; PDGF, platelet-derived growth factor, vWF, von Willebrand's factor.

from falling apart under the shear stress of blood flow.

At the same time that an activated platelet plug is being formed, a number of biochemical reactions occur on the cell surface of the activated platelet. As a result of these reactions, proteins of plasma bind to the activated platelet, and proteolytically cleave one another to generate active **coagulation factors**. These factors, in turn, cause other proteins of plasma to leave the circulation, bind the activated platelet, and be proteolytically cleaved. The cascade ultimately generates the selective protease **thrombin**, which cleaves the plasma protein **fibrinogen** into **fibrin**, which reinforces the initial platelet plug to form a seal that is sufficiently durable to last a period of days (see Figure 19.4).

The biochemical reactions of the clotting pathway are summarized in Figure 19.5. There are two pathways by which clotting can be initiated, and two anti-clotting systems by which it can be controlled. The **intrinsic pathway**, so named because all the components are intrinsic to blood, is initiated by an injury that exposes blood to collagen in the basement membrane of blood vessels. Thus, the stimulus for platelet aggregation also activates clotting. The **extrinsic pathway** requires the release of **tissue thromboplastin** to be activated. Both pathways converge on the activation of factor X.

One anti-clotting system (not shown in Figure 19.5) consists of the anticoagulant factors **antithrombin III**, **protein C**, and **protein S**. These proteins inactivate the procoagulant factors. The degree to which our blood will clot is due to the balance of pro- and anticlotting activity.

A second anti-clotting system involves the protease **plasmin**, formed by the action of thrombin on the precursor **plasminogen** (see Figure 19.5). It operates on a more delayed

FIGURE 19.5. Blood clot formation, its inhibition, and its lysis. Indicated are the intrinsic and extrinsic procoagulant pathways and pathways by which clot formation can be either prevented or lysed (see text). *(Adapted, with permission, from Davoren JB (1997), Blood disorders. In McPhee S et al.,* Pathophysiology of Disease, *2d ed. Stamford, CT, Appleton & Lange, p. 103.)*

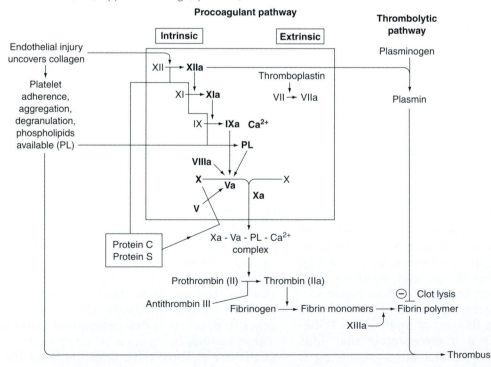

time scale to dissolve clots that were formed a few days earlier and should be in the process of being replaced by fibroblasts forming scar tissue.

There is enough clotting activity in 1 mL of plasma to completely activate all the fibrinogen in the body in under a minute. However, normally, clotting is precisely restricted to the site where it is needed and occurs nowhere else. Several features of the system ensure that blood clotting does not get out of hand:

- The signaling pathways that are set into motion by platelet activation are a fine balance between those that favor and those that oppose clotting (see Figure 19.4).
- The required factors normally require a solid surface where they are brought together in close enough proximity to activate one another. Normally this happens only on an activated platelet. But only a few platelets get activated before the site of collagen exposure is completely covered up.
- The flow of blood constantly dilutes out activated factors.
- The inhibitory pathways were described previously.
- Products released from the activated platelet include platelet-derived growth factor (PDGF), which stimulates migration and proliferation of fibroblasts to carry out definitive repair of the lesion, forming a permanent scar.

Clinical Pearls

○ The normal platelet count (number of platelets per microliter of blood) is 150,000 to 450,000. The bleeding time (a measure of clotting ability) is prolonged (i.e., clot formation is delayed) if platelets are in the 50 to 100,000 range, but there are no clinical consequences except during major surgery or severe trauma. Below 50,000, patients have easy bruising. Below 20,000 platelets per microliter, patients are at risk of serious spontaneous bleeding.

○ Aspirin acetylates and permanently inactivates cyclooxygenase, shifting the balance within an activated platelet in favor of antithrombosis for the duration of the 3- to 5-day lifetime of a platelet. Ibuprofen and other non-steroidal drugs are reversible inhibitors of cyclooxygenase, and thus generally do not have significant effects on blood clotting.

○ Heparin is a *proteoglycan* found on cells that has strong anticoagulant properties and is therefore commonly used for acute anticoagulation. It works by accelerating the action of antithrombin, a coagulation factor inhibitor that binds and inactivates most activated clotting factors (except factor VII).

○ Coumadin (warfarin) is a common chronic anticoagulation drug used to treat patients with inappropriate clot formation. The mechanism by which Coumadin works is to block vitamin K-dependent modifications of clotting factors II, VII, IX, and X in the liver. The factors are still made, but without a modification (addition of an extra carboxyl group to selected glutamic acid residues) needed for their activation.

○ The reasons anticoagulation typically starts with heparin before treatment with Coumadin are that (1) heparin works immediately, whereas Coumadin has no effect on already synthesized clotting factors in the bloodstream, and (2) Coumadin also blocks synthesis of the anticoagulant proteins S and C. Thus, if Coumadin were given by itself without prior anticoagulation with heparin, it might cause a transient procoagulant state in the window of time before its block of clotting factors becomes effective. In practice, typically, Coumadin is often started as soon as heparin is therapeutic, and the heparin is discontinued when the Coumadin becomes therapeutic.

The effects of the two drugs can be distinguished because heparin's primary effect is on the *partial thromboplastin time* (PTT); at therapeutic doses it does not substantially alter the *prothrombin time* (PT).

○ Up to one-half of patients who develop inappropriate clotting (called venous thrombosis) have defects in the normal mechanisms that defend against inappropriate clot formation, including deficiency of protein C or S or antithrombin. Thus, inappropriate clot formation can occur as a result of either anti-clotting deficiency or clotting factor excess.

Review Questions

11. From what cells in the bone marrow are platelets derived?
12. Describe the main steps in the process of clot formation.
13. What lines of defense prevent inappropriate clotting?

Other aspects of innate immunity: complement and interferon

Complement

Complement is a set of proteins in the bloodstream that form an extremely important but non-specific line of defense against organisms that enter the normally sterile internal environment (see Figure 19.6). The **complement cascade** is a set of biochemical reactions that starts with a single abundant serum protein, called C3, that is activated by either of two different routes. Once activated, C3 can be rapidly inactivated with a half-life of 0.1 m if it stays as a free protein in solution or if it

binds to a normal host cell. However, should the activated complement bind to an invader that does not have a defense against it, the activated C3 directs the activation and assembly onto the invader of other complement components in the bloodstream (see Figure 19.6). The result is a chain reaction, known as **complement fixation**, that culminates in one or more of the following outcomes:

- Lysis of the invader cell by formation of a hole in the cell membrane. One of the complement structures assembled by the complement cascade is a *membrane attack complex* that directly brings about injury to the cell on which activated complement has been bound. This mechanism is particularly important for defense against bacteria that are resistant to phagocytosis and against enveloped viruses.
- Release of substances that (1) attract white blood cells and allow them to home in on the would-be pathogen, (2) cause fever (which hurts the invader more than the host), and (3) stimulate release of cytokines and therefore initiate the acute-phase reaction, etc.
- Coating of some pathogens with substances that make them more readily engulfed by phagocytic cells of the immune system (see Sec. 3).
- Binding of complement-coated pathogens to receptors for activated complement on various host immune cells. These receptors trigger a range of additional defense mechanisms, leading to destruction of the invader. These will be discussed in our consideration of the mechanism of action of cytotoxic T lymphocytes (see later).

Mechanisms of complement activation

The **classical pathway of complement activation** involves the ability of antigen-antibody complexes that form on a pathogen to activate complement fixation on that pathogen. This culminates in either direct lysis of the

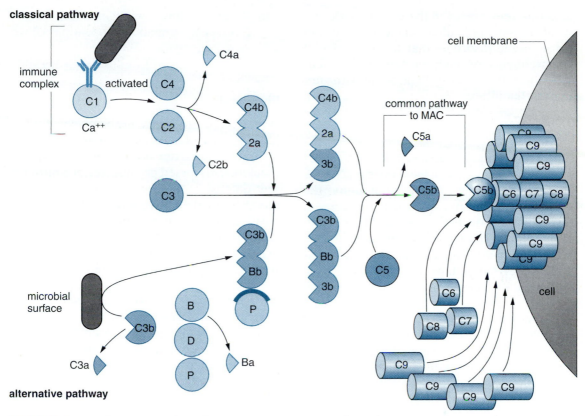

classical pathway

alternative pathway

FIGURE 19.6. Complement cascade and consequences. Activation of complement through the classical and alternative pathways. Soluble proteins of the complement cascade are activated by immune complexes on a pathogen's cell surface directly, resulting in assembly of a multicomponent membrane attack complex that causes lysis of either infected cells or pathogens. *(Adapted, with permission, from Spitznagel JK (1994). Constitutive defenses of the body. In Schaechter M, et al. (eds), Mechanisms of microbial disease, 2d ed. Baltimore, Williams & Wilkins, p 98.)*

pathogen, phagocytosis by immune cells, or killing by cytotoxic T lymphocytes.

The **alternative pathway of complement activation** does not require a specific pathogen to trigger complement activation. Rather, the C3 component of complement is activated spontaneously at a low level in the bloodstream in the absence of a specific target. If no invader is present, the activated C3 is quickly inactivated by other enzymes in the bloodstream. However, if an invader happens to be nearby, the activated complement is ready to bind, which prolongs its half-life, allowing it to recruit the other components and trigger the lethal cascade. Apparently, the needs of host defense are such that the complement system has been selected to be on a veritable hair trigger in order to optimize our well-being over the course of evolution. Indeed, defects in the alternative pathway are associated with severe bacterial infections (see A Case of Physiological Medicine).

Just as a certain number of individuals will suffer from excessive blood clotting as a result of subtle imbalances in the clotting cascade, so also some individuals have allergic and autoimmune disorders that are likely to be a consequence of inappropriate complement activation. Powerful systems come with substantial liabilities.

Interferon

Fibroblasts and epithelial cells (which are often infected by viruses), have the capacity for another dimension of innate immunity, the production of **interferons**, which are secreted proteins that are members of the larger family of cytokines. Interferons activate a number of signaling pathways, culminating in a metabolic state that is hostile to takeover by a viral invader. These anti-viral effects include:

- Activation of ribonucleases that seek out non-host RNAs and degrade them
- Phosphorylation of factors involved in protein synthesis initiation, which inactivates them (viruses effect a takeover of host protein synthesis machinery, so shutting it all down has a distinctly anti-viral effect)
- Activation of various responses of immune cells that target viral-infected cells for destruction

Unlike some of the other cytokines, interferons

- Are made by non-immune cells
- Primarily work locally rather than systemically
- Have effects both on the cells that make them and on immune cells in the neighborhood

Review Questions

14. What are four ways in which complement contributes to host defense?
15. What are the two mechanisms by which complement can be activated?
16. What are three ways in which interferon can impair propagation of a virus?

Phagocytosis

While there are many limbs of constitutive host defense that come into play when an intruder enters the body (e.g., acute-phase reactants, discussed previously), the most potent defense is the class of specialized white blood cells called **phagocytes**. These cells are part of the innate immune system, in that they are not targeted to specific pathogens. When activated by any of a large number of triggers, these cells are targeted to the site of inflammation by the action of various chemoattractants released by the invaders or as part of the inflammatory response. The phagocytes then proceed to engulf and kill various classes of pathogens. The three different types of phagocytic white blood cells, called neutrophils, macrophages, and eosinophils, are discussed here.

Neutrophils

Neutrophils are immune cells that are so named because they stain "neutral" (neither red nor blue) with Wright's stain, a standard dye used in hematology laboratories. Neutrophils arise from stem cells in the bone marrow. After a 2-week period of maturation, they enter the peripheral bloodstream for a few hours before localizing along the blood vessel walls in various tissues, where they await further instructions. Those instructions come in the form of specific chemoattractants, including complement cleavage products and substances made by pathogens. In response to these **chemoattractants**, neutrophils are activated, hone in on the site of intruder entry, and attempt to engulf the pathogen and/or remaining debris to form an intracellular compartment termed a **phago-**

some (see Figure 19.7). The neutrophil then proceeds to release into the phagosome substances that are designed to kill the engulfed intruder. The granules present within the phagocyte are modified **lysosomes** whose contents are activated and released upon fusion with the phagosome to form a **phagolysosome.**

About 10^{10} neutrophils are generated from stem cells daily. The mechanism of phagocytosis is facilitated by proteins called **opsonins** that make the intruder "tasty" to phagocytes. A major role for complement is to serve in this capacity, offsetting various defenses on the part of the pathogen that otherwise impair phagocytosis.

The material released from the granules into the phagolysosome is of several sorts. One type of granule releases various proteases and the enzyme **myeloperoxidase**. A second class of product found in specific neutrophil granules is iron-binding proteins such as lactoferrin (see the discussion of acute-phase reactants), collagenase, and so-called **antimicrobial cationic proteins**.

There are two distinct mechanisms of neutrophil-mediated killing of invaders, one oxygen-dependent, the other oxygen-independent. Oxygen-dependent killing involves bringing together in the phagolysosome enzymes that result in the formation of **hydrogen peroxide** (H_2O_2). H_2O_2 then works with myeloperoxidase to convert chloride ions into hypochlorous ions, the same highly oxidizing substance found in bleach, which destroys the engulfed intruder. However, this mechanism is dependent on a source of oxygen. Sometimes — for example, in deep-seated anaerobic abscesses — oxygen is not present or is used up by microbial or host cell metabolism. In these circumstances, a non-oxygen-dependent mode of killing occurs, using the antimicrobial cationic proteins as a kind of detergent to lyse the membrane of the invader. In general, bacteria of the gut are more likely to include anaerobes that re-

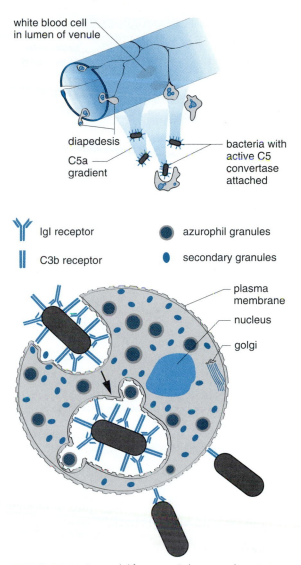

FIGURE 19.7. Neutrophil function. Schematic description of a neutrophil phagocytizing an opsonized bacterium. Specific antibody and complement have coated the bacterium, and the bound IgG and C3b complement proteins have then been recognized by specific receptors on the phagocyte cell surface, allowing phagocytosis. Subsequently, lysosomes and secretory granules containing lysosome-type digestive enzymes fuse to the phagosome to complete the destruction of the engulfed invader.

TABLE 19.3   IMPORTANT ADHESION MOLECULES IN LYMPHOCYTE HOMING

Leukocyte receptor	Leukocyte expression	Endothelial counter-receptor	Function
Selectins			
L-selectin	All	Glycam-1, PSGL-1, others	Rolling
Integrins			
$\alpha M\beta2$ (Mac-1, Mo-1, CD11b/CD18)	Monocytes, PMN, NK	ICAM-1 (CD54)	Firm adhesion
		ICAM-2 (CD102),[a] fibrinogen	Transmigration
$\alpha L\beta2$ (CD11a/CD18)	All	ICAM-1	Firm adhesion
		ICAM-2	Transmigration
$\alpha4\beta1$	All[b]	VCAM-1 (CD106)	Rolling and firm adhesion
$\alpha4\beta7$	Lymphocyte subset	MadCAM	Rolling and firm adhesion
$\alpha v\beta3$	All	PECAM (CD31)	Transmigration
Ig superfamily			
IAP (CD47)	All	Thrombospondin	Transmigration
PECAM	All	PECAM, $\alpha v\beta3$	Transmigration
Others			
PSGL-1	PMN, monocytes, some lymphs	P-selectin (CD62P) L-selectin (CD62L) E-selectin (CD62E)	Rolling
ESL	PMN	E-selectin	Rolling
CD44	All	Hyaluronate	?

[a]The role of Mac-1 interaction with ICAM-2 in transendothelial migration is unknown.
[b]While $\alpha4\beta1$ has an important role in transendothelial migration of monocytes and lymphocytes, its role in PMN transendothelial migration is uncertain.
Abbreviations: NK, natural killer cell; PMN, polymorphonuclear neutrophil.
Reproduced, with permission, from Brown EJ. (1997). Adhesive interactions in the immune system. *Trends Cell Biol* 7:290.

quire this mode of defense, while microbes of the skin are kept in check by oxidative defenses.

Major advances have occurred in recent years in our understanding of the mechanism of white blood cell **homing**, that is, the ability of white blood cells to go to a particular location in the body. It appears that changes in expression of glycoprotein receptors on the endothelium of tissues play a key role in this process. Classes of adhesive glycoproteins (see Table 19.3), including those called **selectins** and **integrins**, can be switched on or off in particular cells to fine-tune the localization and movement of neutrophils either to endothelial cells, across them, or into tissues (see

Sec. 6, Frontiers). It appears that an intricate and poorly understood pathway exists by which various classes of white blood cells travel to and from specific locations in the body, directed by these adhesive proteins.

Macrophages

Macrophages arise from the same stem cell population in the bone marrow that give rise to neutrophils. However, they are distinct in that they leave the bone marrow in a still immature state called a **monocyte** and complete essential aspects of their differentiation in specific tissues. Unlike neutrophils, whose primary function is in innate immunity, macrophages are involved in both innate and acquired immunity (see Sec. 3). Some monocytes form resident **tissue macrophages**. In the liver they are called **Kupffer cells**; in the brain, **microglia**; in the lung, **alveolar macrophages**; in the bone, **osteoclasts**, and so on. They release cytokines, including interleukin-1, that stimulate neutrophil activation and adhesiveness, and greatly enhance the inflammatory response. Other macrophages are recruited to the site of inflammation by signals released from the first wave of neutrophils. Typically, an initial wave of neutrophils arrives on the scene in response to intruder entry, within hours. Then macrophages arrive a day or two later, to join the battle and to play an important role in orchestrating the acquired immune response (see Sec. 3).

Eosinophils

These distinctive white blood cells, so named because they stain red with Wright's stain or Giemsa stain, are very much like neutrophils except that they seem to be used specifically to attack parasites rather than bacteria.

Clinical Pearls

○ Insufficient neutrophils (*neutropenia*), defined as less than 1000 neutrophils per microliter of blood, is a risk factor for serious bacterial infections. Patients whose neutrophil counts fall this low or lower (e.g., because of chemotherapy for cancer) are typically hospitalized and treated with broad-spectrum antibiotics at the first sign of infection (e.g., fever), because normally harmless organisms can become pathogens in the absence of this crucial line of host innate immune defense.

○ Patients with *chronic granulomatous disease* have a defect in oxidative killing of engulfed invaders by phagocytes, as a result of lack of formation of superoxide ions

used to make hydrogen peroxide. Thus, despite their ability to phagocytose normally, they are often unable to kill the intruder. Despite the use of antibiotics, patients with severe cases rarely live beyond childhood, usually succumbing to overwhelming bacterial infections.

○ Some organisms actually make hydrogen peroxide themselves and export it because they lack an endogenous mechanism for its safe inactivation. Thus, when trapped in the phagolysosome, these organisms, which include the common bacterial pathogen *Pneumococcus,* are killed by accumulation of their own toxic waste. Predictably, pneumococci do not cause significant problems for patients with chronic granulomatous disease.

○ Individuals with *Chédiak-Higashi syndrome* have a genetic lesion whose phenotype is that their neutrophils release their granules too soon, i.e., into empty phagolysosomes. As a result, when these cells mature, are activated, and need to actually kill a phagocytized invader, there are no granules left, as they have all been spent earlier in the cell's life.

Review Questions

17. How do neutrophils participate in host defense?
18. Name three different proteins made by neutrophils for host defense.
19. What are two differences between the roles of neutrophils and of macrophages in host defense?
20. What is the role of eosinophils in host defense?

Stress proteins

Intracellular inflammation

Classically, studies of the inflammatory response focused on events that could be monitored outside of cells and did not address the issue of what was going on at the molecular level *within* cells involved in the inflammatory response. We now know that there are profound changes going on within almost all affected cells in response to inflammatory stimuli. These intracellular events are quite distinct from the effects that manifest outside of that cell. This intracellular aspect of the inflammatory response is the domain of **stress proteins**. As stated, these are proteins that generally reside within the cell that makes them, rather than being products secreted from the cell to affect neighboring cells. However, stress proteins induced in one organ can affect other organ systems, and it appears that the immune system monitors the stress protein system rather assiduously (see Sec. 6, Frontiers).

The stress response

When cells are subjected to any of a wide range of stresses, including excessive heat, heavy metals and other toxins, and nutritional deprivation, expression of most genes is turned off. That is, mRNA stops being made from these genes, and existing mRNAs stop being translated. However, transcription of a few genes is actually turned on in response to stress. The proteins encoded by genes are called stress proteins. Expression of stress protein genes appears to be controlled at many levels, including transcription and translation, and intricate mechanisms appear to have evolved to ensure that these defensive proteins are preferentially synthesized in times of stress. Just about every compartment of the cell appears to have its unique set of stress proteins, which falls into several families (see Table 19.4).

It appears that many stress proteins are **molecular chaperones** (see Chap. 2), proteins engaged in shepherding other protein–protein interactions. Thus some stress proteins are present in large amounts even in the non-stressed state. Molecular chaperones are believed to play dozens of different and currently poorly understood roles in cells, a subset of which are involved in stress response. Other roles include the facilitation of protein translocation across specific membranes and its importation into organelles (see Chap. 2), and participation in the pathway of transcriptional activation by steroids and other small biological ligands (see Chaps. 2 and 3).

Synthesis of molecular chaperones is further increased during stress for at least three reasons:

- To accommodate the need to refold proteins that have been partly denatured but are still salvageable
- To hold denatured proteins that are nonsalvageable and need to be degraded — which is better than having them getting in the way, sticking where they shouldn't, causing denaturation of even more proteins
- To facilitate folding of the wave of newly synthesized proteins needed to replace the irreparably denatured proteins

The stress response at the cellular level appears also to be coordinated at the organ system level, since the level of activity of the hypothalamic-pituitary-adrenal axis and of the adrenal medullary catecholamine system affects stress protein expression.

Many of the manipulations observed for the stress response in cultured cells also apply to whole organisms. One of the most dramatic examples of manipulation of the stress response is the phenomenon of **thermotolerance**. When a cell is treated with a sublethal heat stress, then given time to recover, it is able to tolerate a subsequent stress that would have otherwise been lethal. The two stresses can be unrelated, e.g., heat in one case and toxins or nutritional deprivation in the other. This "preconditioning" appears to be due to induction

TABLE 19.4   FAMILIES OF STRESS PROTEINS AND THEIR PATHOPHYSIOLOGICAL SIGNIFICANCE

Name	Size[a]	Bacterial homologue	Locale	Remarks
	kD			
Ubiquitin	8	—	Cytosol/nucleus	Involved in nonlysosomal protein degradation pathway
Hsp 10	10	Gro ES	Mitochondria/chloroplast	Cofactor for Hsp 60
Low-molecular-weight hsp's	20–30	Possible homologues recently identified	Cytosol/nucleus	Proposed regulator of actin cytoskeleton; proposed molecular chaperone
Hsp 47	47	—	Endoplasmic reticulum	Collagen chaperone
Hsp 56	56	—	Cytosol	Part of steroid hormone receptor complex; binds FK506
Hsp 60	60	Gro EL	Mitochondria/chloroplast	Molecular chaperone ("chaperonin")
TCP-1	60	Gro EL	Cytosol/nucleus	Molecular chaperone related to Hsp 60
Hsp 72	70	Dna K	Cytosol/nucleus	Highly stress inducible
Hsp 73	70	Dna K	Cytosol/nucleus	Constitutively expressed molecular chaperone
Grp 75	70	Dna K	Mitochondria/chloroplast	Constitutively expressed molecular chaperone
Grp 78 (BiP)	70	Dna K	Endoplasmic reticulum	Constitutively expressed molecular chaperone
Hsp 90	90	htpG	Cytosol/nucleus	Part of steroid hormone receptor complex; chaperone for retrovirus-encoded tyrosine protein kinases
Hsp 104/110	104/110	Clp family	Cytosol/nucleus	Required to survive severe stress; molecular chaperone

[a]Approximate size by SDS-page, native molecular weight often is very different.
Reproduced, with permission, from Minowada G, Welch WJ. (1995). Clinical implications of the stress response. *J. Clin Invest.* 95:4.

of stress proteins by the sublethal stress that protect against the subsequent, more severe stress. Manipulation of stress proteins constitutes one of the most promising lines of future research in host defense (see Ref. 8).

For reasons that are not at all understood, it appears that the immune system (see Sec. 3) preferentially targets the stress proteins of would-be pathogens. In some cases, the immune reaction to pathogen stress proteins has been shown to be protective against infection. It also appears that immune cells directed against host cell stress proteins are present in individuals with no manifestations of autoimmune disease. This raises the possibility that one surveillance function of the immune system is to recognize excessively or chronically stressed cells and eliminate them. This hypothesis and the notion that stress proteins are a key target in autoimmune dis-

orders remain highly controversial speculations at this time.

Clinical Pearls

○ Survival of skin grafts in reconstructive surgery has been noted to improve if the skin flap is rendered thermotolerant by a pretreatment with sublethal heat (see Ref. 9).
○ The gene for the multidrug resistance p glycoprotein (which is responsible for a substantial amount of the development of chemotherapy resistance on the part of cancers) contains a *heat shock promoter*, suggesting that the appearance of chemotherapy resistance in clinical cancer is a self-protective stress response on the part of the tumor cell.

Review Questions

21. What are stress proteins?
22. Name three conditions that induce production of stress proteins.
23. What are three functions for molecular chaperones during stress?
24. What is thermotolerance?

3. THE ACQUIRED IMMUNE SYSTEM

There are two types of defenses in the body. The first, comprising innate immunity, does not require prior contact with the specific invader. Defenses of this type have been the focus of the preceding section (Sec. 2). Immune defenses of the second type are *antigen-specific*, meaning that they are selectively tailored against a particular structural feature present on a would-be intruder — sort of a molecular "smart bomb," in contrast to the conventional weaponry of innate immunity. All of the antigen-specific forms of immune response are carried out by various subsets of **lymphocytes**, a type of white blood cell (see Table 19.5).

In order to induce a robust defense that is both reliable (will recognize any of the mil-

TABLE 19.5   CATEGORIES OF IMMUNE CELLS

Cell	Surface components	Function
T Lymphocytes	T_3	Involved in cell-mediated immunity
Helper T cells (T_H)	T_4	Recognizes antigen with class II MHC; promotes differentiation of B cells and cytotoxic T cells; activates macrophages
	T-cell receptor complex: α, β dimer associated with T_3	Recognizes antigen with class I MHC; kills antigen-expressing cells
Cytotoxic T cells (CTL)	T_8	
γ/δ T cells	Probably all T_4 and T_8 negative	Respond to commonly encountered microbial antigens perhaps at epithelial boundaries; MHC restriction and function unknown
Suppressor T cells	T_8 Receptor for antigen unknown	Downregulates the activities of other lymphocytes
B lymphocytes	Surface immunoglobulin, Fc receptors, class II MHC	Recognizes antigen directly; differentiates into antibody-producing plasma cells, antigen presentation
Large granular lymphocytes (LGL)		
K cells	Fc receptor	Kills antibody-coated cells (ADCC)
NK cells	Receptor for target "antigen" unknown	Kills cells with some selectivity
Macrophages	Fc receptor, C3 receptor; some have class II MHC; can bind to wide variety of substance via surface "receptors"	Antigen presentation; phagocytosis killing of microbes and tumor cells; secretion of IL-1
Dendritic cells	Fc receptor, C3 receptor, class II MHC	Antigen presentation
Mast cells (tissues) and basophils (blood)	High-affinity receptors for IgE	Allergic responses; histamine release
Neutrophils	Fc receptor, C3 receptor, C5 receptor, and FMLP receptor	Phagocytosis and killing of bacteria, yeast, and fungi
Eosinophils		Phagocytosis and elimination of parasites

Reproduced, with permission, from Ziegler HK, Nairn R (1994). Induced defenses of the body. In Schechter M et al. (eds), *Mechanisms of Microbial Disease*, 2d ed. Baltimore, Williams & Wilkins, p 139.

lions of possible different antigens in the outside world) and antigen-specific, the host must:

- Have had prior contact with that intruder.
- Be able to remember that prior contact and respond in a qualitatively different manner upon subsequent contact because of it. This property is called **memory**.
- Be able to discriminate self from non-self.
- Have a generally effective means of eliminating or suppressing antigen-specific reactions against self.

The acquired immune system of a healthy adult human has all of these characteristics. Lack of any one of them can occur as a result of genetic, developmental, environmental, or degenerative disorders and represents a weak link in host defense that puts the host at risk of disease.

General principles of acquired immunity

The acquired immune response can occur either in soluble form, in which specific immune cells (called **B lymphocytes**) secrete **antibodies**, or in a cell-mediated form, in which specific immune cells (called **T lymphocytes**) recognize specific antigens, usually on cells (see Figure 19.8 and Table 19.6). Antibodies are secreted proteins consisting of two pairs of two proteins, called heavy and light chains, that bind to specific structural features called **epitopes** that define an antigen (see Figure 19.9). Cell-mediated immune responses are more complex than antibody ones in that there can be many different consequences of antigen recognition by a T cell, including differentiation into cytotoxic T cells or into cytokine-secreting T cells that direct various other aspects of the immune response (e.g., the actions of macrophages, B cells, etc.).

Whether the acquired immune response is antibody-mediated or cell-mediated, or both, it is believed to occur by a process of **lymphocyte activation** followed by **clonal selection** (see Figure 19.10). The idea behind clonal selection is that the mature immune system starts out with millions and millions of individual cells and that each can recognize a single epitope. Among them, there are cells that are specific or potentially specific for just about any structure that can occur. When the host is exposed to an antigen for the first time, the specific cell(s) that recognize that antigen respond by undergoing cell division. This is called the **primary immune response**. Thus, where the antigen was first recognized by only one or a few cells, as a result of that first exposure it is now recognized by many cells. Some of those cells become **memory cells** that will respond in the same way the next time the antigen is seen. Others will respond to a second exposure to this specific antigen by differentiation into mature effector cells that either secrete antibodies or carry out cell-mediated responses. This is the **secondary immune response**. The mechanisms that govern which cell will become a long-lived memory cell and which will mature into a short-lived effector cell are unknown, but may involve exposure to different cytokines.

The basis for the primary and secondary immune responses is that each of the millions of immune cells specific for a different antigen has on its surface a receptor that recognizes the antigen against which it is directed. When that receptor is occupied by the specific antigen, the cells are triggered to proliferate. In conjunction with proliferation, the secondary immune response is associated with differentiation into different functional classes of cells (in the case of T cells) and with "fine-tuning" of the specificity of the antibody, so that the most specific possible antibody or T cell is generated and expanded.

Generation of antibody diversity

How is it possible that we have millions and millions of cells directed against specific epitopes that allow us to recognize just about any antigen that we might come across? The

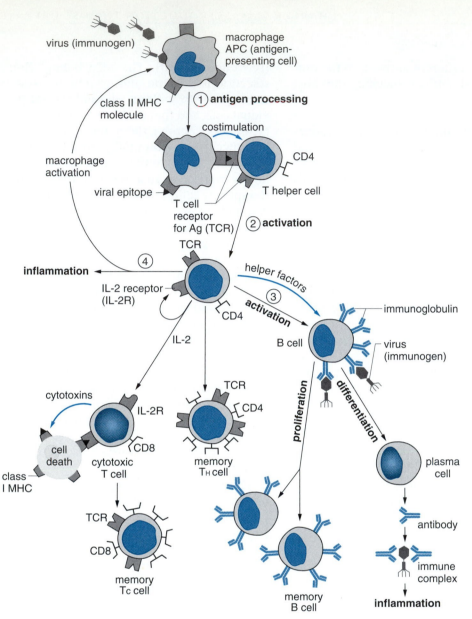

FIGURE 19.8. Sequence of events in the acquired immune response. A macrophage comes across a virus or other source of foreign antigens. Antigen processing occurs, and the macrophage processes the foreign antigens and presents them to a helper T cell. The T cell is activated and undergoes one of several lines of differentiation. One line of mature helper T cells may assist cytotoxic T cells, some of which engage in killing cells that are virus-infected and displaying the appropriate MHC class 1 antigens. Other cytotoxic T cells form memory cells, allowing a more robust response to this antigen in the future. Other helper T cells assist in B-cell activation to increase the immune response and give rise to inflammation. *(Adapted, with permission, from Stites DP, et al. (eds) (1997). Medical Immunology, 9th ed. Stamford, CT, Appleton & Lange, p 66.)*

TABLE 19.6   IMPORTANT SURFACE MOLECULES ON T CELLS

Marker	Major function or significance
T-cell receptor	Antigen binding.
CD3 complex	Signal transduction from T-cell receptor; lineage-specific marker.
CD2, CD5, CD7	Lineage-specific markers.
CD4	Subset-specific marker (mainly on helper cells); interaction with class II MHC proteins.
CD8	Subset-specific marker (mainly on cytotoxic cells); interaction with class I MHC proteins.
CD28	Activation-specific marker; receives B7-mediated costimulation from APC.
CD40 ligand (CD40L)	Activation-specific marker; delivers contact-mediated help to B cells.
IL-2 receptor Class II MHC proteins Transferrin receptor CD25, CD29, CD54, CD69	Other activation-specific markers.
IL-1 receptor IL-6 receptor TNFα receptor	Other cytokine receptors.
Fc receptors	Immunoglobulin binding.
LFA-1, ICAM-1	Cell–cell adhesion molecules.

ABBREVIATIONS: APC = antigen-presenting cell; IL = interleukin; TNF = tumor necrosis factor; LFA = leukocyte functional antigen; ICAM = intercellular adhesion molecule.
Reproduced, with permission, from Parslow T (1997). Lymphocytes and lymphoid tissues. In Stites DP, et al. (eds). *Medical Immunology*, 9th ed. Stamford, CT, Appleton & Lange, p 48.

receptors on the surface of T and B cells are complex proteins (see Figure 19.9A) derived from several genes that underwent rearrangement during the course of development of that organism's immune system. Thus, the general mechanisms that allow genes to recombine during the transmission of genetic information from generation to generation have evolved a specific adaptation that makes the acquired immune system possible. The **heavy chain** is one of the two proteins that comprise an antibody molecule and is related to the structure that serves as a receptor on the T- and B-cell surfaces. The heavy chain gene has several regions that are found in many copies, each slightly different from all others, called the genome (see Figure 19.9A). About 200 genes encode the V region, 10 genes encode the J region, and 4 genes encode the D region. These genes can recombine to make the *variable region*, resulting in a potential diversity of $200 \times 10 \times 4 = 8,000$ antibody specificities for just the heavy chain. For the light chain, about 800 such specificities are found. By combining different heavy chains with different light chains, one gets $8,000 \times 800 = 6,400,000$ different variable-region specificities at the level of the primary response alone. Random mutation occurs during V, D, and J region recombination and during proliferation of any one clone of immune cells in response to antigen, a process called **somatic mutation**, which can generate an additional 10- to 100-fold further increase in diversity of epitope recognition (see Figure 19.11). Finally, each variable region is associated with a constant region that imparts different classes of activity to the antibody, e.g., whether it will be used to defend mucosal surfaces (called secretory IgA) or for initial or subsequent antibody responses in the bloodstream (called IgM and IgG, respectively; see Figure 19.9B).

Now consider what happens in "real time" as a human host with some 10 million potential specificities comes in contact for the first time with an antigen that is recognized, but poorly, by one of them. Because the recognition is poor, the affinity for the receptor is relatively low. Nevertheless, some binding does occur, and some proliferation is stimulated. During the primary response and during subsequent exposure to the antigen, some random somatic mutations will occur that in-

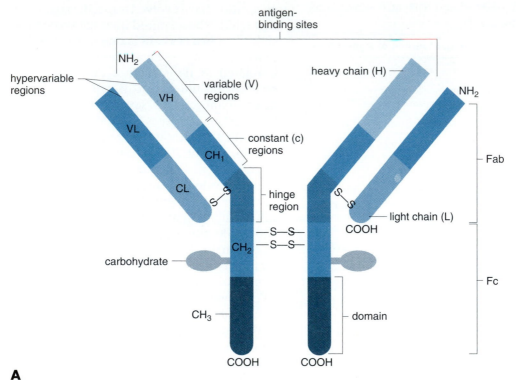

A

FIGURE 19.9. Immunoglobulin structure. *A.* Schematic structure of IgG, showing the heavy and light polypeptide chains and some of their structural features, including the antigen-binding sites that recognize epitopes of foreign proteins and the Fc region, which is recognized by receptors on the phagocyte.

crease the affinity for the receptor. These higher-affinity mutations are selected because they result in more cell proliferation with successive rounds of stimulation by contact with the epitope. Eventually, an antibody with substantially higher affinity than was initially present ends up being selected as the dominant response to the particular antigen. Furthermore, there will be a large number of cells producing this antibody due to proliferation. At each step in the evolution of antibody affinity, some cells terminally differentiate into antibody-secreting plasma cells. At that point, they lose their surface immunoglobulin antigen receptors and become dedicated antibody factories only,

pumping out as much as 2,000 antibody molecules per second.

The relationship between the surface receptor and the specificity of a clone of T lymphocytes is more complex in that it does not involve secreted antibody that looks very much like the surface receptor. Rather, the immature T cell differentiates into one of several types of cells, primarily **helper T cells** or **cytotoxic T cells**, whose functions will be discussed later in this section.

Elimination of reactivity to self

Both B cells and T cells have mechanisms to generate over 10^8 or more different antibody

Isotype	Structure	Concentration in Serum, mg/m;	No. of Heavy Chain Domains	Distinguishing Feature or Functions
IgM	B cell	1.5	5	First in development and response
IgD	B cell	0.03	5	B-cell receptor
IgG		12.5	4	Opsonin, ADCC
IgE	Mast cell or basophil	0.00005	5	Allergic response
IgA	SC	0.05 3.5	4	In secretions (GALT)

B

FIGURE 19.9 — (continued) B. Structures and characteristics of various antibody subclasses. (Reproduced, with permission, from Ziegler HK, Nairn R (1994). Induced defenses of the body. In Schechter M, et al. (eds), Mechanisms of Microbial Disease, 2d ed. Baltimore, Williams & Wilkins, pp 125, 126.)

specificities. These specificities are represented in the antigen receptor that marks the surface of T and B cells. But since this set of specificities covers almost all possible antigens, it includes many that cross-react with self-antigens, which if not eliminated would result in immune attack on various organs. Thus, somehow there must be a means, very early in postnatal development, to identify and eliminate most of these self-reactive clones.

To accomplish this, T lymphocytes are "educated" in the **thymus**, an organ in the upper chest, early in the development of the immune system (see Figure 19.12). In effect, the 10 million specificities of antibodies and T-cell receptors are screened for any reactivity to self, with reactive clones eliminated.

Once this process of selection against self-reactive clones is complete, the thymus undergoes atrophy and degeneration. Although the precise pathway of maturation through the thymus remains to be sorted out, it seems likely that this involves changes in surface markers that allow the immune system to know when a clone has been "certified" as not being directed against self.

In the case of the B lymphocytes and antibody production, a system very similar to that of the thymus for T lymphocytes is found in the chicken, in the form of a gut organ called the bursa of Fabricius (this structure is the origin of the name "B cells"). No equivalent of the bursa is found in mammals, however, and it is assumed that the equivalent process occurs more diffusely through the

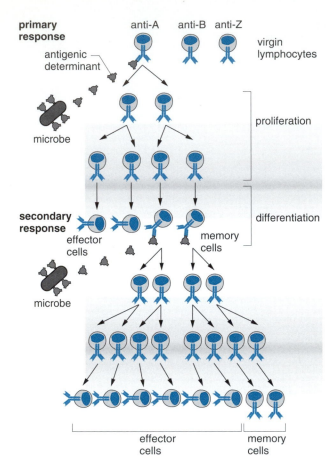

primary response

anti-A   anti-B   anti-Z

antigenic determinant

virgin lymphocytes

microbe

proliferation

secondary response

effector cells

differentiation

memory cells

microbe

effector cells

memory cells

FIGURE 19.10. Clonal selection. When an antigen is seen by the immune system, it binds to clones of lymphocytes with receptors for that antigen. This binding triggers those lymphocytes to proliferate and differentiate (the primary response). Some of those differentiated cells are effector cells that work to eliminate that antigen from the body, while other cells differentiate into memory cells that serve to keep the host in a state of readiness. Should the antigen reappear, the memory cells guarantee that the secondary response will be much more intense and more likely to eliminate the antigen quickly. Note that other lymphocytes with receptors that recognize other antigens (e.g., anti-B and anti-Z at the top of the figure) are not affected by the expansion and differentiation of anti-A cells. The role of antigen-presenting cells is omitted for simplicity. *(Adapted, with permission, from Ziegler HK, Nairn R (1994). Induced defenses of the body. In Schechter M, et al. (eds), Mechanisms of Microbial Disease, 2d ed. Baltimore, Williams & Wilkins, p 117.)*

lymphoid tissue of the GI tract and elsewhere.

T cells play a crucial role in regulation of the function of B cells. Thus, **T suppressor cells** may be able to attenuate or perhaps even terminate a B-cell response. This may be another means of eliminating reactivity to self. Regardless of the mechanisms, when the immune system does not react to a particular antigen, it is said to be **tolerant** of that antigen. These mechanisms of "self" education often result in tolerance.

FIGURE 19.11. *A.* Organization of immunoglobulin genes and generation of diversity. The gene rearrangements that occur during B-cell development and the response to antigen are depicted. DNA segments encoding individual portions of the mature protein are carried separately in the germ line DNA. These gene segments get rearranged in differentiated cells committed to expressing these genes. Once a variable-region gene segment is joined to a constant-region gene segment, the production of different isotypes of antibody allows the same antigen-binding region to be used for different functions. Genes are not drawn to scale, and many details are omitted. *B.* Generation of diversity. Schematic illustration of the mechanism by which a large number of unique immunoglobulin molecules are created (see text). *(Adapted, with permission, from Ziegler HK, Nairn R (1994).Induced defenses of the body. In Schechter M, et al. (eds), Mechanisms of Microbial Disease, 2d ed. Baltimore, Williams & Wilkins, pp 132, 133.)*

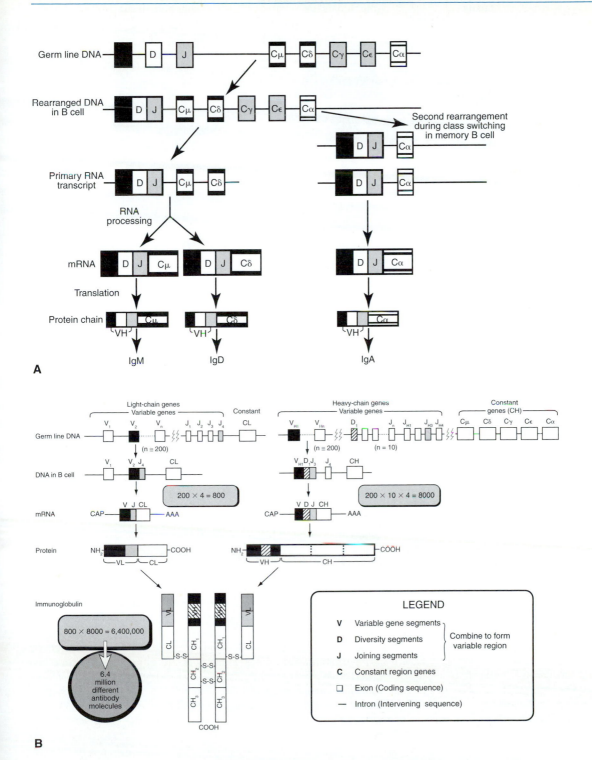

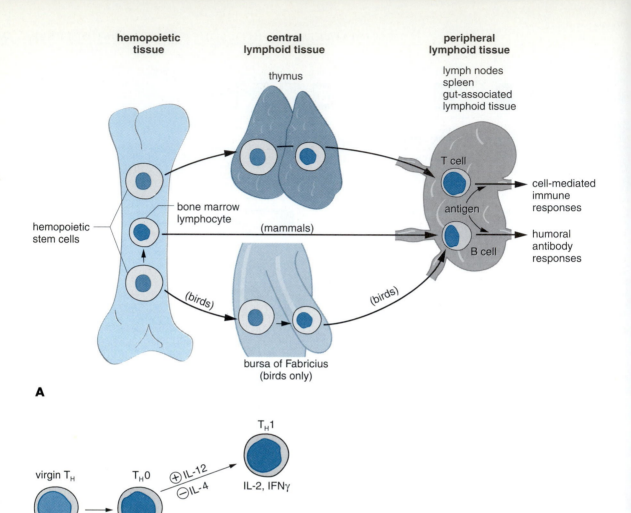

A

B

FIGURE 19.12. Lymphocyte development. *A.* Overall scheme. The development of functional T and B lymphocytes occurs in central or primary lymphoid organs, and the response to antigen takes place in peripheral or secondary lymphoid tissues. B and T lymphocytes have different pathways of development. *B.* Differentiation of helper T cells into T_H1 and T_H2 subsets. Upon initial activation, virgin helper T cells produce IL-2. In the presence of IL-2, a macrophage-derived cytokine, differentiation into T_H1 cells occurs. These cells produce IL-2 and interferon gamma and are effective at enhancing immune response involving phagocytes. In the presence of IL-4, differentiation into T_H2 cells occurs. These cells promote mast cell and eosinophil-mediated responses. Each class of helper T cell inhibits the development of the other. *(A Adapted, with permission, from Ziegler HK, Nairn R (1994). Induced defenses of the body. In Schechter M, et al. (eds). Mechanisms of Microbial Disease, 2d ed. Baltimore, Williams & Wilkins, p 117. B Adapted, with permission, from Stites DP, et al., 1997, Medical Immunology, 9th ed. Stamford, CT, Appleton & Lange, p. 140.)*

Review Questions

25. What are some common and distinctive features of T cells versus B cells?
26. What is the idea behind clonal selection?
27. How is antibody diversity generated?
28. How is reactivity to self normally prevented?

Humoral immunity

Humoral immunity refers to acquired immunity conferred by soluble secreted proteins, i.e., antibodies. The structure of antibody molecules has some distinctive features (see Figure 19.9):

• We have already discussed how various genes recombine to form the coding regions for the heavy and light chains, mixing possible binding sites in such a way that, when all is said and done, there is an antibody capable of reacting to just about anything.
    Because antibodies have two identical binding sites, they are said to be **bivalent**, that is, able to separately bind two copies of whatever antigen they are directed against.
• Despite being bivalent, antibody molecules are *asymmetric*, allowing different regions to perform different functions. In particular, each antibody molecule has, in addition to the variable regions of heavy and light chains that come together to form the antigen-binding "pocket," a region called the Fc region (see Figure 19.9A). Composed of the constant regions of the two heavy chains, the Fc region is responsible for consequences after antibody has bound antigen. It allows the antibody to target the antigen to different fates. Thus, in some cases, the Fc region binds to Fc receptors on the surface of phagocytes, thereby promoting disposal of the antibody-bound invader through phagocytosis.

Different classes of antibodies

Five different kinds of constant regions present in the germline can be used by the mechanisms of generating antibody diversity to build the final gene coding for an individual antibody heavy chain. Each of these **immunoglobulin (Ig) classes** or **isotypes** has a different physiological purpose. Within each class are a number of different subclasses that subserve more selective functions.

IgG antibodies

This is the major class of antibodies in the bloodstream, and the major antibodies represented in the secondary response. IgG consists of a single antibody dimer of two heavy chains, each of which is associated with a copy of (the same) light chain (see Figure 19.9). The several different subclasses of IgG differ in their ability to activate complement (IgG subclass 4 does not), bind Fc receptors (IgG subclasses 1 and 3 do), etc.

IgM antibodies

These are the antibodies generally made as the primary immune response. They form huge pentameric complexes of the standard dimeric antibody, readily activate complement, and promote cross linking of the antigen (see Figure 19.9B). Their large size keeps them in the bloodstream and generally out of tissues. The antigen receptor on B cells is a variant of IgM that is anchored as a dimeric integral membrane protein on the cell surface.

IgD antibodies

These are a quantitatively minor population of antibodies that are believed to play a role as a form of "mature" antigen receptor after certain B cells are beyond the stage where they can be educated as to what is or is not a "self" antigen. Their precise role in the immune response is not clear.

IgA antibodies

These are antibodies of the secretory immune system; they are made in massive quantities that are constantly being released into epithelial secretions. They have a distinctive structure consisting of two antibody dimers associated with a so-called J chain that facilitates assembly and a chain called the "secretory component" that protects IgA from degradation. IgA molecules undergo **transcytosis**, a form of endocytosis that moves individual IgA molecules from the bloodstream, where they are secreted by plasma cells, to the lumen of various epithelia (see Chap. 2). IgA antibodies are a key part of the defense of these highly vulnerable portals of entry into the body.

IgE antibodies

These antibodies are in the lowest concentration normally. They are responsible for allergic reactions, from relatively mild symptoms of "hay fever" to severe **anaphylaxis**. The basis for their involvement in allergic reactions is that certain white blood cells known as **basophils** and **mast cells** have high-affinity receptors for the IgE Fc regions. When IgE is bound, these white blood cells release histamine and other vasoactive substances that promote smooth-muscle contraction, leaking of fluid across capillaries, itching, and other allergic manifestations.

However, IgE also appears to be important in the defense against certain parasites. Eosinophils, the phagocytic cells specific for defense against parasitic infections, have receptors for IgE Fc regions on their surface. Some observers have suggested that susceptibility to allergies is the price we pay for a defense against parasites.

Cellular immunity

Cell-mediated immunity carried out by T cells differs from B-cell-directed antibody defenses in the following ways:

- A maturing T cell can become one of several subsets of cytotoxic T lymphocytes or T helper cells. In the case of B cells, the only terminally differentiated fate is that of an antibody-producing plasma cell.
- T cells recognize the antigen to which they are directed, on cell surfaces in the context of so-called **major histocompatibility complex (MHC) antigens**. The MHC antigens are proteins on the surface of most cells. These MHC antigens allow the immune system to know that the cell is part of "self" and to know if a "self" cell is infected with a virus or otherwise out of control, and therefore should be targeted for destruction. The T-cell antigen receptor is special in that it will recognize antigens only when they are on the surface of a cell and in the context of the correct MHC antigen. These restrictions as to where and when a T cell recognizes its antigen are not observed with B cells, whose receptors and antibody products recognize soluble or bound antigens by themselves, irrespective of MHC or other contexts.
- The developmental pathways are distinctive, with T cells being dependent on the thymus for maturation and differentiation, whereas B cells are not.
- Various other gene products participate in T-cell activation and differentiation. These appear not to be involved in B-cell maturation or function.
- The nature of the T cell antigen receptor, while being part of the immunoglobulin superfamily, is quite different from that of the antigen receptor on B cells. The B-cell antigen receptor is very similar to secreted antibody in structure. There is no secreted form of T-cell receptor, analogous to the way B

cells have antibodies that are similar to their antigen receptors.

Cytotoxic T lymphocytes

Cytotoxic T lymphocytes (CTLs) are the "pit bulls" of the T-cell response. They attack host cells that have been infected with viruses or that harbor intracellular bacteria, by recognizing the foreign antigen on the cell surface in the context of MHC antigens. There are multiple mechanisms by which CTLs kill their target cells. One recently elucidated mechanism is that CTLs (and natural killer cells; see the following discussion) release two important classes of secretory products, called **perforins** and **granzymes**. Perforins are proteases that punch holes in cells targeted by CTLs. Granzymes enter the cell through these holes, and at least one of their modes of action involves activation of apoptosis, resulting in death of the target cell from within. This kind of clever mechanism may explain why CTLs themselves are not damaged by their attack on infected cells and are able to survive and move on to carry out subsequent attacks on other infected cells.

Helper T cells

Helper T cells are classes of mature T cells that serve to stimulate the proliferation of both B cells and CTLs. Initially, when a helper T cell sees the antigen against which it is directed for the first time, it produces the cytokine IL-2 and differentiates into one of two classes of helper T cells, called T_H1 and T_H2. Each of these subsets of helper T cells makes a different array of cytokines that activate different aspects of the immune response that are particularly well suited for attacking one particular type of invader (see the following discussion). In addition to their role in regulation of B cells and CTLs, some helper T cells play an important role in acti-

vating macrophages, particularly their ability to phagocytose microbes and kill cancer cells.

Different subsets of helper T cells promote either cell-mediated or antibody-mediated immunity, in addition to promoting **isotype switching**, that is, expressing a particular antibody specificity in the form of, for example, an IgE antibody rather than as an IgG antibody. Thus, allergic reactions mediated by IgE typically involve the subset of helper T cells called T_H2 cells. Understanding helper T cell development may make immunomodulation (that is, rewiring the immune response from favoring T_H2 to favoring T_H1) possible as a treatment for certain allergic disorders in the future. However, it is overly simplistic to think of T_H2 as a "bad" immune response or of T_H1 as always "good." Some studies suggest that both T_H1 and T_H2 helper T cells contribute to the beta cell destruction in autoimmune diabetes mellitus, for example (see Ref. 10).

Suppressor T cells

The notion that there is a category of **suppressor T cells** that are analogous but opposite in action to helper T cells is controversial and poorly understood. Some workers believe that suppressor T cells decrease or extinguish many of the same activities that helper T cells serve to increase. Suppressor T cells do not use the same antigen receptor as do CTLs and helper T cells, yet their suppressor activities are antigen-specific.

Other lymphocyte subsets

In addition to B and T cells, there are subsets of lymphocytes that are called "null cells" because they have characteristics of neither. Some of these cells appear to be important for various antibody-dependent forms of cell lysis.

Macrophages

Macrophages have already been discussed as part of the innate immune system. However, as or more important than that constitutive role is their role in **antigen presentation**, the process by which the immune system is informed that an intruder has entered the body.

The collaboration between macrophages and T cells is complex. T cells elaborate cytokines that stimulate macrophage functions. Macrophages in turn not only process and present antigens to T cells, they also secrete cytokines.

Natural killer cells

Natural killer (NK) cells are an independent lineage of lymphocytes (see Figure 19.2), derived from a bone marrow stem cell precursor but distinguished from T cells by their ability to release granules and kill cells displaying certain antigens that the individual has never seen before (unlike cytotoxic T lymphocytes, which require prior sensitization for a good response). In molecular terms, NK cells have a distinctive set of receptors that distinguish them from T cells. NK cells make up about 15% of peripheral blood lymphocytes, most of the rest of which are T cells (75%) or B cells (10%). The precise role of NK cells in the web of host defenses remains poorly understood.

MHC antigens and antigen presentation

MHC antigens were first identified because of their importance in transplant survival — transplant recipients will reject tissue from an MHC-incompatible donor. It is believed, however, that the MHC antigens play a much broader role in cell-mediated immunity in terms of antigen presentation.

There are two broad forms of antigen presentation. One involves endogenous antigens, as occur in a virally infected cell. Small peptides derived from viral antigens associate with so-called MHC class I antigens in the endoplasmic reticulum and travel through the secretory pathway (see Chap. 2) to the cell surface. There the combination of viral peptides and MHC I antigens is recognized by the antigen receptor on specific T cells, including CTLs, to generate an immune response, culminating in the destruction of the virally infected cell.

A second form of antigen presentation involves exogenous antigens engulfed by a phagocyte (e.g., a macrophage), which first breaks antigens down and releases from them small peptides that bind to MHC class II antigens and travel to the cell surface for presentation to T lymphocytes. The T lymphocyte whose antigen receptor recognizes the foreign peptide is activated by this interaction, triggering a cell-mediated immune response.

Cytokines

Cytokines are secreted products that affect immune functions. The functions of cytokines include regulation of the growth, development, and activation of the immune system and mediation of the inflammatory response.

In some cases, cytokines are made by immune cells to affect other immune cells or to affect cells outside of the immune system. A good example is the effect of cytokines to increase MHC antigen exposure on the surface of macrophages, thereby boosting their capacity for antigen presentation.

In other cases, cytokines are made by nonimmunologic cells (e.g., the endothelial cells of capillary beds) to affect either immune or other nonimmune cells. A huge number of soluble mediators (over one hundred) have been identified that fulfill the criteria for being cytokines (see a partial list in Table 19.7). Many of them are local mediators of a paracrine or autocrine nature (see Chap. 3), but

TABLE 19.7 CYTOKINES

Human interleukins

Interleukins	Principal cell source	Principal effects
IL-1α and β	Macrophages, other APCs, other somatic cells	Costimulation of APCs and T cells B-cell growth and Ig production Acute-phase response of liver Phagocyte activation Inflammation and fever Hematopoiesis
IL-2	Activated T_H2 cells, T_C cells, NK cells	Proliferation of activated T cells NK and T_C cell functions B-cell proliferation and IgG2 expression
IL-3	T lymphocytes	Growth of early hematopoietic progenitors
IL-4	T_H2 cells, mast cells	B-cell proliferation, IgE expression, and class II MHC-expression T_H2- and T_C-cell proliferation and functions Eosinophil and mast cell growth and function Inhibition of monokine production
IL-5	T_H2 cells, mast cells	Eosinophil growth and function
IL-6	Activated T_H2 cells, APCs, other somatic cells	Synergistic effects with IL-1 or TNF Induces fever Acute-phase response of liver B-cell growth and Ig production
IL-7	Thymic and marrow stromal cells	T and B lymphopoiesis T_C-cell functions
IL-8	Macrophages, other somatic cells	Chemoattractant for neutrophils and T cells Angiogenic
IL-9	Cultured T cells	Some hematopoietic and thymopoietic effects
IL-10	Activated T_H2, CD8 T, and B lymphocytes, macrophages	Inhibition of cytokine production by T_H1 cells, NK cells, and APCs Promotion of B-cell proliferation and antibody responses Suppression of cellular immunity
IL-11	Stromal cells	Synergistic effects on hematopoiesis and thrombopoiesis
IL-12	B cells, macrophages	Proliferation and function of activated T_C and NK cells IFNγ production Promotes T_H1-cell induction; suppresses T_H2-cell functions Promotion of cell-mediated immune responses
IL-13	T_H2 cells	Mimics IL-4 effects
IL-14	T cells, B cells, tumor cells	Proliferation of activated B cells
IL-15	Epithelial cells, monocytes Nonlymphocytic cells	Mimics IL-2 effects
IL-16	CD8+ > CD4+ lymphocytes	Chemoattracts CD4+ cells (T cells, eosinophils and monocytes) Comitogenic for CD4+ T cells

TABLE 19.7   CYTOKINES (*continued*)

Human noninterleukin immunoregulatory cytokines

Interleukins	Principal cell source	Principal effects[a]
TNFα	Activated macrophages, other somatic cells	IL-1-like effects Vascular thrombosis and tumor necrosis
TNFβ	Activated $T_H 1$ cells	IL-1-like and TNF-like effects Development of peripheral lymphoid organs
IFNα and β	Macrophages; neutrophils, other somatic cells	Antiviral effects Induction of class I MHC on all somatic cells Activation of macrophages, NK cells, and "bystander" $CD8^+$ T cells
IFNγ	Activated $T_H 1$ and NK cells	Induction of class I MHC on all somatic cells Induction of class II MHC on APCs and somatic cells Activation of macrophages, neutrophils, and NK cells Promotion of cell-mediated immunity (inhibits $T_H 2$ cells) Induction of high endothelial venules Antiviral effects
TGFβ	Activated T lymphocytes, platelets, macrophages, other somatic cells	Anti-inflammatory (suppression of cytokine production and class II MHC expression) Antiproliferative for myelomonocytic cells and lymphocytes Promotion of B-cell expression of IgA Promotion of fibroblast proliferation and wound healing

[a]All of the listed processes are enhanced unless otherwise indicated.
ABBREVIATIONS: IL = interleukin; Ig = immunoglobulin; APC = antigen-presenting cell; NK = natural killer; IFN = interferon; TNF = tumor necrosis factor; MHC = major histocompatibility complex; TGF = transforming growth factor.
First part of table reproduced, with permission, from Oppenheim JJ, Ruschetti FW (1997). Cytokines. In Stites DP et al. (eds), *Medical Immunology*, 9th ed. Stamford, CT, Appleton & Lange, pp. 147 & 148.

some also have more classical endocrine functions (e.g., action at a distance via the bloodstream). Many cytokines appear redundant in that they partially or completely mimic each other's activities and have effects on many different cell types. As with other local mediators, our understanding of what cytokines do and how they do it is extremely rudimentary, as is our understanding of the adaptive purpose of particular patterns of cytokine secretion.

Like that of other mediators (see Chap. 3), the action of cytokines occurs through receptors. Since these receptors may result in different outcomes depending on the signaling mechanism they are connected to, cytokines can have different effects depending on the cell type they reach.

Families of cytokines and their receptors

In general, cytokines can be grouped as being:

- Immunoregulatory, by virtue of their effect on the activation and differentiation of peripheral lymphocytes and monocytes. Examples of immunoregulatory cytokines are interleukin (IL)-2, IL-4, and transforming growth factor (TGF)β.
- Proinflammatory, based on their production by phagocytes in response to specific infectious agents. Examples of proinflammatory

cytokines are IL-1, IL-6, tumor necrosis factor (TNF) α, and the chemokine family.

• Maturational, due to their effects on the growth and development of immature white blood cells (e.g., in the bone marrow). Examples of maturational cytokines are IL-3, IL-7, and granulocyte-macrophage colony stimulating factor (GM-CSF).

Through the action of cytokines, various signaling pathways get turned on or off in the target cells, resulting in new patterns of cell surface protein expression and new effector functions that literally expand the size and complexity of the immune system to mind-boggling levels of complexity.

The basis for these effects is signal transduction via five broad families of cytokine receptors (see Figure 19.13). Each member of these families activates distinctive protein kinases or transcription factors in signaling cascades that define, through distinctive patterns of gene expression, the specific cell type's complexity. Given our current less than rudimentary understanding of both the concepts and the details of this process, it is easy to understand why immunologic diseases are some of the most frustrating and challenging disorders to understand or treat.

Review Questions

29. Antibody molecules have the characteristic of being individually bivalent and asymmetrical. What is the significance of these features?

30. Describe the structure of an IgG versus an IgM antibody.

31. Name five ways in which cell-mediated immunity differs from antibody-mediated immunity.

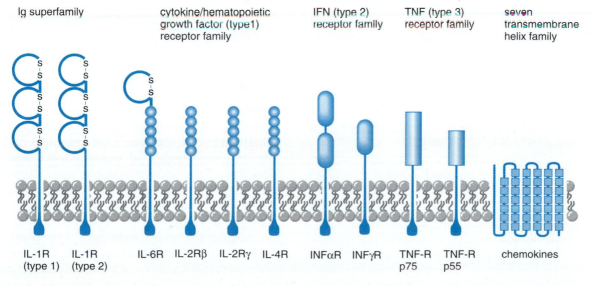

FIGURE 19.13. Families of cytokine receptors. Segregation of cytokine receptors into families is based on similarities in their amino acid sequence and structure. Each family has many members. Specificity of a response to cytokines is determined not only by the cytokine(s) that are present but also by the receptors that are available for them to bind to. (Adapted, with permission, from Haynes BS, Fauci AS (1998). Introduction to the immune system. In Fauci AS, et al. (eds), Harrison's Textbook of Internal Medicine, 14th ed. New York, McGraw-Hill, p 1760.)

32. What are the three subsets of mature T lymphocytes?

33. What is the difference between MHC class I and class II antigen presentation?

34. What are cytokines, who makes them, and what are three categories of functions they perform?

4. HOST DEFENSE HOMEOSTASIS

Regulation of the normal immune response

Host defenses are normally called upon in a highly regulated, fine-tuned manner:

First, white blood cells are attracted to sites where foreign antigens to which they are sensitive have been found.

Second, these antigens are recognized by various specific and nonspecific mechanisms, and complement is activated.

Third, the immune response is directed into one or more of the many possible pathways, and the chosen pathways are amplified to the extent appropriate by cytokines, microbial antigens, and other substances.

Finally, various classes of immune cells arrive on different time scales with a program to kill and then clean up the mess.

Normally, these immune responses are regulated in a number of ways:

- The lifespan of terminally differentiated immune cells is short. A plasma cell, for example, lives for only a few days. Thus the immune response to any individual antigen is self-limited.
- Nonspecific phagocytic cells are constantly engulfing, sequestering, and degrading antigens, thereby removing the very stimuli that set off the immune response.
- Soluble antibodies can occupy all available antigens and thereby cease the stimulation of antigen receptors on the surface of B cells that would otherwise be a continuing trigger to B-cell differentiation into plasma cells.
- Fc receptors on B cells appear to function as a sort of "off signal" that counters the "on signal" mediated by the antigen receptor. Thus, somewhere in the course of the immune response, the equilibrium shifts from expansion to termination.
- Helper T cells regulate the immune response directly, and also through cytokines.
- Antibodies can themselves serve as antigens such that specific antibodies are elicited to the specific binding sites of other specific antibodies. Such antibody-specific antibodies are termed **idiotypes**. The **network theory of immune regulation** proposes that the immune system is in a sort of dynamic equilibrium between antibodies, antibodies to antibodies, antibodies to antibodies to antibodies, etc. (see Figure 19.14). The introduction of a foreign antigen upsets this balance, which is ultimately reestablished and serves to keep the levels of antibodies to antigens that are not physically present at a low level.

Immunodeficiency

A defect in any of the many mechanisms that are part of the immune response, or that participate in boosting the immune response, results in some degree of **immunodeficiency**. Sometimes immunodeficiency is mild, transient, or extremely selective. Other times it is severe or persistent or involves many antigens or antigens that are seen commonly. **Acquired immunodeficiency syndrome** (AIDS), for example, results from a severe

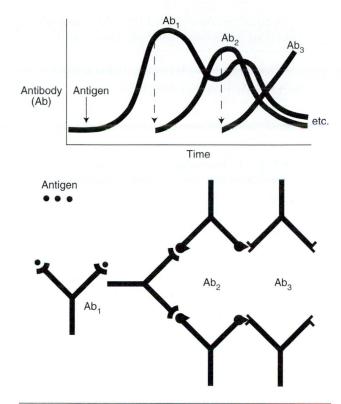

Ab$_1$, directed against antigenic determinant (epitope)
Ab$_2$, directed against idiotypic determinant (idiotope) of Ab$_1$
Ab$_3$, directed against idiotope of Ab$_2$

FIGURE 19.14. Network theory of antibody homeostasis. The top of the figure illustrates that after exposure to an antigen, the body generates an immune response. When that response reaches a high concentration, it is sensed by the immune system and an antibody is made against the variable region of the first set of antibodies. This lowers the amount of the first antibody in solution until an antibody is made to the second, which lowers its concentration and allows the concentration of the first antibody to rise in parallel with the rise in concentration of the antibody against the antibody. Thus the full immune response in an animal is an incredibly complex collection of individual antibodies, including some that dampen each other. How the host integrates all of this information with the needs of the body at any given time is not known. *(Reproduced, with permission, from Ziegler HK, Nairn R (1994). Induced defenses of the body. In Schechter M, et al. (eds), Mechanisms of Microbial Disease, 2d ed. Baltimore, Williams & Wilkins, p 145.)*

immunodeficiency: a lack of helper T cells due to the fact that human immunodeficiency virus (HIV) targets helper T cells for infection via the the distinctive CD4 antigen on their surface. Eventually these cells are killed by the viral infection and the ability of the host to mount an immune response is impaired, resulting in increased susceptibility to the infections that occur in AIDS patients. The normal immune response, which is greatly dependent on CD4+ helper cells, would have prevented these from occurring.

A more selective example of immunodeficiency is the observation that the elderly and individuals who lack a spleen (a key immunologic organ) are at greater risk of pneumococcal pneumonia and hence benefit from vaccination to boost their antibody levels in advance of attack by these organisms.

Finally, it has been observed that individuals may not mount a full immune response to vaccinations given when they are concurrently taking drugs to prevent malaria infection. It is believed that the drugs to prevent malaria infection are also altering in subtle ways the pathways of antigen processing in immune cells. Thus, the normal mechanism by which we respond to immunization may be impaired.

Autoimmunity and hypersensitivity

Conversely, the immune response can be excessive or inappropriately directed against host antigens. As a result of either an excess of normal processes or develement of abnormal ones, host damage can occur.

Autoimmunity

Current concepts, such as the basis for generation of antibody diversity and the network theory, suggest that self vs. nonself discrimination is not an all-or-none response. There are non-host antigens that can look like host antigens under certain circumstances, and there are host antigens that can mimic nonself antigens under certain circumstances. There are probably mechanisms in place to prevent or attenuate certain inappropriate responses. With particular genes, particular exposures, other complicating conditions, and age, any or several of these mechanisms can get out of control, resulting in autoimmune disorders. As with disorders of immunodeficiency, these are not all-or-none conditions, but rather include some that are mild and others that are severe.

Some intracellular host antigens may have never been seen by the immune system, and hence, tolerance was never established. Thus, when injury or illness exposes these antigens, or when the mechanism to actively prevent response to them is impaired, autoimmunity may sometimes result. In other cases, drugs or environmental agents can modify a host antigen to make it look more "foreign" and hence trigger an inappropriate immune response. This immune response may then recognize and react with the native, nonmodified host antigen causing an autoimmune disease.

Hypersensitivity responses

Hypersensitivity responses, also called allergic reactions, are inappropriate secondary immune responses in individuals previously exposed to an antigen (i.e., who have mounted a primary immune response). There are four types of hypersensivity responses, the first three of which are antibody-mediated and the last cell mediated (see Figure 19.15):

- **Type I (immediate) hypersensitivity** is the result of IgE-class antibody binding antigen and then binding to mast cell Fc receptors, with the subsequent release of histamine and other allergic mediators. This includes processes at work in allergic asthma, hay fever, urticaria, and anaphylaxis to insect venoms. It is under the genetic control of the MHC class II genes, which is one reason why some individuals are more susceptible than others.
- **Type II (cytotoxic hypersensitivity)** is due to cell lysis upon antibody binding. It can be complement-mediated or mediated by cytotoxic T lymphocytes. **Transfusion reactions** and **hemolytic anemias** caused by reactions to certain drugs are good examples.
- **Type III (immune-complex-mediated hypersensitivity)** results from immune complex deposition in certain tissues, with complement-mediated cell lysis. This leads to disruption of organ system function and fever. The joints and the kidneys are particularly prominent sites of involvement. Often these types of reactions occur in chronic infections (e.g., by hepatitis B virus, various parasites, etc.).
- **Type IV (delayed hypersensitivity)** occurs 24 to 48 h after antigen exposure. It occurs as a consequence of T-cell activation, cytokine secretion, and a subsequent influx of activated macrophages. Poison ivy reactions and tuberculin skin test reactions are good examples of this form of hypersensitive immune response. **Granuloma formation** in diseases such as TB, histoplasmosis, and lep-

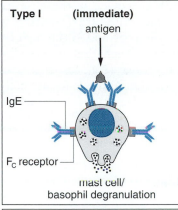

Type I   (immediate)

antigen

IgE

F$_C$ receptor

mast cell/
basophil degranulation

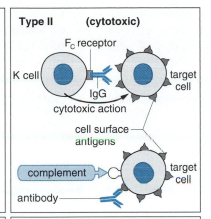

Type II   (cytotoxic)

F$_C$ receptor

K cell

target
cell

IgG
cytotoxic action

cell surface
antigens

complement

target
cell

antibody

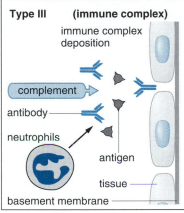

Type III   (immune complex)

immune complex
deposition

complement

antibody

neutrophils

antigen

tissue

basement membrane

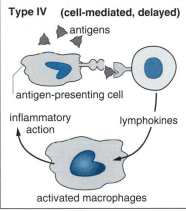

Type IV   (cell-mediated, delayed)

antigens

antigen-presenting cell

inflammatory
action

lymphokines

activated macrophages

FIGURE 19.15. Hypersensitivity responses. These reactions are secondary responses to antigens that occur in an exaggerated or inappropriate form. The responses to different pathogens are observed to favor different inflammatory reactions (see text). *(Adapted, with permission, from Ziegler HK, Nairn R (1994). Induced defenses of the body. In Schechter M, et al. (eds), Mechanisms of Microbial Disease, 2nd ed. Baltimore, Williams & Wilkins, p 148.)*

rosy is an example of a delayed hypersensitivity response.

Immune regulation and natural selection

Why the immune system chooses to go down one path rather than another remains quite mysterious. A more host-destructive response would be desirable if the alternative were that the host would succumb to the invader. On the other hand, if antibiotics and other means of controlling a pathogen are effective, as is often the case today, the milder immune response might be more desirable. However, which course is more desirable could change with time especially if a pathogen gained the upper hand through antibiotic resistance or other mechanisms.

Clinical Pearls

○ In assessing the possibility of serious infection in a patient who has a fever but no obvious localizing signs (e.g., of an abcess), examination of a sample of peripheral blood is often helpful. An elevated white blood count with a predominance of neutrophils, combined with a "shift to the left" reflecting the appearance of not quite completely mature cells, are key findings. These suggest that there is an ongoing bacterial infection sufficiently severe to have called upon the bone marrow to generate a massive outpouring of neutrophils. The importance of the immature forms is that it indicates that the neutrophils present in the bloodstream reflect new cells generated in the bone marrow, not simply old cells that have "demarginated" and left sites on the endothelium to return to the circulation (e.g., as occurs in response to pharmacologic doses of steroids or epinephrine even in the absence of bacterial or other antigens).

○ The spleen is an immunologic organ in which antibodies are produced by B cells and in which large numbers of opsonized bacteria are removed. Lack of a spleen (e.g., due to loss of the spleen following trauma or infarction, as occurs in patients with sickle cell anemia) creates a defect in immune regulation that predisposes to certain severe infections where the normal host defense is particularly dependent on B cell-mediated soluble antibody immunity. In particular, these patients are at high risk of infections with the bacteria *Streptococcus pneumoniae* and the parasite *Babesia.* To protect against the former, all patients without a spleen or with a disease such as sickle cell anemia that will inevitably infarct the spleen should receive vaccination. To protect against the latter, areas where babesiosis is endemic (e.g., Cape Cod, Massachusetts) should be avoided by these individuals.

○ High concentrations of peripheral blood monocytes are seen in certain infections, including TB, lysteriosis, Rocky Mountain spotted fever, malaria, and visceral leischmaniasis. The pathophysiological reasons for this are uncertain.

○ Some infections in some locations are distinctive in that it appears that the host immune response is responsible for far more severe damage than the organism per se. In part this may reflect the fact that the host response evolved in the absence of antibiotics and other treatments. Today, the added help provided the host by these modalities is such that dampening the immune response (e.g., by treatment with steroids) has been shown to distinctly improve the outcome in diseases such as tuberculous meningitis and *Pneumocystis carinii* pneumonia.

Review Questions

35. What are six ways in which the immune response can be regulated?
36. What is immunodeficiency, and what are three different ways in which it can occur?
37. Suggest two different ways in which autoimmunity can develop all of a sudden in an adult who has not had a previous manifestation of autoimmune disease.
38. Describe the four classes of hypersensitivity reactions and give an example of each.

5. HOST-PATHOGEN INTERACTIONS

Host defense exists to prevent infection and other potential sources of demise of the organism. Pathogens, in turn, respond to these defenses with countermeasures selected for their contribution to overcoming host defenses. This "arms race" between host and pathogen continues to this day. In this section we will briefly consider some of the general mechanisms by which hosts and pathogens attempt to overcome or bolster defenses.

Altered receptor recognition

At the outset of this chapter, the point was made that receptors are generally necessary in order for infection to occur. Thus, a pathogen with an altered surface ligand that promotes binding or internalization will probably have higher rates of infection, survival, and reproduction than pathogens with the non-mutated ligand. For example, mutation of a co-receptor that is needed for optimal HIV infection of patients appears to explain the marked resistance of some individuals to HIV infection.

Blocking complement action

A wide range of strategies have been employed by pathogens to overcome complement and other nonspecific destructive factors of the innate immune system:

- Some pathogenic bacteria, such as strains of *Staphylococcus aureus,* are covered with a capsule that masks their complement-activating surface components. In this way, they evade the alternative pathway of complement activation.
- *Meningococcus* promotes its success by somehow managing to get itself coated with the host's IgA antibodies. These antibodies cannot activate complement and also prevent binding of those antibody classes that can activate complement.
- Some strains of bacteria (called gram-negative because of the staining characteristics of their cell surface to Gram's stain) such as salmonella and *Escherichia coli* contain long sugar side chains on their surface that prevent the complement attack complex from getting to the membrane.
- The herpes simplex virus envelope glycoprotein binds complement component C3b, thereby inhibiting activation of complement through the alternative pathway. Small-pox virus, on the other hand, secretes a protein homologous to complement component C4b, and thereby interferes with complement activation through the classical pathway (see Figure 19.6).
- Older individuals of the parasite *Schistosoma mansonii* are more resistant to com-

plement-mediated lysis than young parasites because they have managed to incorporate into their membrane copies of a host protein, called decay accelerating factor, that normally prevents host cells from inadvertently activating the complement cascade.

Resistance to phagocytosis

The importance of phagocytosis in host defense is revealed by the extent to which organisms are willing to go to evade or subvert this host defense mechanism:

- By blocking complement activation, pathogens evade phagocytosis. This is because key activated complement components serve as opsonins, products that improve the efficiency of phagocytosis. Without those opsonins, phagocytosis of certain pathogens is extremely difficult. Furthermore, products released from the pathogen by the complement fixation reaction serve as chemotaxins that attract a horde of phagocytes to ensure that the invader is engulfed.
- Some pathogens paralyze neutrophils by releasing toxins that inhibit neutrophil and monocyte mobility and chemotaxis. This is the mechanism of action of a toxin from *Bordetella pertussis,* the agent responsible for whooping cough. This agent actually makes several toxins that work in different ways.
- Some pathogens fight phagocytes directly, synthesizing leukocidins, proteins that kill the phagocytes (both neutrophils and macrophages) before they can kill the pathogen. Some of the most highly invasive bacterial pathogens, including *Pseudomonas,* group A streptococci, and the *Clostridia* that cause gas gangrene, are examples of leukocidin producers.
- Some invasive strains of *staphylococci* make a protein called protein A that binds the Fc portion of antibodies, which is normally used to promote phagocytosis.

- Some bacteria, including *gonococci, meningococci, haemophilus*, and pathogenic dental *streptococci*, secrete proteases that partly or completely degrade IgA, allowing them to overcome this key line of epithelial defense.
- A particularly clever strategy with many variations is to allow the phagocyte to ingest the bacterium, but then impair the phagocyte's ability to kill, so that the bacterium can grow and reproduce inside the neutrophil, in a protected space. Some parasites, such as the trypanosome that causes Chagas' disease and the rickettsiae of Rocky Mountain spotted fever, manage to escape from the phagosome to the cytoplasm prior to fusion with the lysosome. In the case of rickettsiae, coating of the microbe with antibodies inhibits its ability to escape from the phagosome, suggesting that the rickettsiae must have a receptor for this purpose. The microbes that cause tuberculosis, psittacosis, and Legionnaire's disease manage to block fusion of the phagosome with lysosomes and then proceed to replicate within the phagosome. Leischmania and other parasites are simply resistant to the action of lysosomal enzymes or secrete inhibitors that block these enzymes. Furthermore, these organisms can thrive in extremely acidic (as low as pH 4) environments. Finally, some organisms poison the oxidative mechanism by either breaking down hydrogen peroxide as fast as it is produced or inhibiting the pathway by which high concentrations of reactive oxygen molecules are generated in the phagocyte.

Immune suppression

The most dramatic example of infection-associated immunosuppression is that of HIV resulting in AIDS. This virus manages to secure itself a niche by its ability to use the CD4 antigen on a crucial subset of T lymphocytes as its receptor for entry. The infected cells are killed by the virus, resulting in an immune system-crippling state — which contributes to the ability of the virus to persist.

More subtle examples of immunosuppression by infectious agents have been recognized. For example, tuberculosis is much more common following measles outbreaks, suggesting that measles virus infection is immunosuppressive in a way that increases the risk of developing TB. It seems that for a period of time subsequent to measles infection, B cells decrease antibody production and T cells display impaired delayed hypersensitivity.

In other cases, infecting pathogens suppress the cytokine responses of infected cells. Thus, in the protozoal infection leischmaniasis, an inappropriate cytokine response is believed to be why infected macrophages fail to be appropriately activated or make MHC class I and II products (see Sec. 2), which would otherwise have triggered inflammatory events that would have eradicated the infection.

Immune evasion

In some cases, pathogens evade the immune system without suppressing it. For example, the parasite *Trypanosoma brucei* changes its surface coat more quickly than the host can mount an immune response. Thus the antibody response against the pathogen is never appropriate for the antigen being displayed on the cell surface at that time.

Another approach to immune evasion is simply to lie low until things quiet down. Thus viral latency is the tendency of some viruses to integrate into the genome and lie dormant for extended periods of time, perhaps awaiting a more opportune time to reactivate and once again produce disease. Such times might include windows of relative immune deficiency that might occur as a consequence of other infections or even simple old age.

Manipulation of host signaling pathways

A final observation that is probably relevant to overcoming host defenses is that some bacteria appear to manipulate host signaling pathways. Thus certain virulent strains of *H. pylori*, the bacteria implicated in the development of peptic ulcer disease, make products that appear to have effects on signaling within epithelial cells. The connection between these effects on host signaling and microbe survival is not yet known. Presumably, in some as yet not understood way, these manipulations impair host defense. However, what makes these observations of special interest is that these strains of pathogen are associated with higher incidence of GI tract malignancies, suggesting that a consequence of this manipulation, whether intended by the pathogen or not, is an increased incidence of malignant transformation (see Sec. 6, Frontiers).

Clinical Pearl

○ Knowledge of the mechanisms by which parasites block host defense can be the basis for novel therapeutic approaches. For example, the knowledge that *Leishmania* prevent appropriate cytokine responses suggested that recombinant interferon gamma might promote macrophage activation and thereby enhance patient response to other drugs in visceral leishmaniasis. This actually works!

Review Questions

39. Name six general strategies used by pathogens to evade host defenses.
40. Describe five ways in which pathogens counter complement.

41. Describe five ways in which pathogens avoid destruction by phagocytosis.
42. Give one example (other than HIV and AIDS) of pathogen-mediated immune suppression.
43. Give one example each of two very different means of immune evasion.
44. What is a possible consequence of *H. pylori* manipulation of host signaling pathways?

6. FRONTIERS IN HOST DEFENSE

Limitations of the arms race analogy for host-pathogen interaction

It is often appealing to think of the struggle for survival between the host and potential pathogens as one of an arms race in which the development of a defense raises the selection pressure in favor of developing a new variant of offense that evades the defense, etc. For example, the development of antibiotic resistance is often best conceptualized in this way. However, recent studies in plants suggest that a deeper understanding of host-pathogen interactions may be needed, at least in some cases (see Ref. 11). Contrary to the arms race model, it appears that a dynamic variation in disease susceptibility and resistance genes has been maintained for millions of years in these plants. The authors of this study suggest an alternative "trench warfare" hypothesis to explain the findings. One interpretation might be that some disease susceptibility genes confer selective advantages that are not currently appreciated. Perhaps poorly understood changes in the environment result in a see-saw effect in which the balance may tip one way or the other over time, but not enough to eliminate the susceptibility gene.

Integrins and selectins in host defense

Selectins and **integrins** are cell surface receptors that bring about cell movement and ad-

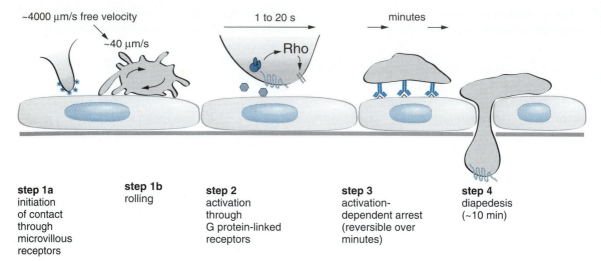

step 1a
initiation
of contact
through
microvillous
receptors

step 1b
rolling

step 2
activation
through
G protein-linked
receptors

step 3
activation-
dependent arrest
(reversible over
minutes)

step 4
diapedesis
(~10 min)

FIGURE 19.16. Neutrophil interactions with the endothelium. Neutrophils, also called polymorphonuclear leukocytes (PMNs), interact with the endothelium in ways that allow them to either roll, attach, or migrate across the cell layer. The nature of these selectin-carbohydrate interactions promotes rolling. However, when inflammation is triggered, the PMNs are activated by exposure to the appropriate cytokines. This results in changes in selectins and their ligands such that the PMNs stop rolling and are localized to the site of inflammation. Further changes in receptors on the cell surface promote migration across the endothelium so that the activated PMNs can enter the fray.

hesion while also regulating signal transduction pathways within cells (see Figure 19.16). These and other families of adhesive proteins are crucial for immune cell recruitment to particular sites and for movement across capillary walls during inflammation (see Table 19.3 and Ref. 12). In brief, selectin-selectin interactions between neutrophils and endothelial cells bring about "rolling" of cells along the endothelium. The effect of cytokines is to convert these interactions into more stable attachments to particular sites on the endothelium involving other families of adhesive proteins. In response to inflammatory mediators, the integrin expression on the neutrophils or on endothelial cells changes, making possible the movement of neutrophils across the endothelium into tissues, where they can do battle with invaders. These changes in the adhesive state of im-

mune cells involve signal transduction-mediated regulation of adhesiveness and complex interactions between many different gene products on the immune cells and the endothelium. Given their central role in immune cell dynamics, it is not surprising that these adhesion molecules should be a tempting target for both sides in the ongoing war between the host and the pathogen. Recent studies have revealed some new examples in both directions.

In the mid 1990s, a number of highly lethal cases of a pulmonary distress syndrome associated with low platelet counts occurred in the southwestern United States. Subsequent study implicated hantavirus, an enveloped virus known to infect rodents, in the human disease. Now work has shown that the infecting hantavirus achieves access to human cells by using as its receptor a specific integrin that is found in high concentrations on respiratory epithelia and platelets (see Ref. 13). The virus seems to interact with the integrins in a more complex manner than some previously defined integrin interactions, which appear to be based on recognition of a simple three-amino-acid residue motif, arginine-glycine-aspartic acid. Furthermore, even cells whose specific integrin is physiologically defective are capable of being infected, suggesting that the virus targets some feature of the integrin distinct from those identified as necessary for *physiological* cell adhesive functions. This work will now set the stage for future attempts to identify the specific binding site and suggests ways in which entry of the virus might be blocked without disrupting integrin function in respiratory or platelet physiology.

The ability of microbes to go from benign bystanders to invasive pathogens is due to a complex interactions of many factors. A surprising recent finding was that a single gene in the fungus *Candida albicans* appears to control adhesion, filamentous growth (a form associated with pathogenicity), and virulence. This gene was noted to have limited similarities to vertebrate integrins, suggesting some possible mechanisms by which the pathogen uses this product to have its way. The fact that this gene is nevertheless quite divergent from host integrins raises the hope that it will be possible to develop drugs that interfere with its function without disrupting essential functions of host integrins (see Ref. 14).

In another study, the role of two different adhesive proteins, called E selectins and P selectins, present on endothelial cells, in the recruitment of eosinophils as part of allergic reactions was studied (see Ref. 15). Recruitment of eosinophils into mouse skin in response to one of two different types of allergic reaction was shown to be dependent on the combination of E and P selectins, as demonstrated by blockage of the reaction by specific monoclonal antibodies. In the case of other allergic reactions, neither E nor P selectins appeared necessary for the recruitment to occur. An antibody to a specific integrin appeared to block both types of allergic reaction. The pattern of adhesive molecules responsible for various allergic reactions should be further resolvable, and small molecules that mimic the interfering effect of antibodies may be identifiable. This and similar studies raise the hope that in the near future it will be possible to selectively block or attenuate subsets of the inflammatory response involved in allergic reactions.

The innate immune system in health and disease

Changes in scientific thinking are driven by both new ideas and new data (see Chap. 1). One example in progress is the way our thinking about the innate immune system continues to evolve. Innate immunity is found even in procaryotes, in whom restriction endonucleases provide a constitutive means of cleaving nonself DNA. Acquired immunity, however, is a development of the last 400 million years found only in cartilaginous and bony fish, amphibians, reptiles, birds, and mammals. It was at one point thought that the innate immune system, being more "primitive," was a less important line of defense. Subsequently it was recognized that this system is still crucial to well-being of the human host, and in some ways is more important than acquired immunity. More recently the "wisdom of evolution" is seen in the realization that the acquired immune system has been interfaced with the innate immune system in the course of evolution (see Ref. 16). Thus, it appears that innate immune components help the acquired system decide the direction in which the immune response ought to proceed (e.g., cell-mediated, T_H1-dependent responses versus antibody-mediated, T_H2-dependent responses) in order to eliminate a particular type of pathogen.

Unfortunately, a complex chain creates the potential for new weak links, and hence, these very features of immunity that make it richer and more sophisticated than one might have imagined are the potential basis for disease. For example, some recent findings suggest that pathogens have exploited the essential nature of innate and acquired immune communication to their own ends (see Ref. 17).

Perhaps a more surprising example is the finding that metabolic syndromes, including those involved in the pathogenesis of diabetes mellitus, appear directly related to disordered innate immunity in the form of the acute-phase response (see Ref. 18). It will be crucial to better understand the basis for this overlap between metabolic disease and host defense. Is it an unfortunate consequence of one set of signals and effectors (e.g., in this case cytokines and lipoproteins) being used for two different purposes (e.g., for both regulation of substrates and for host defense), with the two sometimes working at cross purposes? Or is there is a more profound connection? Apart from the excitement that always accompanies new avenues of investigation, these findings serve to remind us how little we really know about our genes and their relationship to disease.

Vaginal ecology as host defense

The notion that the endogenous microbial flora represents a distinctive line of host defense has already been raised in Chapter 5 and at the outset of this chapter. Recent work suggests that there is a connection between loss of normal vaginal microbial flora and increased susceptibility to heterosexual transmission of HIV disease (see Refs. 20, 21). It appears that normal vaginal microbes include enormous numbers of hydrogen peroxide-producing lactobacilli which maintain a highly toxic environment for a number of pathogens, including HIV. Thus, a change to a non-lactobacillus vaginal microflora may not only be responsible for low-grade bacterial and fungal infections but also increase the risk of HIV infection. Normalizing female microbial flora may be an important non-pharmacologic basis for enhancing HIV resistance. This is another good example of how a pharmacologically driven focus of medicine may overlook simple and inexpensive ways of health maintenance through reestablishment of homeostasis. Diet and lifestyle-based intervention toward this goal are especially important in the developing countries, where the spread of HIV is rampant and resources for drug therapy are negligible.

Immunization against Alzheimer's disease?

Despite important progress in understanding many of its features, both the normal physiological function and the fundamental pathologic mechanism involved in Alzheimer's disease remain a matter of speculation (see Chap. 18). In particular, it has been debated whether amyloid plaques composed of β amyloid peptide, which are found in the brain in Alzheimer's disease, are a cause or simply a consequence of the pathologic process. Recently it was found that immunization of mice with partially purifed β amyloid peptide results in disappearance of CNS plaques and prevention of injury in a strain of mice that develop plaques similar to those observed in Alzheimer's disease (see Ref. 22). It remains to be seen whether application of this approach to humans will actually prevent Alzheimer's disease — without causing something else just as bad. While understanding a process is wonderful, more often than not, clinicians are thankful when (hopefully) something they have done has helped to make the patient better, whether or not the physiology or pathophysiology of the process is understood.

7. HOW DOES NORMAL PHYSIOLOGY PROVIDE INSIGHT INTO THE INITIAL CASE PRESENTATION?

Wall tension resulting from an overly full bladder can result in ischemia of tissues, which in turn seems to predispose to infection. Which mechanisms of host defense are being impaired by ischemia is not exactly clear.

Host tissues are formidable barriers to invasion, in part because even the potential portals of entry, such as the mucous membranes of the urogenital tract, are constantly bathed in IgA and other defensive secretions. The introduction of an indwelling Foley provides a foreign body on which bacteria can colonize and spread into the bladder. The use of antibiotics will fail to eradicate these invaders and instead will select for antibiotic-resistant species.

With severe underlying defects relevant to immunity, as is the case in this individual with a neurogenic bladder, frequent intermittent catheterization is far superior to an indwelling Foley in that it allows emptying of the bladder and prevention of excessive bladder distention and ischemia, without the risks of infection posed by a constantly present foreign body. This story is a reminder that antibiotics only serve as an adjunct to host defense mechanisms and cannot substitute for them.

You can explain to Mr. F. that the indwelling Foley catheter bypasses his body's barriers to the entry of bacteria and provides a safe haven on which bacteria can grow and eventually spread. The resistant organisms are a consequence of the selection pressure from frequent antibiotic use. Attempting to eliminate the colonization by a change of antibiotics will probably not prevent him from developing another urinary tract infection and will increase the chance that such a subsequent infection will have an even broader spectrum of antibiotic resistance than previously. Avoiding indwelling Foley catheters, avoiding bladder distention, thorough intermittent catheterization (i.e., using sterile technique to insert the catheter three times a day to empty his bladder and then right away removing the catheter), and enhancing his immune functions through good nutrition and avoidance of severe stress will be far more helpful.

SUMMARY AND REVIEW OF KEY CONCEPTS

1. Given how harsh the world is, it is amazing that we survive at all. Recent human history represents the greatest shift ever in the battle with pathogens in favor of the host. However, the struggle is not over — and probably never will be. Either natural or human-made catastrophes or the gradual power of natural selection aided and abetted by irresponsible human actions may well turn the tide against us in the future.

2. There are five broad lines of host defense: (1) external barriers (mechanical, environmental, anatomic); (2) innate immunity; (3) acquired immunity; (4) intracellular defenses, including stress proteins; and (5) systemic, immune-dampening mechanisms such as the adrenal glucocorticoids. All of these systems interact with one another and give a graded, multifaceted, integrated response to invaders, manifested as acute and then chronic inflammation.

3. Innate immunity includes: (1) complement, (2) phagocytosis, (3) acute-phase reactants, including binding proteins that deny invaders the crucial nutrient iron and lipoproteins that serve as sinks for disposal of hydrophobic substances, including toxins, and (4) the self-limiting nature of various biochemical cascades.

4. Acquired immunity is of two broad sorts: antibody-mediated and cell-mediated, carried out by two sets of lymphocytes, B and T, respectively, that work together.

5. The acquired immune system is characterized by the capacity for memory and selection. Antibodies are soluble, bivalent, and asymmetrical. T cells are more complex in their differentiation, forming various subsets of helper cells, suppressor cells, and cytotoxic cells. Diversity is acquired by recombination, somatic mutation, and clonal selection. Antigen receptors on the cell surface of T and B cells are coupled to immune stimulation, cell proliferation, and differentiation. Some cells remain as memory cells, allowing the host to respond in the future to that antigen, more vigorously than the first time. The MHC antigens and the mechanism of antigen presentation are crucial for informing the immune system of the nature of an intrusion.

6. In addition to lymphocytes (B, T, and other), white blood cells include neutrophils, monocytes, macrophages, eosinophils, and basophils, each of which mediate particular subsets of events of innate and acquired immunity. Neutrophils are entirely part of the innate immune system, while macrophages and eosinophils are involved in both innate and acquired immunity.

7. A link between innate and acquired immunity is the role of cytokines as inducers and activators of cells in both limbs of the immune response. Besides being inducers and activators of cells of the immune response, cytokines are mediators of other aspects of inflammation and are factors for growth, development, and differentiation of white blood cells in the bone marrow and elsewhere.

8. Pathogens have developed a wide range of means of subverting the immune response, including (1) blocking complement, (2) blocking phagocytosis and its usual conse-quences, (3) suppressing the immune response, and (4) evading acquired immunity and elsewhere.

9. The immune response is sufficiently fearsome that unless it is carefully controlled, it can do more harm than good. Autoimmunity and allergic reactions are examples of where the immune system inadvertently does harm.

A CASE OF PHYSIOLOGICAL MEDICINE

B.D. is a 22-year-old Princeton-educated journalist who presented to the emergency room with "the worst headache of my life." His father had had meningitis as a child, a point that was appreciated only days later, in retrospect. On physical exam, Mr. D. was noted to have an extremely high fever, a stiff neck, and photophobia (difficulty looking at bright lights). Blood studies showed an elevated white blood count with a "left shift," consistent with a serious bacterial infection. A curious pattern of red spots was noted over his body. Mr. D.'s mental status was completely clear, and he struck all of the staff as a particularly urbane, educated, and witty individual. Indeed, his engaging demeanor lulled them into a greater degree of complacency than might have been appropriate in view of subsequent developments — he seemed "too well" to be really sick.

The clinical picture led the examining clinician to note that Mr. D.'s presentation was consistent with meningitis (infection of the lining of the brain) noting also that the rash was classic for *meningococcal meningitis*, a particularly aggressive infection. Thus the decision was made to obtain a sample of cerebrospinal fluid (CSF) by performing a lumbar puncture (inserting a small needle into the back into the epidural space; see Chap. 18). Unfortunately, someone had the bright idea of first sending Mr. D. off for a routine chest x-ray, figuring that there was no rush to perform the lumbar puncture "since the patient looked like he was doing fine." Luckily, half an hour later, the student volunteer in the emergency room that night, who had delivered the patient to the x-ray department, decided to check up on him. The x-ray technician said that the patient was nowhere to be found. After a brief search, the student found Mr. D. on the floor of an adjacent corridor. In stark contrast to his clinical picture less than an hour earlier, Mr. D. was now disoriented, combative, and quite ill appearing. Help was summoned, the rapid progression of his meningitis was appreciated, and antibiotics were started immediately. A lumbar puncture was performed, which confirmed meningococcal meningitis, with intracellular microbes noted on examination of white blood cells in Mr. D.'s CSF.

Mr. D. was admitted to the intensive care unit, where he proceeded to become hypotensive and to lapse into a coma. Antibiotic coverage was broadened. By the next day sensitivity of the organism to the original regimen was confirmed. Gradually, over a period of days, Mr. D. improved, with slow clearing of his mental status. Even one month afterward, he continued to have some mild memory deficits. More detailed investigation revealed that Mr. D. had a complement deficiency inherited from his father.

QUESTIONS

1. What are the major lines of host defense against a bacterial infection?
2. Suggest a mechanism by which Mr. D. developed meningitis.
3. What lessons about infectious disease should the staff have learned from this case?
4. What is the significance of Mr. D.'s complement deficiency?

ANSWERS

1. First, mechanical, environmental, and anatomic barriers that keep organisms out of the normally sterile internal environment.

   Second, the innate immune system, including complement, neutrophil phagocytosis, and the acute-phase response.

   Third, various modes of acquired immunity, including antibodies and cell-mediated responses.
2. Somehow, the organism must have managed to invade the bloodstream. This organism usually colonizes the respiratory tract, but exactly how it manages to invade the bloodstream is still unclear. Once invasion of the bloodstream has been achieved, seeding of the organism into the brain can occur. The meninges are cell layers that form a lining for the brain; hence, an inflammatory response involving them (e.g., including an infection) is termed a meningitis.
3. It can be very difficult to assess the state of the host defenses and how close they are to collapse. Hence, it is important to be attentive to warning signs. In this case, Mr. D. had subtle signs that the infection was serious (elevated white blood count and left shift), a sign that it had spread (symptoms of meningitis), a sign that the organism involved might be a particularly vicious one (the rash of meningiococcernia), and a family history consistent with a hereditary deficiency in host defense. However, the staff was fooled by "how good the patient looked." Luckily, the enquiring student volunteer saved the day. Had antibiotics been initiated immediately upon making the presumptive diagnosis in the emergency department (i.e., one hour earlier), Mr. D.'s course might have been substantially ameliorated. Had they been further delayed, even briefly (i.e., if the

student had not gone to check up on him), he would probably have suffered major, irreversible neurologic damage, and might even have died. An important aspect of being a good clinician is knowing when the usually reliable "eyeball test" of "how good the patient looks" is not to be trusted.

4. A crucial line of innate immunity was impaired, due to a familial genetic mutation, allowing the organism to get an initial foothold such that Mr. D. could have rapidly succumbed.

References and suggested readings

GENERAL REFERENCES

1. Stites DP, et al. (eds) (1997). *Medical Immunology,* 9th ed. Stamford, CT, Appleton & Lange.
2. Schechter M, et al. (eds) (1994). *Mechanisms of Microbial Disease,* 2d ed. Baltimore, Williams & Wilkins.
3. Fauci A, et al. (eds) (1998). *Harrison's Textbook of Internal Medicine,* 14th ed. New York, McGraw-Hill.
4. McPhee S, et al. (eds) (1997). *Pathophysiology of Disease: An Introduction to Clinical Medicine,* 2d ed. Stamford, CT, Appleton & Lange.
5. Singer AJ, Clark RAF (1999). Cutaneous wound healing. *N Engl J Med* 341:738–741.
6. Weinberg ED (1996). Iron withholding: A defense against viral infections. *Biometals* 9:393–399.
7. Feingold KR, Grunfeld C (1997). Lipoproteins: Are they important components of host defense? *Hepatology* 26:1685–1686.
8. Minowada G, Welch WJ (1995). Clinical implications of the stress response. *J Clin Invest* 95:3–12.
9. Koenig WJ, et al. (1992). Improving acute skin-flap survival through stress conditioning using heat shock and recovery. *Plast Reconstr Surg* 90:659–664.
10. Almawi WY, et al. (1999). T helper type 1 and 2 cytokines mediate the onset and progression of type I (insulin-dependent) diabetes. *J Clin Endocrinol Metab* 84:1497–1502.

FRONTIERS REFERENCES

11. Stahl EA, et al. (1999). Dynamics of disease resistance polymorphism at the Rpm1 locus of arabidopsis. *Nature* 400:667–671.
12. Brown EJ (1997). Adhesive interactions in the immune system. *Trends Cell Biol* 7:289–295.
13. Gavrilovskaya IN, et al. (1998). beta3 Integrins mediate the cellular entry of hantaviruses that cause respiratory failure. *Proc Natl Acad Sci U S A* 95:7074–7079.
14. Gale CA, et al. (1998). Linkage of adhesion, filamentous growth, and virulence in C. albicans to a single gene, INT1. *Science* 279:1355–1358.
15. Teixeira MM (1998). Contribution of endothelial selectins and alpha 4 integrins to eosinophil trafficking in allergic and nonallergic inflammatory reactions in skin. *J Immunol* 161:2516–2523.
16. Fearon DT, Locksley RM (1998). The instructive role of innate immunity in the acquired immune response. *Science* 272:50–54.
17. Gooding LR (1992). Virus proteins that counteract host immune defenses. *Cell* 71:5–7.
18. Pickup JC, et al. (1997). NIDDM as a disease of the innate immune system: Association of acute-phase reactants and interleukin-6 with metabolic syndrome X. *Diabetologia* 40:1286–1292.
19. Hillier SL (1998). The vaginal microbial ecosystem and resistance to HIV disease. *AIDS Res Hum Retroviruses* 14:S17–22.
20. Brainard J (1998). HIV's quiet accomplice? Imbalances in vaginal flora may link to the AIDS epidemic. *Science News* 154:158–159.
21. Butcher EC, Picker LJ (1996). Lymphocyte homing and homeostasis. *Science* 272:60–63.
22. Schenk D, et al. (1999). Immunization with amyloid-beta attenuates Alzheimer-disease-like pathology in the PDAPP mouse. *Nature* 400:173–177.

ORGAN SYSTEM INTEGRATION

20

1. INTRODUCTION TO ORGAN SYSTEM INTEGRATION

The approach of this textbook has been to divide the body into various component organ systems and provide a focused discussion of each from a generalist's perspective. However, categorization by organ system does not always correspond well to the reality of human physiological function or disease pathogenesis, which can cut across systems as we define them, have consequences that involve multiple organ systems, or result from the cumulative effect of many different influences on any one organ system.

Often, our current understanding about how two organ systems interact under normal homeostatic conditions can instruct us on what can go wrong in disease. For example, an appreciation of the normal enterohepatic circulation of bile allows us to anticipate diarrhea, steatorrhea, malabsorption, and fat-soluble vitamin deficiencies (and their consequences, such as prolonged bleeding due to lack of vitamin K) in a patient with liver disease. It also helps us remember that (and understand why) a patient with inflammation or resection of the terminal ileum (where bile acids are reabsorbed) is at risk of developing a similar syndrome.

While physiology can be extremely useful in thinking through the basis for a patient's presentation, one should never make the mistake of assuming that the patient who does not present in the expected way cannot have any particular problem. This is because our understanding of organ systems is far from complete. Variables that, in our wildest imagination, are not thought to be involved in a given physiological function or disease process may someday be found to be crucial — and to account for the anomalous patient or presentation. There is no foolproof approach to diagnosis, and there is no substitute for meticulous attention to detail.

New developments often reveal homeostasis to be a far more complex and rich set of interactions than we might have previously believed. Thus, the recent demonstration (see Ref. 1) that intestinal epithelial cells express both thyroid-stimulating hormone (TSH) and receptors for thyrotropin-releasing hormone (TRH) and that T lymphocytes in the intestine express TSH receptor suggests the existence of a self-contained local TRH-TSH paracrine network for intestinal T-cell homeostasis. This seems likely to be crucial for a better understanding of autoimmune disorders of the intestine (see Chaps. 5 and 12). At the moment, however, it is nothing more than a novel observation whose physiological and pathophysiological significance is fundamentally unknown.

The purpose of this chapter is to briefly indicate some of the variables that affect how the organ systems covered in this book interact with each other normally, and to identify some general implications for disease.

Perspectives on organ system integration

One way to see the importance of organ system interactions is to consider how loss of function of one organ system affects other organs of the body (see Table 20.1).

Another way to view organ system integration is as a means of accounting for what we *do not* know about individual organ system functions. This way of thinking may be of particular value for the reader who is unable to completely accept the view (put forward in Chapter 1) that facts are *not* what science and medicine are supposed to be about. Given the nature of different functioning parts interacting to make the whole, ascribing the unknown to interactions with other organ systems is generally a safe bet.

What is physiological medicine?

Physiological medicine is clinical practice that pays special attention to the ways in

TABLE 20.1 ORGAN SYSTEM INTEGRATION GRID

	Liver	GI	Ep	Cv	Resp	Renal	Febp	Hyp	Thy	Ad	Ca	Ma	Fe	Pr	Neuro	Defense
liver	—	16	31	46	61	76	91	106	121	136	151	166	181	196	211	226
GI	1	—	32	47	62	77	92	107	122	137	152	167	182	197	212	227
ep	2	17	—	48	63	78	93	108	123	138	153	168	183	198	213	228
cv	3	18	33	—	64	79	94	109	124	139	154	169	184	199	214	229
resp	4	19	34	49	—	80	95	110	125	140	155	170	185	200	215	230
renal	5	20	35	50	65	—	96	111	126	141	156	171	186	201	216	231
febp	6	21	36	51	66	81	—	112	127	142	157	172	187	202	217	232
hyp	7	22	37	52	67	82	97	—	128	143	158	173	188	203	218	233
thy	8	23	38	53	68	83	98	113	—	144	159	174	189	204	219	234
ad	9	24	39	54	69	84	99	114	129	—	160	175	190	205	220	235
ca	10	25	40	55	70	85	100	115	130	145	—	176	191	206	221	236
ma	11	26	41	56	71	86	101	116	131	146	161	—	192	207	222	237
fe	12	27	42	57	72	87	102	117	132	147	162	177	—	208	223	238
preg	13	28	43	58	73	88	103	118	133	148	163	178	193	—	224	239
neuro	14	29	44	59	74	89	104	119	134	149	164	179	194	209	—	240
defense	15	30	45	60	75	90	105	120	135	150	165	180	195	210	225	—

The reader can use this grid to develop for him- or herself a systematic recapitulation of organ system interactions during the course of review of preceding chapters. Simply list for each number all interactions between the indicated organ systems you can find.

ABBREVIATIONS: GI = gastrointestinal system; ep = endocrine pancreas; cv = cardiovascular system; resp = respiratory system; renal = kidney; febp = fluid, electrolyte, and blood pressure homeostasis; hyp = hypothalamus and pituitary gland; thy = thyroid gland; ad = adrenal gland; ca = calcium and mineral metabolism; ma = male reproductive system; fe = female reproductive system; preg = pregnancy and physiology of the neonate; neuro = nervous system; defense = host defense systems.

which organ systems normally interact with one another. Not only does such an emphasis help the clinician identify and prioritize the interventions that need to be carried out to support a patient with a dysfunctional organ, it also helps focus therapy on the desired endpoint of *restoration of homeostasis*, to the greatest extent possible. Thus, to continue the analogy developed previously, a patient presenting with diarrhea and malabsorption following surgery for resection of part of the ileum would be treated with bile-acid-binding resins and a diet whose fat content was restricted to medium-chain triglycerides that can be absorbed without the help of bile. Furthermore, the clinician will be particularly attuned to the possibility of fat-soluble vitamin deficiencies in such a patient. In this case, therapy is driven by our knowledge of enterohepatic circulation and the likely consequences of its disruption. Of course, it is likely that more will be learned over time about the role of bile and other means of manipulating its flow, and the therapeutic recommendations will probably change in the future. At any given point in time, however, interventions must be made based on the current hypothesis, but with caution, in the recognition that current knowledge is not certain.

The practice of physiological medicine

Generalist clinicians practicing physiological medicine need to systematically consider the possible ways in which:

- Dysfunction of one organ system might affect others.
- Disordered homeostasis might manifest as new disease of a specific organ system.

Ideally, we would identify disease early enough to reestablish homeostasis without resorting to pharmacologic intervention. That is why it is so important to talk to patients regarding diet and lifestyle changes *while they are still healthy.*

However, it is often the case that patients come to medical attention when disease processes are sufficiently advanced that pharmacologic intervention is deemed necessary. The challenge at that point is to achieve three goals:

- Treat the disease in the context of the patient as a whole.
- Anticipate and avoid or minimize complications and side effects, especially those that are rooted in the normal physiology of organ system interactions and therefore could have been anticipated.
- Attempt to reestablish homeostasis.

A distinguishing assumption of this physiological approach to medicine is the recognition that our understanding of human physiology, now and for the foreseeable future, is modest at best, when compared to the power homeostatic mechanisms have achieved through millions and millions of years of natural selection. In particular, these limitations have some specific consequences for clinical practice:

- We cannot easily distinguish whether an intervention that we know can be helpful in some cases will be helpful or harmful in any particular case.
- We do not know the boundaries that define, for any individual patient, when a potentially helpful intervention becomes harmful.

Given this state of ignorance, the prudent approach will often be to intervene pharmacologically for the shortest reasonable period of time, and to attempt to "hand off" to homeostatic mechanisms at the earliest possible juncture.

Clinical Pearl

○ When a patient develops acute bacterial gastroenteritis, it is often more effective to provide fluid replacement than to try and stop the diarrhea, since diarrhea serves the useful purpose of elimination of the pathogen or toxin. Taking an agent to combat diarrhea, which is just the symptom of the underlying disorder, often prolongs the otherwise self-limited disorder.

Review Questions

1. What is physiological medicine?
2. What are the goals of the practice of physiological medicine?
3. What are some important consequences of our current, limited understanding of human physiology?

Case Presentation: Multiorgan Failure in the Intensive Care Unit

JB is a 54-year-old homeless alcoholic who has had numerous previous visits to the emergency room for alcohol intoxication, alcohol withdrawal, and minor trauma. Early this morning he was picked up by paramedics, who found him lying on the sidewalk in a torrential downpour. In the ER, he was noted to have an altered mental status, which was ascribed at first to intoxication, until his blood alcohol level came back at less than 0.02% (0.08% is the legal limit for driving). He was also observed to be hypothermic, with a temperature of 35°C, and to have a white blood count of 16,000 with neutrophil predominance and a "left shift." The initial chest x-ray was read as normal.

Because of concern about his hypothermia in the setting of an elevated white blood count with no obvious source of infection, the patient was admitted for observation. During the night he was noted to become more combative, and a blood gas revealed marked hypoxia, with blood gas determination being pH, 7.2; P_{CO_2}, 60; P_{O_2}, 45 on 5 L of O_2 by nose.

The patient was transferred to the ICU, where his respiratory status rapidly deteriorated, resulting in emergency intubation for respiratory failure. Blood cultures were drawn, a lumbar puncture to obtain cerebrospinal fluid (CSF) was performed, and broad-spectrum antibiotics were started. He was noted to be febrile to a temperature of 40°C with a falling white blood count, down to 2.0 by the next day, at which point cultures of blood and CSF were positive for *Streptococcus pneumoniae* sensitive to penicillin.

Despite adequate levels of antibiotics, the patient had an inexorable downhill course. His chest x-ray was consistent with the adult respiratory distress syndrome (ARDS), and his lungs were stiff and difficult to ventilate. He developed a pneumothorax and required a chest tube. He was noted to be hypotensive and required pressor drugs to maintain his blood pressure in a reasonable range. He developed acute renal failure, and dialysis was instituted. Cardiac irritability was noted, with runs of ventricular tachycardia despite antiarrhythmic therapy. His finger and toe tips were noted to have become necrotic, presumably from the systemic pressor therapy. On the fifth hospital day, he had a cardiac arrest from which he could not be resuscitated.

This case of sepsis syndrome illustrates the gravity of multiorgan system failure, where therapy of one dysfunctional organ can cause injury to another. The mortality of pneumococcal sepsis remains extremely high even in the best of settings.

2. KEY VARIABLES IN MEDICAL PHYSIOLOGY

Genes

Our genes are the basis for our traits (see Table 20.2). However, this truism tends to obscure some complicating and some mysterious features of human genetics that must be kept in mind. In Chapter 2 we presented

TABLE 20.2 INHERITED DISEASES WITH INCREASED FREQUENCY IN PARTICULAR ETHNIC GROUPS

Ethnic group	Simply inherited disorder
African blacks	Hemoglobinopathies, especially Hb S, Hb C, persistent Hb F, α and β thalassemia Glucose-6-phosphate dehydrogenase deficiency
Armenians	Familial Mediterranean fever
Ashkenazi Jews	Abetalipoproteinemia Bloom's syndrome Dystonia musculorum deformans (recessive form) Gaucher's disease (adult form) Tay-Sachs disease Breast ovarian cancer BRCA1 (specific mutation)
Chinese	α Thalassemia Glucose-6-phosphate dehydrogenase deficiency Adult lactase deficiency
Eskimos (Inuit)	Pseudocholinesterase deficiency Congenital adrenal hyperplasia
Finns	Congenital nephrosis Aspartylglucosaminuria
French Canadians	Tyrosinemia Familial hypercholesterolemia
Japanese	Acatalasemia
Lebanese	Familial hypercholesterolemia
Mediterranean peoples (Italians, Greeks, Sephardic Jews)	β Thalassemia Glucose-6-phosphate dehydrogenase deficiency Familial Mediterranean fever Glycogen storage disease, type III
Europeans	Cystic fibrosis
Scandinavians	α_1-antitrypsin deficiency LCAT (lecithin:cholesterol acyltransferase) deficiency
South African whites	Porphyria variegata Familial hypercholesterolemia

Reproduced, with permission, from Beaudet AL (1998). Genetics and disease. In Fauci A, et al. (eds), *Harrison's Textbook of Internal Medicine,* 14th ed. New York, McGraw-Hill, p 389.

some of the simple core principles of modern Mendelian genetics. However, in Chapter 1 we made the argument that science deals in theories, hypotheses, and experiments, not facts. Thus, while the simple principles of modern genetics are the best current overall explanations for heritable phenomena, and do indeed explain a lot, they are historically specific and do not account for everything. New findings will, inevitably, challenge and ultimately enrich our thinking about human genetics. **Epigenetics** is a term used to describe genetic phenomena that cannot be simply explained using Mendelian genetics. It is not possible for us (or anyone else) to predict in advance which currently anomalous observations, including those of epigenetics, will pave the way for major advances in thinking. But that such revolutions in thinking will occur, we are confident. Let us mention just a few of the current hints that modern genetics is not going to be solely a mopping-up operation culminating in the sequencing of the human genome:

- Coding sequences account for only about 1% of the 3 billion base pairs of DNA in the human genome. The remaining 99% are repetitive sequences of *unknown function*. This humbling fact alone should lead us to be more appreciative of the huge gaps in our current level of understanding of human biology.
- Mutations are not always stable. Sometimes "premutations" occur that, while having no phenotype, appear to predispose future generations to other mutations that cause certain diseases. The best examples are the so-called **triplet repeat diseases**, including Huntington's disease, in which variable expansion of these DNA sequences can occur, resulting, by currently mysterious means, in disease. The same phenomenon might underlie currently unknown aspects of normal physiology, of which only the disease-associated manifestations are currently appreciated.
- Inheritance of two copies of one autosomal allele from one parent rather than one from each parent appears to occur in the T locus of mice and possibly also in humans.
- Imprinting, whereby the allele for a particular gene from the mother (or the father) is silent. Thus, mutations in the sole expressed gene cannot be compensated for by a normal gene from the other parent. This rare occurrence is believed to contribute to some rare genetic disorders such as Prader-Willi syndrome (presenting with diabetes, obesity, mental retardation, and behavioral disorders).

The significance of these and other "anomalous" observations is twofold.

First, they suggest that some diseases come about through the expression of many genes interacting in complex and poorly understood ways. Even when a disease is due to a "simple" genetic defect, the manifestations of that disease in patients varies tremendously, presumably in part as a function of other genes with which the mutant gene product interacts, directly or indirectly. Hence understanding these anomalous observations may be the key to understanding major dimensions of human disease, not just the one in a million genetic defects that demonstrate the existence of poorly understood biological phenomena.

Second, these complexities should lead to further caution in the application of pharmacologic intervention to the correction of physiological disorders. Studies will generally not have been large enough, or carried out for a long enough time, to rule out the possibility of complex and delayed interactions that could do the patient harm. In part, differences between patients in this regard may have a genetic basis (see Table 20.3).

Sex

While sex is, at least in humans, an aspect of genetics, in that it depends on whether an X or a Y chromosome was inherited from one's father, we mention it separately from other genetic influences on physiology. This is because it is a factor that historically has not received appropriate consideration and appreciation. Thus, many studies have been carried out on male subjects alone, with the conclusions uncritically generalized to all humans. One way to redress this sexist historical oversight is to heighten awareness of this issue by today's students.

The dominant physiological basis for differences in physiology between males and females in humans is the influence of the high levels of estrogen and progesterone from development through menopause. However, additional potential bases for sex differences in physiology could include

- Non-Mendelian features of genetics, including imprinting.

TABLE 20.3 EFFECTS OF GENES ON DRUG INTERACTIONS

Disorder	Molecular abnormality	Mode of inheritance	Frequency	Clinical effect	Drugs producing abnormal response
Slow inactivation of isoniazid	Isoniazid acetylase in liver	Autosomal recessive	50% of U.S. population	Polyneuritis	Isoniazid, sulfamethazine, sulfamaprine, phenelzine, dapsone, hydralazine
Suxamethonium sensitivity	Pseudocholinesterase in plasma	Autosomal recessive	Several mutant alleles: most common affects 1 in 2500	Apnea	Suxamethonium, succinylcholine
Malignant hyperthermia	Ryanodine receptor	Autosomal dominant	1 in 20,000 anesthetized patients	Severe, hyperpyrexia, muscle rigidity, death	Such anesthetics as halothane, succinylcholine, methoxyflurane, ether, cyclopropane
Debrisoquine sensitivity	Cytochrome P450, CYP2D6	Autosomal recessive	5–10%; range 0–18% in ethnic groups	Toxicity of drugs, e.g., postural hypotension	Antiarrythmics, beta blockers, neuroleptics, tricyclic antidepressants
Glucose-6-phosphate dehydrogenase deficiency	Glucose-6-phosphate dehydrogenase in erythrocytes	X-linked recessive	~1 × 10^8 affected persons in world; common in persons of African, Mediterranean, Asiatic origin; multiple mutant alleles	Hemolysis	Analgesics, sulfonamides, antimalarials, nitrofurantoin, other drugs

Reproduced, with permission, from Beaudet AL (1998). Genetics and disease. In Fauci A, et al. (eds). *Harrison's Textbook of Internal Medicine,* 14th ed. New York, McGraw-Hill, p 388.

• Structural differences, e.g., in the brain, perhaps as a consequence of development in different hormonal environments. In certain birds, for example, learning of songs appears to be influenced by both hormonal and nonhormonal factors (see Ref. 2).

Sex-specific features of physiology are a major aspect of Chapters 15 to 17.

Review Questions

4. Name four observations that suggest that human genetics is more complex than might be inferred from simple Mendelian principles.

5. Suggest two implications of anomalous observations in human genetics, as they might relate to treatment of patients.

6. Why should sex differences in physiology be emphasized more than any other genetically determined differences?

Environment

Physiology does not occur in a vacuum. Evolution is driven by the environment, which is the agent of natural selection. The characteristics of a person's location (i.e., his or her environment) influences that person's development, functions, aging, diseases, and, ultimately, cause of death. At earlier points in human history, features of the environment that more often resulted in an early death would have provided *selection pressure* favoring survival of individuals with mutations that confer resistance. Even when individuals die beyond the reproductive years, the importance of older individuals for survival of the young could be expected to impact selection for resistance to certain diseases in the postreproductive years.

In modern societies, both of these would-be environmental selection pressures are modified by the nature of the health care system. Thus, rather than serving as a driving force of natural selection, environmental and other causes of illness are more likely to manifest today as individuals presenting in need of medical care. Thus the importance of the environment for medical physiology is in the recognition that some environments are better than others, in terms of fostering homeostasis, resistance to disease, fulfillment of intellectual and physical capabilities, etc. For a society to be able to afford to provide the best possible health care to all of its members, it must foster environments in which people are more likely to be healthy.

As with the complex interplay of genes (see the previous discussion), our current concepts of organ system function and homeostasis are sufficiently crude that we cannot fully appreciate or predict the impact of the environment on these variables. Hence concerns about toxic exposures in the environment may be appropriate even when they have yet to be substantiated by a conservative interpretation of the evidence (see Ref. 3). Table 20.4 indicates some of the established or strongly suspected connections between environmental toxins and organ system dysfunction. Table 20.5 indicates some of the human-caused environmental contaminants that have been found to be carcinogenic.

Lifestyle and habits

In many ways, lifestyle and habits can be lumped together under the category of environment, as variables that influence physiology and homeostasis. Effective communica-

TABLE 20.4   ENVIRONMENTAL TOXINS AND ORGAN SYSTEM DYSFUNCTION

Organ system dysfunction	Environmental toxin
Respiratory disease	Asbestos
Cancer	Radiation, benzene, asbestos
Coronary disease	Carbon disulfide, carbon monoxide
Hepatitis/chronic liver disease	Alcohol, carbon tetrachloride
Kidney disease	Hydrocarbons
Peripheral neuropathy	Organic solvents, lead, arsenic
Neuropsychiatric symptoms	Organic solvents, heavy metals
Teratogenesis and reproductive problems	Polychlorinated biphenyls, heavy metals
Immunosuppression, autoimmunity, and hypersensitivity	Mercury, organic solvents

tion with patients is crucial if these and other causes of ill health are to be addressed effectively by health care providers. Thus, lobbying for (and getting patients to lobby for) enforcement of existing laws and enactment of better laws governing safe disposal of industrial wastes and other means of diminishing the burden of environmental hazards is one way for a clinician to directly affect the low-level environmental burden of toxins and carcinogens we all face on a daily basis. Similarly, cigarette smoking and other aspects of unhealthy lifestyles and habits can also often be modifed effectively by communication with patients (see A Case of Physiological Medicine at the end of this chapter).

An important dimension of that communication is the use of physiology to provide a *rationale* by which the patient can understand and remember the clinician's recommendations.

Clinical Pearls

○ Patients with xeroderma pigmentosum have a defect in DNA repair that renders them particularly sensitive to the carcinogenic effects of ultraviolet sunlight.

TABLE 20.5 CARCINOGENS IN THE ENVIRONMENT

Aflatoxins	Estrogen, nonsteroidal
Aluminum production	Estrogen, steroidal
4-Aminobiphenyl	Furniture and cabinet working
Analgesic mixtures containing phenacetin	Hematite mining, underground, with exposure to radon
Arsenic and arsenic compounds	Iron and steel founding
Asbestos	Isopropyl alcohol manufacture, strong-acid process
Auramine manufacture	Magenta manufacture
Azathioprine	Melphalan
Benzene	8-Methoxypsoralen (Methoxsalen) plus ultraviolet radiation
Benzidine	
Betel quid with tobacco	Mineral oils, untreated and mildly treated
N,N-bis(2-chloroethyl)-2-naphthylamine (Chlornaphazine)	MOPP (combined therapy with nitrogen mustard, vincristine, procarbazine, and prednisone) and other combined chemotherapy including alkylating agents
Bis(chloromethyl)ether and chloromethyl methyl ether (technical-grade)	
Boot and shoe manufacture and repair	Mustard gas (sulfur mustard)
1,4-Butanediol dimethanesulfonate (Myleran)	2-Naphthylamine
Chlorambucil	Nickel and nickel compounds
1-(2-Chloroethyl)-3-(4-methylcyclohexyl)-1-nitrosourea (methyl-CCNU)	Oral contraceptives, combined
	Oral contraceptives, sequential
Chromium compounds, hexavalent	Rubber industry
Coal gasification	Shale oils
Coal-tar pitches	Soots
Coal tars	Talc-containing asbestiform fibers
Coke production	
Cyclophosphamide	Tobacco products, smokeless
Diethylstilbestrol	Tobacco smoke
Erionite	Treosulfan
Estrogen replacement therapy	Vinyl chloride

Reproduced, with permission, from Hu H, Speizer FE (1998). Influence of environmental and occupational hazards on disease. In Fauci A, et al. (eds), *Harrison's Textbook of Internal Medicine*, 14th ed. New York, McGraw-Hill, p 2522.

○ Patients with galactosemia are deficient in the enzymes of galactose metabolism. Ingestion of galactose by these patients causes mental retardation, liver disease, and cataracts. The treatment is a milk-free diet until completion of neurologic development. Soy products are generally well tolerated because soy galactose is not readily digested and absorbed.

Nutrition

What we eat is another aspect of our "environment" that has enormous importance in human disease. Nutrition influences physiology in several ways that will be briefly discussed.

First, a certain minimum amount of essential nutrients is needed to prevent the development of specific deficiency diseases. Exactly what those amounts are has been controversial. In some cases (see Ref. 4), the current recommendations (see Tables 20.6A and B) have been viewed as too high (e.g., for protein) or too low (e.g., for vitamin C). In the case of vitamin C and the B complex vitamins, the concept of biochemical individuality discussed in Chapter 1 has been suggested as a basis for large differences in individual requirements.

Regardless, a diet lacking some minimum level of these nutrients will create an increased risk of development of deficiency disease, which, in turn, will lower features such as host resistance to infection, energy level, and intellectual functioning, and thus be nonadaptive.

Second, an excess of nutrients is in many ways more harmful than a mild deficiency. In part this is a reflection of the fact that, through most of human history, our ancestors faced the risk of famine, starvation, and lack of food rather than food excess. Thus, we have been selected for extremely efficient mechanisms to conserve calories and store food when it happens to be plentiful. However, we are not as good at burning away any excess (see Chap. 11). It is particularly noteworthy that the only intervention that consistently slows aging in animals is *caloric restriction*.

TABLE 20.6A ESSENTIAL NUTRIENTS OF THE BODY

Category	Age (years) or condition	Weight (kg)	Weight (lb)	Height (cm)	Height (in)	Protein (g)	Vitamin A (mg RE)	Vitamin D (mg)	Vitamin E (mg α-TE)	Vitamin K (mg)	Vitamin C (mg)	Thiamine (mg)	Riboflavin (mg)	Niacin (mg NE)	Vitamin B₆ (mg)	Folate (µg)	Vitamin B₁₂ (µg)	Calcium (mg)	Phosphorus (mg)	Magnesium (mg)	Iron (mg)	Zinc (mg)	Iodine (µg)	Selenium (µg)
Males	15–18	66	145	176	69	59	1,000	10	10	65	60	1.5	1.8	20	2.0	200	2.0	1,200	1,200	400	12	15	150	50
	19–24	72	160	177	70	58	1,000	10	10	70	60	1.5	1.7	19	2.0	200	2.0	1,200	1,200	350	10	15	150	70
	25–50	79	174	176	70	63	1,000	5	10	80	60	1.5	1.7	19	2.0	200	2.0	800	800	350	10	15	150	70
	51+	77	170	173	68	63	1,000	5	10	80	60	1.2	1.4	15	2.0	200	2.0	800	800	350	10	15	150	70
Females	15–18	55	120	163	64	44	800	10	8	55	60	1.1	1.3	15	1.5	180	2.0	1,200	1,200	300	15	12	150	50
	19–24	58	128	164	65	46	800	10	8	60	60	1.1	1.3	15	1.6	180	2.0	1,200	1,200	280	15	12	150	55
	25–50	63	138	163	64	50	800	5	8	65	60	1.1	1.3	15	1.6	180	2.0	800	800	280	15	12	150	55
	51+	65	143	160	63	50	800	5	8	65	60	1.0	1.2	13	1.6	180	2.0	800	800	280	10	12	150	55
Pregnant						60	800	10	10	65	70	1.5	1.6	17	2.2	400	2.2	1,200	1,200	320	30	15	175	65
Lactating	1st 6 months					65	1,300	10	12	65	95	1.6	1.8	20	2.1	280	2.6	1,200	1,200	355	15	19	200	75
	2nd 6 months					62	1,200	10	11	65	90	1.6	1.7	20	2.1	260	2.6	1,200	1,200	340	15	16	200	75

Reproduced from National Research Council: *Recommended Dietary Allowances*, 10th ed. National Academy of Sciences, 1989.

TABLE 20.6B　ESSENTIAL MACROMINERALS: SUMMARY OF MAJOR CHARACTERISTICS

Elements	Functions	Deficiency disease or symptoms	Toxicity disease or symptoms[a]
Calcium	Constituent of bones, teeth; regulation of nerve, muscle function	Children: rickets Adults: osteomalacia. May contribute to osteoporosis	Occurs with excess absorption due to hypervitaminosis D or hypercalcemia due to hyperparathyroidism or other causes of hypercalcemia
Phosphorus	Constituent of bones, teeth, ATP, phosphorylated metabolic intermediates. Nucleic acids	Children: rickets Adults: osteomalacia	Low serum Ca^{2+} : P ratio stimulates secondary hyperparathyroidism; may lead to bone loss
Sodium	Principal cation in extracellular fluid. Regulates plasma volume, acid-base balance, nerve and muscle function, Na^+-K^+-ATPase	Unknown on normal diet, secondary to injury or illness	Hypertension (in susceptible individuals)
Potassium	Principal cation in intracellular fluid; nerve and muscle function, Na^+-K^+-ATPase	Occurs secondary to illness, injury, or diuretic therapy; muscular weakness, paralysis, mental confusion	Cardiac arrest, small bowel ulcers
Chloride	Fluid and electrolyte balance; gastric fluid	Infants fed salt-free formula. Secondary to vomiting, diuretic therapy, renal disease	Cardiac arrest, small bowel ulcers
Magnesium	Constituent of bones, teeth; enzyme cofactor (kinases, etc.)	Secondary to malabsorption or diarrhea, alcoholism	Depressed deep tendon reflexes and respiration

[a] Excess mineral intake produces toxic symptoms. Unless otherwise specified, symptoms include nonspecific nausea, diarrhea and irritability.
Reproduced, with permission, from Murray RK et al. (1988) *Harper's Biochemistry*, 21st ed. Stamford, CT, Appleton & Lange.

Third, in addition to the *quantities* of nutrients consumed, we must be concerned with their *qualitative* features. Thus, lack of fiber in the diet is associated with GI tract dysfunction, manifesting first as **constipation** and culminating in **diverticular disease**. Whether carbohydrates are consumed in complex form or as simple sugars affects their absorption from the GI tract and, in turn, dictates the ease with which the endocrine pancreas is able to maintain blood glucose. Thus, as the homeostatic reserve falls (due to either old age, insulin resistance, or some other reason), the nature of the diet affects the ability to maintain blood glucose control. Thus also, deviations from the optimum diet subject various organ systems to stress at the cellular level (see Chap. 19). In the case of blood glucose control, cell stress manifests as beta cell exhaustion, apoptosis, glucose toxicity, etc. (see Chap. 6).

Whether maladaptive features of the diet such as lack of fiber, caloric excess, etc., actually result in any particular manifestation of disease in a given period of time depends on numerous variables. These variables include

1. Complex interactions with the products of various genes
2. Homeostatic reserve of various organ systems

3. Other aspects of stress in the environment (e.g., the presence of ongoing infection, levels of reactive oxygen species in cigarette smoke).

Exactly how these variables interact and whether there are others that are as (or more) important are not currently known (another basis for uncertainty in medicine).

Consequences of nutritional deficiencies

There are numerous consequences of nutritional deficiencies. **Protein-calorie malnutrition** occurs when either intake of amino acids is insufficient to meet minimal protein synthetic needs (the disorder called **kwashiorkor**) or total energy intake is inadequate for minimum needs (the disorder called **murasmus**). This can occur through simple starvation in areas afflicted with war or famine, or in complex disease states of individual patients, characterized by malabsorption, diarrhea, and glucosuria. In addition, a variety of conditions — including fever, surgery, neoplasia, and burns — are associated with increased nutritional needs to fuel a hypermetabolic state.

The manifestations of nutritional deficiencies are entirely consistent with expectation: weight loss, growth failure, and organ atrophy. When nutritional deprivation is severe, hypoalbuminemia due to deficient hepatic protein synthesis can occur. This in turn results in edema and ascites formation due to inadequate plasma oncotic pressure.

A second category of nutritional deficiency is lack of specific micronutrients in the setting of adequate quantities of protein and energy substrate intake. These deficiency disorders give rise to a range of syndromes whose physiological basis remains, generally, poorly understood (see Table 20.7). This should serve as a further reminder of the lack of sophistication of our understanding of the ideal human diet in particular and of human physiology in general.

Finally, a number of drugs are known to affect absorption and other aspects of human nutrition (see Table 20.8). Again, in most cases, the molecular mechanisms involved, and often the physiological processes being affected, are not fully understood.

Clinical Pearls

○ A diet high in complex carbohydrates with no concentrated sweets is recommended for patients with diabetes mellitus. This is because the patient with diabetes mellitus does not have the functional reserve of an individual with a normal endocrine pancreas, and neither insulin injections nor oral hypoglycemic agents (which either stimulate insulin secretion or promote glucose utilization) are able to adequately compensate. Thus, achieving slow and steady glucose absorption by manipulating the diet makes blood glucose easier to control.

○ Tuberculosis is an example of a disease that manifests in many different ways in different individuals, depending on subtle features of the state of the host's immune system. Less than 10% of people infected with TB are aware of the initial infection or have any disease within the first 5 years. It appears that cellular immunity generally holds the disease in check, but is often unable to irradicate the organism. Depending on genes (the HLA type Bev-15 is particularly susceptible), the state of nutrition, and other features that affect immune response, varying degrees of effort must be exerted by the host to contain the infection. Sometimes activation of cytokines results in profound weight loss and debilitation as part of the host's war of attrition against the stubborn invader.

TABLE 20.7 DEFICIENCY DISEASES

Clinical sign	Nutrient deficiency	Clinical sign	Nutrient deficiency
Hair		**Mouth (cont'd)**	
Transverse depigmentation	Protein, copper	Atrophic lingual papillae	Niacin, iron, riboflavin folate, vitamin B_{12}
Easily pluckable	Protein		
Sparse and thin	Protein, zinc, biotin	Hypogeusia	Zinc, vitamin A
Skin		Tongue fissuring	Niacin
Dry, scaling	Zinc, vitamin A, essential fatty acids	**Neck**	
		Goiter	Iodine
Flaky paint dermatitis	Protein, niacin, riboflavin	**Chest**	
Follicular hyperkeratosis	Vitamins A and C	Thoracic rosary	Vitamin D
Perifollicular petechiae	Vitamin C	**Heart**	
Petechiae, purpura	Vitamins C and K	High-output failure	Thiamin
Pigmentation, desquamation	Niacin	Decreased output	Protein-calorie
Nasolabial seborrhea	Niacin, riboflavin, pyridoxine	**Abdomen**	
Pallor	Iron, folate, vitamin B_{12}, copper	Hepatosplenomegaly	Protein-calorie
Scrotal/vulvar dermatoses	Riboflavin	Distention	Protein-calorie
Subcutaneous fat loss	Calorie	Diarrhea	Niacin, folate, vitamin B
Nails		**Extremities**	
Spooning	Iron	Muscle tenderness, pain	Thiamin, vitamin C
Transverse lines, ridging	Protein-calorie	Muscle wasting	Protein-calorie
Head		Edema	Protein, thiamin
Temporal muscle wasting	Protein-calorie	Bone tenderness	Vitamin D, vitamin C, calcium, phosphorus
Parotid enlargement	Protein		
Eyes		**Neurologic**	
Night blindness	Vitamin A, zinc	Hyporeflexia	Thiamin
Corneal vascularization	Riboflavin	Decreased position and vibratory sense	Vitamin B_{12}, thiamin
Xerosis, Bitot spots, keratomalacia	Vitamin A		
Conjunctival inflammation	Riboflavin	Paresthesias	Vitamin B_{12}, thiamin, niacin
Mouth		Confabulation, disorientation	Thiamin
Glossitis (scarlet, raw)	Niacin, pyridoxine, riboflavin, vitamin B_{12}, folate	Dementia	Niacin
		Ophthalmoplegia	Thiamin, phosphorus
Bleeding gums	Vitamin C, riboflavin	Tetany	Calcium, magnesium
Cheilosis	Riboflavin	**Other**	
Angular stomatitis	Riboflavin, iron	Delayed wound healing	Zinc, protein-calorie, vitamin C

Reproduced, with permission, from Baron RB (1998). Nutrition. In Tierney LM, et al. (eds), *Current Medical Diagnosis and Treatment 1998.* Stamford, CT, Appleton & Lange, p 1158.

Sometimes the infection is walled off; other times tremendous tissue destruction as a result of activated macrophages occurs. Sometimes the disease is held in check for years before progressing. Sometimes dissemination throughout the body, with foci of infection in the bone or elsewhere, can occur. Reactivation takes place when the balance tips in favor of the organism over the host defense, often decades after initial infection, as a result of even a very slight diminution of immune function (e.g., with age, treatment with glucocorticoids, other illnesses, etc.).

TABLE 20.8 DRUG EFFECTS ON NUTRITION

Drug	Effect
Analgesics and anti-inflammatories	
Salicylates	Decrease serum ascorbic acid; increase urinary loss of ascorbic acid, potassium, and amino acids
Sulfasalazine	Impairs folate absorption and antagonizes folate supplementation
Antacids	
Aluminum antacids	Decrease absorption of phosphate and vitamin A
H_2 blockers	Decrease iron and vitamin B_{12} absorption
Octreotide acetate	Hypo- and hyperglycemia; decreases fat and carotene absorption
Anticonvulsants	
Phenobarbital	Decreases serum folate; increases vitamin D and vitamin K turnover and may cause deficiency
Phenytoin	Decreases serum folate; increases vitamin D and vitamin K turnover and may cause deficiency
Primidone	Decreases serum folate and vitamins B_6, B_{12}; decreases calcium absorption; increases vitamin D and vitamin K turnover and may cause deficiency
Antimicrobials	
Neomycin	Binds bile acids and decreases absorption of fat, carotene; of vitamins A, D, K, and B_{12}; and of potassium, sodium, calcium, nitrogen
Amphotericin B	Decreases serum magnesium and potassium
Aminosalicylic acid	Increases absorption of folate, vitamin B_{12}, iron, cholesterol, fat
Chloramphenicol	Increases need for vitamins B_2, B_6, B_{12}; increases serum iron
Penicillin	Hypokalemia; renal potassium wasting
Tetracycline	Calcium, iron, magnesium inhibit drug absorption; decreases vitamin K synthesis
Cycloserine	May decrease absorption of calcium, magnesium; may decrease serum folate and vitamins B_6, B_{12}; decreases protein synthesis
Isoniazid	Vitamin B_6 antagonist; may cause deficiency
Sulfonamides	Decrease absorption of folate; decrease serum folate, iron
Nitrofurantoin	Decreases serum folate
Pyrimethamine	Decreases serum B_{12} and folate
Antimitotics	
Methotrexate	Decreases activation of folate
Colchicine	Decreases absorption of vitamin B_{12}, carotene, fat, sodium, potassium, cholesterol, lactose, nitrogen
Cathartics	
Phenolphthalein	Malabsorption, hypokalemia; deficiency of vitamin D, calcium
Mineral oil	Malabsorption; decreased absorption of vitamins A, D, K
Diuretics	Some cause hypokalemia, hypomagnesemia; may increase urinary excretion of vitamins B_1, B_6; calcium, magnesium, potassium
Hypocholesterolemics	
Cholestyramine	Binds bile acids; decreases absorption of fat, carotene; vitamins A, D, K, B_{12}; folate, iron
Clofibrate	Decreases absorption of carotene, vitamin B_{12}, iron, glucose
Hypotensives	
Hydralazine	Vitamin B_6 deficiency
Captopril	May cause hyponatremia, hyperkalemia; decreases taste acuity
Oral contraceptives	Vitamin B_6, folate deficiency; may increase the need for other nutrients

Reproduced, with permission, from Baron RB (1998). Nutrition. In Tierney LM, et al. (eds), *Current Medical Diagnosis and Treatment 1998*. Stamford, CT, Appleton & Lange, p 1154.

TABLE 20.9 PHYSIOLOGICAL CHANGES WITH AGE

Organ/system	Age-related physiologic change[a]	Consequences of age-related physiologic change	Consequences of disease, not age
General	↑ Body fat	↑ Volume of distribution for fat-soluble drugs	Obesity
	↓ Total body water	↓ Volume of distribution for water-soluble drugs	Anorexia
Eyes/ears	Presbyopia Lens opacification	↓ Accommodation ↑ Susceptibility to glare Need for increased illumination	Blindness
	↓ High-frequency acuity	Difficulty discriminating words if background noise is present	Deafness
Endocrine	Impaired glucose homeostasis	↑ Glucose level in response to acute illness	Diabetes mellitus
	↓ Thyroxine clearance (and production)	↓ T_4 dose required in hypothyroidism	Thyroid dysfunction
	↑ ADH, ↓ renin, and ↓ aldosterone ↓ Testosterone		↓ Na⁻, ↑ K⁺ Impotence
	↓ Vitamin D absorption and activation	Osteopenia	Osteomalacia, fracture
Respiratory	↓ Lung elasticity and ↑ chest wall stiffness	Ventilation/perfusion mismatch and ↓ PO_2	Dyspnea, hypoxia
Cardiovascular	↓ Arterial compliance and ↑ systolic BP → LVH	Hypotensive response to ↑ HR, volume depletion, or loss of atrial contraction	Syncope
	↓ β-adrenergic responsiveness	↓ Cardiac output and HR response to stress	Heart failure
	↓ Baroreceptor sensitivity and ↓ SA node automaticity	Impaired blood pressure response to standing, volume depletion	Heart block
Gastrointestinal	↓ Hepatic function ↓ Gastric acidity	Delayed metabolism of some drugs ↓ Ca⁺ absorption on empty stomach	Cirrhosis Osteoporosis, B_{12} deficiency
	↓ Colonic motility ↓ Anorectal function	Constipation	Fecal impaction Fecal incontinence
Hematologic/ immune system	↓ Bone marrow reserve(?)		Anemia
	↓ T cell function ↑ Autoantibodies	False-negative PPD response False-positive rheumatoid factor, antinuclear antibody	Autoimmune disease
Renal	↓ GFR ↓ Urine concentration/dilution (see also "Endocrine")	Impaired excretion of some drugs Delayed response to salt or fluid restriction/overload; nocturia	↑ Serum creatinine ↓ ↑ Na⁻
Genitourinary	Vaginal/urethral mucosal atrophy Prostate enlargement	Dyspareunia, bacteriuria ↑ Residual urine volume	Symptomatic UTI Urinary incontinence; urinary retention
Musculoskeletal	↓ Lean body mass, muscle ↓ Bone density	Osteopenia	Functional impairment Hip fracture
Nervous system	Brain atrophy ↓ Brain catechol synthesis ↓ Brain dopaminergic synthesis ↓ Righting reflexes ↓ Stage 4 sleep	Benign senescent forgetfulness Stiffer gait ↑ Body sway Early wakening, insomnia	Dementia, delirium Depression Parkinson's disease Falls Sleep apnea

[a] Changes generally observed in healthy elderly subjects free of symptoms and detectable disease in the organ system studied. The changes are usually important only when the system is stressed or other factors are added (e.g., drugs, disease, or environmental challenge); they rarely result in symptoms otherwise.

ABBREVIATIONS: T_2, thyroxine; BP, blood pressure; HR, heart rate; ADH, antidiuretic hormone; GFR, glomerular filtration rate. Reproduced, with permission, from Resnick NM (1998). Geriatric medicine. In Fauci A, et al. (eds), *Harrison's Textbook of Internal Medicine*, 14th ed. New York, McGraw-Hill, p 38.

Review Questions

7. Suggest a basis for distinguishing life-style and habits from other aspects of the environment that have an impact on physiology and disease.
8. What are three aspects of nutrition that have an impact on physiology?
9. What are some potential consequences of deviation from an optimal diet?
10. What features might modify the consequences of deviation from an optimal diet?

Age

Theories of aging were briefly discussed in Chapter 1. The principle that age results in a diminution of functional reserve in every organ system was presented (see Chap. 1). A detailed compilation of the changes in the structure and function of various organ systems is beyond the scope of this book. However, Table 20.9 presents some of the key physiological changes that occur in old age.

Clinical Pearls

○ New disease in the elderly most often affects the organ systems with the least physiological reserve. Thus, hyperthyroidism often presents with atrial fibrillation and mental status changes rather than with exopthalmos, goiter, or tremor.
○ Since the brain is an organ system whose functional reserve is often most compromised in the elderly, altered mental status is a common presentation of many different disorders, including infection and cardiovascular and musculoskeletal disease. Additionally, the causes of symptoms in a given organ system in the elderly are often different from those in younger individuals. Thus, acute confusion is less often due to a brain lesion, depression is less often

due to a primary psychiatric disorder, syncope is less often due to heart disease, and incontinence is less often due to bladder dysfunction than would be the case in a younger patient.
○ Side effects of drugs occur at lower doses in the elderly, as a result of the decreased physiological and homeostatic reserve.
○ Since many homeostatic mechanisms are impaired with advanced age, improvement of contributing factors often results in a marked improvement in a patient's overall quality of life, even when the underlying disease process is irreversible. A good example is that the cognitive impairment in patients with Alzheimer's disease will often worsen dramatically with hearing or visual impairment, or with other disorders such as heart failure, depression, infection, or electrolyte abnormalities. Often, when these other causes are uncovered and treated, the patient's mental status returns to its recent (but still deteriorating) baseline.

3. OUR EVOLUTIONARY HERITAGE

Anything but the most cursory consideration of the implications of evolution for an understanding of physiology and its application to modern medicine would go beyond the scope of this book. Briefly, we wish to emphasize three points.

First, a consideration of evolution provides a valuable, humbling perspective from which health professionals should consider human health and disease. We are not the only way life has or could have evolved on earth. Indeed, our branch on the tree of life is a rather minor one (see Figure 20.1). We are just the product of the selection pressures of certain environments on what came before us. The extent to which we are in continuity with our ancestors is remarkable, as illustrated by the

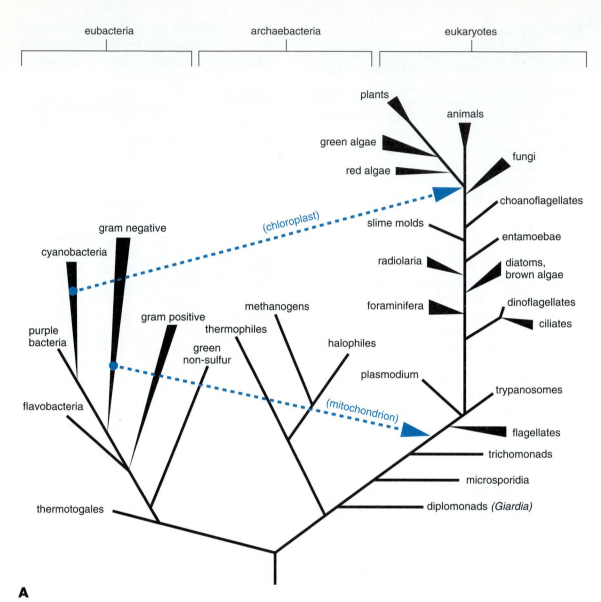

A

FIGURE 20.1. Humans' place on the evolutionary tree. *A.* The three major kingdoms of living organisms and their major branches. *B.* Correlation of the major geological, paleontological, and cellular events in evolution. At the left, time in millions of years from the present is indicated; on the right, some biological innovations are indicated. *(Adapted from Gerhart J, Kirschner M (1997). Cells, Embryos, and Evolution. Malden, MA, Blackwell Science.)*

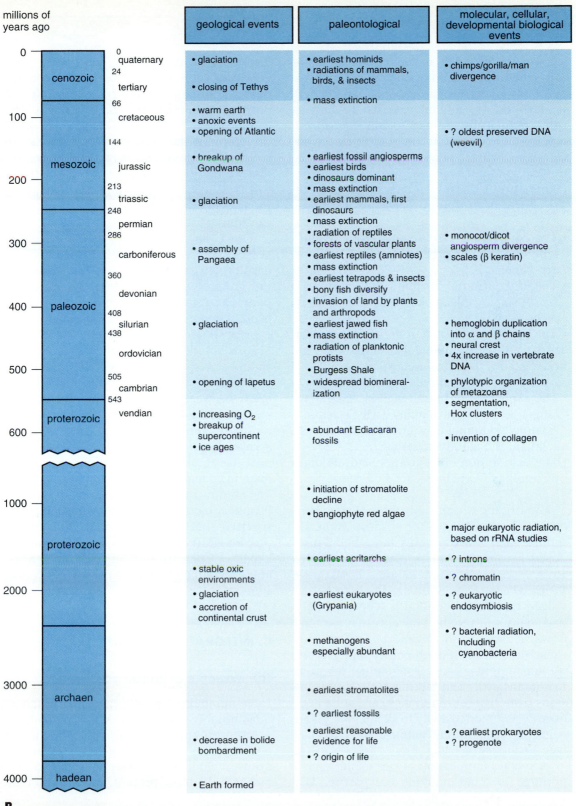

B

FIGURE 20.1 — (*continued*)

similarities between us and other animals (e.g., the organization of our internal organs and body plan); this provides an intellectual justification for animal research to understand human disease and for the use of cell culture and cell-free techniques to gain conceptual insight into how organ systems work.

On the other hand, we also represent the culmination of several remarkable leaps in the course of evolution. These leaps include

- The development of the eukaryotic phenotype (e.g., versus procaryotes such as modern bacteria)
- The organization of multicellularity (e.g., versus single-celled eukaryotes such as yeast or protozoans)
- The further entrainment and regulation of organ systems implied by homeothermia (i.e., maintenance of a constant body temperature, unlike reptiles or amphibians)
- The expansion of brain function, leading to language and tool making (which remain relatively rudimentary in even our closest relative, the chimpanzee)
- The elaboration of civilization, culture, and technology over the last 50,000 years.

Exactly how each of these leaps was achieved remains a matter of speculation, although cogent hypotheses have been proposed for many of them (see, for example, Refs. 5 to 8). At least in some cases, new forms of gene regulation are likely to be involved (see Refs. 9 and 10). It seems likely that many will require concepts that we cannot articulate or understand at present. Because these leaps remain poorly understood, we must apply insights from animal research to humans with great caution. Indeed, conclusions from one set of humans cannot be necessarily assumed to apply to all humans, given concepts such as biochemical individuality (see Frontiers of Chap. 2).

A second implication of our evolutionary heritage is mind-numbing *complexity*. We have seen in earlier chapters how a given gene product is used and reused in the course of evolution, in different places for different purposes (see also Sec. 5, Frontiers). That complexity is further compounded at each of the leaps in the product of evolution previously described. This may account for much that we do not understand about health and disease and once again suggests that we approach pharmacotherapy of disease with caution.

Third, an evolutionary perspective suggests that health care should involve a reliance on normal function and homeostasis to the greatest extent possible. Whatever the body can reasonably be expected to do for itself, it should do for itself. The patient who can eat should generally not be fed by intravenous solution. The patient who can walk should generally be encouraged to do so. The patient on mechanical ventilation should generally be weaned from that support as soon as possible, so that he or she can breathe on his or her own. Each of those generally accepted principles of modern medical practice has multiple justifications related to avoiding complications, optimizing quality of life, minimizing cost, and so forth. It is probably not coincidental that an evolutionary perspective that recognizes that homeostatic, physiological mechanisms are generally far ahead of our current best (or even foreseeable) technology comes to the same conclusions.

4. INTEGRATION OF COMPLEX EFFECTS

The example of cancer cachexia

In a number of pathologic circumstances, most notably cancer and AIDS, patients develop profound cachexia (weight loss). This phenomenon involves a number of mechanisms, including loss of appetite and abnormal carbohydrate, protein, and lipid metabo-

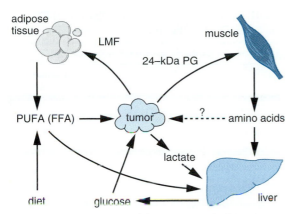

FIGURE 20.2. Some possible ways in which a cancer can subvert homeostasis to its own ends, resulting in cachexia. About half of all solid tumors cause a syndrome of cachexia in patients. This syndrome is characterized by the catabolism of skeletal muscle protein and adipose tissue triglycerides. A proteoglycan (PG) made by the cancer appears to mediate the protein catabolism in skeletal muscle, while other lipid-mobilizing factors (LMF) act to enhance free fatty acid release from adipose tissue. Finally, anaerobic metabolism in the tumor itself generates lactate, which the liver converts to glucose, further providing for the needs of the cancer. Polyunsaturated fatty acids = PUFA; free fatty acids = FFA. *(Adapted, with permission, from Nabel GJ, Grunfeld C (1996). Calories lost — another mediator of cancer cachexia. Nature Med 2:397–400.)*

lism. An understanding of it requires an integration of concepts covered in Chapters 3, 4, 11, and 19 and serves as a model for how knowledge of physiological mechanisms can facilitate an understanding of the pathologic twist that occurs in disease.

Some of these effects, including the production of cytokines such as tumor necrosis factor, upregulation of leptin, etc., appear to be part of a war of attrition initiated by the host to retard the advance of the cancer (see Ref. 11). However, other effects appear to be a counteroffensive on the part of the cancer to confound the defenses of the host (see Refs. 12 and 13). At least three mechanisms have been identified by which some cancer

cells integrate the metabolism of the liver, adipose tissue, and muscle to their advantage (see Figure 20.2):

- Production of low-molecular-weight proteoglycans that specifically trigger protein degradation and amino acid release from muscle, thereby providing fuel substrates for the tumor.
- Production of lactate through anaerobic metabolism in the tumor. The lactate flows to the liver and is converted via gluconeogenesis into glucose, which also supplies fuel to the tumor.
- Production of lipid-mobilizing factors that stimulate adipose tissue breakdown with release of various free fatty acids such as linoleic and acrachidonic acid, which promote tumor growth through various signaling mechanisms.

This is a case where the cancer appears to subvert normal host defenses and turn them on their heads, indicative of the complexity of — and surprises in store with — organ system interactions in health and disease.

Review Questions

11. What are two mechanisms by which host factors induce cachexia in cancer patients?
12. What are some of the products made by cancer cells that induce cachexia?

The example of cigarette smoking

The effects of cigarette smoking on normal physiology are devastating (see Ref. 14). Four general mechanisms are believed to be involved:

- Smoke enhances oxidation, which is chemically analogous to burning of tissues. Furthermore, oxidative inactivation of α_1 antitrypsin by smoke specifically strips the body of a crucial defense against terribly injurious substances (e.g., neutrophil elastase) that are being dumped in the lungs in response to smoke-induced irritation. In effect, the oxidative effects of smoking subject all recipients of smoke — including secondhand smoke — to a form of accelerated, premature aging. Individuals who seem to be able to smoke without ill effect in terms of the development of shortness of breath and other signs of emphysema may have genetically higher levels of α_1 antitrypsin, but this does not protect them against the other, more insidious effects of smoking via the other mechanisms.

- Smoke causes low-grade carbon monoxide poisoning in those who inhale — not enough to kill you immediately, but equivalent to a form of slow strangulation of all of your tissues (because it is carried throughout the bloodstream) by impairing the capacity of blood to provide them oxygen.
- Nicotine induces alteration in catecholamines, blood endorphins, glucose, fatty acids, vasopressin, and other substances in the bloodstream and in the brain. This wreaks havoc on the pattern of complex signaling that your body uses to maintain homeostasis.
- Carcinogens in smoke serve as initiators and/or promoters of malignant transformation.

Consequences of smoking

Through disruption of normal physiology via the mechanisms previously outlined, smoking causes two broad groups of diseases. Some of these, summarized in Table 20.10, are major causes of death, including

- Emphysema
- Coronary artery disease, atherosclerosis, and stroke
- Lung cancer

TABLE 20.10   CAUSES OF MORBIDITY AND MORTALITY RELATED TO CIGARETTE SMOKING

Fatal diseases positively associated with smoking[a]

Disorder		Relative risk (smoker/ nonsmokers)
(i) Increased risk largely or entirely caused by smoking Cancer of:		
Lung	M	22.4
	F	11.9
Upper respiratory sites	M	24.5
	F	5.6
Bladder and other urinary organs	M	2.9
	F	2.6
Pancreas	M	2.1
	F	2.3
Ischemic heart disease	M	1.9
	F	1.8
Aortic aneurysm[‡]	M	4.1
	F	4.6
Chronic obstructive pulmonary disease	M	9.7
	F	10.5
(ii) Increased risk partly caused by smoking Cancer of:		
Esophagus	M	7.6
	F	10.3
Kidney	M	3.0
	F	1.4
Cerebrovascular lesions	M	2.2
	F	1.8
(iii) Increased risk due to confounding Cancer of cervix	F	2.1
All diseases excluding those in category (iii)	M	3.2
	F	2.4
All diseases excluding those in categories (ii) or (iii)	M	3.4
	F	2.7

Nonfatal diseases positively associated with smoking

(i) Increased risk largely or entirely caused by smoking Peripheral vascular disease (age 45–74 years)	2.0
(ii) Increased risk partly caused by smoking	
Cataracts (men aged 40–84 years)	2.2
Crohn's disease	2.1
Gastric ulcer (aged 20–61 years, Norway)	3.4
Duodenal ulcer (aged 20–61 years, Norway)	4.1
Hip fracture (aged ≥ 65 years)	1.3
Periodontitis (aged 19–40 years)[Prevalence]	3.0
Macular degeneration	NA
Deafness	NA
Facial wrinkles	2.6
Renal failure	NA
Dementia	2.2–2.3

[a] Relative risks taken from the American Cancer Study (CPSII).
NA = not available.
From Wald NJ, Hackshaw AK (1996). Cigarette smoking: An epidemiological overview. *Br Med Bull* 52:3–11.

Other disorders associated with smoking (see Table 20.10) are causes of disability, pain, and suffering, but generally not death; these include

- Association with gum disease and poor response of gum disease to treatment — meaning that smokers' teeth are more likely to fall out at a young age (see Ref. 16)
- Association with hearing and vision loss — meaning that smokers are more likely to go deaf or blind at a younger age (see Refs. 17 and 18)
- Association with the occurrence of ectopic pregnancy — meaning that the risk of a failed pregnancy and intraabdominal catastrophe is increased (see Ref. 18)
- Association with increased wrinkling of skin (see Ref. 19)
- Association with the development of dementia and Alzheimer's disease (see Ref. 20)
- Association with the development of kidney disease (see Ref. 21)

Some patients are not moved by the risk of death, perhaps because of denial, because it is too distant a consequence, or for other reasons. On the other hand, those same individuals may find the thought of losing their teeth or their hearing or of developing wrinkled skin to be of far greater emotional concern — sufficient perhaps to effect change in behavior.

It is often difficult for a patient to remember the clinician's pronouncements and recommendations once he or she has returned home from the clinician's office. This may be in part because the recommendations are heard as a jumble of disconnected points. However, when they are told as part of the logical story of smoking's varied and devastating effects on normal physiology, they are much harder to forget.

Review Questions

13. What are some causes of death related to smoking?
14. What are some causes of misery (but not death) related to smoking?
15. What are four mechanisms by which smoking is believed to have injurious effects on many tissues, if not on every tissue in the body?

5. FRONTIERS IN ORGAN SYSTEM INTEGRATION

The integrated response to hypoxia

Recent years have seen remarkable progress in our molecular understanding of the cellular response to lack of oxygen, also known as **hypoxia** (see Ref. 9). It appears that higher eukaryotes have a universal **oxygen sensor** that, much like the oxygen-hemoglobin interaction, exists in both oxygenated and deoxygenated forms with an **allosteric transition** from one to the other dependent on oxygenation. Oxygenated, the sensor is inactive. In the deoxygenated form, it appears to trigger a cascade of phosphorylation events that activate a signal transduction pathway; this culminates in increased activity of a specific transcription factor called HIF-1 that governs expression of genes in response to hypoxia (see Figure 20.3). The range of consequences of activation of HIF-1 via the oxygen sensor include

- Adaptation to anaerobic metabolism
- Erythropoiesis (synthesis of red blood cells)
- Angiogenesis (proliferation of blood vessels in hypoxic tissues)
- Vasodilation (increasing blood flow in existing blood vessels of hypoxic tissue)
- Increased respiratory rate (to maximize oxygen saturation of hemoglobin and elimination of carbon dioxide)

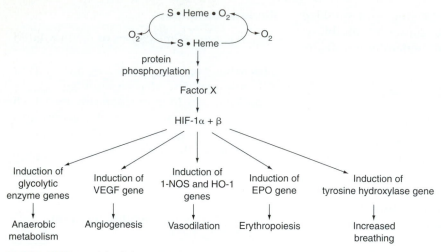

FIGURE 20.3. Model of the HIF-1 hypoxia response pathway. At normal tissue oxygen tension, O_2 is bound to a hemeprotein oxygen sensor (S. Heme). When oxygen levels drop, oxygen dissociates, causing a change in the sensor that triggers a protein phsophorylation signaling pathway, which activates a hypothetical regulator (Factor X) and increases expression of the HIF-1α and 1β subunits. The HIF-1 α/β heterodimer binds and activates expression of various genes, including those encoding glycolytic enzymes (for anaerobic metabolism), growth factors such as VEGF needed for angiogenesis, inducible nitric oxide synthesase and heme oxygenase-1 (which produce vasodilators), erythropoietin (to make more red blood cells), and tyrosine hydroxylase (an enzyme involved in dopamine production, which increases respiratory rate). These genes help an organism survive at low oxygen tension and trigger a homeostatic response to correct the hypoxia. Some of these genes are induced in all tissues; others are triggered by hypoxia in some tissues but not others, suggesting that other factors, with a tissue-specific distribution, are also necessary for their expression. (Adapted, with permission, from Guillemin K, Krasnow MA [1997]. The hypoxic response: Huffing and HIFing. Cell 89:9–12.)

A remarkable feature of this system is that somehow, different tissues know to activate some but not necessarily all of the genes that can respond to HIF-1. Thus, expression of the gene for erythropoietin, the hormone involved in red blood cell production, occurs only in the liver and kidney. Presumably other factors will be found that work in concert with HIF-1 to confer such tissue- and development-specific expression.

The implications of this newly appreciated pathway of normal physiology are also remarkable. The cellular response to hypoxia differs depending on severity and tissue type involved; responses range from shutdown of nonessential cellular functions to p53-mediated activation of apoptosis (see Chap. 2). If we understood these responses and how to selectively activate them, we might be able to rescue ischemic tissues and develop a new approach to the killing of cancer cells. Interestingly, simple unicellular eukaryotes such as yeast do not have the HIF-1 gene that is so universal in higher eukaryotes, suggesting that this is one of the pathways that may account for distinctive features of higher eukaryotic biology (i.e., the leaps discussed in Sec. 3 above).

Array technology, epigenetics, and the human genome project

Successes such as the progress in molecular understanding of the hypoxic response discussed previously have given rise to a new optimism concerning the potential of molecular biology for changing the nature of health care and the quality of our lives (and for making some people a lot of money in the process).

Programs are now underway to completely sequence the 3 billion base pairs of DNA in the human genome. A by-product of these efforts will be a tremendous advance in the pace of drug development and a far more sophisticated characterization of the particular sets of genes expressed in response to particular circumstances, environments, etc. For example, the development of DNA array chips (e.g., see Ref. 22) will eventually allow cells, animals, and even humans to be screened to identify every single quantitative change in mRNA concentration for every gene in particular tissues of patients who respond well (or poorly) or have side effects to a drug. Implicitly, this may allow us to know why patients did or did not respond in one way versus another, and thus focus medical therapy on those patients who will most benefit.

There are, however, potential limitations to this logic. Transcriptional control, while the best understood, is certainly not the only level of regulation of gene expression. What is left after all regulation through changes in levels of mRNAs has been understood in quantitative terms may still be a large part of biological regulation (see, for example, Ref. 10). Subtle aspects of the details of many if not all complex signaling pathways may involve regulation at the translational or post-translational level.

As another example, consider epigenetic mechanisms — that is, gene expression controlled at the level of DNA and or RNA by currently mysterious means (see Ref. 23). These may prove to be more than special cases and oddities, but rather are central features of disease processes or aspects that contribute important features needed to understand drug effects. Although epigenetic mechanism will surely prove to be perfectly explainable in terms of chemical reactions involving proteins, lipids, and nucleic acids, their widespread involvement in human biology may make it impossible to come to simple conclusions simply by analysis of changes in transcript levels using DNA array technology.

These arguments are not meant to suggest that these new technologies will not have an enormous impact on science or medicine. Rather, they are made solely to remind us that history does not end with today, tomorrow, or the next day. New understanding begets new questions, which subplant the old questions as the most important ones. Our current understanding, by definition, cannot fathom what the future will bring. And yet, the science and medicine of today can be based only on what we think we know today. Our only plea is that scientists and clinicians alike not forget that today's insights will probably be viewed as but a humble way station in the development of human thought and action.

Holistic nutrition

Perhaps one of the least understood, and clinically most important, areas of normal physiology is that of human nutrition. The human diet has undergone dramatic change in the last century. Traditional diets have been substantially replaced by "fast foods." Food that has been processed (removing fiber and some trace nutrients) and to which artificial supplements have been added are standard features of the diet for large fractions of the population. The full impact of these changes on health and disease remains unknown and most likely will take decades, at best, to be understood. Given that the eating habits of populations are likely to continue to change rapidly and are likely to be influenced by a host of confounding variables, such as other aspects of the environment, age, and genetic factors, evidence for an optimal human diet may be a long way off.

Lacking clear-cut evidence, an interesting approach is to return to traditional diets as an indicator of the kinds of foods on which we historically evolved. These traditional diets were typically far higher in fiber and in diversity of plant products consumed, and lower in protein, fat, simple sugars, and artificial supplements, than the typical diet of the modern world. Cogent arguments have been made that a return to such diets might mitigate many of the minor and major ailments of modern society that may be connected in complex ways to the dietary changes of the last century (see Ref. 4). Such an approach to human nutrition emphasizes obtaining needed nutrients primarily through a wide variety of plant products. This allows the body to use, to the greatest extent possible, its homeostatic mechanisms to meet its nutritional needs. Conceptually this approach is quite different from the current focus on quantities of protein, fat, and caloric intake as the end-points by which diet is measured.

Humans and *Helicobacter pylori*: a symbiotic relationship?

Conventional thinking has it that *H. pylori* is a pathogen to be eradicated on sight. The basis for this view is that a clear case has been made for the involvement of *H. pylori* in the pathogenesis of peptic ulcer disease, and that it may possibly be involved in other disorders such as gastric ulcer and gastric cancer. However, it appears that this particular host-microbe relationship is more complex than explained by a simple "us" vs. "them," "good" vs. "bad" dichotomy (see Ref. 24). *H. pylori* has evolved in humans and their ancestors for millions of years. During this time, adaptation may have resulted in mutual benefits such that elimination of *H. pylori* results in GI tract dysfunction and a higher risk of developing esophageal disease. Homeostasis in this case may involve a balance between different strains of *H. pylori* such that protective effects on esophageal disease balance the risk of gastric and duodenal disease. This sort of thinking, which places us in the continuum of evolution of life on earth, is quintessential physiological medicine.

Conservation of genes and the evolution of complex behavior

We have already pointed out the unsolved mystery of how to account for the difference between humans and chimpanzees based on a mere 1 to 2% difference in our DNA sequences. Indeed, each of the leaps in evolution that we have discussed poses a similar mystery in understanding the transition from an earlier form of life in which that complexity does not occur. Recently, a remarkable experiment was performed that illustrates how evolution reuses genetic material for widely divergent purposes. Vasopressin, a gene product involved in triggering water channel movement to the plasma membrane in the distal renal tubule and collecting duct, and also in regulation of blood pressure (see Chap. 10), has also been implicated in complex animal behavior. Two different species of field rodents (called voles) are known to display radically different forms of social behavior. The prairie vole is highly social and monogamous, while the mountain vole is highly asocial and promiscuous. When laboratory mice were generated that were transgenic (see Chap. 2) for a specific isoform of the prairie vole vasopressin receptor, they were found to take on the social behaviors of the prairie vole, and those behaviors were further heightened by central administration of vasopressin (see Ref. 25). Thus, nature manages to achieve enormous economies by reuse of "old" proteins in creative ways that cut across organ systems, in this case the brain and the kidney, behavior and fluid homeostasis.

6. HOW NORMAL PHYSIOLOGY PROVIDES INSIGHT INTO THE INITIAL CASE

Mr. B's history of alcoholism provides several strikes against him. First, he is a debilitated, immunocompromised host whose ability to fend off pathogens is impaired. Second, as an alcoholic, he is at greater risk of inhaling vomited stomach contents (a condition known as aspiration), which can lead to severe lung inflammation and pneumonia. Third, his recent history lulls the clinicians into a misplaced complacency. Just another drunk. But not really.

The body, when losing the battle with an invader, activates cytokines at levels that are dangerous to the host. Various organs and lines of defense cannot function optimally as the pH and oxygenation drop. Mental status change is an early sign, but could also indicate more selective involvement of the brain in the disease process.

The fall in Mr. B's white blood cells is a worrisome sign. Sometimes this just represents the immunosuppressive effects triggered by a viral infection. However, sometimes it is a sign that Mr B's defenses have been overwhelmed by the invader and worse is yet to come.

Once he presented to the emergency room, Mr. B's only chance of survival involved the kind of intensive (and expensive) medical intervention observed here. Sometimes it will be life-saving. Sometimes it is simply not enough (for poorly understood genetic and environmental reasons, or perhaps the nature of the infecting organism, or simply bad luck).

It is notable that once multiorgan system failure was underway, treatments that were intended to benefit Mr. B probably contributed to his demise. For example, the pressors being used to maintain his blood pressure in the face of cytokine-mediated collapse resulted in ischemia of his fingers, toes, and, presumably, other organs, such as the heart and kidneys.

The take-home messages of this case are twofold:

1. Disease is a lot cheaper to prevent than to treat. If this person had received effective rehabilitation from alcoholism, his story might have had a different outcome. A far smaller expenditure of resources to address the underlying social problem that set him up for illness might have bolstered host defenses sufficiently to prevent this hospitalization and others.
2. When homeostasis is lost, the patient will probably succumb, despite the best of care and regardless of the susceptibility of the infecting organism to the antibiotics used.

SUMMARY AND REVIEW OF KEY CONCEPTS

1. Often a consideration of our current understanding of how two organ systems interact under normal homeostatic conditions can instruct us on what can go wrong in disease.
2. It is often clear from the manifestations of their interaction that our understanding of organ systems is quite limited. New developments often reveal homeostasis to be a

far more complex and rich set of interactions than we might have previously believed.

3. Physiological medicine is clinical practice that pays special attention to the ways in which organ systems normally interact with one another.

4. Modern genetics is not going to be solely a mopping-up operation culminating in the sequencing of the human genome. That will be just one more step in the unending task of understanding ourselves. Between currently described phenomena called epigenetics and mechanisms that are likely to be discovered in the future, many concepts currently not in hand are likely to prove crucial to the practice of physiological medicine in the future.

5. Some key variables that affect the function and interplay of organ systems are genes; sex; the environment, including lifestyle, habits, and nutrition; and aging.

6. Cachexia in patients with cancer is an example of complex interactions involving multiple organ systems by which cancer cells turn the body's own homeostatic mechanisms against itself.

7. Cigarette smoking is a good example of a habit that wreaks havoc with many physiological organ system interactions by (1) enhanced oxidation, a form of accelerated aging; (2) carbon monoxide poisoning, a form of strangulation; (3) nicotine addiction; and (4) tumor initiation and promotion (carcinogenesis).

8. Patients often do not appreciate that cigarette smoking can do more than just kill you: It can make your life miserable through effects such as tooth and hearing loss, dementia, and cosmetic disfigurement.

9. Some frontiers in organ system integration: Recent progress in deciphering the physiological response to hypoxia is a shining example of the promise of the molecular future. However, the future may not be as simple as the present would have us believe it could be. Novel concepts of human nutrition emphasize our evolutionary and cultural heritage over simple applications of science or technology. The view of host vs. pathogen may be too simplistic. Certain organisms such as *H. pylori*, with which we have coevolved for millions of years, are likely to be protective against some disorders while predisposing to others. The challenge is to better understand these relationships under homeostatic conditions, not just for the paradigm of host–pathogen interactions that is the subject of the reference cited, but for all aspects of human health and disease.

A CASE OF PHYSIOLOGICAL MEDICINE

It is another busy day in your family practice clinic. In the course of the day, you see two alcoholics, three smokers, and two adolescents that represent the diversity of expression of human disease.

The first alcoholic is a 60-year-old man who is a self-described "two-fisted drinker," consuming no less than a fifth of scotch daily for the last 45 years. While he has some of the stigmata of chronic alcohol use (e.g., Dupuytren's contractures of the hands, vascular spiders, testicular atrophy), his liver is of normal size, neither shrunken (as often occurs in cirrhosis) nor swollen or tender (as often occurs with acute inflammation). His bilirubin is only slightly elevated; his serum concentrations of liver enzymes are mildly elevated; he has no obvious ascites on physical examination, only mild episodes of abdominal pain, no blood in his stool, and only mild elevation of serum amylase.

The second alcoholic is a 40-year-old man with a history of one six-pack of beer consumption per day for about 10 years. He presented to the clinic with new-onset abdominal swelling, jaundice, and excruciating abdominal pain. His amylase is 1200; his bilirubin is 12. He appears to have acute hepatitis and acute pancreatitis. Ultrasound examination of his liver reveals portal hypertension and a fatty liver.

All three smokers you saw today have a history of smoking one to two packs per day for 20 years or more.

The first is a 42-year-old sales executive who presented with a chronic cough and on chest x-ray has a right lung mass. Needle biopsy has just confirmed the worst: squamous cell carcinoma of the lung. Other studies suggest that metastatic disease is widespread. This patient's prognosis is dismal. He probably will not live to the end of the year.

The second smoker is a 52-year-old man who stopped smoking 5 years ago because his shortness of breath was interfering with his life-style. Unfortunately, the damage to his lungs has progressed, and he is now an oxygen-dependent pulmonary cripple. His passion in life was playing the piano — which he can no longer do because of shortness of breath with minimal exertion. His FEV1 is 0.3 L. His baseline Po_2 off oxygen is 45 mmHg. For him, life has become a matter of survival in pain; he is dyspneic at rest, unable to sleep for more than a few minutes without being awakened by a sense of strangulation, with trips to the bathroom representing a real challenge of endurance. Now despondent, he has decided to go back to smoking, saying that he hopes it will kill him off and end his misery.

The third smoker is a 72-year-old who has smoked since age 16. While he admits that he "can't run like I used to," his life appears not to have been directly impaired by smoking, which he continues to do to the tune of one to two packs per day. On closer history, however, you find that his spouse and son — both nonsmokers — died 10 years and 1 year ago, respectively, of lung cancer. Quite probably, they were victims of life with a human chimney. He feels that he is alone in the world, is depressed, and misses his departed family members terribly.

Your final two patients of the day were adolescents. The first, a boy of 16, has been your patient ever since he broke his arm at age 10. He admits to weekly alcohol drinking binges with friends. Bright and arrogant, his goal is to be a lawyer — and he can't wait for the drinking parties at college. His parents seem unconcerned by this alarming behavior. Their attitude is, "boys will be boys."

The second is a rebellious 15-year-old girl whom you have followed since birth — in fact, you delivered her! She has started smoking — because it is cool. Her parents are exasperated, and their communication with their daughter is at its nadir.

You have a good rapport with each of these seven patients. The challenge is how to leverage your relationship with them to help them understand and change habits (drinking and smoking) that are adversely affecting their health and the health of those around them.

QUESTIONS

1. How might the interaction of genes and environment be different in the three alcohol consumers?
2. How might you explain the effects of smoking in a way that would be effective for each of the four smokers?
3. What variables might account for the difference in presentation of the different drinkers?
4. What variables might account for the differences in presentation of the different smokers?

ANSWERS

1. The first individual had genes that probably have allowed him to avoid the worst consequences of alcoholism. However, it is likely that he is experiencing more subtle effects of alcohol on the brain, bone marrow, etc., that will impinge on his quality of life in the future. Thus, what he is gaining in the short term is probably coming at a price: He may be squandering the potential for an even longer and healthier old age.

   The second individual is unfortunate in being, apparently, particularly susceptible to hepatic and pancreatic inflammation. Perhaps some day this will be shown to have an immunologic basis. However, currently little is known as to the nature of the genetic versus environmental features that govern these different responses to acute and chronic alcohol use.

   The adolescent binge drinker may have a genetic predisposition to alcoholism. By preventing the development of habits early, potential problems can be addressed far more effectively.

2. Perhaps discussion of the cosmetic and "not cool" aspects of smoking-related disability (e.g., loss of sight, hearing, and teeth) would have more of an impact on the first and third smokers. Perhaps a survey of the range of different ways in which smoking can kill might impress patients who would otherwise end up like the second smoker.

3. Genes (including those of the immune system), environment (including nutrition or other habits), or other poorly understood factors.

4. Genes (including those of the immune system, level of expression of α_1 antitrypsin, activity of neutrophil elastase, etc.), environment (including other exposures to chemical carcinogens and causes of lung inflammation), or other poorly understood factors.

References and suggested readings

GENERAL REFERENCES

1. Wang J, et al. (1997). Local hormone networks and intestinal T cell homeostasis. *Science* 275:1937–1939.
2. Schlinger BA (1997). Sex steroids and their actions on the birdsong system. *J Neurobiol* 33:619–631.
3. Colborn T, et al. (1996). *Our Stolen Future.* New York, Penguin.
4. Lingappa YR, Lingappa BT (1992). *Wholesome Nutrition.* Worcester, MA, Ecobiology Foundation International.
5. Gerhart J, Kirschner M (1997). *Cells, Embryos, and Evolution.* Malden, MA, Blackwell Science.
6. Margulis L (1998). *Symbiotic Planet.* New York, Basic Books.
7. Rose MR (1999). *Darwin's Spectre.* Princeton, NJ, Princeton University Press.
8. Gould SJ (1989). *Wonderful Life.* New York, Norton.
9. Guillemin K, Krasnow MA (1997). The hypoxic response: Huffing and HIFing. *Cell* 89:9–12.
10. Hegde R, Lingappa VR (1999). Regulation of protein biogenesis at the ER. *Trends Cell Biol* 9:132–136.
11. Grunfeld C, et al. (1996). Endotoxin and cytokines induce expression of leptin, the ob gene product in hamsters. *J Clin Invest* 97:2152–2157.
12. Nabel GJ, Grunfeld C (1996). Calories lost — another mediator of cancer cachexia. *Nature Med* 2:397–400.
13. Todorov PT, et al. (1998). Purification and characterization of a tumor lipid-mobilizing factor. *Cancer Res* 58:2353–2358.
14. Slotkin TA (1998). Fetal nicotine or cocaine exposure: Which one is worse? *J Pharmacol Exp Ther* 285:931–945.
15. Rossing MA (1998). Genetic influences on smoking: Candidate genes. *Environ Health Perspect* 106:231–238.

16. Chan D (1998). Cigarette smoking and age-related macular degeneration. *Optom Vis Sci* 75:476–484.

17. Kornman KS, di Giovine FS (1998). Genetic variations in cytokine expression: A risk factor for severity of adult periodontitis. *Ann Periodontol* 3:327–338.

18. Saraiya M, et al. (1998). Cigarette smoking as a risk factor for ectopic pregnancy. *Am J Obstet Gynecol* 178:493–498.

19. Castelo-Branco C, et al. (1998). Facial wrinkling in postmenopausal women. Effects of smoking status and hormone replacement therapy. *Maturitas* 29:75–86.

20. Ott A, et al. (1998). Smoking and risk of dementia and Alzheimer's disease in a population-based cohort study: The Rotterdam Study. *Lancet* 351:1840–1843.

21. Gambaro G, et al. (1998). Renal impairment in chronic cigarette smokers. *J Am Soc Nephrol* 9:562–567.

FRONTIERS REFERENCES

22. DiRisi J, et al. (1997). Exploring the metabolic and genetic control of gene expression on a genomic scale. *Science* 278:680–686.

23. Lewin B (1998). The mystique of epigenetics. *Cell* 93:301–303.

24. Blaser MJ (1999). Hypothesis: The changing relationships of *helicobacter pylori* and humans: Implications for health and disease. *J Infect Dis* 179:1523–1530.

25. Young LJ et al. (1999). Increased affiliative response to vasopressin in mice expression the V1a receptor from a monogamous vole. *Nature* 400:766–768.

GLOSSARY OF TERMS

A-kinase (cyclic AMP–dependent protein kinase) Enzyme that phosphorylates target proteins in response to a rise in intracellular cyclic AMP. First identified in skeletal muscle as part of the pathway of regulation of glycogen breakdown in response to adrenaline.

Absorption Transport across an epithelium, typically from the lumenal side into the bloodstream.

Acetyl coenzyme A (acetyl CoA) An important metabolite consisting of a thioester of coenzyme A and acetic acid. The acetyl group can be generated from carbohydrates, fatty acids or amino acids and serves to move 2 carbon units into the tricarboxylic acid cycle, or to modify proteins and other substances, or can be used to make steroids and other compounds.

Acetylcholine Neurotransmitter that functions at cholinergic chemical synapses, found both in the brain and in the peripheral nervous system. It is the neurotransmitter at vertebrate neuromuscular junctions.

Achalasia Failure of the smooth muscle fibers of the gastrointestinal tract to relax, most commonly observed for the esophagus and the lower esophageal sphincter, due to degeneration of ganglion cells in the wall of the organ.

Acid A molecule that can donate a proton in solution.

Acidosis Any condition in which there is an excess of acid or depletion of base in the body resulting in a decrease in blood pH.

Acinar tissue Tissue made of small saclike dilations, particularly those found in various glands that deliver secretions into an exocrine duct.

Acinus (of the liver) A functional unit of liver tissue as defined by its blood supply. Thus a liver acinus is supplied by a terminal branch of the portal vein and of the hepatic artery and drained by a terminal branch of the bile duct.

Acquired immunity The components of the immune system in which memory of first contact with a pathogen allows heightened specific response in the form of antibodies or cell-mediated responses upon subsequent contact.

Acrosomal reaction A sequence of structural changes that occur in spermatozoa when they are in the vicinity of an ovum in the oviduct or uterine tube, believed to facilitate entry of a spermatozoon into the ovum during fertilization.

Acrosome The caplike, membrane-bound structure containing lysosomal enzymes that is found at the anterior portion of a spermatozoon and which facilitates entry of spermatozoa into ova during fertilization.

Actin filament A helical protein filament formed by the polymerization of globular actin molecules. A major constituent of the cytoskeleton of all eukaryotic cells and part of the contractile apparatus of skeletal muscle.

Action potential Self-propagating waves of electrical excitation at the plasma membrane that are the basis for transmission of signals along nerves and muscles.

Activation energy Extra energy that must be possessed by atoms or molecules in addition to their ground-state energy if they are to undergo a particular chemical reaction.

Active transport Movement of a molecule across a membrane or other barrier driven by energy other than that stored in the concentration gradient or electrochemical gradient of the transported molecule.

Activin A protein hormone made by the Sertoli cells in the male and granulosa cells in the female that stimulates the secretion of follicle-stimulating hormone and is involved in other complex interactions.

Adaptation Adjustment of sensitivity following repeated stimulation. This is the mechanism that allows a system to react to small changes, even against a high background level of stimulation.

Addison's disease Adrenal failure resulting in a syndrome of hypotension, weakness, hyperpigmentation, electrolyte abnormalities, and susceptibility to stress due to lack of adrenal cortical hormones.

Adenylate cyclase (adenyl cyclase) The enzyme which forms cyclic AMP from ATP. Activation of adenylate cyclase occurs in response to a variety of hormones and is a key step in signal transduction and intracellular signalling.

Adenoma A benign tumor of epithelial origin.

Adenosine A purine nucleoside with diverse cellular functions. Adenosine containing nucleotides are involved in transfer of chemical energy (e.g., in the form of ATP) and are a structural component of RNA. Adenosine is also the ligand for receptors that make it a powerful local mediator.

Adrenal cortex The outer part of the adrenal gland, where glucocorticoids and other steroids are made.

Adrenal medulla The center of the adrenal gland, where catecholamines are made.

Adrenaline See epinephrine.

Adrenergic receptor A member of the class of receptors activated by catecholamines such as norepinephrine and epinephrine.

Adrenocorticotropic hormone (ACTH, corticotropin) A pituitary hormone central to the body's response to stress. This 39-amino-acid peptide is generated from a larger precursor (proopiomelanocortin) by processing. ACTH stimulates the production of corticosteroids and is under feedback control by cortisol.

Aerobic A process that requires or occurs in the presence of oxygen.

Afferent The subset of nerves that conducts electrical impulses from peripheral tissues back to the central nervous system.

Affinity The property of specific binding between molecular structures.

Afterload The pressure against which the ventricle must work to eject blood during systole of the cardiac cycle.

Aging Growing old, which manifests, in organisms, as gradual, progressive loss of physiological function.

Agonist An analog of a hormone that is capable of binding to that hormone's receptor and inducing action that mimics the effects of the natural hormone.

Albumin The major plasma protein (60% of the total); it is responsible for much of the plasma colloidal osmotic pressure and serves as a transport protein for small hydrophobic molecules in the bloodstream.

Aldosterone A steroid hormone derived from cholesterol that is the major mineralocorticoid secreted by the adrenal cortex. It plays an important role in fluid and electrolyte homeostasis, promoting sodium, bicarbonate (and secondarily, water) retention, and potassium and hydrogen ion secretion. Its secretion is stimulated by potassium ions and angiotensin II.

Alkalosis A pathologic condition resulting from accumulation of base, or from the loss of acid in the body fluids, characterized by decrease in hydrogen ion concentration and an increase in pH.

Allele One of a set of alternative forms of a gene. In a diploid cell, each gene will have two alleles, each occupying the same position (locus) on homologous chromosomes.

Allelic polymorphisms Differences in the sequence of a particular gene that occur in a population, but that are not associated with a clinical disease.

Allopathy The system on which the practice of Western medicine is based, presently dominated by a reductionist approach to understanding the pathophysiology of disease and emphasizing the use of drugs to treat disease.

Allostery The ability of a macromolecule to have its reactivity with another molecule altered by combination with a third molecule or the enzyme inhibition exercised by such alteration.

Alpha-1-antitrypsin A liver synthesized plasma protein with broad protease-inhibiting properties, lack of which results in development of emphysema.

Alveolar-to-arterial gradient (A-a gradient) The gradient of gas, usually oxygen, between blood and the air in the alveolus.

Amenorrhea Abnormal cessation of, or failure to develop, menstrual bleeding.

Amino acid An organic molecule containing both an amino group and a carboxyl group. Those that serve as the building blocks of proteins are α amino acids, having both the amino and carboxyl groups linked to the same carbon atom.

γ-Aminobutyric acid (GABA) An amino acid formed in the metabolism of L-glutamic acid, it is the principal inhibitory neurotransmitter in the brain but is also found in several extraneural tissues, including the kidneys and pancreas. In the brain, it is released from some presynaptic cells upon depolarization. Through receptor binding it modulates membrane chloride permeability and inhibits postsynaptic cell firing.

Ammonia NH_3.

Ammonium The unstable radical NH_4^+.

Amnion A thin but tough membrane of embryonic development derived from the trophoblast that contains the embryo and fetus.

Amorphic A genetic mutation resulting in complete loss of function of the encoded protein.

Ampulla of Vater The location where the common bile duct joins the major pancreatic duct just prior to their emerging into the duodenum.

Amylase A group of digestive enzymes, forms of which are made by the salivary gland and the pancreas, that catalyze hydrolysis of starch into simpler compounds.

Amyloid Proteinaceous material with distinctive staining properties seen in plaque-like deposits in various histologic preparations. A marker for a variety of chronic degenerative disease states.

Anabolic Biosynthetic reactions in a cell in which large molecules are made from smaller ones.

Anaerobic A cell, organism, or metabolic process that functions in the absence of oxygen.

Androgen 19 carbon steroid hormones including testosterone and dihydrotestosterone that are derived from cholesterol and promote masculinization.

Aneurysm A defect in the wall of a heart chamber or blood vessel resulting in a sac-like outpouching. An aneurysm can rupture or be the site of formation of a blood clot, both of which can have catastrophic consequences.

Angina pectoris (angina) Chest, left arm or jaw pain, pressure or tightness, due to insufficient blood flow to cardiac muscle, often precipitated by exertion or excitement.

Angiogenic Having to do with the blood vessel and its development.

Angiotensin I An intermediate generated from angiotensinogen by the enzyme renin. Angiotensin I is subsequently converted to angiotensin II, a potent vasoconstrictor and stimulus of aldosterone secretion.

Angiotensin II An octapeptide hormone generated by the action of angiotensin-converting enzyme (ACE) on angiotensin I in vascular endothelium, chiefly in the lungs. It is a powerful vasopressor and stimulator of aldosterone secretion and also functions as a neurotransmitter. It raises blood pressure and diminishes fluid loss in the kidney by restricting blood flow.

Angiotensin converting enzyme An enzyme that catalyzes the cleavage of a dipeptide of the C-terminal end of the oligopeptide angiotensin I to form the activated angiotensin II.

Anion An ion carrying a negative charge reflecting the presence of excess electrons.

Anion gap A calculated parameter (blood sodium − [chloride + bicarbonate]) that indicates the levels of organic acids and other substances (unmeasured anions) in the bloodstream, which can be elevated in certain pathological conditions.

Anorexia The general pathological condition in which an individual has lost the desire for food.

Antagonist An analog of a hormone that blocks hormone action by preventing hormone binding or by binding but not activating the receptor.

Antibody A protein produced by B lymphocytes as a major limb of the host defense response to a foreign molecule or invading organism. Often binds to the foreign molecule or cell extremely tightly, thereby inactivating it or marking it for destruction by phagocytosis or complement-induced lysis.

Antidiuretic hormone (ADH) See vasopressin.

Antioxidant The class of small substances such as ascorbate that can provide electrons to quench electron-poor reactive oxygen species that would otherwise react with and damage proteins or other important macromolecules.

Aortic stenosis A pathological condition in which the opening of the aortic valve is incomplete or otherwise narrowed, causing obstruction to blood flow out of the heart.

Aphagia Inability to swallow.

Apical The tip of a cell, structure, or organ. The apical surface of an epithelial cell is the exposed free surface, often facing a glandular lumen and opposite to the basal surface, which rests on the basal lamina that separates the epithelium from other tissue.

Apolipoprotein B An hepatically synthesized protein that is a major component of very low density lipoprotein particles (VLDL) and the sole protein component of LDL particles. Uptake of LDL into the liver is mediated by apolipoprotein B-specific receptors.

Apoptosis A cellular suicide program manifest throughout metazoan development and physiology. Most cells respond to specific triggers that shift a balance of factors in favor of apoptosis. The resulting cascade of enzyme activation culminates in a highly programmed form of cell death, typically without an inflammatory immune response.

Aquaporins Channels that transport water from the renal tubular lumen to the bloodstream.

Aqueous Water-containing.

Arachidonic acid A polyunsaturated 20-carbon essential fatty acid occurring in animal fats and also formed by biosynthesis from dietary linoleic acid. It is a precursor in the biosynthesis of leukotrienes, prostaglandins, and thromboxanes.

Arachnoid villi Small projections of the arachnoid protruding into the superior sagittal sinus, through which cerebrospinal fluid is reabsorbed into the blood in the venous system.

Aromatase The cellular enzyme that catalyses the conversion of androgens to estrogens.

Arteriosclerosis Vascular diseases in which the arterial wall is thickened and has lost its compliance.

Ascites The accumulation of extravasated fluid in the abdominal cavity in excess of the capacity of the lymphatic system to return it to the circulation.

Association constant (binding constant, K_m) A measure of the extent of a reversible association between two molecules.

Asterixis A characteristic finding in liver failure and other causes of metabolic encephalopathy in which toxic substances interfere with the ability to maintain sustained contraction of muscle groups. Most readily demonstrable by asking the patient to cock back their wrists and "hold up traffic", resulting in a characteristic intermittent jerking motion.

Astrocyte Ectodermally derived cells associated with neurons that serve a wide range of metabolic, immunologic, structural and nutritional supportive roles in neuronal function.

Atelectasis A failure of a lung or a portion of a lung to expand, e.g. due to a mucous plug obstructing the airway.

Atherosclerosis A subset of arteriosclerosis characterized by the presence of atheromas, or plaques, containing cholesterol. These lesions form within the intima and inner media of large and medium-sized arteries, causing turbulence, obstructing blood flow and serving as a nidus for clot formation.

Atresia Involution and atrophy, usually as a result of programmed cell death. Specifically used to refer to the process by which nondominant follicles are eliminated during the female reproductive menstrual cycle.

Atrial natriuretic peptide (ANP, atrial natriuretic factor, ANF, atriopeptin) A hormone involved in a variety of functions that contribute to excretion of sodium in the urine as part of renal and cardiovascular homeostasis. ANP is made as a larger precursor in atrial myocytes and released in response to atrial stretch or volume overload.

Atrophy Decrease in size of a cell, tissue or organ as a result of lack of use.

Autocrine A local mediator released by a cell that has its own receptors that are activated by the mediator.

Autoimmune disease A disorder in which the immune system mistakes self-structures for foreign invaders that must be attacked and destroyed.

Automaticity The capacity of certain specialized "pacemaker" cells to initiate an action potential by spontaneous depolarization, in the absence of an external stimulus.

Autonomic nervous system The components of the nervous system specialized for largely involuntary regulation of tissue and organ system function. The components of the autonomic nervous system are the sympathetic, parasympathetic and enteric nervous system.

Autoregulation The ability of cellular systems to detect and adjust their activity in response to changes in the environment brought about by their actions, typically due to negative feedback mechanisms.

Avogadro's number The number of molecules in a mole, 6.0235×10 to the 23rd power, named after the Italian physicist who was one of the first to recognize its significance. This number of molecules is equal in weight, in grams, to the molecular weight of the substance.

Axon The process extending from the cell body of a neuron that transmits impulses to other cells including muscles, glands, and other neurons.

B lymphocyte The class of cells of the immune system that can differentiate into antibody-producing cells when appropriately stimulated.

Baroreceptors Receptors, usually in the walls of blood vessels, that sense changes in blood pressure and transmit that information to the central nervous system.

Basal The surface of a cell opposite the apical surface, typically associated with the basement membrane.

Basement membrane The extracellular matrix and connective tissue layer typically found abutting the basal surface of epithelia.

Basolateral The non-apical sides of an epithelial cell, including typically, the surface in contact with the basement membrane.

Basophil A class of white blood cells that release vasoactive amines (e.g., histamine and seratonin) when stimulated.

Benign A condition that is not associated with a high rate of bad clinical outcomes; with respect to tumors, one that tends not to spread from the initial site; non-malignant.

Bile A fluid substance secreted by hepatocytes via the bile canaliculus, stored in the gall bladder and eventually flowing into the small intestine via the bile ducts. It is alkaline due to a high content of bicarbonate, brownish green to yellow in color, and bitter to taste. The constituents of bile include bile salts, cholesterol, phospholipids, bilirubin and electrolytes.

Bilirubin One of a series of pigments derived from metabolism of heme by reticuloendothelial cells that is normally cleared from the bloodstream by conjugation and export in bile. Failure to export bile results in a yellowing of the eyes and skin termed jaundice, due to the accumulation of bilirubin and other pigments.

Binding constant A measurement of the tendency of a molecule to bind to another (e.g., a ligand to a receptor).

Biochemical individuality The observation that individuals within a population display substantial variation in biochemical pathways or their regulation, resulting in significant differences from one individual to the next in side effects to drugs, nutritional requirements, and other physiological and pathophysiological features.

Biological plausibility An explanation for a statistical association that makes sense in terms of our current understanding of biological mechanisms. Thus, for example, the association of peptic ulcer disease with *Helicobacter pylori* infection is consistent with our understanding that this organism can infect epithelial cells of the gastric mucosa and bring about changes that predispose to the development of ulcers.

Biological response modifier Molecules released by cells that bind receptors and activate signal transduction mechanisms. Unlike hormones, they do not travel long distances into the bloodstream, but are present in low quantities or are quickly degraded and affect only receptors on cells in the immediate neighborhood of their production.

Blastocyst The mammalian embryo at the post-morula stage. It has a fluid-filled cavity like a blastula, but unlike it, the blastocyst has multiple layers of cells.

Blastula An early stage of development in an animal embryo characterized by the presence of a single layer of cells surrounding a fluid-filled cavity.

Blood The fluid by which the diverse organ systems of the body communicate and exchange materials and signals, without which complex multicellular animals could not exist (see Chap. 19).

Blood-brain barrier The difficulty entering the brain encountered by many substances in the blood stream. Its molecular basis lies in the presence of tight junctions between the endothelial cells that make up the capillary walls.

Bombesin A peptide found in the brain and gut that serves important signaling functions of a paracrine or autocrine nature.

Bowman's space The space within the glomerulus between the tuft of capillaries and Bowman's capsule that is contiguous with the lumen of the renal tubule.

Bradydysrhythmia (bradyarrhythmia, bradycardia) The slowing of the heart rate to less than 60 beats per minute in an adult.

Bradykinin A nine amino acid residue

peptide produced in various inflammatory reactions by activation of kinins, that is a potent vasodilator, increases vascular permeability, stimulates pain receptors, and causes contraction of a variety of extravascular smooth muscles.

Brunner's glands Glands in the submucous layer of the duodenal wall which lead to the crypts of Lieberkuhn. Among their secretory products is the hormone urogastrone.

Buccal mucosa Mucosa lining the inside of the cheek.

Buffer Something in a system that tends to prevent or diminish external forces that would otherwise bring about changes in that system. Specifically often used to refer to a chemical with a tendency to donate or accept protons which serves to prevent or diminish a change in hydrogen ion concentration (pH) in a solution (e.g., in blood).

C kinase Calcium-dependent protein kinase that, when activated by diacylglycerol and an increase in the concentration of calcium, phosphorylates target proteins on specific serine and threonine residues.

C-reactive protein (CRP) An acute phase reactant protein (induced by systemic inflammatory syndromes) that is a member of the family of globulins secreted by the liver.

Cachexia A state of profound weight loss and malnutrition often seen in patients with terminal cancer.

Calcitonin A 32-amino-acid polypeptide hormone synthesized by the parafollicular cells of the thyroid gland that responds to hypercalcemia by lowering plasma calcium and phosphate levels, inhibiting bone resorption, and generally as an antagonist to parathyroid hormone. However its clinical signficance is less clear.

Calmodulin A ubiquitous calcium-binding protein whose binding to other proteins is governed by changes in intracellular calcium concentration. Its binding modifies the activity of many target enzymes and membrane transport proteins.

Cancer A class of disorders that have in common some aberration of the normal mechanisms of cell growth control.

Capacitation The poorly understood process by which sperm achieve the ability to fertilize an egg that typically occurs during the process of transport down the uterine tube.

Carbohydrate A general term for sugars and related compounds containing carbon, hydrogen, and oxygen, usually with the empirical formula (CH_2O).

Cardiac output Volume of blood ejected from the heart per unit time (e.g. liters/min).

Cardiomyopathy Primary, noninflammatory disease of the heart muscle.

Cardiovascular system The organ system comprising the heart and blood vessels by which blood circulates throughout the body (see Chapters 7 and 10).

Cartilage Connective tissue, often working in concert with bones, that makes possible muscle movement of the body as a whole, as well as of individual organ systems.

Caspase A family of proteolytic enzymes activated as part of the final common pathway of programmed cell death.

Catabolic Enzyme-catalyzed reactions in a cell by which complex molecules are degraded to simpler ones with release of energy. Intermediates in these reactions are sometimes called catabolites.

Catalyst A substance unchanged in a chemical reaction that increases the rate of the chemical reaction.

Catecholamine One of a group of amines that activate receptors in the autonomic nervous system and other locations. Examples include dopamine, norepinephrine, and epinephrine.

Cation A positively charged ion reflecting an insufficient supply of electrons.

Cell The smallest unit of life, defined as the smallest scale of organization at which the capacity to carry out functions needed for reproduction occurs.

Cell cycle The reproductive cycle of the

cell; the orderly sequence of events by which the cell duplicates its contents and divides into two.

Cell-mediated immunity Immunity mediated by T lymphocytes either by direct contact or by release of toxic substances. Examples of cell-mediated immunity include delayed hypersensitivity reactions, systemic response to viral and bacterial infections, contact dermatitis, granulomatous reactions, allograft rejection, and graft-versus host reactions.

Cerebrospinal fluid A fluid formed by the choroid plexus that circulates through the ventricles and subarachnoid space of the brain before entering the venous drainage.

Channel A conduit allowing large numbers of specific molecules to flow down the concentration gradient for that substance, through a hole that they create across the biological membrane.

Chaperone A protein that helps other proteins avoid misfolding, thereby facilitating their proper folding.

Chemokine A local mediator of the immune system.

Chemoreceptor A receptor or sense organ sensitive to chemical changes, such as the carotid body, which responds to low blood oxygen content by triggering increased respiration and blood pressure.

Chemotaxis Movement or orientation of a cell in response to a chemical concentration gradient. Most white blood cells exhibit chemotaxis in response to a wide variety of substances released at sites of inflammation.

Chief cells 1. Cells found in the lower portions of the gastric glands of the stomach that secrete the protease pepsin. 2. The most abundant cells in the parathyroid gland whose secretory product is parathyroid hormone.

Chirality Molecular asymmetry in three dimensions. Otherwise identical molecules can appear as mirror images, which are labeled "L" (levo = left) and "D" (dextro =

right) and are not interchangeable in biological systems.

Cholecystokinin (CCK) A polypeptide hormone secreted from both the brain (hypothalamus) and the gut (duodenal mucosa). In the brain, CCK is a neurotransmitter involved in satiety; in the gut, CCK stimulates contraction of the gallbladder (with release of bile) and secretion of pancreatic enzymes.

Cholestasis Cessation of bile flow most often due to inflammation and injury to hepatocytes or obstruction of bile ducts within or outside of the liver.

Cholesterol A hydrophobic lipid molecule that is a major constituent of biological membranes and is the precursor for both steroid hormones and bile acids. In excess, it plays an important role in the pathogenesis of atherosclerosis and coronary artery disease.

Cholinergic Stimulated, activated, or transmitted by choline (acetylcholine); a term applied to the sympathetic and parasympathetic nerve fibers that liberate acetylcholine at a synapse when a nerve impulse passes, or an agent that produces that effect. Also known as parasympathomimetic.

Chorion The mesoderm-lined membrane composed of trophoblastic cells that forms a protective outer layer for the embryo.

Chorionic villi Projections of the chorion into the endometrium of the uterus through which maternal fetal exchange takes place.

Chromosome Structure composed of a very long DNA molecule and associated proteins that carries hereditary information of an organism. Especially evident in cells undergoing mitosis when each chromosome becomes condensed.

Chylomicron The subset of lipoprotein particles produced in the small intestine after a fat-rich meal and used to transport exogenous (dietary) cholesterol and triglycerides. Chylomicron remnants are cleared from the bloodstream by the liver through the process of receptor-mediated endocytosis.

Chyme The well-homogenized slurry generated from ingested food by the combined action of gastric acid, enzymes and motility.

Ciracadian Recurring phenomena or rhythms of the body that occur with a periodicity of approximately 24 hrs.

Circumventricular organs Several small structures located around the edges of the third and fourth ventricles that lack the regular blood-brain barrier and thus serve as significant sites for neural-endocrine interactions.

Cirrhosis End-stage disease characterized by the presence of fibrous scar tissue disrupting the architecture of the liver.

Citric acid cycle (tricarboxylic acid or TCA cycle; Krebs cycle) The central metabolic pathway found in all aerobic organisms in which acetyl groups derived from food molecules are oxidized to CO_2 and H_2O. Localized within mitochondria in eukaryotic cells.

Clinical judgment The combination of the art of clinical medicine, including communication, attention to detail, and intuition, with scientific knowledge, as applied to the clinical care of individual patients.

Coding region (of mRNA) The region between the untranslated regions that encodes the triplet nucleotide codon sequence that will be translated as an amino acid sequence for a protein.

Colloid As a general term, referring to a proteinaceous solution; as a specific term referring to the iodinate thyroglobulin found in the thyroid follicular lumen which is converted into thyroid hormone by reuptake and proteolysis in thyroid follicular epithelial cells.

Coma An unconscious state from which a patient is unarousable even upon vigorous or painful stimulation.

Complement A group of proteins found in blood plasma which are activated by either antigen-antibody complexes or by microorganisms. When activated, complement components participate in immune-mediated destruction and stimulate phagocytosis (e.g., of bacteria and other invaders).

Complementary nucleotide sequence Two nucleic acid sequences forming a perfect base-paired double helix with each other.

Compliance The ability of an object to be stretched or distended; the opposite of stiffness.

Concentration The amount of a substance in a given volume.

Concepts Common principles that emerge from a consideration of the unifying features of individual conclusions from a large body of experimental data.

Congestive heart failure A syndrome in which forward output of blood from the heart is inadequate. Depending on whether it is the left or the right heart or both which are failing, and the rapidity with which the syndrome develops, it may be manifest as either peripheral edema (right sided failure) or elevated pulmonary vascular pressures with extravasation of fluid into the lungs, impairing oxygenation (left sided failure), or both.

Conjugation In genetics, the process by which compatible bacteria exchange genetic material, an important reason for the spread of antibiotic resistance. In liver physiology, the covalent chemical modification of hydrophobic drugs with hydrophilic sugars and other compounds in phase II drug metabolism.

Connective tissue Tissue that serves to protect, delimit, and demarcate various tissues.

Constitutive Produced in constant amount; the opposite of regulated. Constitutive secretion, for example, occurs continuously without requiring an external stimulus.

Corpus luteum A luteinizing hormone-dependent, progesterone-producing structure which develops in an ovarian follicle subsequent to discharge of its mature ovum.

Cortical bone The compact structure of calcium and phosphate salts that makes up the shaft of a bone and surrounds the marrow.

Corticospinal tract (pyramidal tract) The major motor neuron pathway, composed of nerves arising in the sensorimotor regions of the cerebral cortex, synapsing with motor neurons in the brainstem, and decussating (crossing) in the pyramids of the medulla.

Corticotropin See adrenocorticotropic hormone.

Corticoptropin releasing hormone (CRH) A peptide secreted from the median eminence of the hypothalamus into the pituitary portal circulation that binds to specific receptors on the corticotroph cells of the anterior pituitary and stimulates the secretion of corticotropin which is a stimulus of cortisol secretion by the adrenal cortex. CRH is also synthesized by other organ systems where it serves as a neurotransmitter and paracrine local mediator.

Cortisol A steroid hormone secreted as part of the stress response, cortisol is the major endogenous glucocorticoid in humans. It is synthesized in the zona fasiculata and reticulata of the adrenal cortex in response to stimulation from corticotropin. Cortisol elevates blood glucose and promotes protein breakdown and central redistribution of fat, and has mineralocorticoid activity. It is also a regulator of the immune system.

Covalent bond A chemical bond in which two atoms within a molecule share one or more electrons. Breaking these bonds requires a relatively large input of energy.

Crackles Abnormal sounds heard on auscultation of the lungs, primarily heard during inspiration, occurring in congestive heart failure and other conditions. Also called rales.

Cranial nerves The twelve pairs of nerves emanating from the base of the brain that leave the cranial cavity through various openings in the skull. Together with the spinal nerves and the autonomic nervous system, they comprise the peripheral nervous system.

Cross-talk Hormone activation of a variety of different second messenger signal transduction pathways that may reinforce or cancel out other ligand-activated receptor pathways. Steroid hormones can also form homo- and heterodimers, giving hybrid molecules with unique transcriptional activation characteristics.

Crypts of Lieberkuhn Intestinal glands.

Crystalloid A non-proteinaceous electrolyte solution capable of transport through animal cell membranes.

Cushing's syndrome A condition of glucocorticoid excess due typically to pituitary or adrenal tumors or to excessive glucocorticoid intake. The signs and symptoms of Cushing's syndrome include moon facies, fat redistribution from the extremities to the face, neck and trunk, hypertension, diabetes mellitus, amenorrhea, abdominal pain and stria, muscle wasting and weakness.

Cyclic AMP A nucleotide that is generated from ATP in response to hormonal stimulation of cell-surface receptors. Cyclic AMP acts as a signaling molecule by activating A-kinase; it is hydrolyzed to AMP by a phosphodiesterase.

Cyclin A protein that periodically rises and falls in concentration in step with the eucaryotic cell cycle. Cyclins activate crucial protein kinases (called cyclin-dependent protein kinases) and thereby help control progression from one stage of the cell cycle to the next.

Cyclin-dependent protein kinase (Cdk protein) A protein kinase that has to be complexed with a cyclin protein in order to act; different Cdk-cyclin complexes are thought to trigger different steps in the cell division cycle by phosphorylating specific target proteins.

Cyclooxygenase (COX) An enzyme that converts arachidonic acid into prostaglandin H, an unstable intermediate.

Cyclooxygenase pathway A pathway in which free arachidonic acid is converted into thromboxanes, prostaglandins, and prostacyclins.

Cystic fibrosis An autosomal recessive disorder characterized by a defect in the gene encoding the cystic fibrosis transmembrane regulator (CFTR), which controls epithelial chloride transport. As a result of this defect, patients develop pulmonary disease with chronic bacterial colonization and pancreatic insufficiency.

Cytochrome Colored, heme-containing protein that transfers electrons during cellular respiration and photosynthesis.

Cytochrome P450 A heme-containing enzyme involved in metabolic transformation of compounds in the endoplasmic reticulum and mitochondria of animal cells. It is of particular importance in steroid hormone metabolism and oxidation reactions of drug detoxification.

Cytokine An extracellular signaling protein or peptide that acts as a local mediator in cell-cell communication. Functions include regulation of the growth, development, and activation of the immune system and mediation of the inflammatory response.

Cytoplasm Contents of a cell that are contained within its plasma membrane but, in the case of eukaryotic cells, outside the nucleus and other membrane-delimited structures.

Cytosol The contents of the cytoplasm, excluding organelles. It is a gel-like liquid within the cell.

Cytotoxic T lymphocytes (CTLs) Ferocious warriors of the immune system, members of the T lymphocyte class, that recognize and kill target cells displaying the antigen against which the cytotoxic T lymphocyte's antigen receptors are directed. A component of cell-mediated immunity.

Cytotrophoblast The inner cell layer of the trophoblast of the early embryo.

Dalton A standard unit of molecular mass. Approximately equal to the mass of a hydrogen atom (1.66×10^{-24} g).

Data Empirical findings about some aspect of the environment.

Decidua The endometrium of the uterus during pregnancy.

Decidua basalis The maternal part of the placenta.

Decidual cells Stromal cells of the endometrium of the pregnant uterus, modified by the influence of progesterone, that appear in the late luteal phase and have paracine interactions with the developing embryo.

Decussate The crossing over of fiber tracts of the central nervous system from one side of the body to the other.

Deduction Deriving a conclusion by reasoning from accepted principles. Deduction or deductive knowledge includes, for example, mathematical truths about which there is certainty because they are so defined.

Denature To dramatically change the conformation of a protein or nucleic acid by heating or by exposure to chemicals, usually resulting in the loss of biological function.

Dendrite Elongated, tree-like processes of a neuron that receive information from the environment or from other neurons.

Deoxyribonucleic acid (DNA) A chemical composed of nucleotides that is used by cells to encode information and is the molecular basis for inheritable characteristics. Thus, genes are made of DNA.

Depolarization The transient loss or reversal of membrane potential in cells upon triggering of an action potential.

Dermatome The area of skin on the body surface whose sensory nerve endings emanate from a single spinal nerve root.

Desensitization Adjustment of sensitivity following repeated stimulation such that the response elicited is less than previously observed for the same stimulus.

Developmental program A program of function in an organism that results in growth or change, not homeostasis.

Dexamethasone A synthetic glucocorticoid whose affinity for the glucocorticoid receptor is 25 to 100 times greater than that of cortisol.

Diabetes insipidus A metabolic disorder caused by injury of the posterior pituitary that results in a deficient quantity of antidiuretic hormone (ADH) being released and thus in failure of tubular reabsorption of water in the kidney. As a result, a large amount of dilute urine is excreted, followed by dehydration and great thirst.

Diabetes mellitus A complex set of disorders that have in common absolute or relative insulin deficiency resulting in impaired carbohydrate metabolism manifest as an elevation in the fasting blood glucose concentration.

Diacylglycerol (DAG) A cleavage product of phosphatidylinositol biphosphate (PIP$_2$) that has profound effects on cell signaling.

Dialysis (Hemodialysis) The process of removal of diffusable substances, for example from blood, by exchange with a crystalloid solution across a semipermeable membrane.

Diapedesis The outward passage through intact vessel walls of cellular elements of the blood.

Diastole The window of time between the first and second heart sounds during which ventricular filling occurs.

Diffusion The process by which molecules move from regions of high concentration to regions of low concentration by random molecular motion.

Diffusion gradient The maximum difference in the concentration of a substance in different parts of a solution.

Dihydrotestosterone (DHT) An androgenic hormone generated in peripheral tissues as a result of the action of enzyme 5alpha-reductase on testosterone. DHT is responsible for virilization during embryonic development, for most male secondary sexual characteristics at puberty, and for aspects of adult male sexual function.

Dihydroxy Prefix referring to any compound that includes two molecules of the hydroxy (OH) radical.

Dioxin A highly toxic by-product of polychlorinated biphenyl compound (PCB) production. PCBs were once widely used as insulators.

2,3-Diphosphoglycerate (2,3-bisphosphoglycerate) A salt or ester of diphosphoglyceric acid; it is contained in red blood cells, where it plays a role in liberating oxygen from hemoglobin in the peripheral circulation. It is also an intermediate in the conversion of 3-phosphoglycerate to 2-phosphoglycerate in glycolysis.

Diplotene The first stage of the first prophase of meiosis, characterized by onset of separation between the chromosomes.

Disseminated intravascular coagulation (DIC) A disorder characterized by reduction in the elements involved in blood coagulation as a result of their utilization in widespread blood clotting within the vessels.

Disulfide bond A covalent linkage formed between two sulfhydryl groups on cysteines. It is a common way to join two proteins or to link together different parts of the same protein in the extracellular space.

Diuresis An increase in the rate of urine flow out of the body

Diuretic A pharmaceutical that, when absorbed, promotes diuresis.

Diverticular disease Disease, commonly of the colon, caused by formation of a circumscribed pouch or sac occurring normally or created by herniation of the lining mucous membrane through a defect in the muscular coat.

Dominant The member of a pair of alleles that is expressed in the phenotype of an organism while the other allele is not, even though both are present. Also refers to the phenotype expressed by a dominant allele.

Dopamine A catecholamine intermediate in the synthesis of norepinephrine, resulting from decarboxylation of dopa, which has its own specific receptors and acts as a neurotransmitter in both the central and peripheral nervous systems.

Dorsal Pertaining to the back or a position more toward the back.

Dorsal root ganglion The ganglion found on the posterior root of each spinal nerve, composed of the unipolar nerve cell bodies of the sensory neurons of the nerve.

Dumping syndrome A complex of symptoms including varying degrees of nausea, weakness, sweating, diarrhea and syncope that develops, typically after meals, in patients who have undergone partial gastrectomy.

Duodenum The first or proximal portion of the small intestine, extending from the pylorus to the jejunum.

Dura mater The tough, fibrous outer membrane covering the brain and spinal cord.

Dynein A member of a large family of motor proteins that use the energy of ATP to move along a microtubule.

Dynorphin A family of endogenous peptides with affinity for opiate receptors.

Dysmenorrhea Pain during menstrual bleeding.

Dysphagia Painful swallowing.

Dyspnea Difficult or labored breathing.

Dysrhythmia An abnormal cardiac rhythm.

Echocardiogram (echocardiograph) Noninvasive sound wave study of the motion of the heart that allows detection of abnormalities in wall motion or valvular function and determination of the fraction of blood ejected during the cardiac cycle.

Eclampsia Seizures in a pregnant woman with preeclampsia.

Edema Excessive interstitial (extracellular, extravascular) fluid in tissues, in excess of the capacity of the lymphatic drainage for return to the venous system.

Efferent Conveying or conducting away from a center. A nerve that carries impulses from the central nervous system toward the periphery.

Efflux An outflowing.

Effusion Accumulation of fluid in a cavity or space in excess of normal volumes, usually due to inflammatory reaction or elevated hydrostatic pressure in blood vessels. Typically referring to fluid collections between the layers of the pleura of the lungs (a pleural effusion) or the pericardium of the heart (a pericardial effusion).

Eicosanoid A structural category of local mediators that is derived from lipids such as arachidonic acid; it includes the prostaglandins, thromboxanes, and leukotrienes.

Ejection fraction The proportion of the volume of blood in the ventricles at the end of diastole that is ejected during systole; it is the stroke volume divided by the end-diastolic volume, usually expressed as a percentage, normally 57 to 73%.

Electrocardiogram A recording of the electrical potential caused by the excitation of the heart muscle during the course of the cardiac cycle, as detected from defined positions at the body surface.

Electrochemical gradient The driving force that causes an ion to move across a membrane as a result of the combined influence of a difference in its concentration on the two sides of the membrane and the electric charge difference across the membrane.

Electrolyte A substance that dissociates into ions when in solution, and thus becomes capable of conducting electricity; an ionic solute.

Electroneutrality An equivalence of positive and negative charges.

Endocrine glands Organs of the body specialized for the secretion of hormones into the bloodstream.

Endocytosis Uptake of material into a cell by an invagination of the plasma membrane and its internalization in a membrane-bounded vesicle.

Endometriosis A pathological condition in which endometrial tissue is found in locations other than the lining of the uterus. The cyclical response of this ectopic tissue to hormones can be very painful.

Endometrium The inner histological layer of the uterus which undergoes cyclical development, maturation and sloughing in response to hormonal changes of the menstrual cycle.

Endoplasmic reticulum (ER) A labyrinthine, membrane-bounded compartment in the cytoplasm of eukaryotic cells where lipids are synthesized and most membrane-bound and secretory proteins are made. The ER is the first compartment in the secretory pathway.

Endorphin Peptides derived from proopiomelanocortin that have affinity for opiate receptors and are powerful analgesics.

Endothelin A 21 amino acid polypeptide produced by endothelial cells and other sources that has been implicated in various signalling functions in different organs of the body including as a vasoconstrictor and as a neurotransmitter.

Endothelium The mesoderm derived layer of epithelial cells that make up the walls of blood and lymphatic vessels.

Energy The capacity to do work.

Enkephalin A family of peptide neurotransmitters with affinity for opiate receptors that, like the endorphins, has analgesic activity.

Enteric nervous system (ENS) The enteric plexus, the autonomic innervation of the gastrointestinal tract, considered separately from the autonomic nervous system because it has independent local reflex activity. Composed of the myenteric plexus and the submucosal plexus.

Enterochromaffin cells (ECL) Basal granular cells where serotonin is synthesized and stored.

Enterocyte Epithelial cells of the intestinal lumen.

Enterohepatic circulation The pathway of flow of bile from synthesis in hepatocytes, secretion into the bile canaliculus, storage in the gallbladder, release into the GI tract lumen to reabsorption from the terminal ileum into the portal blood flow. This returns bile acids to the liver where they are extracted from the blood and transferred back into the bile canaliculus.

Entropy A measure of the degree of disorder in a system; the higher the entropy, the greater the disorder.

Enzyme A biological catalyst, usually a protein, that can increase the rate of a chemical reaction by lowering its activation energy.

Enzyme induction Increased synthesis of an enzyme in response to a stimulus.

Epidermal growth factor A mitogenic polypeptide produced by many cell types that promotes growth and differentiation and is essential in embryogenesis and important in wound healing.

Epinephrine (adrenaline) A hormone released by chromaffin cells in the adrenal gland and by some neurons in response to stress. It produces "fight or flight" responses, including increased heart rate.

Epiphyseal plate The island of cartilage located between the epiphysis and the shaft of the bone whose growth allows bone length to increase.

Epistemology The study of knowledge, including what it is and how we get it.

Epitope A structural feature of an antigen that is recognized by an antibody.

Equilibrium Balance. When used specifically in a physicochemical context, it refers to the distribution of reactants and products after a chemical reaction has gone to completion under standard conditions.

Equilibrium constant (K_{eq}) Ratio of forward and reverse rate constants for a reaction; equal to the association constant.

Erythropoetin The renal hormone that is an important regulator of red blood cell production by the bone marrow.

Estradiol A powerful member of the family of estrogen steroids that plays a crucial role in the menstrual cycle and maintenance of reproductive and other organs in the female.

Estrogen A general term for 18 carbon steroids involved in female reproductive physiology.

Estrone An oxidation product of estradiol. It is less potent than estradiol but is metabolically convertible to it. It is secreted by the ovary but is primarily produced from peripheral metabolism of estradiol and androstenedione.

Eukaryote A living organism composed of one or more cells with a distinct nucleus and cytoplasm.

Exocrine Secretions directed out of the body via a duct.

Exocytosis The process by which most molecules are secreted from a eukaryotic cell. These molecules are packaged in membrane-bounded vesicles that fuse with the plasma membrane, releasing their contents to the outside.

Extrapyramidal motor system Those regions of the brain defined functionally, that are not part of the pyramidal tract but which control and modify motor activites, including the basal ganglia, striatum, substantia nigra.

Extravasation Escape of fluids (e.g., of blood from a vessel into tissues).

Exudate An effusion containing cellular and proteinaceous debris suggestive of an intense inflammatory reaction.

Facilitated diffusion Movement of molecules down their concentration gradient at faster than their spontaneous rate of movement across a membrane bilayer by virtue of their affinity for transporters that bind them on one side, shuttle them across the membrane and release them on the other side.

Facts Statements that are true.

Fatty acid A compound such as palmitic acid that has a carboxylic acid attached to a long hydrocarbon chain. Used as a major source of energy during metabolism and as a starting point for the synthesis of phospholipids.

Ferritin The major intracellular storage form of iron in the body. Comprised of a complex of iron and the high affinity iron-binding protein apoferritin.

Fibrin A major constituent of blood clots formed by the proteolysis of fibrinogen by thrombin.

Fibrinogen A fraction of human plasma that is converted into insoluble fibrin in the presence of thrombin.

Fibrosis A response to injury in which functional tissues are replaced by scar tissue composed of fibroblasts with resulting diminution and impairment of organ system functions.

First law of thermodynamics Energy can be neither created nor destroyed.

Fixed acid An acid that cannot be removed as a gas by the lung and hence must be removed by the kidneys via the urine.

Follicle stimulating hormone (FSH) One of two polypeptide hormones made by the gonadotropes of the anterior pituitary gland in response to stimulation by gonadotropin-releasing hormone from the hypothalamus. FSH stimulates ovarian follicular growth and development in the female and spermatogenesis in males.

Frank-Starling curve The relationship of cardiac output to ventricular filling at various degrees of cardiac muscle contractility in cardiovascular physiology. This relationship reflects the observation that, as atrial pressure and venous return increase, initially, there is a proportional increase in cardiac output, as stretch of muscle fibers makes their function more efficient. However, as cardiac muscle fibers are stretched further, output does not increase and eventually, decreases, as the efficiency of over-stretched cardiac muscle fiber contraction starts to diminish.

Free energy (*G*) Energy that can be extracted from a system to drive reactions. It takes into account both energy and entropy. It reflects the tendency of chemical reactions to proceed spontaneously.

Free radical A group of atoms that enters into and goes out of chemical combination without change, forms one of the fundamental constituents of a molecule, and is extremely reactive; it has a very short half-life and carries an unpaired electron.

Futile cycle Pathways of biochemical reactions that are exactly opposite in their reactants and products such that, when their activity is equal, the only outcome is the consumption of ATP and the generation of heat.

G Cell Endocrine cells in the mucosa of the pyloric region of the stomach, whose secretory products include gastrin.

G Protein Any of a large group of cytoplasmic GTP-binding proteins that play crucial roles as regulators of signal transduction Classically, G proteins are heterotrimers activated by binding of a hormone to its transmembrane receptor.

GIP A polypeptide hormone synthesized by cells in the mucosa of the GI tract that triggers insulin secretion in response to food composition.

Gallbladder The sac-like structure adjacent to the liver in which bile is stored.

Gamma-aminobutyric acid (GABA) A metabolite of the amino acid glutamate which is the major inhibitory neurotransmitter in the brain.

Ganglion A group of nerve cell bodies located outside the central nervous system, or certain nuclear groups within the brain or spinal cord.

Gastrin A GI tract polypeptide hormone released into the bloodstream by the G cells of the pyloric glands in the gastric antrum, that is a powerful stimulus to acid secretion by the parietal cells.

Gastritis Inflammation of the epithelial lining of the stomach.

Gastrocolic reflex The increased intestinal peristalsis observed when food enters the stomach when it is empty.

Gastrointestinal tract The system of organs that carries out the digestion and absorp-tion of desired substances from food and the elimination of waste. Organs include the esophagus, stomach, small and large intestines, and accessory organs of gastrointestinal function, such as the pancreas and gall bladder (see Chap. 5).

Gastroparesis Paralysis or disorder motility of the stomach, often due to disorders of the enteric nervous system.

Gene expression The manifestation of information encoded in an organism's genome at different times, in different tissues, and in different amounts to produce a phenotype, usually due to the synthesis of a protein.

Genome The sum total of all genetic information carried by a cell or an organism.

Genotype The genes of an individual cell or organism.

Germ cell The mature or immature reproductive cells; ovum in the female, sperm in the male.

Glial cell A nonneural cell of the supportive tissues of the central nervous system; there are three types: astrocytes, oligodendrocytes, and microglia.

Glomerulus A tuft of capillaries in the kidney, projecting into the expanded capsule of each renal tubule.

Glucagon A polypeptide hormone secreted by the pancreatic alpha cells that increases blood glucose concentration.

Glucokinase An enzyme that catalyzes the phosphorylation of D-glucose at the 6 carbon. It is specific for glucose.

Gluconeogenesis The biochemical pathway by which non-carbohydrate molecules such as amino acids, lactate and glycerol are converted into glucose.

Glucose-dependent insulinotropic peptide (GIP) A gastrointestinal hormone that stimulates anticipatory insulin release upon sensing food composition. It explains why an oral load of glucose stimulates more insulin secretion than the equivalent amount of glucose given intravenously.

Glutathione A widely distributed tripeptide that functions as a major intracellular reducing agent and is involved in drug detoxification.

Glycentin A precursor protein that encodes one of the enteroglucagon-related peptides of the GI tract.

Glycocalyx Refers to the "coat" of glycoproteins and glycolipids that is displayed on the plasma membrane of many cells of the body.

Glycogen A large polysaccharide that is highly branched. It constitutes the major carbohydrate reserve in animals, is stored primarily in liver and muscle, and is synthesized and degraded for energy as demanded.

Glycogenolysis The biochemical pathway by which glycogen is broken down into glucose.

Glycolysis A widely used metabolic pathway in the cytosol in which sugars are incompletely degraded without the use of oxygen, resulting in production of ATP.

Goblet cell Mucus secreting cell found in the epithelia of the GI and respiratory tract.

Golgi apparatus A set of vesicular compartments of the secretory pathway within eukaryotic cells. Maturation of sugars on glycoproteins is one of the many activities that take place in the Golgi apparatus.

Gonadotrope A cell in the anterior pituitary that synthesizes and secretes follicle-stimulating hormone (FSH) and luteinizing hormone (LH) in response to gonadotropin-releasing hormone activation of receptors on its surface.

Gonadotroph See follicle-stimulating hormone and luteinizing hormone.

Gonadotropin-releasing hormone (GnRH) A hypothalamic peptide released into the pituitary portal circulation whose effect is to trigger LH and FSH secretion from gonadotrope cells of the anterior pituitary.

Granulation tissue Healthy vascular tissue formed during normal wound healing

Granuloma A nodular collection of mononuclear immune cells due to chronic inflammation in response to a number of different infectious and non-infectious disease processes including tuberculosis and sacoidosis.

Granulosa cells The cells within an ovarian follicle that surround and nourish an oocyte, which develop into the lutein cells of the corpus luteum after ovulation.

Growth hormone (somatotropin) A polypeptide hormone secreted into the systemic circulation by somatotropes of the anterior pituitary gland, which stimulates growth through effects on organ, cartilage and skeletal growth and on carbohydrate, protein and lipid metabolism.

GTPase activity The enzymatic activity that results in hydrolysis of guanosine triphosphate (GTP).

Guaiac An indicator reagent that turns blue in the presence of heme and an oxidizing developer solution. This test is commonly used to identify occult gastrointestinal bleeding by collecting and testing samples of a patient's stools.

Haploid Having only one set of chromosomes, as in a sperm cell or a bacterium.

Haptoglobin An acute phase reactant hemoglobin-binding protein in plasma whose action is responsible for preventing loss of free hemoglobin in the urine.

Haustra Characteristic outpouching of the wall of the colon as a consequence of the location and dynamic contraction state of circular GI tract smooth muscle.

Helicobacter pylori A gram-negative microaerophilic bacteria associated with chronic inflammation of the stomach and development of gastritis, ulcers, and possibly cancer.

Helper T cells Differentiated T lymphocytes whose help is required for the production of antibodies against most T-dependent antigens.

Hematocrit The percentage of the volume of whole blood composed of red blood cells.

Heme A cyclic organic molecule containing an iron atom that carries oxygen in hemoglobin and carries an electron in cytochromes.

Hemochromatosis A disorder due to deposition of hemosiderin, an intracellular storage form of iron, in the parenchymal cells, causing tissue damage and dysfunction of the liver, pancreas, heart, and pituitary.

Hemodialysis Mechanical filtration of blood by removal of low molecular weight substances that can cross a semipermeable membrane.

Hepatic encephalopathy A distinctive change in brain function as a result of liver disease, typically associated with asterixis.

Hepatocyte A liver parenchymal cell.

Herniation The forcing of the abnormal protrusion of an organ or other body structure through a defect or natural opening in a covering, membrane, muscle or bone.

Hexokinase An enzyme that catalyzes the phosphorylation of hexose (6-carbon sugar) at the 6 carbon. It exists in all tissues and as various isoforms. The liver isoform is specific for glucose and is termed glucokinase.

High-density lipoprotein (HDL) A class of lipoproteins that promote transport of cholesterol from extrahepatic tissue to the liver for excretion in the bile. HDL is synthesized by the liver.

High-pressure liquid chromatography (HPLC) A technique whereby substances are separated under high pressure by their physical properties based on interaction with resins that compose a column. This differs from conventional chromatography, where flow is by gravity, in that higher pressures allow better resolution of similar substances with less diffusion.

Hirschsprung's disease Congenital megacolon.

Hirsutism The presence of an abnormally large amount of body hair typically in a male pattern of distribution.

Histamine A small molecule derived from the amino acid histidine, released from mast cells and basophils in allergic reactions. It causes irritation, itching, dilation of blood vessels, and contraction of smooth muscle.

Homeostasis The tendency of physiological systems to resist deviation from a normal range.

Homeothermy The ability of certain multicellular organisms to maintain their body temperature in the face of substantial changes of temperature in the environment.

Hormone A chemical substance produced in the body that has a specific regulatory effect on the activity of certain cells or a certain organ or organs.

Hormone-sensitive lipase An enzyme in adipose tissue that is inhibited by insulin. In the absence of insulin, it hydrolyzes stored triglycerides in adipose tissue into free fatty acids and glycerol.

Human chorionic gonadotropin (HCG) An LH-like hormone secreted from syncytiotrophoblasts of the developing embryo that supports the corpus luteum during the first several weeks of pregnancy until the placenta's ability to produce progesterone has been fully developed.

Human life cycle The time span comprising human prenatal life, birth, infancy, childhood, adolescence, adulthood, and old age, culminating in death.

Human placental lactogen (HPL), human chorionic somatomammotropin (hCS) A growth hormone–like protein hormone made by the syncytiotrophoblasts of the placenta that has growth-promoting activity and antagonizes maternal insulin in pregnancy.

Humoral immunity The branch of the immune system that involves the production of antibodies and other factors carried in the bloodstream.

Hyaluronidase Enzymes whose action results in the breakdown of hyaluronic acid, a major component of the glycocalyx and extracellular matrix in various tissues and organs.

Hydrogen bond An ionic interaction between various biologically important polar molecules, most notably water (see Figure 2.1).

Hydrolase Any enzyme whose mechanism of action involves the cleavage of chemical bonds through the addition of a molecule of water. This includes proteases, phosphatases, esterases, glycosidases, lipases, nucleotidases.

Hydrolysis Cleavage of a covalent bond in a molecule with accompanying addition of water, $-H$ being added to one product of the cleavage and $-OH$ to the other.

Hydrophilic Water loving; soluble in water.

Hydrophobic interaction A biologically important noncovalent interaction in which nonpolar molecules or parts of molecules are unable to form hydrogen bonds with surrounding water. These molecules or parts of molecules will then preferentially associate with each other. See Figure 2.1.

Hydrostatic pressure The pressure (e.g., across a membrane) due to the water in the system. For example, the distribution of fluid across the vasculature is determined by a balance of forces including the hydrostatic pressure tending to push water out and the oncotic pressure tending to pull water in.

Hydroxyapatite An inorganic compound composed of calcium and phosphate salts found in the matrix of bone and teeth that gives them rigidity.

Hypercapnia Elevated levels of carbon dioxide in the blood stream.

Hyperglycemia High blood sugar.

Hyperinsulinemia An elevated concentration of insulin in blood plasma.

Hyperlipidemia Elevated concentrations of lipids in blood plasma.

Hypermorphic A genetic mutation resulting in a gain in function of the encoded protein.

Hyperphagia Excessive eating.

Hyperplasia Increased number and rate of multiplication of cells in normal tissue. When self-limited, hyperplasia is often a physiological response. However, when prolonged, hyperplasia can be a precursor to the development of pathological processes such as cancer.

Hypertension Persistently high arterial blood pressure.

Hypertonic The quality in any medium of having a sufficiently high concentration of solutes to cause water to move out of a cell through osmosis.

Hypertrophy The enlargement or overgrowth of an organ or part as a result of an increase in the size of its constituent cells.

Hyperventilation Abnormally prolonged, rapid, and/or deep breathing that results in an increased amount of air entering the alveoli of the lungs, causing reduced carbon dioxide tension and eventually alkalosis.

Hypoglycemia Low blood sugar.

Hypomorphic A genetic mutation resulting in partial loss of function of the encoded protein.

Hypotension Low blood pressure.

Hypothalamus The ventral part of the diencephalon that forms the floor of the third ventricle, making up less than 1% of the brain. It includes many nuclei that are involved in mechanisms that activate, control, and integrate the peripheral autonomic mechanisms, endocrine activity, and many somatic functions, such as water balance, sleep, food intake, body temperature, and development. It is structurally and functionally connected to the pituitary gland.

Hypothermia Low body temperature.

Hypothyroidism Deficiency of thyroid activity.

Hypotonic The quality in any medium of having a sufficiently low concentration of solutes to cause water to move into a cell through osmosis.

Iatrogenic disease An adverse condition resulting from medical treatment.

Idiotype The set of antigenic determinants that distinguish one antibody from another.

Ileum The third and last portion of the small intestine from the end of the jejunum to the cecum.

Immune system An organ system that includes the spleen, bone marrow, lymph nodes, and specialized immune cells that reside in most organs or travel between organs and in blood and participate in specific and nonspecific forms of host defense (see Chap. 19).

Immunoglobulin The protein family that make up the structure of antibodies.

In vitro A term used by biochemists to refer to processes taking place in an isolated cell-free extract and used by cell biologists to refer to cells growing in culture rather than as part of an organism.

Incidence The rate of new cases of a specific disease occurring during a certain period of time.

Induction A way of getting knowledge by generalizing from experience. For example, we come to know that elephants have trunks by seeing a few elephants and noting that they all have trunks. We do not need to see every single elephant on earth in order to come to that general conclusion. This knowledge is not formally certain, but it is extremely likely to be true. In contrast, deduction or deductive knowledge includes, for example, mathematical truths about which there is certainty because they are so defined. A different use of the term induction refers to the mechanism by which one process (e.g., during development) is brought about by another.

Inflammation Acute or chronic immune response to tissue injury or infection characterized by pain, redness, heat, and swelling due to increased blood flow, vascular permeability, and migration of leukocytes.

Influx An inflowing.

Information Specific interpretations of data, within a generally accepted paradigm, that seem likely to be valid.

Inhibin A glycoprotein made by Sertoli cells in the male and granulosa cells in the female that inhibits pituitary follicle-stimulating hormone (FSH) secretion and has other complex and poorly understood functions as a local mediator in the testes and the ovary.

Innate immunity Immune mechanisms that do not require prior exposure to a pathogen to be fully effective.

Inositol-1,4,5-triphosphate (IP$_3$) A cleavage product of phosphatidyl-inositol biphosphate (PIP$_2$) that has profound effects on cell signaling.

Insulin A polypeptide hormone that is secreted by beta cells in the pancreas and helps regulate glucose metabolism in animals.

Integrin A family of integral membrane proteins that function as cell adhesion receptors.

Intercalated disks Dense bands running between myocardial cells both transversely and longitudinally, forming a stepped configuration.

Interferon A form of nonspecific antiviral host defense mediated by a family of proteins that activates processes that interfere with viral gene expression.

Interleukin Any of a family of secreted proteins termed cytokines and lymphokines that is involved in local interactions between immune cells.

Interleukin-6 (IL-6) A specific lymphokine produced by activated T cells, fibroblasts and macrophages that promotes B lymphocyte differentiation and immunoglobulin production.

Intermediate filament A fibrous protein filament that forms ropelike networks in animal cells. One of the three most prominent types of cytoskeletal filaments.

Interneuron Neurons that connect two other neurons, typically located between primary sensory neurons and motor neurons.

Iodide Any binary compound of iodine; the ion of iodine with a negative charge.

Iodine A halogen element, atomic number 53.

Ionic bond Cohesion between two atoms, one with a positive charge, the other with a negative charge. One type of noncovalent interaction or bond.

Ischemia Deficiency of blood, and the oxygen it carries, in a part of the body.

Ischemic cardiomyopathy Heart failure with left ventricular dilation caused by ischemic heart disease.

Islets of Langerhans Clusters of hormone-secreting cells scattered throughout the pancreas, composed of alpha cells, which secrete glucagon; beta cells, which secrete insulin; and delta cells, which secrete somatostatin.

Isoform Any of a group of two or more different proteins that have the same sequence but different shapes or modifications. In the case of enzymes, they may have the same catalytic action but different chemical, physical, or immunologic characteristics.

Isotope Atoms with the same nuclear charge (i.e., number of protons and electrons) but different nuclear mass (due to the presence of varying numbers of neutrons). Isotopes have the same chemical properties but are distinguishable from one another and thus have powerful technological applications (e.g., in radioimmunoassays).

Isotype Different subfamilies of the larger family of immunoglobulin proteins (i.e., heavy chains or light chains), that differ in their constant regions. Thus, IgG and IgM are different immunoglobulin isotypes.

Jaundice Yellow discoloration of the skin and eyes due to abnormal elevation or accumulation of bilirubin in the blood and tissues.

Jejunum The second part of the small intestine following the duodenum and continuing to the ileum.

Juxtaglomerular cells (juxtaglomerular apparatus) Structure located at the beginning of the afferent glomerular arteriole that secretes renin and is involved in renal autoregulation.

Kallikrein A proteolytic enzyme found in blood plasma that cleaves kininogens to form kinins and activates plasminogen.

Ketoacidosis Fall in blood pH due to accumulation of large concentrations of ketones, usually due to excessive fatty acid oxidation and dehydration. Classically seen in mild form during starvation and in severe form in patients with insulin-dependent diabetes mellitus who have not taken insulin for a prolonged period of time.

Ketone Any of a large class of organic compounds containing the carbonyl group, $C=O$, with the carbonyl group within the carbon chain.

Kidneys The organs that filter blood, regulating its composition, and form urine (see Chaps. 9 and 10).

Kinase One of the enzymes that catalyze the transfer of a high-energy group from a donor (usually ATP) to an acceptor; they are named according to the acceptor.

Kinesin One type of motor protein that uses the energy of ATP to move along a microtubule.

Kinetic energy The energy of molecular motion.

Kinetic proofreading A way of improving the fidelity of protein synthesis by having an elongation factor introduce a timed delay in chain elongation. During that time, an incorrect aminoacyl tRNA is more likely to dissociate and leave the ribosome.

Kinetics The study of the rate at which reactions occur. Biological and physiological systems have special means (e.g., through the action of enzymes) of altering the kinetics of various chemical reactions, which is one of the reasons why life, as we know it, is possible.

Kininogen The circulating protein precursor of bradykinin, a locally vasodilating peptide.

Krebs cycle The central metabolic pathway found in all aerobic organisms, in which acetyl groups derived from food molecules are oxidized to CO_2 and H_2O. It occurs in mitochondria in eukaryotic cells and is dependent on oxygen.

Kupffer cells Phagocytic cells that line the walls of the sinusoids of the liver, making up a part of the reticuloendothelial system.

Lactic acid An end product of glycolysis generated during anaerobic metabolism.

Lactotroph A prolactin-secreting cell.

Lacuna A small pit or hollow cavity.

Lamina propria The connective tissue layer lining the GI tract located under the epithelial basement membrane.

Law of mass action The tendency of reactants to drive a reaction in the direction that establishes equilibrium.

Leptin A hormone secreted by adipocytes in response to a particular level of triglyeride storage that results in lowered levels of neuropeptide Y in the hypothalamus and triggers the sense of satiety.

Leukocyte Any white blood cell.

Leukotrienes One of several classes of local mediators derived from the lipid arachidonic acid.

Leydig cells Stromal cells of the testis that make androgens, analogous to the thecal cells of the ovary.

Ligand Any molecule that binds to a specific site on a protein or other molecule.

Linoleic acid A polyunsaturated 18-carbon fatty acid occurring in some fish oils and many seed-derived oils. It is an essential fatty acid that cannot by synthesized by animal tissues and must be obtained in the diet. It is used in the formation of prostaglandins.

Lipase An enzyme that catalyzes the cleavage of fatty acids from the glycerol moiety of a triglyceride.

Lipid An organic molecule that is insoluble in water but dissolves readily in nonpolar organic solvents. Lipids include fatty acids and steroids and are a source of body fuel and an important constituent of cellular membranes.

Lipid peroxidation The process by which oxidation (loss of electron density by addition of oxygen to a molecule or removal of a hydrogen) alters lipids.

Lipocortin A calcium-binding protein believed to mediate the anti-inflammatory action of glucocorticoids.

Lipophilic Lipid or fat loving; soluble in lipids.

Lipoprotein A lipoprotein complex that allows lipids to be transported in the bloodstream. There are several specific types including very low density lipoproteins (VLDL), low density lipoproteins (LDL), high density lipoproteins (HDL) and chylomycrons, characterized by distinctive lipid and protein composition and therefore density.

Lipoxygenase pathway A pathway in which free arachidonic acid is converted into products, which include leukotrienes.

Liver An organ involved in filtering blood for many different purposes, including defense and metabolism (see Chap. 4). The liver also provides substances such as bile and many of the proteins found in blood.

Lobule (in the liver) A unit of hepatic architecture; each is a polygon of liver tissue with a central vein at its center and portal canals peripherally at the corners.

Local mediators Molecules released by cells that bind receptors and activate signal transduction mechanisms. Unlike classical hormones, they do not travel long distances in the bloodstream, but are present in low quantities or are quickly degraded and therefore affect only cells in the immediate neighborhood in which they are produced.

Loop of Henle A part of the nephron located between the proximal and distal tubules.

Low density lipoprotein (LDL) A specific subclass of lipoproteins generated from VLDL secreted by the liver, which provide cholesterol to other tissues via the bloodstream before being recycled back to the liver.

Lupus erythematosus A complex and poorly understood immunological disorder characterized by the presence of elevated titers of auto-antibodies including some directed against DNA. Lupus can present with skin manifestations and damage to various organs including the brain and kidney.

Luteinization The process by which a postovulatory ovarian follicle is transformed into a corpus luteum, in which the granulosa cells produce progesterone in response to luteinizing hormone (LH).

Luteinizing hormone (LH) An anterior pituitary hormone which is involved in promoting estrogen and progesterone production by the ovary and testosterone production by the testis.

Lymphocyte Mononuclear, nonphagocytic white blood cells involved in humoral immunity (B cells) or cell mediated immunity (T cells).

Lysosome In eukaryotic cells, a membrane-bound organelle containing digestive enzymes.

Macromolecule A molecule, such as a protein, nucleic acid, or polysaccharide, usually a polymer of simpler constituents, with a mass of thousands of Daltons.

Macrophage Mononuclear phagocytic cells of the immune system.

Macrosomia Abnormally large for gestational age fetal size.

Macula densa A zone of cells in the distal renal tubule that detects and responds to changes in tubular sodium concentration.

Major histocompatibility complex (MHC) antigens Systems of tissue antigens that distinguish self from nonself and are involved in transplant rejection.

Malignant A characteristic of tumors and tumor cells reflecting the degree to which they are invasive and/or are able to undergo metastasis. A malignant tumor is a cancer.

Mass spectrometry A physical technique for determining the mass, and therefore the composition, of chemical substances. Because the components of a complex macromolecule are made up of atoms of defined mass; if you know the precise mass of the chemical constituents that make up a complex substance, you can figure out its composition. A mass spectrometer is an instrument that subjects substances to acceleration in a curved magnetic field. The extent to which they are deflected by that magnetic field allows calculation of their mass.

Mast cell Connective tissue cells that participate in allergic responses through release of histamine upon activation.

Medial longitudinal fasciculus (MLF) A fiber tract extending between the mesencephalon and the upper part of the spinal cord that connects the vestibular nuclei with motor nuclei, chiefly those of the third, fourth, sixth, and eleventh cranial nerves.

Medulla The most interior portion of an organ. In the brain, the **medulla oblongata** is the truncated cone of nerve tissue with important collections of nerve cells that deal with vital functions such as respiration, circulation, and special senses.

Megakaryocyte Giant cells of the bone marrow. Mature platelets are released from their cytoplasm.

Meiosis A special type of cell division by which eggs and sperm cells are produced, involving a diminution by half in the amount of genetic material. It comprises two successive nuclear divisions with only one round of DNA replication, which produces four haploid daughter cells from an initial diploid cell.

Melanocyte-stimulating hormone A melanotropic peptide derived from proopiomelanocortin and released by the intermediate lobe of the pituitary gland. The acylated forms cause the dispersion of pigment granules of melanocytes, while the non-acylated forms are neurotransmitters.

Melatonin A hormone secreted by the pineal gland that increases with exposure to light and that influences hormone production and in humans is implicated in the regulation of sleep, mood, puberty, and ovarian cycles.

Membrane A structure composed of a double layer of lipid molecules and associated proteins that encloses all cells and, in eukaryotic cells, many organelles.

Memory cells Subsets of T and B lymphocytes that have been sensitized by prior exposure to a specific antigen, which allow the organism to respond more quickly and vigorously to subsequent challenge by the same antigen.

Menarche The time of onset of menstrual function.

Mendelian genetics Basic principles of heredity that derive from the work of Gregor Mendel.

Mesangial cells Myoepithelial cells found in the mesangium of the glomerulus that respond to angiotensin II, make prostaglandins and may play an important role in renal hemodynamics.

Mesangium The matrix of cells and connective tissue that helps to support the capillary loops in a renal glomerulus.

Mesenchyme Cells of the embryonic mesoderm that give rise to connective tissue and blood vessels.

Mesentery Folds of the peritoneum that attach the small intestine to the inner wall of the peritoneal space.

Metastasis The spread of cancer cells from their site of origin to other sites in the body.

Methionine A sulfur-containing amino acid.

Microglia Small, nonneural, macrophage-derived cells in the brain that act as phagocytes to engulf waste products and invaders.

Microtubule A long, cylindrical structure composed of the protein tubulin. It is one of the three major classes of filaments of the cytoskeleton.

Migrating motor complex A cyclic pattern of peristalsis in the stomach that occurs during fasting and sweeps indigestibles out of the stomach and through the gastrointestinal tract.

Mineralocorticoid A steroid hormone in-

volved in fluid and electrolyte regulation through its affects on renal ion transport. The major mineralicorticoid is aldosterone, which is synthesized by the zona glomerulosa of the adrenal cortex under the influence of potassium and angiotensin II.

Mitochondria Membrane-bounded organelles, about the size of a bacterium, that carry out fatty acid oxidation, oxidative phosphorylation, and produce most of the ATP in eukaryotic cells.

Mitogen A substance that induces cellular proliferation.

Mitosis The process of eukaryotic cell division resulting in diploid daughter cells.

Molarity The number of moles of a solute per liter of solution.

Mole M grams of a substance, where M is the relative molecular mass (molecular weight); this will be 6×10^{23} molecules of the substance.

Molecular chaperone A protein that helps other proteins avoid misfolding pathways that would produce inactive or aggregated states.

Monocyte A mononuclear phagocytic leukocyte. Monocytes are formed in the bone marrow and transported to tissues such as the lungs and liver, where they develop into macrophages.

Motilin A polypeptide hormone secreted by endocrine cells of the GI tract that has the effect of increasing intestinal motility.

Mucopolysaccharide Glycosaminoglycan, any of several high-molecular-weight linear polysaccharides having disaccharide repeating units and other distinguishing features. They include chondroitin sulfates, dermatan sulfates, heparin sulfate, keratan sulfates, and hyaluronic acid.

Mucosa Mucous membrane; often refers to the innermost layer of the gastrointestinal tract.

Multimeric protein An assembly of protein molecules physically associated with each other.

Muscarinic receptor An acetylcholine receptor that is stimulated by the alkaloid muscarine and blocked by atropine; these receptors are found on autonomic effector cells and on central neurons in the thalamus and cerebral cortex.

Muscle Tissue that makes possible movement of the body as a whole, as well as of individual organ systems themselves, often working in concert with bones.

Muscularis A muscle layer or coat.

Mutation Heritable change in the nucleotide sequence of a chromosome.

Myelin sheath The electrical insulation around the axons of certain neurons that greatly speeds the conduction of nerve impulses. It is fomed by concentric layers of the plasma membrane of oligodendrocytes adjacent to the myelinated neuron.

Myoepithelial cells Modified contractile smooth muscle cells, believed to be of ectodermal origin, located around and between certain glandular exocrine cells. It is assumed that contraction of these cells helps express secretion from the gland into the duct.

Myosin A type of motor protein that uses ATP to drive movements along actin filaments.

Natriuresis Renal sodium loss.

Natural killer (NK) cells Cells of the innate immune system that carry out cytotoxic reactions against particular targets in the absence of prior sensitization.

Necrosis Death of individual cells or groups of cells, usually as a result of external injury.

Negative feedback A response by which an output from a system triggers a decrease in the stimulus that triggered the output.

Neomorphic A genetic mutation resulting in acquisition of a new property of the encoded protein.

Nephron The anatomical and physiological unit of renal function comprised of the glomerulus and renal tubule associated with a blood supply defined by the flow through the afferent and efferent arterioles.

Nervous system The brain, spinal cord, peripheral nerves, and tissues in other organ systems that are specialized for rapid transmission of signals (see Chap. 18). Within the nervous system are the special senses: sight, hearing, taste, and smell.

Neuroendocrine axis A coordinated system involving the nervous and endocrine systems and hormones such as vasopressin that are elaborated in neurons or neuron-like cells. The term refers also to cascades of hormones from the hypothalamus, pituitary gland, and endocrine end organ that directs specific changes in the activity of various target tissues.

Neurogenic shock Loss of blood pressure due to vasodilation in response to trauma to, or the effect of toxic products on, the nervous system.

Neuroglycopenia The acute affects of extremely low blood glucose on the brain, resulting in impaired brain function and accelerated neuronal cell death. If recurrent, this can result in impaired intellect and altered personality.

Neuromuscular junction The junction between a nerve and a muscle.

Neuron A conducting cell of the nervous system.

Neuropathy A functional disturbance or pathologic change in the peripheral nervous system.

Neuropeptide Y A peptide neurotransmitter of particular importance in the basal ganglia, thalamus, and hypothalamus, and in the dorsal horn of the spinal cord. Its functions include vasoconstriction and regulation of satiety.

Neurotransmitter A small molecule secreted by the presynaptic nerve cell at a synapse to relay a signal to the postsynaptic cell. Examples include acetylcholine, glutamate, γ-aminobutyric acid (GABA), glycine, and many neuropeptides.

Neutrophil (polymorphonuclear leukocyte, PMN) A granule-containing leukocyte having a nucleus with three to five lobes and having the properties of chemotaxis, adherence to immune complexes, and phagocytosis.

Nicotinic receptor An acetylcholine receptor found in the autonomic nervous system, on striated muscle, and on spinal central neurons that is stimulated initially and blocked at high doses by the alkaloid nicotine.

Nitric oxide A gas composed of nitrogen and oxygen (NO), formed by enzymes called nitric oxide synthases, that is an important local mediator and intracellular second messenger of signaling.

Noncovalent interaction Relatively weak interaction between atoms and molecules that do not share electrons; noncovalent bonds take 20 times less energy to break than covalent bonds.

Norepinephrine A naturally occurring catecholamine neurohormone, a major neurotransmitter of the sympathetic nervous system and a powerful stimulus of constriction of capillaries and arteries.

Nuclear envelope The double membrane surrounding the nucleus. It consists of outer and inner membranes perforated by nuclear pores.

Nuclear lamina The fibrous layer of the inner surface of the inner nuclear membrane, made up of a network of intermediate filaments.

Nuclear pore A channel through the nuclear envelope that allows selected molecules to move between the nucleus and the cytoplasm.

Nucleoside triphosphate A molecule composed of a nucleoside (a purine or pyrimidine base linked to either a ribose or a deoxyribose sugar) and three phosphate groups. These molecules are principal carriers of energy in cells.

Nucleotide A nucleoside with one or more phosphate groups joined in ester linkages to the sugar moity. DNA and RNA are polymers of nucleotides.

Nucleus A prominent membrane-bounded organelle in a eukaryotic cell, containing DNA organized into chromosomes.

Obtundation Altered consciousness as in a comatose state.

Occam's razor The idea that, all else being equal, the simplest hypothesis that fits the data is the most appropriate one.

Odynophagia Painful swallowing.

Oligodendrocyte A nonneural cell of ectodermal origin that forms part of the glia of the central nervous system; projections of the surface membranes of these cells fan out and coil around the axons of many neurons to form myelin sheaths in the white matter.

Oncogene One of a large number of genes that can help make a cell cancerous. Typically, a mutant form of a normal gene (protooncogene) involved in the control of cell growth or division.

Oncotic pressure The osmotic pressure due to the presence of proteins (e.g., in blood) that tends to offset hydrostatic pressure and contributes to the balance of distribution of fluid between the vasculature and the interstitial space.

Oocyte A developing egg cell in the female.

Oogonia Primordial germ cells in the fetal ovary that proliferate rapidly through mitosis, then near the time of birth become primary oocytes by entering into the prophase of meiosis.

Opiate See Opiod.

Opiod Natural or synthetic substance that binds to the same receptors as does the pain-relieving drug morphine. The endogenous opiates include the dynorphins, endorphins and enkephalins.

Opsonin Any substance that binds to particulate antigens and induces their phagocytosis by macrophages and neutrophils. The term usually refers to two types of substances, opsonizing antibodies and certain complement fragments, both of which trigger phagocytosis by binding to specific cell-surface and other receptors.

Organ A group of tissues that work together to carry out a particular role in survival of the organism.

Organ systems Coordinated groups of organs that carry out particular functions.

Organelle A membrane-bounded structure, such as mitochondria, found in cells.

Organic Carbon containing.

Organify To attach an element to carbon-containing compounds.

Osmolality An expression of the concentration of an osmotically active substance in units of osmoles of the substance per kilogram of solution.

Osmolarity An expression of the concentration of an osmotically active substance in units of osmoles of the substance per liter of solution.

Osmoreceptor Specialized neurons of the hypothalamus that detect increases in osmolarity and trigger water-seeking behavior and the release of antidiuretic hormones to conserve body water.

Osmosis Net movement of water molecules across a semipermeable membrane, driven by a difference in the concentration of the solute on either side. The membrane must be permeable to water but not to the solute molecules.

Osmotic diuresis Increased excretion of water in the urine resulting from the presence of nonabsorbable or poorly absorbable, osmotically active substances (mannitol, urea, glucose, etc.) in the renal tubules.

Osmotic pressure Pressure that must be exerted on the high solute concentration side of a semipermeable membrane to prevent the flow of water across the membrane as a result of osmosis; it is proportional to the osmolality of the solution.

Osteoblast A fibroblast-derived differen-

tiated cell that synthesizes and secretes bone matrix proteins.

Osteoclast A multinuclear differentiated cell involved in the absorption and removal of bone.

Osteoporosis Reduction in the amount of bone mass, which can lead to fracture after minimal trauma.

Oxidation Loss of electrons from an atom, as occurs during the addition of oxygen to a molecule or when hydrogen is removed. The opposite of reduction.

Oxidative phosphorylation The process in bacteria and mitochondria in which ATP formation is driven by the transfer of electrons from food molecules to molecular oxygen. It involves the intermediate generation of a pH gradient across a membrane.

Oxytocin An octapeptide made in the hypothalamus and stored in the posterior lobe of the pituitary gland. It has uterine-contracting and milk-ejecting actions and contributes to the second stage of labor.

Pacemaker A cell or structure that sets the pace at which a phenomenon occurs.

Palliative therapy Treatment intended to relieve symptoms, but not to cure disease; used in terminally ill patients or when treatment is futile, unavailable, unwanted, or exceedingly risky.

Paracrine A type of intercellular communication in which a hormone binds to receptors on cells in the immediate neighborhood of the cell from which it was secreted rather than traveling via the bloodstream to act at a distance, as in classical endocrine systems.

Paradigm A view of the world in which certain concepts make sense. For example, modern science often operates under the reductionist paradigm that all disease can ultimately be explained by an understanding of molecular and cellular biological mechanisms.

Parafollicular cell An ovoid cell with an irregular nucleus and many dark cytoplasmic granules, located along with the principal cells of the thyroid follicles, that elaborates the polypeptide hormone calcitonin.

Paraneoplastic syndrome A disease state resulting from the biological effects of hormones or other products made by cancers.

Parasympathetic nervous system (PSNS) The part of the autonomic nervous system whose ganglia are at, or close to, the organs innervated, including heart, the smooth muscle and glands of the head and neck, and the thoracic, abdominal and pelvic viscera.

Parathyroid hormone (PTH) A polypeptide hormone secreted by the parathyroid glands, whose action defends blood calcium concentration by direct and indirect effects on bone, gut, and kidney.

Parenchyma The functional cells of an organ, as distinguished from the cells that make up its framework.

Parietal cells Large cells in the stomach mucosa that secrete hydrochloric acid and produce intrinsic factor.

Pathophysiological knowledge The set of reproducible observations as to how organ systems respond to various stimuli over time, organized into working hypotheses about organ system dysfunction and disease.

Pathway A set of enzymes that act in concert, with the product of the first enzyme serving as the reactant for the reaction catalyzed by the second enzyme, and so on.

Pepsin The enzyme of gastric juice that catalyzes the hydrolysis of proteins into polypeptides.

Peptide bond A chemical bond between the carbonyl group of one amino acid and the amino group of a second amino acid—a special form of amide linkage.

Peptidergic Having to do with peptides.

Perfusion Flow (e.g., of blood) through an organ.

Periosteum A specialized connective tissue covering all bones and cells with bone-forming potential. The outer layer is a network of dense connective tissue containing blood vessels, and the deep layer is composed of more loosely arranged collagenous bundles with spindle-shaped connective tissue cells.

Periphery The rest of the body outside a region of interest.

Peristalsis The wormlike movement by which the gastrointestinal tract propels its contents, consisting of a wave of contraction, both circular and longitudinal, passing along the tube.

Peritoneum The serous membrane lining the walls of the abdominal and pelvic cavities and the organs contained within.

Peroxidase An enzyme that catalyzes the oxidation of organic substrates by hydrogen peroxide, which is reduced to water.

Peyer's patches Follicular aggregates of lymphoid tissue, especially in the ileum.

Phagocyte Any cell capable of engulfing microorganisms or particulate matter. Phagocytes of the immune system recognize and ingest targets coated with antibodies or complement for which they have receptors.

Phagocytosis Endocytosis of particulate matter.

Phenotype The observable characteristics of a cell or organism.

Phosphatase An enzyme that removes a phosphate group from a molecule by hydrolysis of an esterified phosphoric acid with liberation of inorganic phosphate.

Phosphatidylinositol One of a family of lipids containing phosphorylated inositol derivatives. Although quantitatively minor components of the plasma membrane, they are important in signal transduction in eukaryotic cells.

Phosphatidylinositol biphosphate (PIP$_2$) A lipid in the plasma membrane cleaved by an enzyme activated by G protein, resulting in two products with profound effects on cell signaling, inositol-1,4,5-triphosphate (IP$_3$) and diacylglycerol (DAG).

Phosphatidylinositol pathway The pathway in which G protein activation by cell surface receptors results in an alteration of the activity of an enzyme that cleaves phosphatidylinositol biphosphate (PIP_2), generating two products with profound effects on cell signaling, inositol-1,4,5-triphosphate (IP_3) and diacylglycerol (DAG).

Phosphodiester bond A covalent chemical bond formed when two hydroxyl groups are linked in ester linkage to the same phosphate group, such as adjacent nucleotides in RNA or DNA.

Phospholipase C A member of a family of enzymes that catalyzes the hydrolysis of the phosphoric ester bond of a membrane phospholipid. The products of the reaction are a phosphorylated alcohol and diacylglycerol.

Physiological knowledge The set of reproducible observations as to how organ systems respond to particular stimuli over time, organized into working hypotheses about organ system function.

Pinocytic vesicle A vesicle formed and internalized during the course of non-receptor-mediated endocytosis.

Pinocytosis A subset of endocytosis that is not receptor mediated, by which cells sample the fluid in their environment through invagination, pinching off, and internalization of pinocytic vesicles.

Pituitary gland An epithelial gland located at the base of the brain, attached by a stalk to the hypothalamus, from which it receives an important neural and vascular outflow. The anterior lobe has distinct populations of cells, each uniquely involved in the synthesis of particular polypeptide hormones. The posterior lobe is composed of neurons whose cell bodies lie in the hypothalamus, but whose terminals in the pituitary release peptide hormones in the circulation.

Placebo effect The observation that patients often get substantial symptomatic improvement from treatments that have no known pharmacologic basis.

Placental lactogen (hPL) A polypeptide hormone secreted by the placenta that enters the maternal circulation. It has growth-promoting activity, is immunologically similar to human growth hormone, and counters maternal insulin activity during pregnancy.

Plasma The fluid portion of the blood, after removal of cells, in which proteins and solutes are dissolved. Plasma differs from serum in that it is the fluid portion of blood in the absence of clotting, whereas serum is the fluid portion after formation, retraction, and removal of clot.

Plasma cells Terminally differentiated cells of the B lymphocyte lineage that produce antibodies.

Plasma membrane The membrane that surrounds a living cell.

Plasmin A proteolytic enzyme made from a larger inactive precursor called plasminogen that is found in plasma. When cleaved by plasminogen activators, plasminogen is converted to the active protease plasmin that catalyzes the hydrolysis of peptide bonds on the carboxyl side of lysine or arginine residues of fibrin, an important step in breaking up clots and establishing clotting homeostasis.

Plasminogen The inactive precursor of plasmin.

Platelet A disk-shaped cellular structure in the blood that is formed in the megakaryocyte and released from its cytoplasm in clusters. It is chiefly involved in blood coagulation. Platelets lack a nucleus but contain active enzymes and mitochondria.

Plexus A network of vessels or nerves. **Myenteric plexus** A nerve plexus within the muscular layers of the intestines that directs gut motility. **Submucosal plexus** A nerve plexus within the submucosal layers of the intestines that directs intestinal motility.

Plicae circulares Round folds, especially in the jejunum.

Polar molecule A molecule in which different parts of the molecule have a relatively positive (electron-poor) or negative (electron-rich) charge.

Polycystic ovary syndrome A clinical symptom complex associated with ovaries containing multiple small follicular cysts and characterized by decreased menstruation, infertility, overweight, and hirsutism. There are elevated testosterone and luteinizing hormone (LH) and reduced testosterone-binding globulin levels in the blood.

Polymorphism See allelic polymorphism.

Polymorphonuclear leukocyte (PMN, neutrophil) A granular leukocyte having a nucleus with three to five lobes and having the properties of chemotaxis, adherence to immune complexes, and phagocytosis.

Polyol pathway (sorbitol pathway) The pathway through which sorbitol accumulates within cells, changes their osmolarity, and decreases their concentration of myoinositol, an important signal transduction precursor of the phosphatidylinositol pathway. The resultant disordered signal transduction may result in a cascade of abnormalities in different tissues.

Polypeptide A linear polymer composed of multiple amino acids. Proteins are large polypeptides, and the two terms can be used interchangeably.

Polyploid A cell or an organism that contains more than two sets of homologous chromosomes.

Polyribosome (polysome) An mRNA molecule to which are attached a number of ribosomes engaged in protein synthesis.

Portal triad (hepatic triad) The grouping of a portal venule, hepatic arteriole, and bile canaliculus enclosed in a sheathlike structure at the angles of liver lobules.

Positive feedback A feedback system in which an output from a system triggers an increase in the input that triggered the output. This is often seen in systems involving development and maturation.

Potential energy Stored energy in various forms.

Preeclampsia A syndrome of hypertension, edema and proteinuria that can occur as a complication of pregnancy.

Pregnenolone The product of cleavage of the side chain from cholesterol generated in the mitochondria as an intermediate in steroid hormone biogenesis.

Preload End-diastolic ventricular volume, usually referred to with respect to its effect on the contractility of the heart. As preload goes up, to a point, cardiac output goes up.

Progesterone The principal progestational hormone of the body, synthesized by the corpus luteum, placenta, and adrenal cortex; it prepares the uterus for the fertilized ovum and maintains an optimal intrauterine environment for sustaining pregnancy.

Prokaryote A single-celled organism such as bacteria that lacks a well-defined, membrane-enclosed nucleus.

Prolactin Hormone secreted by lactotrope cells of the anterior pituitary, under negative regulation by dopamine from the hypothalamus. In humans, prolactin promotes mammary gland (breast) development and milk production.

Prostacyclins A subset of eicosanoid local mediators related to the prostaglandins.

Prostaglandin (PG) Local mediators, so named because they were originally (erroneously) believed to be produced by the prostate gland, which have a wide range of effects on many different tissues, and which are derived from the 20 carbon fatty acid arachidonic acid.

Protease An enzyme that cleaves peptide bonds in a protein.

Protein trafficking The movement of proteins from one compartment to another, e.g., during protein secretion or endocytosis.

Proteins Molecules composed of strings of amino acid residues. Proteins are the primary way in which information encoded in genes is expressed.

Proteolysis Cleavage of a peptide bond by

insertion of a water molecule, catalysed by acids, bases, or enzymes.

Proton pump inhibitors Drugs whose mechanism of action is to inhibit the H^+,K^+-ATPase that serves as a proton pump in the plasma membrane of an acid-producing parietal cell.

Protooncogenes Cellular genes whose dysregulation can result in uncontrolled proliferation. Typically, integration of viral DNA, spontaneous mutation, or recombination events are responsible for activation of protooncogenes.

Pulmonary edema Accumulation of fluid in the pulmonary airspaces as a result of increased hydrostatic pressure (e.g., due to heart failure) or elevated vascular permeability (e.g., due to inflammation or septic shock).

Pulmonary embolism Blockage of a branch of the pulmonary artery (e.g., by a blood clot) resulting in ventilation and perfusion mismatch.

Pulmonary hypertension Elevated pulmonary artery pressure (above 30 mm Hg systolic, 12 mm Hg diastolic).

Pump A type of transporter that can move a substance against its concentration gradient, either by hydrolyzing ATP or by linking the transport to that of another substance flowing down its concentration gradient.

Pyramidal tract (corticospinal tract) The major motor neuron pathway, composed of nerves arising in the sensorimotor regions of the cerebral cortex, synapsing with motor neurons in the brainstem, and decussating (crossing) in the pyramids of the medulla.

Pyrogen Any substance that produces fever.

Radioimmunoassay A way of indirectly measuring the concentration of a substance in a sample by the ability of that substance to bind to a receptor or antibody. It is based on the principle that competition for binding gives a close approximation of concentration (making certain assumptions) and can be easily measured if receptor- (or antibody-)

bound material can be separated from the fraction that is free (see Chap. 3).

Rales Abnormal sounds heard on auscultation of the lungs, primarily during inspiration, occurring in congestive heart failure, pneumonia, and other conditions, sounding like and also called crackles.

Reactive oxygen substrate (ROS) Highly reactive oxygen-containing compounds that can react with and covalently modify proteins and thereby damage a cell. Also called reactive oxygen species.

Receptor A protein that binds a specific signaling molecule (ligand) and initiates a response in the cell. Cell-surface receptors are located in the plasma membrane, with their ligand-binding site exposed to the external medium. Intracellular receptors, such as steroid hormone receptors, bind ligands that diffuse into the cell across the plasma membrane.

Receptor-ligand interaction Binding of a receptor protein to the substance for which it has affinity.

Recessive Refers to the member of a pair of alleles that fails to be expressed in the phenotype of an organism when the dominant member is present. Also refers to the phenotype of an individual that has two recessive alleles.

Recombination The generation of new gene combinations by crossing over between homologous chromosomes.

Redox Oxidation-reduction. The chemical reaction whereby electrons are removed (oxidation) from atoms of the substance being oxidized and transferred to atoms being reduced (reduction).

5α-reductase An enzyme that catalyzes the irreversible reduction of testosterone to dihydrotestosterone.

Reduction Addition of electron density to an atom, as occurs during the addition of hydrogen to a molecule or the removal of oxygen from it. The opposite of oxidation.

Relaxin A water-soluble polypeptide produced in the corpus luteum and pregnant uterus, it produces relaxation of the pubic symphysis and dilation of the uterine cervix in some animal species.

Renin An enzyme secreted by the juxtaglomerular apparatus of the kidney for the purpose of blood pressure regulation, that cleaves circulating angiotensinogen to generate angiotensin I, which is then cleaved by angiotensin converting enzyme to generate angiotensin II, a potent vasoconstrictor.

Reproductive system The various organs and structures that are involved in production, storage, delivery, and fertilization of germ cells and support the growth of the fetus in a manner that allows propagation of the species (see Chaps. 15 and 16).

Reticuloendothelial system A group of cells (e.g., in the liver and spleen), including macrophages, and certain specialized endothelial cells and fibroblasts, with phagocytic properties that ingest bacteria and other debris that happens to enter the circulation.

Retinopathy An inflammatory or degenerative condition of the retina. Often seen as a chronic complication of diabetes mellitus.

Retroperitoneal Behind the peritoneum. The kidney is an example of a retroperitoneal organ.

Reverse T3 (triiodothyronine) A form of thyroid hormone lacking any known biological activity that is generated from thyroxine as part of thyroid hormone homeostasis.

Rhabdomyolysis Disintegration of striated muscle fibers often due to pressure or crush injury, with excretion of myoglobin in the urine and risk of acute renal failure.

Ribonucleic acid (RNA) A chemical structurally very similar to DNA, made of long strings of nucleotides, that is used for a variety of specialized purposes in cells, including the transfer of information from long-lived repository form to a short-lived usable form. RNA also plays a structural role in some multiprotein complexes.

Ribosome A particle composed of ribosomal RNAs and ribosomal proteins that associates with messenger RNA and catalyzes the synthesis of protein.

Rostral A term related to location within the central nervous system. In the spinal cord this refers to a location higher up; in the brain it refers to more anterior (forward) structures.

Ruffled membrane A specialized membrane structure produced by osteoclasts that functions like a lysosome, secreting acid and enzymes that dissolve the isolated bone surface and degrade the component proteins.

S_3 The third heart sound, heard in diastole as a result of early, rapid filling of a ventricle, as occurs in congestive heart failure.

Sarcoplasmic reticulum (SR) A special form of nonribosome-bearing reticular membranes found in the sarcoplasm of striated muscle and making up a system of smooth-surfaced tubules forming a plexus around each myofibril.

Schwann cell A form of oligodendrocyte that wraps its plasma membrane around axons of selected neurons to form myelinated nerve fibers.

Scientific knowledge Data and working hypotheses derived by the scientific method, reinforced by subjecting those data and hypotheses to reinspection in light of new technology, data, or insights in the future.

Scientific method The way information is gathered within the reductionist paradigm. Its response to any question involves formulating a testable hypothesis, carrying out experimental tests of that hypothesis, and revising the hypothesis based on the results of the experimental tests and other factors.

Second law of thermodynamics The entropy (randomness or disorder) of the universe as a whole always increases.

Second messenger A small molecule that is formed in or released into the cytosol in response to an extracellular signal and helps to relay the signal to the interior of the cell. Examples include cyclic AMP, IP_3, and Ca^{2+}.

Secretagogue Any substance that has the capacity to stimulate secretion of some other substance.

Secretin A gut hormone secreted from the duodenal and jejunal mucosa in response to the entry of acidic chyme from the stomach. Secretin in turn stimulates secretion of alkaline fluid from the exocrine pancreas to neutralize intestinal pH to achieve conditions compatible with enzymatic digestion of food.

Secretion In renal physiology, transport from the bloodstream into the tubular lumen. In biosynthesis, the release of exported proteins (e.g., hormones) from cells by exocytosis.

Secretory granules or vesicles Membrane-bounded organelles within cells that are used to store secretory proteins and ferry them to their final destination (e.g., release them outside of a cell by fusion of the secretory granule membrane with the plasma membrane). Their darkly staining contents make these organelles visible in light microscopy as small solid objects.

Secretory pathway The complex movement of newly synthesized secretory and membrane proteins from their site of synthesis to their final destination often culminating in secretion.

Selectin Any of a family of cell adhesion molecules that function to mediate the binding of leukocytes to the vascular endothelium.

Semipermeable membrane A membrane permeable to water but not to solute molecules in the water.

Sepsis A life-threatening systemic inflammatory syndrome triggered by the presence of overwhelming infection or microorganism-derived toxins.

Serosa A serous membrane that comprises the outer most layer of the GI tract furthest from the lumen.

Serotonin A monoamine vasoconstrictor with many physiological properties, including inhibiting gastric secretion, stimulating smooth muscle, and serving as a central neurotransmitter. It is also a precursor of melatonin.

Sertoli cells Cells that comprise the seminiferous tubules of the testes providing support and nutrition for developing sperm, analogous in many ways to the role of granulosa cells in development of the ovum.

Shock Any condition resulting in cardiovascular collapse and loss of blood pressure associated with failure to perfuse the crucial organs of the body.

Side-chain cleavage enzyme A mitochondrial enzyme involved in steroid biochemistry that carries out the early step of conversion of cholesterol to pregnenolone by removing the 4-carbon side chain present on the cholesterol molecule. This is the rate-limiting step in the synthesis of most steroids.

Sign Evidence, usually physical, of a disease that is perceptible to the examiner.

Signal sequence The short sequence of amino acids that targets newly synthesized protein to and across the membrane of the endoplasmic reticulum.

Signal transduction Relaying of a signal by converting it from one physical or chemical form to another. In cell biology, the process by which a cell converts an extracellular signal into an intracellular response.

Signaling pathway A pathway of cellular activity involving concerted changes in the activity of sets of enzymes that serve a particular biochemical purpose. It is triggered by the binding and activation of a receptor.

Sinusoid A terminal blood channel consisting of a large, irregular anastomosing vessel lined with endothelium (e.g., in the liver).

Skeleton The hard calcium–phosphate matrix around which organ systems are suspended (see Chap. 14). The bones that make up the skeleton provide crucial support for all other organ systems.

Skin The outer covering of the body. Skin not only protects the internal environment from external physical assault (e.g., evaporation and dehydration) but is a barrier to invasion of pathogens.

Sodium-potassium ATPase (sodium pump, Na^+,K^+-ATPase) A transmembrane carrier protein found in the plasma membrane of most animal cells that pumps sodium out of and potassium into the cell, using the energy derived from ATP hydrolysis.

Somatomedin Any of several peptides found in plasma, complexed with binding proteins, that stimulate cellular growth and replication, particularly in bone and muscle, and have insulin-like biological activities.

Somatostatin Any of several tetradecapeptides produced primarily in the hypothalamus, the GI tract, and by the delta cells of the pancreatic islets, that inhibit release of pituitary hormones and insulin and glucagon in the pancreas, of gastrin in the gastric mucosa, of secretin by the intestinal mucosa, and of other hormones.

Somatotropin See growth hormone.

Spermatagonia Undifferentiated germ cells of a male.

Spermatazoon A mature male germ cell.

Sphincter Structures composed of circular smooth muscle demarcating various regions of the GI tract, characterized by a state of tonic contraction. During periods of transient relaxation, sphincters allow the passage of material along the GI tract.

Sphincter of Oddi. The sphincter at the termination of the common bile duct and pancreatic duct where they traverse the wall of the duodenum, through which bile and pancreatic secretions enter the GI tract lumen.

Spillover A hormone's binding to and activation of receptors other than its usual target, for which it has a lower affinity and with which it does not significantly interact at the concentrations normally found in the bloodstream. This often occurs in the situation of an unusually high concentration of the hormone.

Spirometry Measurement of various aspects of lung and airway mechanics.

Splanchnic Pertaining to the internal abdominal organs (e.g., liver and GI tract).

Splicing (of RNA) Modification of an RNA transcript in which internal regions can be removed.

Starling forces Forces that contribute to movement through a capillary membrane. They include capillary pressure, interstitial fluid pressure, plasma colloid oncotic pressure, and interstitial fluid colloid osmotic pressure.

Starling's law of the heart Relationship of the force of cardiac ventricular muscle contraction to the degree of stretch of the muscle fibers (e.g., due to increased preload).

Stellate cells (of the liver) Members of the family of reticuloendothelial cells in the liver characterized by the presence of a droplet of vitamin A in their cytoplasm, implicated in the pathophysiology of cirrhosis.

Stenosis Narrowing of a passage way, for example of blood flow through the aortic valve (aortic stenosis) or of the lumen of the GI tract at the piloric sphincter (pyloric stenosis).

Steroid A hydrophobic molecule related to cholesterol. Many important hormones, such as estrogen and testosterone, are steroids.

Steroidogenic acute regulatory protein (StAR protein) A gene product stimulated by adrenocorticotropic hormone (ACTH) that moves a pool of cholesterol from the outer to the inner mitochondrial membrane, making the cholesterol accessible to cytochrome P450, which is the rate-limiting step in steroid biogenesis.

Stoichiometry Pertaining to the numerical correspondence of one thing with another (e.g., one to one in the case of small and large subunits that compose the ribosome; three to two in the case of the number of sodium atoms pumped out for potassium ions pumped in, by sodium potassium ATPase).

Stress protein A member of the family of

cellular proteins whose synthesis is increased in times of stress.

Stress response The ability of a subset of proteins to increase its expression during stress.

Striated muscle Any muscle whose fibers are divided by transverse bands into striations.

Stroma The supporting connective tissue of an organ in which the functional cells are embedded.

Submucosa The layer of areolar connective tissue beneath the mucous membrane.

Substrate The molecule on which an enzyme acts.

Superoxide dismutase An oxidoreductase catalysing the reduction of superoxide anions to hydrogen peroxide.

Suppressor T cells A subset of differentiated T lymphocytes that impairs expression of subsets of the immune response (e.g., through suppression of antibody production or cell-mediated immunity).

Suprachiasmic nucleus A small nucleus in the supraoptic region of the hypothalamus that generates circadian rhythms, including those involving the hormone melatonin from the pineal gland.

Surface tension The resistance that acts to preserve the integrity of a surface, such as the resistance to rupture possessed by the surface film of a liquid, or the strain upon the surface of a liquid in contact with another substance with which it does not mix.

Surfactant In pulmonary physiology, a mixture of phospholipids (mainly lecithin and sphingomyelin) secreted by the alveolar type II cells into the alveoli and respiratory air passages that reduces the surface tension of pulmonary fluids and thus contributes to the elastic properties of pulmonary tissue.

Sympathetic nervous system (SNS) The part of the autonomic nervous system whose preganglionic fibers emanate from the thoracolumbar portion of the spinal cord. The sympathetic ganglia lie close to the spinal cord and give rise to postganglionic fibers that ennervate the blood vessels, smooth muscle and glands of the head and neck, and the thoracic, abdominal and pelvic organs.

Symptom Evidence of a disease that is perceived by the patient.

Synapse Communicating cell-cell junction that allows signals to pass from a nerve cell to another cell. In a chemical synapse, the signal is carried by a diffusible neurotransmitter; in an electrical synapse, a direct connection is made between the cytoplasm of the two cells via gap junctions.

Syncope Transient loss of consciousness (e.g., due to a brief period of hypoperfusion of the brain).

Syncytiotrophoblast The outer layer of the ectodermal from which the placenta develops, which produces proteins, peptides, and steroids.

Syncytium A mass of cytoplasm containing many nuclei enclosed by a single plasma membrane. Typically the result either of cell fusion or of a series of incomplete division cycles in which the nuclei divide but the cell does not.

Syndrome of inappropriate ADH secretion (SIADH) A common syndrome of excessive antidiuretic hormone secretion resulting in hyponatremia and inappropriately elevated urine osmolality in the absence of volume depletion (in which case it would be appropriate). Commonly caused by a variety of different pulmonary and CNS diseases, including head trauma. Water restriction, which causes mild dehydration, makes the spontaneous ADH secretion appropriate.

System A set of interacting parts that work together.

Systole The period of the cardiac cycle during which the ventricles contract.

T lymphocyte A lymphocyte dependent on maturation in the thymus, primarily responsible for cell-mediated immunity.

T tubule The system of invaginating transverse intracellular tubules emanating from the plasma membrane of skeletal and cardiac muscle, that provide a pathway for the near simultaneous activation of all myofibrils in the muscle cell which makes efficient, concerted muscle contraction possible.

Tachydysrhythmia (tachyarrhythmia, tachycardia) Abnormally rapid heart rate, usually more than 100 beats per minute in an adult.

Taeniae coli Three thickened bands along the length of the colon composed of longitudinal muscle fibers.

TCA cycle See tricarboxylic acid cycle.

Technology The tools derived from an application of concepts and theories to the need for practical applications.

Teleology A useful storytelling technique whereby events that occurred through natural selection are presented as if they occurred for a purpose.

Testosterone The major androgen made by the Leydig cells of the testes in response to stimulation by luteinizing hormone.

Tetany Spontaneous tonic muscular contractions, typically occurring when there is a fall in extracellular ionized calcium concentrations, resulting in neuromuscular hyperexcitability.

Thecal cells Androgen-secreting cells that make up the stroma of the ovary. Follicles are embedded in the ovarian stroma, separated from thecal cells by a basement membrane.

Theory A hypothesis that has stood the tests of time and experimentation and has grown to encompass a wide range of experimental phenomena from which many testable hypotheses spanning various fields have emerged.

Thermodynamics The study of the distribution between reactants and products, or equilibrium, that is achieved when a reaction has gone to completion.

Thermogenesis The production of heat within the animal body.

Thrombin The enzyme derived from prothrombin that cleaves fibrinogen into fibrin.

Thrombolysis The process by which blood clots are dissolved, involving the action of the serum protease plasmin on fibrin.

Thrombophlebitis Inflammation of a vein associated with blood clot formation.

Thrombosis The formation of a blood clot.

Thromboxanes A subclass of eicosanoid local mediators.

Thrombus A blood clot, consisting of platelets entrapped within a crosslinked fibrin meshwork.

Thyroid-stimulating hormone (TSH, thyrotropin) A two-subunit glycoprotein hormone of the anterior pituitary that promotes the growth of, sustains, and stimulates hormone secretion from the thyroid gland.

Thyroglobulin A high molecular glycoprotein that serves as the precursor of thyroid hormone. After iodination, thyroglobulin is stored in the thyroid follicular lumen as colloid until it is taken up and digested by proteases to release active thyroid hormones (T_3 and T_4).

Thyroxine (T_4) The major form of thyroid hormone released from the thyroid gland. It is an precursor of tri-iodothyronine (T_3), the more active form of thyroid hormone affecting energy consumption and metabolism of most organs in the body.

Tidal volume The amount of gas that is inspired and expired during one cycle of gentle breathing normally about 500 mL in an adult.

Tight junction A cell-cell junction that seals adjacent epithelial cells together, preventing the passage by diffusion of most dissolved molecules from one side of the epithelial sheet to the other.

Tissues Groups of cells of similar function.

Tonic Characterized by continuous presence; e.g., tonic stimulation maintains closure of a sphincter.

Tonicity The concentration of solutes that are not freely permeable across the plasma membranes of most cells, the effective osmotic pressure equivalent.

Trabecular bone A spongy network with a large surface area that makes up the center of bones and is the site of most active calcium turnover.

Transamination A biochemical reaction in which amino groups are transferred from an amino acid to an alpha keto acid creating a new amino acid and a new alpha keto acid. This reaction allows shuttling of amino groups without having to generate the highly toxic free ammonium ion.

Trans-Golgi network (TGN) A compartment at the end of the Golgi apparatus from which sorting of vesicles by destination takes place.

Transcription (of DNA) The copying of one strand of DNA into a complementary RNA sequence by the enzyme RNA polymerase.

Transcription factor Any protein required to initiate or regulate transcription in eukaryotes. Includes both gene regulatory proteins and general transcription factors.

Transcytosis A specialized form of endocytosis to transport IgA and IgM across the intestinal epithelium.

Transfer RNA (tRNA) A set of small RNA molecules used in protein synthesis as an interface (adaptor) between mRNA and amino acids. Each type of tRNA molecule is covalently linked to a particular amino acid and is used to achieve fidelity of protein synthesis.

Transferrin A serum protein that binds and transports iron.

Translation (of RNA) The process by which the sequence of nucleotides in a messenger RNA molecule directs the incorporation of amino acids into protein; occurs on a ribosome.

Translocation Movement of a substance across a barrier. It often refers specifically to movement of newly synthesized proteins across the membrane of the endoplasmic reticulum in the early steps of the secretory pathway.

Translocation channel The specialized aqueous proteinaceous pore through which newly synthesized proteins move to the lumen of the endoplasmic reticulum.

Transporter A molecule that binds a substance on one side of a membrane and then undergoes a conformational change that allows the molecule to cross to the other side of the membrane.

Transudate A fluid substance that has passed through a membrane or been extruded from the blood as a result of hydrodynamic forces. A transudate, in contrast to an exudate, is characterized by high fluidity and a low content of protein, cells, or solid materials derived from cells.

Tricarboxylic acid cycle The central metabolic pathway found in all aerobic organisms in which acetyl groups derived from food molecules are oxidized to CO_2 and H_2O. Occurs in mitochondria in eukaryotic cells and requires oxygen.

Triglyceride Glycerol ester of fatty acids. The main constituent of fat droplets in animal tissues (where the fatty acids are saturated) and of vegetable oil (where the fatty acids are mainly unsaturated).

Triiodothyronine (T_3) A thyroid hormone, mostly produced by the deiodination of thyroxine (T_4) in the peripheral tissues, chiefly the liver. It is 10 times more active as a transcription activator than T_4.

Trophoblast A two cell layer of ectodermal tissue on the outside of the blastocyst from which the placenta will develop.

Trypsin A protease of the class containing a serine residue in the active site that cleaves peptide bonds on the carboxyl side of either arginine or lysine. Trypsin is secreted by the exocrine pancreas in precursor form, trypsinogen which is subsequently activated in the lumen of the duodenum as part of the program of digestion.

Trypsinogen The inactive precursor from

which active trypsin is derived by proteolytic cleavage.

Tumor promoters Nongenetic ways in which malignant transformation can be favored. These include physical injury and chemical toxins.

Tumor suppressor genes Genes that normally act as triggers of pathways that prevent inappropriate oncogene activation, often by activating the apoptotic pathway.

Tyrosine An amino acid used for protein synthesis that is derived metabolically from phenylalanine. Tyrosine serves as a biosynthetic precursor for thyroid hormones, catecholamines, and melanin.

Tyrosine kinase Protein-tyrosine kinase, an enzyme that phosphorylates a protein on tyrosine residues, as opposed to serine and or threonine residues, which can also be phosphorylated.

Uncoupling protein A class of proteins in the inner mitochondrial membrane that dissipates the proton gradient resulting from the action of the respiratory chain, as a result of which oxidation of substrates in the TCA cycle is uncoupled from the phosphorylation of ADP to ATP, and energy is lost as heat.

Untranslated regions Regions at both ends of an mRNA that play an important role in regulating when mRNA is to be used and how long-lived it will be.

Urea The endproduct of the urea cycle by which toxic free ammonia groups are converted into a less toxic form that is readily excreted by the kidneys.

Urea cycle A series of metabolic reactions occurring in the liver by which ammonia is converted to urea using cyclically regenerated ornithine as a carrier.

Uremia The signs and symptoms of chronic renal failure. It occurs due to the toxic effects of elevated blood levels of urea and other compounds excreted by the normal kidney.

Urodilatin An ANP-like local mediator made by the distal renal tubule in response to a rise in blood pressure or circulating volume.

Vagal Due to stimulation from the vagus nerve.

Vagotomy Surgical transection of the vagus nerve.

Vagus nerve The tenth cranial nerve, arising from the medulla; it supplies sensory fibers to the ear, tongue, pharynx, and larynx; motor fibers to the pharynx, larynx, and esophagus; and parasympathetic and visceral afferent fibers to thoracic and abdominal viscera.

Van der Waals interaction A type of noncovalent interaction between molecules.

Vapor pressure Movement of molecules at equilibrium between liquid and gaseous phases.

Varices Enlarged, tortuous veins, arteries, or lymphatic vessels.

Vasa recta The hairpin loop capillaries of the kidney that dip down into the medullary interstitium, making possible the countercurrent multiplier mechanism of concentration.

Vasoactive intestinal polypeptide (VIP) A peptide gastrointestinal (GI) hormone with secretin-like effects on the pancreas that may also affect GI blood blow and gut motility.

Vasoconstriction A decrease in the caliber of blood vessels due to contraction of smooth muscle in the vessel wall.

Vasodilation An increase in the caliber of blood vessels due to relaxation of smooth muscle in the vessel wall.

Vasomotor Descriptive of forces that affect the caliber of a blood vessel, usually through effects on vascular smooth muscle.

Vasopressin (antidiuretic hormone, ADH) An octapeptide hormone formed in the hypothalamus and stored in the posterior lobe of the pituitary that stimulates the contraction of the muscular tissue of the capillaries and arterioles, raising the blood pressure. It promotes contraction of the intestinal musculature and increases peristalsis, and it exerts some contractile influence on the uterus.

Ventilation The process of exchange of air between the lungs and the ambient air.

Very-low-density lipoprotein (VLDL) A class of lipoproteins, synthesized in the liver, that transport triglycerides from the intestine and liver to adipose and muscle tissues. They contain primarily triglycerides in their lipid cores, with some cholesterol.

Vesicle A small, membrane-bound, organelle in the cytoplasm of a eukaryotic cell.

Virilization The consequences of excessive androgens in the female, resulting in development of male secondary sexual characteristics.

Vitamin D Two steroid compounds, 1,25-dihydrocholecalciferol (D_3), which is synthesized in the skin and is active as a hormone, and ergocalciferol (D_2), which is the usual dietary supplement. It is released in response to low serum calcium and functions to increase gastrointestinal tract calcium absorption and to promote calcium deposition in bone.

Volatile acid An acid that in animals can be excreted as a gas via the lungs, such as CO_2.

Vomiting The forcible expulsion of the contents of the stomach through the mouth.

Wild type The normal, nonmutant form of an organism or gene; the form found in nature (in the wild).

Wolff-Chaikoff block The inhibition of the organification of iodine in the presence of excess iodide. This is a transient phenomenon, overcome in about a week by negative-feedback loops involving iodide transport within the thyroid.

Working hypothesis An assumption based on data.

Zygote A diploid cell produced by fusion of a male and a female gamete; a fertilized egg.

INDEX

Note: Page numbers followed by *f* refer to figures; page numbers followed by *t* refer to tables.

ISBN 0-07-038128-3
90000
9 780070 381285